CONTENTS IN BRIEF

15th EDITION

STRUCTURE & FUNCTION OF THE BODY

Kevin T. Patton, PhD
Founding Professor of Life Science, Emeritus Faculty
St. Charles Community College
Cottleville, Missouri
Professor of Human Anatomy & Physiology Instruction
New York Chiropractic College
Seneca Falls, New York

Gary A. Thibodeau, PhD
Chancellor Emeritus
Professor Emeritus of Biology
University of Wisconsin—River Falls
River Falls, Wisconsin

ELSEVIER

ELSEVIER

3251 Riverport Lane
St. Louis, Missouri 63043

STRUCTURE & FUNCTION OF THE BODY,
FIFTEENTH EDITION

Softcover ISBN: 978-0-323-34112-7
Hardcover ISBN: 978-0-323-35725-8

Library of Congress Cataloging-in-Publication Data

Thibodeau, Gary A., 1938- , author.
Structure & function of the body / Kevin T. Patton, Gary A. Thibodeau.
-- 15th edition.
p. ; cm.
Structure and function of the body
Author's names reversed on previous edition.
Includes bibliographical references and index.
ISBN 978-0-323-34112-7 (pbk. : alk. paper)
I. Patton, Kevin T., author. II. Title. III. Title: Structure and function of the body.
[DNLM: 1. Physiological Phenomena. 2. Anatomy. QT 104]
QP34.5
612--dc23

2015036370

Executive Content Strategist: Kellie White
Content Development Manager: Laurie Gower
Senior Content Development Specialist: Karen C. Turner
Publishing Services Manager: Jeffrey Patterson
Book Production Specialist: Carol O'Connell
Design Direction: Brian Salisbury

Printed in Canada
Last digit is the print number: 9 8 7 6 5

ABOUT THE AUTHORS

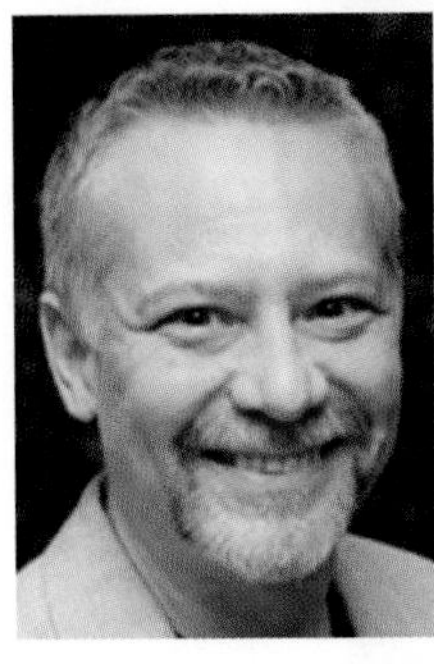

Kevin Patton has taught anatomy and physiology to high school, community college, university, and graduate students from various backgrounds for more than three decades. He has earned several citations for teaching anatomy and physiology, including the Missouri Governor's Award for Excellence in Teaching. His teaching experience has helped him produce a text that will be easier to understand for all students. "One thing I've learned," says Kevin, "is that most of us learn scientific concepts more easily when we can *see* what's going on." His talent for using imagery to teach is evident throughout this edition, with its improved illustration program.

Kevin found that the work that led him to a PhD in vertebrate anatomy and physiology instilled in him an appreciation for the "big picture" of human structure and function. He also has a keen interest in the science of learning, which is reflected in the enhanced pedagogical design of this edition.

Kevin's interest in promoting excellence in teaching anatomy and physiology has led him to take an active role in the Human Anatomy and Physiology Society (HAPS). He serves as HAPS President Emeritus and was the founding Director of HAPS Institute (HAPS-I), a professional continuing education program for anatomy and physiology teachers. As a founding faculty member of a Master of Science in Anatomy & Physiology Instruction, he currently mentors those who are preparing to teach A&P or improve their skills. Kevin also produces several online resources for A&P students and teachers, including *theAPstudent.org* and *theAPprofessor.org*.

To my family and friends, who never let me forget the joys of discovery, adventure, and good humor.

To the many teachers who taught me more by who they were than by what they said.

To my students, who help me keep the joy of learning fresh and exciting.

Kevin T. Patton

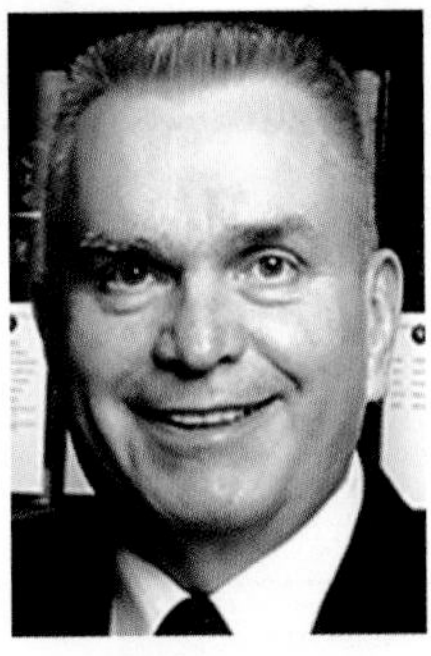

Gary Thibodeau has been teaching anatomy and physiology for more than three decades. Since 1975, *Structure & Function of the Body* has been a logical extension of his interest and commitment to education. Gary's teaching style encourages active interaction with students, and he uses a variety of teaching methodologies—a style that has been incorporated into every aspect of this edition. He is considered a pioneer in the introduction of collaborative learning strategies to the teaching of anatomy and physiology. His focus continues to be successful, student-centered learning—leveraged by text, Web-based, and ancillary teaching materials.

Gary is active in numerous professional organizations, including the Human Anatomy and Physiology Society (HAPS), the American Association of Anatomists, and the American Association for the Advancement of Science (AAAS). His biography is included in numerous publications, including *Who's Who in America, Who's Who in American Education, Outstanding Educators in America, American Men and Women of Science,* and *Who's Who in Medicine and Healthcare.*

While earning master's degrees in both zoology and pharmacology, and a PhD in physiology, Gary says that he became "fascinated by the connectedness of the life sciences." That fascination has led to this edition's unifying themes, which focus on how each concept fits into the "big picture" of the human body.

To my parents, M.A. Thibodeau and Florence Thibodeau, who had a deep respect for education at all levels and who truly believed that you never give up being a student.

To my wife, Emogene, an ever-generous and uncommonly discerning critic, for her love, support, and encouragement over the years.

To my children, Douglas and Beth, for making it all worthwhile.

To my grandchildren, Allan Gary Foster and Johanna Lorraine Foster, for proving to me that you really can learn something new every day.

Gary A. Thibodeau

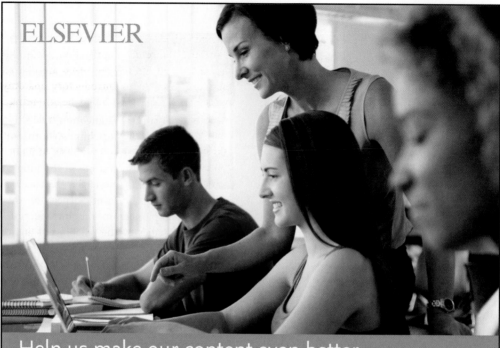

PREFACE

The true quality of a textbook is best measured by how well it supports, promotes, and encourages both good teaching and effective learning. The 15th edition of *Structure & Function of the Body* is a new text with a long tradition of excellence. It is based on profound respect for both the teacher and the student. That respect is coupled with an excitement for the subject matter honed by both authors during decades of teaching anatomy and physiology.

We have listened carefully to input from users of previous editions. We know that teachers use different techniques to convey ideas, present difficult concepts, or explain how applications of principles of anatomy and physiology can affect, for example, health, diverse personal interests of students in the class, or other areas of biology. Students, of course, learn in different ways, at different paces, and for different reasons. Success for some is largely predicated on readability of the text; others are more visual in their learning and rely heavily on excellent illustrations; still others learn best in groups and by verbal review of concepts. A good text must be flexible enough to help accommodate, not hinder, these differing needs of both teacher and student.

Success in both teaching and learning is, in many ways, determined by how effective we are at transforming information into knowledge. This is especially true in anatomy and physiology, where both student and teacher are now being confronted with an enormous accumulation of factual information. *Structure & Function of the Body* is intended to help transform that information into a coherent knowledge base. It is written at an appropriate level to help students with divergent needs and learning styles to unify information, stimulate critical thinking, and hopefully acquire a taste for knowledge about the wonders of the human body. The new edition is designed for ease of use and improved reading comprehension. It will encourage students to explore, question, and look for relationships not only between related facts in a single discipline but also among fields of academic inquiry and personal experience.

This 15th edition of *Structure & Function of the Body* retains many features that have proved successful in several decades of classroom use; however, as an updated text, it presents a wealth of carefully selected new content in both anatomy and physiology, as well as pedagogical enhancements that will better serve the needs of today's instructors and students. The writing style and depth of coverage are intended to challenge, reward, and reinforce introductory students as they grasp and assimilate important concepts.

During the revision of this text, each change in content and organization was evaluated by anatomy and physiology teachers working in the field—teachers currently assisting students to learn about human structure and function for the first time. The result is a text that students will read, one designed to help the teacher teach and the student learn. It is particularly suited to introductory anatomy and physiology courses in nursing and allied health–related programs. Emphasis is on material required for entry into more advanced courses, completion of professional licensing examinations, and successful application of information in a practical, work-related environment.

Unifying Themes

Structure & Function of the Body is dominated by two major unifying themes. First, structure and function complement one another in the normal, healthy human body. Second, nearly all structure and function in the body can be explained in terms of keeping conditions in the internal environment relatively constant—in homeostasis. Repeated emphasis of these principles encourages students to integrate otherwise isolated factual information into a cohesive and understandable whole. As a result, anatomy and physiology emerge as living and dynamic topics of personal interest and importance to the student.

Organization and Content

The 22 chapters of *Structure & Function of the Body* present the core material of anatomy and physiology most important for introductory students. The selection of appropriate information in both disciplines eliminates the confusing mix of nonessential and overly specialized material that unfortunately accompanies basic information in many introductory textbooks. Information is presented in a way that makes it easy for students to know and understand what is important.

Further, pedagogical aids in each chapter identify learning objectives and then reinforce successful mastery of this clearly identified core material. The sequencing of chapters in the book follows a course organization most commonly used in teaching at the undergraduate level. However, because each chapter is self-contained, instructors have the flexibility to alter the sequence of material to fit personal teaching preferences or the special content or time constraints of their courses or students.

At every level of organization, both within and among chapters, care has been taken to couple structural information with important functional concepts. In each chapter of the text, appropriate physiological content balances the anatomical information that is presented. As a result, the student has a more integrated understanding of human structure and function. Throughout the text, examples that stress the complementarity of structure and function have been consciously selected to emphasize the importance of homeostasis as a unifying concept.

Acquiring and using the terms so necessary for the study of anatomy and physiology can be difficult for many students—both native speakers and English-language learners. To assist students in this area, new terms are introduced in a word list *before* they read each chapter, as recommended by learning and reading specialists.

The organization of chapters and paragraphs allows students to both "read" and "raid" this book easily to learn essential concepts of human structure and function. One long chapter covering both cell biology and tissues has been split in this edition into two shorter, more focused chapters. Similarly, long passages within many of the chapters were subdivided into smaller sections with new subheadings. These steps help the reader to more easily construct their own conceptual framework as they read—and they help students find what they are looking for when they raid the book for specific bits of knowledge. Every chapter also uses skillfully designed visuals to reinforce written information with sensory input.

The style of presentation of material in this text and its readability, accuracy, and level of coverage have been carefully developed to meet the needs of undergraduate students taking an introductory course in anatomy and physiology. *Structure & Function of the Body* remains an introductory textbook—a teaching book rather than a reference text. No textbook can replace the direction and stimulation provided by an enthusiastic teacher to a curious and involved student. A good textbook, however, can and should be enjoyable to read and helpful to both.

Pedagogical Features

Structure & Function of the Body is a student-oriented text. Written in a very readable style, it has numerous pedagogical aids that maintain interest and motivation. Every chapter contains the following elements that facilitate learning and the retention of information in the most effective manner.

Chapter outline: An overview outline introduces each chapter and enables the student to preview the content and direction of the chapter at the major concept level before the detailed reading.

Chapter objectives: The opening page of each chapter contains several measurable objectives for the student. Each objective clearly identifies for the student, before he or she reads the chapter, what the key goals should be and what information should be mastered.

Embedded study hints: New to this edition are embedded hints that advise students on how to best use the pedagogical elements of the text to their advantage. These "shortcuts" based on the science of learning help students develop advanced stills in textbook comprehension and student success.

Hint

Rational word lists: Key terms are now introduced in a newly enhanced word list that begins at the start of each chapter. Each term has a simple pronunciation guide that helps students become familiar with the new combinations of syllables, so that beginning students can avoid tripping over them while reading the chapter. Each listed term is also broken into word parts, each defined in English, to help students become accustomed to—and comfortable with—the language of science and medicine. In previous editions, simple word lists at the end of each chapter did not include all the key terms of the chapter highlighted in boldface. The new comprehensive word lists make sure that all complex terms that may be new to the reader are seen and pronounced before each chapter is read. Both native English speakers and English-language learners (ELL) benefit by using these word lists as suggested.

Quick Check questions: The popular Quick Check feature provides a way for students to check their basic reading comprehension at the end of each passage that they have read. Quick Checks each consist of a few questions and are scattered at appropriate points throughout the text of each chapter. The questions are *simple,* meant only to check whether the student read and understood the main points of each passage.

QUICK CHECK

AnimationDirect: In each chapter, boxes with a special icon point the reader to animations of important principles available in AnimationDirect, which is included in the online Evolve resources. AnimationDirect features brief animated sequences that demonstrate concepts that are not easily illustrated in static diagrams. For this edition, many of the animations are new. These animations help put a student's understanding in motion and thus help solidify learning.

e

Boxed sidebars

Boxed information appears in every chapter. We have grouped these sidebar features into four categories:

- Health and Well-Being
- Clinical Application
- Research, Issues, and Trends
- Science Applications

The sidebars increase student interest and thus motivate student learning. They also help students apply information learned in the course to help them develop critical thinking skills.

Carefully selected clinical examples are included in each chapter of the book to help students understand that the disease process is a disruption in homeostasis and a breakdown of the normal integration of form and function. We use clinical examples to reinforce the concepts of how disease affects normal function and how therapies can restore normal function. We have found in our own teaching that such examples stimulate student interest.

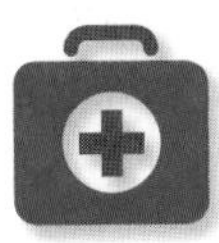

Boxed information highlighting health and wellness issues reinforces the basic concepts of human structure and function by applying them in practical ways to current problems in public health, athletics, and fitness.

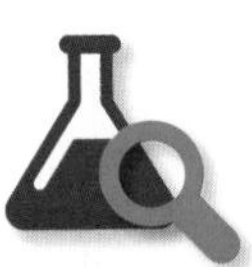

Select boxed essays on issues and trends in research and medicine will spark an interest in the dynamic fields of science, technology, and ethics that underlie the modern arena of human biology.

Science Applications boxes feature possible career paths that use the concepts taught in this text. These career paths are mentioned in the context of the work of an important global figure in the history of scientific endeavor. Such information will further motivate learning by illustrating its practical applications and will stimulate students to think about their own career choices.

Outline summaries: Extensive and detailed end-of-chapter summaries in outline format provide excellent guides for students as they review the text materials when preparing for examinations. Many students also find these detailed guides useful as a chapter preview in conjunction with the chapter outline. Audio chapter summaries are also available on the accompanying Evolve website.

Active Learning

New to this edition is an end-of-chapter section titled *Active Learning*. This section includes the following components:

Study tips: Each Active Learning section includes a list of specific tips, hints, and activities on how to most effectively and actively study the concepts of that chapter. In previous editions, similar tips were found at the start of each chapter. Student feedback informed us that because the tips describe particular concepts learned later in the chapter, they make more sense to the reader after reading the entire chapter.

Review questions: Subjective review questions at the end of each chapter allow students to use a narrative format to discuss concepts and synthesize important chapter information for review by the instructor. The answers to these review questions are available in the Instructor's Resource Manual that accompanies the text.

Critical thinking questions: Review questions that encourage students to use critical thinking skills are highlighted at the end of each chapter. Answers to these questions are also found in the Instructor's Resource Manual.

Chapter tests: Objective-type chapter test questions are included at the end of each chapter. They serve as quick checks for the recall and mastery of important subject matter. They are also designed as aids to increase the retention of information. Answers to all chapter test questions are provided at the end of the text.

Appendices

Body mass index (BMI): A brief overview of the body mass index and how it is used to assess risk for weight-related health conditions is included as a separate appendix that can be used in the introduction to the body in Chapter 1, the study of tissues in Chapter 4, the study of nutrition and metabolism in Chapter 17, or anywhere else the student or teacher finds it useful.

Common Medical Abbreviations, Prefixes, and Suffixes: Common word parts used in scientific and medical terminology are grouped as prefixes, suffixes, and roots to complement the word-study approach used in the chapter word lists and throughout the text narrative. Common medical abbreviations further assist students in mastering the vocabulary of anatomy and physiology.

Glossary: Every boldface term and most of the italicized terms used in the book are clearly defined and a simple pronunciation guide provided.

Index: A comprehensive topic index serves as a ready reference for locating information when "raiding" the textbook during study.

Illustrations

A major strength of *Structure & Function of the Body* has always been the exceptional quality, accuracy, and beauty of the illustration program. This edition features a continued refreshing and enhancement of the art program. The truest test of any illustration is how effectively it can complement and strengthen written information found in the text and how successfully it can be used by the student as a learning tool. Extensive use has been made of full-color illustrations, micrographs, and dissection photographs throughout the text. Each illustration is carefully referred to in the text and is designed to support the text discussion. Many new and enhanced illustrations appear in this edition of the textbook. Many of the new illustrations have moved complex information from the legend to small boxes within the illustration. Learning science has shown that this approach reduces cognitive load for the reader—thus enhancing learning effectiveness.

Continuing in this edition of *Structure & Function of the Body* is the careful use of anatomical rosettes in all anatomical illustrations (see the Anatomical Directions page at the beginning of the book for an illustration of this useful element). These rosettes, like the compass rosettes found on geographical maps, orient the user to the direction, or orientation, of the figure by pointing which way is left and which way is right—directions that in anatomy may appear backward to the beginning student. As with map users, the need for these rosettes will diminish as one becomes more familiar with "the territory" of the human body.

Clear View of the Human Body

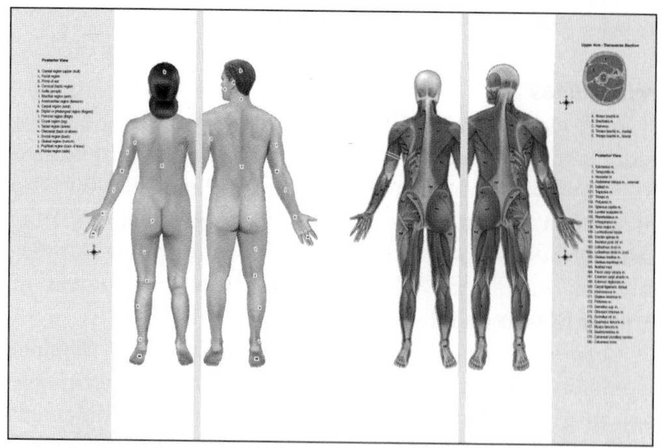

We are particularly excited to once again present a full-color, semitransparent model of the body called the ***Clear View of the Human Body.*** Located around Chapter 5 in the textbook, this feature permits the virtual dissection of male and female human bodies along several different planes. Developed by Kevin Patton and Paul Krieger, this tool helps learners assimilate their knowledge of the complex structure of the human body. It also helps students visualize human anatomy in the manner of today's clinical and scientific body-imaging technology. New to this edition are additional illustrations of the body exterior, with additional labels of important regions and structures.

Digital Learning Tools

A wide variety of multisensory learning tools are available at *evolve.elsevier.com/PattonThibodeau/humanbody:*

- New **Active Concept Maps** take complicated processes or structures and break them down into individual steps or components, using narration and animation to guide students through the topic.
- **Audio chapter summaries** for each chapter in the book are a student favorite. These concise, narrated overviews are called out at the start of each chapter Outline Summary and can be accessed on the Evolve website. Students can listen to the audio files on their computers or download them to their portable device so they can either preview or review chapter content while on the go.
- Throughout the text, special **Animation-Direct** icons alert the reader to animations that can be accessed on the Evolve website. These cover a wide range of topics and body systems.
- More than 350 **Self-Test Questions** allow students to get instant feedback on what you've learned in each chapter.
- The **Body Spectrum Electronic Anatomy Coloring Book** is one of our most popular interactive features on Evolve. Using a visual-kinesthetic approach, this tool simplifies the way students learn anatomy and medical terminology by offering more than 70 detailed anatomy illustrations that can be colored online or printed out to color and study offline.
- The **Panorama of Anatomy and Physiology** has interactive exercises, quizzes, and activities that reinforce key anatomy & physiology concepts.
- Not sure how a term is pronounced? Listen to the proper pronunciation with the **Audio Glossary**!
- **FAQs**—Frequently Asked Questions—by students, along with answers from the authors.

Online Resources for Instructors

Instructors can get access to a number of teaching tools on Evolve, available at: *evolve.elsevier.com/PattonThibodeau/humanbody:*

TEACH Instructor Resource Manual

TEACH has been completely updated and revised for this edition. The TEACH lesson plans help instructors prepare for class and make full use of the rich array of ancillaries and resources that come with the textbook. The content covered in each textbook chapter is divided across one or more lesson plans, each designed to occupy 50 minutes of class time. Lesson plans are organized into easily understandable sections that are each tied to the chapter learning objectives:

- **Instructor Preparation:** This section provides a checklist of all the things you need to do to prepare for class, including a list of all the items that you need to bring to class to perform any activity or demonstration included in the lesson plan, and all pertinent key terms covered in that lesson.
- **Student Preparation:** Textbook readings, study guide exercises, online activities, and other applicable homework assignments for each lesson are provided here along with an overall estimated completion time.
- **The 50-Minute Lesson Plan:** A lecture description with pertinent teaching points for each learning objective that reflects the chapter lecture slides that come as part of TEACH is included, as well as classroom activities and online activities, one or more critical thinking questions, and time estimates for the classroom lecture and activities.
- **Assessment Plan:** To ensure that your students have mastered all the objectives, the new TEACH includes a separate "Assessment Plan" section. An easy-to-use table maps each assessment tool to the lesson plans and chapter objectives so you can see all your assessment options—by chapter, by lesson, and by objective—and choose accordingly.

Test Bank

An electronic test bank of more than 3900 questions with answers—revised and updated for this edition—gives instructors an easy way to test students' comprehension of text material and create comprehensive exams for students.

Image Collection

The image collection includes nearly 400 anatomy and physiology images from the text, available in jpeg and PowerPoint formats, with and without labels and with and without lead lines. Use these images to enhance the visual elements of your lectures, discussions, case studies, quizzes, tests, handouts, and more.

Changes to the 15th Edition

Compiled by the author during the revision process of this textbook, this detailed list includes updates in the textbook since the last edition. These include major changes, such as the split of one chapter into two, to smaller but still important details, such as changes in key terms. This document will help in planning as you upgrade from the 14th edition to the new 15th edition of *Structure & Function of the Body*. Updates and teaching tips are also posted at *PattonSF.org*.

Supplements

The supplements package has been carefully planned and developed to assist instructors and to enhance their use of the text. Each supplement has been thoroughly reviewed by many of the same instructors who reviewed the text.

- *Study Guide.* Written by Linda Swisher, it provides students with additional self-study aids, including chapter overviews, topic reviews, and application and labeling exercises (such as matching, crossword puzzles, fill in the blank, and multiple choice), as well as answers in the back of the guide.
- *Anatomy and Physiology Online for Structure & Function of the Body.* This optional tool is a 22-module online course that brings A&P to life and helps you understand the most important concepts presented in *Structure & Function of the Body.* It includes over 100 animations, 250 interactive exercises, and quizzes and exams to assess student comprehension. Available on the Evolve website.
- *Survival Guide for Anatomy & Physiology.* An entertaining and easy-to-read set of tips, shortcuts, and advice, this "survival kit" helps students achieve success in anatomy and physiology.

A Word of Thanks

Many people have contributed to the development and success of *Structure & Function of the Body.* We extend our thanks and deep appreciation to the various students and classroom instructors who have provided us with helpful suggestions following their use of earlier editions of this text.

A special thanks to contributor Linda Swisher, who helped us improve the learning opportunities in every single chapter of the book. Thanks once again to Ed Calcaterra for his many previous contributions to this text. A specific thank you goes to the following clinicians, researchers, and instructors who critiqued in detail the previous editions of this text or various drafts of the revision. Their invaluable comments were instrumental in the development of this new edition.

Bert Atsma
Union County College
Cranford, New Jersey

Ethel J. Avery
Trenholm State Technical College
Montgomery, Alabama

Gail Balser, RN, BSN, MSN
Lakeland, Florida

Joan I. Barber, PhD
Delaware Technical & Community College
Newark, Delaware

Barbara Barger
Clarion County Career Center
Shippenville, Pennsylvania

Blythe A. Batten, RN, BS, BSN
Pinellas Technical Education Center
St. Petersburg, Florida

Rachel Beecham, PhD
Mississippi Valley State University
Itta Bena, Mississippi

Kristi Bertrand, MPH, CMA (AAMA), CPC, PBT (ASCP)
The Medical Institute of Kentucky
Lexington, Kentucky

Jackie Brittingham
Simpson College
Indianola, Iowa

Kristin Bruzzini, PhD
Maryville University
St. Louis, Missouri

Donna J. Burleson, RN, MS, MSN
Cisco Junior College
Abilene, Texas

Ed Calcaterra, BS, MEd
Instructor, DeSmet Jesuit High School
Creve Coeur, Missouri

Jeanne Calvert, BA, MS
University of Saint Francis
Fort Wayne, Indiana

Dale Charles, MS, RN, ACLS, CPR
Spencerian College
Louisville, Kentucky

Lydia R. Chavana
South Texas Vo-Tech Institute
McAllen, Texas

Linda C. Cole, RN, MSN, CS, FNP
Saint Charles Community College
Cottleville, Missouri

Maria Conn
Mayo State Vo-Tech School
Pikeville, Kentucky

Janie Corbitt, RN, MLS
Central Georgia Technical College
Milledgeville, Georgia

Linda M. Crum
University of Tennessee Medical Center
Knoxville, Tennessee

Joseph Devine
Allied Health Careers
Austin, Texas

Edna M. Dilmore
Bessemer State Technical College
Bessemer, Alabama

Camille DiLullo, PhD
Philadelphia College of Osteopathic Medicine
Philadelphia, Pennsylvania

Kathleen Reilly Dolin, MS, RN
Northampton Community College
Bethlehem, Pennsylvania

Marian Doyle, MS
Northampton Community College
Fogelsville, Pennsylvania

Kathy J. Dusthimer, MSN, RN, FNP-BC
Black Hawk College
Moline, Illinois

Cammie Emory
Bossier Parish Community College
Benton, Louisiana

David Evans, PhD, FRES
Penn College
Williamsport, Pennsylvania

Penny Fauber, RN, BSN, MS, PhD
Dabney S. Lancaster Community College
Clifton Forge, Virginia

Jerry S. Findley, BS, MA
South Plains College
Levelland, Texas

Sally Flesch, PhD, RN
Black Hawk College
Moline, Illinois

Michael Harman, MS
Lone Star College – North Harris
Houston, Texas

Gary Heisermann, PhD
Boston University
Boston, Massachusetts

Ann Henninger, PhD
Wartburg College
Waverly, Iowa

Elizabeth Hodgson, MS
York College of Pennsylvania
York, Pennsylvania

Denise L. Kampfhenkel, RN, BSN
Schreiner University
Kerrville, Texas

Rebecca Kartje, MD, MBA, WTCS certified
Nicolet College
Rhinelander, Wisconsin

Patricia Laing-Arie
Meridian Technology Center
Stillwater, Oklahoma

Anne Lilly
Santa Rosa Junior College
Santa Rosa, California

Melanie S. MacNeil, MS, PhD
Brock University
St. Catharines, Ontario, Canada

Evie Mann
National College
Florence, Kentucky

Dan Matusiak, PhD
St. Dominic High School
O'Fallon, Missouri

Richard E. McKeeby
Union County College
Cranford, New Jersey

Michael A. Minardo, DC, MS
Manhattan College and College of Mount Saint Vincent
Riverdale, New York

Michael Murrow
George Washington University
Annapolis, Maryland

Tanya Nix, MBA, BSB, AAS/Surgical Technology
Northeast Texas Community College
Mount Pleasant, Texas

Amy Obringer, PhD
University of Saint Francis
Fort Wayne, Indiana

Susan Caley Opsal, MS
Illinois Valley Community College
Oglesby, Illinois

Keith R. Orloff
California Paramedical and Technical College
Long Beach, California

Vijay L. Parkash, MD, MSHCA
Broward College, South Campus
Pembroke Pines, Florida

Christine Payne
Sarasota County Technical Institute
Sarasota, Florida

Jessica Petersen
Pensacola State College
Pensacola, Florida

Roberta Pohlman, PhD
Wright State University
Dayton, Ohio

Krista Rompolski, MS, PhD, NSCA-CPT
Drexel University
Philadelphia, Pennsylvania

Ann Senisi Scott
Nassau Tech VOCES
Westbury, New York

Gerry Silverstein, PhD
University of Vermont
Burlington, Vermont

Kathleen Stockman
Delaware Technical & Community College
Newark, Delaware

Anna M. Strand
Gogebic Community College
Ironwood, Michigan

Kent R. Thomas, PhD
Wichita State University
Wichita, Kansas

Karin VanMeter, PhD
Iowa State University
Ames, Iowa

Eugene R. Volz
Sacramento City College
Sacramento, California

Amy Way
Lock Haven University
Clearfield, Pennsylvania

Margaret Weck, DA
St. Louis College of Pharmacy
St. Louis, Missouri

Iris Wilkelhake
Southeast Community College
Lincoln, Nebraska

Steve Wood, MS, ABD
Lone Star College
Houston, Texas

Thanks are due to all the people at Elsevier who have worked with us on this new edition. We wish especially to acknowledge the support and efforts of Kellie White, Executive Content Strategist; Karen Turner, Senior Content Development Specialist; Jeffrey Patterson, Publishing Services Manager; Carol O'Connell, Project Manager; and Brian Salisbury, Designer; all of whom were instrumental in bringing this edition to successful completion.

Kevin T. Patton
Gary A. Thibodeau

CONTENTS

17 Nutrition and Metabolism, 394

18 Urinary System, 408

19 Fluid and Electrolyte Balance, 428

20 Acid-Base Balance, 444

21 Reproductive Systems, 458

STRUCTURE & FUNCTION
OF THE BODY

Introduction to the Body

OUTLINE

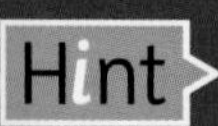

Scan this outline before you begin to read the chapter, as a preview of how the concepts are organized.

OBJECTIVES

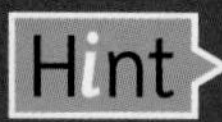

Before reading the chapter, review these goals for your learning.

After you have completed this chapter, you should be able to:

1. Define the terms *anatomy* and *physiology*.
2. Describe the process used to form scientific theories.
3. List and discuss in order of increasing complexity the levels of organization of the body.
4. Define the terms *anatomical position, supine,* and *prone.*
5. List and define the principal directional terms and sections (planes) used in describing the body and the relationship of body parts to one another.
6. List the major cavities of the body and the subdivisions of each.
7. List the nine abdominopelvic regions and the abdominopelvic quadrants.
8. Discuss and contrast the axial and the appendicular subdivisions of the body. Identify a number of specific anatomical regions in each area.
9. Explain the meaning of the term *homeostasis* and give an example of a typical homeostatic mechanism.

CHAPTER 1

There are many wonders in our world, but none is more wondrous than the human body. This is a textbook about that incomparable structure. It deals with two very distinct and yet interrelated sciences: **anatomy** and **physiology.**

As a science, anatomy is often defined as the study of the structure of an organism and the relationships of its parts. The word *anatomy* is derived from two word parts that mean "cutting apart." Anatomists learn about the structure of the human body by cutting it apart. This process, called **dissection,** is still the principal technique used to isolate and study the structural components or parts of the human body.

Physiology, on the other hand, is the study of the functions of living organisms and their parts. Physiologists use scientific experimentation to tease out how each activity of the body works, how it is regulated, and how it fits into the complex, coordinated operation of the whole human organism.

In the chapters that follow, you will see again and again that anatomical parts have structures exactly suited to perform specific functions. Each has a particular size, shape, form, or position in the body related directly to its ability to perform a unique and specialized activity. This principle—that *structure fits function*—is the key to understanding all of human biology.

LANGUAGE OF SCIENCE AND MEDICINE

Hint Before reading the chapter, say each of these terms out loud. This will help you to avoid stumbling over them as you read.

abdominal
(ab-DOM-ih-nal)
[*abdomin-* **belly,** *-al* **relating to**]

abdominal cavity
(ab-DOM-ih-nal KAV-ih-tee)
[*abdomin-* **belly,** *-al* **relating to,** *cav-* **hollow,** *-ity* **state**]

abdominopelvic cavity
(ab-DOM-ih-no-PEL-vik KAV-ih-tee)
[*abdomin-* **belly,** *-pelv-* **basin,** *cav-* **hollow,** *-ity* **state**]

abdominopelvic quadrant
(ab-DOM-ih-no-PEL-vik KWOD-rant)
[*abdomin-* **belly,** *-pelv-* **basin,** *cav-* **hollow,** *-ity* **state,** *-quad-* **four**]

abdominopelvic region
(ab-DOM-ih-no-PEL-vik REE-jun)
[*abdomin-* **belly,** *-pelv-* **basin,** *-ic* **relating to**]

allied health professions
(AL-eyed helth pro-FESH-unz)

anatomical position
(an-ah-TOM-i-kal poh-ZISH-un)
[*ana-* **apart,** *-tom-* **cut,** *-ical-* **relating to,** *posit-* **place,** *-tion* **state**]

anatomist
(ah-NAT-oh-mist)
[*ana-* **apart,** *-tom-* **cut,** *-ist* **agent**]

anatomy
(ah-NAT-oh-mee)
[*ana-* **apart,** *-tom-* **cut,** *-y* **action**]

antebrachial
(an-tee-BRAY-kee-al)
[*ante-* **front,** *-brachi-* **arm,** *-al* **relating to**]

anterior
(an-TEER-ee-or)
[*ante-* **front,** *-er-* **more,** *-or* **quality**]

Continued on p. 16

Scientific Method

What we often call the **scientific method** is merely a systematic approach to discovery. Although there is no single method for scientific discovery, many scientists follow the steps outlined in **Figure 1-1** to discover the concepts of human biology discussed in this textbook.

First, one makes a tentative explanation, called a **hypothesis.** A hypothesis is a reasonable guess based on previous informal observations or on previously tested explanations.

After a hypothesis has been proposed, it must be tested. This testing process is called **experimentation.** Scientific experiments are designed to be as simple as possible, to avoid the possibility of errors. Often, **experimental controls** are used to ensure that the test situation is not affecting the results. For example, if a new cancer drug is being tested, half of the test subjects will get the drug and half of the subjects will be given a harmless substitute. The group getting the drug is called the *test group*, and the group getting the substitute is called the *control group*. If both groups improve, or if only the control group improves, the drug's effectiveness hasn't been demonstrated. If the test group improves, but the control group does not, the hypothesis that the drug works is tentatively accepted as true. Experimentation requires accurate measurement and recording of data, along with logical interpretations of the data.

If the results of experimentation support the original hypothesis, it is tentatively accepted as true, and the researcher moves on to the next step. If the data do not support the hypothesis, the researcher tentatively rejects the hypothesis. Knowing which hypotheses are untrue is as valuable as knowing which hypotheses are true.

Initial experimental results are published in scientific journals so that other researchers can benefit from them and verify them. If experimental results cannot be reproduced by other scientists, then the hypothesis is not widely accepted. If a hypothesis withstands this rigorous retesting, the level of confidence in the hypothesis increases. A hypothesis that has gained a high level of confidence is called a **theory** or **law.**

Why is it important to know the steps of experimentation and developing theories if your main interest is a career in science applications—such as a health career? It is hard to grasp concepts fully if you do not understand how they were discovered and how they can change after additional experimentation. The facts presented in this textbook are among the latest theories of how the body is built and how it functions. As methods of imaging the body and measuring functional processes improve, we find new data that cause us to replace old theories with newer ones.

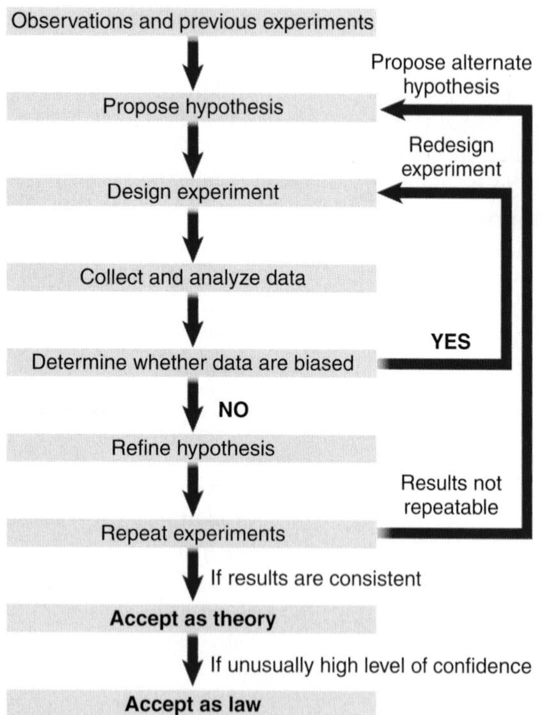

FIGURE 1-1 Scientific method. In this classic example, initial observations or results from other experiments may lead to formation of a new hypothesis. As more testing is done, eliminating outside influences or biases and ensuring consistent results, scientists begin to have more confidence in the principle and call it a theory or law.

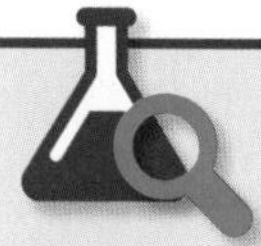

RESEARCH, ISSUES, AND TRENDS

METRIC SYSTEM

Scientists, many government agencies, and increasing numbers of American industries are using or moving toward the conversion of our system of English measurements to the metric system. The metric system is a decimal system in which measurement of length is based on the *meter* (39.37 inches), and weight or mass is based on the *gram* (about 454 grams equal a pound).

A micrometer is one millionth of a meter. (*Micron* is another name for micrometer.) In the metric system, the units of length are as follows:

1 kilometer = 1000 meters
1 meter (m) = 39.37 inches
1 centimeter (cm) = 1/100 m
1 millimeter (mm) = 1/1000 m
1 micrometer (μm) or micron (μ) = 1/1,000,000 m
1 nanometer (nm) = 1/1,000,000,000 m
1 Angstrom (Å) = 1/10,000,000,000 m

Approximately equal to 1 inch:

2.5 cm
25 mm
25,000 μm
25,000,000 nm

Levels of Organization

Before you begin the study of the many structures and functions of the human body, it is important to think about how those parts are organized and how they might logically fit together into a functioning whole.

Examine **Figure 1-2**. It illustrates the differing **levels of organization** that influence body structure and function. Note that the levels of organization progress from the least complex (chemical level) to the most complex (organism level). Because you already know that "structure fits function," it should not surprise you that the highly complex and coordinated functions of the whole body can be understood by discovering the many basic processes that occur in the smaller parts, such as organs, tissues, and cells.

Organization is one of the most important characteristics of body structure. Even the word *organism,* used to denote a living thing, implies organization.

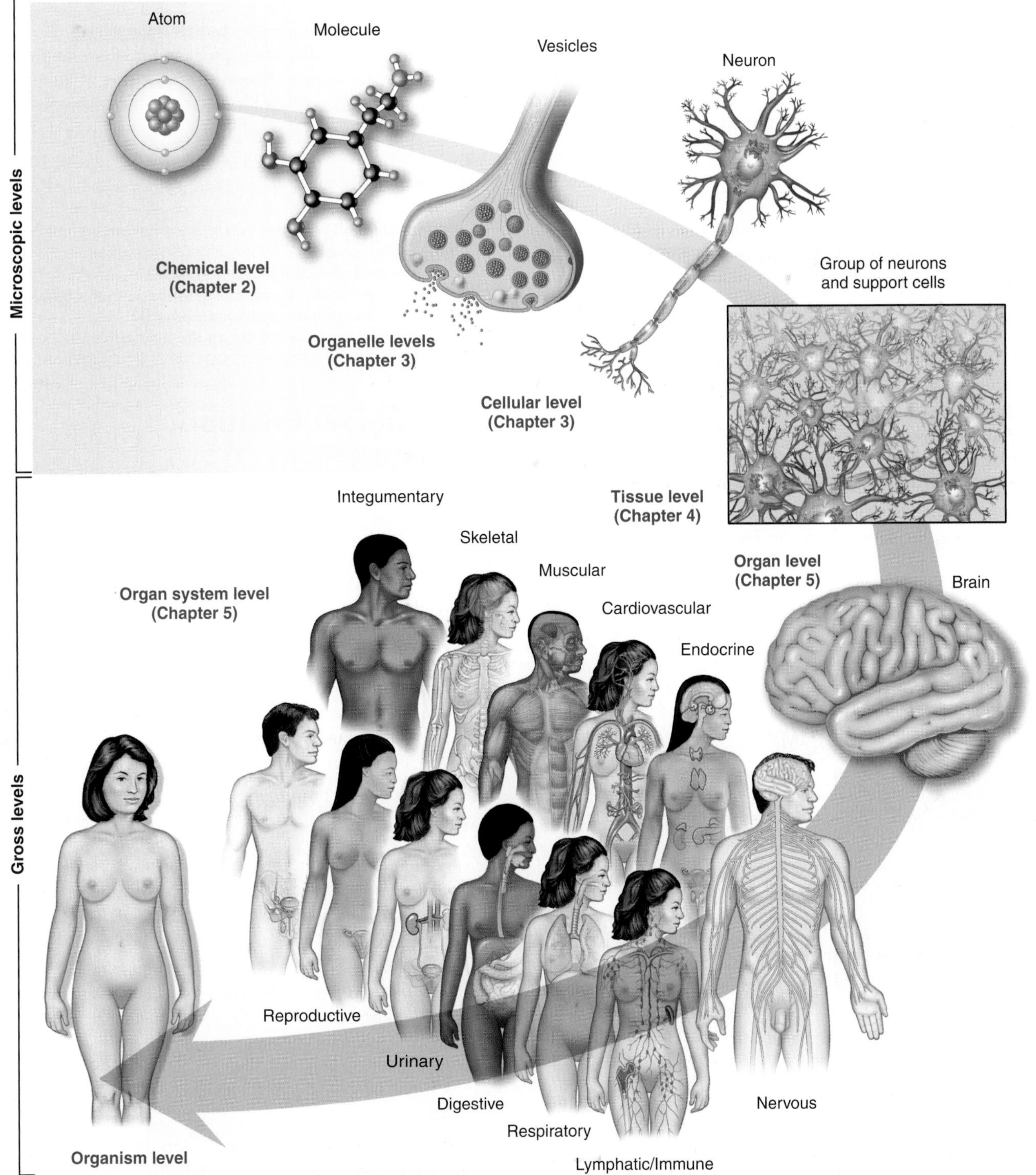

FIGURE 1-2 Levels of organization in the body. Atoms, molecules, and cells can ordinarily be seen only with a microscope, but the gross (large) structures of tissues, organs, systems, and the whole organism can be seen easily with the unaided eye.

Although the body is a single structure, it is made up of trillions of smaller structures—each with its own functions. Atoms and molecules are often referred to as the **chemical level** of organization. The existence of life depends on the proper amounts and proportions of many chemical substances in the cells of the body.

Many of the physical and chemical phenomena that play important roles in the life process are reviewed in Chapter 2. Such information provides an understanding of the physical basis for life and for the study of the next levels of organization so important in the study of anatomy and physiology—cells, tissues, organs, and systems.

Cells are considered to be the smallest "living" units of structure and function in our body. Although long recognized as the simplest units of living matter, cells are far from simple. They are extremely complex, a fact you will discover in Chapter 3.

Tissues are somewhat more complex than cells. By definition a tissue is an organization of many cells that act together to perform a common function. The cells of a tissue may be of several types but all are working together in some way to produce the structural and functional qualities of the tissue. Cells of a tissue are often held together and surrounded by varying amounts and varieties of gluelike, nonliving intercellular substances. The varied properties of different tissues are explored in Chapter 4.

Organs are larger and more complex than tissues. An organ is a group of several different kinds of tissues arranged in way that allow them to act as a unit to perform a special function. For instance, the brain shown in **Figure 1-2** is an example of organization at the organ level. Unlike microscopic molecules and cells, some tissues and most organs are gross (large) structures that can be seen easily without a microscope.

Systems are the most complex units that make up the body. A system is an organization of varying numbers and kinds of organs that can work together to perform complex functions for the body. All of the organs of the nervous system shown in **Figure 1-2** function to monitor and regulate the overall functioning of the body.

The *body as a whole*—the human **organism**—is all the atoms, molecules, cells, tissues, organs, and systems that you will study in subsequent chapters of this text. Although capable of being dissected or broken down into many parts, the body is a unified and complex assembly of structurally and functionally interactive components, each working together to ensure healthy survival.

QUICK CHECK

1. What is *anatomy*? What is *physiology*?
2. What are the major levels of organization in the body?
3. How is a tissue different than an organ?
4. Explain the principle "structure fits function."

Anatomical Position

Discussions about the body, the way it moves, its posture, or the relationship of one area to another assume that the body as a whole is in a specific position called the **anatomical position.** In this reference position (**Figure 1-3**) the body is in

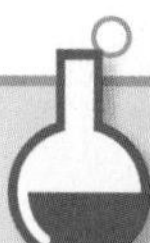

SCIENCE APPLICATIONS

MODERN ANATOMY

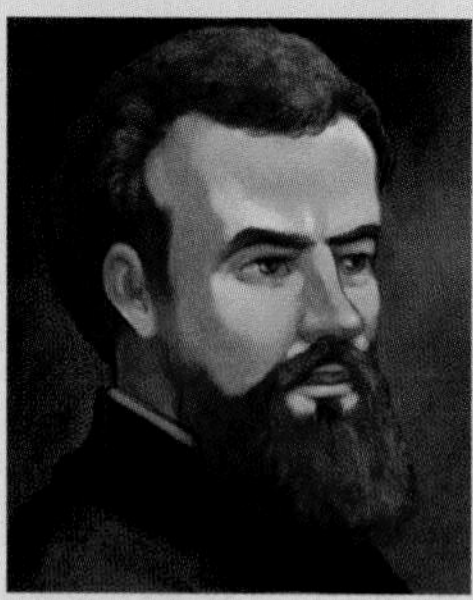

Andreas Vesalius (1514-1546)

Anatomists study the structure of the human body. Modern anatomy started during the Renaissance in Europe with the Flemish scientist Andreas Vesalius *(left)* and his contemporaries. Vesalius was the first to apply a scientific method (see the text on p. 4) to the study of the human body. Most anatomists still dissect *cadavers* (preserved human remains). However, today many anatomists also use imaging technologies such as x-rays, computerized scans, and even digitized photographs of thin slices of the body as you can see in the figure from the National Library of Medicine's Visible Human Project. Such digitized images can be reconstructed into dissectible, three-dimensional body views by computers.

Applications of modern anatomy are also found in the fields of **forensic science, anthropology, medicine** and **allied health professions,** *sports* and *athletics, dance,* and even *art* and *computerized animation.*

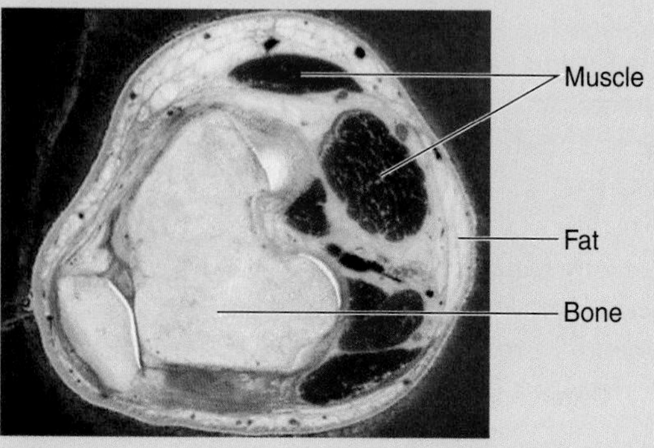

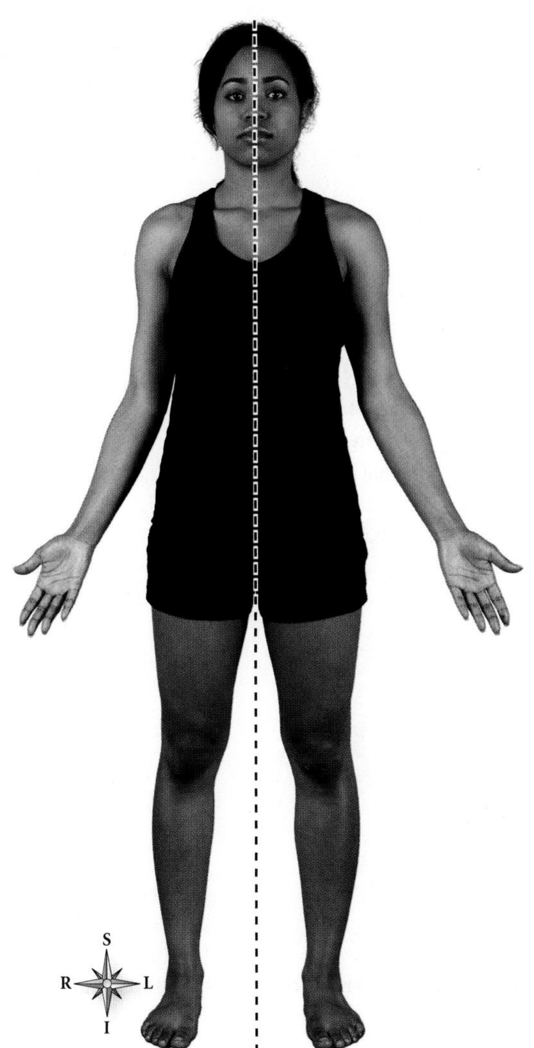

FIGURE 1-3 Anatomical position. The body is in an erect or standing posture with the arms at the sides and the palms forward. The head and feet also point forward. The dashed line shows the axis of the body's external *bilateral symmetry,* in which the right and left sides of the body are mirror images of each other. The anatomical compass rosette is explained in the text at the end of this page.

an erect or standing posture with the arms at the sides and palms turned forward. The head also points forward, as do the feet, which are aligned at the toe and set slightly apart. The broken line along the middle, or *median,* of the body demonstrates that the body has external *bilateral symmetry*—that is, the left and right sides of the body roughly mirror each other.

The anatomical position is a reference position that gives meaning to the directional terms used to describe the body parts and regions. In other words, you need to know the anatomical position so that you know how to apply *directional terms* correctly regardless of the particular position of the body being described.

Supine and **prone** are terms used to describe the position of the body when it is not in the anatomical position. In the supine position the body is lying face upward, and in the prone position the body is lying face downward.

Anatomical Directions

When studying the body, it is often helpful to know where an organ is in relation to other structures.

Directional Terms

The following **directional terms** are used in describing relative positions of body parts. To help you understand them better, they are listed in sets of opposite pairs.

1. **Superior** and **inferior** (Figure 1-4)—*superior* means "toward the head," and *inferior* means "toward the feet." *Superior* also means "upper" or "above," and *inferior* means "lower" or "below." For example, the lungs are located superior to the diaphragm, whereas the stomach is located inferior to it. (Check Figure 1-8 on p. 11 if you are not sure where these organs are.)
2. **Anterior** and **posterior** (see Figure 1-4)—*anterior* means "front" or "in front of." *Posterior* means "back" or "in back of." In humans, who walk in an upright position, *ventral* (toward the belly) can be used in place of anterior, and *dorsal* (toward the back) can be used for posterior. For example, the nose is on the anterior surface of the body, and the shoulder blades are on its posterior surface.
3. **Medial** and **lateral** (see Figure 1-4)—*medial* means "toward the midline of the body." *Lateral* means "toward the side of the body or away from its midline." For example, the great toe is at the medial side of the foot, and the little toe is at its lateral side. The heart lies medial to the lungs, and the lungs lie lateral to the heart.
4. **Proximal** and **distal** (see Figure 1-4)—*proximal* means "toward or nearest the trunk of the body, or nearest the point of origin of one of its parts." *Distal* means "away from or farthest from the trunk or the point of origin of a body part." For example, the elbow lies at the proximal end of the forearm, whereas the hand lies at its distal end. Likewise, the distal portion of a kidney tubule is more distant from the tubule origin than is the proximal part of the kidney tubule.
5. **Superficial** and **deep**—*superficial* means nearer the surface. *Deep* means farther away from the body surface. For example, the skin of the arm is superficial to the muscles below it, and the bone of the arm is deep to the muscles that surround and cover it.

Anatomical Compass Rosette

To make the reading of anatomical figures a little easier for you, we have used an anatomical compass rosette throughout this book. On many figures, you will see a small compass rosette like you might see on a geographical map. Instead of being labeled **N, S, E,** or **W,** the anatomical compass rosette is labeled with abbreviated anatomical directions. For example, in

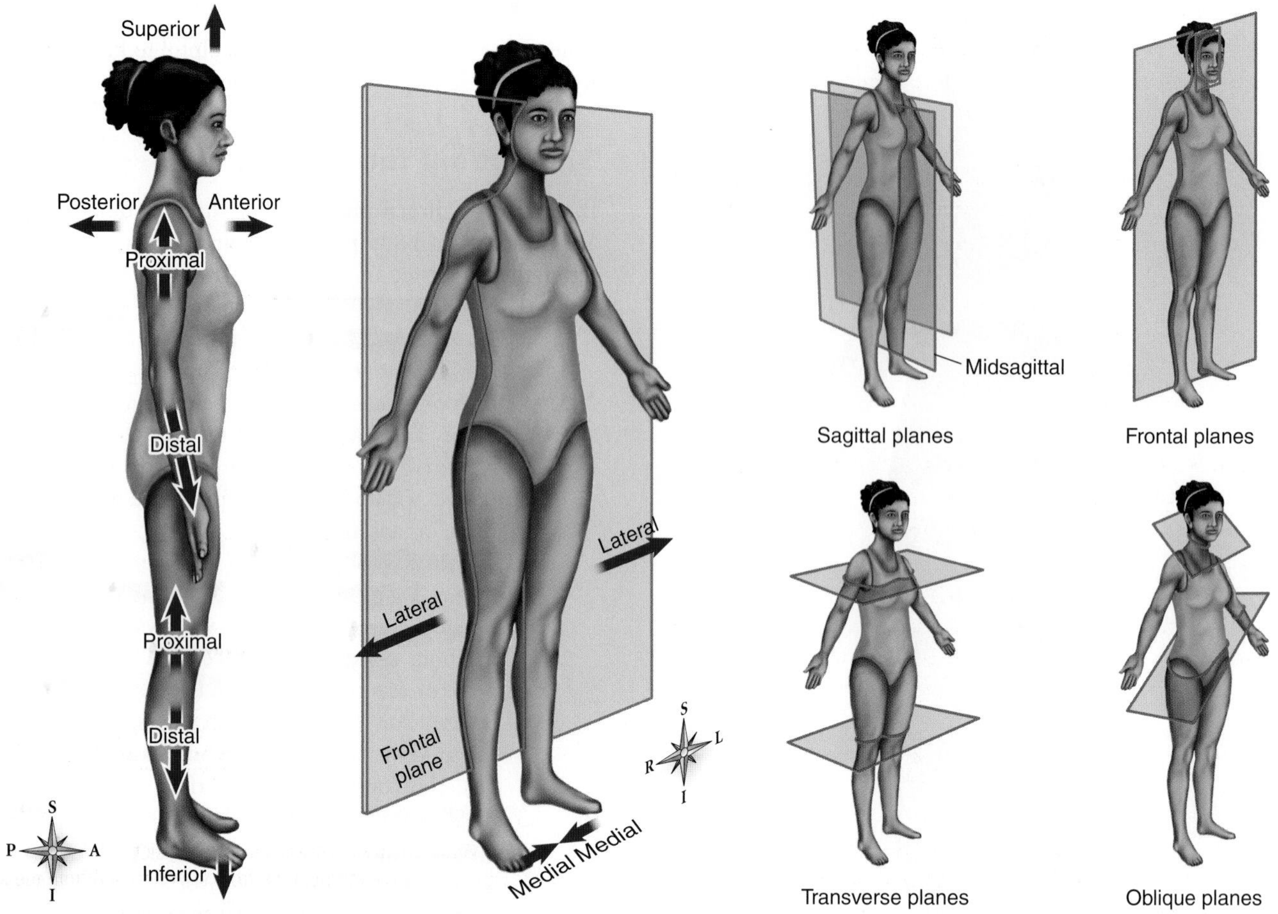

FIGURE 1-4 Directions and planes of the body. The arrows show anatomical directions and the blue plates show examples of body planes along which cuts or sections are made in visualizing the structure of the body.

Figure 1-3, the rosette is labeled **S** (for superior) on top and **I** (for inferior) on the bottom. Notice that in Figure 1-3 the rosette shows **R** (right) on the subject's right, not your right. Now look at the rosettes in Figure 1-4 and compare them to the body positions shown.

Here are the directional abbreviations used with the rosettes in this book:

A = Anterior
D = Distal
I = Inferior
(opposite M) L = Lateral
(opposite R) L = Left
M = Medial
(opposite A) P = Posterior
(opposite D) P = Proximal
R = Right
S = Superior

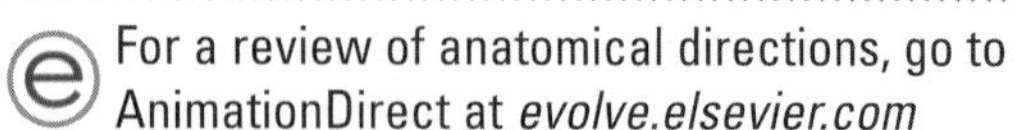

For a review of anatomical directions, go to AnimationDirect at *evolve.elsevier.com*

QUICK CHECK

1. What is the anatomical position?
2. Why are the anatomical directions listed in pairs?

Planes of the Body

To facilitate the study of individual organs or the body as a whole, it is often useful to subdivide or "cut" it into smaller segments. This can be done with actual cuts in a dissection, or it can be done virtually, as in medical imaging in computed tomography (CT) or magnetic resonance imaging (MRI) scans. To understand such a cut—also called a **section**—one must imagine a body being divided by an imaginary flat plate called a **plane.**

Because many anatomical sections, cut along specific planes of the body, are used in anatomical studies and medical imaging, we describe them here. As you read the following descriptions, identify each type of plane in Figure 1-4.

1. **Sagittal plane**—a sagittal cut or section runs along a lengthwise plane running from front to back. It

divides the body or any of its parts into right and left sides. The **midsagittal plane** shown in Figure 1-4 is a unique type of sagittal plane that divides the body into two *equal halves*.

2. **Frontal plane**—a frontal plane *(coronal plane)* is a lengthwise plane running from side to side. As you can see in Figure 1-4, a frontal plane divides the body or any of its parts into anterior and posterior (front and back) portions.
3. **Transverse plane**—a transverse plane is a *horizontal* or crosswise plane. Such a plane (see Figure 1-4) divides the body or any of its parts into upper and lower portions.

Sometimes it is helpful to make a cut along a plane that is not parallel to the planes we have already mentioned. Such diagonal cuts are made along **oblique planes,** which you can see illustrated in Figure 1-4.

Besides using planes to cut the body into various sections, we sometimes use planes to describe movement. For example, one rotates the head in a transverse plane, and one can move a finger along both a sagittal plane and along a frontal plane.

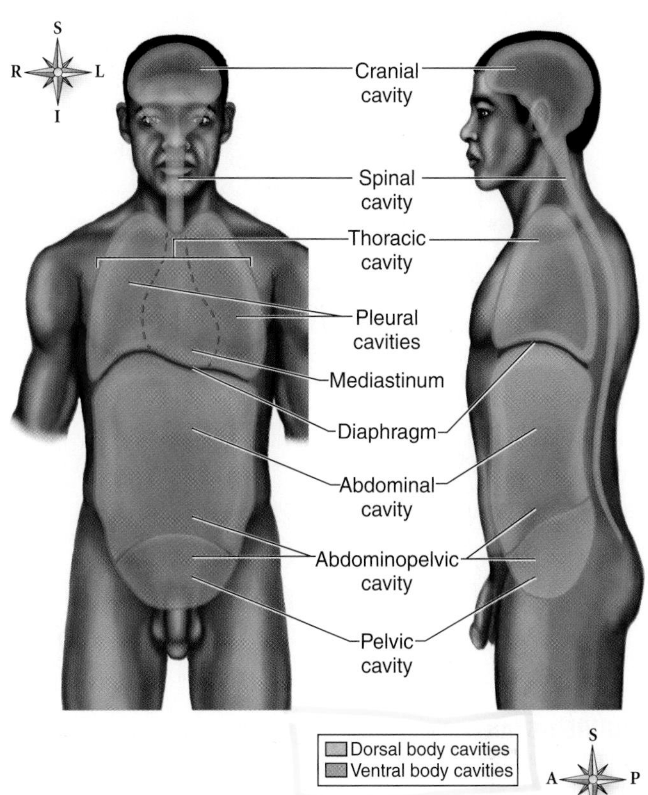

FIGURE 1-5 Body cavities. Location and subdivisions of the dorsal and ventral body cavities as viewed from the front (anterior) and from the side (lateral).

Body Cavities

Contrary to its external appearance, the body is not a solid structure. It is made up of open spaces or cavities that in turn contain compact, well-ordered arrangements of internal organs. The two major body cavities are called the **dorsal body cavities** and **ventral body cavities.** The location and outlines of the major body cavities are illustrated in Figure 1-5.

Dorsal Cavities

The dorsal cavities shown in Figure 1-5 include the space inside the skull that contains the brain. It is called the **cranial cavity.** The space inside the spinal column is called the **spinal cavity.** It contains the spinal cord. The cranial and spinal cavities are *dorsal cavities because they are located in a dorsal position in the body.*

Ventral Cavities

The *ventral cavities* are located in a ventral position in the body.

Thoracic and Abdominopelvic Cavities

The upper ventral cavities include the **thoracic cavity,** a space that you may think of as your chest cavity. Its midportion is a subdivision of the thoracic cavity, called the **mediastinum.** The lateral subdivisions of the thoracic cavity are called the right and left **pleural cavities.**

The lower ventral cavities in Figure 1-5 include an **abdominal cavity** and a **pelvic cavity.** Actually, they form only one cavity, the **abdominopelvic cavity,** because no physical partition separates them. In Figure 1-5 a faint line shows the approximate point of separation between the abdominal and pelvic subdivisions. Notice, however, that an actual physical partition separates the thoracic cavity above from the abdominopelvic cavity below. This muscular sheet is the **diaphragm.** It is dome-shaped and is the most important muscle for breathing.

Abdominopelvic Quadrants and Regions

To make it easier to locate organs in the large abdominopelvic cavity, anatomists have divided the abdominopelvic cavity into four **abdominopelvic quadrants:**

1. Right upper (or right superior) quadrant
2. Right lower (or right inferior) quadrant
3. Left upper (or left superior) quadrant
4. Left lower (or left inferior) quadrant

As you can see in Figure 1-6, the midsagittal and transverse planes, which were described in the previous section, pass through the navel (umbilicus) and divide the abdominopelvic region into the four quadrants. This method of subdividing the abdominopelvic cavity is frequently used by health professionals and is useful for locating the origin of pain or describing the location of a tumor or other abnormality.

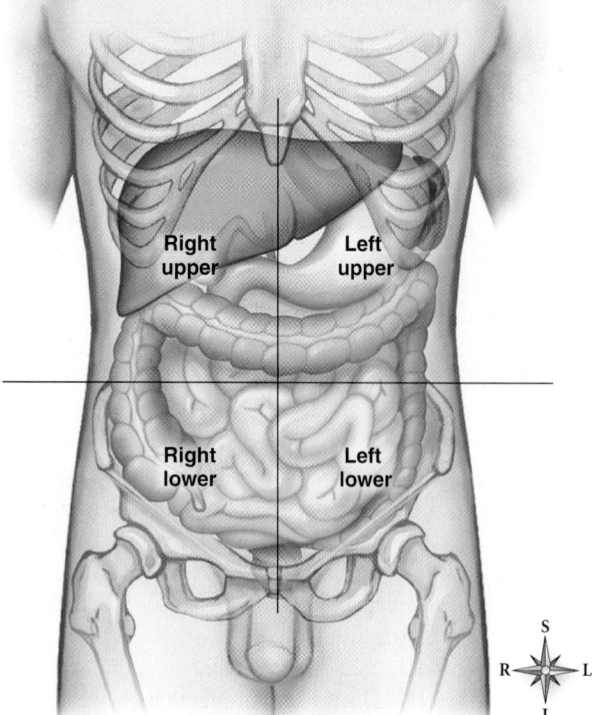

FIGURE 1-6 Abdominopelvic quadrants. Diagram showing location of internal organs within four abdominal quadrants.

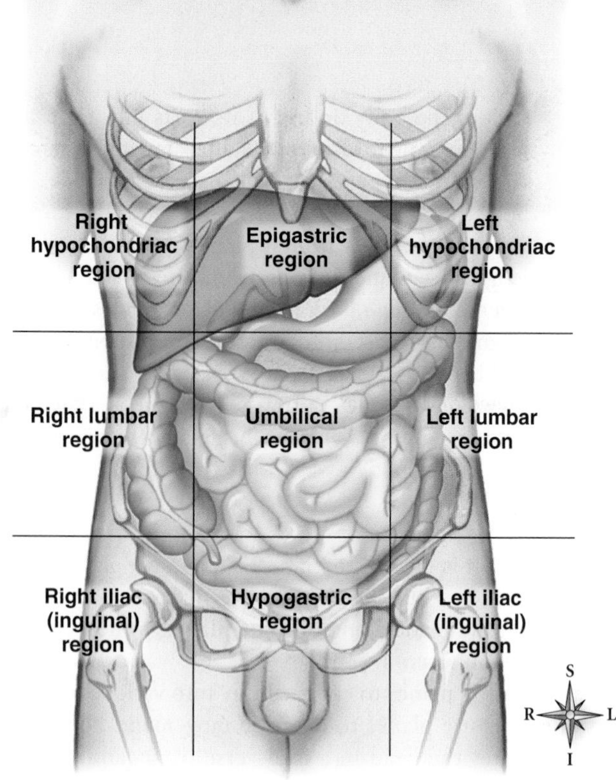

FIGURE 1-7 Abdominopelvic regions. The most superficial organs are shown. Look at **Figure 1-8** (p. 11). Can you identify the deeper structures in each region?

You may notice that terms like *upper* and *lower* are often used to name quadrants, which may seem overly informal compared with the more technical terms *superior* and *inferior.* However, this practice reflects the usage found in many clinical environments, where a mix of informal and technical terminology is commonly encountered.

Another and perhaps more precise way to divide the abdominopelvic cavity is shown in **Figure 1-7**. Here, the abdominopelvic cavity is subdivided into nine abdominopelvic regions defined as follows:

1. **Upper abdominopelvic regions**—the **right hypochondriac** and **left hypochondriac regions** and the **epigastric region** lie above an imaginary line across the abdomen at the level of the ninth rib cartilages.
2. **Middle abdominopelvic regions**—the **right lumbar** and **left lumbar regions** and the **umbilical region** lie below an imaginary line across the abdomen at the level of the ninth rib cartilages and above an imaginary line across the abdomen at the top of the hip bones.
3. **Lower abdominopelvic regions**—the **right iliac** and **left iliac regions** (also called **inguinal regions**) and the **hypogastric region** lie below an imaginary line across the abdomen at the level of the top of the hip bones.

Some of the organs in the largest body cavities are visible in **Figure 1-8** and are listed in **Table 1-1**. Find each body cavity in a model of the human body if you have access to one. Try to identify the organs in each cavity, and try to visualize their locations in your own body. Study **Figure 1-5** and **Figure 1-8**.

QUICK CHECK

1. What is meant by a *section* of the body?
2. What are the two major cavities of the body?
3. What is the difference between the *abdominal cavity* and the *abdominopelvic cavity*?
4. What is the difference between *right upper quadrant* and *right superior quadrant*?

TABLE 1-1 Body Cavities

BODY CAVITY	ORGAN(S)
Ventral Body Cavities	
Thoracic Cavity	
Mediastinum	Trachea, heart, blood vessels
Pleural cavities	Lungs
Abdominopelvic Cavity	
Abdominal cavity	Liver, gallbladder, stomach, spleen, pancreas, small intestine, parts of large intestine
Pelvic cavity	Lower (sigmoid) colon, rectum, urinary bladder, reproductive organs
Dorsal Body Cavities	
Cranial cavity	Brain
Spinal cavity	Spinal cord

Body Regions

To recognize an object, you usually first notice its overall structure and form. For example, a car is recognized as a car before the specific details of its tires, grill, or wheel covers are noted. Recognition of the human form also occurs as you first identify overall shape and basic outline. However, for more specific identification to occur, details of size, shape, and appearance of individual body areas must be described. Individuals differ in overall appearance because specific body areas such as the face or torso have unique identifying characteristics. Detailed descriptions of the human form require that specific regions be identified and appropriate terms be used to describe them.

The ability to identify and correctly describe specific body areas is particularly important in the health sciences. For a patient to complain of pain in the head is not as specific and therefore not as useful to a physician or nurse as a more specific and localized description. Saying that the pain is facial provides additional information and helps to more specifically identify the area of pain. By using correct anatomical terms such as forehead, cheek, or chin to describe the area of pain, attention can be focused even more quickly on the specific anatomical area that may need attention. Familiarize yourself with the more common terms used to describe specific body regions identified in **Figure 1-9** and listed in **Table 1-2**.

The body as a whole can be subdivided into two major portions or components: **axial** and **appendicular.** The axial portion of the body consists of the head, neck, and torso or trunk. The appendicular portion consists of the upper and lower extremities (or limbs).

Each major axial and appendicular area is subdivided as shown in **Figure 1-9**. Note, for example, that the torso is composed of thoracic, abdominal, and pelvic areas, and the upper extremity is divided into arm, forearm, wrist, and hand components. Although most terms used to describe gross body regions are well understood, misuse is

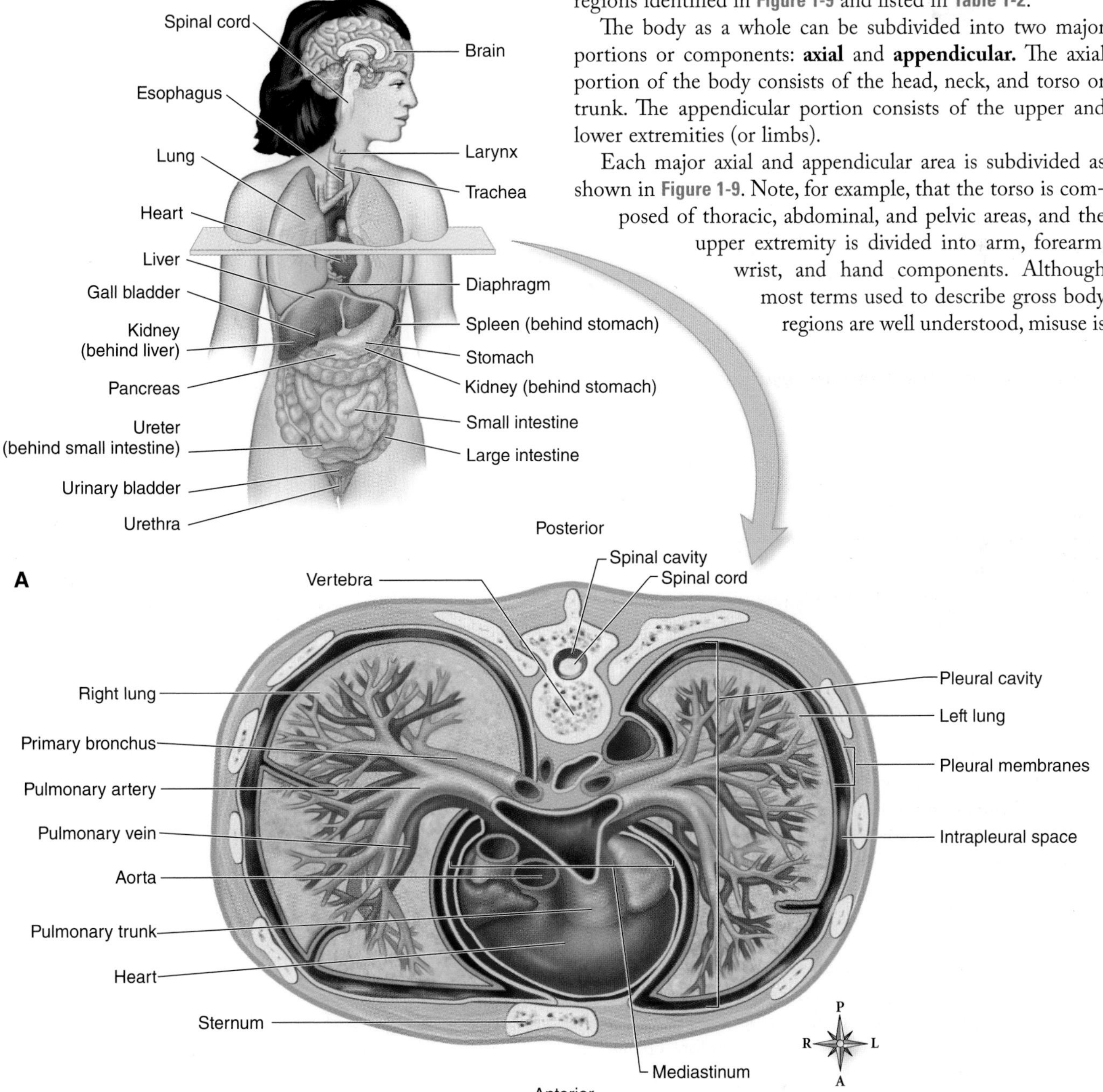

FIGURE 1-8 Organs of the major body cavities. A, A view from the front. **B,** Transverse section viewed from above.

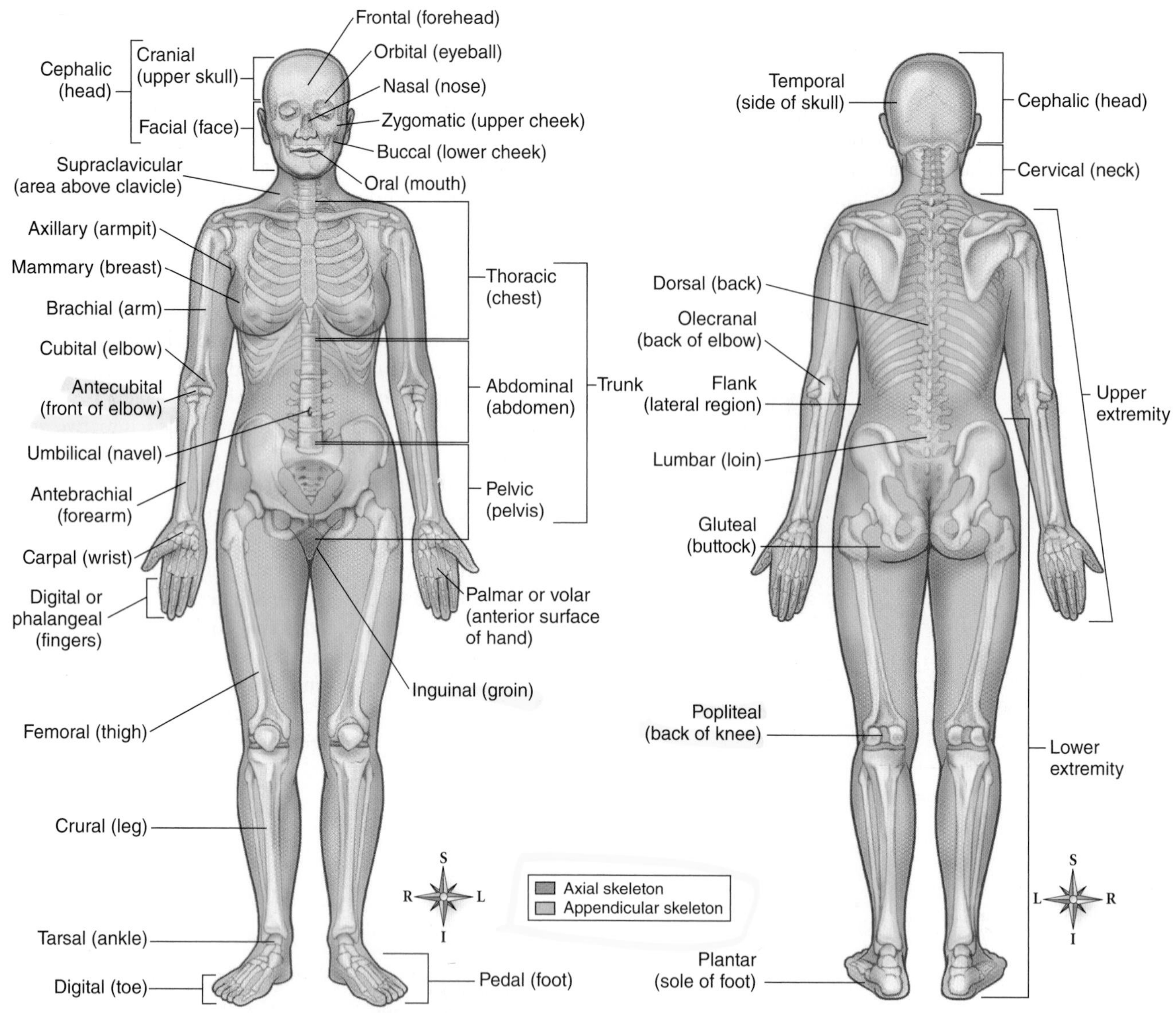

FIGURE 1-9 Axial and appendicular divisions of the body. Specific body regions are labeled (examples in parentheses). For example, the cephalic region includes the head. Notice how the axial and appendicular regions of the body frame are distinguished by contrasting colors.

common. The word *leg* is a good example: it refers to the area of the lower extremity between the knee and ankle and not to the entire lower extremity.

The structure of each person's body is unique. Even identical twins have some variations in the size, shape, and texture of various tissues and organs. The structure of the body also changes in many ways and at varying rates during a lifetime. Before young adulthood, the body develops and grows. After young adulthood, the body gradually undergoes changes related to aging. For example, with the reduced activity of the body as one advances through older adulthood, many body organs and tissues decrease in size and therefore change in their functions. A degenerative process that results from disuse is called **atrophy.** In many cases, atrophy can be reversed with therapy. Some tissues simply lose their elasticity or ability to regenerate as we get older. Nearly every chapter of this book refers to a few of the changes that occur through the life cycle.

QUICK CHECK

1. What is the difference between the *axial* portion of the body and the *appendicular* portion of the body?
2. What are some of the regions of the upper extremity and lower extremity?

The Balance of Body Functions

Homeostasis

Although they may have very different structures, all living organisms maintain mechanisms that ensure survival of the body and success in propagating its genes through its offspring.

TABLE 1-2 Descriptive Terms for Body Regions

AREA OR BODY REGION	EXAMPLE
Abdominal region	Anterior torso below diaphragm
Antebrachial region	Forearm
Axillary region	Armpit
Brachial region	Arm
Buccal region	Cheek
Carpal region	Wrist
Cephalic region	Head
Cervical region	Neck
Cranial region	Skull
Crural region	Leg
Cubital region	Elbow*
Cutaneous region	Skin (or body surface)
Digital region	Fingers or toes
Dorsal region	Back
Facial region	Face
Frontal region	Forehead
Nasal region	Nose
Oral region	Mouth
Orbital region *or* **ophthalmic region**	Eyes
Zygomatic region	Upper cheek
Femoral region	Thigh
Gluteal region	Buttock
Inguinal region	Groin
Lumbar region	Lower back between ribs and pelvis
Mammary region	Breast
Occipital region	Back of lower skull
Olecranal region	Back of elbow
Palmar region	Palm of hand
Pedal region	Foot
Pelvic region	Lower portion of torso
Perineal region	Area (perineum) between anus and genitals
Plantar region	Sole of foot
Popliteal region	Area behind knee
Supraclavicular region	Area above clavicle
Tarsal region	Ankle
Temporal region	Side of skull
Thoracic region	Chest
Umbilical region	Area around navel or umbilicus
Volar region	Palm or sole

*The term *cubital* may also be used to refer to the forearm.

Survival depends on the body maintaining relatively constant conditions within the body. **Homeostasis** is what physiologists call the relative constancy of the internal environment. The cells of the body live in an internal environment made up mostly of water combined with salts and other dissolved substances.

Like fish in a fishbowl, the cells are able to survive only if the conditions of their watery environment remain relatively stable—that is, only if conditions stay within a narrow range. The temperature, salt content, acid level (pH), fluid volume and pressure, oxygen concentration, and other vital conditions must remain within acceptable limits. To maintain a narrow range of water conditions in a fishbowl, one may add a heater, an air pump, and filters. Likewise, the body has mechanisms that act as heaters, air pumps, and the like, to maintain the relatively stable conditions of its internal fluid environment (**Figure 1-10**).

Because the activities of cells and external disturbances are always shifting the conditions inside the body, fluctuations

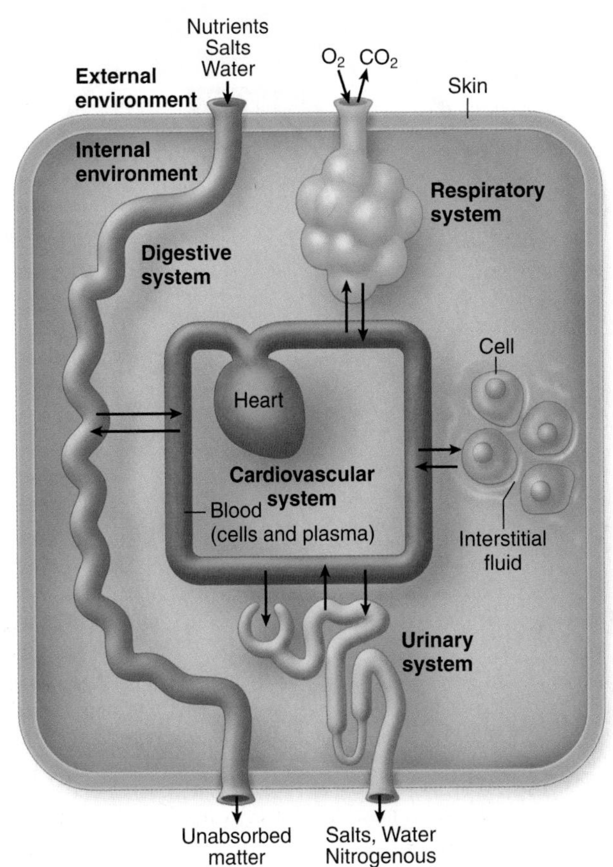

FIGURE 1-10 Diagram of the body's internal environment. The human body is like a bag of fluid separated from the external environment. Tubes, such as the digestive tract and respiratory tract, bring the external environment to deeper parts of the bag where substances can be absorbed into the internal fluid environment or excreted into the external environment. All the "accessories" somehow help maintain a constant environment inside the bag that allows the cells that live there to survive.

occur frequently. Therefore, the body must constantly work to maintain or restore stability, or homeostasis. For example, the heat generated by muscle activity during exercise may cause the body's temperature to rise above normal. The body must then release sweat, which evaporates and cools the body back to a normal temperature.

Feedback Control

To accomplish such self-regulation, a highly complex and integrated communication control system is required. The basic type of control system in the body is called a **feedback loop.**

The idea of a feedback loop is borrowed from engineering. **Figure 1-11**, *A*, shows how an engineer would describe the feedback loop that maintains stability of temperature in a building. Cold winds outside a building may cause a decrease in building temperature below normal. A **sensor,** in this case a thermometer, detects the change in temperature. Information from the sensor *feeds back* to a **control center**—a thermostat in this example—that compares the actual temperature with the normal temperature and responds by activating the building's furnace. The furnace is called an **effector** because it has an effect on the controlled condition (temperature). Because the sensor continually feeds information back to the control center, the furnace will be automatically shut off when the temperature has returned to normal.

As you can see in **Figure 1-11**, *B*, the body uses a similar feedback loop in restoring body temperature when a person becomes chilled. Nerve endings that act as temperature sensors feed information to a control center in the brain that compares actual body temperature to normal body temperature. In response to a chill, the brain sends nerve signals to muscles that shiver. Shivering produces heat that increases our body temperature. We stop shivering when feedback

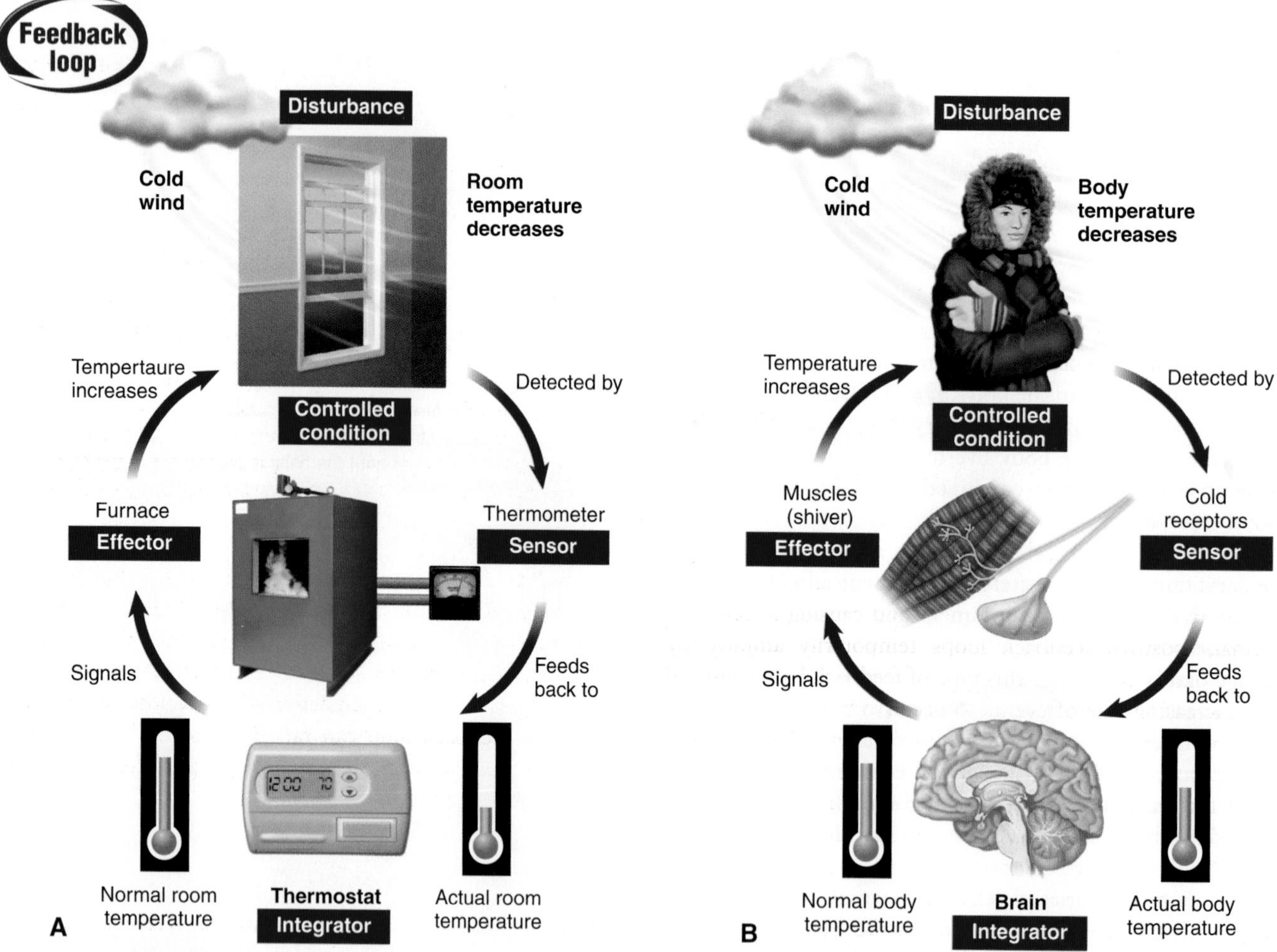

FIGURE 1-11 Negative feedback loops. A, An engineer's diagram showing how a relatively constant room temperature (controlled condition) can be maintained. A thermostat (control center) receives feedback information from a thermometer (sensor) and responds by counteracting a change from normal by activating a furnace (effector). **B,** A physiologist's diagram showing how a relatively constant body temperature (controlled condition) can be maintained. The brain (control center) receives feedback information from nerve endings called cold receptors (sensors) and responds by counteracting a change from normal by activating shivering by muscles (effectors), which increases body temperature.

information tells the brain that body temperature has increased to normal.

Negative Feedback

Feedback loops such as those shown in Figure 1-11 are called **negative feedback loops** because they oppose, or negate, a change in a controlled condition. Most homeostatic control loops in the body involve negative feedback because reversing changes back toward a normal value tends to stabilize conditions—exactly what homeostasis is all about.

Think about the opposite circumstance of that shown in Figure 1-11, as when we become overheated during hot weather. Temperature receptors detect a body temperature higher than normal, and the brain sends signals to the sweat glands to cool us down through evaporation. Thus the conditions are reversed and balance is restored.

Another example of a negative feedback loop occurs when increasing blood carbon dioxide concentration caused by muscles producing additional carbon dioxide during exercise is counteracted by an increase in breathing to bring the blood carbon dioxide level back down to normal. An additional example is the excretion of larger than usual volumes of urine when the volume of fluid in the body is greater than the normal, ideal amount.

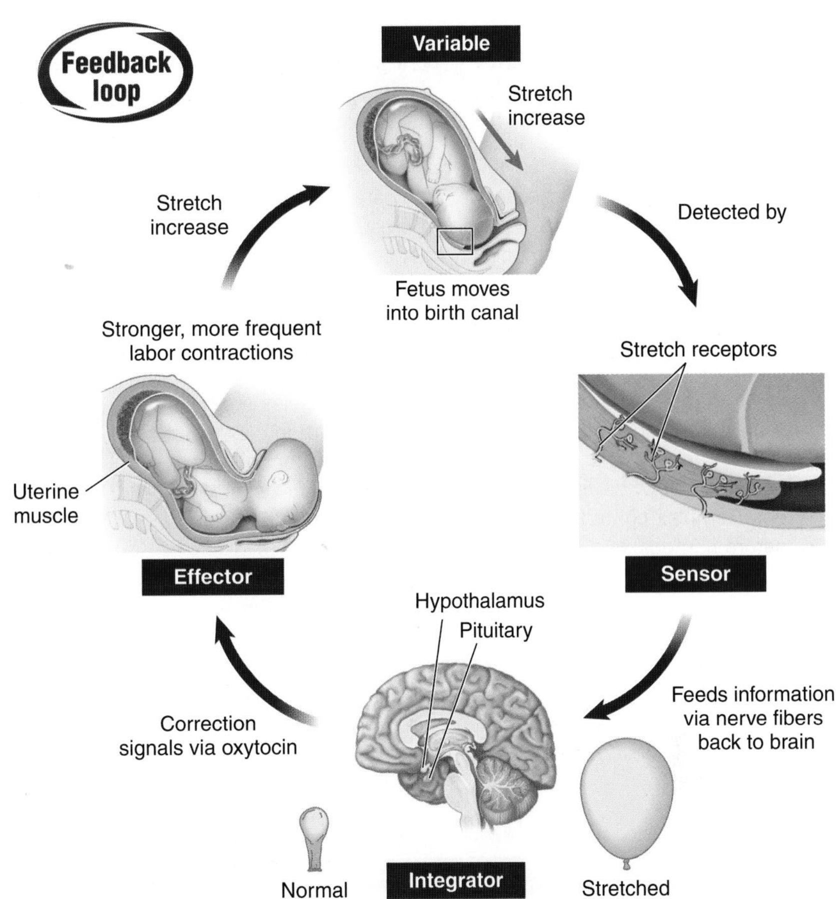

FIGURE 1-12 Positive feedback loop. An example of positive feedback occurs when a baby is born. As the baby is pushed from the womb (uterus) into the birth canal (vagina), stretch receptors detect the movement of the baby. Stretch information is fed back to the brain, triggering the pituitary gland to secrete a hormone called oxytocin (OT). OT travels through the bloodstream to the uterus, where it stimulates stronger contractions. Stronger contractions push the baby farther along the birth canal, thereby increasing stretch and stimulating the release of more OT. Uterine contractions quickly get stronger and stronger until the baby is pushed out of the body, and the positive feedback loop is broken. OT also can be injected therapeutically by a physician to stimulate labor contractions.

Positive Feedback

Although not common, **positive feedback loops** exist in the body and are sometimes also involved in normal function. Positive feedback control loops are stimulatory. Instead of opposing a change in the internal environment and causing a "return to normal," positive feedback loops temporarily amplify the change that is occurring. This type of feedback loop causes an ever-increasing rate of events to occur until something stops the process. An example of a positive feedback loop includes the events that cause rapid increases in uterine contractions before the birth of a baby (Figure 1-12). Another example is the increasingly rapid sticking together of blood cells called *platelets* to form a plug that begins formation of a blood clot.

In each of these cases, the process increases rapidly until the positive feedback loop is stopped suddenly by the birth of a baby or the formation of a clot. In the long run, such normal positive feedback events also help maintain constancy of the internal environment.

However, negative feedback can abnormally turn into positive feedback, possibly causing a deadly shift in body function. For example, severe bleeding may cause a drop in blood pressure (needed for continued blood flow), so the heart beats faster to increase the blood pressure back to normal, while also increasing the loss of blood, which causes a further drop in blood pressure and an even faster heart rate in an ever-increasing cycle. The amplification of blood loss caused by this positive feedback loop can rapidly turn deadly. To stop the positive feedback loop, one could apply pressure to the wound to stop or slow the loss of blood.

Normal Fluctuations

It is important to realize that normal homeostatic control mechanisms can only maintain a *relative* constancy. All homeostatically controlled conditions in the body do not remain absolutely constant. Rather, conditions normally fluctuate near a normal, ideal value. Thus body temperature, for example, rarely remains exactly the same for very long. It usually fluctuates up and down near a person's normal body temperature.

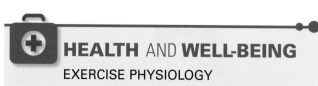

HEALTH AND WELL-BEING

EXERCISE PHYSIOLOGY

Exercise physiologists study the effects of exercise on the body organ systems. For example, many are interested in the complex control mechanisms that preserve or restore homeostasis during or immediately after periods of strenuous physical activity. Exercise, defined as any significant use of skeletal muscles, is a normal activity with beneficial results. However, exercise temporarily disrupts the internal environment—a situation that requires homeostatic mechanisms to restore stability. For example, when muscles are worked, the core body temperature rises and carbon dioxide levels in the blood increase. These and many other body functions quickly deviate from "normal ranges" that exist at rest. Complex control mechanisms must then "kick in" to restore homeostasis.

As a scientific discipline, exercise physiology attempts to explain many body processes in terms of how they function to restore homeostasis during and after exercise. Exercise physiology has many practical applications in therapy and rehabilitation, athletics, occupational health, and general wellness. This specialty concerns itself with the function of the whole body, not just one or two body systems.

Because all organs function to help maintain homeostatic balance, we discuss negative and positive feedback mechanisms often throughout the remaining chapters of this book.

Before leaving this brief introduction to physiology, we must pause to state an important principle: the ability to maintain the balance of body functions is related to age. During childhood, homeostatic functions gradually become more and more efficient and effective. They operate with maximum efficiency and effectiveness during young adulthood. During late adulthood and old age, they gradually become less and less efficient and effective.

Changes and functions occurring during the early years are called *developmental processes*. Those occurring after young adulthood are called *aging processes*. In general, developmental processes improve efficiency of functions. Aging processes usually diminish them.

QUICK CHECK

1. Why is *homeostasis* also called "balance" of body function?
2. What is a *feedback loop* and how does it work?
3. How does *negative feedback* differ from *positive feedback*?
4. How can negative feedback abnormally turn into positive feedback?

LANGUAGE OF SCIENCE AND MEDICINE *(continued from p. 3)*

anthropology
(an-thro-POL-oh-jee)
[*anthropo-* **human,** *-log-* **words (study of),** *-y* **activity**]

appendicular
(ah-pen-DIK-yoo-lar)
[*append-* **hang upon,** *-ic-* **relating to,** *-ul-* **little,** *-ar* **relating to**]

atrophy
(AT-roh-fee)
[*a-* **without,** *-troph-* **nourishment,** *-y* **state**]

axial
(AK-see-all)
[*axi-* **axis,** *-al* **relating to**]

axillary
(AK-sil-layr-ee)
[*axilla-* **wing,** *-ary* **relating to**]

brachial
(BRAY-kee-al)
[*brachi-* **arm,** *-al* **relating to**]

buccal
(BUK-al)
[*bucca-* **cheek,** *-al* **relating to**]

carpal
(KAR-pul)
[*carp-* **wrist,** *-al* **relating to**]

cell
(sel)
[*cell* **storeroom**]

cephalic
(seh-FAL-ik)
[*cephal-* **head,** *-ic* **relating to**]

cervical
(SER-vih-kal)
[*cervic-* **neck,** *-al* **relating to**]

chemical level
(KEM-ih-kal LEV-el)
[*chem-* **alchemy,** *-ical* **relating to**]

control center
(kon-TROHL SEN-ter)

cranial
(KRAY-nee-al)
[*crani-* **skull,** *-al* **relating to**]

cranial cavity
(KRAY-nee-al KAV-ih-tee)
[*crani-* **skull,** *-al* **relating to,** *cav-* **hollow,** *-ity* **state**]

crural
(KROOR-al)
[*crur-* **leg,** *-al* **relating to**]

cubital
(KYOO-bih-tal)
[*cubit-* **elbow,** *-al* **relating to**]

cutaneous
(kyoo-TAYN-ee-us)
[*cut-* **skin,** *-aneous* **relating to**]

deep

diaphragm
(DYE-ah-fram)
[*dia-* **across,** *-phrag-* **enclose**]

digital
(DIJ-ih-tal)
[*digit-* **finger or toe,** *-al* **relating to**]

directional term

dissection
(dih-SEK-shun)
[*dissect-* **to cut apart,** *-tion* **process**]

distal
(DIS-tal)
[*dist-* **distance,** *-al* **relating to**]

dorsal
(DOR-sal)
[*dors-* **back,** *-al* **relating to**]

dorsal body cavity
(DOR-sal BOD-ee KAV-ih-tee)
[*dors-* **back,** *-al* **relating to,** *cav-* **hollow,** *-ity* **state**]

effector
(ef-FEK-tor)
[*effect-* **accomplish,** *-or* **agent**]

epigastric region
(ep-ih-GAS-trik)
[*epi-* **upon,** *gastr-* **stomach,** *-ic* **relating to]**

exercise physiologist
(EK-ser-syze fiz-ee-OL-oh-jist)
[*physio-* **nature (function),** *-o-* **combining form,** *-log-* **words (study of),** *-ist* **agent]**

experimental control
(eks-payr-ih-MEN-tel kon-TROL)
[*ex-* **out of,** *-peri-* **tested,** *-ment-* **thing,** *-al* **relating to]**

experimentation
(eks-payr-ih-men-TAY-shun)
[*ex-* **out of,** *-peri-* **tested,** *-ment-* **thing,** *-tion* **process]**

facial
(FAY-shal)
[*faci-* **face,** *-al* **relating to]**

feedback loop
(FEED-bak loop)

femoral
(FEM-or-al)
[*femor-* **thigh,** *-al* **relating to]**

forensic science
(foh-REN-zik SYE-ens)
[*forens-* **of the public forum,** *-ic* **relating to,** *scienc-* **knowledge]**

frontal
(FRON-tal)

frontal plane
(FRUN-tal playn)
[*front-* **forehead,** *-al* **relating to,** *plan-* **flat surface]**

gluteal
(GLOO-tee-al)
[*glut-* **buttocks,** *-al* **relating to]**

homeostasis
(hoh-me-oh-STAY-sis)
[*homeo-* **same or equal,** *-stasis* **standing still]**

hypochondriac region
(hye-poh-KON-dree-ak REE-jun)
[*hypo-* **under or below,** *-chondr-* **cartilage,** *-ac* **relating to]**

hypogastric region
(hye-poh-GAST-rik)
[*hypo-* **under or below,** *gastr-* **stomach,** *-ic* **relating to]**

hypothesis
(hye-POTH-eh-sis)
[*hypo-* **under or below,** *-thesis* **placing or proposition]**

iliac region
(ILL-ee-ak)
[*ilia-* **loin or gut (ileum),** *-ac* **relating to]**

inferior
(in-FEER-ee-or)
[*infer-* **lower,** *-or* **quality]**

inguinal
(ING-gwih-nal)
[*inguin-* **groin,** *-al* **relating to]**

lateral
(LAT-er-al)
[*later-* **side,** *-al* **relating to]**

law

levels of organization
(LEV-elz ov or-gan-i-ZAY-shun)

lumbar
(LUM-bar)
[*lumb-* **loin,** *-ar* **relating to]**

lumbar region
(LUM-bar, REE-jun)
[*lumb-* **loin,** *-ar* **relating to]**

mammary
(MAM-mah-ree)
[*mamma-* **breast,** *-ry* **relating to]**

medial
(MEE-dee-al)
[*media-* **middle,** *-al* **relating to]**

mediastinum
(mee-dee-as-TYE-num)
[*mediastin-* **midway,** *-um* **thing]**

medicine
(MED-ih-sin)
[*med-* **heal,** *-ic-* **relating to,** *-ine* **of or like]**

midsagittal plane
(mid-SAJ-ih-tal playn)
[*mid-* **middle,** *-sagitta-* **arrow,** *-al* **relating to,** *plan-* **flat surface]**

nasal
(NAY-zal)
[*nas-* **nose,** *-al* **relating to]**

negative feedback
(NEG-ah-tiv FEED-bak)
[*nega-* **deny,** *-tive* **relating to]**

oblique plane
(oh-BLEEK playn)
[*obliq-* **slanted,** *plan-* **flat surface]**

occipital
(ok-SIP-it-al)
[*occipit-* **back of head,** *-al* **relating to]**

olecranal
(oh-LEK-rah-non)
[*olecran-* **elbow,** *-al* **relating to]**

ophthalmic
(op-THAL-mik)
[*oph-* **eye or vision,** *-thalm-* **inner chamber,** *-ic* **relating to]**

oral
(OR-al)
[*or-* **mouth,** *-al* **relating to]**

orbital
(OR-bih-tal)
[*orbi-* **circle,** *-al* **relating to]**

organ
(OR-gan)
[*organ* **tool or instrument]**

organism
(OR-gah-niz-im)
[*organ-* **instrument,** *-ism* **condition]**

palmar
(PAHL-mar)
[*palm-* **palm of hand,** *-ar* **relating to]**

pedal
(PEED-al)
[*ped-* **foot,** *-al* **relating to]**

pelvic
(PEL-vik)
[*pelvi-* **basin,** *-ic* **relating to]**

pelvic cavity
(PEL-vik KAV-ih-tee)
[*pelvi-* **basin,** *-ic* **relating to,** *cav-* **hollow,** *-ity* **state]**

perineal
(payr-ih-NEE-al)
[*peri-* **around,** *-ine-* **excrete (perineum),** *-al* **relating to]**

physiology
(fiz-ee-OL-oh-jee)
[*physio-* **nature (function),** *-o-* **combining form,** *-log-* **words (study of),** *-y* **activity]**

plane
(playn)
[*plan-* **flat surface]**

plantar
(PLAN-tar)
[*planta-* **sole of foot,** *-ar* **relating to]**

pleural cavity
(PLOOR-al KAV-ih-tee)
[*pleura-* **rib,** *-al* **relating to,** *cav-* **hollow,** *-ity* **state]**

popliteal
(pop-lih-TEE-al)
[*poplit-* **back of knee,** *-al* **relating to]**

positive feedback
(POZ-it-iv FEED-bak)
[*posit-* **to place or amplify,** *-tive* **relating to]**

posterior
(pos-TEER-ee-or)
[*poster-* **behind,** *-or* **quality]**

prone
(prohn)
[*prone* **lying face down]**

proximal
(PROK-si-mal)
[*proxima-* **near,** *-al* **relating to]**

sagittal plane
(SAJ-i-tal playn)
[*sagitta-* **arrow,** *-al* **relating to,** *plan-* **flat surface]**

scientific method
(sye-en-TIF-ik METH-od)

section
(SEK-shun)
[*sect-* **cut,** *-ion* **process or state]**

sensor
(SEN-sor)
[*sens-* **feel,** *-or* **relating to**]

spinal cavity
(SPY-nal KAV-ih-tee)
[*spin-* **backbone,** *-al* **relating to,** *cav-* **hollow,** *-ity* **state**]

superficial
(soo-per-FISH-al)
[*super-* **over or above,** *-fici-* **face,** *-al* **relating to**]

superior
(soo-PEER-ee-or)
[*super-* **over or above,** *-or* **quality**]

supine
(SOO-pyne)
[*supin-* **lying on the back**]

supraclavicular
(soo-prah-klah-VIK-yoo-lar)
[*supra-* **above or over,** *-clavi-* **key,** *-ul-* **little,** *-ar* **relating to**]

system
(SIS-tem)
[*system* **organized whole**]

tarsal
(TAR-sal)
[*tars-* **ankle,** *-al* **relating to**]

temporal
(TEM-poh-ral)
[*tempora-* **temple (of head),** *-al* **relating to**]

theory
(THEE-ah-ree)
[*theor-* **look at,** *-y* **act of**]

thoracic
(thoh-RASS-ik)
[*thorac-* **chest (thorax),** *-ic* **relating to**]

thoracic cavity
(thoh-RASS-ik KAV-it-ee)
[*thorac-* **chest (thorax),** *-ic* **relating to,** *cav-* **hollow,** *-ity* **state**]

tissue
(TISH-yoo)
[*tissu-* **fabric**]

transverse plane
(TRANS-vers playn)
[*trans-* **across or through,** *-vers* **turn,** *plan-* **flat surface**]

umbilical
(um-BIL-ih-kul)
[*umbilic-* **navel,** *-al* **relating to**]

ventral body cavity
(VEN-tral BOD-ee KAV-ih-tee)
[*ventr-* **belly,** *-al* **relating to,** *cav-* **hollow,** *-ity* **state**]

volar
(VOH-lar)
[*vola-* **hollow of hand,** *-ar* **relating to**]

zygomatic
(zye-goh-MAT-ik)
[*zygo-* **union or yoke,** *-ic* **relating to**]

❑ OUTLINE SUMMARY

To download a digital audio version of the chapter summary for use with your device, access the ***Audio Chapter Summaries*** *online at evolve.elsevier.com.*

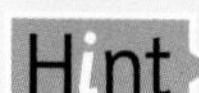

Scan this summary after reading the chapter to help you reinforce the key concepts. Later, use the summary as a quick review before your class or before a test.

Scientific Method

A. Science involves logical inquiry based on experimentation (see **Figure 1-1**)
   1. Hypothesis — idea or principle to be tested in experiments
   2. Experiment — series of tests of a hypothesis; a controlled experiment eliminates biases or outside influences
   3. Theory or law — a hypothesis that has been proved by experiments to have a high degree of confidence
B. The process of science is active and changing as new experiments add new knowledge

Levels of Organization

A. Organization is the most important characteristic of body structure
B. The body as a whole is a unit constructed of the following smaller units (see **Figure 1-2**):
   1. Atoms and molecules — chemical level
   2. Cells — the smallest structural units; organizations of various chemicals
   3. Tissues — organizations of similar cells
   4. Organs — organizations of different kinds of tissues
   5. Systems — organizations of many different kinds of organs
   6. Organism — organization of all systems together, forming a whole body

Anatomical Position

A. Reference position in which the body stands erect with the arms at the sides and palms turned forward (see **Figure 1-3**)
B. Anatomical position gives meaning to directional terms

Anatomical Directions

A. Superior — toward the head, upper, above
B. Inferior — toward the feet, lower, below
C. Anterior — front, in front of (same as ventral in humans)
D. Posterior — back, in back of (same as dorsal in humans)
E. Medial — toward the midline of a structure
F. Lateral — away from the midline or toward the side of a structure
G. Proximal — toward or nearest the trunk, or nearest the point of origin of a structure
H. Distal — away from or farthest from the trunk, or farthest from a structure's point of origin
I. Superficial — nearer the body surface
J. Deep — farther away from the body surface

Planes of the Body (see **Figure 1-4**)

A. Sagittal plane — lengthwise plane that divides a structure into right and left sections
   1. Midsagittal plane — sagittal plane that divides the body into two equal halves
B. Frontal (coronal) plane — lengthwise plane that divides a structure into anterior and posterior sections
C. Transverse plane — horizontal plane that divides a structure into upper and lower sections
D. Oblique plane — any plane that is not parallel to any of the planes listed above, thus producing a slanted section

Body Cavities (see **Figure 1-5, Table 1-1**)

A. Dorsal cavities
   1. Cranial cavity contains brain
   2. Spinal cavity contains spinal cord
B. Ventral cavities
   1. Thoracic cavity
      a. Mediastinum — midportion of thoracic cavity; heart and trachea are located in mediastinum
      b. Pleural cavities — right lung is located in right pleural cavity, left lung is in left pleural cavity
   2. Abdominopelvic cavity
      a. Abdominal cavity contains stomach, intestines, liver, gallbladder, pancreas, and spleen
      b. Pelvic cavity contains reproductive organs, urinary bladder, and lowest part of intestine
      c. Abdominopelvic subdivisions
         (1) Four abdominopelvic quadrants (see **Figure 1-6**)
         (2) Nine abdominopelvic regions (see **Figure 1-7**)
C. Organs of the major body cavities can be seen in **Figure 1-8**

Body Regions (see **Figure 1-9, Table 1-2**)

A. Axial region — head, neck, and torso or trunk
B. Appendicular region — upper and lower extremities
C. Body structure and function vary among individuals and also throughout an individual's life span; atrophy (decrease in size) occurs when an organ is not used

The Balance of Body Functions

A. Survival of the individual and of the genes that make up the body is of the utmost importance
B. Survival depends on the maintenance or restoration of homeostasis (relative constancy of the internal environment)
   1. The internal environment is a fluid that must be kept stable by the operation of various organ systems (**Figure 1-10**)
   2. The body uses stabilizing negative feedback loops (**Figure 1-11**) and, less often, amplifying positive feedback loops to maintain or restore homeostasis (**Figure 1-12**)
   3. Feedback loops involve a sensor, a control center, and an effector
   4. Negative feedback loops can turn into positive feedback loops during injury or disease, possibly causing a deadly shift in body function
C. All organs function to maintain homeostasis
D. Ability to maintain balance of body functions is related to age. Peak efficiency occurs during young adulthood, and diminishing efficiency of many functions begins after young adulthood

❑ ACTIVE LEARNING

STUDY TIPS

Hint *Use these tips to achieve success in meeting your learning goals.*

1. A number of topics are introduced in this chapter that will be important throughout the rest of the course.
2. One of your first steps should be mastering the new terminology of each chapter. Read the new terms listed at the beginning of each chapter out loud before attempting to read or learn each new topic. Use the pronunciation guides provided, saying each term several times to "get it into" your working memory. Pay attention to word parts, too; they'll help you master the terminology of science and medicine more quickly. (For more terminology tips, see *my-ap.us/fsboS2*.)
3. Homeostasis is an important concept when studying the human body. The word itself tells you what it means: *homeo* means "the same," *stasis* means "staying." Homeostasis is the balance the body tries to maintain by making sure its internal environment "stays the same." Make sure you understand this concept. (For more tips on homeostasis, see *my-ap.us/rs3KqV*.)
4. Another important topic introduced in this chapter is the structural levels of organization. The lower levels are the building blocks on which the upper levels depend. As various disease processes are explained in later chapters, notice how many of these processes cause failure at the chemical or cellular level and how this failure affects organs, systems, and even the body as a whole.
5. Become familiar with the directional terms; you will see them in almost every diagram in the text. The terms also are used in naming several body structures (for example, superior vena cava, distal convoluted tubule). The terms are fairly easy to learn because they are presented in opposite pairs, so if you learn one term, you almost always automatically know its opposite. Flash cards will help you learn them. (For more on using flashcards effectively, see *my-ap.us/LzuowE*. See *my-ap.us/K9GtVc* for more tips on learning directions.)
6. **Table 1-2** and the Glossary are helpful resources to keep in mind when you see an unfamiliar term.
7. In your study group, try to come up with examples of negative feedback loops that help maintain a balance. Be creative; don't just use the furnace example. Go over your directional-term flash cards or photocopy **Figure 1-4** and then blacken out the terms so you and your fellow students can use the illustration to quiz each other. Go over the questions at the end of the chapter and discuss possible test questions.

Review Questions

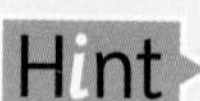
Write out the answers to these questions after reading the chapter and reviewing the Chapter Summary. If you simply think through the answer without writing it down, you won't retain much of your new learning.

1. Define anatomy and physiology.
2. Describe the process used to form scientific theories.
3. List and explain the levels of organization in a living thing.
4. Describe the anatomical position.
5. Name and explain the three planes or sections of the body.
6. List two organs of the mediastinum, two organs of the abdominal cavity, and two organs of the pelvic cavity.
7. From the upper left to the lower right, list the nine regions of the abdominopelvic cavity.
8. Name the two subdivisions of the dorsal cavity. What structures does each contain?
9. Explain the difference between the terms *lower extremity, thigh*, and *leg*.
10. Name the major areas that are included in the axial portion of the body.
11. List four conditions in the cell that must be kept in homeostatic balance.
12. List the three parts of a negative feedback loop and give the function of each.

Critical Thinking

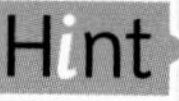
After finishing the Review Questions, write out the answers to these more in-depth questions to help you apply your new knowledge. Go back to sections of the chapter that relate to concepts that you find difficult.

13. Name a structure that is inferior to the heart, superior to the heart, anterior to the heart, posterior to the heart, and lateral to the heart.
14. The maintenance of body temperature and the birth of a baby are two body functions that are regulated by feedback loops. Explain the different feedback loops that regulate each process.
15. If a person complained of a pain in the epigastric region, what organs could be involved?
16. Consider some casual observation that you have made that might lead to the formation of a hypothesis. Explain how you could determine if your hypothesis is true or not. What would have to take place for your hypothesis to be accepted by others as fact?

Chapter Test

Hint *After studying the chapter, test your mastery by responding to these items. Try to answer them without looking up the answers. Then, verify the answers using the key in Appendix C at the back of this book.*

1. ________ is a term derived from two Greek words meaning "cutting up."
2. ________ means the study of the function of living organisms and their parts.
3. A hypothesis that has been rigorously tested can be called a ________ or ________.
4. ________, ________, ________, ________, and ________ are the five organizational levels of a living thing.
5. ________ and ________ are terms used to describe the body position when it is not in anatomical position.
6. A ________ section cuts the body or any of its parts into upper and lower portions.
7. A ________ section cuts the body or any of its parts into front and back portions.
8. A ________ section cuts the body or any of its parts into left and right portions.
9. If the body is cut into equal right and left sides, the cut is called a ________ section or plane.
10. In addition to using planes to cut the body into various sections, we sometimes use planes to describe ________.
11. The body portion that consists of the head, neck, and torso is called the ________ portion.
12. The body portion that consists of the upper and lower extremities is the ________ portion.
13. The two major cavities of the body are the:
    a. thoracic and abdominal
    b. abdominal and pelvic
    c. dorsal and ventral
    d. anterior and posterior
14. The structure that divides the thoracic cavity from the abdominal cavity is the:
    a. mediastinum
    b. diaphragm
    c. lungs
    d. stomach
15. The epigastric region of the abdominopelvic cavity:
    a. is inferior to the umbilical region
    b. is lateral to the umbilical region
    c. is medial to the umbilical region
    d. none of the above
16. The hypogastric region of the abdominopelvic cavity is:
    a. inferior to the umbilical region
    b. lateral to the left iliac region
    c. medial to the right iliac region
    d. both a and c
17. Which of the following is an example of a positive feedback loop?
    a. maintaining a constant body temperature
    b. contractions of the uterus during childbirth
    c. maintaining a constant volume of water in the body
    d. both a and c
18. The excretion of larger than usual volumes of urine when the volume of fluid in the body is greater than normal is an example of:
    a. positive feedback
    b. negative feedback
    c. normal fluctuation
    d. both b and c

Match each of the directional terms in Column B with its opposite term in Column A.

Column A		Column B
19. ________	superior	a. posterior
20. ________	distal	b. superficial
21. ________	anterior	c. medial
22. ________	lateral	d. proximal
23. ________	deep	e. inferior

Chemistry of Life

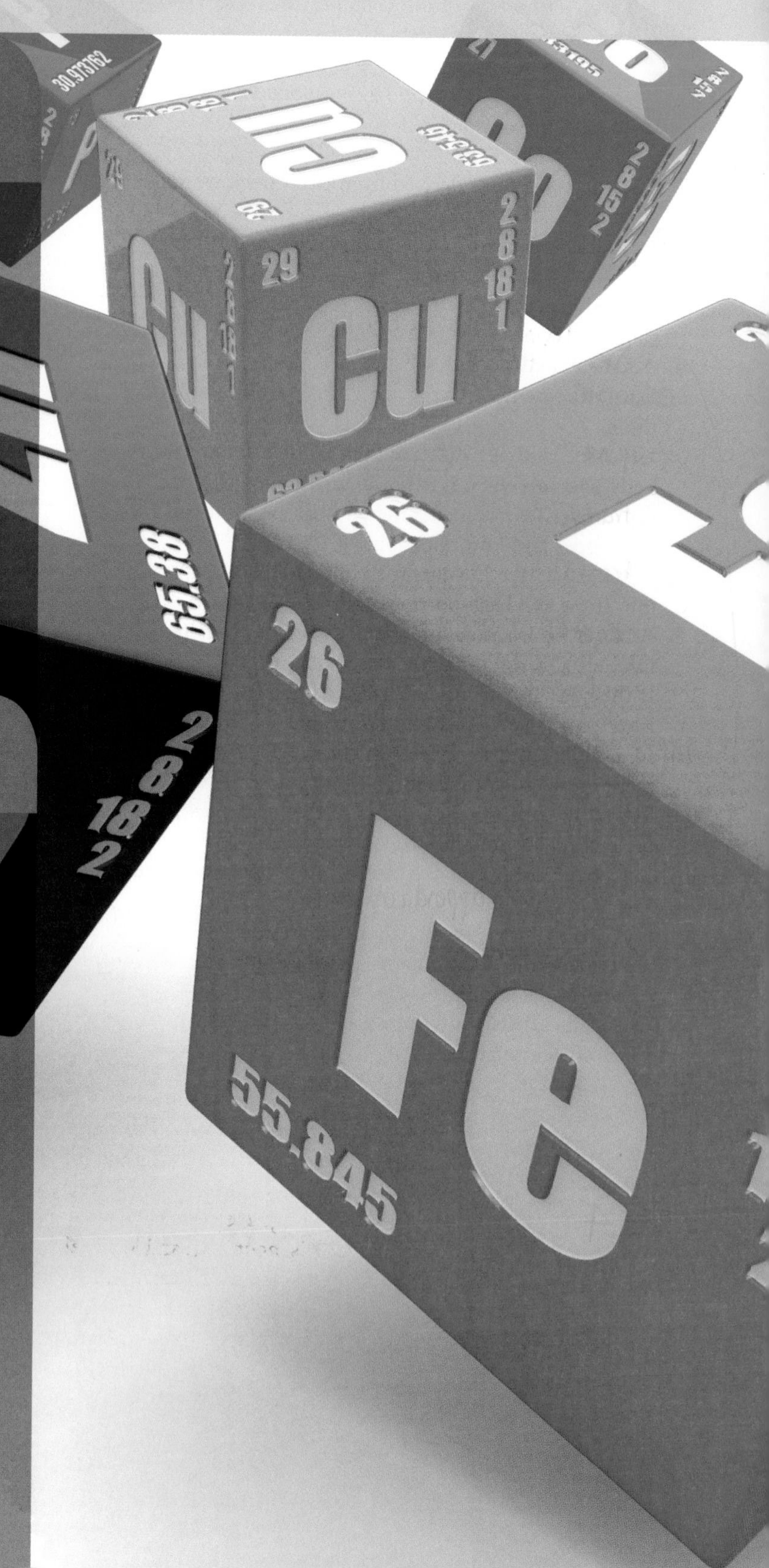

OUTLINE

Hint *Scan this outline before you begin to read the chapter, as a preview of how the concepts are organized.*

OBJECTIVES

Hint *Before reading the chapter, review these goals for your learning.*

After you have completed this chapter, you should be able to:

1. List and define the levels of chemical organization, including *atom, element, molecule,* and *compound.*
2. Describe the structure of an atom.
3. Compare and contrast major types of chemical bonding.
4. Distinguish between organic and inorganic chemical compounds.
5. Discuss the chemical characteristics of water.
6. Explain the concept of pH.
7. Discuss the structure and function of the following types of organic molecules: carbohydrate, lipid, protein, and nucleic acid.

CHAPTER 2

Life is full of chemistry, and the more we learn about chemicals and their structures, the better we can understand chemical processes in the human body. The digestion of food, the formation of bone tissue, and the contraction of a muscle are all chemical processes. Thus the basic principles of anatomy and physiology are ultimately based on principles of chemistry. A whole field of science, **biochemistry,** is devoted to studying the chemical aspects of life. To truly understand the human body, it is important to understand a few basic facts about biochemistry, the chemistry of life. The best place to begin is with the building blocks of matter.

Levels of Chemical Organization

Matter is anything that occupies space and has mass. Biochemists classify matter into several levels of organization for easier study. The smallest unit of matter is the **atom.** Atoms are used to build more complicated substances in the body. In the body, most chemicals are in the form of **molecules.** Molecules are particles of matter that are composed of one or more atoms. Atoms are considered to be the basic units of matter. So a good place to start is with the atom.

Atoms

Atoms are so small they can be observed only with very sophisticated equipment. For example, *tunneling microscopes and atomic force microscopes (AFMs)* can produce pictures of individual atoms (**Figure 2-1**). Atoms are composed of several kinds of *subatomic particles:* **protons, electrons,** and **neutrons.** At the core of each atom is a **nucleus** composed of positively charged protons and uncharged neutrons. The number of protons in the nucleus is an atom's **atomic number.** The number of protons and neutrons combined is the atom's **atomic mass.**

Negatively charged electrons surround the nucleus at a distance. If an atom is neutral (carries no electrical charge), there is one electron for every proton. Electrons don't stay still. Instead, electrons keep darting about within certain limits called **orbitals.** Each orbital can hold two electrons. Even though the name orbital

LANGUAGE OF **SCIENCE AND MEDICINE**

Hint Before reading the chapter, say each of these terms out loud. This will help you to avoid stumbling over them as you read.

acid
(ASS-id)

acidosis
(ass-ih-DOH-sis)
[*acid-* **sour,** *-osis* **condition**]

adenine
(AD-eh-neen)
[*aden-* **gland,** *-ine* **chemical**]

adenosine triphosphate (ATP)
(ah-DEN-oh-seen try-FOS-fayt)
[*adenos-* **shortened from** ***adenine-ribose,*** *-ine* **chemical,** *tri-* **three,** *-phosph-* **phosphorus,** *-ate* **oxygen**]

alkaline
(AL-kah-lin)
[*alkal-* **ashes,** *-ine* **relating to**]

alkalosis
(al-kah-LOH-sis)
[*alkal-* **ashes,** *-osis* **condition**]

amino acid
(ah-MEE-noh ASS-id)
[*amino* **NH_2,** *acid* **sour**]

aqueous solution
(AY-kwee-us)
[*aqu-* **water,** *-ous* **relating to**]

atherosclerosis
(ath-er-oh-skleh-ROH-sis)
[*ather-* **porridge,** *-sclero-* **harden,** *-osis* **condition**]

atom
(AT-om)
[*atom* **indivisible**]

atomic mass
(ah-TOM-ik)
[*atom-* **indivisible,** *-ic* **relating to**]

atomic number
(ah-TOM-ik)
[*atom-* **indivisible,** *-ic* **relating to**]

Continued on p. 34

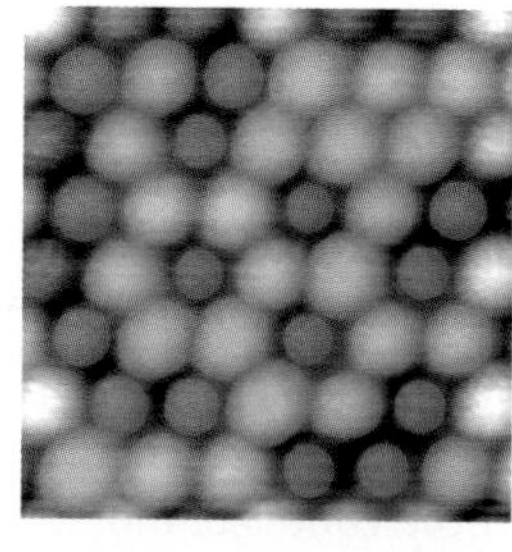

FIGURE 2-1 Atoms. A group of cloud-like atoms in a crystal as pictured by atomic force microscopy (AFM). Added colors highlight different kinds of atoms.

implies that their electrons move around in elliptical orbits, and are even pictured that way in some atomic models, electrons actually move about in chaotic, unpredictable paths.

Orbitals are arranged into **energy levels** (shells), depending on their distance from the nucleus. The farther an orbital extends from the nucleus, the higher its energy level is. The energy level closest to the nucleus has one orbital, so it can hold two electrons. The next energy level has up to four orbitals, so it can hold eight electrons. **Figure 2-2** shows a **carbon (C)** atom. Notice that the first energy level (the innermost shell) contains two electrons and the outer energy level contains four electrons. The outer energy level of a carbon atom could hold up to four more electrons (for a total of eight). The number of electrons in the outer energy level of an atom determines how it behaves chemically (that is, how it may unite with other atoms). This behavior, called *chemical bonding*, is discussed later in this chapter.

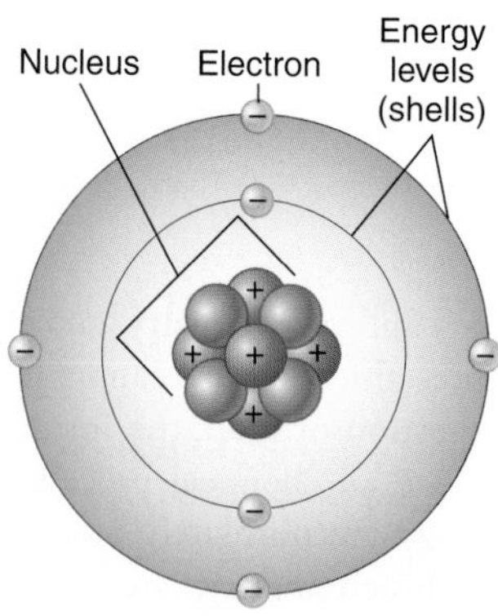

FIGURE 2-2 A model of the atom. The nucleus—protons (+) and neutrons—is at the core. Electrons inhabit outer regions called *energy levels*. This is a carbon atom, a fact that is determined by the number of its protons. All carbon atoms (and only carbon atoms) have six protons. Because there are only four electrons in the outer energy level, which can hold up to eight electrons, this carbon atom will share electrons with other atoms so that its outer energy level becomes full. (One proton and two neutrons in the nucleus are not visible in this illustration.)

Elements, Molecules, and Compounds

Substances can be classified as **elements** or **compounds.** Elements are pure substances, composed of only one of more than a hundred types of atoms that exist in nature. Four kinds of atoms (***oxygen, carbon, hydrogen,*** and ***nitrogen***) make up about 96% of the human body, but there are traces of about 20 other elements in the body. **Table 2-1** lists some of the major elements in the body. **Table 2-1** also gives for each element its universal chemical *symbol*—the abbreviation used by chemists worldwide.

Atoms usually unite with each other to form larger chemical units called *molecules.* Some molecules are made of several atoms of the same element. **Compounds** are substances whose molecules have more than one element in them. In order to describe which atoms are present in a compound, a chemical *formula* is used. The *formula* for a compound contains symbols that represent each element in the molecule. The number of atoms of each element in the molecule is expressed as a subscript after the elemental symbol. For example, each molecule of the compound **carbon dioxide** has one carbon (C) atom and two oxygen (O) atoms; thus its molecular formula is CO_2.

TABLE 2-1 Important Elements in the Human Body

ELEMENT	SYMBOL	NUMBER OF PROTONS IN NUCLEUS	NUMBER OF ELECTRONS IN OUTER SHELL*
Major Elements (Greater Than 96% of Body Weight)			
Oxygen	O	8	6
Carbon	C	6	4
Hydrogen	H	1	1
Nitrogen	N	7	5
Trace Elements (Examples of More Than 20 Trace Elements Found in the Body)			
Calcium	Ca	20	2
Phosphorus	P	15	5
Sodium (Latin *natrium*)	Na	11	1
Potassium (Latin *kalium*)	K	19	1
Chlorine	Cl	17	7
Iodine	I	53	7

*Maximum is eight, except for hydrogen. The maximum for that element is two.

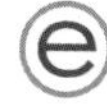
To learn more about molecule formation, go to AnimationDirect at *evolve.elsevier.com.*

QUICK CHECK

1. What kinds of particles make up matter?
2. What is a compound? An element?
3. What is an energy level?
4. What are the four kinds of atoms that make up the majority of the human body?

Chemical Bonding

Chemical bonds form to make atoms more stable. An atom is said to be chemically stable when its outer energy level is "full" (that is, when its energy shells have the maximum number of electrons they can hold). All but a handful of atoms have room for more electrons in their outermost energy level. A basic chemical principle states that

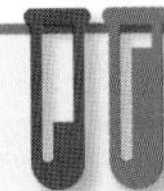

CLINICAL APPLICATION

RADIOACTIVE ISOTOPES

Each element is unique because of the number of protons it has. In short, each element has its own *atomic number.* However, atoms of the same element can have different numbers of neutrons. Two atoms that have the same atomic number but different atomic masses are **isotopes** of the same element. An example is hydrogen. Hydrogen has three isotopes: ^{1}H (the most common isotope), ^{2}H, and ^{3}H. The figure shows that each different isotope has only one proton but different numbers of neutrons.

Some isotopes have unstable nuclei that radiate (give off) particles. Radiation particles include protons, neutrons, electrons, and altered versions of these normal subatomic particles. An isotope that emits radiation is called a **radioactive isotope**.

Radioactive isotopes of common elements are sometimes used in *nuclear medicine* to evaluate the function of body parts. Radioactive iodine (^{125}I) put into the body and taken up by the thyroid gland gives off radiation that can be easily measured. Thus the rate of thyroid activity can be determined. Images of internal organs can be formed by radiation scanners that plot out the location of injected or ingested radioactive isotopes. For example, radioactive technetium (^{99}Tc) is commonly used to image the liver and spleen. The radioactive isotopes ^{13}N, ^{15}O, and ^{11}C are often used to study the brain in a technique called the *PET scan.*

Radiation can damage cells. Exposure to high levels of radiation may cause cells to develop into cancer cells. Higher levels of radiation completely destroy tissues, causing *radiation sickness.* Low doses of radioactive substances are sometimes given to cancer patients to destroy cancer cells. The side effects of these treatments result from the unavoidable destruction of normal cells with the cancer cells.

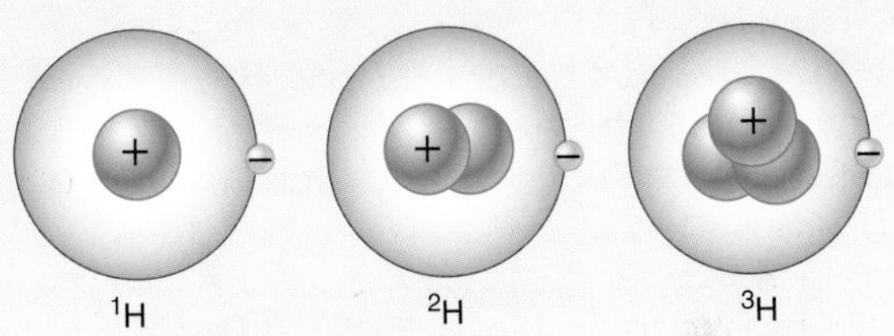

atoms react with one another in ways to make their outermost energy level full. To do this, atoms can share, donate, or borrow electrons.

For example, a hydrogen atom has one electron and one proton. Its single energy shell has one electron but can hold two, so it is not full. If two hydrogen atoms "share" their single electrons with each other, then both will have full energy shells, making them more stable as a molecule than either would be as an atom. This is an example of how atoms **bond** to form molecules. Other atoms may donate or borrow electrons until the outermost energy level is full and then form crystals.

Ionic Bonds

One common way in which atoms make their outermost energy level full is to form **ionic bonds** with other atoms. An ionic bond forms between an atom that has only one or two electrons in the outermost level (that would normally hold eight) and an atom that needs only one or two electrons to fill its outer level. The atom with one or two electrons simply "donates" its outer shell electrons to the one that needs one or two.

For example, as you can see in **Table 2-1**, the sodium (Na) atom has one electron in its outer level and the chlorine (Cl) atom has seven. Both need to have eight electrons to fill their outer shell. **Figure 2-3**, *A*, shows how sodium and chlorine form an ionic bond when sodium "donates" the electron in its outer shell to chlorine. Now both atoms have full outer shells (although sodium's outer shell is now one energy level lower). Because the sodium atom lost an electron, it now has one more proton than it has electrons. This makes it a positive ***ion***, an electrically charged atom. Chlorine has received an electron to become a negative ion called the *chloride* ion. Because oppositely charged particles attract one another, the sodium and chloride ions are drawn together to form a sodium chloride (NaCl) crystal—common table salt (**Figure 2-3**, *B*). The crystal is held together by ionic bonds.

Ionic compounds usually dissolve easily in water because water molecules are attracted to ions and wedge between the ions—thus forcing them apart. When this happens, we say the compounds **dissociate** to form free ions. Compounds that form ions when dissolved in water are called **electrolytes**.

The formula of an ion always shows its charge by a "+" or "–" superscript after the chemical symbol. Thus the sodium ion is Na^{+}, and the chloride ion is Cl^{-}. Calcium (Ca) atoms lose two electrons when they form ions, so the calcium ion is written as Ca^{++}.

Because the body's internal environment is mostly water, we find many dissolved ions in the body. Specific ions have important roles to play in muscle contraction, nerve signaling, and other vital functions. **Table 2-2** lists some of the more important ions present in body fluids. Many of these ions will be discussed in later chapters. Chapter 19 describes mechanisms that maintain the homeostasis of the electrolytes throughout the body.

Covalent Bonds

Atoms also may fill their energy levels by sharing electrons rather than donating or receiving them. When atoms share electrons, then a **covalent bond** forms. For example, **Figure 2-4**

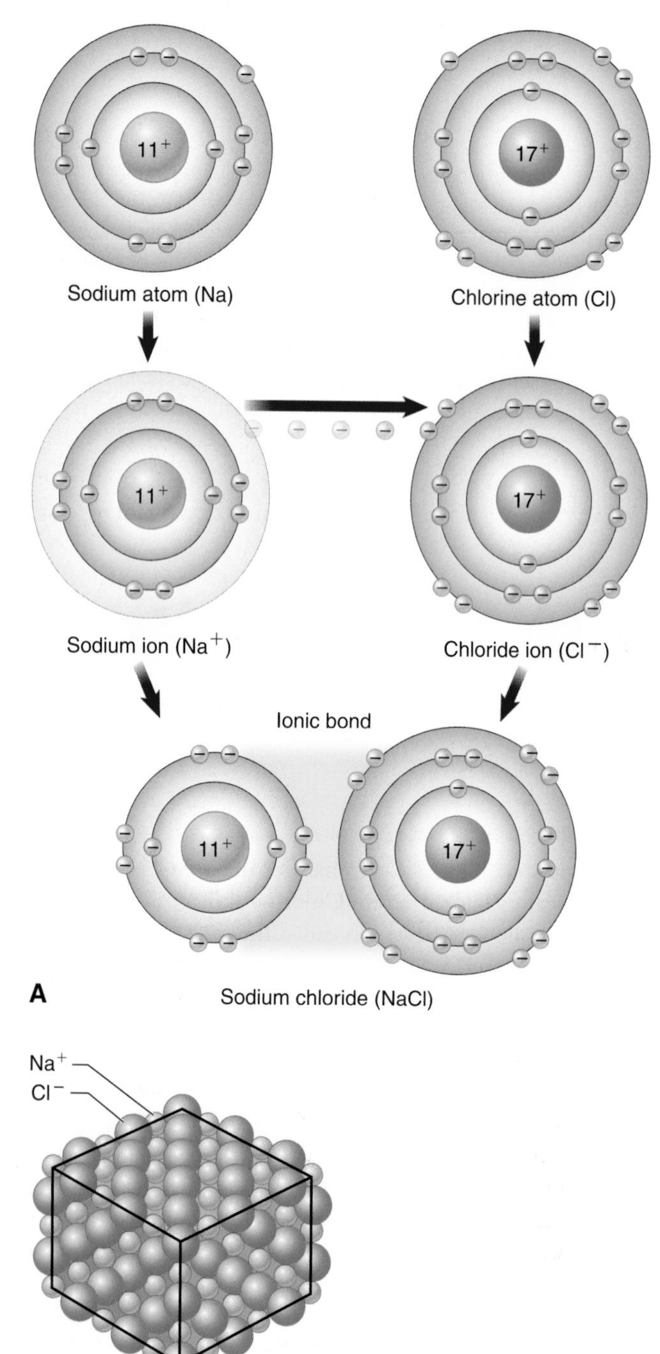

FIGURE 2-3 **Ionic bonding. A,** The sodium atom donates the single electron in its outer energy level to a chlorine atom having seven electrons in its outer level. Now both have eight electrons in their outer shells. Because the electron/proton ratio changes, the sodium atom becomes a positive sodium ion. The chlorine atom becomes a negative chloride ion. The positive-negative attraction between these oppositely charged ions is called an *ionic bond.* **B,** A cube-shaped crystal of sodium chloride (table salt).

shows how two hydrogen atoms may move together closely so that their energy levels overlap. Each energy level contributes its one electron to the sharing relationship. That way, both outer levels have access to both electrons. Because atoms involved in a covalent bond must stay close to each other, it is not surprising that covalent bonds are not easily broken. Covalent bonds normally do not break apart in water.

TABLE 2-2 Important Ions in Human Body Fluids

NAME	SYMBOL
Sodium	Na^{+}
Chloride	Cl^{-}
Potassium (Latin *kalium*)	K^{+}
Calcium	Ca^{++}
Hydrogen	H^{+}
Magnesium	Mg^{++}
Hydroxide	OH^{-}
Phosphate	$PO_4^{\equiv}$

Carbon, nitrogen, oxygen, and hydrogen almost always share electrons to form covalent bonds, making this type of bonding important in the human body. Covalent bonding is used to form all of the major organic compounds found in the body.

Hydrogen Bonds

A kind of weak attraction that helps hold your body's substance together is the **hydrogen bond.** Slight electrical charges may develop in different regions of a molecule when tiny hydrogen atoms are not able to equally share their electrons in a covalent bond. Oppositely charged ends of various molecules then electrically attract one another (**Figure 2-5**).

Hydrogen bonds do not form new molecules, but instead provide subtle forces that help a large molecule stay in a particular shape. They may also help hold together neighboring molecules. For example, hydrogen bonds help hold proteins in

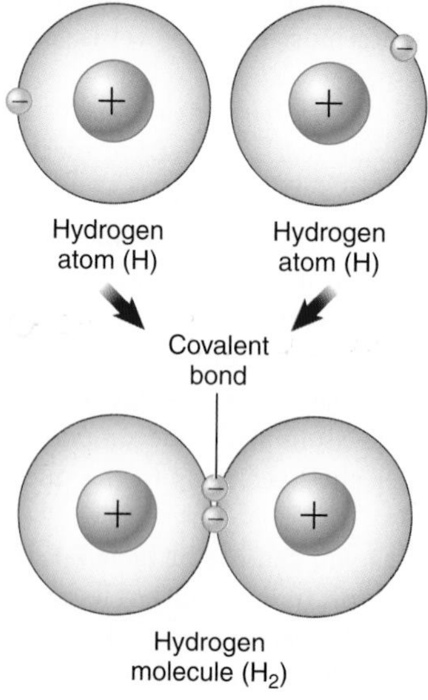

FIGURE 2-4 **Covalent bonding.** Two hydrogen atoms move together, overlapping their energy levels. Although neither gains nor loses an electron, the atoms share the electrons, forming a covalent bond.

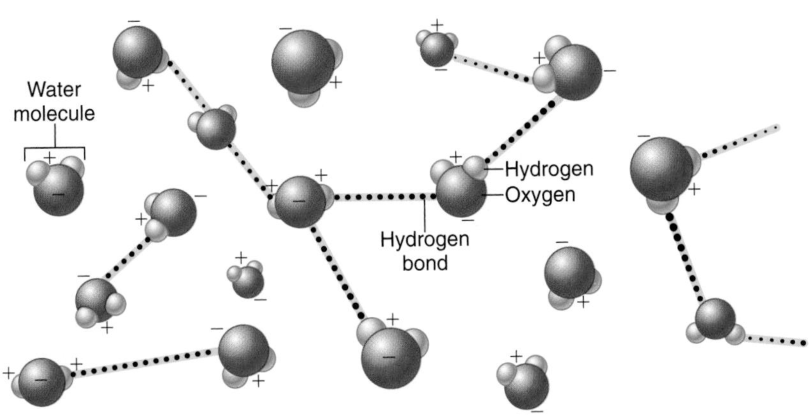

FIGURE 2-5 Hydrogen bonds. Because the tiny hydrogen atoms in water cannot share their electrons equally with a large oxygen atom, the water molecule develops slightly different charges at each end. Like weak magnets, the water molecules form temporary attachments (hydrogen bonds) that give liquid water its slightly gluelike properties.

their complex folded shapes (see **Figure 2-12** on p. 31). Hydrogen bonds also keep water molecules loosely joined together, giving water a weak gluelike quality that helps hold your body together (see **Figure 2-5**).

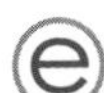
To learn more about chemical bonding, go to AnimationDirect at *evolve.elsevier.com*.

QUICK CHECK

1. How is an ion formed?
2. What is meant by an electrolyte *dissociating* in water?
3. What is covalent chemical bonding?
4. Why are hydrogen bonds important?
5. How is the charge of an ion indicated in a formula?

Inorganic Chemistry

In living organisms, there are two kinds of compounds: **organic** and **inorganic.** Organic compounds are composed of molecules that contain carbon-carbon (C–C) covalent bonds, carbon-hydrogen (C–H) covalent bonds, or both. Few inorganic compounds have carbon atoms in them, and none have C–C or C–H bonds. Organic molecules are generally larger and more complex than inorganic molecules. The human body has both kinds of compounds because both are equally important to the chemistry of life. We will discuss the chemistry of inorganic compounds first and then move on to some of the important types of organic compounds.

Water

Although it is an inorganic compound, **water** is essential to life. Water is the most abundant compound in the body, found in and around each cell. Its slightly gluelike properties help hold the tissues of the body together.

Solutions

Water is the **solvent** in which most other compounds or **solutes** are dissolved. When water is the solvent for a *mixture* (a blend of two or more kinds of molecules), the mixture is called an **aqueous solution.** An aqueous solution containing common salt (NaCl) and other molecules forms the "internal sea" of the body.

Water molecules not only compose the basic internal environment of the body but also participate in many important *chemical reactions.* Chemical reactions are interactions among molecules in which atoms regroup into new combinations.

Water Chemistry

Dehydration synthesis is a common type of chemical reaction in the body. In any kind of synthesis reaction, the **reactants** combine to form a larger **product.** In dehydration synthesis, reactants combine only after two hydrogen (H) atoms and an oxygen (O) atom are removed. These leftover H and O atoms come together, forming H_2O, or water. As **Figure 2-6** shows, the result is both the large product molecule and a water molecule. Just as dehydration of a cell is a loss of water from the cell and dehydration of the body is loss of fluid from the entire internal environment, dehydration synthesis is a reaction in which water is lost from the reactants.

Another common reaction in the body, **hydrolysis,** also involves water. In this reaction, water *(hydro-)* disrupts the bonds in large molecules, causing them to be broken down into smaller molecules *(lysis).* Hydrolysis is virtually the reverse of dehydration synthesis, as **Figure 2-6** shows.

All of the major types of organic compounds discussed later in this chapter are formed in water and use water (dehydration synthesis). All four organic molecule types are broken apart in water and use water (hydrolysis). Clearly, water is an important substance in the body!

Chemical reactions always involve energy transfers. Energy is required to build the molecules. Some of that energy is

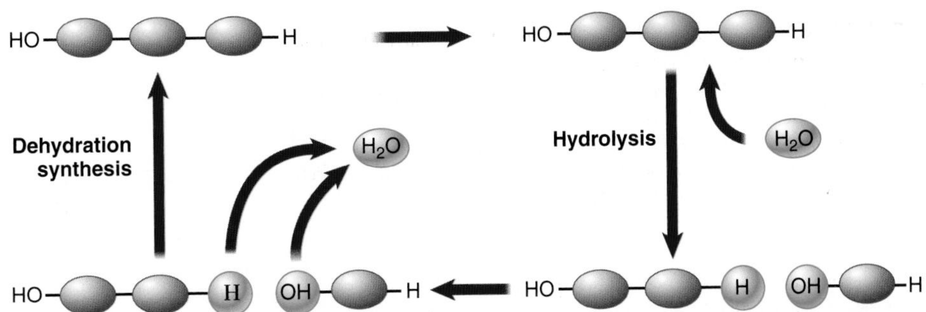

FIGURE 2-6 Water-based chemistry. Dehydration synthesis *(left)* is a reaction in which small molecules are assembled into large molecules by removing water (H and O atoms). Hydrolysis *(right)* operates in the reverse direction. H and O from water are added as large molecules are broken down into small molecules.

stored as potential energy in the chemical bonds. The stored energy can then be released when the chemical bonds in the molecule are later broken apart. For example, a molecule called *adenosine triphosphate (ATP)* breaks apart in the muscle cells to yield the energy needed for muscle contraction (see **Figure 2-15** on p. 33).

Chemists often use a *chemical equation* to represent a chemical reaction. In a chemical equation, the reactants are separated from the products by an arrow ($\longrightarrow$) showing the "direction" of the reaction. Reactants are separated from each other and products are separated from each other by addition signs (+). Thus the reaction *potassium and chloride combine to form potassium chloride* can be expressed as the equation:

$$K^+ + Cl^- \longrightarrow KCl$$

The single arrow ($\longrightarrow$) is used for equations that occur in only one direction. For example, when hydrochloric acid (HCl) is dissolved in water, all of it dissociates to form H^+ and Cl^-:

$$HCl \longrightarrow H^+ + Cl^-$$

The double arrow ($\longleftrightarrow$) is used for reactions that happen in "both directions" at the same time. When carbonic acid (H_2CO_3) dissolves in water, some of it dissociates into H^+ (hydrogen ion) and HCO_3^- (bicarbonate), but not all of it. As additional ions dissociate, previously dissociated ions bond together again, forming H_2CO_3:

$$H_2CO_3 \longleftrightarrow H^+ + HCO_3^-$$

In short, the double arrow indicates that at any instant in time both reactants and products are present in the solution at the same time.

Acids, Bases, and Salts

Besides water, many other inorganic compounds are important in the chemistry of life. For example, acids and bases are compounds that profoundly affect chemical reactions in the body. As explained in more detail at the beginning of Chapter 20, a few water molecules dissociate to form the H^+ ion and the OH^- (hydroxide) ion:

$$H_2O \longleftrightarrow H^+ + OH^-$$

Acids

In pure water, the balance between these two ions is equal. However, when an **acid** such as hydrochloric acid (HCl) dissociates into H^+ and Cl^-, it shifts this balance in favor of excess H^+ ions.

In the blood, carbon dioxide (CO_2) forms carbonic acid (H_2CO_3) when it dissolves in water. Some of the carbonic acid then dissociates to form H^+ ions and HCO_3^- (bicarbonate) ions, producing an excess of H^+ ions in the blood. Thus high CO_2 levels in the blood make the blood more acidic.

Bases

Bases, or **alkaline** compounds, on the other hand, shift the balance in the opposite direction. For example, sodium hydroxide (NaOH) is a base that forms OH^- ions but no H^+ ions.

Looking at it simply, acids are compounds that produce an excess of H^+ ions, and bases are compounds that produce an excess of OH^- ions (or a decrease in H^+).

pH

The relative H^+ concentration is a measure of how acidic or basic a solution is. The H^+ concentration is usually expressed in units of **pH.** The formula used to calculate pH units gives a value of 7 to pure water. A higher pH value indicates a low relative concentration of H^+—a base. A lower pH value indicates a higher H^+ concentration—an acid.

Figure 2-7 shows a scale of pH from 0 to 14. Notice that when the pH of a solution is less than 7, the scale "tips" toward the side marked "high H^+." When the pH is more than 7, the scale "tips" toward the side marked "low H^+." pH units increase or decrease by factors of 10. Thus a pH 5 solution has 10 times the H^+ concentration of a pH 6 solution. A pH 4 solution has 100 times the H^+ concentration of a pH 6 solution.

A *strong acid* is an acid that completely, or almost completely, dissociates to form H^+ ions. Strong acids are indicated by very low pH values—far below pH 7. A *weak acid,* on the other hand, dissociates very little and therefore produces few excess H^+ ions in solution. Weak acids have a pH value just below 7.

Likewise, *strong bases* produce a very low relative H^+ concentration and have a very high pH value—far above 7. *Weak*

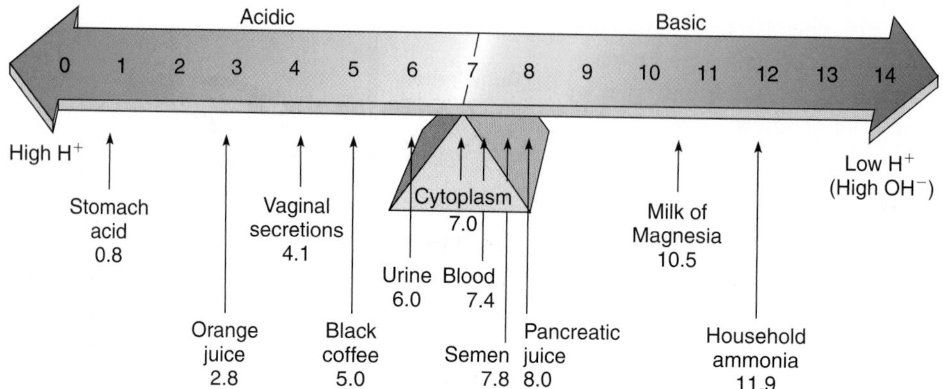

FIGURE 2-7 The pH scale. The H^+ concentration is balanced with the OH^- concentration at pH 7. At values above 7 (low H^+), the scale tips in the basic direction. At values below 7 (high H^+), the scale tips toward the acidic side.

bases produce an H^+ concentration a bit lower than pure water and thus have a pH value just a bit higher than 7.

Salts

When a strong acid and a strong base mix, excess H^+ ions may combine with the excess OH^- ions to form water. That is, they may neutralize each other. The remaining ions usually form neutral ionic compounds called ***salts.*** For example:

$$\underset{\text{acid}}{HCl} + \underset{\text{base}}{NaOH} \rightarrow H^+ + Cl^- + Na^+ + OH^- \rightarrow \underset{\text{water}}{H_2O} + \underset{\text{salt}}{NaCl}$$

Homeostasis of pH

The pH of body fluids affects body chemistry so greatly that normal body function can be maintained only within a narrow range of pH. **Acidosis** (low blood pH) and **alkalosis** (high blood pH) are equally dangerous and thankfully rarely occur because of the homeostatic mechanisms of the body.

The body can remove excess H^+ ions by excreting them in the urine (see Chapter 18). Another way to remove acid is by increasing the loss of CO_2 (an acid) by way of the respiratory system (see Chapter 15).

A third way to adjust the body's pH is by using **buffers**—chemicals in the blood that maintain pH. Buffers maintain pH balance by preventing sudden changes in the H^+ ion concentration. Buffers do this by forming a chemical system that neutralizes acids and bases as they are added to a solution.

The mechanisms by which the body maintains pH homeostasis, or acid-base balance, are discussed further in Chapter 20.

QUICK CHECK

1. What is an organic compound?
2. What are the chemical characteristics of water?
3. What is the difference between dehydration synthesis and hydrolysis?
4. Explain the concept of pH.
5. Does an acid have a low or high pH? Does a base have a low or high pH?
6. What is the difference between alkalosis and acidosis? What prevents these conditions from occurring frequently in the body?

Organic Chemistry

Organic compounds are much more complex than inorganic compounds. In this section, we describe the basic structure and function of each major type of organic compound found in the body: **carbohydrates, lipids** (fats), **proteins,** and **nucleic acids.** All four of these organic compounds are formed by dehydration synthesis reactions. Conversely, their bonds can be broken by hydrolysis.

Table 2-3 summarizes the structure and the function of each type of organic compound. Refer to this table as you read through the descriptions that follow.

Carbohydrates

The name *carbohydrate* literally means "carbon (C) and water (H_2O)," signifying the types of atoms that form carbohydrate molecules.

TABLE 2-3 Major Types of Organic Compounds

EXAMPLE	COMPONENTS	FUNCTIONS
Carbohydrate		
Monosaccharide (glucose, galactose, fructose)	Single monosaccharide unit	Used as a source of energy; used to build other carbohydrates
Disaccharide (sucrose, lactose, maltose)	Two monosaccharide units	Can be broken into monosaccharides
Polysaccharide (glycogen, starch)	Many monosaccharide units	Used to store monosaccharides (thus to store energy)
Lipid		
Triglyceride	One glycerol, three fatty acids	Stores energy; provides protective structural padding
Phospholipid	Phosphorus-containing unit, two fatty acids	Forms cell membranes
Cholesterol	Four carbon rings at core	Transports lipids; stabilizes cell membranes; is basis of steroid hormones
Protein		
Structural proteins	Amino acids	Form structures of the body (fibers)
Functional proteins (enzymes, hormones)	Amino acids	Facilitate chemical reactions; send signals; regulate functions
Nucleic Acid		
Deoxyribonucleic acid (DNA)	Nucleotides (contain deoxyribose)	Contains information (genetic code) for making proteins
Ribonucleic acid (RNA)	Nucleotides (contain ribose)	Serves as a copy of a portion of the genetic code during protein synthesis
Adenosine triphosphate (ATP)	Modified nucleotide (ribose, adenine, and three phosphates)	Transfers energy from nutrient molecules to power work in the cell

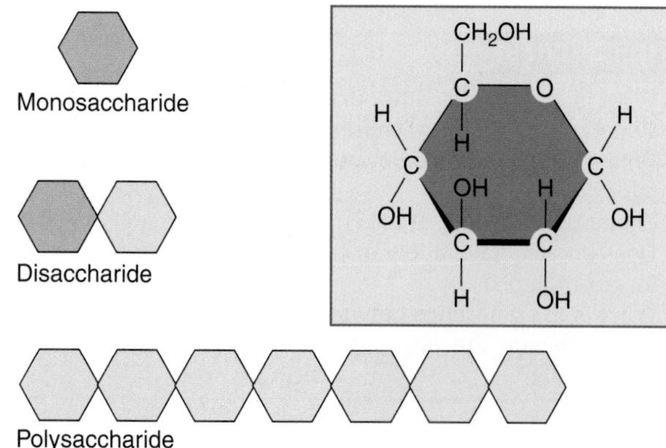

FIGURE 2-8 Carbohydrates. Monosaccharides are single carbohydrate units joined by dehydration synthesis to form disaccharides and polysaccharides. The detailed chemical structure of the monosaccharide glucose is shown in the inset.

The basic unit of carbohydrate molecules is called a **monosaccharide** (Figure 2-8). Glucose (dextrose) is an important monosaccharide in the body. Cells use it as their primary source of energy (see Chapter 17).

A molecule made of two saccharide units is a double sugar, or **disaccharide.** The disaccharides sucrose (table sugar) and lactose (milk sugar) are important dietary carbohydrates. After they are eaten, the body breaks them apart, or digests them, to form monosaccharides that can be used as cellular fuel.

Many saccharide units joined together form **polysaccharides.** Examples of polysaccharides are **glycogen** and *starch*. Glycogen is the polysaccharide of glucose that the human body stores. Plants store glucose as starch. Each glycogen molecule is a chain of glucose molecules joined together. Liver cells and muscle cells form glycogen when there is an excess of glucose in the blood, thus putting them into "storage" for later use. When we eat plants, we can break apart their starch molecules to get glucose.

Carbohydrates have potential energy stored in their bonds. When the bonds are broken in cells, the energy is released and then trapped by the cell's chemistry to do work. Chapter 17 explains more about the process by which the body extracts energy from carbohydrates and other nutrient molecules.

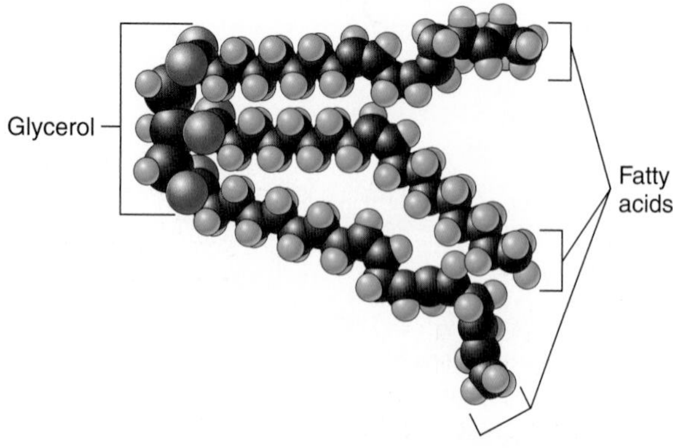

FIGURE 2-9 Triglyceride. Each triglyceride is composed of three fatty acid units attached to a glycerol unit.

Lipids

Lipids are fats and oils. Fats are lipids that are solid at room temperature, such as the fat in butter and lard. Oils, such as corn oil and olive oil, are liquid at room temperature. There are several important types of lipids in the body:

1. **Triglycerides** are lipid molecules formed by a *glycerol* unit or "head" joined to three *fatty acid "tails"* (Figure 2-9). Like carbohydrates, their bonds can be broken apart to yield energy (see Chapter 17). Thus triglycerides are useful in storing energy in cells for later use. Triglycerides stored in fat tissue also provide helpful "padding" around organs and under the skin to stabilize and protect body structures.
2. **Phospholipids** are similar to triglycerides but, as their name implies, have phosphorus-containing units called *phosphates* in them. The phosphate at the base of the glycerol head attracts water. Two fatty acid tails repel water. Figure 2-10, *A*, shows the head and double tail of the phospholipid molecule. This structure allows them to form a stable *bilayer* in water that forms the foundation for the cell membrane. In Figure 2-10, *B*, the water-attracting heads face the water and the water-repelling tails face away from the water (and toward each other).

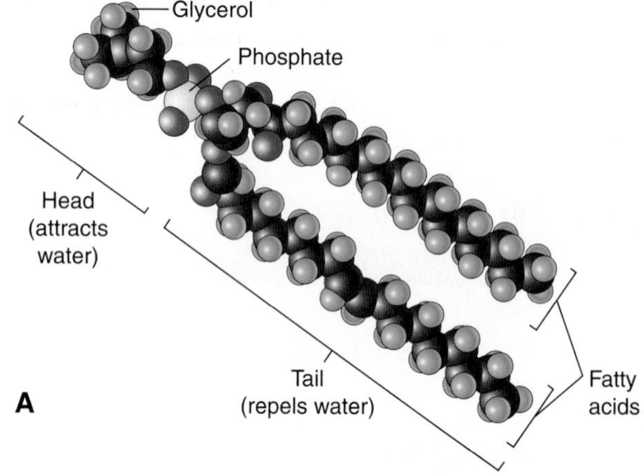

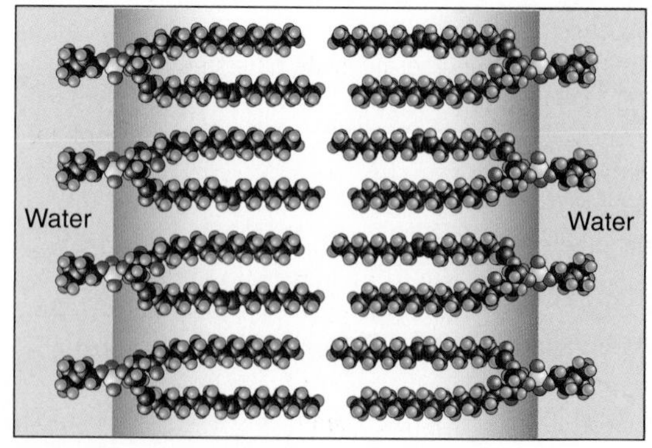

FIGURE 2-10 Phospholipids. A, Each phospholipid molecule has a phosphorus-containing "head" that attracts water and a lipid "tail" that repels water. **B,** Because the tails repel water, phospholipid molecules often arrange themselves so that their tails face away from water. The stable structure that results is a bilayer sheet forming a small bubble.

Cholesterol

Cortisol
(a steroid hormone)

FIGURE 2-11 Cholesterol. Cholesterol *(left)* has a steroid structure, represented here as four yellow rings. Changes to the side groups can convert cholesterol to cortisol *(shown)* or other steroid hormones.

3. **Cholesterol** is a *steroid* lipid (a multiple ring structure) that performs several important functions in the body. It combines with phospholipids in the cell membrane to help stabilize its bilayer structure. As Chapter 11 explains, the body also uses cholesterol as a starting point in making *steroid hormones* such as estrogen, testosterone, and cortisone (cortisol) (**Figure 2-11**).

Proteins

Proteins are very large molecules composed of basic units called **amino acids.** In addition to containing carbon, hydrogen, and oxygen, all amino acids contain nitrogen (N). There are many different amino acids used in cells to build proteins. By means of a process described fully in Chapter 3, a particular sequence of different amino acids is strung together and held by **peptide bonds.**

CLINICAL APPLICATION

BLOOD LIPOPROTEINS

A lipid such as cholesterol can travel in the blood only after it has attached to a protein molecule, forming a lipoprotein. Some of these molecules are called *high-density lipoproteins (HDLs)* because they have a high density of protein (more protein than lipid). Another type of molecule contains less protein (and more lipid), so it is called *low-density lipoprotein (LDL)*.

The cholesterol in LDLs is often called "bad" cholesterol because high blood levels of LDL are associated with **atherosclerosis,** a life-threatening blockage of arteries. LDLs carry cholesterol to *cells,* including the cells that line blood vessels. HDLs, on the other hand, carry "good" cholesterol *away from cells* and toward the liver for elimination from the body. A high proportion of HDL in the blood is associated with a low risk of developing atherosclerosis. Factors such as cigarette smoking decrease HDL levels and thus contribute to risk of atherosclerosis. Factors such as exercise increase HDL levels and thus decrease the risk of atherosclerosis.

Positive-negative attractions between different atoms in the long amino acid strand cause it to coil on itself again and again to form its highly complex shape. Folded proteins may combine with other folded proteins to form even larger, more complicated shapes. The complex, three-dimensional molecule that results is a protein molecule (**Figure 2-12**).

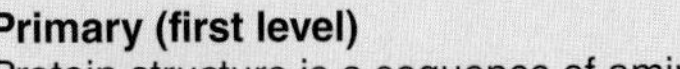

Primary (first level)
Protein structure is a sequence of amino acids in a chain.

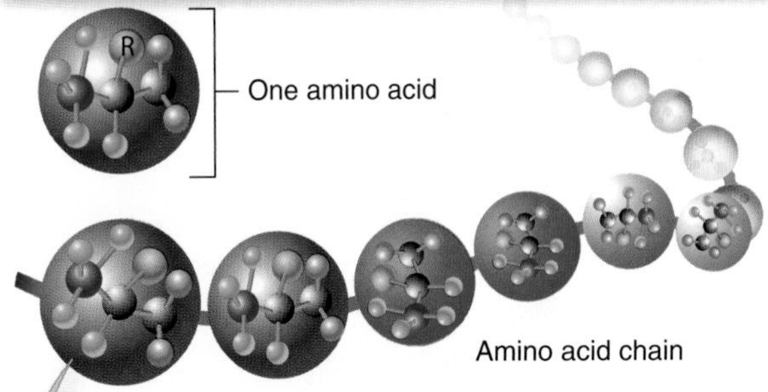

Secondary (second level)
Protein structure is formed by folding and twisting of amino acid chain.

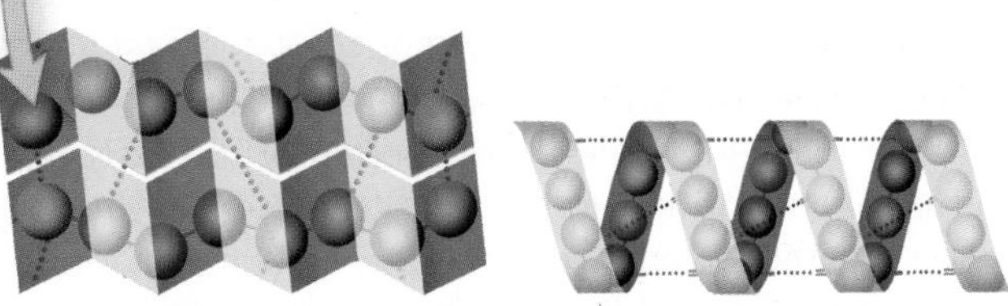

Tertiary (third level)
Protein structure is formed when the twists and folds of the secondary structure fold again to form a larger 3-dimensional structure.

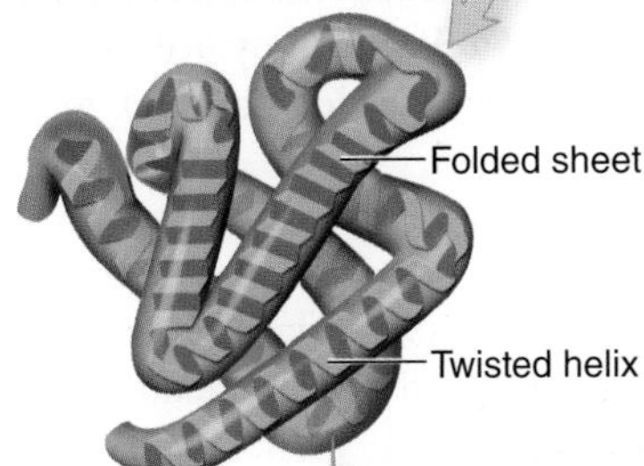

Quaternary (fourth level)
Protein structure is a protein consisting of more than one folded amino acid chain.

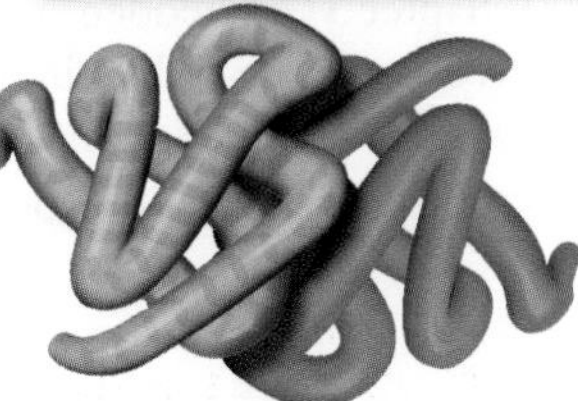

FIGURE 2-12 Protein. Protein molecules are large, complex molecules formed by one or more twisted and folded strands of amino acids. Each amino acid is connected to the next amino acid by covalent peptide bonds. This diagram shows how amino acids form strands that fold, and then fold again, into highly complex shapes.

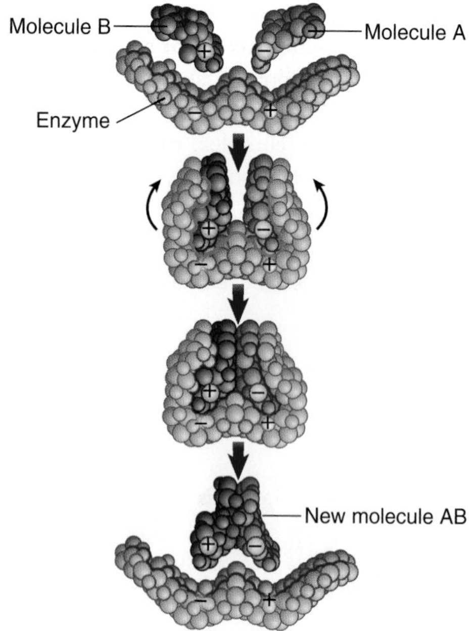

FIGURE 2-13 Enzyme action. Enzymes are functional proteins whose molecular shape allows them to catalyze chemical reactions. Molecules *A* and *B* are brought together by the enzyme to form a larger molecule, *AB.*

The folded shape of a protein molecule determines its role in body chemistry. **Structural proteins** are shaped in ways that allow them to form essential structures of the body. Collagen, a protein with a fiber shape, holds most of the body tissues together. Keratin, another structural protein, forms a network of waterproof fibers in the outer layer of the skin.

Functional proteins have shapes that enable them to participate in chemical processes of the body. Functional proteins include some of the hormones, growth factors, cell membrane channels and receptors, and enzymes.

Enzymes are chemical catalysts. This means that they help a chemical reaction occur but are not reactants or products themselves. They participate in chemical reactions but are not changed by the reactions. Enzymes are vital to body chemistry. No reaction in the body occurs fast enough unless the specific enzymes needed for that reaction are present.

Figure 2-13 illustrates how shape is important to the function of enzyme molecules. Each enzyme has a shape that "fits" the specific *substrate* molecules it works on much as a key fits specific locks. This explanation of enzyme action is sometimes called the **lock-and-key model.** Notice that, unlike most keys, the enzyme is dynamic and changes its shape when it encounters a substrate to more exactly fit.

Proteins can bond with other organic compounds and form "mixed" molecules. For example, *glycoproteins* (described in Chapter 3) embedded in cell membranes and *proteoglycans* between cells (described in Chapter 4) are proteins with sugars attached. *Lipoproteins* are lipid-protein combinations (as described in the Blood Lipoproteins box).

TABLE 2-4 Components of Nucleotides

NUCLEOTIDE	DNA	RNA
Sugar	Deoxyribose	Ribose
Phosphate	Phosphate	Phosphate
Nitrogen base	Cytosine	Cytosine
	Guanine	Guanine
	Adenine	Adenine
	Thymine	Uracil

Nucleic Acids

The two forms of nucleic acid are **deoxyribonucleic acid (DNA)** and **ribonucleic acid (RNA).** As outlined in Chapter 3, the basic building blocks of nucleic acids are called **nucleotides.**

Each nucleotide consists of a *phosphate unit,* a sugar (*ribose* or *deoxyribose*), and a *nitrogen base.* DNA nucleotide bases include **adenine, thymine, guanine,** and **cytosine.** RNA uses the same set of bases, except for the substitution of ***uracil*** for thymine (Table 2-4).

Nucleotides bind to one another to form strands or other structures. In the DNA molecule, nucleotides are arranged in a twisted, double strand called a **double helix** (Figure 2-14).

The sequence of different nucleotides along the DNA double helix is the "master code" for assembling proteins and other nucleic acids. *Messenger RNA (mRNA)* molecules have a sequence that forms a temporary "working copy" of a portion of the DNA code called a *gene.* The code in nucleic acids ultimately directs the entire symphony of living chemistry.

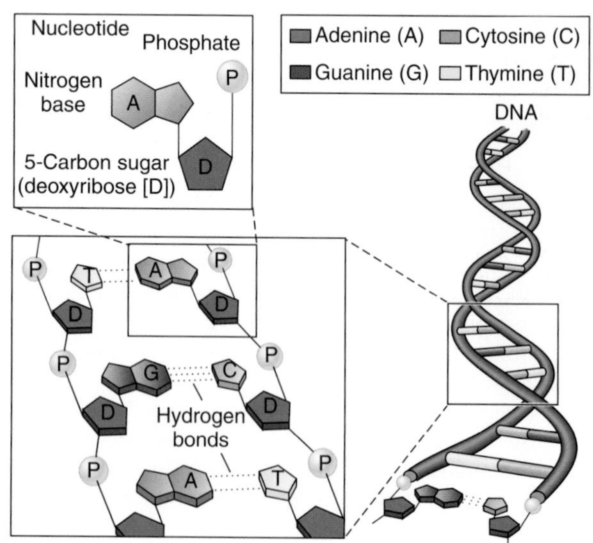

FIGURE 2-14 DNA. Deoxyribonucleic acid (DNA), like all nucleic acids, is composed of units called *nucleotides.* Each nucleotide has a phosphate, a sugar, and a nitrogen base. In DNA, the nucleotides are arranged in a double helix formation as you can see in the simple structural models on the left.

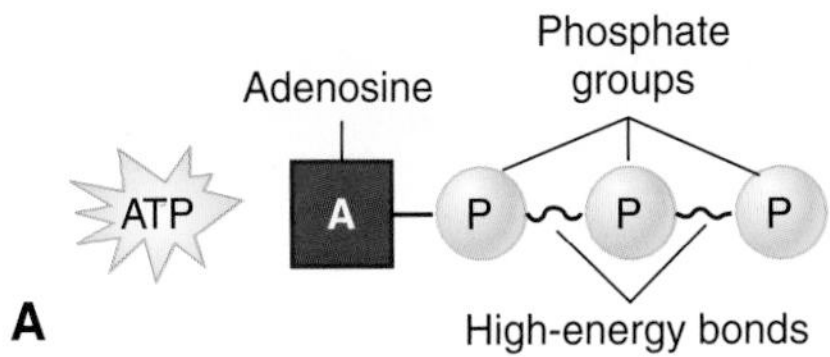

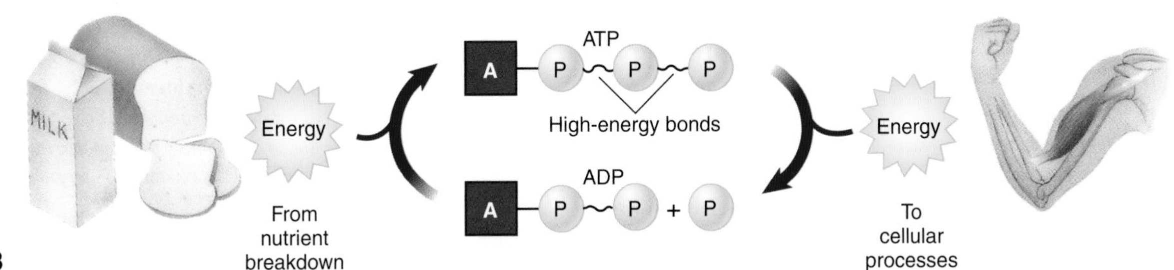

FIGURE 2-15 ATP. A, Structure of adenosine triphosphate (ATP). Because the adenosine group is made up of a sugar (ribose) and a base (adenine), ATP is really a nucleotide with added phosphates. **B,** The role of ATP in transferring energy from nutrient molecules to cellular processes. *ADP,* Adenosine diphosphate.

A modified nucleotide called **adenosine triphosphate (ATP)** plays an important energy-transfer role in the body. As Figure 2-15 shows adenosine (a base and a sugar) has not just one phosphate, as in a standard nucleotide, but instead has three phosphates. The "extra" phosphates have relatively unstable "high-energy" bonds that require a great amount of energy (from nutrients) to form, and release, great energy when broken. When a phosphate breaks off—forming *adenosine diphosphate (ADP)*—the energy released is used to do work in cells. Thus ATP acts as a sort of energy-transfer "battery" that picks up energy from nutrients and then quickly makes the energy available to cellular processes. Chapter 17 outlines details of how ATP works in the cells.

QUICK CHECK

1. Which types of organic molecules do these subunits form? Monosaccharides? Fatty acids? Amino acids? Nucleotides?
2. Why is the structure of protein molecules important?
3. What is the role of DNA in the body?
4. What is the role of ATP in the body?
5. What are enzymes? Explain the importance of enzymes in the body.
6. How does organic chemistry differ from inorganic chemistry?

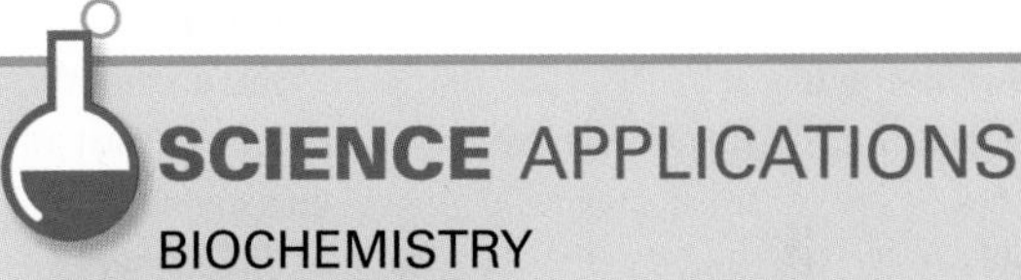

SCIENCE APPLICATIONS

BIOCHEMISTRY

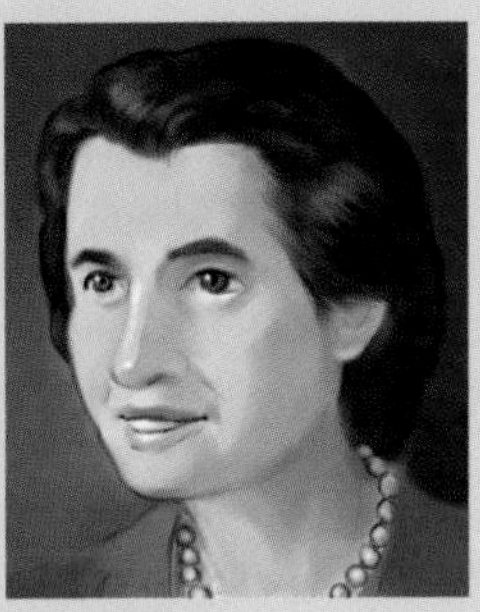

Rosalind Franklin (1920-1958)

British scientist Rosalind Franklin was one of the leading **biochemists** of the modern age. Franklin used x-rays to cast shadows through DNA to analyze its structure. When she was only 32 years old, she discovered the unusual helical (spiral) structure of the DNA molecule and how the sugars and phosphates form an outer backbone to the molecule (see Figure 2-14). Her breakthrough helped James Watson, Francis Crick, and Maurice Wilkins finally work out the structure and function of DNA in 1953 and thus crack the "code of life." The three men received a Nobel Prize for their achievement in 1962, but Franklin's early death from cancer in 1958 prevented her from sharing in the credit for one of the greatest discoveries of all time.

Biochemists continue to make important discoveries that increase our understanding of human structure and function. Aided by **laboratory technicians** and *lab assistants*, biochemists also find ways to help other professionals apply biochemistry to solve everyday problems. For example, **clinical laboratory technicians** analyze samples from the bodies of patients for signs of health or disease. Others who use biochemistry as a basis for their work include **nuclear medicine technologists, pharmacists** and **pharmacy technicians, dietitians,** *forensic investigators,* **genetic counselors**, and *science journalists*.

LANGUAGE OF SCIENCE AND MEDICINE (continued from p. 23)

base
(bays)
[*base* **foundation**]

biochemist
(bye-oh-KEM-ist)
[*bio-* **life,** *-chem-* **alchemy,** *-ist* **agent**]

biochemistry
(bye-oh-KEM-is-tree)
[*bio-* **life,** *-chem-* **alchemy,** *-ist* **agent,** *-ry* **practice of**]

bond
[*bond-* **band**]

buffer
(BUFF-er)
[*buffe-* **cushion,** *-er* **actor**]

carbohydrate
(kar-boh-HYE-drayt)
[*carbo-* **carbon,** *-hydr-* **hydrogen,** *-ate* **oxygen**]

carbon
(KAR-bun)
[*carbon* **coal**]

carbon dioxide
(KAR-bun dye-AHK-syde)
[*carbon* **coal,** *di-* **two,** *-ox-* **sharp (oxygen),** *-ide* **chemical**]

cholesterol
(koh-LESS-ter-ol)
[*chole-* **bile,** *-stero-* **solid,** *-ol* **oil**]

clinical laboratory technician
(KLIN-i-kal LAB-rah-tor-ee tek-NISH-en)
[*clin-* **sickbed,** *-ic* **relating to,** *-al* **relating to,** *labor-* **work,** *-tory* **place of activity,** *techn-* **art or skill,** *-ic* **relating to,** *-ian* **practitioner**]

compound
(KOM-pound)
[*compound* **put together**]

covalent bond
(ko-VAYL-ent)
[*co-* **with,** *-valen* **power,** *bond* **band**]

cytosine
(SYE-toh-seen)
[*cyto-* **cell,** *-os-* **sugar,** *-ine* **like**]

dehydration synthesis
(dee-hye-DRAY-shun SIN-the-sis)
[*de-* **from,** *-hydrat-* **water,** *-tion* **process,** *synthesis* **putting together**]

deoxyribonucleic acid (DNA)
(dee-ok-see-rye-boh-nook-lay-ik AS-id)
[*de-* **removed,** *-oxy-* **oxygen,** *-ribo-* **ribose (sugar),** *-nucle-* **nucleus (kernel),** *-ic* **relating to,** *acid* **sour**]

dietitian
(dye-eh-TISH-en)
[*diet-* **way of living,** *-itian* **practitioner**]

disaccharide
(dye-SAK-ah-ride)
[*di-* **two,** *-sacchar-* **sugar,** *-ide* **chemical**]

dissociate
(dih-SOH-see-ayt)
[*dis-* **apart,** *-socia-* **unite,** *-ate* **action**]

double helix
(HEE-lix)
[*helix* **spiral**]

electrolyte
(eh-LEK-troh-lyte)
[*electro-* **electricity,** *-lyt* **loosening**]

electron
(eh-LEK-tron)
[*electr-* **electric,** *-on* **unit**]

element
(EL-eh-ment)
[*element* **first principle**]

energy level
(EN-er-gee)
[*en-* **in,** *-erg-* **work,** *-y* **state**]

enzyme
(EN-zyme)
[*en-* **in,** *-zyme* **ferment**]

functional protein
(FUNK-shen-al PRO-teen)
[*function-* **to perform,** *-al* **relating to,** *prote-* **primary,** *-in* **substance**]

genetic counselor
(jeh-NET-ik KOWN-se-lor)
[*gene-* **produce,** *-ic* **relating to,** *counsel-* **advise or plan,** *-or* **agent**]

glycogen
(GLYE-koh-jen)
[*glyco-* **sweet,** *-gen* **produce**]

guanine
(GWAH-neen)
[*guan-* **guano,** *-ine* **like**]

hydrogen
(HYE-droh-jen)
[*hydro-* **water,** *-gen* **produce**]

hydrogen bond
(HYE-droh-jen)
[*hydro-* **water,** *-gen* **produce,** *bond* **band**]

hydrolysis
(hye-DROHL-ih-sis)
[*hydro-* **water,** *-lysis* **loosening**]

inorganic compound
(in-or-GAN-ik KOM-pound)
[*in-* **not,** *-organic* **natural,** *compound* **to assemble**]

ion
(EYE-on)
[*ion* **to go**]

ionic bond
(eye-ON-ik)
[*ion* **to go,** *-ic* **relating to,** *bond* **band**]

isotope
(EYE-so-tohp)
[*iso-* **equal,** *-tope* **place**]

laboratory technician
(LAB-rah-tor-ee tek-NISH-en)
[*labor-* **work,** *-tory* **place of activity,** *techn-* **art or skill,** *-ic* **relating to,** *-ian* **practitioner**]

lipid
(LIP-id)
[*lip-* **fat,** *-id* **form**]

lock-and-key model
(lok and kee MAHD-el)

matter
(MAT-er)
[*matter* **something from which something is made**]

molecule
(MOL-eh-kyool)
[*mole-* **mass,** *-cul* **small**]

monosaccharide
(mon-oh-SAK-ah-ride)
[*mono-* **one,** *-sacchar-* **sugar,** *-ide* **chemical**]

neutron
(NOO-tron)
[*neuter-* **neither,** *-on* **unit**]

nitrogen
(NYE-troh-jen)
[*nitro-* **soda,** *-gen* **produce**]

nuclear medicine technologist
(NOO-klee-ar MED-ih-sin tek-NOL-oh-jist)
[*nucle-* **nut or kernel,** *-ar* **relating to,** *techn-* **art or skill,** *-log-* **words (study of),** *-ist* **agent**]

nucleic acid
(noo-KLAY-ik AS-id)
[*nucle-* **nut kernel,** *-ic* **relating to,** *acid* **sour**]

nucleotide
(NOO-klee-oh-tyde)
[*nucleo-* **nut or kernel,** *-ide* **chemical**]

nucleus
(NOO-klee-us)
[*nucleus* **kernel**]

orbital
(OR-bih-tal)
[*orb-* **circle, disk, ring,** *-al* **relating to**]

organic compound
(or-GAN-ik KOM pound)
[*organ-* **tool or instrument,** *-ic* **relating to,** *compound* **to assemble**]

oxygen
(AHK-sih-jen)
[*oxy-* **sharp,** *-gen* **produce**]

peptide bond
(PEP-tyde)
[*pept-* **digest,** *-ide* **chemical**]

pH
[abbreviation for *potenz* **power,** *hydrogen* **hydrogen**]

pharmacist
(FAR-mah-sist)
[*pharmac-* **drug,** *-ist* **agent**]

pharmacy technician
(FAR-mah-see tek-NISH-en)
[*pharmac-* **drug,** *-y* **location of activity,** *techn-* **art or skill,** *-ic* **relating to,** *-ian* **practitioner**]

phospholipid
(fos-foh-LIP-id)
[*phospho-* **phosphorus,** *-lip-* **fat,** *-id* **form**]

polysaccharide
(pahl-ee-SAK-ah-ride)
[*poly-* **many,** *-sacchar-* **sugar,** *-ide* **chemical**]

product

protein
(PRO-teen)
[*prote-* **primary,** *-in* **substance**]

proton
(PROH-ton)
[*proto-* **first,** *-on* **elementary atomic particle**]

radioactive isotope
(ray-dee-oh-AK-tiv EYE-soh-tope)
[*radi-o* **send out rays,** *iso-* **equal,** *-tope* **place**]

reactant
(ree-AK-tant)
[*re-* **again,** *-act-* **act,** *-ant* **agent**]

ribonucleic acid (RNA)
(rye-boh-noo-KLAY-ik ASS-id)
[*ribo-* **ribose (sugar),** *-nucle-* **nucleus,** *-ic* **pertaining to,** *acid* **sour**]

salt
(sawlt)

solute
(SOL-yoot)
[*solut* **dissolved**]

solvent
(SOL-vent)
[*solv-* **dissolve,** *-ent* **agent**]

structural protein
(STRUK-shur-al PRO-teen)
[*structura-* **arrangement,** *-al* **relating to,** *prote-* **primary,** *-in* **substance**]

thymine
(THYE-meen)
[*thym-* **thymus,** *-ine* **like**]

triglyceride
(try-GLI-seh-ryde)
[*tri-* **three,** *-glycer-* **sweet,** *-ide* **chemical**]

uracil
(YOOR-ah-sil)
[*ura-* **urea,** *-il* **chemical**]

water

❑ OUTLINE SUMMARY

To download a digital audio version of the chapter summary for use with your device, access the ***Audio Chapter Summaries*** *online at evolve.elsevier.com.*

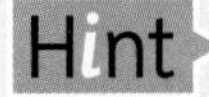

Scan this summary after reading the chapter to help you reinforce the key concepts. Later, use the summary as a quick review before your class or before a test.

Levels of Chemical Organization

A. Atoms (see **Figure 2-1** and **Figure 2-2**)
   1. Nucleus — central core of atom
      a. Proton — positively charged particle in nucleus
      b. Neutron — uncharged particle in nucleus
      c. Atomic number — number of protons in the nucleus; determines the type of atom
      d. Atomic mass — number of protons and neutrons combined
   2. Energy levels — regions surrounding atomic nucleus that contain electrons
      a. Electron — negatively charged particle
      b. May contain up to eight electrons in each level
      c. Energy increases with distance from nucleus
B. Elements, molecules, and compounds
   1. Element — a pure substance; made up of only one kind of atom
   2. Molecule — a group of atoms bound together in a group
   3. Compound — substances whose molecules have more than one kind of atom

Chemical Bonding

A. Chemical bonds form to make atoms more stable
   1. Atoms react with one another in ways that make their outermost energy level full
   2. Atoms may share electrons, or donate or borrow them to become stable
B. Ionic bonds (see **Figure 2-3**)
   1. Ions form when an atom gains or loses electrons in its outer energy level to become stable
      a. Positive ion — has lost electrons; indicated by superscript positive sign(s), as in Na^+ or Ca^{++}
      b. Negative ion — has gained electrons; indicated by superscript negative sign(s), as in Cl^-
   2. Ionic bonds form when oppositely charged ions attract each other because of electrical attraction
   3. Electrolyte — molecule that dissociates (breaks apart) in water to form individual ions; an ionic compound
C. Covalent bonds (see **Figure 2-4**)
   1. Covalent bonds form when atoms share their outer energy to fill up and thus become stable
   2. Covalent bonds do not ordinarily easily dissociate in water
D. Hydrogen bonds
   1. Weak forces that hold molecules in folded shapes (see **Figure 2-12**) or in groups (see **Figure 2-5**)
   2. Do *not* form new molecules

Inorganic Chemistry

A. *Organic* molecules contain carbon-carbon covalent bonds or carbon-hydrogen covalent bonds; *inorganic* molecules do not
B. Examples of inorganic molecules: water and some acids, bases, and salts
C. Water
  1. Water is essential to life
  2. Water's slightly gluelike nature helps hold the body together
  3. Water is a solvent (liquid into which solutes are dissolved), forming aqueous solutions in the body
  4. Water is involved in chemical reactions (see **Figure 2-6**)
    a. Dehydration synthesis — chemical reaction in which water is removed from small molecules so they can be strung together to form a larger molecule
    b. Hydrolysis — chemical reaction in which water is added to the subunits of a large molecule to break it apart into smaller molecules
    c. All the major organic molecules are formed through dehydration synthesis and are broken apart by hydrolysis
    d. Chemical reactions always involve energy transfers, as when energy is used to build ATP molecules
    e. Chemical equations show how reactants interact to form products; arrows separate the reactants from the products
D. Acids, bases, and salts
  1. Water molecules dissociate to form equal amounts of H^+ (hydrogen ion) and OH^- (hydroxide ion)
  2. Acid — substance that shifts the H^+/OH^- balance in favor of H^+; opposite of base
  3. Base — substance that shifts the H^+/OH^- balance against H^+; also known as an alkaline; opposite of acid
  4. pH — mathematical expression of relative H^+ concentration in an aqueous solution (see **Figure 2-7**)
    a. A pH value of 7 is neutral (neither acid nor base)
    b. pH values above 7 are basic; pH values below 7 are acidic
  5. Neutralization occurs when acids and bases mix and form salts
  6. pH imbalance occurs when blood pH is too high (alkalosis) or too low (acidosis); homeostasis restores and maintains pH balance in the body
  7. Buffers are chemical systems that absorb excess acids or bases and thus help maintain a relatively stable pH

Organic Chemistry

A. Carbohydrates — sugars and complex carbohydrates (see **Figure 2-8**)
  1. Contain carbon (C), hydrogen (H), oxygen (O)
  2. Made up of six-carbon subunits called *monosaccharides* or single sugars (e.g., glucose)
  3. Disaccharide — double sugar made up of two monosaccharide units (e.g., sucrose, lactose)
  4. Polysaccharide — complex carbohydrate made up of many monosaccharide units (e.g., glycogen made up of many glucose units)
  5. Function of carbohydrates is to store energy for later use
B. Lipids — fats and oils
  1. Triglycerides (see **Figure 2-9**)
    a. Made up of one glycerol unit and three fatty acids
    b. Store energy for later use
  2. Phospholipids (see **Figure 2-10**)
    a. Similar to triglyceride structure, except with only two fatty acids, and with a phosphorus-containing group attached to glycerol
    b. The head attracts water and the double tail does not, thus forming stable double layers (bilayers) in water
    c. Form membranes of cells
  3. Cholesterol (see **Figure 2-11**)
    a. Molecules have a steroid structure made up of multiple rings
    b. Cholesterol stabilizes the phospholipid tails in cellular membranes and is also converted into steroid hormones by the body
C. Proteins
  1. Very large molecules made up of different amino acids held together in long, folded chains by peptide bonds (see **Figure 2-12**)
  2. Structural proteins
    a. Form various structures of the body
    b. Collagen is a fibrous protein that holds many tissues together
    c. Keratin forms tough, waterproof fibers in the outer layer of the skin
  3. Functional proteins
    a. Participate in chemical processes of the body
    b. Examples: hormones, cell membrane channels and receptors, enzymes
    c. Enzymes (see **Figure 2-13**)
      (1) Catalysts — help chemical reactions occur
      (2) Lock-and-key model — each enzyme fits a particular molecule that it acts on as a key fits into a lock
  4. Proteins can combine with other organic molecules to form glycoproteins, proteoglycans, or lipoproteins

Chapter Test

Hint *After studying the chapter, test your mastery by responding to these items. Try to answer them without looking up the answers. Then, verify the answers using the key in Appendix C at the back of this book.*

1. ________ is anything that occupies space and has mass.
2. Molecules are made up of particles called ________.
3. Positively charged particles within the nucleus of an atom are called ________.
4. Electrons inhabit regions of the atoms called ________ levels.
5. Substances with molecules having more than one kind of atom are called ________.
6. A(n) ________ chemical bond occurs when atoms share electrons.
7. The symbol K^+ represents the potassium ________.
8. A compound that dissociates in water to form ions is called a(n) ________.
9. Molecules that have a carbon-carbon bond in them are classified as ________ compounds.
10. In saltwater, salt is the solute and water is the ________.
11. When water is used to build up small molecules into larger molecules, the process is called ________.
12. ________ are solutions that have an excess of hydrogen ions.
13. Blood contains chemicals called ________ that maintain a stable pH.

Match each type of compound in Column B with the corresponding example given in Column A.

Column A		Column B
14. ________	glycogen	a. salt
15. ________	collagen	b. acid
16. ________	RNA	c. base
17. ________	cholesterol	d. carbohydrate
18. ________	NaCl	e. lipid
19. ________	NaOH	f. protein
20. ________	HCl	g. nucleic acid

21. An ion is formed when
    a. electrons are shared
    b. electrons remain in place
    c. electrons are gained or lost
    d. neutrons are added to the nucleus
22. In the equation $H_2O + CO_2 \rightarrow H^+ + HCO_3^-$, which of these is a reactant?
    a. CO_2
    b. HCO_3^-
    c. O_2
    d. $\rightarrow$
23. Which of these chemical subunits is found in DNA?
    a. uracil
    b. ribose
    c. amino acid
    d. deoxyribose
24. Which of these represents an acid?
    a. pH 7.5
    b. pH 6.1
    c. pH 9.0
    d. pH 7.0
25. Steroid hormones are:
    a. carbohydrates
    b. proteins
    c. lipids
    d. nucleic acids

Cells

OUTLINE

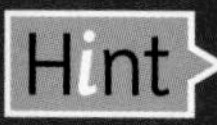

Scan this outline before you begin to read the chapter, as a preview of how the concepts are organized.

OBJECTIVES

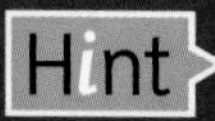

Before reading the chapter, review these goals for your learning.

After you have completed this chapter, you should be able to:

1. Identify and discuss the basic structure and function of the three major components of a cell.
2. List and briefly discuss the functions of the primary cellular organelles.
3. Compare the major passive and active transport processes that act to move substances through cell membranes.
4. Compare and discuss DNA and RNA and their function in protein synthesis.
5. Discuss the stages of mitosis and explain the importance of cellular reproduction.

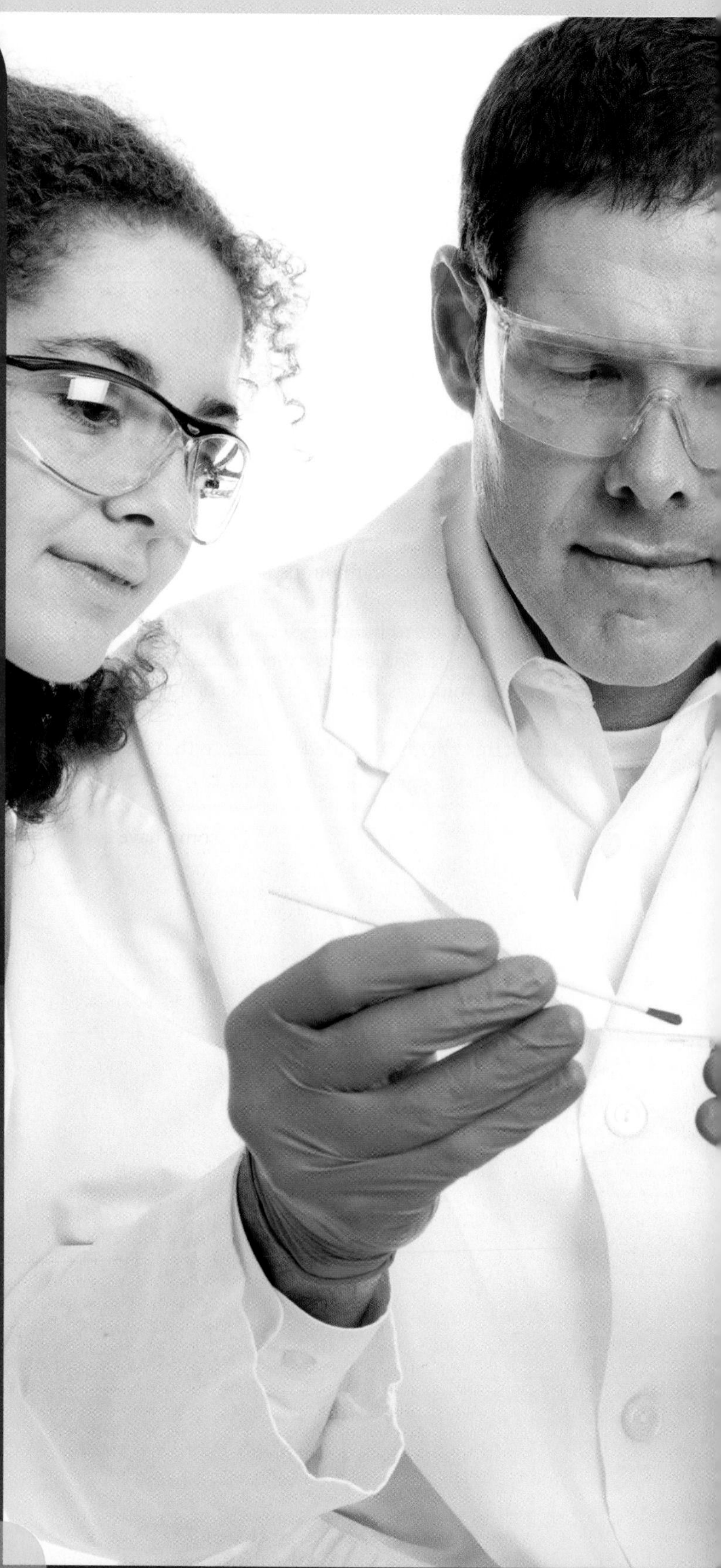

CHAPTER 3

About 300 years ago Robert Hooke looked through his microscope, one of the very early, somewhat primitive ones, at some plant material. What he saw must have surprised him. Instead of a single magnified piece of plant material, he saw many small spaces created by cell walls. Because they reminded him of miniature storerooms or "cells," that is what he called them: *cells*. Since Hooke's time, thousands of individuals have examined thousands of plant and animal specimens and found them all, without exception, to be composed of cells. This fact, that cells are the smallest structural units of living things, has become the foundation of modern biology.

Many living things are so simple that they consist of just one cell. The human body, however, is so complex that it consists not of a few thousand or millions or even billions of cells but of many trillions of them. This chapter discusses the basic concepts of cell structure and function.

Overview of Cells

Size and Shape

Human cells are microscopic in size; that is, they can be seen only when magnified by a microscope. However, they vary considerably in size. An ovum (female sex cell), for example, has a diameter of about 150 micrometers, but red blood cells have a diameter of only 7.5 micrometers. Cells differ even more notably in shape than in size. Some are flat, some are brick-shaped, some are threadlike, and some have irregular shapes.

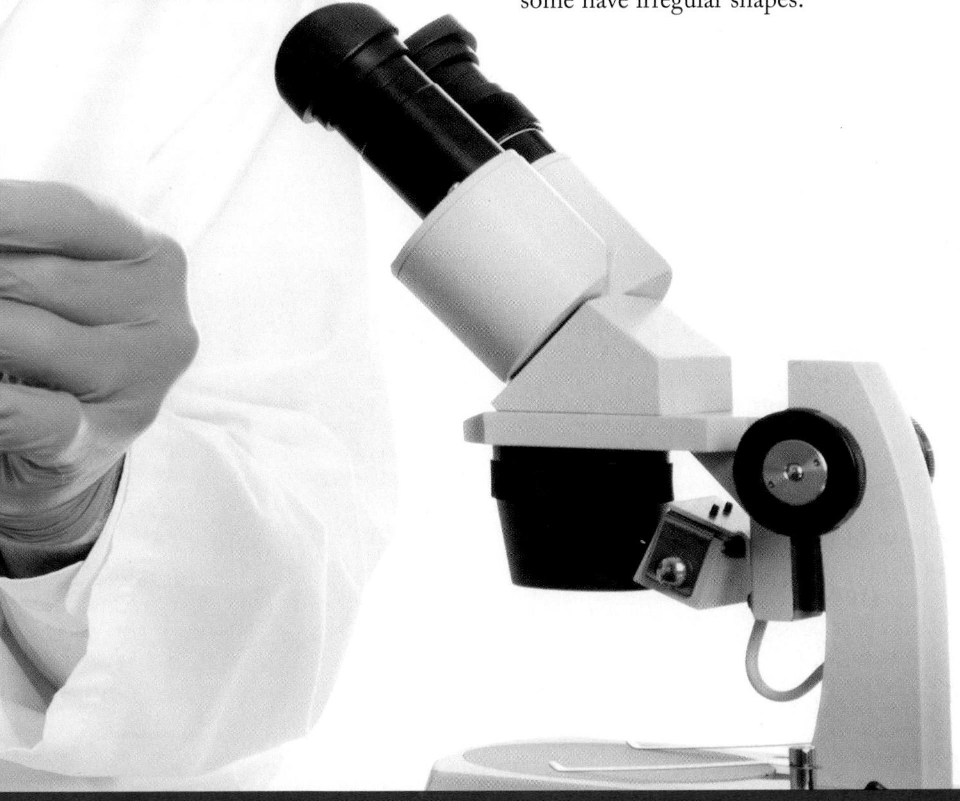

LANGUAGE OF **SCIENCE** AND **MEDICINE**

Hint **Before reading the chapter, say each of these terms out loud. This will help you to avoid stumbling over them as you read.**

active transport
(AK-tiv TRANZ-port)
[*act-* **move,** *-ive* **relating to,** *trans-* **across,** *-port* **carry**]

adenosine triphosphate (ATP)
(ah-DEN-oh-seen try-FOS-fayt)
[*adenos-* shortened from *adenine-* **ribose,** *-ine* **chemical,** *tri-* **three,** *-phosph-* **phosphorus,** *-ate* **oxygen**]

anaphase
(AN-ah-fayz)
[*ana-* **apart,** *-phase* **stage**]

apoptosis
(app-oh-TOH-sis *or* app-op-TOH-sis)
[*apo-* **away,** *-ptosis* **falling**]

benign tumors
(bee-NYNE TOO-mer)
[*benign* **kind**]

centriole
(SEN-tree-ohl)
[*centr-* **center,** *-ole* **small**]

centromere
(SEN-troh-meer)
[*centr-* **center,** *-mere* **part**]

centrosome
(SEN-troh-sohm)
[*centr-* **center,** *-som* **body**]

chromatid
(KROH-mah-tid)
[*chrom-* **color,** *-id* **structure or body**]

chromatin granule
(KROH-mah-tin GRAN-yool)
[*chrom-* **color,** *-in* **substance,** *gran-* **grain,** *-ule* **little**]

chromosome
(KROH-meh-sohm)
[*chrom-* **color,** *-som-* **body**]

Continued on p. 59

Composition

Cells contain **cytoplasm**—the living substance that exists only in cells. The term *cyto* is a Greek combining form and denotes a relationship to a cell. Each cell in the body is surrounded by a thin membrane, the *plasma membrane.* This membrane separates the cell contents from the dilute saltwater solution called **interstitial fluid (IF),** or simply *tissue fluid,* which bathes every cell in the body. Numerous specialized structures called *organelles,* which are described in subsequent sections of this chapter, are contained within the cytoplasm of each cell. A small, circular body called the *nucleus* is also inside the cell.

Parts of the Cell

The three main parts of a cell are:

1. Plasma membrane
2. Cytoplasm
3. Nucleus

The plasma membrane surrounds the entire cell, forming its outer boundary. The cytoplasm is all the living material inside the cell (except the nucleus). The nucleus is a large, membrane-bound structure in most cells that contains the genetic code.

Plasma Membrane

As the name suggests, the **plasma membrane** is the membrane that encloses the cytoplasm and forms the outer boundary of the cell. It is an incredibly delicate structure—only about 7 nm (nanometers) or 3/10,000,000 of an inch thick! Yet it has a precise, orderly structure (**Figure 3-1**). Two layers of phosphate-containing fat molecules called **phospholipids** form a fluid framework for the plasma membrane. Another kind of fat molecule called *cholesterol* is also a component of the plasma membrane. Cholesterol helps stabilize the phospholipid molecules to prevent breakage of the plasma membrane.

Note in **Figure 3-1** that protein molecules dot the surfaces of the membrane and many extend all the way through the phospholipid framework.

Despite its seeming fragility, the plasma membrane is strong enough to keep the cell whole and intact. It also performs other life-preserving functions for the cell. It serves as a well-guarded gateway between the fluid inside the cell and the fluid around it. Certain substances move through it, by way of transporter channels and carriers, but it bars the passage of other substances.

The plasma membrane even functions as a communication device. In what way, you may wonder? Some of the proteins on the membrane's outer surface serve as receptors for certain other molecules when these other molecules contact the proteins. In other words, certain molecules bind to certain receptor proteins. For example, some hormones (chemicals secreted into blood from ductless glands) bind to membrane receptors, and a change in cell functions follows. We might therefore think of such hormones as chemical messages, communicated to cells by binding to their cytoplasmic membrane receptors.

The plasma membrane also identifies a cell as being part of one particular individual. Some of its surface proteins serve as positive identification tags because they occur only in the cells of that individual. A practical application of this fact is made in *tissue typing,* a procedure performed before an organ from

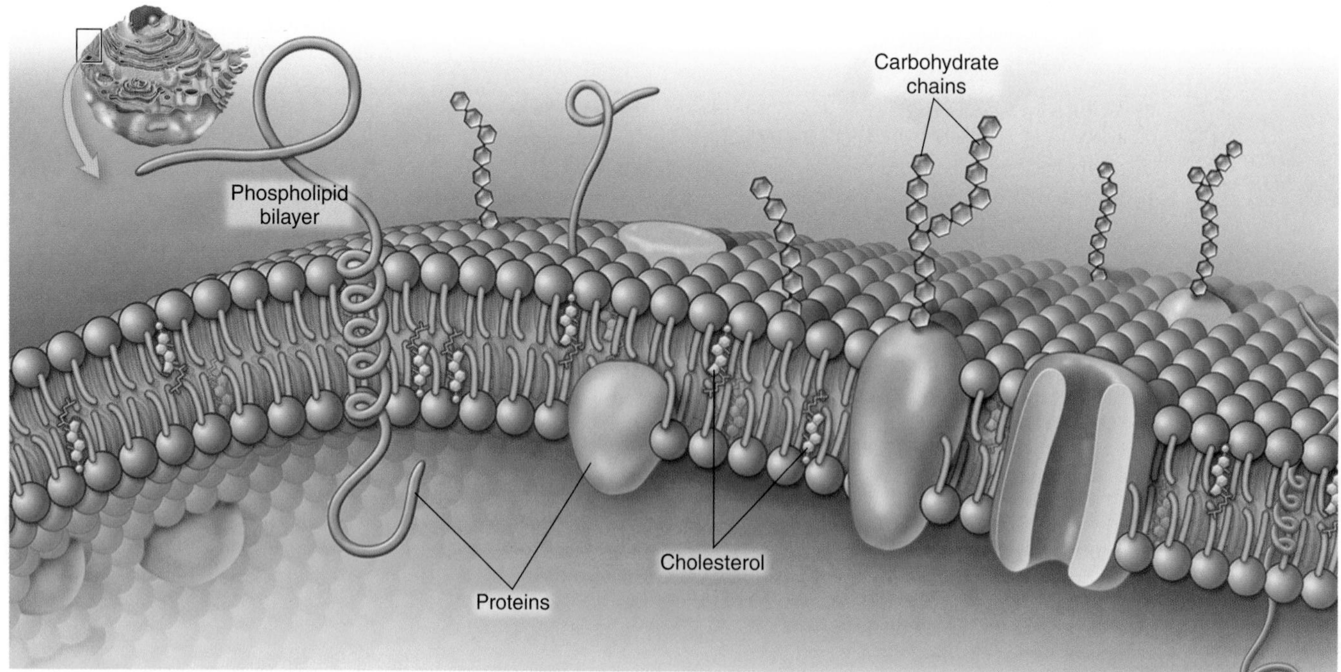

FIGURE 3-1 Structure of the plasma membrane. Note that protein molecules may penetrate completely through the two layers of phospholipid molecules.

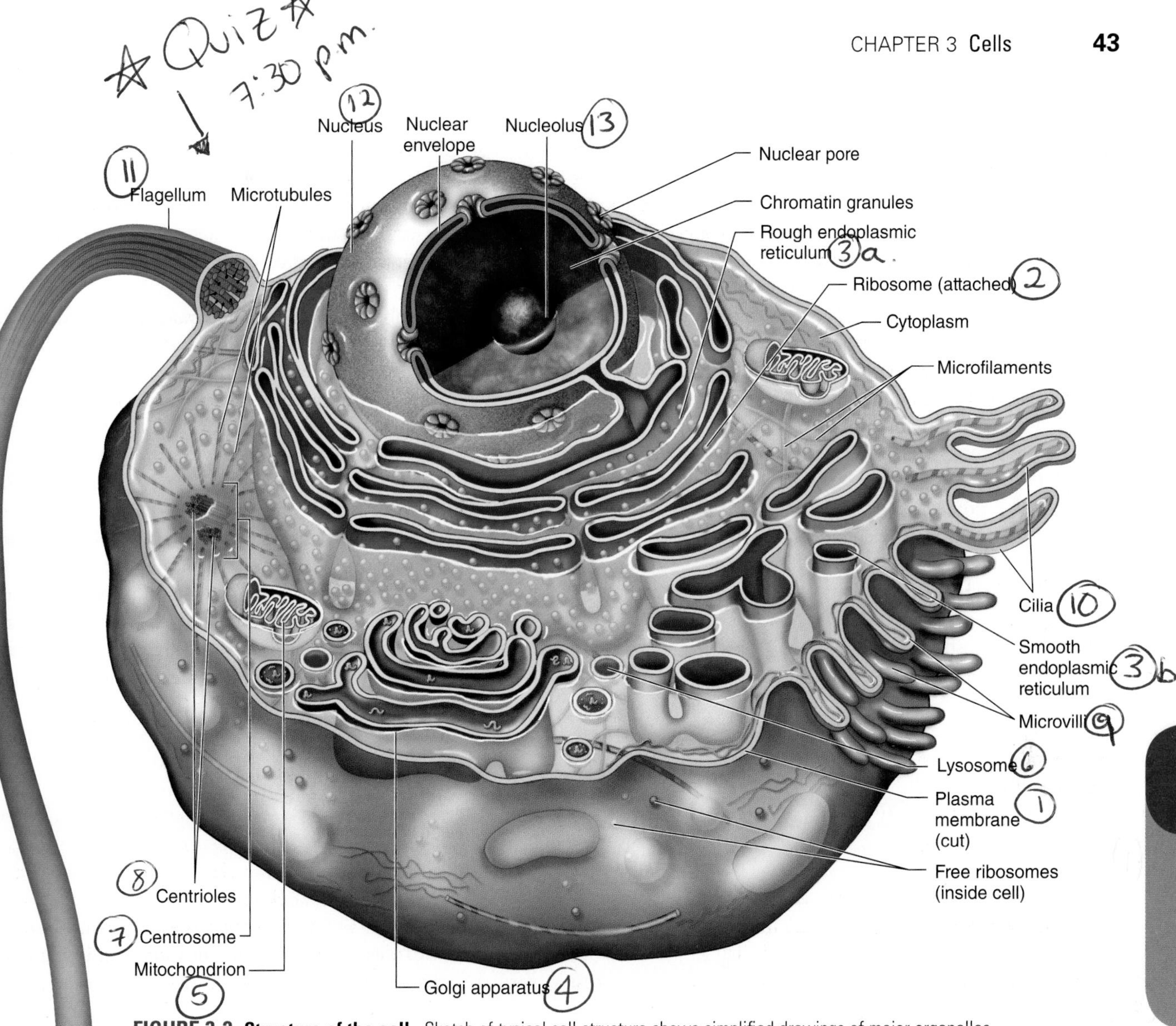

FIGURE 3-2 Structure of the cell. Sketch of typical cell structure shows simplified drawings of major organelles.

one individual is transplanted into another. Carbohydrate chains attached to the surface of cells often play a role in the identification of cell types.

Another function of membrane proteins is as transporters that move various substances across the membrane. Such movement across cellular membranes is discussed in detail later in this chapter (see p. 48).

Cytoplasm

Cytoplasm is the internal living material of cells. It fills the space between the plasma membrane and the nucleus, which can be seen in Figure 3-2 as a round or spherical structure in the center of the cell. Numerous small structures are part of the cytoplasm, along with the fluid that serves as the interior environment of each cell. As a group, the small structures that make up much of the cytoplasm are called **organelles.** This name means "little organs," an appropriate name because they function for the cell just as organs function for the body.

In Figure 3-2 you can see small threadlike structures scattered around in the cytoplasm. You can see only a few of the many threads that make up the **cytoskeleton,** or "cell skeleton." Thin threadlike filaments in this framework are called *microfilaments*. Tiny, hollow tubes called *microtubules* are also important.

Like the body's framework of bones and muscles, the cytoskeleton provides support and movement. The various organelles are not just floating around randomly. They are instead being held (or moved) by the fibers and *molecular motors* of the cytoskeleton. When a cell moves, or when organelles within a cell move, it is actually the parts of the cytoskeleton that are pulling or pushing membranes and organelles.

Look again at **Figure 3-2**. Notice how many different kinds of structures you can see in the cytoplasm of this cell. A little more than a generation ago, most of these organelles were unknown. We now know of many types of organelles, only a few of which are shown here. They are so small that they are invisible even when magnified 1000 times by a light microscope. The advent of electron microscopes in the early twentieth century finally brought them into view by magnifying them many thousands of times. Next we briefly discuss the following organelles, all of which are found in cytoplasm (**Table 3-1**):

1. Ribosomes
2. Endoplasmic reticulum
3. Golgi apparatus
4. Mitochondria
5. Lysosomes
6. Centrosome
7. Cell extensions

Ribosomes

Organelles called **ribosomes,** shown as dots in **Figure 3-2**, are tiny particles found throughout the cell. They are each made up of two tiny subunits constructed mostly of a special kind of RNA called *ribosomal RNA (rRNA)*.

Some ribosomes are found temporarily attached to a network of membranous canals called *endoplasmic reticulum (ER)*. Ribosomes also may be free in the cytoplasm. Ribosomes perform a very complex function—they make enzymes and other protein compounds. Thus they are aptly nicknamed "protein factories."

Endoplasmic Reticulum

An **endoplasmic reticulum (ER)** is a system of membranes forming a network of connecting sacs and canals that wind back and forth through a cell's cytoplasm, from the nucleus almost to the plasma membrane. The tubular passageways or canals in the ER carry proteins and other substances through the cytoplasm of the cell from one area to another.

TABLE 3-1 Major Cell Parts

CELL PART	STRUCTURE	FUNCTION(S)
Plasma membrane	Phospholipid bilayer studded with proteins	Serves as the boundary of the cell; protein and carbohydrate molecules on the outer surface of plasma membrane perform various functions; for example, they serve as markers that identify cells of each individual, as receptor molecules for certain hormones, or transporters to move substances through the membrane
Ribosomes	Tiny particles, each made up of rRNA subunits	Synthesize proteins; a cell's "protein factories"
Endoplasmic reticulum (ER)	Membranous network of interconnected canals and sacs, some with ribosomes attached (rough ER) and some without attachments (smooth ER)	Rough ER receives and transports synthesized proteins (from ribosomes); smooth ER synthesizes lipids and certain carbohydrates
Golgi apparatus	Stack of flattened, membranous sacs	Chemically processes, then packages substances from the ER
Mitochondria	Membranous capsules containing a large, folded internal membrane encrusted with enzymes	ATP synthesis; a cell's "power plants" or "battery chargers"
Lysosome	"Bubble" of hydrolysis enzymes encased by membrane	A cell's "digestive bag," it breaks apart large molecules
Centrosome	Area near nucleus without a visible boundary; contains centrioles	Organizes microtubules of the cytoskeleton
Centrioles	Pair of hollow cylinders at right angles to each other, each made up of tiny tubules within the centrosome	Help organize and move chromosomes during cell reproduction
Microvilli	Tiny cell surface extensions supported internally by microfilaments	Increase surface area of plasma membrane for efficiency of absorption
Cilia	Hairlike cell surface extensions supported by an internal cylinder made of microtubules (longer than microvilli)	Sensory "antennae" to detect conditions outside the cell; some cilia also move substances over surface of the cell
Flagellum	Long whiplike projection on the sperm; similar to a cilium but much longer	The only example in humans is the "tail" of a sperm cell, propelling the sperm through fluids
Nucleus	Double-membraned, spherical envelope containing DNA strands	Contains DNA, which dictates protein synthesis, thereby playing an essential role in other cell activities such as transport, metabolism, growth, and heredity
Nucleolus	Dense region of the nucleus	Makes subunits that form ribosomes

There are two types of ER: *rough* and *smooth*.

Rough ER gets its name from the many ribosomes that are attached to its outer surface, giving it a rough texture similar to sandpaper. As ribosomes make their proteins, they may attach to the rough ER and insert the protein into the interior of the ER.

The ER then begins folding the new proteins and transports them to areas in which chemical processing takes place. These areas of the ER are so full of molecules that ribosomes have no room into which they can pass their proteins and so they do not attach. The absence of attached ribosomes gives this type of ER a smooth texture. Fats, carbohydrates, and proteins that make up cellular membrane material are manufactured in smooth ER. Thus the smooth ER makes a new membrane for the cell.

To sum up: rough ER receives, folds, and transports newly made proteins, and smooth ER makes a new membrane.

Golgi Apparatus

The **Golgi apparatus** consists of tiny, flattened sacs stacked on one another near the nucleus. Little bubbles, or sacs, break off the smooth ER and carry new proteins and other compounds to the sacs of the Golgi apparatus (**Figure 3-3**). These little sacs, also called **vesicles,** fuse with the Golgi sacs and allow the contents of both to mingle.

The Golgi apparatus chemically processes the molecules from the ER by continuing the folding of proteins begun in the ER and combining them with other molecules to form quaternary proteins (see **Figure 2-12**, p. 31) or combinations such as glycoproteins (carbohydrate/protein combinations).

The Golgi apparatus then packages the processed molecules into new little vesicles that pinch off and pull away from the Golgi apparatus, moving slowly outward to the plasma

FIGURE 3-3 The cell's protein export system. The Golgi apparatus processes and packages protein molecules delivered from the endoplasmic reticulum by small vesicles. Some vesicles migrate to the plasma membrane to secrete the final products, and other vesicles remain inside the cell for a time and serve as storage vessels for the substance to be secreted. *ER,* Endoplasmic reticulum.

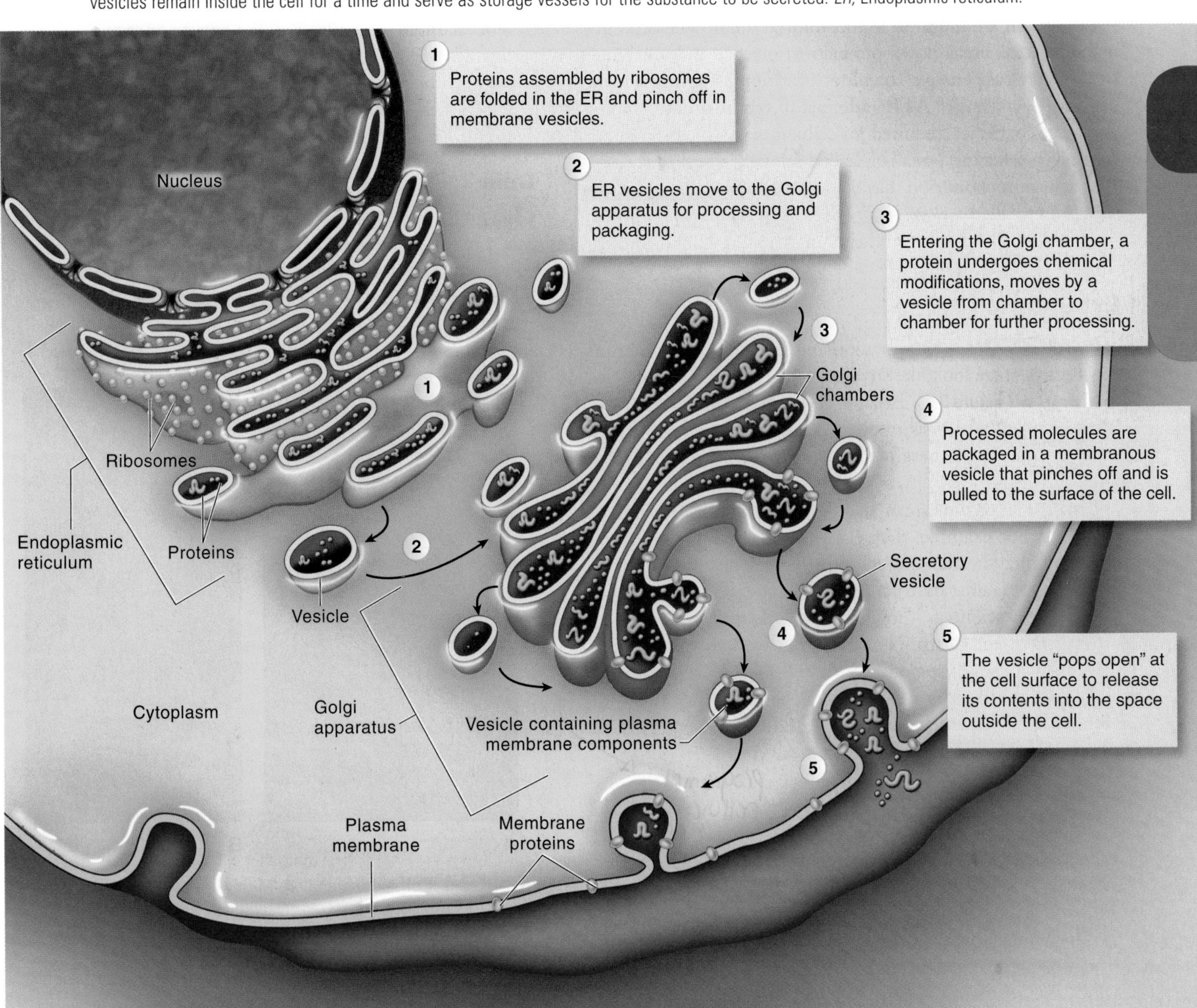

membrane. Each vesicle fuses with the plasma membrane, opens to the outside of the cell, and releases its contents.

An example of a Golgi apparatus product is the slippery substance called *mucus.* If we wanted to nickname the Golgi apparatus, we might call it the cell's "chemical processing and packaging center."

Mitochondria

The **mitochondrion** is another kind of organelle in all cells. Mitochondria are so tiny that a lineup of 15,000 or more of them would fill a space only about 2.5 cm (1 inch long). Two membranous sacs, one inside the other, compose a single mitochondrion. The inner membrane forms folds that look like miniature incomplete partitions. Within a mitochondrion's fragile membranes, complex, energy-converting chemical reactions occur continuously. Because these reactions supply most of the power for cellular work, mitochondria have been nicknamed the cell's "power plants."

Enzymes (molecules that promote specific chemical reactions), which are found in mitochondrial membranes and inner substance, break down products of glucose and other nutrients to release energy. The mitochondrion uses this released energy to "recharge" **ATP (adenosine triphosphate)** molecules, the "batteries" required for cellular work (see p. 33). This energy-transferring process is called *cellular respiration.*

Each mitochondrion has its own tiny DNA molecule, sometimes called a *mitochondrial chromosome,* which contains information for building and running the mitochondrion.

Lysosomes

The **lysosomes** are membranous-walled organelles that in their active stage look like small sacs, often with tiny particles in them (see **Figure 3-2**). Because lysosomes contain enzymes that promote hydrolysis, they can break apart (digest) large nutrient molecules. Therefore, they have the nickname "digestive bags."

Lysosomal enzymes can also digest substances other than nutrients. For example, they can digest and thereby destroy microbes that invade the cell. Thus lysosomes can help to protect cells against destruction by microbes.

Formerly, scientists thought lysosomes were involved in programmed cell death. Now, however, we know a different set of mechanisms is responsible for "cell suicide," or **apoptosis,** which makes space for newer cells. When apoptosis does not occur normally, the cell may remain and cause overgrowth of the tissue—possibly producing a tumor.

Centrosome

The **centrosome** is a region of cytoplasm near the nucleus of each cell. It serves as the *microtubule-organizing center* of the cell, thus playing an important role in organizing and moving the structures within the cell.

Centrioles are paired organelles found within the centrosome. Two of these rod-shaped structures exist in every cell. They are arranged so that they lie at right angles to each other (see **Figure 3-2**). Each centriole is composed of microtubules that play an important role in forming a tapered framework or "spindle" that moves chromosomes during cell division, as we shall see later in this chapter.

The centrosome also plays a role in forming and organizing the cell's cytoskeleton, including some of a cell's outward extensions.

Cell Extensions

Most cells have various indentations and extensions that serve many different functions. Here we describe three of the major types of cell extensions.

Microvilli

Microvilli are small, fingerlike projections of the plasma membrane of some cells (**Figure 3-4,** *A*). These projections increase the surface area of the cell and thus increase its ability to absorb substances.

For example, cells that line the small intestine are covered with microvilli that increase the absorption rate of nutrients into the blood. Microvilli have microfilaments inside them that produce wobbly movement and thus make absorption even more efficient.

Cilia

Cilia are extremely fine, hairlike extensions on the exposed or free surfaces of cells. Cilia are larger than microvilli and possess inner microtubules that support them and enable them to move (see **Figure 3-4,** *A*). Every cell has at least one cilium.

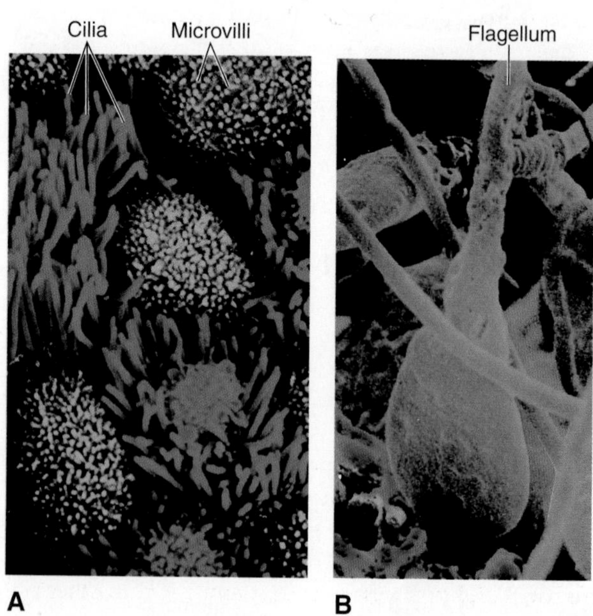

FIGURE 3-4 Cell extensions. A, Microvilli *(light blue)* are small, fingerlike extensions of the plasma membrane that increase the surface area for absorption. Cilia *(darker blue)* are longer than microvilli and move back and forth, pushing fluids along the surface. **B,** The tail-like flagellum that propels each sperm cell is so long that it does not fit into the photograph at this magnification.

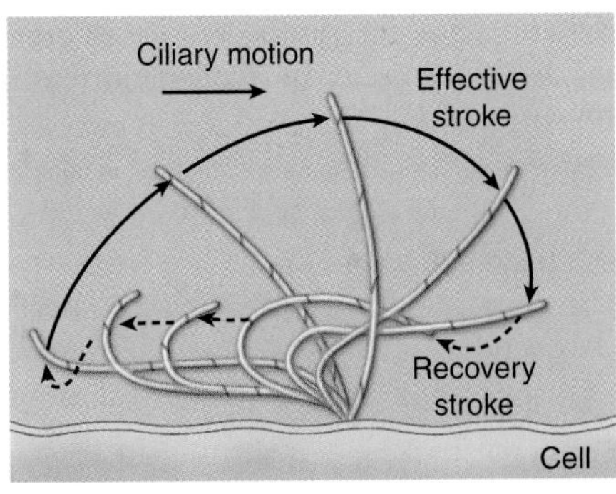

Cilium

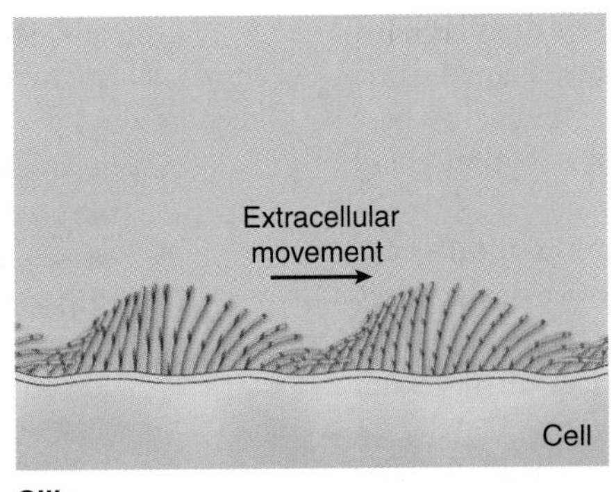

Cilia

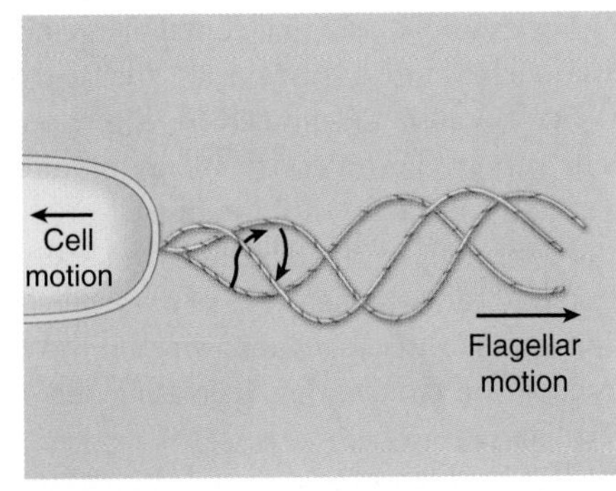

Flagellum

FIGURE 3-5 Movement patterns. In humans, cilia *(left and middle)* found in groups on stationary cells beat in a coordinated oarlike pattern to push fluid and particles in the extracellular fluid along the outer cell surface. A flagellum *(right)* produces wave-like movements, which propels a sperm cell forward—like the tail of an eel.

All cilia act like an insect's antenna, allowing the cell to sense its surroundings. For example, the hairlike cilia in the taste buds of the mouth can detect different chemicals by taste.

Some cells have hundreds of cilia capable of moving together in a wavelike fashion (Figure 3-5). By moving as a group in one direction, the cilia can propel mucus over the surfaces of cells that line the respiratory or reproductive tubes.

Flagella

A **flagellum** is a single projection extending from the cell surface. Flagella are structurally similar to cilia but much longer. Like cilia, flagella can move. The cylinder of microtubules inside the flagellum moves in a way that whips the flagellum around like a propeller, pushing the cell forward (see Figure 3-5).

In a human, the only example of a flagellum is the "tail" of the male sperm cell (see Figure 3-4, *B*). Wiggling movements of the flagellum make it possible for sperm to "swim" or move toward the ovum after they are deposited in the female reproductive tract.

Nucleus

Central Structure of a Cell

Viewed under a light microscope, the **nucleus** of a cell looks like a very simple structure—just a small sphere in the central portion of the cell. In certain specialized cells, the nucleus may be pushed to one side, perhaps compressed a bit into a more flattened shape.

However, its simple appearance belies the complex and critical role the nucleus plays in cell function. The nucleus contains most of the cell's genetic information, which ultimately controls every organelle in the cytoplasm. It also controls the complex process of cell reproduction. In other words, the nucleus must function properly for a cell to accomplish its normal activities and be able to duplicate itself.

Note that the cell nucleus in Figure 3-2 is surrounded by a **nuclear envelope** made up of two separate membranes. The nuclear envelope has many tiny openings called *nuclear pores* that permit large molecules to move into and out of the nucleus. The nuclear envelope encloses a special type of cell material in the nucleus called **nucleoplasm.** Nucleoplasm contains a number of structures, with two of the most important shown in Figure 3-2. They are the nucleolus and the chromatin granules.

Nucleolus

The **nucleolus** is a dense region of the nuclear material that is critical in protein formation because it is where the cell makes the subunits that form ribosomes. The ribosome subunits then migrate through the nuclear envelope into the cytoplasm of the cell to form ribosomes, which produce proteins.

Chromatin and Chromosomes

Chromatin granules in the nucleus are made of proteins around which are wound segments of the long, threadlike molecules called *DNA,* or *deoxyribonucleic acid.* DNA is the genetic material often described as the chemical "cookbook" of the body. Because it contains the code for building both structural proteins and functional proteins, DNA determines everything from gender and metabolic rate to body build and hair color in every human being.

During cell division, DNA molecules become tightly coiled. They then look like short, compact structures and are called **chromosomes.**

Each cell of the body contains a total of 46 different DNA molecules in its nucleus and one copy of a forty-seventh DNA molecule in each of its mitochondria. The importance and function of DNA is explained in greater detail in the section on cell reproduction later in this chapter.

Relationship of Cell Structure and Function

Every human cell performs certain functions. Some maintain the cell's survival, and others help maintain the body's survival. In many instances, the number and type of organelles within cells cause cells to differ dramatically in terms of their specialized functions.

For example, cells that contain large numbers of mitochondria, such as heart muscle cells, are capable of sustained work. Why? Because the numerous mitochondria found in these cells supply the necessary energy required for rhythmic and ongoing contractions of the heart.

Movement of the flagellum of a sperm cell is another example of the way each type of organelle has a particular function. The sperm's flagellum propels it through the reproductive tract of the female, thus increasing the chances of successful fertilization.

This is how and why organizational structure at the cellular level is so important for function in living organisms. Examples in every chapter of the text illustrate how structure and function are intimately related at every level of body organization.

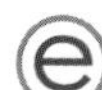
To learn more about cell structures and their functions, go to AnimationDirect at *evolve.elsevier.com.*

QUICK CHECK

1. What is the molecular composition of the plasma membrane of the cell?
2. What is cytoplasm? What is contained within the cytoplasm?
3. What are the primary organelles of the cell? What are the functions of these organelles?
4. Which two kinds of cell structures contain DNA?

Movement of Substances Through Cell Membranes

Types of Membrane Transport

The plasma membrane in every healthy cell separates the contents of the cell from the tissue fluid that surrounds it. At the same time the membrane must permit certain substances to enter the cell and allow others to leave. Heavy traffic moves continuously in both directions through cell membranes. Molecules of water, nutrients, gases, wastes, and many other substances stream in and out of all cells in endless procession.

A number of different **transport processes** allow this mass movement of substances into and out of cells. These transport processes are classified under two general headings:

1. **Passive transport** processes
2. **Active transport** processes

As implied by the name, active transport processes require the expenditure of energy by the cell, and passive transport processes do not. The energy required for active transport processes is obtained from **ATP.** ATP is produced in the mitochondria using energy from nutrients and is capable of releasing that energy to do work in the cell. For active transport processes to occur, the breakdown of ATP and the use of the released energy are required.

The details of active and passive transport of substances across cell membranes are much easier to understand if you keep in mind the following two key facts:

1. In passive transport processes, no cellular energy is required to move substances from a high concentration to a low concentration.
2. In active transport processes, cellular energy is required to move substances from a low concentration to a high concentration.

Passive Transport Processes

The primary passive transport processes that move substances through membranes include the following:

1. Diffusion
2. Osmosis
3. Dialysis
4. Filtration

Scientists describe the movement of substances in passive systems as going "down a concentration gradient." This means that substances in passive systems move from a region of high concentration to a region of low concentration until they reach equal proportions on both sides of the membrane. As you read the next few paragraphs, refer to **Table 3-2**, which summarizes important information about passive transport processes.

Diffusion

Diffusion—a good example of a passive transport process—is the process by which substances scatter themselves evenly throughout an available space. The system does not require additional energy for this movement. Diffusion can thus be described as a trend of movement of particles down a concentration gradient—that is, from an area of high concentration toward an area of lower concentration.

To demonstrate diffusion of particles throughout a fluid, perform this simple experiment the next time you pour yourself a cup of coffee or tea (**Figure 3-6**). Place some sugar on a teaspoon and lower it gently to the bottom of the cup. Let it stand for 2 or 3 minutes, and then, holding the cup steady, take a sip off the top. It will taste sweet. Why? Because some of the sugar molecules will have diffused from the area of high concentration near the mound of sugar at the bottom of the cup to the area of low concentration at the top of the cup—thus sweetening the entire solution.

Assume that the tea is brewed using a tea bag made of shredded tea leaves inside a pouch of porous filter paper. One can easily watch the diffusion of dark pigment particles from a concentrated area inside the tea bag to the less concentrated area in the water outside the tea bag. Thus the pigment particles moved through a membrane (the paper) by diffusion, that is, the tendency to spread out and create a uniform concentration or *equilibrium.*

The key to diffusion across a membrane is the presence of pores big enough for the particles to pass through. In cell

TABLE 3-2 Passive Transport Processes

PROCESS	DESCRIPTION	EXAMPLES
Diffusion	Movement of particles through a membrane from an area of high concentration to an area of low concentration—that is, down the concentration gradient	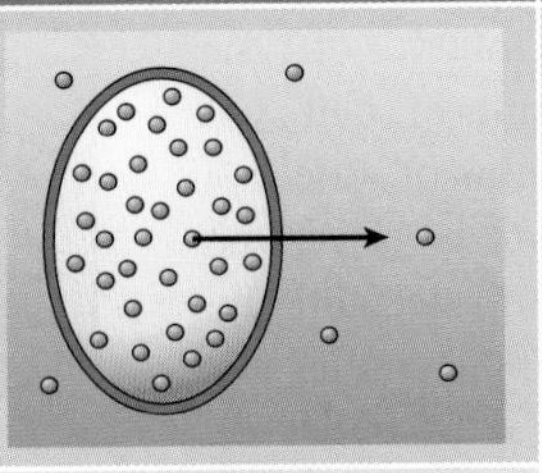 Movement of carbon dioxide out of all cells; movement of sodium ions into nerve cells as they conduct an impulse
Osmosis	Passive movement of water through a selectively permeable membrane in the presence of at least one impermeant solute	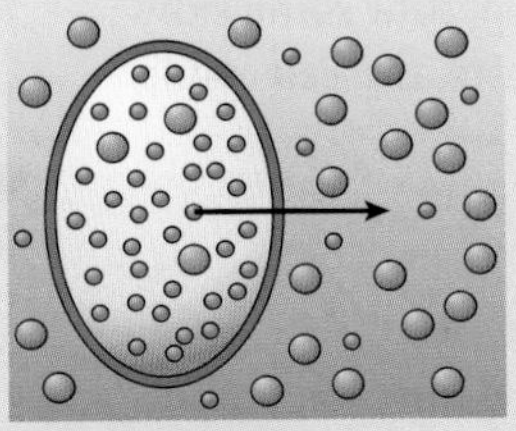 Movement of water molecules into and out of cells to correct imbalances in water concentration
Filtration	Movement of water and small solute particles, but not larger particles, through a filtration membrane; movement occurs from area of high pressure to area of low pressure High pressure / Low pressure	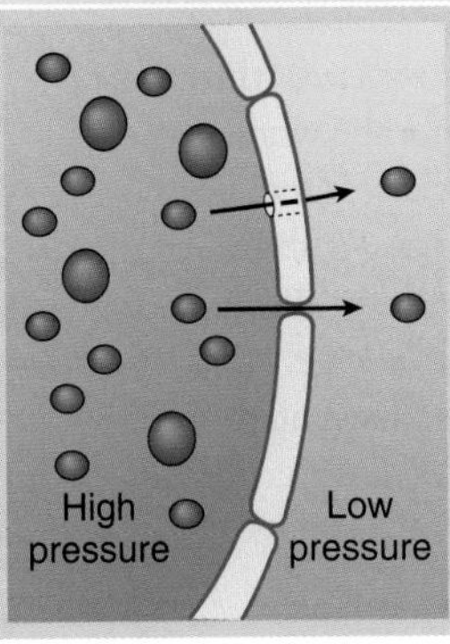 In the kidney, movement of water and small solutes from blood vessels but lack of movement by blood proteins and blood cells; begins the formation of urine

membranes, most molecules cannot pass through the membrane unless there are gateways that permit it. Various protein channels act as gated doorways that permit certain molecules to diffuse through them. Other protein structures act as carriers that bind to the particles and carry them through to the other side of the membrane. Without these transporters, most **solutes** (substances dissolved in the water) could not diffuse through cell membranes.

The process of diffusion is shown in **Figure 3-7**. Note that both substances diffuse rapidly through the porous membrane in both directions. However, as indicated by the purple arrows, more of the solute (dissolved substance) moves out of the 20% solution, where the concentration is higher, into the 10% solution, where the concentration is lower, than in the opposite

Lump of sugar

Time

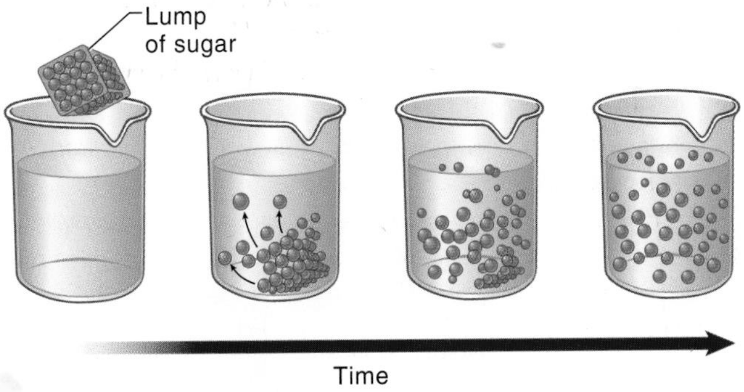

FIGURE 3-6 Diffusion. The molecules of a lump of sugar are very densely packed when they enter the water. As sugar molecules collide frequently in the area of high concentration, they gradually spread away from each other—toward the area of lower concentration. Eventually, the sugar molecules become evenly distributed.

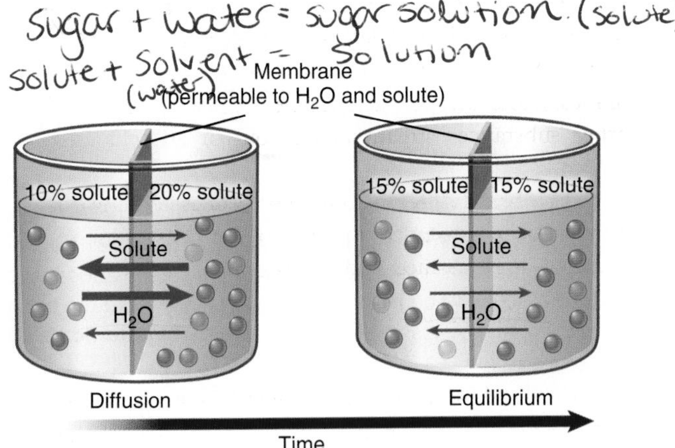

FIGURE 3-7 Diffusion through a membrane. Note that the membrane is permeable to the purple solute particles and to water molecules and that it separates a 10% solution of purple solute particles from a 20% solution of purple particles. The container on the left shows the two solutions separated by the membrane at the start of diffusion. The container on the right shows the result of diffusion over time.

direction. This is an example of movement down a concentration gradient.

The result? Equilibration (balancing) of the concentrations of the two solutions occurs after an interval of time. After this equilibrium is reached, equal amounts of solute will diffuse in both directions, as will equal amounts of water.

The plasma membrane of a cell is said to be selectively permeable because it permits the passage of certain substances but not others. That is, it has specific channels and carriers to allow diffusion of specific kinds of molecules. This is a necessary property if the cell is to permit some substances, such as nutrients, to gain entrance to the cell while excluding others.

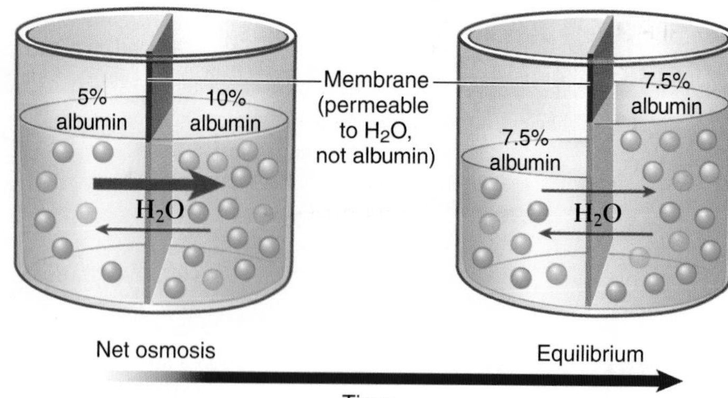

FIGURE 3-8 Osmosis. The solute albumin cannot cross the semipermeable membrane, but water can. The resulting movement of water (only) produces equilibration of the solutions, as water moves away from the side where it is most abundant and toward the solution with more solute particles. Osmosis also causes a shift in fluid volume and pressure (osmotic pressure).

Osmosis

Osmosis is a special case of passive transport. It is in many ways similar to diffusion, but is thought to involve unique mechanisms at the pores of cell membranes.

Osmosis is the passive movement of *water molecules* through water channels in a selectively permeable membrane when some of the *solute* cannot cross the membrane (because there are no open channels or carriers for that solute). Figure 3-8 shows that osmosis moves water in a direction that results in dilution of solution to a type of equilibrium called *osmotic balance.*

In osmosis, because water moves into a space but there is no exchange of solutes, a change in fluid pressure may result. Such fluid pressure is called *osmotic pressure.*

Dialysis

In a process called **dialysis,** some solutes move across a selectively permeable membrane by diffusion and other solutes do not (Figure 3-9). Thus, dialysis results in an uneven distribution of various solutes.

Dialysis is often used as a medical procedure in which blood is pumped through membranous tubing bathed in a solution that mimics normal body fluids. Because the small

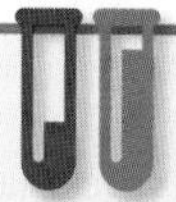

CLINICAL APPLICATION

OSMOTIC BALANCE

The internal fluid environment of the body is mostly a weak solution of salts such as NaCl and other solutes—as is the solution inside each cell of the body. Osmotic balance is maintained through homeostasis. However, disruptions of homeostasis can cause potentially dangerous movement of water and resulting shifts in pressure. Here, we explore examples of what can go wrong.

A salt solution is said to be **isotonic** (*iso* = equal) if it contains the same concentration of salt normally found in a living red blood cell, which measures 0.9% NaCl. Salt particles (Na^+ and Cl^- ions) do not cross the plasma membrane easily, so salt solutions that differ in concentrations from the cell's fluid will promote the osmosis of water one way or the other. A solution that contains a higher level of salt than the cell does (above 0.9%) is said to be **hypertonic** (*hyper* = above) to the cell and one containing less salt (below 0.9%) is **hypotonic** (*hypo* = below) to the cell.

With what you now know about filtration, diffusion, and osmosis, can you predict what would occur if red blood cells were placed in isotonic, hypotonic, and hypertonic solutions?

Examine the figures. Note that red blood cells placed in isotonic solution remain unchanged because there is no effective difference in salt or water concentrations. The movement of water into and out of the cells is about equal. This is not the case with red cells placed in hypertonic salt solution. They immediately lose water from their cytoplasm into the surrounding salty solution, and they shrink. This process is called **crenation** because under a microscope, these cells appear to have a crenated (scalloped) border.

The opposite occurs if red cells are placed in a hypotonic solution. They swell as water enters the cell from the surrounding dilute solution. Eventually the cells break or **lyse,** and the hemoglobin they contain is released into the surrounding solution.

Hypotonic solution (cells lyse)

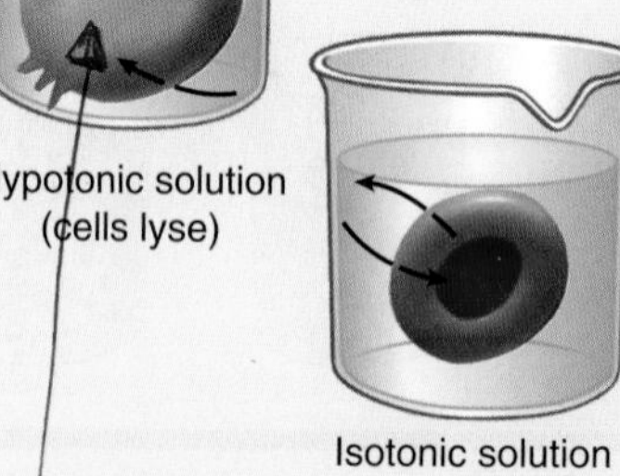

Isotonic solution

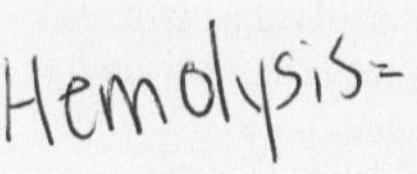

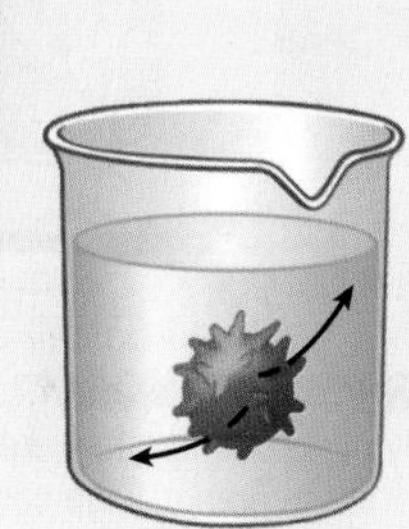

Hypertonic solution (cells crenate)

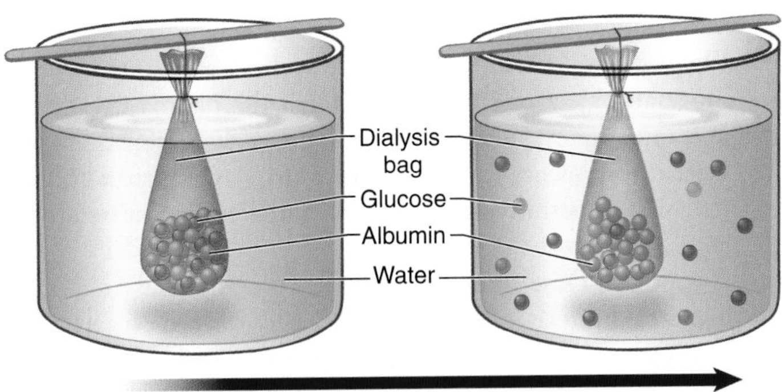

FIGURE 3-9 Dialysis. A membrane bag containing glucose, water, and albumin (protein) molecules is suspended in pure water. Over time, the smaller solute molecules (glucose) diffuse out of the bag. The larger solute molecules (albumin) remain trapped in the bag because the bag is impermeable to them. Thus dialysis results in separation of small and large solute particles.

waste molecules normally removed by the kidney diffuse into the bath solution, but the larger proteins in the blood cannot diffuse, such dialysis can safely "clean" the blood of waste.

Another strategy is to instead pump the bath solution into the fluid space of the abdominopelvic cavity to accept the blood's wastes by dialysis. After some time, the "dirty" solution is then pumped back out of the body.

These dialysis procedures can be used when the kidney is not functioning efficiently.

Filtration

Filtration is the movement of water and solutes through a membrane as a result of a pushing force that is greater on one side of the membrane than on the other side. The force is called *hydrostatic pressure,* which is simply the force or weight of a fluid pushing against some surface (an example is blood pressure, in which blood pushes against vessel walls).

A principle concerning filtration that is of great physiological importance is that it always occurs *down* a hydrostatic pressure gradient. This means that when two fluids have unequal hydrostatic pressures and are separated by a membrane, water and diffusible solutes or particles (those to which the membrane is permeable) will filter out of the solution that has the higher hydrostatic pressure into the solution that has the lower hydrostatic pressure.

Filtration is partly responsible for moving water and small solutes from blood into the fluid spaces of the body's tissues. Filtration is one of the processes responsible for urine formation in the kidney. Wastes are filtered out of the blood into the kidney tubules because of a difference in hydrostatic pressure.

To learn more about passive transport, go to AnimationDirect at *evolve.elsevier.com.*

Active Transport Processes

Active transport is the uphill movement of a substance through a living cell membrane. *Uphill* means "up a concentration gradient" (that is, from a lower to a higher concentration). The energy required for this movement is obtained from ATP. Because the formation and breakdown of ATP require complex cellular activity, active transport mechanisms can take place only through living membranes. **Table 3-3** summarizes active transport processes.

TABLE 3-3 Active Transport Processes

PROCESS	DESCRIPTION	EXAMPLES
Ion pump	Movement of solute particles from an area of low concentration to an area of high concentration (up the concentration gradient) by means of a carrier protein structure (ATP)	In muscle cells, pumping of nearly all calcium ions to special compartments—or out of the cell
Phagocytosis	Movement of cells or other large particles into cell by trapping it in a section of plasma membrane that pinches off inside the cell	Trapping of bacterial cells by phagocytic white blood cells
Pinocytosis	Movement of fluid and dissolved molecules into a cell by trapping them in a section of plasma membrane that pinches off inside the cell	Trapping of large protein molecules by some body cells

Ion Pumps

A complex membrane component called the *ion pump* makes possible a number of active transport mechanisms. An ion pump is an example of a protein structure in the cell membrane called a *carrier*. The ion pump uses energy from ATP to actively move ions across cell membranes *against* their concentration gradients. *Pump* is an appropriate term because it suggests that active transport moves a substance in an uphill direction just as a water pump, for example, moves water uphill.

An ion pump is specific to one particular kind of ion. Therefore, different ion pumps are required to move different types of ions. For example, sodium pumps move sodium ions only. Likewise, calcium pumps move calcium ions, and potassium pumps move potassium ions.

Some ion pumps are "coupled" to one another so that two or more different substances may be moved through the cell membrane at one time. For example, the **sodium-potassium pump,** shown in **Figure 3-10**, pumps sodium ions out of a cell while it pumps potassium ions into the cell. Because both ions are moved against their concentration gradients, this pump creates a high sodium concentration outside the cell and a high potassium concentration inside the cell. Such a pump is required to remove sodium from the inside of a nerve cell after it has rushed in as a result of the passage of a nerve impulse. Some ion pumps are coupled with other specific carriers that transport glucose, amino acids, and other substances. However, there are no transporter pumps for moving water. Water can move only passively by osmosis.

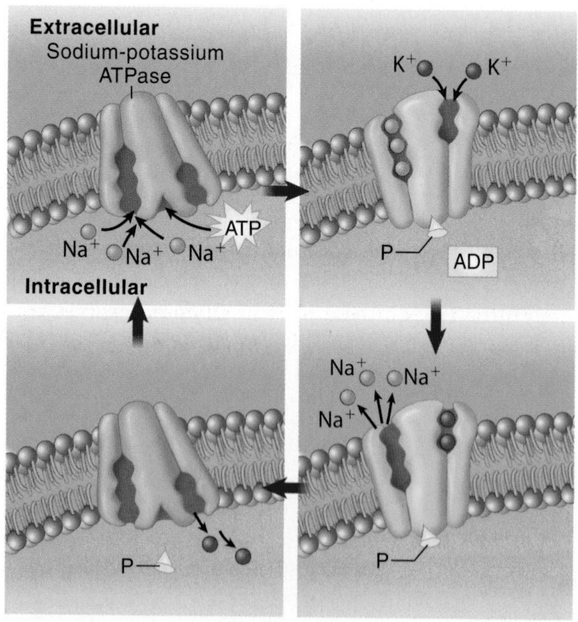

FIGURE 3-10 Sodium-potassium pump. Three sodium ions (Na^+) are pumped out of the cell and two potassium ions (K^+) are pumped into the cell during one pumping cycle of this carrier molecule. ATP is broken down in the process so that the energy freed from ATP can be used to pump the ions.

Phagocytosis

Phagocytosis is another example of how a cell can actively move an object or substance through the plasma membrane and into the cytoplasm. The term *phagocytosis* comes from a Greek word meaning "to eat." The word is appropriate because this process permits a cell to engulf and literally "eat" relatively large particles.

Certain white blood cells can use phagocytosis to destroy invading bacteria and chunks of debris from tissue damage. During this process the cytoskeleton extends the cell's plasma membrane to form a pocket around the particles to be moved into the cell and thus encloses the material in a vesicle. Movements of the cytoskeleton pull the vesicle deeper into the cell.

Once inside the cytoplasm, the phagocytic vesicle fuses with a lysosome containing digestive enzymes and the particles are broken apart (**Figure 3-11**).

Pinocytosis

Pinocytosis is an active transport mechanism used to incorporate fluids or dissolved substances into cells by trapping them in a pocket of plasma membrane that pinches off inside the cell. Again, the term is appropriate because the word part *pino-* comes from the Greek word meaning "drink."

Because the cytoskeleton uses energy from ATP to produce the movements of pinocytosis and phagocytosis, these processes are active transport mechanisms.

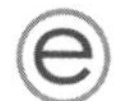
To learn more about active transport, go to AnimationDirect at *evolve.elsevier.com*.

QUICK CHECK

1. What is the difference between a passive transport process and an active transport process?
2. Briefly explain the following primary passive transport processes: (1) diffusion, (2) osmosis, (3) dialysis, (4) filtration.
3. How does an ion pump work? Is it an active or passive transport process?
4. How do phagocytosis and pinocytosis differ?

Cell Growth and Reproduction

Cell Growth

For normal growth and maintenance, the cell must continually produce the many diverse structural and functional proteins needed for human life. The functional proteins then synthesize carbohydrates and lipids and help regulate all cell functions.

The two *nucleic acids* **deoxyribonucleic acid (DNA)** and **ribonucleic acid (RNA)** play crucial roles in directing protein synthesis in each cell. We start our story of cell growth and reproduction with these amazing molecules.

DNA

Chromosomes, which are composed largely of DNA, contain the information needed to make all the proteins of the

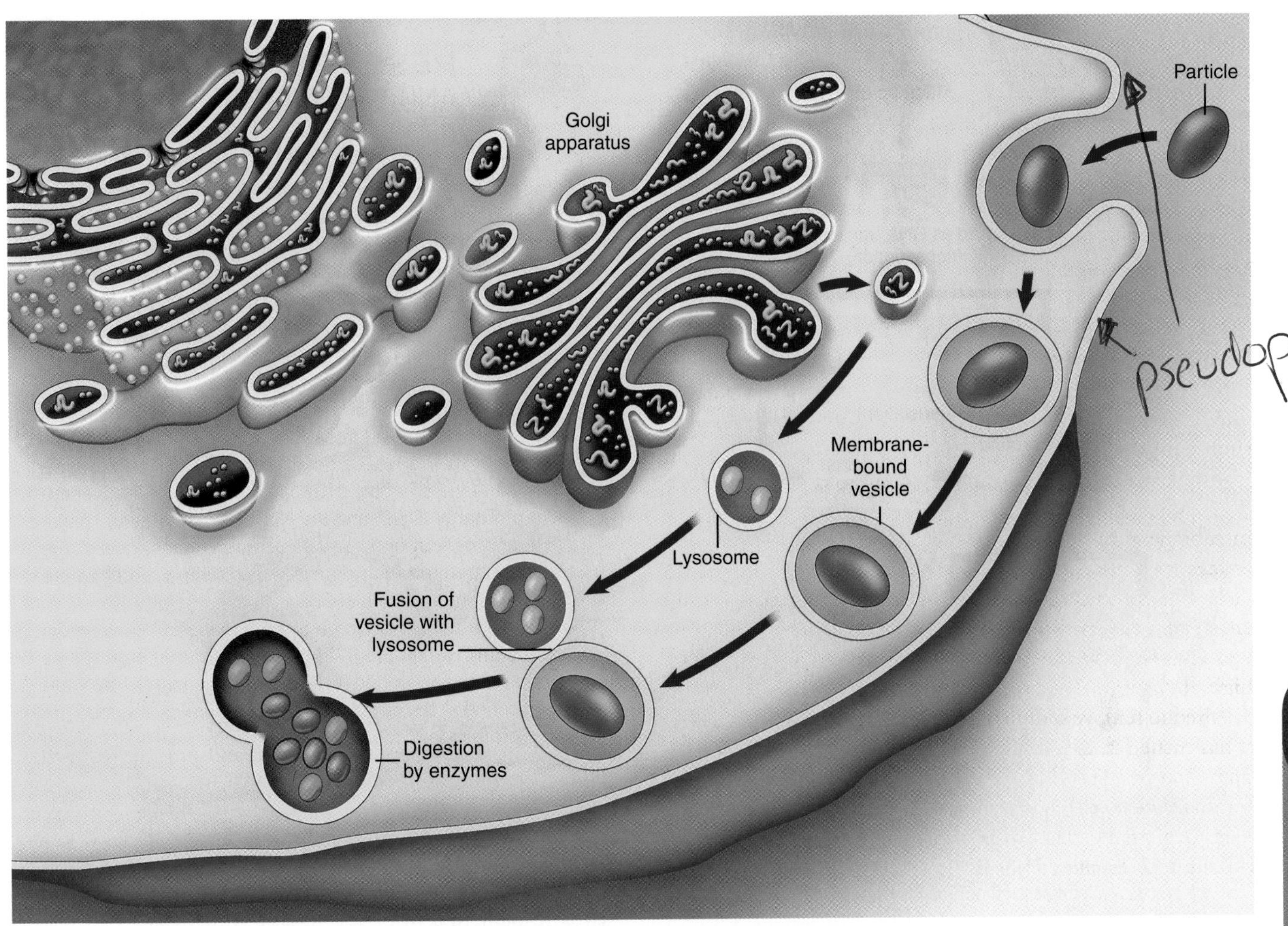

FIGURE 3-11 Phagocytosis. The cell's cytoskeleton reaches out and engulfs a particle, forming a vesicle. Cytoskeletal movements pull the vesicle containing the particle into the cytoplasm, where it fuses with a lysosome. Enzymes from the lysosome break down (digest) the particle. Pinocytosis works in a similar way, except that fluids (not large particles) are engulfed and brought into the cell.

cells—the information that allows a cell to live and function normally. The *genetic code* contained in segments of the DNA molecules that are called **genes** ultimately determines the structure and function of all cells (**Figure 3-12**). This coded information can be transmitted to generations of cells and eventually to offspring.

Structurally, the DNA molecule resembles a long, narrow ladder made of a pliable material. It is twisted round and round its axis, taking on the shape of a double helix (see **Figure 2-14**, p. 32). Each DNA molecule is made of many smaller units called *nucleotides*. Each nucleotide is made up of a sugar, a phosphate, and a base (**Table 3-4**). The bases are adenine, thymine, guanine, and cytosine. These nitrogen-containing chemicals are called *bases* because by themselves they have a high pH, and chemicals with a high pH are called "bases" (see pp. 28-29 for a discussion of acids and bases).

As you can see in **Figure 2-14** (p. 32), each step in the DNA ladder consists of a pair of bases. Only two combinations of bases occur, and the same two bases *always* pair off with each other in a DNA molecule. Adenine always binds to thymine, and cytosine always binds to guanine. This characteristic of DNA structure is called **complementary base pairing.**

A ***gene*** is a specific segment of base pairs in a chromosome. Although the types of base pairs in all chromosomes are the same, the order or *sequence* of base pairs is not the same. This

TABLE 3-4 Components of Nucleotides

NUCLEOTIDE	DNA	RNA
Sugar	Deoxyribose	Ribose
Phosphate	Phosphate	Phosphate
Nitrogen base	Cytosine	Cytosine
	Guanine	Guanine
	Adenine	Adenine
	Thymine	Uracil

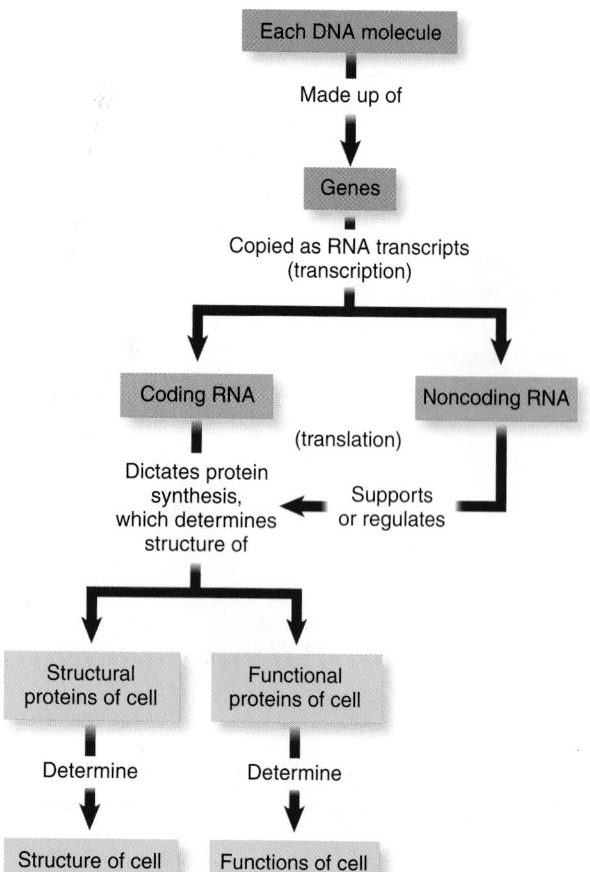

FIGURE 3-12 Function of genes. Genes copied from DNA are copied to RNA in a process called transcription. The RNA transcripts are then used in a process called translation, in which a code that determines the sequence of amino acids is translated to form a protein. The structure of the resulting protein determines the role of the protein in body structure and function—and ultimately, the structure and function of the body.

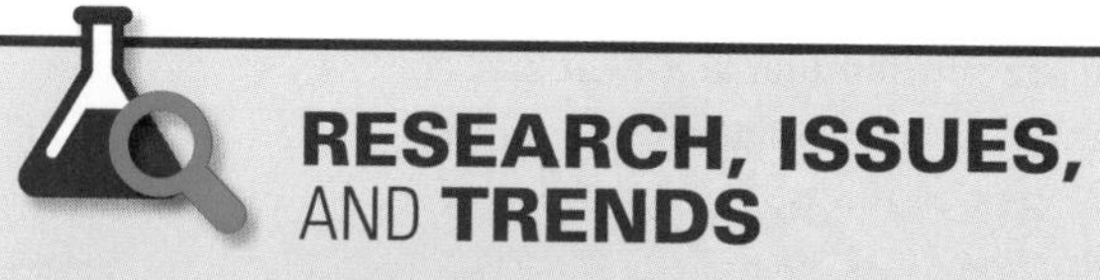

RESEARCH, ISSUES, AND TRENDS

HUMAN GENOME

All of the DNA in each cell of the body is called the **genome.** Intense, coordinated effort by scientists has mapped all the gene locations in the human genome. Efforts at reading the different genetic codes possible at each location are still under way. Much of the work of mapping the human genome was done as part of the Human Genome Project (HGP), which was started in 1990.

Besides producing a complete human genetic map and developing tools of genetic mapping, a field called *genomics,* HGP also addresses the ethical, legal, and social issues that may arise—a notable first for such a massive scientific research effort. HGP is sponsored by the Department of Energy (DOE) and the National Institutes of Health (NIH), and its first director was James Watson, one of the scientists credited with originally discovering the structure of the DNA molecule in 1953.

With the human genome already mapped, many scientists are still working to fill in the details of the many genes and gene variants found in the human genome. Many are also working in the related field of *proteomics,* the study of all the proteins encoded by each of the genes of the human genome.

fact has tremendous functional importance because it is the sequence of base pairs in each gene of each chromosome that determines the genetic code.

Most genes direct the synthesis of at least one kind of protein molecule. Each protein may function, for example, as an enzyme, a structural component of a cell, or a specific hormone. Or it may combine with other protein molecules, or even with carbohydrates or lipids, to form any number of large, complex molecules such as quaternary proteins, glycoproteins, proteoglycans, or lipoproteins.

The enzymes and other functional molecules produced by protein synthesis facilitate and regulate cellular chemical reactions that drive all the functions of cells—and thereby all the functions of the body.

In humans having 46 nuclear chromosomes and one kind of mitochondrial chromosome in each body cell, DNA has a content of genetic information totaling about 3 *billion* base pairs in perhaps 19,000 or so protein-coding genes. Sections of DNA that do not code for protein structure have other functions, which include regulation of turning genes on and off and regulating protein synthesis. This means that over a billion bits of information are inherited from each of our two biological parents. Is it any wonder, then, with all of this genetic information packed into each of our cells, that we are such complex organisms?

RNA

The genetic information contained in protein-coding genes is capable of "directing" the synthesis of a specific protein. Some genes instead contain information needed to build regulatory types of RNA molecules.

Regulatory RNA molecules act as functional molecules that affect some of the chemical processes in a cell. For example, *ribosomal RNA (rRNA)* molecules form most of the ribosome's protein-synthesizing structure and other RNA molecules that serve as temporary working copies of genetic code.

Most of the DNA, with its genetic code that dictates directions for protein synthesis, is contained in the nucleus of the cell. The actual process of protein synthesis, however, occurs at ribosomes in the cytoplasm and on ER. Another nucleic acid, RNA, copies this genetic information from the nucleus and carries it to the cytoplasm. RNA may also be an end product formed in the nucleus using the DNA code and transported out to the cytoplasm, where it regulates various functions of the cell.

If you are not familiar with the chemical structure of proteins or nucleic acids, you may want to review Chapter 2 before continuing in this chapter.

Both RNA and DNA are composed of *nucleotide* subunits made up of a sugar, a phosphate, and one of four bases. RNA subunits, however, contain a different sugar and base component. In RNA nucleotide subunits, the base uracil substitutes for the base thymine. The types of RNA discussed here are all single-stranded molecules, not double-stranded like DNA. However, short, double-stranded RNA molecules also exist in nature.

Protein Synthesis

The process of transferring genetic information from the nucleus into the cytoplasm, where proteins are actually produced, requires completion of two steps: **transcription** and **translation.**

Transcription

During **transcription** the double-stranded DNA molecule separates or unwinds, and a type of RNA called **messenger RNA (mRNA)** is formed (**Figure 3-13**, *Step 1*). Each strand of mRNA is a duplicate or copy of a particular gene sequence along one of the newly separated DNA spirals. The messenger RNA is said to have been "transcribed" or copied from its DNA mold or template. The mRNA then functions as a temporary "working copy" of a gene from DNA. The mRNA transcripts pass from the nucleus to the cytoplasm to direct protein synthesis in the ribosomes and ER (**Figure 3-13**, *Step 2*).

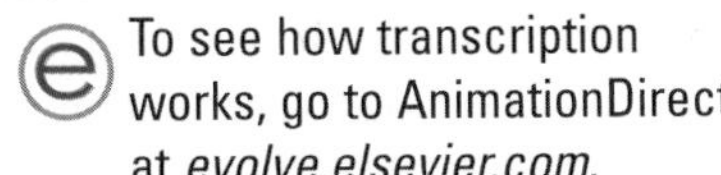

To see how transcription works, go to AnimationDirect at *evolve.elsevier.com.*

Translation

Translation is the process of "translating" the genetic code in the mRNA transcript to synthesize a protein. Translation occurs within ribosomes, which attach around the mRNA strands in the cytoplasm. The ribosomes move along the mRNA transcript and "read" the information encoded there to direct the choice and sequencing of the appropriate chemical building blocks called *amino acids.*

1 Protein synthesis begins with transcription, a process in which an mRNA molecule forms along one gene sequence of a DNA molecule within the cell's nucleus. As it is formed, the mRNA molecule separates from the DNA molecule.
Nucleus (site of transcription)
DNA
mRNA
Nuclear envelope
2 The mRNA transcript then leaves the nucleus through the large nuclear pores.
mRNA transported out of nucleus
Nuclear pores
Small ribosome unit
Large ribosome unit
3 Outside the nucleus, ribosome subunits attach to the beginning of the mRNA molecule and begin the process of translation.
Growing polypeptide chain
Peptide bonds
Anticodon (mRNA binding site)
tRNA
Amino acid binding site
Cytoplasm (site of translation)
Peptide bond forming
Amino acids
Codon
Direction of ribosome advance
4 In translation, tRNA molecules bring specific amino acids, encoded by each mRNA codon, into place at the ribosome site. As the amino acids are brought into the proper sequence, they are joined together by peptide bonds to form long strands called polypeptides.
Transcription
Translation

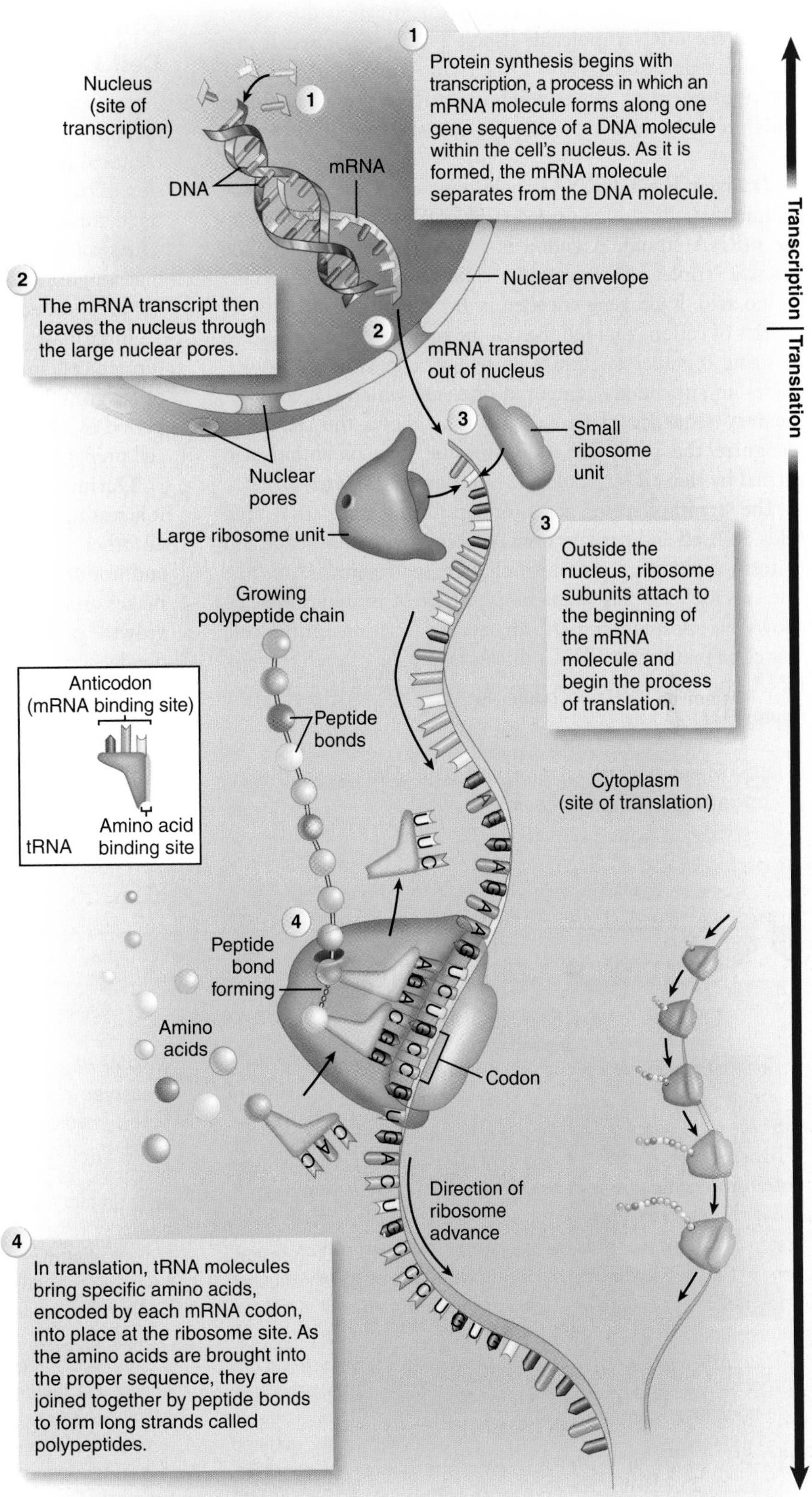

FIGURE 3-13 Protein synthesis. Steps show transcription of the DNA code to mRNA and subsequent translation of the mRNA at the ribosome to assemble a polypeptide. Several polypeptide chains may be needed to make a complete protein molecule. *DNA,* Deoxyribonucleic acid; *mRNA,* messenger RNA (ribonucleic acid); *tRNA,* transfer RNA.

First, the two subunits of a ribosome attach at the beginning of the mRNA molecule (**Figure 3-13**, *Step 3*). Recall that ribosomes are made mostly of RNA-ribosomal RNA (rRNA). The ribosome then moves down the mRNA strand as amino acids are assembled into their proper sequence (**Figure 3-13**, *Step 4*).

Transfer RNA (tRNA) molecules assist the process by bringing specific amino acids in to "dock" at each **codon** along the mRNA strand. A codon is a series of three nucleotide bases, a "triplet," that acts as a code representing a specific amino acid. Each gene encoded in the mRNA is made up of a series of codons that tell the cell the sequence of amino acids to string together to form a protein strand. Each tRNA includes an anticodon segment at one end, which is a complementary sequence of three bases that allows the tRNA to recognize the particular codon for the type of amino acid carried by that tRNA molecule (see **Figure 3-13**, *inset*).

The strand of amino acids formed during translation then folds on itself and perhaps even combines with another strand to form a complete protein molecule (see **Figure 2-12**, p. 31). The specific, complex shape of each type of protein molecule allows the molecule to perform specific functions in the cell. It is clear that because DNA directs the shape of each protein, DNA also directs the function of each protein in a cell (see **Figure 3-12**).

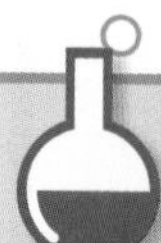

To see how translation works, go to AnimationDirect at *evolve.elsevier.com.*

Cell Reproduction

Cell Life Cycle

The process of cell reproduction is one part of the cell's life cycle. It involves the division of the cell into two genetically identical daughter cells. Cell reproduction thus requires division of the nucleus—a process called **mitosis**—and division of the cytoplasm.

As you can see in **Figure 3-14**, when a cell is not dividing, but instead going about its usual functions, it is in a period of its life cycle called **interphase**.

Interphase includes the initial growing stages of a newly formed cell, in which a cell is busy with protein synthesis and other growth and maintenance functions. This initial growth period of interphase is followed by a period during which the cell prepares for possible cell division.

During interphase, the cell is said to be "resting." However, it is resting only from the standpoint of active cell division. In all other aspects it is exceedingly active. During interphase and just before mitosis begins, the DNA of each chromosome makes an identical copy of itself. The cell then enters another growth period of interphase before it begins to actively divide.

DNA Replication

DNA molecules are somewhat unusual in that, unlike most molecules in nature, they can make identical copies of themselves—a process called **DNA replication.** Before a cell

SCIENCE APPLICATIONS

GENETICS AND GENOMICS

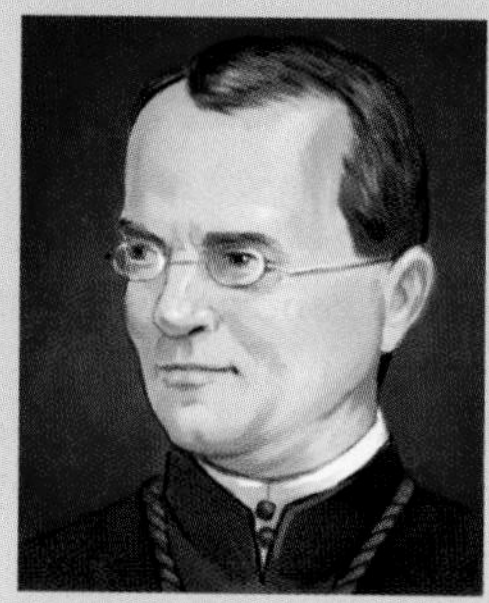

Gregor Mendel (1822-1884)

The Moravian-German Gregor Mendel was born to peasant farmers who taught him how plants and animals are bred for specific traits. Mendel's acceptance into a monastery allowed him to study the science that would later help him understand the mechanism of inheritance of biological traits.

Convinced that "particles" in the cells of the parents were responsible for inheritance of traits, Mendel carried out the now famous experiments with several generations of pea plants. In his report *Experiments with Plant Hybrids* Mendel outlined what has become the foundation of the science of **genetics.** Not only did he reveal the presence of genetic particles (which are now called *genes*) and the basic patterns of how they are transmitted to offspring, but also he set in motion two important movements in modern biology.

First, Mendel was among the first to use mathematical analysis to support his theory about inheritance. Mendel's work pioneered the systematic use of mathematics, quantified measurements, and applied statistics in biological research. Today, medical researchers often enlist the help of *statisticians, mathematicians, computer programmers,* and others in designing experiments, analyzing data, and interpreting results. In fact a whole field, sometimes called *bio-mathematics,* has now emerged to apply the principles of mathematics to biological study.

Second, Mendel was the first to discover how the biological mechanisms of inheritance worked in living organisms. This, of course, led to the science of genetics. Many disciplines have since grown from the study and application of genetics. For example, **genetic counselors** use principles of genetics to advise clients who wish to produce offspring but are worried about possible genetic disorders. *Agricultural scientists* use genetic principles in refining hybrid crop plants and livestock. **Genetic engineers** develop ways to manipulate the genetic code to produce a variety of therapies and enhanced biological characteristics of agricultural products. *Genomics scientists* analyze the genetic codes of organisms to help us better understand structure and function, which may lead to better treatments for genetic disorders.

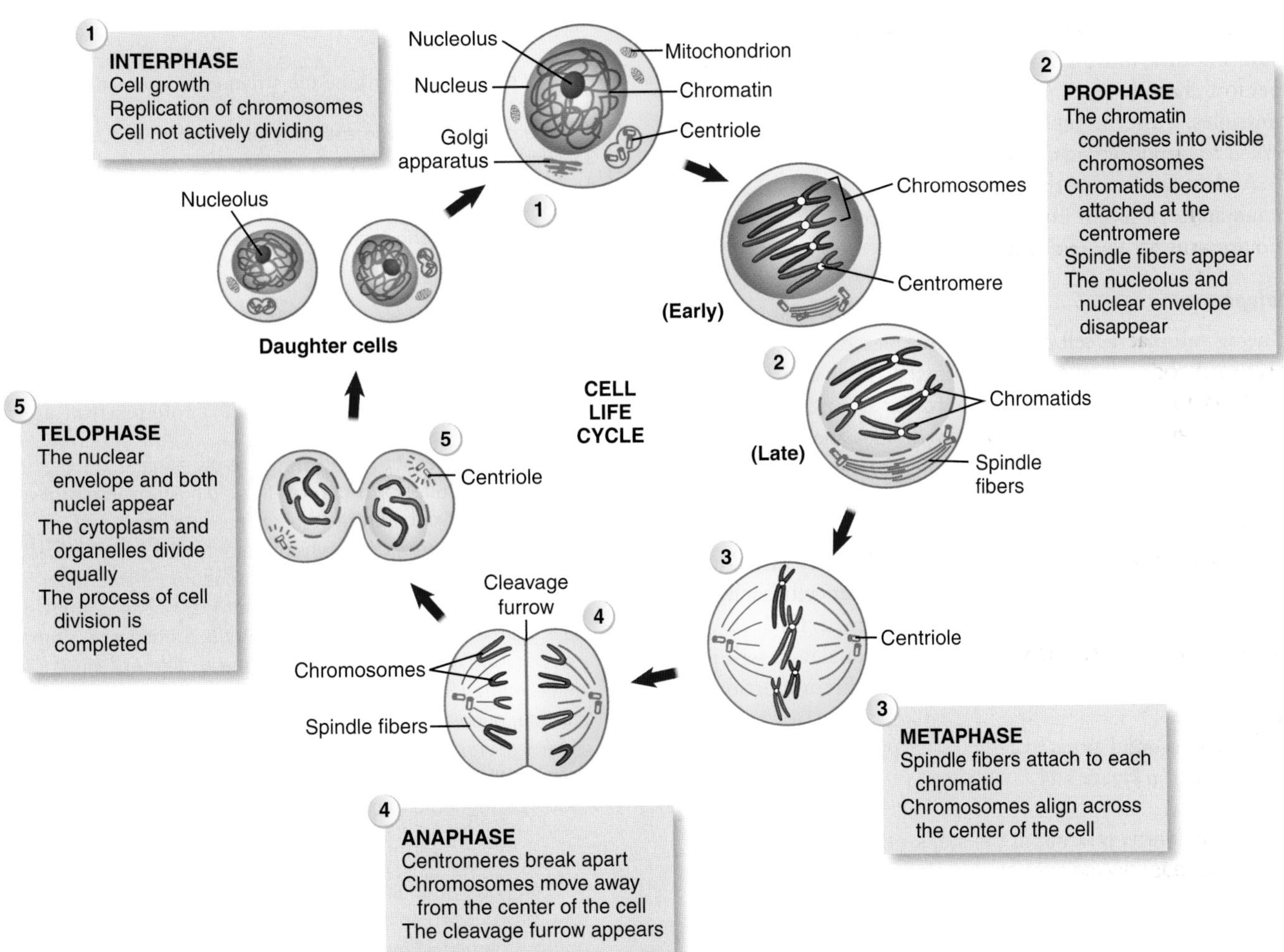

FIGURE 3-14 Cell life cycle. Interphase is followed by the four phases of mitosis, at the end of which the resulting daughter cells enter interphase. For simplicity, only four chromosomes per cell are shown in the diagram.

divides to form two new cells, each DNA molecule in its nucleus forms another DNA molecule just like itself.

When a DNA molecule is not replicating, it has the shape of a tightly coiled double helix. As it begins replication, short segments of the DNA molecule uncoil, and the two strands of the molecule pull apart between their base pairs. The separated strands therefore contain unpaired bases.

Each unpaired base in each of the two separated strands attracts its complementary base (in the nucleoplasm) and binds to it. Specifically, each adenine attracts and binds to a thymine, and each cytosine attracts and binds to a guanine. These steps are repeated over and over throughout the length of the DNA molecule. Thus each half of a DNA molecule becomes a whole DNA molecule identical to the original DNA molecule.

After DNA replication is complete, the cell continues to grow until it is ready for the first phase of mitosis.

Mitosis

Mitosis is the process of dividing the replicated genetic material—the DNA—of the nucleus in an orderly way so that each resulting daughter cell has a complete identical set.

Prophase

Look at Figure 3-14 and note the changes that identify the first stage of mitosis, **prophase**. The chromatin becomes "organized." Chromosomes in the nucleus have formed two strands called **chromatids**. Note that the two chromatids are held together by a beadlike structure called the **centromere**. In the cytoplasm the centrioles are moving away from each other as a network of tubules called **spindle fibers** forms between them. These spindle fibers serve as "guidewires" and assist the chromosomes to move toward opposite ends of the cell later in mitosis.

Metaphase

By the time **metaphase** begins, the nuclear envelope and nucleolus have disappeared. Note in Figure 3-14 the chromosomes have aligned themselves across the center of the cell. Also, the centrioles have migrated to opposite ends of the cell, and spindle fibers are attached to each chromatid.

Anaphase

As **anaphase** begins, the beadlike centromeres, which were holding the paired chromatids together, break apart. As a result, the individual chromatids, identified once again as chromosomes, move away from the center of the cell. Movement of chromosomes occurs along spindle fibers toward the centrioles. Note in **Figure 3-14** that chromosomes are being pulled to opposite ends of the cell.

A **cleavage furrow** that begins to divide the plasma membrane and cytoplasm into two daughter cells can be seen for the first time at the end of anaphase.

Telophase

During **telophase**, cell division is completed. Two nuclei appear, and chromosomes become less distinct and appear to break up. As the nuclear envelope forms around the chromatin, the cleavage furrow completely divides the cell into two parts. The division of the plasma membrane and cytoplasm surrounding the nucleus is called **cytokinesis.**

Before division is complete, each nucleus is surrounded by cytoplasm in which organelles have been equally distributed. By the end of telophase, two separate daughter cells, each having identical genetic characteristics, are formed. Each daughter cell is now in interphase, is fully functional, and will perhaps itself undergo mitotic cell division (cell reproduction) in the future.

Now is a good time to review the phases of the cell life cycle shown in **Figure 3-14**.

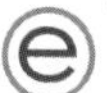
To learn more about the steps of cell division, go to AnimationDirect at *evolve.elsevier.com*.

Results of Cell Division

Mitotic cell division results in the production of identical new cells. During developmental years, the addition of cells helps tissues and organs grow in size. During such periods of body growth, mitosis also allows groups of similar cells to **differentiate,** or develop into different *tissues*. In the adult, mitosis replaces cells that have become less functional with age or have been damaged or destroyed by illness or injury.

If the body loses its ability to control the cell life cycle—cell growth, reproduction, differentiation, and death—an abnormal mass of proliferating cells develops. This mass is a **neoplasm.** Neoplasms may be relatively harmless growths called **benign tumors** or dangerous and **malignant** cancerous growths.

QUICK CHECK

1. How do genes determine the structure and function of the body?
2. Where is genetic information stored in the cell?
3. What are the main steps to making a protein in the cell?
4. What are the four phases of mitotic cell division?
5. What is the interphase period of a cell? What is the importance of this period in the life cycle of a cell?

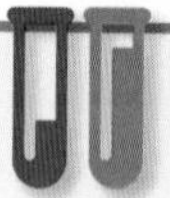

CLINICAL APPLICATION

STEM CELLS

Scientists all over the world are currently engaged in intensive research efforts to unravel the biological secrets of a special kind of undifferentiated cell called a **stem cell.**

Embryonic stem cells, which are obtained from a developing embryo, can be isolated and cultured in the laboratory. Using complex research methods, these primitive cells can then be stimulated to produce additional stem cells or be "directed" to produce many different kinds of differentiated daughter cell types including nerve, blood, muscle, and various types of glandular tissue.

Adult stem cells are undifferentiated cells found scattered within mature tissues throughout the body. Current research suggests that all adult tissues have some of these undifferentiated cells that are capable of producing any of the specialized cell types within its particular tissue.

Injections of adult bone marrow stem cells is a therapy now being used to treat patients with leukemia or bone marrow damaged by toxins or high-dose x-ray. Current research suggests that some adult stem cells, like embryonic stem cells, can be coaxed into producing a variety of different types of cells.

Stem cell research has produced exciting advances in biology that will continue to have a profound impact on human health. Already, stem cell therapies for treating Parkinson disease, stroke, diabetes, and spinal cord injury, to name only a few, are being investigated by medical scientists. Some scientists are using stem cells to build entire new organs and other structures.

Although many scientific and ethical questions remain unanswered, the potential now exists for cell, tissue, and organ "engineering" that may well permit repair or total replacement of diseased or damaged organs in a functioning organ system.

LANGUAGE OF SCIENCE AND MEDICINE (continued from p. 41)

cilium
(SIL-ee-um)
pl., cilia
(SIL-ee-ah)
[*cili-* **eyelid,** *-um* **thing**]

cleavage furrow
(KLEE-vij FUR-oh)
[*cleav-* **split,** *-age* **state,** *furrow* **trench**]

codon
(KOH-don)
[*cod-* **book,** *-on* **thing**]

complementary base pairing
(kom-pleh-MEN-tah-ree bays PAIR-ing)
[*comple-* **complete,** *-ment-* **process,** *-ary* **relating to**]

crenation
(kreh-NAY-shun)
[*crenat-* **scalloped or notched,** *-ation* **process**]

cytokinesis
(sye-toh-kin-EE-sis)
[*cyto-* **cell,** *-kinesis* **movement**]

cytoplasm
(SYE-toh-plaz-em)
[*cyto-* **cell,** *-plasm* **to mold**]

cytoskeleton
(sye-toh-SKEL-eh-ton)
[*cyto-* **cell,** *-skeleto* **dried body**]

deoxyribonucleic acid (DNA)
(dee-ok-see-rye-boh-nook-lay-ik AS-id)
[*de-* **removed,** *-oxy-* **oxygen,** *-nucle-* **nucleus (kernel),** *-ic* **relating to,** *acid* **sour**]

dialysis
(dye-AL-ih-sis)
[*dia-* **apart,** *-lysis* **loosening**]

differentiate
(dif-er-EN-shee-ayt)
[*different-* **difference,** *-ate* **action**]

diffusion
(dih-FYOO-shun)
[*dis-* **apart,** *-fus-* **flow,** *-tion* **process**]

DNA replication
(dee en ay rep-lih-KAY-shun)
[*re-* **again,** *-plic-* **fold,** *-ation* **process**]

endoplasmic reticulum (ER)
(en-doh-PLAZ-mik reh-TIK-yoo-lum)
[*endo-* **inward or within,** *-plasm-* **to mold,** *-ic* **relating to,** *ret-* **net,** *-ic-* **relating to,** *-ul-* **little,** *-um* **thing**]

filtration
(fil-TRAY-shun)
[*filtr-* **strain,** *-ation* **process**]

flagellum
(flah-JEL-um)
pl., flagella
(flah-JEL-ah)
[*flagellum* **whip**]

gene
(jeen)
[*gen-* **produce or generate**]

genetic counselor
(jeh-NET-ik KOWN-sel-er)
[*gene-* **produce,** *-ic* **relating to**]

genetic engineer
(jeh-NET-ik en-juh-NEER)
[*gene-* **produce,** *-ic* **relating to,** *engin-* **devise or design,** *-eer* **practitioner**]

genetics
(jeh-NET-iks)
[*gene-* **produce,** *-ic* **relating to**]

genome
(JEE-nohm)
[*gen-* **produce (gene),** *-ome* **entire collection**]

Golgi apparatus
(GOL-jee ap-ah-RA-tus)
[*Camillo Golgi* **Italian histologist**]

hypertonic
(hye-per-TON-ik)
[*hyper-* **excessive,** *-ton-* **tension,** *-ic* **relating to**]

hypotonic
(hye-poh-TON-ik)
[*hypo-* **under or below,** *-ton-* **tension,** *-ic* **relating to**]

interphase
(IN-ter-fayz)
[*inter-* **between,** *-phase* **stage**]

interstitial fluid
(in-ter-STISH-al FLOO-id)
[*inter-* **between,** *-stit-* **stand,** *-al* **relating to**]

isotonic
(eye-soh-TON-ik)
[*iso-* **equal,** *-ton-* **tension,** *-ic* **relating to**]

lyse
(lyze)
[*lysis* **loosening**]

lysosome
(LYE-so-sohm)
[*lyso-* **dissolution,** *-som* **body**]

malignant tumor
(mah-LIG-nant TOO-mer)
[*malign* **bad,** *-ant* **state;** *tumor* **swelling**]

messenger RNA (mRNA)
(MES-en-jer ar en ay)
[*RNA-* **ribonucleic acid**]

metaphase
(MET-ah-fayz)
[*meta-* **change (place),** *-phase* **stage**]

microvillus
(my-kroh-VIL-us)
pl., microvilli
(my-kroh-VIL-eye or my-kroh-VIL-ee)
[*micro-* **small,** *-villus* **shaggy hair**]

mitochondrion
(my-toh-KON-dree-on)
pl., mitochondria
(my-toh-KON-dree-ah)
[*mito-* **thread,** *-chondrion* **granule**]

mitosis
(my-TOH-sis)
[*mitos-* **thread,** *-osis* **process**]

neoplasm
(NEE-oh-plaz-em)
[*neo-* **new,** *-plasm* **formation**]

nuclear envelope
(NOO-klee-ar)
[*nucle-* **nucleus (kernel),** *-ar* **relating to**]

nucleolus
(noo-KLEE-oh-lus)
[*nucleo-* **nucleus (kernel),** *-olus* **little**]

nucleoplasm
(NOO-klee-oh-plaz-im)
[*nucleo-* **nucleus (kernel),** *-plasm* **substance**]

nucleus
(NOO-klee-us)
[*nucleus* **kernel**]

organelle
(or-gah-NEL)
[*organ-* **tool or instrument,** *-elle* **small**]

osmosis
(os-MO-sis)
[*osmos-* **push,** *-osis* **process**]

passive transport
(PAS-iv TRANZ-port)
[*pass-* **submit,** *-ive* **relating to,** *trans-* **across,** *-port* **carry**]

phagocytosis
(fag-oh-sye-TOH-sis)
[*phago-* **eat,** *-cyte-* **cell,** *-osis* **process**]

phospholipid
(fos-fo-LIP-id)
[*phospho-* **phosphorus,** *-lip-* **fat,** *-id* **form**]

pinocytosis
(pin-oh-sye-TOH-sis)
[*pino-* **drink,** *-cyto-* **cell,** *-osis* **process**]

plasma membrane
(PLAZ-mah)
[*plasma* **substance,** *membrane* **thin skin**]

prophase
(PRO-fayz)
[*pro-* **first,** *-phase* **stage**]

ribonucleic acid (RNA)
(rye-boh-noo-KLAY-ik AS-id)
[*ribo-* **ribose (sugar),** *nucle-* **nucleus,** *-ic* **pertaining to,** *acid* **sour]**

ribosome
(RYE-boh-sohm)
[*ribo-* **ribose or RNA,** *-som-* **body]**

sodium-potassium pump
(SO-dee-um poh-TAS-ee-um)
[*sod-* **soda,** *-um* **thing or substance,** *potass-* **potash,** *-um* **thing or substance]**

solute
(SOL-yoot)
[*solut* **dissolved]**

spindle fiber
(SPIN-dul FYE-ber)

stem cell
(stem sel)
[*stem* **tree trunk,** *cell* **storeroom]**

telophase
(TEL-oh-fayz or TEE-loh-fayz)
[*telo-* **end,** *-phase* **stage]**

transcription
(tranz-KRIP-shun)
[*trans-* **across,** *-script-* **write,** *-tion* **process]**

transfer RNA (tRNA)
(TRANZ-fer ar en ay)
[*trans-* **across,** *-fer* **carry,** *RNA* **ribonucleic acid]**

translation
(tranz-LAY-shun)
[*translat-* **bring over,** *-tion* **process]**

transport process
(TRANZ-port PRO-ses)
[*trans-* **across,** *-port* **carry]**

vesicle
(VES-ih-kul)
[*vesic-* **blister,** *-cle* **little]**

OUTLINE SUMMARY

To download a digital audio version of the chapter summary for use with your device, access the ***Audio Chapter Summaries*** *online at evolve.elsevier.com.*

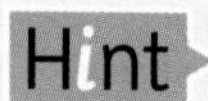

Scan this summary after reading the chapter to help you reinforce the key concepts. Later, use the summary as a quick review before your class or before a test.

Cells

A. Size and shape
   1. Human cells vary considerably in size; all are microscopic
   2. Cells differ notably in shape
B. Composition
   1. Cells contain cytoplasm, a substance found only in cells
   2. Organelles are specialized structures within the cytoplasm
   3. Cell interior is surrounded by plasma membrane

Parts of the Cell

A. Plasma membrane forms (see **Figure 3-1**)
   1. Forms outer boundary of cell
   2. Composed of thin, two-layered membrane of phospholipids and embedded with proteins
   3. Is selectively permeable
B. Cytoplasm (see **Figure 3-2**)
   1. All cell substance from the nucleus to the plasma membrane
   2. Cytoskeleton — internal framework of cell
      a. Made up of microfilaments and microtubules
      b. Provides support and movement of cell and organelles
      c. Other cell parts
C. Ribosomes
   1. Made of two tiny subunits of mostly ribosomal RNA (rRNA)
   2. May attach to rough ER or lie free in cytoplasm
   3. Manufacture enzymes and other proteins; often called *protein factories*
D. Endoplasmic reticulum (ER)
   1. Network of connecting sacs and canals
   2. Carries substances through cytoplasm
   3. Rough ER collects, folds, and transports proteins made by ribosomes
   4. Smooth ER synthesizes chemicals; makes new membrane
E. Golgi apparatus (see **Figure 3-3**)
   1. Group of flattened sacs near nucleus
   2. Collects chemicals into vesicles that move from the smooth ER outward to the plasma membrane
   3. Called the *chemical processing and packaging center*
F. Mitochondria
   1. Composed of inner and outer membranous sacs
   2. Involved with energy-releasing chemical reactions (cellular respiration)
   3. Often called *power plants* of the cell
   4. Each mitochondrion contains one DNA molecule
G. Lysosomes
   1. Membrane-enclosed packets containing digestive enzymes
   2. Have protective function (eat microbes)
   3. Formerly thought to be responsible for apoptosis (programmed cell death)

H. Centrosome
1. Microtubule-organizing region of the cytoskeleton near the nucleus
2. Centrioles — paired organelles that lie at right angles to each other within the centrosome and function in moving chromosomes during cell reproduction

I. Cell extensions (see **Figure 3-4**)
1. Microvilli — short extensions of the plasma membrane that increase surface area and produce slight movements that enhance absorption by the cell
2. Cilia — hairlike extensions with inner microtubules found on free or exposed surfaces of all cells; serve sensory functions, but some are also capable of moving together in a wavelike fashion to propel mucus across a surface (see **Figure 3-5**)
3. Flagella — single projections (much longer than cilia) that act as "tails" of sperm cells

J. Nucleus
1. Controls cell because it contains most of the genetic code (genome), instructions for making proteins, which in turn determine cell structure and function
2. Component structures include nuclear envelope, nucleoplasm, nucleolus, and chromatin granules
3. DNA molecules become tightly coiled chromosomes during cell division
4. 46 nuclear chromosomes contain DNA, which contains genetic code

Relationship of Cell Structure and Function

A. Every human cell has a designated function: some help maintain the cell, and others regulate life processes

B. Specialized functions of a cell differ depending on number and type of organelles

Movements of Substances Through Cell Membranes

A. Types of membrane transport
1. Transport processes move substances into and out of cells
2. Types of transport
   a. Passive transport — do not require the cell to expend energy
   b. Active transport — require the cell to expend energy (from ATP)

B. Passive transport processes
1. Passive transport processes do not require added energy and result in movement "down a concentration gradient"
2. Diffusion
   a. Substances scatter themselves evenly throughout an available space, the particles moving from high to low concentration (see **Figure 3-6**)
   b. Solute particles may thus move through channels or carriers in a membrane to reach an equilibrium (equality of concentration) of solution on both sides of the membrane (see **Figure 3-7**)
   c. Passive process — it is unnecessary to add energy to the system
3. Osmosis (see **Figure 3-8**)
   a. Passive movement of water molecules when some solutes cannot cross the membrane
   b. Similar to diffusion, water moves in a direction that produces an equilibrium
   c. Because water moves, but not all the solutes, osmotic pressure may change across the membrane
4. Dialysis — some solutes move across a selectively permeable membrane by diffusion and other solutes do not, thus resulting in uneven distribution of solute types (see **Figure 3-9**)
5. Filtration — movement of water and solutes caused by hydrostatic pressure on one side of membrane

C. Active transport processes
1. Active transport processes occur only in living cells; movement of substances is "up the concentration gradient"; requires energy from ATP
2. Ion pumps (see **Figure 3-10**)
   a. An ion pump is a protein complex in the cell membrane
   b. Ion pumps use energy from ATP to move substances across cell membranes against their concentration gradients
   c. Examples: sodium-potassium pump, calcium pump
   d. Some ion pumps work with other carriers so that glucose or amino acids are transported along with ions
3. Phagocytosis and pinocytosis
   a. Phagocytosis ("cell eating") engulfs large particles in a vesicle as a protective mechanism often used to destroy bacteria or debris from tissue damage (see **Figure 3-11**)
   b. Pinocytosis ("cell drinking") engulfs fluids or dissolved substances into cells
   c. Both are active transport mechanisms because they require cell energy (from ATP) to move the cytoskeleton in a way that engulfs material and pulls it into the cell

Cell Growth and Reproduction

A. Cell growth
1. Proteins determine the structure and function of cells
2. Protein synthesis is directed by two nucleic acids: deoxyribonucleic acid (DNA) and ribonucleic acid (RNA)
3. DNA
   a. Make up 46 chromosomes contained in cell nucleus

b. Large molecule shaped like a spiral staircase; sugar (deoxyribose) and phosphate units compose sides of the molecule; base pairs (adenine-thymine or guanine-cytosine) compose "steps" (see **Figure 2-14**, p. 32)
c. Base pairings always the same (complementary base pairing), but the sequence of base pairs differs in different DNA molecule
d. A gene is a specific sequence of base pairs within a DNA molecule
e. Genes dictate formation of enzymes and other proteins by ribosomes, thereby indirectly determining a cell's structure and functions (see **Figure 3-12**)

4. RNA
   a. RNA molecules are made from genes that do not code directly for proteins
   b. RNA molecules regulate cell processes, such as protein synthesis
   c. RNA subunits are made up of nucleotides, but have ribose as their sugar and have the base uracil instead of thymine
5. Protein synthesis — occurs in cytoplasm; thus genetic information must pass from the nucleus to the cytoplasm (see **Figure 3-13**)
   a. Transcription
      (1) Double-stranded DNA separates to form messenger RNA (mRNA)
      (2) Each strand of mRNA is a copy (transcript) of a particular gene (base-pair sequence) from a segment of DNA
   b. mRNA molecules pass from the nucleus to the cytoplasm where they direct protein synthesis in ribosomes and ER
   c. Translation
      (1) Translation of code in mRNA transcript to synthesize proteins in cytoplasm in ribosomes
      (2) Codon — a series of three nucleotide bases in mRNA that acts as a code for a specific amino acid
      (3) tRNA— carries a specific amino acid and has an anticodon, which is 3-base sequence that complements the mRNA codon that signifies that amino acid
      (4) tRNA brings amino acids into place along the mRNA strand where it is held by a ribosome, thus forming a strand of amino acids

B. Cell reproduction
1. Cell life cycle — includes reproduction of cell involving division of the nucleus (mitosis) and the cytoplasm
   a. Two daughter cells result from the division
   b. Interphase — period of life cycle when the cell is not actively dividing
2. DNA replication — process by which each half of a DNA molecule becomes a whole molecule identical to the original DNA molecule; precedes mitosis
3. Mitosis — process in cell division that distributes identical nuclear chromosomes (DNA molecules) to each new cell formed when the original cell divides (see **Figure 3-14**)
   a. Prophase — first stage
      (1) Chromatin granules become organized
      (2) Chromosomes (pairs of linked chromatids) appear
      (3) Centrioles move away from nucleus
      (4) Nuclear envelope disappears, freeing genetic material
      (5) Spindle fibers appear
   b. Metaphase — second stage
      (1) Chromosomes align across center of cell
      (2) Spindle fibers attach themselves to each chromatid
   c. Anaphase — third stage
      (1) Centromeres break apart
      (2) Separated chromatids now called *chromosomes*
      (3) Chromosomes are pulled to opposite ends of cell
      (4) Cleavage furrow develops at end of anaphase
   d. Telophase — fourth stage
      (1) Cell division is completed
      (2) Nuclei appear in daughter cells
      (3) Nuclear envelope and nucleoli appear
      (4) Cytoplasm is divided (cytokinesis)
   e. Daughter cells become fully functional, thus ending mitosis and entering interphase
4. Results of cell division
   a. Two identical cells result from cell division, growing tissues or replacing old or damaged cells
   b. Differentiation — process by which daughter cells can specialize and form different kinds of tissue
   c. Abnormalities of mitotic division can produce benign or malignant neoplasms (tumors)

❑ ACTIVE LEARNING

STUDY TIPS

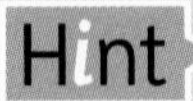

Use these tips to achieve success in meeting your learning goals.

Chapter 3 should be a review of your previous general biology course. Most of what is in this chapter should sound familiar.

1. The section on cell structure begins with the plasma membrane. It is made up mostly of phospholipids, but the most important part of the membrane structure is the proteins embedded in the phospholipids. They play important roles in a number of systems in the body such as the nervous and endocrine systems.
2. The organelles may seem to have strange-sounding names. Use the vocabulary list with the word origins in this chapter to help you determine the meaning of each organelle name. Flash cards would be helpful in learning these new terms.
3. The transport processes of osmosis and dialysis are special cases of diffusion—osmosis with water and dialysis with solutes. Filtration uses a pressure rather than a concentration difference to move substances.
4. *Phagocytosis* and *pinocytosis* are descriptions of what the cell is doing. *Phago* means "to eat," *pino* means "to drink," *cyto* means "cell," and *sis* means "condition."
5. When studying protein synthesis, keep the goal of the process in mind. The cell wants a protein made, the DNA has the plans, but the ribosome is the factory. The DNA needs to tell the ribosome what to build (transcription), and the factory needs to put the protein together in the correct order (translation).
6. Use flash cards to study the phases of mitosis; remember that the phases are based on what is happening to the chromosomes. There are many online resources that illustrate the phases of mitosis. These resources include animations that can help you better understand what occurs in each phase of mitosis.
7. Make and use flash cards to learn the terms used to describe changes in cell growth and reproduction.
8. In your study group, review the flash cards for the organelles, mitosis, and changes in cell growth and reproduction. Be sure to discuss steps in protein synthesis and the cell transport processes. Go over the questions at the end of the chapter and discuss possible test questions.

Review Questions

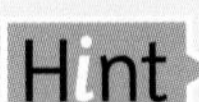

Write out the answers to these questions after reading the chapter and reviewing the Chapter Summary. If you simply think through the answer without writing it down, you won't retain much of your new learning.

1. Describe the structure of the plasma membrane, cytoplasm, and nucleus.
2. List the functions of the plasma membrane, cytoplasm, and nucleus.
3. Name the function of the following organelles: *ribosome, endoplasmic reticulum, Golgi apparatus, mitochondria, lysosomes, centrosome, centrioles, microvilli, cilia,* and *flagella.*
4. List the function of the *nucleus* and *nucleolus.*
5. Explain the difference between *chromatin granules* and *chromosomes.*
6. Describe the processes of *osmosis, diffusion, dialysis,* and *filtration.*
7. Describe the functioning of the *ion pump* and explain the process of *phagocytosis* and *pinocytosis.*
8. Define *gene* and *genome.*
9. Describe the process of transcription.
10. Describe the process of translation.
11. List and briefly describe the four stages in active cell division (mitosis).
12. Explain the importance of cellular reproduction.
13. Name an important event that occurs in mitosis during interphase.
14. Describe the role of DNA and RNA in protein synthesis.

Critical Thinking

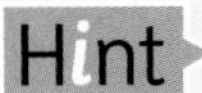

After finishing the Review Questions, write out the answers to these more in-depth questions to help you apply your new knowledge. Go back to sections of the chapter that relate to concepts that you find difficult.

15. Explain what would happen if a cell containing 97% water were placed in a 10% salt solution.
16. If one side of a DNA molecule had a base sequence of adenine-adenine-guanine-cytosine-thymine-cytosine-thymine, what would the sequence of bases on the opposite side of the molecule be?
17. If a molecule of mRNA were made from the base sequence in Question 16, what would be the sequence of bases in the RNA?

Chapter Test

Hint *After studying the chapter, test your mastery by responding to these items. Try to answer them without looking up the answers. Then, verify the answers using the key in Appendix C at the back of this book.*

1. ________ and ________ are two fat-based molecules that make up part of the structure of the plasma membrane.
2. ________ is a term that refers to small structures inside the cell. It means "little organs."
3. ________ is the movement of substances across a cell membrane using cell energy, whereas ________ is the movement of substances across the cell membrane without using cell energy.
4. ________ refers to the movement of fluids or dissolved molecules into the cell by trapping them in the plasma membrane.
5. ________ and ________ are the two nucleic acids that are involved in transcription.
6. ________ is the process in protein synthesis that uses the information in mRNA to build a protein molecule.
7. ________ is the process that forms the mRNA molecule.
8. ________ is a segment of base pairs in a chromosome.
9. ________ is the total genetic information package in a cell.
10. ________ are active transport mechanisms that move charged particles against their concentration gradient to concentrate them on one side of a plasma membrane.
11. Which of the following is a form of passive transport?
    a. filtration
    b. dialysis
    c. osmosis
    d. all of these are forms of passive transport
12. During this stage of mitosis, the chromosomes move away from the center of the cell:
    a. interphase
    b. metaphase
    c. anaphase
    d. telophase
13. During this stage of the cell cycle, the DNA in the nucleus replicates:
    a. interphase
    b. metaphase
    c. prophase
    d. telophase
14. During this stage of mitosis, the chromosomes align in the center of the cell:
    a. interphase
    b. metaphase
    c. prophase
    d. telophase
15. During this stage of mitosis, the chromatin condenses into chromosomes:
    a. interphase
    b. metaphase
    c. prophase
    d. telophase
16. During this stage of mitosis, the nuclear envelope and nuclei reappear:
    a. interphase
    b. prophase
    c. anaphase
    d. telophase

Match each function in Column B with the proper cell structure in Column A.

Column A	Column B
17. ______ Ribosome	a. A long cell projection used to propel sperm cells
18. ______ Endoplasmic reticulum	b. Bags of digestive enzymes in the cell
19. ______ Golgi apparatus	c. Tubelike passages that carry substances through the cytoplasm
20. ______ Mitochondria	d. Short hairlike structures on the free surface of some cells
21. ______ Lysosomes	e. Chemically process and package substances from the endoplasmic reticulum
22. ______ Flagella	f. Directs protein synthesis; the brain of the cell
23. ______ Cilia	g. "Protein factories" in the cell, made of RNA
24. ______ Nucleus	h. Small structure in the nucleus; helps in the formation of ribosomes
25. ______ Nucleoli	i. "Powerhouse" of the cell; most of the cell's ATP is formed here

Tissues

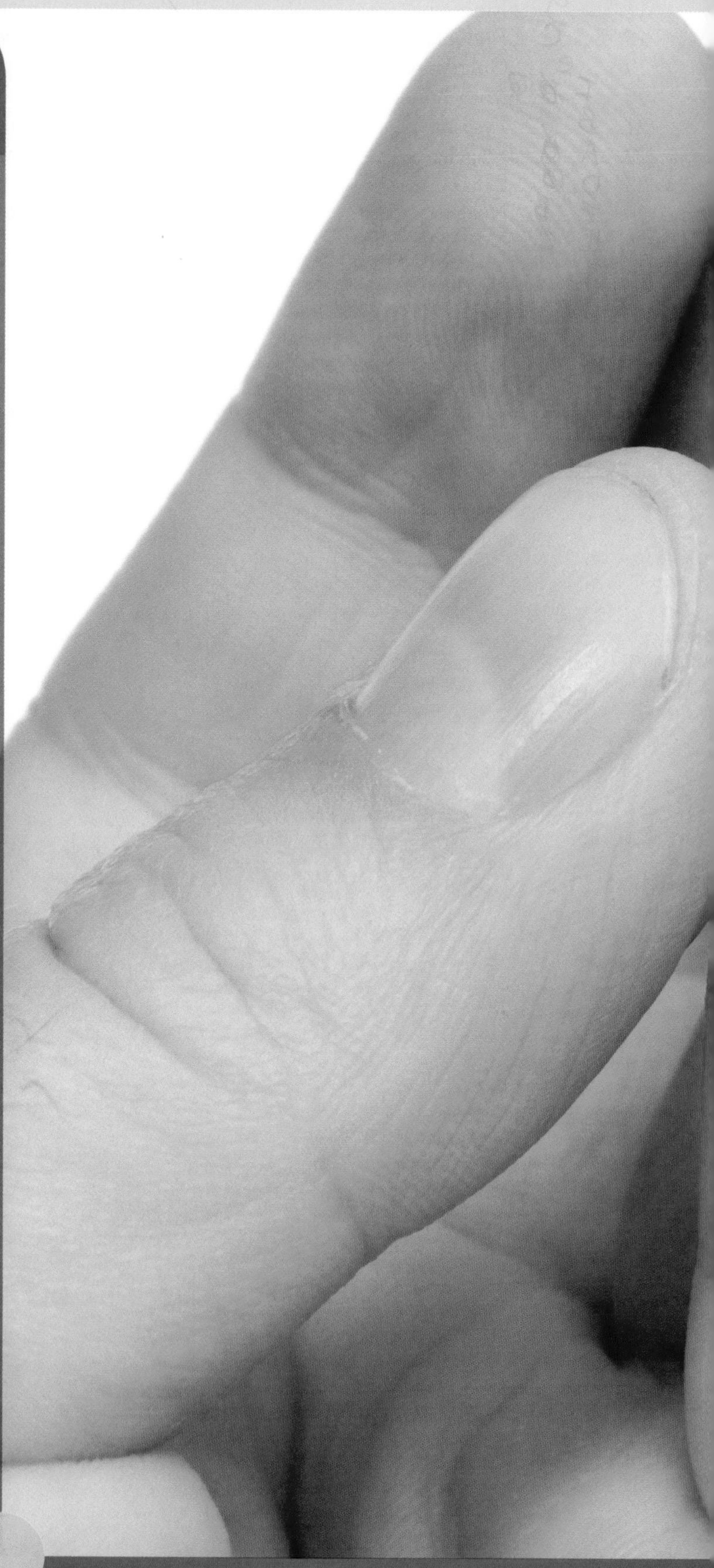

OUTLINE

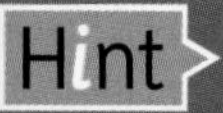

Scan this outline before you begin to read the chapter, as a preview of how the concepts are organized.

OBJECTIVES

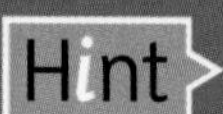

Before reading the chapter, review these goals for your learning.

After you have completed this chapter, you should be able to:

1. Define matrix (extracellular matrix) and discuss how it may affect the function of a tissue.
2. Explain how epithelial tissue is categorized by shape and arrangement of cells.
3. List and briefly discuss the major types of connective tissue.
4. Compare and contrast the three major types of muscle tissue.
5. Describe the function of nervous tissue and list the three structural components of a neuron.

CHAPTER 4

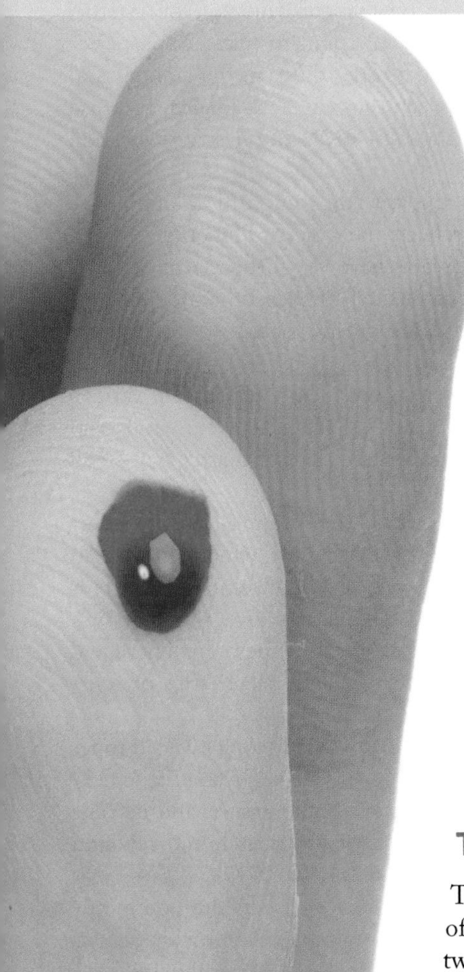

We explored cells in the previous chapter, and now we turn our attention to the various *groupings* of cells called **tissues.** The arrangement of cells in one tissue may form a thin sheet only one cell deep, whereas the cells of another tissue may form huge masses containing millions of cells. Tissues are the "fabric" of the body, and like the various fabrics that make up a garment, each tissue of an organ specializes in performing unique functions that help the organ do its job. This collaborative functioning of tissues within our body's organs maintains homeostatic balance and thus is vital to our survival.

In this chapter, we briefly survey the major kinds of tissues that form the organs of the body. As we progress through later chapters, we will revisit each of these tissue types and explore more detail about their locations, structures, and functions.

Introduction to Tissues

Tissue Types

Tissues differ from each other in the size and shape of their cells, in the amount and kind of material between the cells, and in the special functions they perform to help maintain the body's survival. In **Table 4-1** through **Table 4-3**, you will find a listing of the four major tissues and the various subtypes of each. The tables also include the structure of each subtype along with examples of the location of the tissues and a primary function of each tissue type.

LANGUAGE OF **SCIENCE** AND **MEDICINE**

Hint Before reading the chapter, say each of these terms out loud. This will help you to avoid stumbling over them as you read.

adipose
(AD-ih-pohs)
[*adipo-* **fat,** *-ose* **full of**]

areolar connective tissue
(ah-REE-oh-lar, koh-NEK-tiv TISH-yoo)
[*are-* **open space,** *-ola-* **little,** *-ar* **relating to,** *con-* **together,** *-nect-* **bind,** *-ive* **relating to,** *tissue* **fabric**]

axon
(AK-son)
[*axon* **axle**]

basement membrane
(BAYS-ment MEM-brayn)
[*base-* **base,** *-ment* **thing,** *membrane* **thin skin**]

cardiac muscle tissue
(KAR-dee-ak MUSS-el TISH-yoo)
[*cardi-* **heart,** *-ac* **relating to,** *mus-* **mouse,** *-cle* **small,** *tissue* **fabric**]

cell body
(sel BOD-ee)
[*cell* **storeroom,** *body* **body**]

chondrocyte
(KON-droh-syte)
[*chondro-* **cartilage,** *-cyte* **cell**]

collagen
(KAHL-ah-jen)
[*colla-* **glue,** *-gen* **produce**]

connective tissue
(koh-NEK-tiv TISH-yoo)
[*con-* **together,** *-nect-* **bind,** *-ive* **relating to,** *tissue* **fabric**]

cytologist
(SYE-TOL-oh-jist)
[*cyt-* **cell,** *-log-* **words (study of),** *-ist* **agent**]

Continued on p. 79

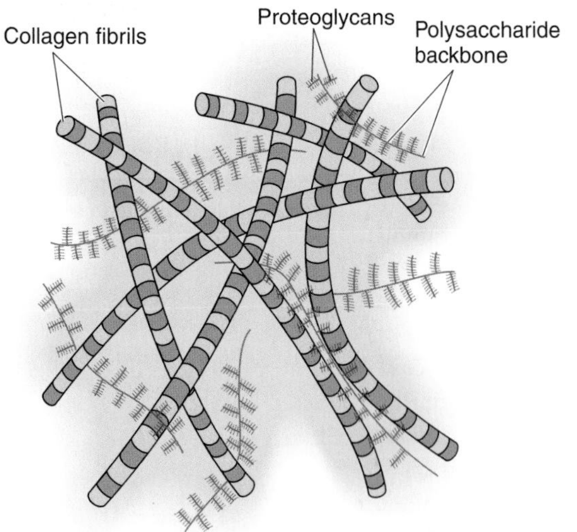

FIGURE 4-1 Extracellular matrix. The matrix is outside of cells, forming a connecting gel that contributes to the overall function of the tissue. This example illustrates thick, ropelike collagen fibrils interspersed with proteoglycan (protein-carbohydrate) structures attached to polysaccharide backbones—all surrounded by water. The collagen gives tissue strength, and the polysaccharide-proteoglycan structures absorb shocks. (Collagen is naturally white, but is often stained pink to make it more visible in microscopic studies.)

The four main kinds of tissues that compose the body's many organs follow:

1. Epithelial tissue—forms sheets that cover or line the body
2. Connective tissue—provides structural and functional support
3. Muscle tissue—contracts to produce movement
4. Nervous tissue—senses, conducts, and processes information

Matrix

Recall from Chapter 1 that a central principle of human physiology is homeostasis—the relative constancy of the internal fluid environment. This fluid environment fills the spaces between the cells of the body. Tissues differ in the amount and kind of fluid material between the cells—the **matrix.** It is also called the *extracellular matrix (ECM)* to emphasize its location between cells.

The matrix varies in amount and composition among the various tissues—which reflects the variety of functions among tissue types. Epithelial tissues have very little matrix because the cells are so closely connected to each other. Connective tissues, on the other hand, are mostly matrix—with the cells few and far between.

Matrix is like jelly, made up of mostly water with various interlocking fibers that thicken it (**Figure 4-1**). The kinds and amounts of fibers can produce a variety of matrix types—all with different functions.

The thin watery matrix of blood—plasma—has no fibers at all (except when forming a blood clot), which allows it to remain free-flowing. The tissue of tendons and ligaments is dense with strong, twisted fibers that give the matrix a thick, ropelike quality. Bone's matrix fibers are encrusted with mineral crystals to give it the characteristics of reinforced concrete.

Collagen is a protein that forms microscopic twisted ropes within the matrix of many tissues. Collagen gives a tissue flexible strength. **Elastin** is present in some tissues, and its rubbery quality gives tissues the ability to stretch and rebound easily.

Various *polysaccharides* and **proteoglycans** are commonly found in a tissue's matrix. These molecules can provide various functions such as linking among cells, absorbing shocks, regulation of tissue function, and lubrication.

TABLE 4-1 Epithelial Tissues

TISSUE	STRUCTURE	LOCATION(S)	FUNCTION(S)
Simple squamous	Single layer of flattened cells	Alveoli of lungs	Diffusion of respiratory gases between alveolar air and blood
		Lining of blood and lymphatic vessels	Diffusion, filtration, and osmosis
Stratified squamous	Many layers; outermost layer(s) are flattened cells	Surface of lining of mouth and esophagus	Protection
		Surface of skin (epidermis)	Protection
Simple cuboidal	Single layer of cells that are as tall as they are wide	Glands, kidney tubules	Secretion, absorption
Simple columnar	Single layer of tall, narrow cells	Surface layer of lining of stomach, intestines, parts of respiratory tract	Protection, secretion, transport (absorption)
Pseudostratified	Single layer of tall cells that wedge together to appear as if there are two or more layers	Surface of lining of trachea	Protection
Stratified transitional	Many layers of varying transitional shapes, capable of stretching	Urinary bladder	Protection

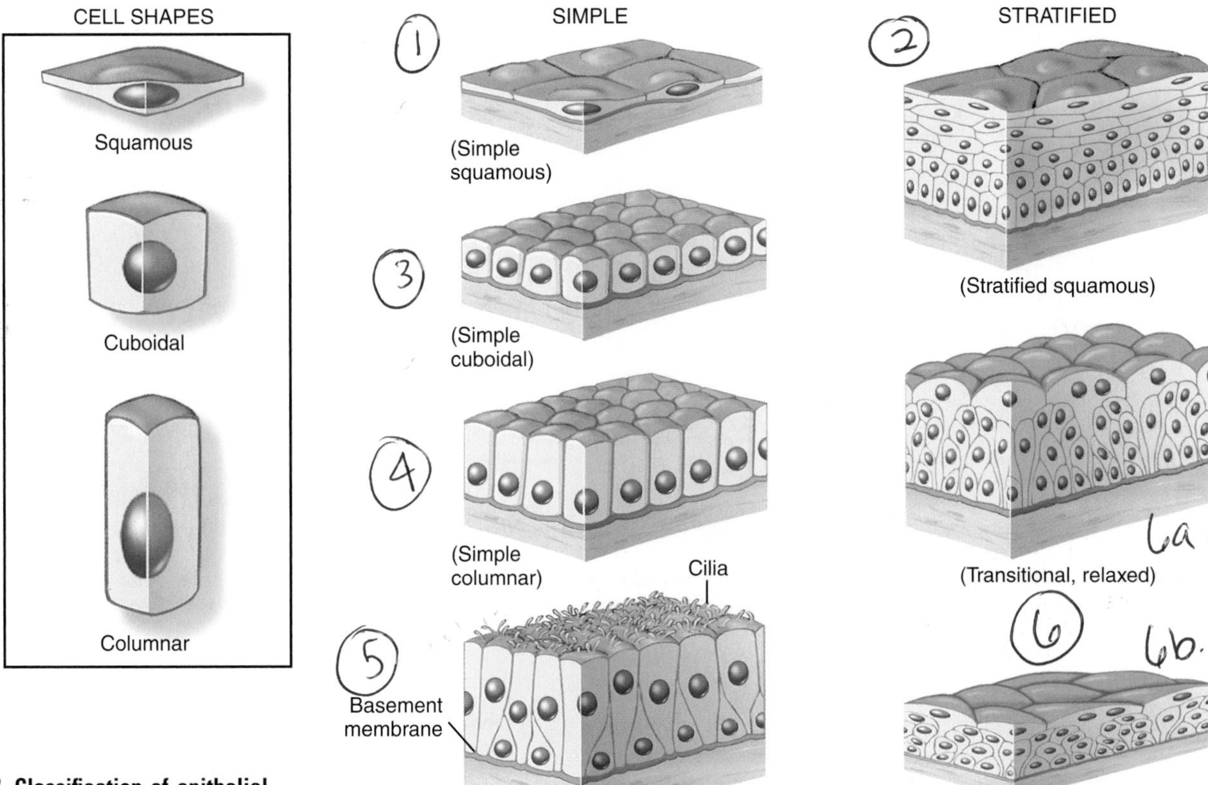

FIGURE 4-2 Classification of epithelial tissues. The tissues are classified according to the shape and arrangement of cells.

Epithelial Tissue

Introduction to Epithelial Tissue

Epithelial tissue covers the body and many of its parts (Table 4-1). It also lines various parts of the body. Because epithelial cells are packed close together with little or no intercellular material between them, they form continuous sheets that contain no blood vessels. Examine Figure 4-2. It illustrates how this large group of tissues can be subdivided according to the *shape* and *arrangement* of the cells found in each type.

Shape of Cells

If classified according to shape, epithelial cells are identified as:

1. Squamous—flat and scalelike
2. Cuboidal—cube-shaped
3. Columnar—higher than they are wide
4. Transitional—varying shapes that can stretch

Arrangement of Cells

If categorized according to arrangement of cells, epithelial tissue can be classified as:

1. Simple—single layer of cells of the same shape
2. Stratified—many layers of cells; named for the shape of cells in the outer layer

Several types of epithelium are described in the paragraphs that follow and are illustrated in Figures 4-3 to 4-8.

Squamous Epithelium

Simple Squamous Epithelium

Simple squamous epithelium consists of a single layer of very thin and irregularly shaped cells. Because of the thin structure of simple squamous epithelium, substances can readily pass through its cells, making transport its special function. Absorption of oxygen into the blood, for example, takes place through the simple squamous epithelium that forms the tiny air sacs in the lungs (Figure 4-3).

Stratified Squamous Epithelium

Stratified squamous epithelium (Figure 4-4) consists of several layers of closely packed cells, an arrangement that makes this tissue especially adept at protection. For instance, stratified squamous epithelial tissue protects the body against invasion by microorganisms. Most microbes cannot work their way through a barrier of stratified squamous tissue such as that which composes the surface of skin and of mucous membranes.

One way of preventing infections, therefore, is to take good care of your skin. Do not let it become cracked from chapping, and guard against cuts and scratches.

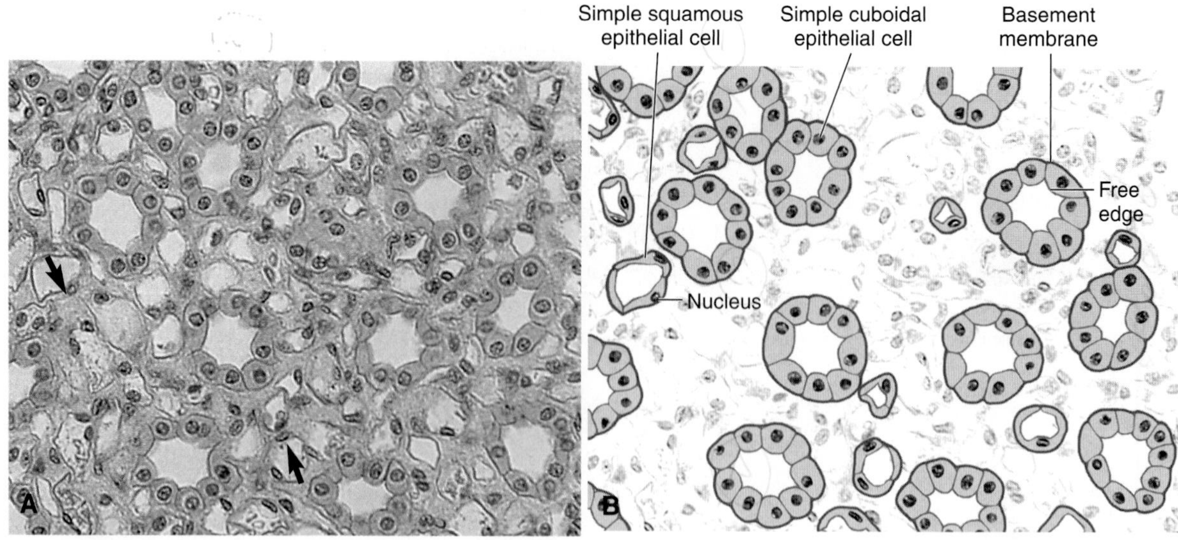

FIGURE 4-3 Simple squamous and simple cuboidal epithelium. A, Photomicrograph shows thin simple squamous epithelium forming some tubules *(arrows)* and simple cuboidal epithelium forming the walls of other tubules. **B,** Sketch of photomicrograph.

Cuboidal Epithelium

Simple cuboidal epithelium is a single layer of cells that are, on average, about as high as they are wide—thus exhibiting a cube shape. This tissue does not form protective coverings but instead forms tubules or other groupings adapted for secretory activity (**Figure 4-5**), which is why they appear to form ringlike arrangements in cross section (see **Figure 4-3**). These secretory cuboidal cells usually function in tubes or clusters of secretory cells commonly called **glands.**

Glands of the body may be classified as **exocrine** if they release their secretion through a duct or as **endocrine** if they release their secretion directly by diffusion into the bloodstream. Examples of glandular secretions include saliva produced by the salivary glands; digestive juices, sweat, or perspiration; and hormones such as those secreted by the pituitary

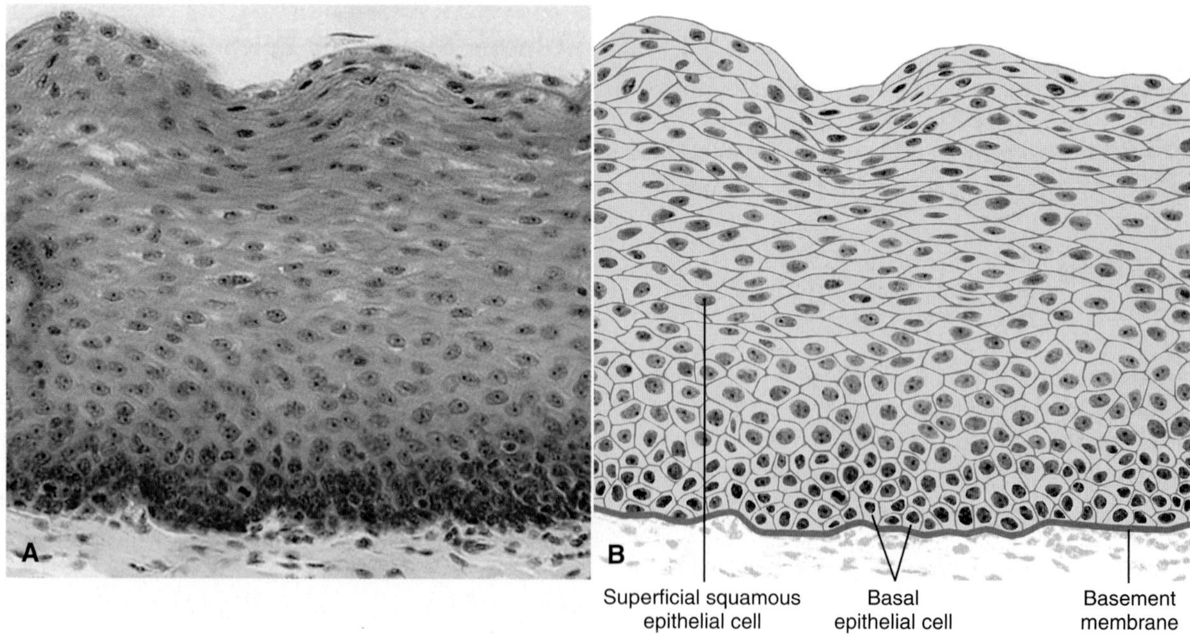

FIGURE 4-4 Stratified squamous epithelium. A, Photomicrograph. **B,** Sketch of the photomicrograph. Note the many layers of epithelial cells and the flattened (squamous) cells in the outer layers.

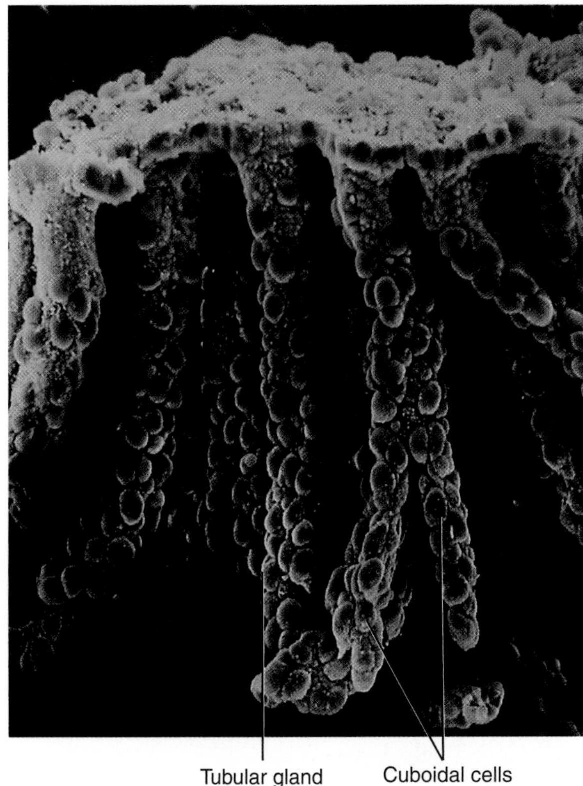

FIGURE 4-5 Simple cuboidal epithelium. This scanning electron micrograph shows how a single layer of cuboidal cells can form glands. The secreting cells arrange themselves into single or branched tubules that open onto a surface—the lining of the stomach in this case.

or thyroid glands. Simple cuboidal epithelium also forms the tubules that form urine in the kidneys.

In some glands, cuboidal epithelium occurs in more than one layer. Such *stratified cuboidal epithelium* may be found in the sweat gland ducts.

Simple Columnar Epithelium

Simple columnar epithelium can be found lining the inner surface of the stomach, intestines, and some areas of the respiratory and reproductive tracts. In Figure 4-6 the simple columnar cells are arranged in a single layer lining the inner surface of the colon or large intestine. These epithelial cells are taller than they are wide, and the nuclei are located toward the bottom of each cell. The "open spaces" among the cells are **goblet cells** that produce mucus. The regular columnar-shaped cells specialize in absorption.

Pseudostratified Epithelium

Pseudostratified epithelium, illustrated in Figure 4-7, is typical of that which lines the trachea or windpipe. Look carefully at the illustration. Note that each cell actually touches the gluelike **basement membrane** that lies under all epithelial tissues. Although the epithelium in Figure 4-7 appears to be several cell layers thick, it is not. This is why it is called *pseudo* (or false) stratified epithelium.

The cilia that extend from the cells are capable of moving in unison (see Figure 3-5, p. 47). In doing so, the cilia move mucus along the lining surface of the trachea, thus affording protection against entry of dust or foreign particles into the lungs.

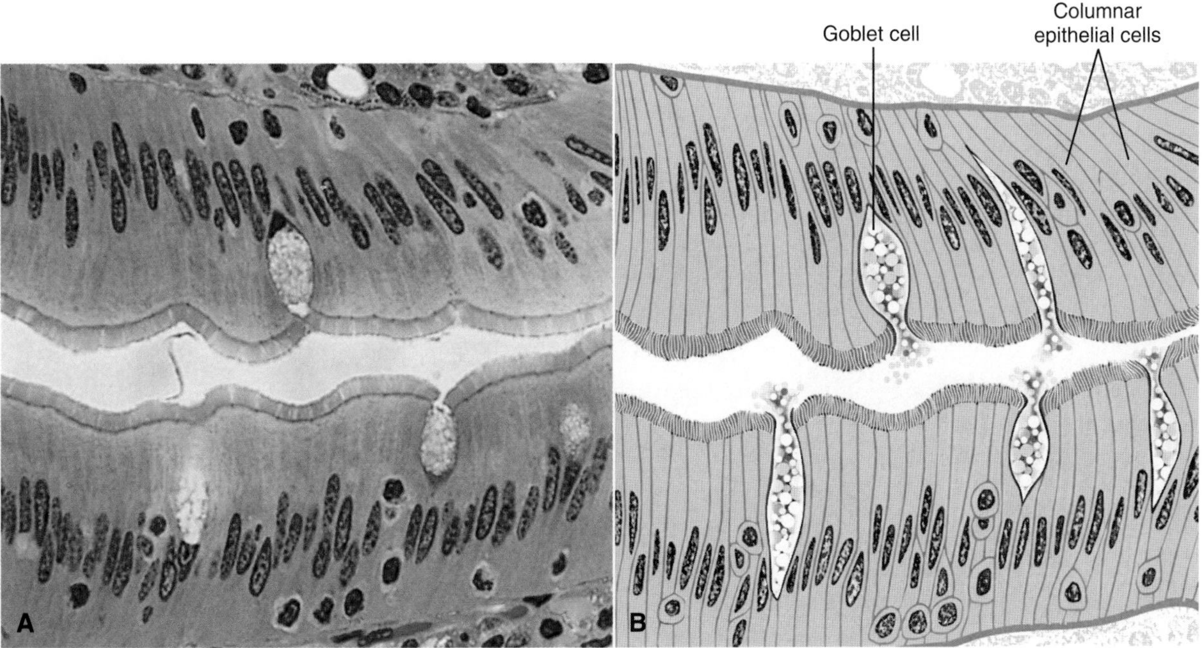

FIGURE 4-6 Simple columnar epithelium. A, Photomicrograph. **B,** Sketch of the photomicrograph. Note the oblong nuclei in all the cells and the goblet or mucus-producing cells that are present.

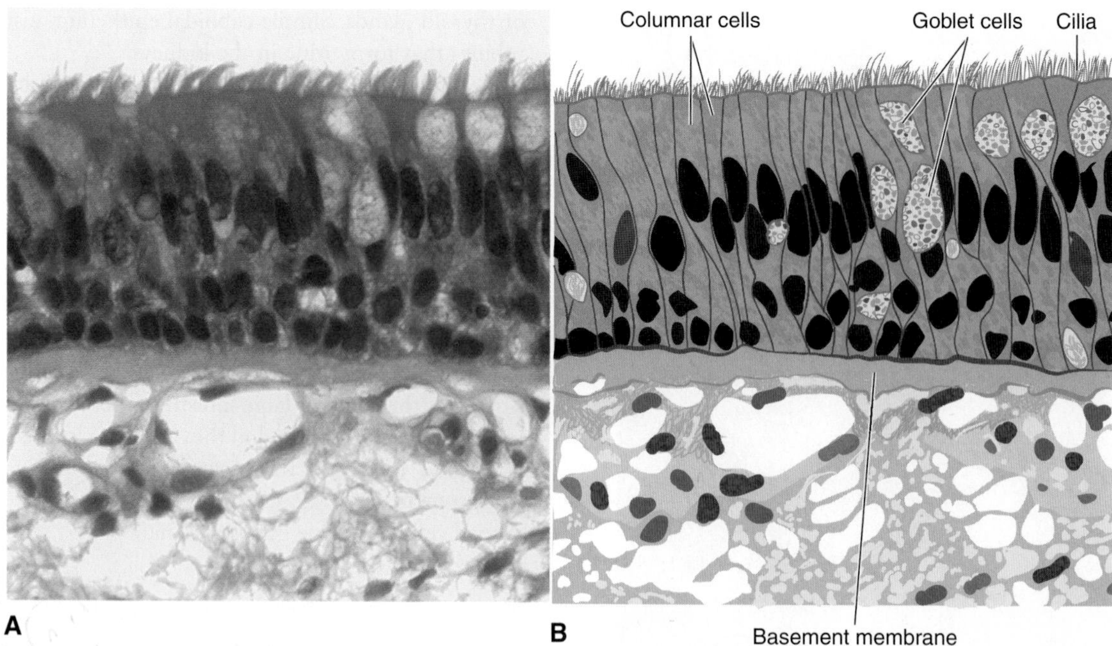

FIGURE 4-7 Pseudostratified columnar epithelium. A, Photomicrograph. The arrangement of nuclei makes this specimen seem stratified, but it is not because each cell reaches the basement membrane, thus forming just one layer. **B,** Sketch of the micrograph. Note the presence of goblet cells and cilia.

Transitional Epithelium

Stratified transitional epithelium is typically found in body areas subjected to stress and must be able to stretch. In many instances, up to 10 layers of differently shaped cells of varying sizes are present in the absence of stretching. When stretching occurs, the epithelial sheet expands, the number of cell layers decreases, and cell shape changes from roughly cuboidal to nearly squamous (flat) in appearance.

An example is the wall of the urinary bladder. The ability of transitional epithelium to stretch easily without damage keeps the bladder wall from tearing as urine fills the bladder. Stratified transitional epithelium is shown in **Figure 4-2** and **Figure 4-8**.

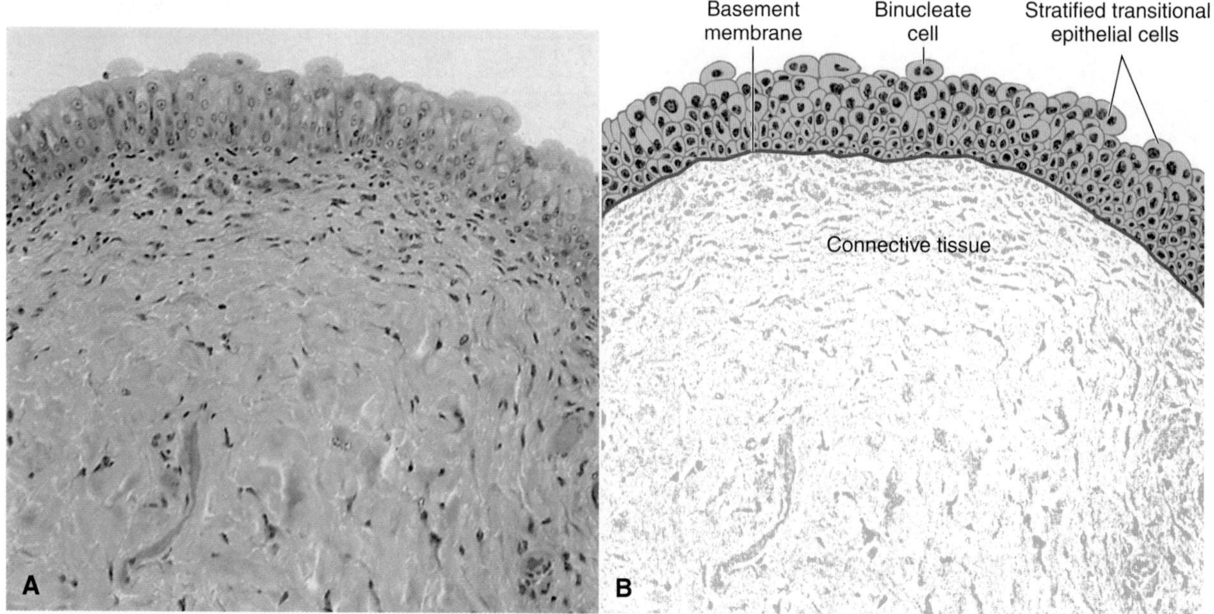

FIGURE 4-8 Stratified transitional epithelium. A, Photomicrograph of tissue lining the urinary bladder wall. **B,** Sketch of the photomicrograph. Note the many layers of epithelial cells of various shapes in this relaxed (unstretched) specimen.

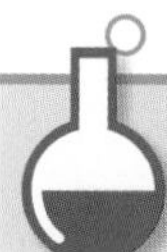

SCIENCE APPLICATIONS
MICROSCOPY

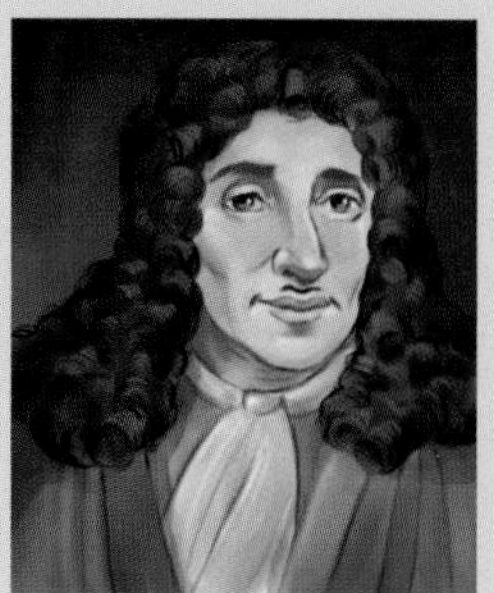
Antonie van Leeuwenhoek (1632-1723)

Until the very hour of his death in 1723, the Dutch drapery merchant Antonie van Leeuwenhoek *(left)* spent most of his 91 years pursuing adventures with the hundreds of microscopes he had built or collected. Using what were, even then, very simple lenses or combinations of lenses, van Leeuwenhoek discovered a whole world of tiny structures he called "animalcules" in body fluids. Although scientists a century later would declare that all living organisms are made up of cells, van Leeuwenhoek was the first to see and describe human blood cells (see **Figure 4-15** on p. 77), human sperm cells, and many other cells and tissues of the body. He was also the first to observe many microscopic organisms that live on or in the human body, many of which are capable of producing disease.

Scientists today use light microscopes that are much more advanced than those of van Leeuwenhoek's time. Some of the most modern microscopes, called *electron microscopes,* use electron beams instead of light to produce images of very high magnification (see **Figure 4-5** on p. 71). Both **cytologists** (cell biologists) and **histologists** (tissue biologists) use microscopes to research the fine structure and function of the human body.

A wide variety of professions have found practical applications for microscopy. Most health professionals use microscopes, or at least images produced with microscopes, to perform routine duties. For example, *clinical laboratory technicians* and **pathologists** frequently use microscopes to assess the health of human cells and tissues. Outside of the health sciences, professionals such as *law enforcement investigators, archaeologists, anthropologists,* and **paleontologists** often use microscopes to further their study of human and animal tissues.

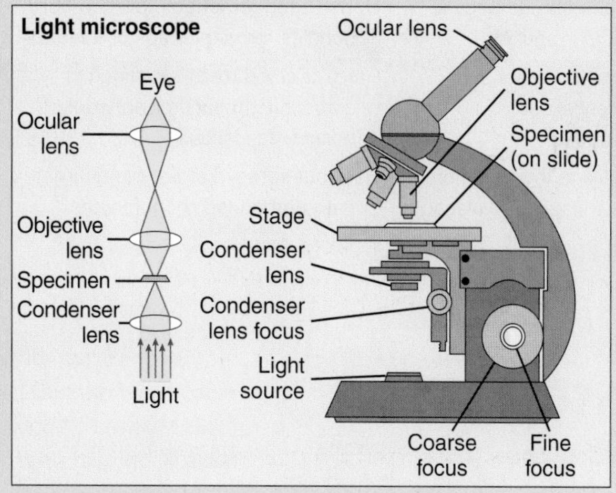

Connective Tissue

Introduction to Connective Tissue

Connective tissue is the most abundant and widely distributed tissue in the body (**Table 4-2**). It also exists in more varied forms than any of the other tissue types. It is found in skin, membranes, muscles, bones, nerves, and all internal organs. Connective tissue exists as delicate, paper-thin webs that hold internal organs together and give them shape. It also exists as strong and tough cords, rigid bones, and even in the form of a fluid—blood.

The functions of connective tissue are as varied as its structure and appearance. It connects tissues to each other and forms a supporting framework for the body as a whole and for its individual organs. As blood, it transports substances throughout the body. Several other kinds of connective tissue function to defend us against microbes and other invaders.

Cells and Matrix

Connective tissue differs from epithelial tissue in the arrangement and variety of its cells and in the amount and kinds of extracellular matrix found between its cells. In addition to the relatively few cells embedded in the matrix of most types of connective tissue, varying numbers and kinds of fibers are also present.

The structural quality and appearance of the matrix and fibers determine the qualities of each type of connective tissue. The matrix of blood, for example, is a liquid, but other types of connective tissue, such as cartilage, have the consistency of firm rubber. The matrix of bone is hard and rigid, although the matrix of connective tissues such as tendons and ligaments is strong and flexible.

Types of Connective Tissue

The following list identifies a number of the major types of connective tissue in the body. Notice that the list is organized by category. Photomicrographs of representative types are provided in the following pages.

A. Fibrous (connective tissue proper)
   1. Loose fibrous (areolar)
   2. Adipose (fat)
      a. White
      b. Brown
   3. Reticular
   4. Dense fibrous
      a. Regular
      b. Irregular

TABLE 4-2 Connective Tissues

TISSUE	STRUCTURE	LOCATION(S)	FUNCTION(S)
Loose fibrous (areolar)	Loose arrangement of collagen fibers, elastic fibers, and cells	Area between other tissues and organs (fascia)	Connection
Adipose (white and brown fat)	Cells contain triglyceride vesicles	**White Fat**	
		Area under skin; padding at various points	Protection, insulation, support, nutrient reserve, regulation
		Brown Fat	
		Pockets within white fat of neck and torso	Heat production, regulation
Reticular	Network of fine collagen (reticular) fibers	Bone marrow, spleen, lymph nodes, cancellous bone cavities	Supports blood-producing cells and immune cells
Dense fibrous (regular and irregular)	Dense arrangement of collagen fiber bundles forming straps or sheets	Tendons, ligaments, skin (deep layer), fascia, scar tissue	Flexible but strong connection
Bone (compact and cancellous)	Hard, calcified matrix arranged in osteons (compact) or network of beams (cancellous)	Skeleton	Support, protection
Cartilage (hyaline, fibrocartilage, and elastic)	Hard but somewhat flexible gel matrix with embedded chondrocytes	**Hyaline**	
		Part of nasal septum, area covering surfaces of bones at joints, larynx wall, rings in trachea, and bronchi	Firm but flexible support
		Fibrocartilage	
		Disks between vertebrae and in knee joint	Withstands pressure
		Elastic	
		External ear	Flexible support
Blood	Liquid matrix with flowing red and white cells	Blood vessels	Transportation
Hematopoietic	Liquid matrix with dense arrangement of blood cell–producing cells	Red bone marrow	Blood cell formation

B. Bone
   1. Compact
   2. Cancellous
C. Cartilage
   1. Hyaline
   2. Fibrocartilage
   3. Elastic
D. Blood
E. Hematopoietic tissue

Fibrous Connective Tissue

Loose Fibrous Connective Tissue (Areolar)

Loose fibrous connective tissue is the most widely distributed of all connective tissue types. It is the "glue" that helps keep the organs of the body together. Also called ***areolar tissue***, it consists of webs of fibers and of a variety of cells embedded in a loose matrix of soft, sticky gel (**Figure 4-9**).

Some of the fibers are made of **collagen,** a strong but flexible fibrous protein. Some are stretchy fibers made of rubbery **elastin** proteins. These *elastic fibers* help tissues return to a shorter length after having been stretched, as in the loose tissue beneath the skin.

It is mainly areolar tissue that makes up the **fascia** of the body. Fascia is the fibrous material that helps bind the skin, muscles, bones, and other organs of the body together.

Adipose Tissue

When it begins to store lipids, areolar tissue can develop into **adipose tissue**, or **fat tissue.** In **Figure 4-10**, numerous vesicles have formed inside the adipose cells where large quantities of triglyceride lipids accumulate. These clear lipid-storage vesicles scatter light like so many snowflakes, giving ordinary adipose tissue a whitish appearance—giving it the alternate name *white fat.* The triglycerides move into storage after a meal and out of storage as energy-producing nutrients are needed by other tissues.

A special kind of adipose tissue called *brown fat* actually burns its fuel when the body is cold to produce heat. This heat, along with shivering by muscles, helps restore homeostasis of body temperature (see **Figure 1-11**, p. 14).

All types of adipose tissue also secrete hormones that help regulate metabolism and fuel storage in the body.

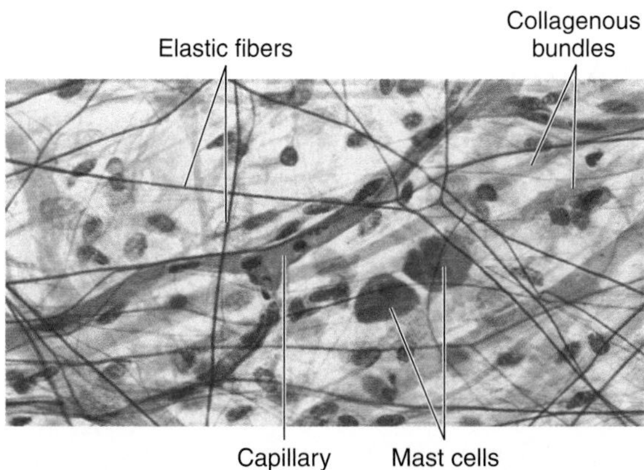

FIGURE 4-9 Loose fibrous (areolar) connective tissue. Notice how the staining used renders the bundles of collagen pink and the elastin fibers dark purple. Compare the loose arrangement of fibers here with those in **Figure 4-12**.

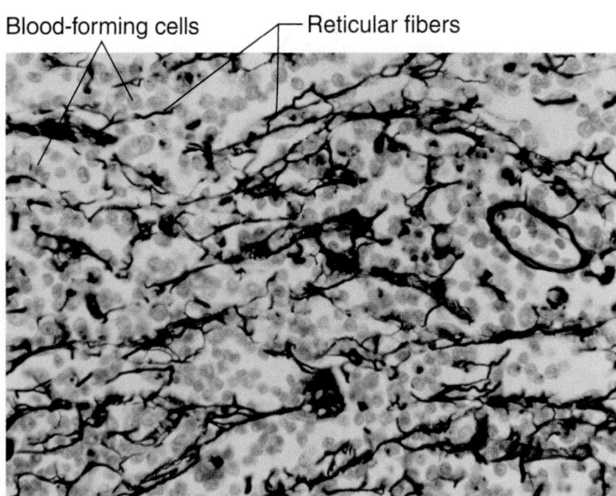

FIGURE 4-11 Reticular connective tissue. The supportive framework of reticular fibers is stained black in this section of a lymph node. Note also the faint blood cells and blood-forming (hematopoietic) cells within the network of fibers.

Reticular Tissue

Another type of fibrous connective tissue called **reticular tissue** has thin, delicate webs of collagen fibers called *reticular fibers.* The word *reticular* means "netlike," and it aptly describes the netlike structure of this tissue, as you can see in **Figure 4-11**.

Reticular tissue is found in bone marrow, for example, where it helps support cells of the blood-forming *hematopoietic tissue*. It is also found in the spleen and lymph nodes, where it supports developing cells of the immune system.

Dense Fibrous Connective Tissue

Dense fibrous connective tissue consists mainly of thick bundles of strong, white **collagen** fibers that are packed closely together. A few fiber-producing cells are scattered among the bundles.

Regular dense fibrous connective tissue has its collagen fiber bundles arranged in roughly parallel rows (**Figure 4-12**). This type of connective tissue makes up tendons—the strong straps that connect muscle to bone. It provides great strength and flexibility, but it cannot stretch. Such characteristics are ideal for these structures that anchor our muscles to our bones.

Irregular dense fibrous connective tissue has its collagen arranged in a chaotic swirl of tangled bundles. This type of tissue forms the tough sheets in the deepest layer of the skin. It forms a tough, flexible support to the epithelial superficial layer of the skin. Although the swirled pattern of fiber bundles allows the skin to stretch a little, overstretching the skin often causes tears in the irregular fibrous tissue called *stretch marks.*

Bone

The matrix of bone is hard because it has a dense packing of collagen bundles encrusted with mineral crystals containing calcium. Bones are a storage area for calcium and provide support and protection for the body.

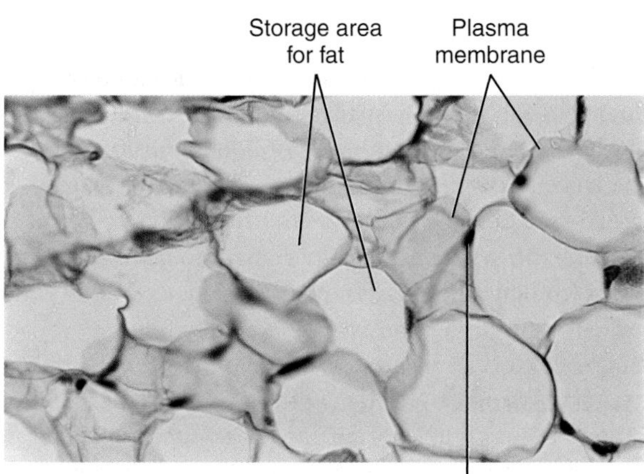

FIGURE 4-10 Adipose tissue. Photomicrograph showing the large lipid storage spaces inside the adipose cells of white fat.

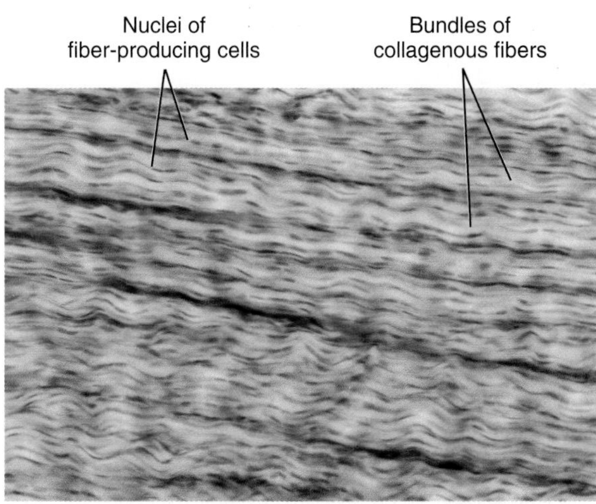

FIGURE 4-12 Dense fibrous connective tissue. Bundles of wavy collagen fibers are roughly parallel to one another in dense regular tissue. Dark nuclei of fiber-producing cells are also visible in this sample from a tendon.

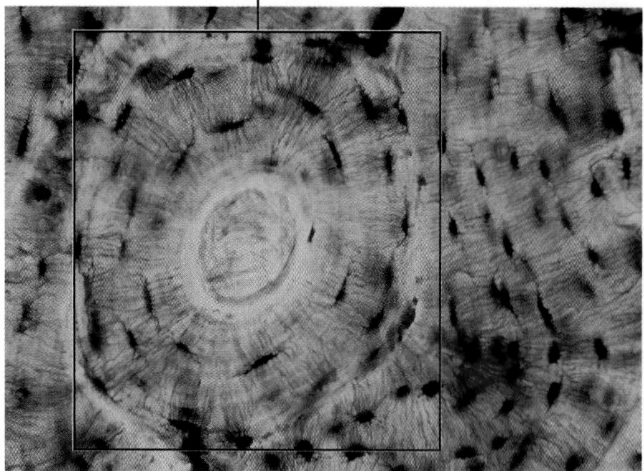

FIGURE 4-13 Bone tissue. Photomicrograph of a chip of compact bone. A cylindrical structural unit of bone, known as an *osteon* (haversian system), is seen in this cross section.

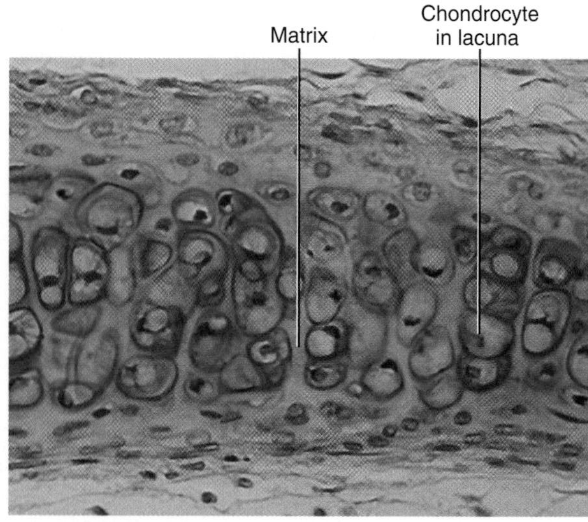

FIGURE 4-14 Cartilage. Photomicrograph showing the chondrocytes distributed throughout the gel-like matrix of hyaline cartilage.

The solid form of bone that makes up the outer walls of bones in the skeleton is called *compact bone*. Compact bone is made up of numerous structural building blocks called **osteons** or **haversian systems**. When compact bone is viewed under a microscope, we can see these circular arrangements of calcified matrix and cells that give bone its characteristic appearance (**Figure 4-13**).

Inside each bone is a type of bone called *cancellous bone* or *spongy bone*. The term *cancellous* refers to something that is made up of a lattice. The term applies to this bone type because it is a chaotic lattice of branching beams. Like a bath sponge, the lattice forms many, interconnected hollow spaces—giving this bone type the name *spongy*. These beams are nearly as hard as compact bone; however, spongy bone cannot be compressed like a wet bath sponge. In fact, the crisscrossing pattern of the bony lattice adds strength—just like the crossed beams that often support roofs of buildings.

The spaces within cancellous bone are filled with blood-forming hematopoietic tissue or adipose tissue.

Cartilage

Unlike bone, the collagen bundles of the matrix are not encrusted with hard minerals. Instead, cartilage matrix has the consistency of a firm plastic or a gristlelike gel. Cartilage cells, which are called **chondrocytes**, are located in many tiny spaces distributed throughout the matrix—giving this tissue the appearance of Swiss cheese (**Figure 4-14**). There are three major types of cartilage.

Hyaline Cartilage

Hyaline cartilage has a moderate amount of collagen in its gel matrix, giving it a translucent, glasslike appearance. The name *hyaline* means "glassy." This is the most common type of cartilage in the body. It is found in the support rings of the respiratory tubes and covering the ends of bones that form joints.

Fibrocartilage

Fibrocartilage is the strongest and most durable type of cartilage. The matrix is rigid and filled with a dense packing of strong collagen fibers. Fibrocartilage disks serve as shock absorbers between adjacent vertebrae and in the knee joint.

Elastic Cartilage

Elastic cartilage contains few collagen fibers but large numbers of very fine elastic fibers that give the matrix material a high degree of flexibility. This type of cartilage is found in the external ear and in the voice box, or larynx.

Blood Tissue

Blood is perhaps the most unusual form of connective tissue because its matrix—blood *plasma*—is liquid. It has transportation and protective functions in the body. *Red blood cells, white blood cells,* and *platelets* are the cell types common to blood (**Figure 4-15**).

Hematopoietic Tissue

Hematopoietic tissue is the bloodlike connective tissue found in the red marrow cavities of bones and in organs such as the spleen, tonsils, and lymph nodes (see **Figure 4-11**). This type of tissue is responsible for the formation of blood cells and lymphatic system cells important in our defense against disease (see **Table 4-2**).

QUICK CHECK

1. What is the difference between simple and stratified epithelial tissue? Between squamous and cuboidal epithelial tissue?
2. Which main tissue type of the body is mostly matrix?
3. What are the primary forms of connective tissue?

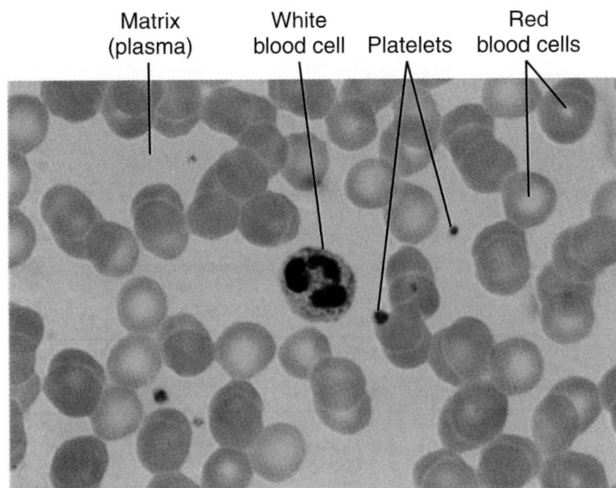

FIGURE 4-15 Blood. Photomicrograph of a human blood smear. This smear shows a white blood cell surrounded by a number of smaller red blood cells and tiny platelets. The liquid matrix of this tissue is also called *plasma.*

Muscle Tissue

Introduction to Muscle Tissue

Muscle cells are the movement specialists of the body. They have a higher degree of contractility (ability to shorten or contract) than any other tissue cells. Besides producing movement, muscle tissue can also maintain contraction to provide stability—and even body heat. Unfortunately, injured muscle cells are often slow to heal and often are replaced by fibrous scar tissue if injured.

There are three kinds of muscle tissue: **skeletal muscle tissue, cardiac muscle tissue,** and **smooth muscle tissue** (**Table 4-3**).

Skeletal Muscle Tissue

Skeletal or striated muscle is called voluntary because willed or *voluntary* control of skeletal muscle contractions is possible. Note in **Figure 4-16** that, when viewed under a microscope, skeletal muscle is characterized by many cross striations and many nuclei per cell. Individual cells are long and threadlike and are often called *fibers.*

Skeletal muscles are attached to bones and, when contracted, produce voluntary and controlled body movements.

Cardiac Muscle Tissue

Cardiac muscle forms the walls of the heart, and the regular but involuntary contractions of cardiac muscle produce the heartbeat. Under the light microscope (**Figure 4-17**), cardiac muscle fibers have faint cross striations (as in skeletal muscle) and thicker dark bands called *intercalated disks.*

Cardiac muscle fibers branch and connect to various other cardiac fiber branches to produce a three-dimensional, interlocking mass of contractile tissue.

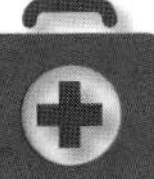

HEALTH AND WELL-BEING

TISSUES AND FITNESS

Achieving and maintaining an ideal body weight is a health-conscious goal. However, a better indicator of health and fitness is body composition. Exercise physiologists assess body composition to identify the percentage of the body made of lean tissue and the percentage made of fat. Body-fat percentage is often determined by using calipers to measure the thickness of skin folds at certain places on the body.

A person with low body weight may still have a high ratio of fat to muscle, an unhealthy condition. In this case the individual is "underweight" but "overfat." In other words, fitness depends more on the percentage and ratio of specific tissue types than the overall amount of tissue present.

Therefore one goal of a good fitness program is a desirable body-fat percentage. For men, the ideal is 12% to 18%, and for women, the ideal is 18% to 24%. Because fat contains stored energy (measured in calories), a low fat percentage means a low energy reserve. High body-fat percentages are associated with several life-threatening conditions, including cardiovascular disease, diabetes, and cancer. A balanced diet and an exercise program ensure that the ratio of fat to muscle tissue stays at a level appropriate for maintaining homeostasis.

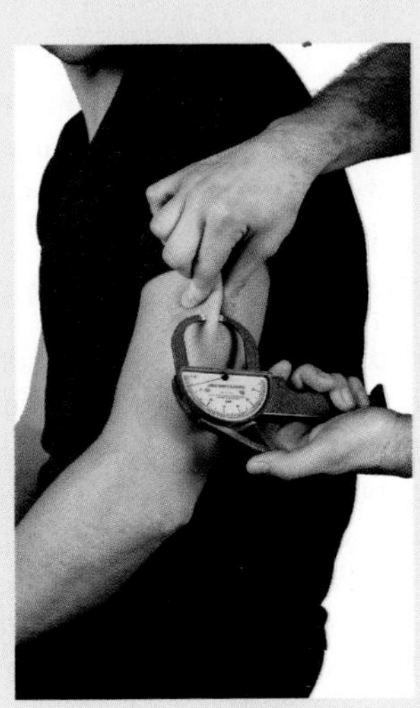

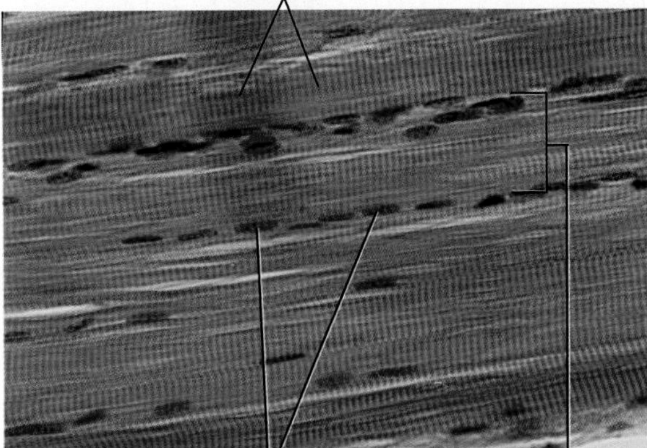

FIGURE 4-16 Skeletal muscle. Photomicrograph showing the striations of the muscle cell fibers in longitudinal section.

TABLE 4-3 Muscle and Nervous Tissues

TISSUE	STRUCTURE	LOCATION(S)	FUNCTION(S)
Muscle			
Skeletal (striated voluntary)	Long, threadlike cells with multiple nuclei and striations	Muscles that attach to bones	Maintenance of posture, movement of bones produces body heat
		Eyeball muscles	Eye movements
		Upper third of esophagus	First part of swallowing
Cardiac (striated involuntary)	Branching, interconnected cylinders with faint striations	Wall of heart	Contraction of heart
Smooth (non-striated involuntary or visceral)	Threadlike cells with single nuclei and no striations	Walls of tubular viscera of digestive, respiratory, and genitourinary tracts	Movement of substances along respective tracts
		Walls of blood vessels and large lymphatic vessels	Changing of diameter of vessels
		Ducts of glands	Movement of substances along ducts
		Intrinsic eye muscles (iris and ciliary body)	Changing of diameter of pupils and shape of lens
		Arrector muscles of hairs	Erection of hairs (goose pimples)
Nervous			
	Nerve cells with large cell bodies and thin fiberlike extensions; supportive glial cells also present	Brain, spinal cord, nerves	Irritability, conduction

Smooth Muscle Tissue

Smooth (visceral) muscle is said to be involuntary because it is not under conscious or willful control. Under a microscope (**Figure 4-18**), smooth muscle cells are seen as long, narrow fibers but not nearly as long as skeletal or striated fibers. Individual smooth muscle cells appear smooth (that is, without cross striations) and have only one nucleus per fiber.

Smooth muscle helps form the walls of blood vessels and hollow organs such as the intestines and other tube-shaped structures in the body. Contractions of smooth (visceral) muscle propel material through the digestive tract and help regulate the diameter of blood vessels. Contraction of smooth muscle in the tubes of the respiratory system, such as the bronchioles in the lungs, can impair breathing and result in asthma attacks and labored respiration.

Nervous Tissue

The function of nervous tissue is to provide rapid communication between body structures and control of body functions (see **Table 4-3**). Nervous tissue consists of two kinds of cells:

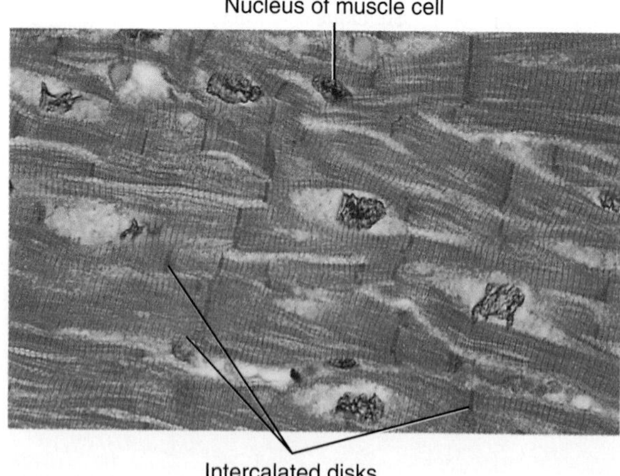

FIGURE 4-17 Cardiac muscle. Photomicrograph showing the branched, lightly striated fibers. The darker bands, called *intercalated disks,* which are characteristic of cardiac muscle, are easily identified in this tissue section.

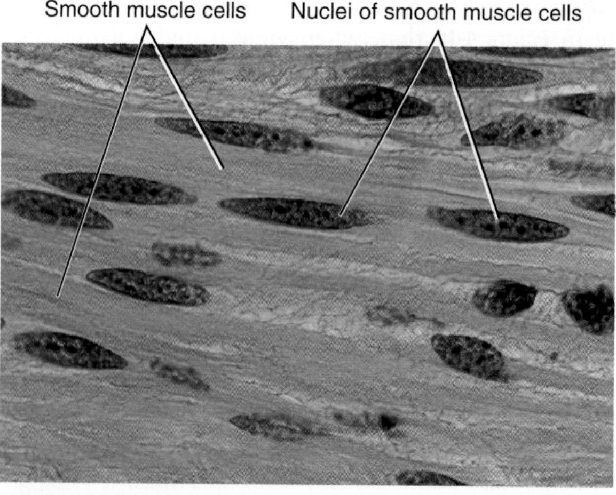

FIGURE 4-18 Smooth muscle. Photomicrograph, longitudinal section. Note the central placement of nuclei in the spindle-shaped smooth muscle fibers.

nerve cells, or **neurons**, which are the conducting units of the system, and special connecting and supporting cells called **glia** or **neuroglia.**

All neurons are characterized by a **cell body** and two types of processes: (1) one **axon,** which transmits a nerve impulse away from the cell body, and (2) one or more **dendrites**, which carry impulses toward the cell body. The large neurons in **Figure 4-19** have many dendrites extending from the cell body.

QUICK CHECK

1. What are the structure and functions of the three main types of muscle tissue?
2. What are the two main types of cells found in nervous tissue? What are their functions?
3. What are the three structural components of a neuron?
4. What are the three primary types of cartilage?

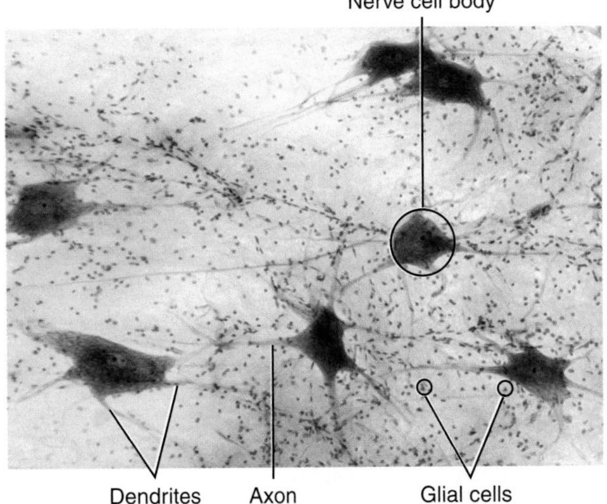

FIGURE 4-19 Nervous tissue. Photomicrograph of neurons and glia in a smear of the spinal cord. The neurons in this slide display characteristic cell bodies and multiple cell processes. Nuclei of glia are visible as dark dots surrounding the neuron.

LANGUAGE OF SCIENCE AND MEDICINE *(continued from p. 67)*

dendrite
(DEN-dryte)
[*dendr-* **tree,** *-ite* **part (branch) of**]

dense fibrous connective tissue
(dens FYE-brus koh-NEK-tiv TISH-yoo)
[*dense* **thick,** *fibro-* **fiber,** *-ous* **relating to,** *con-* **together,** *-nect-* **bind,** *-ive* **relating to,** *tissue* **fabric**]

elastic cartilage
(eh-LAS-tik KAR-tih-lij)
[*elast-* **drive or propel,** *-ic* **relating to,** *cartilag* **cartilage**]

elastin
(eh-LAS-tin)
[*elast-* **strike or beat out,** *-in* **substance**]

endocrine
(EN-doh-krin)
[*endo-* **within,** *-crin* **secrete**]

epithelial tissue
(ep-ih-THEE-lee-al TISH-yoo)
[*epi-* **on or upon,** *-theli-* **nipple,** *-al* **relating to,** *tissue* **fabric**]

exocrine
(EKS-oh-krin)
[*exo-* **outside or outward,** *-crin* **secrete**]

fascia
(FASH-ee-ah)
[*fascia* **band or bundle**]

fat tissue
(fat TISH-yoo)
[*tissue* **fabric**]

fibrocartilage
(fye-broh-KAR-tih-lij)
[*fibr-* **thread or fiber,** *-cartilag* **cartilage**]

gland
(gland)
[*gland* **acorn**]

glia
(GLEE-ah)
[*glia* **glue**]

goblet cell
(GOB-let sel)
[*goblet* **small bowl,** *cell* **storeroom**]

haversian systems
(hah-VER-zhun or HAV-er-zhun SIS-tem)
[*Clopton Havers* **English physician,** *-ian* **relating to**]

hematopoietic tissue
(hee-mah-toh-poy-ET-ik TISH yoo)
[*hema-* **blood,** *-poie-* **to make,** *-ic* **relating to,** *tissue* **fabric**]

histologist
(hih-STOL-oh-jist)
[*histo-* **tissue,** *-log-* **words (study of),** *-ist* **agent**]

hyaline cartilage
(HYE-ah-lin KAR-tih-lij)
[*hyal-* **glass,** *-ine* **of or like,** *cartilag-* **cartilage**]

loose fibrous connective tissue
(LOOS FYE-brus kon-NEK-tiv TISH-yoo)
[*fibr-* **thread or fiber,** *-ous* **relating to,** *con-* **together,** *-nect-* **bind,** *-ive* **relating to,** *tissu-* **fabric**]

matrix
(MAY-triks)
[*matrix* **womb**]

neuroglia
(noo-ROG-lee-ah or noo-roh-GLEE-ah)
sing., neuroglial cell
(noo-ROG-lee-al or noo-roh-GLEE-al sel)
[*neuro-* **nerve,** *-glia* **glue**]

neuron
(NOO-ron)
[*neur-* **string or nerve,** *-on* **unit**]

osteon
(AHS-tee-on)
[*osteo-* **bone,** *-on* **unit**]

paleontologist
(pay-lee-un-TOL-oh-jist)
[*paleo-* **ancient,** *-onto-* **being,** *-log-* **words (study of),** *-ist* **agent**]

pathologist
(pah-THOL-oh-jist)
[*patho-* **disease,** *-log-* **words (study of),** *-ist* **agent**]

proteoglycan
(PRO-tee-oh-GLYE-kan)
[*proteo-* **protein,** *-glycan* **polysaccharide (from** *-glyc-* **sweet)**]

pseudostratified epithelium
(SOOD-oh-STRAT-ih-fyed ep-ih-THEE-lee-um)
[*pseudo-* **false,** *-strati-* **layer,** *-fied* **made,** *epi-* **on or upon,** *theli-* **nipple,** *-um* **thing**]

reticular tissue
(reh-TIK-yoo-lar TISH-yoo)
[*ret-* **net,** *-ic-* **relating to,** *-ul-* **little,** *-ar* **characterized by,** *tissue* **fabric**]

simple columnar epithelium
(SIM-pel koh-LUM-nar ep-ih-THEE-lee-um)
[*simple* **not mixed,** *column-* **column,** *-ar* **relating to,** *epi-* **on,** *-theli-* **nipple,** *-um* **thing**]

simple cuboidal epithelium
(SIM-pel KYOO-boyd-al ep-ih-THEE-lee-um)
[*simple* **not mixed,** *cub-* **cube,** *-oid* **like,** *-al* **relating to,** *epi-* **on,** *-theli-* **nipple,** *-um* **thing**]

simple squamous epithelium
(SIM-pel SKWAY-muss ep-ih-THEE-lee-um)
[*simple* **not mixed,** *squam-* **scale,** *-ous* **characterized by,** *epi-* **on,** *-theli-* **nipple,** *-um* **thing**]

skeletal muscle tissue
(SKEL-et-al MUSS-el TISH-yoo)
[*skelet-* **dried body,** *-al* **relating to,** *mus-* **mouse,** *-cle* **small,** *tissue* **fabric**]

smooth muscle tissue
(smoothe MUSS-el TISH-yoo)
[*smooth* **smooth,** *mus-* **mouse,** *-cle* **small,** *tissue* **fabric**]

stratified squamous epithelium
(STRAT-ih-fyde SKWAY-muss ep-ih-THEE-lee-um)
[*strati-* **layer,** *-fied* **made,** *squam-* **scale,** *-ous* **characterized by,** *epi-* **on,** *-theli-* **nipple,** *-um* **thing**]

stratified transitional epithelium
(STRAT-ih-fyde tran-ZISH-en-al ep-ih-THEE-lee-um)
[*strati-* **layer,** *-fied* **made,** *trans-* **across,** *-tion-* **process,** *-al* **relating to,** *epi-* **on,** *-theli-* **nipple,** *-um* **thing**]

tissue
(TISH-yoo)
[*tissue* **fabric**]

❑ OUTLINE SUMMARY

To download a digital audio version of the chapter summary for use with your device, access the ***Audio Chapter Summaries*** *online at evolve.elsevier.com.*

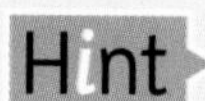

Scan this summary after reading the chapter to help you reinforce the key concepts. Later, use the summary as a quick review before your class or before a test.

Introduction to Tissues

A. Four main tissue types
  1. Epithelial tissue — forms sheets that cover or line the body
  2. Connective tissue — provides structural and functional support
  3. Muscle tissue — contracts to produce movement
  4. Nervous tissue — senses, conducts, and processes information

B. Matrix — also called extracellular matrix (ECM)
  1. Internal fluid environment of the body, surrounding cells of each tissue
  2. Mostly water, but also often contains fibers and other substances that give it thick, jellylike consistency (see **Figure 4-1**)
     a. Collagen — protein that forms twisted ropelike fibers that provide flexible strength to tissue
     b. Elastin — rubbery protein that provides elastic stretch and rebound in tissues
     c. Polysaccharides and proteoglycans help link cells, absorb shock, regulate function, and lubricate

Epithelial Tissue

A. Introduction to epithelial tissue (see **Table 4-1**)
  1. Covers body and lines body cavities
  2. Cells packed closely together with little matrix
  3. Classified by shape of cells (see **Figure 4-2**)
     a. Squamous — flat and scalelike
     b. Cuboidal — cube-shaped
     c. Columnar — higher than they are wide
     d. Transitional — varying shapes that can stretch
  4. Also classified by arrangement of cells into one or more layers: simple or stratified

B. Squamous epithelium
  1. Simple squamous epithelium — single layer of scalelike cells adapted for transport (e.g., absorption) (see **Figure 4-3**)
  2. Stratified squamous epithelium — several layers of closely packed cells specializing in protection (see **Figure 4-4**)

C. Cuboidal epithelium
  1. Simple cuboidal epithelium — single layer of cubelike cells often specialized for secretory activity; may secrete into ducts, directly into blood, and on body surface (see **Figure 4-3** and **Figure 4-5**)
  2. Stratified cuboidal epithelium— two or more layers of cubelike cells, sometimes found in sweat glands and other locations

D. Columnar epithelium
  1. Simple columnar epithelium — tall, columnlike cells arranged in a single layer; contain mucus-producing goblet cells; specialized for absorption (see **Figure 4-6**)
  2. Pseudostratified epithelium — single layer of distorted columnar cells; each cell touches basement membrane (see **Figure 4-7**)

E. Transitional epithelium
   1. Stratified transitional epithelium — up to 10 layers of roughly cuboidal cells that distort to squamous shape when stretched (see **Figure 4-8**)
   2. Found in body areas that stretch, such as urinary bladder

Connective Tissue

A. Introduction to connective tissue (see **Table 4-2**)
   1. Most abundant and widely distributed tissue in body, with many different types, appearances, and functions
   2. Relatively few cells in extracellular matrix between tissue cells
   3. Types
      a. Fibrous — loose fibrous (areolar), adipose (fat), reticular, dense fibrous
      b. Bone — compact and cancellous (spongy)
      c. Cartilage — hyaline, fibrocartilage, elastic
      d. Blood
      e. Hematopoietic tissue
B. Fibrous connective tissue
   1. Loose fibrous connective tissue (areolar) — fibrous glue (fascia) that holds organs together; collagenous and elastic fibers, plus a variety of cell types (see **Figure 4-9**)
   2. Adipose (fat) tissue — white fat stores lipids (triglycerides); brown fat produces heat; both types regulate metabolism (see **Figure 4-10**)
   3. Reticular tissue — delicate net of collagen fibers, as in bone marrow (see **Figure 4-11**)
   4. Dense fibrous tissue — bundles of strong collagen fibers, densely packed
      a. Regular — parallel collagen bundles; example is tendon (see **Figure 4-12**)
      b. Irregular — chaotic, swirling collagen bundles; example is deep layer of skin
C. Bone tissue — matrix is collagen bundles encrusted with calcium mineral crystals
   1. Compact bone — made up of cylindrical osteons (haversian systems); forms outer walls of bones
   2. Cancellous bone — made up of thin, crisscrossing beams of bone; found inside bones; also called *spongy bone*
   3. Bone functions in support and protection (see **Figure 4-13**)
D. Cartilage tissue — matrix is consistency of gristlelike gel; chondrocyte is cell type (see **Figure 4-14**)
   1. Hyaline cartilage — moderate amount of collagen in matrix; forms a flexible gel
   2. Fibrocartilage — matrix is very dense with collagen; forms very tough, hard gel
   3. Elastic cartilage — matrix has some collagen with elastin; forms a soft, elastic gel
E. Blood tissue — matrix is fluid plasma; cell types include RBCs, WBCs, and platelets; functions are transportation and protection (see **Figure 4-15**)
F. Hematopoietic tissue — blood-forming tissue with a liquid matrix

Muscle Tissue

A. Muscle tissue contracts to provide movement or stability; produces body heat (see **Table 4-3**)
B. Skeletal muscle tissue — attaches to bones; also called *striated* or *voluntary*; control is voluntary; striations apparent when viewed under a microscope (see **Figure 4-16**)
C. Cardiac muscle tissue — also called *striated involuntary*; composes heart wall; ordinarily cannot control contractions (see **Figure 4-17**)
D. Smooth muscle tissue — also called *nonstriated (visceral)* or *involuntary*; no cross striations; found in blood vessels and other tube-shaped organs (**Figure 4-18**)

Nervous Tissue

A. Function — rapid communication between body structures and control of body functions (see **Table 4-3**)
B. Neurons (see **Figure 4-19**)
   1. Conduction cells
   2. All neurons have cell body and two types of processes: axon and dendrite
      a. Axon (one) carries nerve impulse away from cell body
      b. Dendrites (one or more) carry nerve impulse toward the cell body
C. Glia (neuroglia) — supportive and connecting cells

❑ ACTIVE LEARNING

STUDY TIPS

Hint *Use these tips to achieve success in meeting your learning goals.*

Chapter 4 should be a review of your previous general biology course. Most of what is in this chapter should sound familiar.

1. Tissue identification may seem a bit overwhelming at first glance. But if you look for "key characteristics" as you study each one, it becomes easier. See *my-ap.us/learntissues* for advice.
2. Tissue types can be practiced easily using flash cards using photos copied from the text. Epithelial tissues cover or protect tissues. An important characteristic of connective tissues is the matrix surrounding the cells.
3. To understand the shape of epithelial cells, you can use a soda can analogy. Imagine a soda can that has been completely smashed. This would represent a squamous-shaped cell. A soda can that has only been smashed half way would represent a cuboidal-shaped cell. A soda can that has not been smashed would represent a columnar-shaped cell. Soda cans arranged together in all of these shapes would represent stratified transitional epithelium.
4. Since membranous epithelium covers the body or lines a cavity, there is always an exposed space in microscopic specimens. After you have identified the exposed space, classify the shape (squamous, cuboidal, or columnar) of the cells. Then determine the number of layers (simple or stratified). Develop a concept map that depicts the different epithelial tissues. Use **Table 4-1** and include the locations of these tissues in the body.
5. When classifying connective tissues, pay close attention to the matrix. Identify whether the matrix is fibrous protein, protein that is ground substance, or fluid. Use available resources (textbook, lab manual, atlas, or Internet sources) to familiarize yourself with the differences among these matrices. Develop a *concept map* that depicts the different connective tissues. Use **Table 4-2** and include the locations of these tissues in the body. (To learn about concept mapping, go to *my-ap.us/MExHCf*).
6. Familiarize yourself with the unique characteristics that define each type of muscle tissue. Refer to **Table 4-3**. Construct a *T-chart* that lists the different muscle tissues and their locations.
7. The use of flash cards or review cards is an excellent strategy to learn the various types of tissues. There are many online sources that have tissue images. Obtain photos or illustrations of the different types of tissues. Place the photo or illustration on one side of an index card. On the opposite side of the card, put the name of the tissue. You can also add additional information such as unique characteristics or location in the body.
8. Draw a concept map showing how the various types of tissue are categorized.
9. In your study groups, quiz each other on tissues, perhaps using photos from books and online sources.
10. Go over the Review Questions and discuss possible test questions.

Review Questions

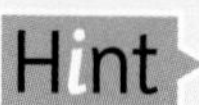

Write out the answers to these questions after reading the chapter and reviewing the Chapter Summary. If you simply think through the answer without writing it down, you won't retain much of your new learning.

1. Name and briefly describe the functions of the four main types of tissue.
2. Describe extracellular matrix and how it may affect the function of tissue.
3. Name and briefly describe the structure and function of three epithelial tissues.
4. Name and describe the primary connective tissues.
5. Name and describe the three muscle tissues.
6. Name the two types of nervous tissue cells. Which is a conductive cell type, and which acts as a support cell?
7. Name the three primary structures of a neuron and explain the function of the nerve cell processes.

Critical Thinking

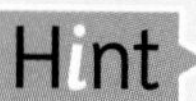

After finishing the Review Questions, write out the answers to these more in-depth questions to help you apply your new knowledge. Go back to sections of the chapter that relate to concepts that you find difficult.

8. Explain what is meant by tissue typing. Why has this become so important in recent years?
9. Christy is a body builder who is obsessed with her physique. She exercises daily and eats a low-fat diet. A personal trainer has assessed her body fat at 12%. Is she too lean, too fat, or just right? Explain the relationship between her body-fat percentage and lifestyle.
10. Chad is a middle-aged, sedentary man who smokes 2 packs a day and is complaining of a chronic, annoying cough. After a series of tests, he is diagnosed with lung cancer. Which type of epithelial tissues might be involved in this diagnosis?

Chapter Test

Hint *After studying the chapter, test your mastery by responding to these items. Try to answer them without looking up the answers. Then, verify the answers using the key in Appendix C at the back of this book.*

1. ________ tissue provides structural and functional support.
2. The fluid material between the cells is called the ________.
3. ________ is present in some tissues and gives them the ability to stretch and rebound easily.
4. Glands that release their secretion into the bloodstream are known as ________.
5. Bubble-filled structures among simple columnar epithelial cells that produce mucus are ________ cells.
6. The type and quality of the ________ and fibers between cells determine the qualities of each type of connective tissue.
7. Loose fibrous connective tissue is also called ________.
8. A special kind of adipose tissue called ________ actually burns its fuel when the body is cold to produce heat.
9. Blood forming tissue is ________.
10. Dense fibrous connective tissue consists mainly of thick bundles of strong, white ________ fibers that are packed closely together.
11. Compact bone is made up of structural building blocks known as ________ or ________.
12. Skeletal muscle is:
    a. smooth
    b. involuntary
    c. identified under a microscope by branching muscle fibers
    d. attached to bones
13. Neuroglia are:
    a. nerve cells
    b. a type of dendrites
    c. a type of axon
    d. special connecting and supporting cells of nervous tissue
14. Which of the following is *not* a classification of epithelial cell shapes?
    a. squamous
    b. basal
    c. cuboidal
    d. transitional
15. ________ is a protein that forms microscopic twisted ropes within the matrix of many tissues and gives a tissue flexible strength.
    a. proteoglycans
    b. polysaccharides
    c. collagen
    d. elastin
16. Stratified transitional epithelium is typically found in body areas:
    a. subjected to stress
    b. requiring transport
    c. requiring protection
    d. requiring the formation of tubules
17. An example of a fluid form of connective tissue is:
    a. water
    b. blood
    c. saline
    d. perspiration
18. Cancellous bone is also referred to as:
    a. osteons
    b. haversian systems
    c. cartilage
    d. spongy bone
19. The strongest and most durable type of cartilage is:
    a. hyaline
    b. fibrocartilage
    c. elastic
    d. chondrocyte
20. Smooth muscle:
    a. is found in the heart
    b. produces voluntary body movements
    c. has multiple nuclei per cell
    d. helps form the walls of blood vessels and hollow organs

Match each function in Column B with the proper answer in Column A.

Column A	Column B
21. cartilage	a. gland
22. exocrine	b. cardiac muscle
23. fascia	c. matrix
24. blood plasma	d. mainly areolar tissue
25. intercalated disks	e. chondrocytes

Organ Systems

OUTLINE

Hint *Scan this outline before you begin to read the chapter, as a preview of how the concepts are organized.*

OBJECTIVES

Hint *Before reading the chapter, review these goals for your learning.*

After you have completed this chapter, you should be able to:

1. Define and contrast the terms *organ* and *organ system.*
2. List the major organ systems of the body.
3. Identify and locate the major organs of each major organ system.
4. Briefly describe the major functions of each major organ system.

CHAPTER 5

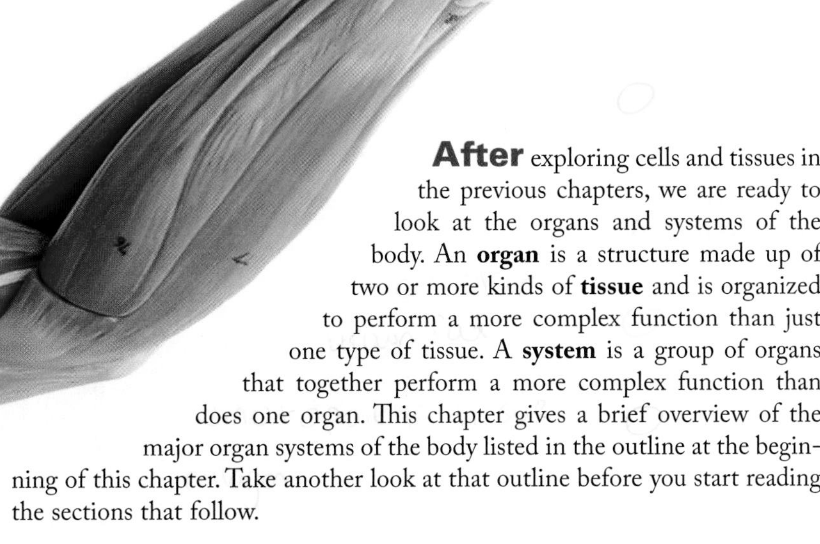

After exploring cells and tissues in the previous chapters, we are ready to look at the organs and systems of the body. An **organ** is a structure made up of two or more kinds of **tissue** and is organized to perform a more complex function than just one type of tissue. A **system** is a group of organs that together perform a more complex function than does one organ. This chapter gives a brief overview of the major organ systems of the body listed in the outline at the beginning of this chapter. Take another look at that outline before you start reading the sections that follow.

This overview of body systems provides the foundation needed to see the "big picture" of human structure and function as we later reveal the details of each system. As you progress through your detailed study of the major organ systems in the chapters that follow, it will be possible to view the body not just as an assembly of individual parts but as an integrated and functioning whole.

LANGUAGE OF SCIENCE AND MEDICINE

Hint Before reading the chapter, say each of these terms out loud. This will help you to avoid stumbling over them as you read.

adrenal gland
(ah-DREE-nal gland)
[*ad-* **toward,** *-ren-* **kidney,** *-al* **relating to,** *gland* **acorn**]

alimentary canal
(al-eh-MEN-tar-ee kah-NAL)
[*aliment-* **nourishment,** *-ary* **relating to,** *canal* **channel**]

alveolus
(al-VEE-oh-lus)
pl., alveoli
(al-VEE-oh-lye)
[*alve-* **hollow,** *-olus* **little**]

antibody
(AN-tih-bod-ee)
[*anti-* **against,** *-body,* **body**]

artery
(AR-ter-ee)
[*arteri-* **vessel**]

bronchus
(BRONG-kus)
pl., bronchi
(BRONG-kye)
[*bronchus* **windpipe**]

capillary
(KAP-ih-layr-ee)
[*capill-* **hair,** *-ary* **relating to**]

cardiac muscle
(KAR-dee-ak MUSS-el)
[*cardi-* **heart,** *-ic* **relating to,** *mus-* **mouse,** *-cle* **little**]

cardiovascular system
(kar-dee-oh-VAS-kyoo-lar SIS-tem)
[*cardio-* **heart,** *-vas-* **vessel,** *-ular* **relating to,** *system* **organized whole**]

Continued on p. 96

Organ Systems

Integumentary System

The **integumentary system** includes only one organ: the skin (Figure 5-1). In most adults, the skin alone weighs 20 pounds or more, accounting for about 16% of total body weight and making it the body's heaviest organ.

Although the integumentary system has only one organ, that one organ, the skin or **integument,** has many millions of *appendages* (structures attached to a main part) and glands. These skin structures include the hair, nails, and sweat- and oil-producing glands. The skin includes many microscopic sense receptors, making it the largest sensory organ of the body. Skin sense receptors permit the body to respond to pain, pressure, touch, texture, vibration, and changes in temperature.

The integumentary system is crucial to survival. Its primary function is *protection.* The skin protects underlying tissue against invasion by harmful bacteria, bars entry of most chemicals, and minimizes the chances of mechanical injury to underlying structures. In addition, the skin regulates body temperature by sweating and by controlling blood flow and therefore heat loss at the body surface. The skin also synthesizes important chemicals, such as vitamin D, and functions as a sophisticated sense organ for temperature, touch, pressure, pain, vibration, and more.

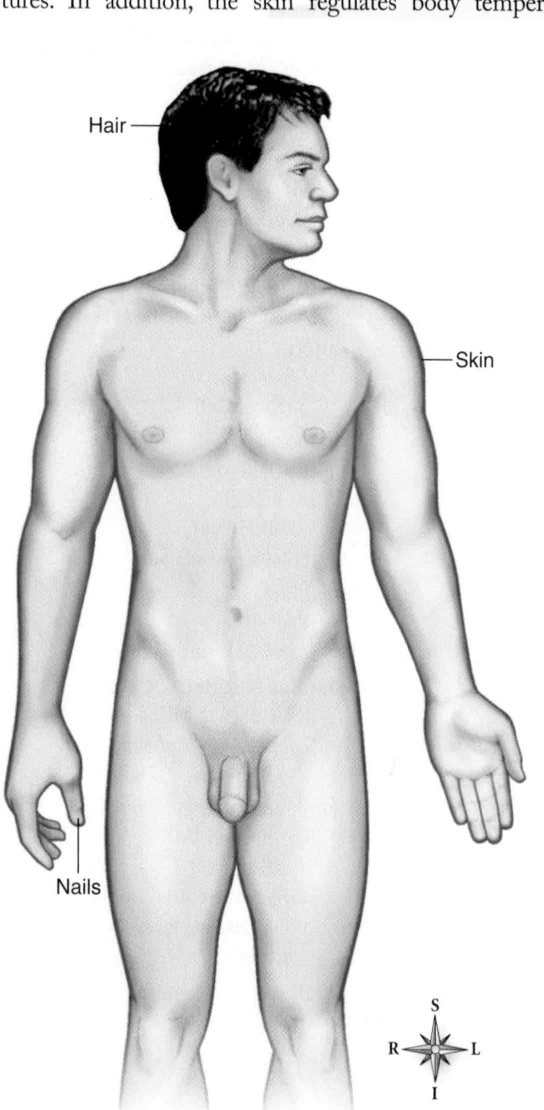

FIGURE 5-1 Integumentary system.

Skeletal System

Bones are the primary organs of the skeletal system. Figure 5-2 shows examples of the 206 individually named bones found in the **skeletal system.** Each individual also has some variable

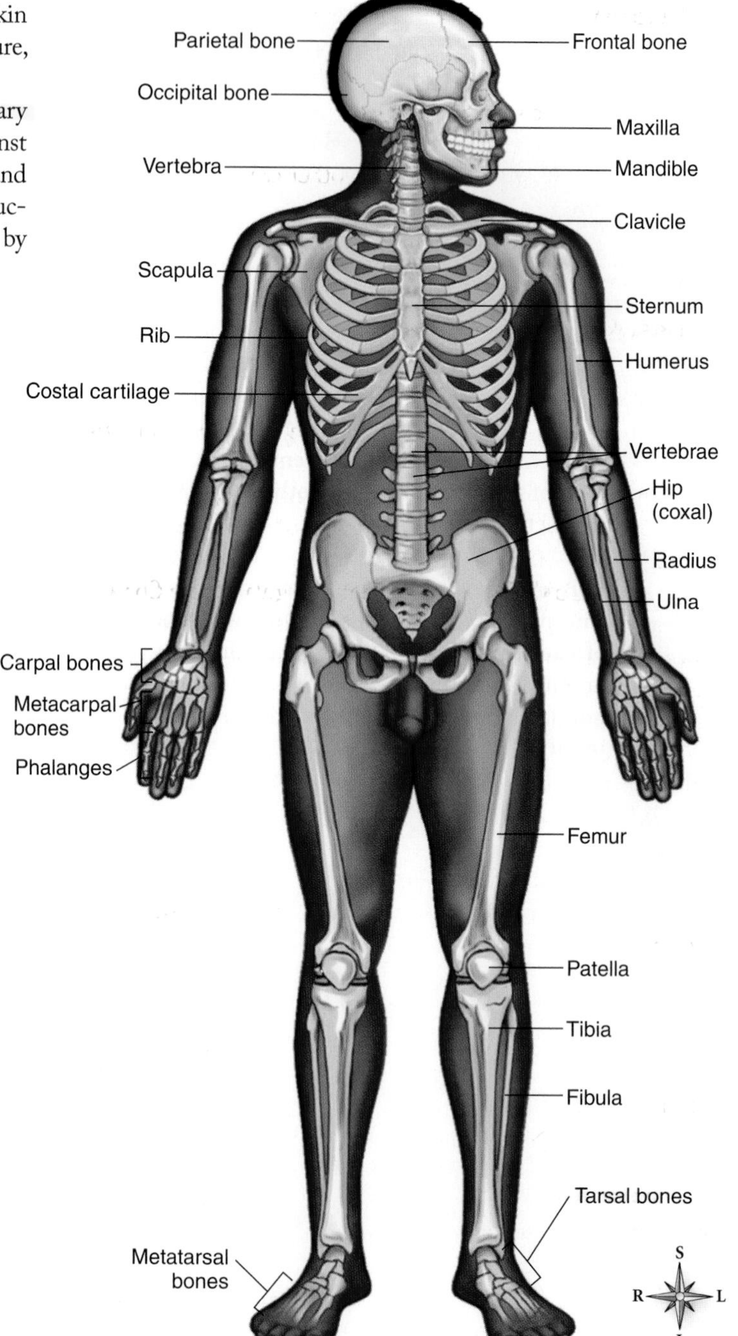

FIGURE 5-2 Skeletal system.

bones that differ from person to person and do not have specific names.

The skeletal system includes not only bones but also related tissues such as cartilage. Cartilage can cushion bones that are linked together and can act as the connection between one bone and another. Look at the large cartilage bands (costal cartilage) that connect the ribs to the sternum in **Figure 5-2**.

Ligaments are bands of fibrous connective tissue that help hold bones together. Connections between two or more bones are called **joints.** The moveable joints between bones make various movements of individual body parts possible. Without movable joints, our bodies would be rigid, immobile hulks.

The skeleton provides protection and a supporting framework for the brain and other internal organs. Without bones and their joints, the body could not move in the way it does. Bones also serve as storage areas for important minerals such as calcium and phosphorus. The formation of blood cells in the red marrow of certain bones is another crucial function of the skeletal system.

Muscular System

Skeletal Muscles

Individual skeletal muscles are the organs of the **muscular system.** Muscles are made up of mostly **skeletal muscle** tissue. Also called **voluntary muscle,** this tissue has the ability to contract when stimulated by conscious nerve regulation. Although movement of the body is the primary function of the muscular system, it also maintains stability of our posture (body position) and provides heat to maintain our body temperature.

A **tendon** is a dense strap or sheet of regular dense fibrous connective tissue. A tendon is part of a muscle organ that attaches the muscle to a bone (or to another muscle). The anterior tibialis tendon of the leg labeled in **Figure 5-3** shows how tendons attach muscles to bones.

When stimulated by a nervous impulse, skeletal muscle tissue shortens or contracts. Voluntary movement occurs when skeletal muscles shorten—a function of the way muscles are attached to bones and the way bones articulate (join) with one another in joints. Sometimes it is useful to think of this cooperative functioning of the bones and muscles as the *skeletomuscular system.*

Muscles of Other Systems

In addition to skeletal muscle organs of the muscular system, the body contains other types of muscle tissue that form parts of organs in other systems of the body.

For example, **smooth muscle** tissue is found in the walls of hollow organs such as the stomach and small intestine. Smooth muscles help move fluids through organs and often form valves that regulate when fluids may move from one section of a hollow organ to another.

A third type of muscle tissue is the **cardiac muscle** in the wall of the heart. By contracting, it pumps blood through the circulatory system. Some cardiac muscle cells in the heart generate the rhythm of the heartbeat.

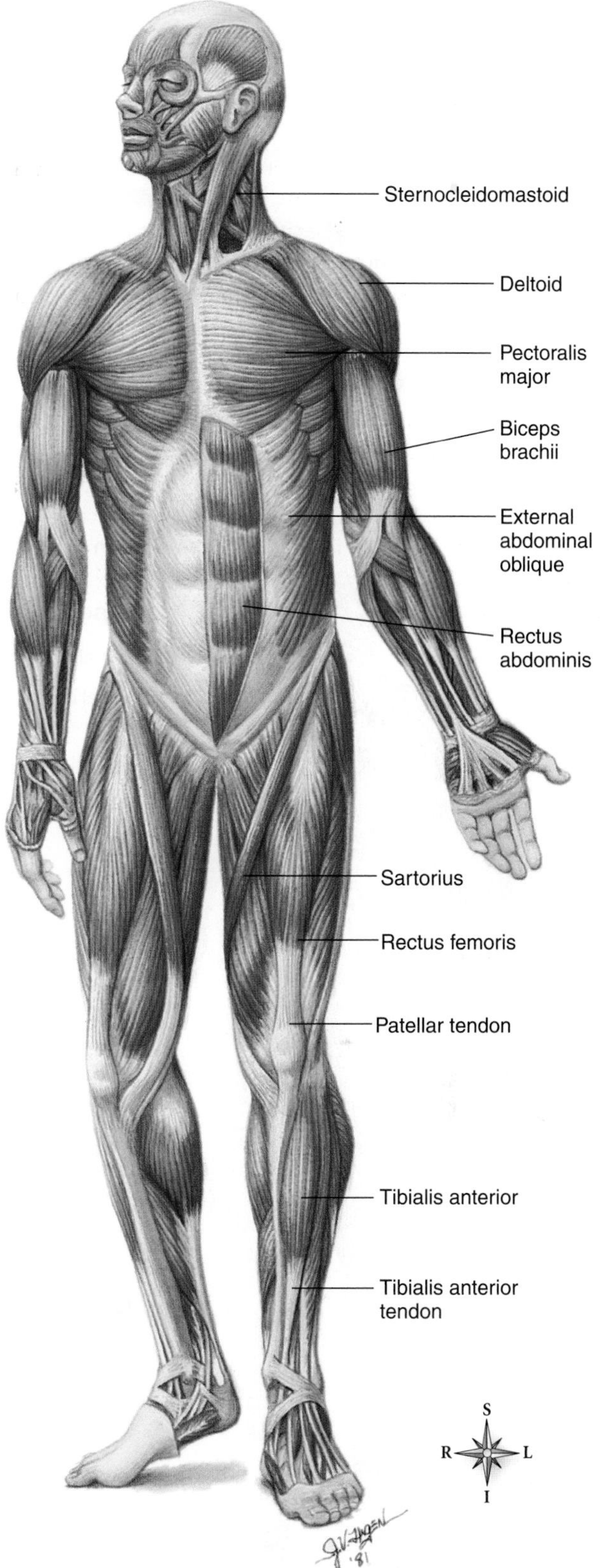

FIGURE 5-3 Muscular system.

Smooth and cardiac muscle tissues are **involuntary** because they are regulated by subconscious mechanisms.

Nervous System

The brain, spinal cord, and nerves are the organs of the **nervous system** (Figure 5-4). The brain and spinal cord make up the **central nervous system (CNS).** These two organs provide the central control of the whole nervous system.

The *cranial nerves* extend from the brain and the *spinal nerves* extend from the spinal cord. The cranial and spinal nerves, and all their branches, make up the **peripheral nervous system (PNS).** The word *peripheral* means "around the boundary," a good term for the nerve branches that extend all the way to the farthest boundaries of the body.

The extensive networking of the components of the nervous system makes it possible for this complex system to perform its primary functions. These include the following:

1. Communication to and from body organs
2. Integration of body functions
3. Control of body functions
4. Detection of sensory stimuli

These functions are performed by signals called **nerve impulses.** In general, the functions of the nervous system result in rapid activity that lasts usually for a short duration. For example, we can chew our food normally, walk, and perform coordinated muscular movements only if our nervous system functions properly. The nerve impulses permit the rapid and precise control of diverse body functions. Other types of nerve impulses cause glands to secrete hormones or other fluids.

In addition, elements of the peripheral nervous system can recognize certain **stimuli,** such as heat, light, sound, pressure, or temperature, that affect the body. When stimulated, these **sense organs** (discussed in Chapter 10) generate nerve impulses that travel to the brain or spinal cord where analysis or relay occurs and, if needed, appropriate action is initiated.

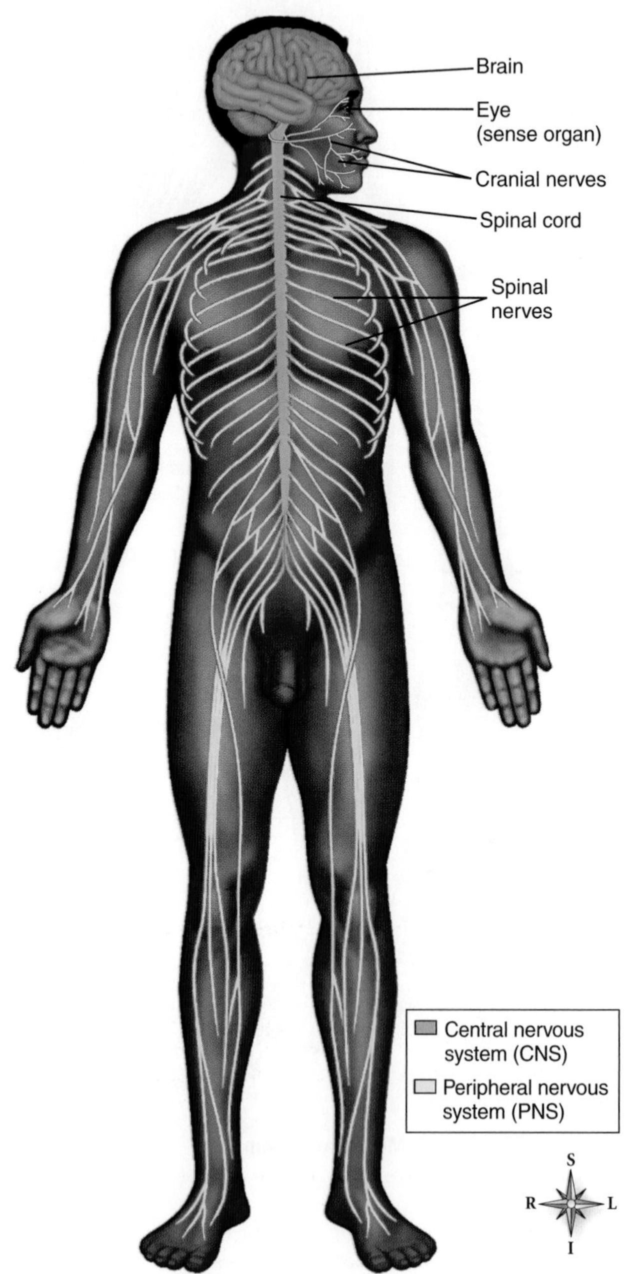

FIGURE 5-4 Nervous system.

Endocrine System

The **endocrine system** is composed of glands that secrete chemicals known as **hormones** directly into the blood. Sometimes called *ductless glands,* the organs of the endocrine system perform the same general functions as the nervous system: communication, integration, and control. The nervous system provides rapid, brief control by fast-traveling nerve impulses. The endocrine system provides slower but longer-lasting control by hormone secretion. For example, secretion of growth hormone controls the rate of development over long periods of gradual growth.

It is no wonder that the nervous and endocrine systems are sometimes thought of as one large regulatory system—the *neuroendocrine system.*

In addition to controlling growth, hormones are the main regulators of metabolism, reproduction, and other body activities. They play important roles in fluid and electrolyte balance and acid-base balance. The various roles of major hormones are integrated into discussions throughout the rest of this book.

As you can see in Figure 5-5, endocrine glands are widely distributed throughout the body. But this is not the complete picture—endocrine glands are far more numerous and widespread than is shown here. We look at just a few of the major endocrine glands.

The **pituitary gland, pineal gland,** and **hypothalamus** are located in the skull. The **thyroid gland** and **parathyroid glands** are in the neck, and the **thymus gland** is in the thoracic cavity, specifically in the mediastinum (see Figure 1-5, p. 9). The **adrenal glands** and **pancreas** are found in the abdominal cavity.

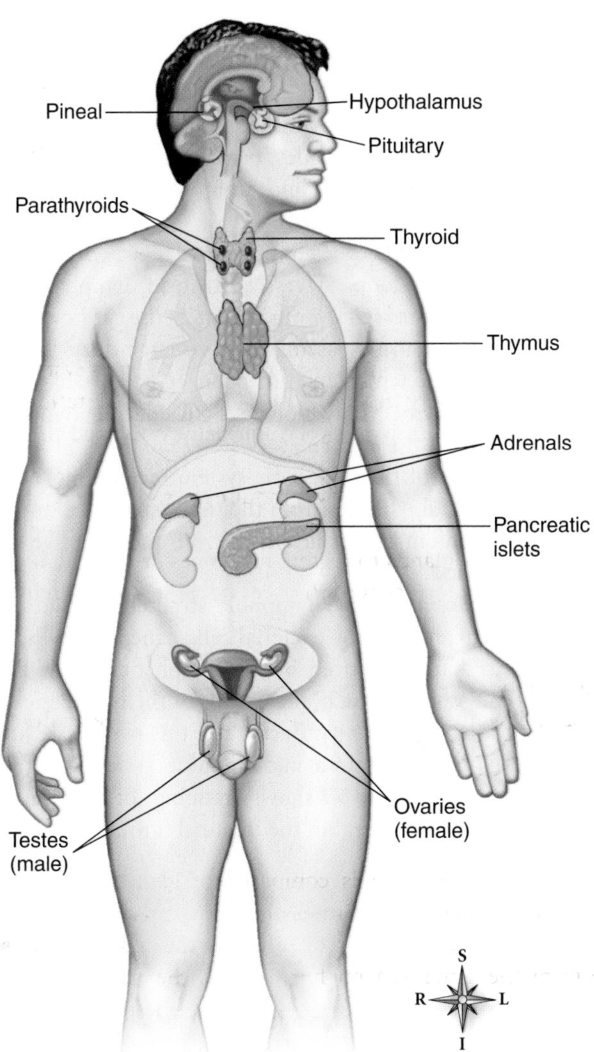

FIGURE 5-5 Endocrine system.

Note in Figure 5-5 that some reproductive glands (ovaries in the female and the testes in the male) also function as endocrine glands.

Cardiovascular System

The **cardiovascular system** consists of the heart and a closed system of vessels made up of **arteries, veins,** and **capillaries** (Figure 5-6). As the name implies, blood contained in this system is pumped by the heart around a closed circle, or circuit, of vessels as it passes through the body. The cardiovascular system is sometimes called the **circulatory system.**

The primary function of the cardiovascular or circulatory system is *transportation.* The need for an efficient transportation system in the body is critical. Transportation needs include continuous movement of oxygen and carbon dioxide, nutrients, hormones, and other important substances. Wastes produced by the cells are released into the bloodstream on an ongoing basis and are transported by the blood to the excretory organs. The cardiovascular system also helps regulate body temperature by distributing heat throughout the body and by assisting in retaining or releasing heat from the body by regulating blood flow near the body surface. Some cells of the cardiovascular system also function in defense of the body by way of immunity.

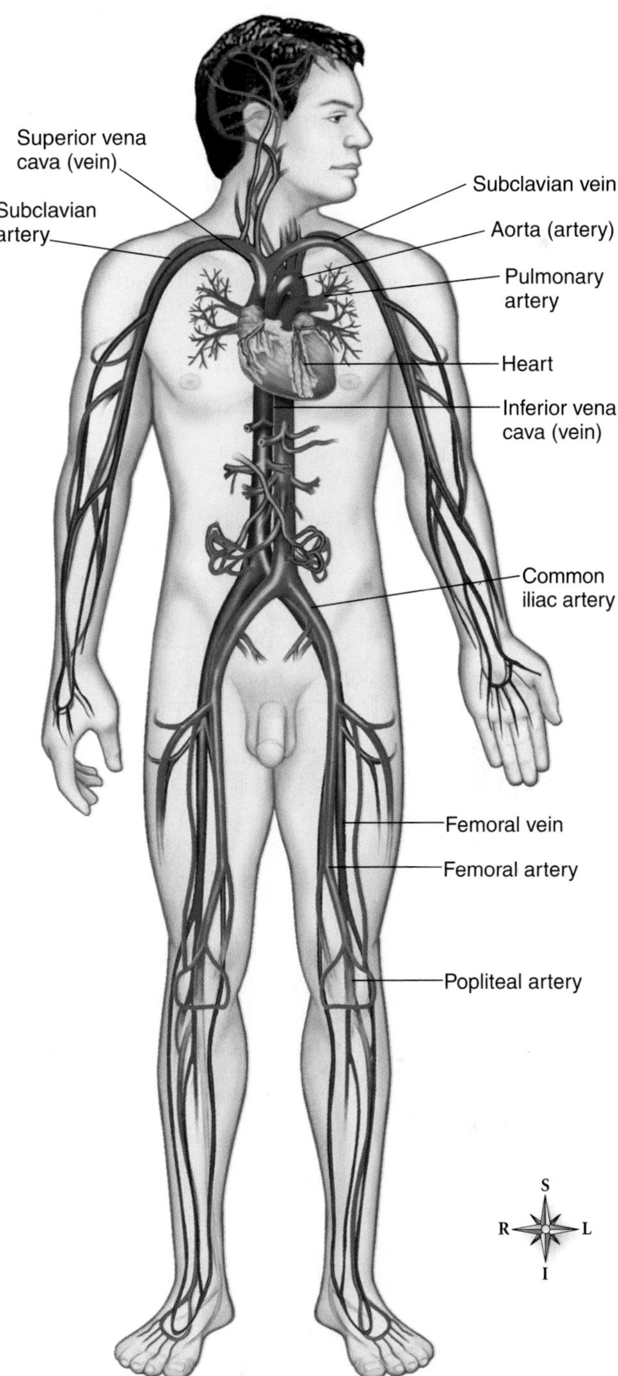

FIGURE 5-6 Cardiovascular (circulatory) system.

QUICK CHECK

1. What is the largest organ in the integumentary system?
2. What are the organs of the skeletal system?
3. What are the major functions of the nervous system?
4. What organs make up the cardiovascular system?

Lymphatic and Immune Systems

Lymphatic System

The **lymphatic system** is composed of **lymphatic vessels** together with other lymphatic organs made up of masses of defensive cells often called *lymphoid tissue.* These lymphoid organs include the **lymph nodes, tonsils, thymus gland**, and **spleen** (**Figure 5-7**). Note that the thymus functions as an endocrine gland and as a lymphatic organ. Although it is part of the skeletal system, *red bone marrow* is often considered to also be a lymphoid structure.

Instead of containing blood, the lymphatic vessels are filled with **lymph,** a watery fluid that contains lymphocytes, proteins, and some fatty molecules, but no red blood cells. The lymph is formed from the fluid around the body cells and diffuses into the lymph vessels.

Unlike blood, lymph does not circulate repeatedly through a closed circuit, or loop, of vessels. Instead, lymph flowing through lymphatic vessels eventually enters the cardiovascular, or circulatory, system by passing through large ducts, such as the **thoracic duct,** which in turn connect with veins in the upper thoracic cavity. Many biologists consider the lymphatic system to be part of the circulatory system.

The functions of the lymphatic system include movement of fluids and small particles from the tissue spaces around the cells and movement of fats absorbed from the digestive tract back to the blood.

Lymph nodes and other lymphoid structures act as small filters that trap and destroy bacterial cells, cancerous cells, and other debris that are carried by the lymph fluid as it flows through the tissues. As such, the organs of the lymphatic system play a role in immunity. Because of this overlap of functions, the lymphatic system and immune system are often discussed together. **Figure 5-7** shows groupings of lymph nodes in the axillary (armpit) and in the inguinal (groin) areas of the body.

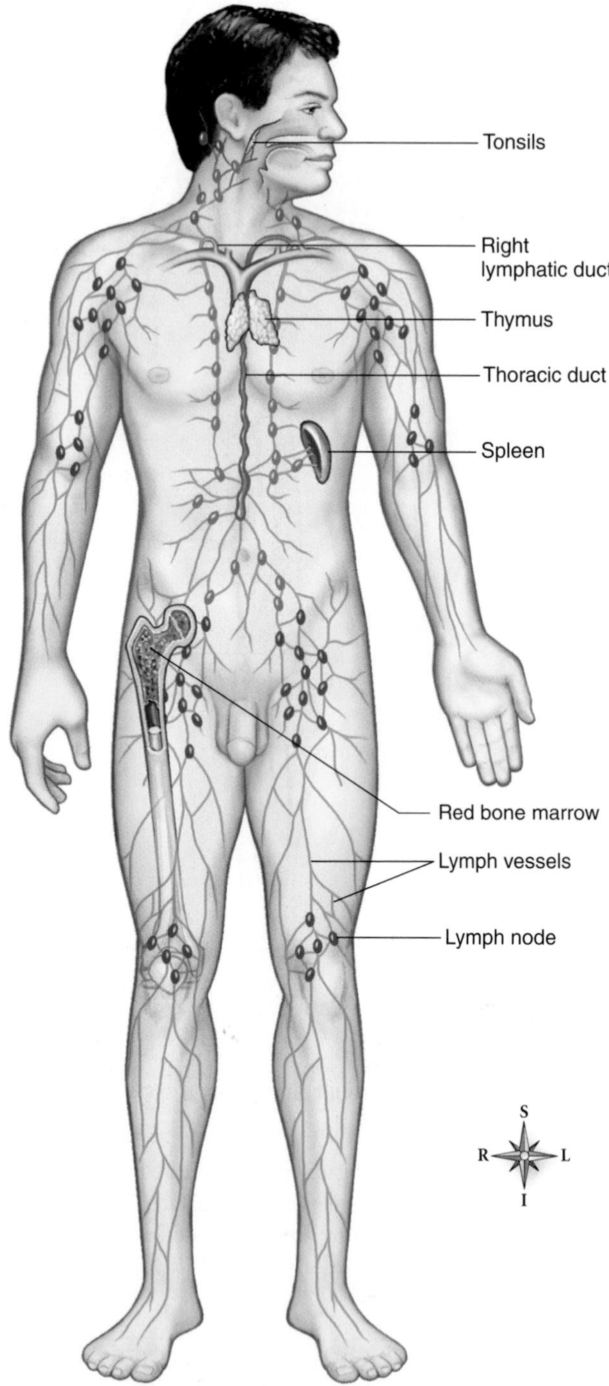

FIGURE 5-7 Lymphatic system.

Immune System

All of the body's defense systems together make up the **immune system.** It protects us from disease-causing microorganisms, harmful toxins, transplanted tissue cells, and any of our own cells that have turned malignant or cancerous. The immune system also helps us react appropriately to various irritants and injuries.

The immune system is composed of protective cells (such as phagocytes) and various types of defensive protein molecules (produced by secretory immune cells). Some immune system cells have the ability to attack, engulf, and destroy harmful bacteria directly by phagocytosis. Other more numerous immune system cells secrete protein compounds called **antibodies** and **complements.** These substances produce chemical reactions that help protect the body from many harmful agents.

The lymphatic and immune systems, which are linked to each other and to the cardiovascular system, are discussed in Chapter 14.

Respiratory System

The major organs of the **respiratory system** include the **nose, pharynx** (throat), **larynx** (voice box), **trachea** (windpipe), **bronchi,** and **lungs** (**Figure 5-8**). Together these organs facilitate the movement of air into the tiny, thin-walled sacs of the lungs called **alveoli.**

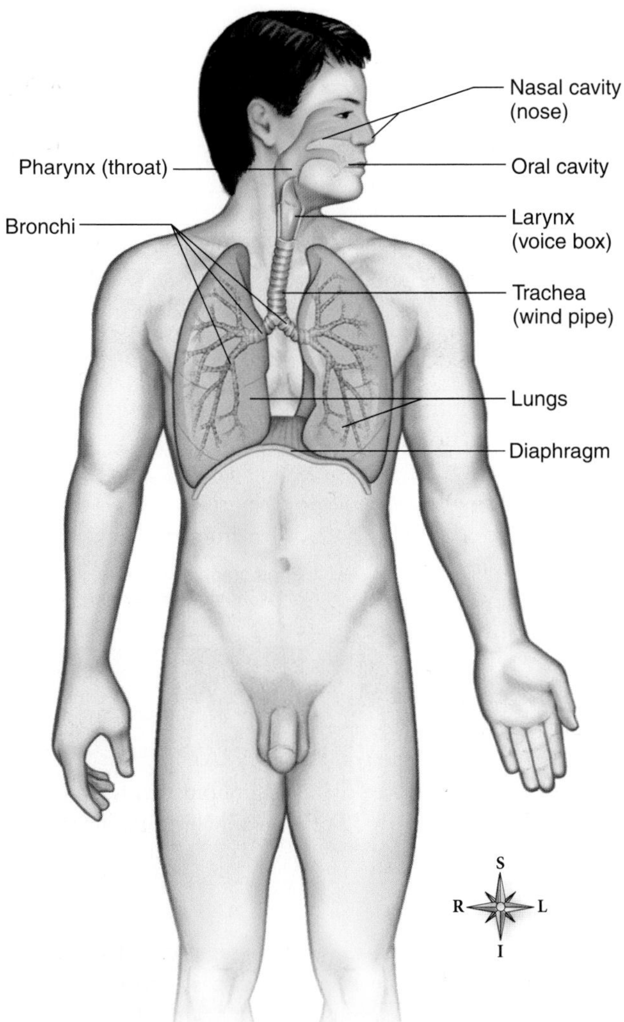

FIGURE 5-8 Respiratory system.

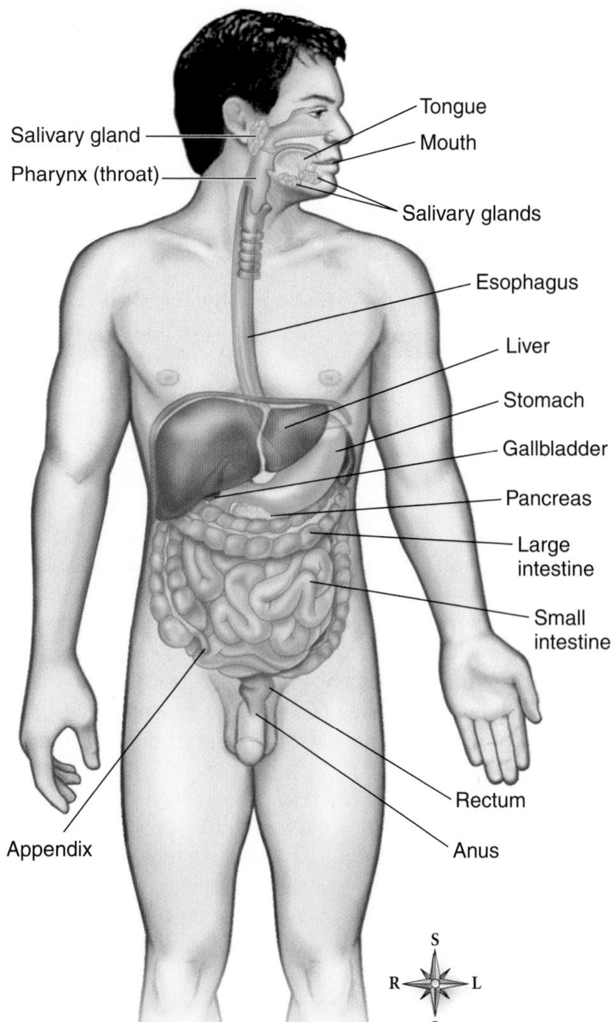

FIGURE 5-9 Digestive system.

In the alveoli, oxygen from the air is exchanged for unneeded carbon dioxide. Carbon dioxide is carried to the lungs by the blood so it can be eliminated from the body. Figure 5-8 also shows the *diaphragm,* which is a sheet of muscle that plays a major role in inflating the lungs during breathing.

The organs of the respiratory system perform a number of functions in addition to permitting movement of air into the alveoli. For example, if you live in a cold or dry environment, incoming air can be warmed and humidified as it passes over the lining of the respiratory air passages. In addition, inhaled irritants such as pollen or dust passing through the respiratory tubes can be trapped in the sticky mucus that covers the lining of many respiratory passages and then eliminated from the body.

The respiratory system also is involved in regulating the acid-base balance of the body—a function that is discussed in Chapter 20.

Digestive System

The organs of the **digestive system** (Figure 5-9) are often separated into two groups: the *primary organs* and the *secondary* or *accessory organs*. They work together to ensure proper digestion and absorption of nutrients—and elimination of waste.

The primary organs of digestion form the digestive tract. They include the mouth, pharynx, esophagus, stomach, small intestine, large intestine, rectum, and anal canal. The accessory organs of digestion may attach to the digestive tract (or be inside it). Accessory digestive organs include the teeth, salivary glands, tongue, liver, gallbladder, pancreas, and appendix.

The digestive tract is a tube, open at both ends. It is also called the **alimentary canal,** a major part of which is the **gastrointestinal (GI) tract.** Food that enters the alimentary canal is digested, its nutrients are absorbed, and the undigested residue is eliminated from the body as waste material called **feces.**

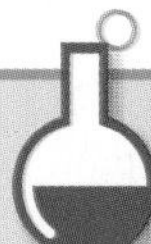

SCIENCE APPLICATIONS

RADIOGRAPHY

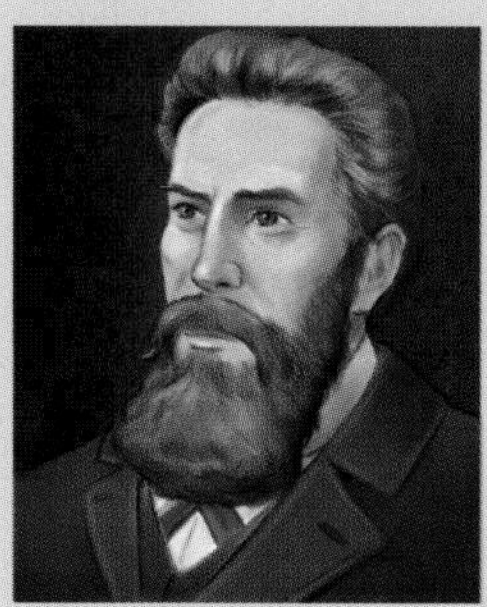
Wilhelm Röntgen (1845-1923)

In 1895, the German physicist Wilhelm Röntgen (RENT-gun) made one of the most important medical discoveries of the modern age: radiographic imaging of the body. **Radiography,** or x-ray photography, is the oldest and still the most widely used method of noninvasive imaging of internal body structures and earned Röntgen a Nobel Prize. While studying the effects of electricity passing through gas under low pressures, Röntgen accidentally discovered x-rays when they caused a plate coated with special chemicals to glow. Not long after that, he showed that they could produce shadows of internal organs such as bones on photographic film. His first, and most famous, radiograph was of his wife Bertha's hand. Although a little fuzzy, it clearly showed Bertha's finger bones and the outline of her ring. When this radiograph was published by a Vienna newspaper, the entire world became instantly aware of his breakthrough discovery.

The figure at right shows how radiography works. A source of waves in the x band of the radiation spectrum beams the x-rays through a body and to a piece of photographic film or phosphorescent screen. The resulting image shows the outlines of bones and other dense structures that absorb the x-rays. As the figure shows, one way to make soft, hollow structures such as digestive organs more visible is to use radiopaque contrast material. For example, barium sulfate (which absorbs x-rays) can be introduced into the colon to make it more visible in a radiograph.

Today, many variations of Röntgen's invention are used to study internal organs without having to cut into the body. For example, computed tomography (CT) scanning is a modern, computerized type of x-ray photography. **Radiological technologists** are health professionals whose chief responsibility is to make radiographs, and **radiologists** are responsible for interpreting these images. Many *medical, veterinary,* and *dental professionals* rely on these images and interpretations in their diagnosis, assessment, and treatment of patients. In addition, radiography is used in many *industrial* and *investigative* settings—even by *archaeologists* studying mummies.

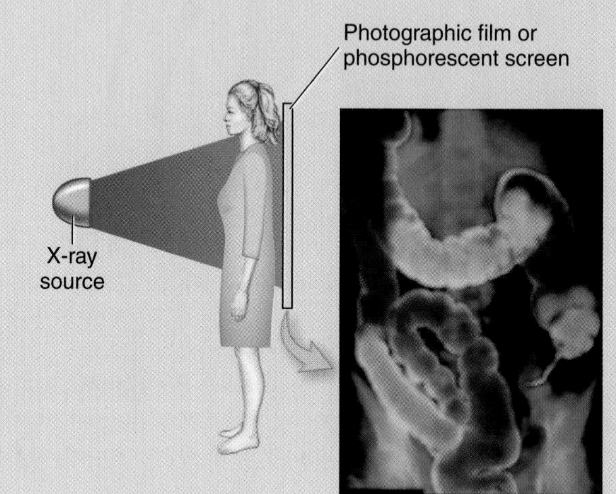

Urinary System

The organs of the **urinary system** include the **kidneys, ureters, urinary bladder,** and **urethra.**

The kidneys (**Figure 5-10**) filter out, or "clear," the blood of the waste products continually produced by the metabolism of nutrients in the body cells. The kidneys also play an important role in maintaining the electrolyte, water, and acid-base balances in the body.

The waste product produced by the kidneys is called **urine.** After it is produced by the kidneys, urine flows out of the kidneys, through the ureters, and into the urinary bladder where it is temporarily stored. Urine passes from the bladder to the outside of the body through the urethra. In the male the urethra passes through the penis and has a double function—it transports both urine and semen (seminal fluid). Therefore it has urinary and reproductive purposes. In the female the urinary and reproductive passages are completely separate, so the urethra performs only a urinary function.

Other organs, in addition to the organs of the urinary system, also are involved in the elimination of body wastes. Undigested food residues and metabolic wastes are eliminated from the intestinal tract as feces, and the lungs rid the body of carbon dioxide. The skin also serves an excretory function by eliminating water and some salts in sweat.

Reproductive Systems

The normal function of the **reproductive system** is different from the normal function of other organ systems of the body. The proper functioning of the reproductive systems ensures survival, not of the individual but of the genes. In addition, production of the hormones that permit the development of sexual characteristics also affects other structures and functions of the body.

This chapter continues on p. 93, after the Clear View insert.

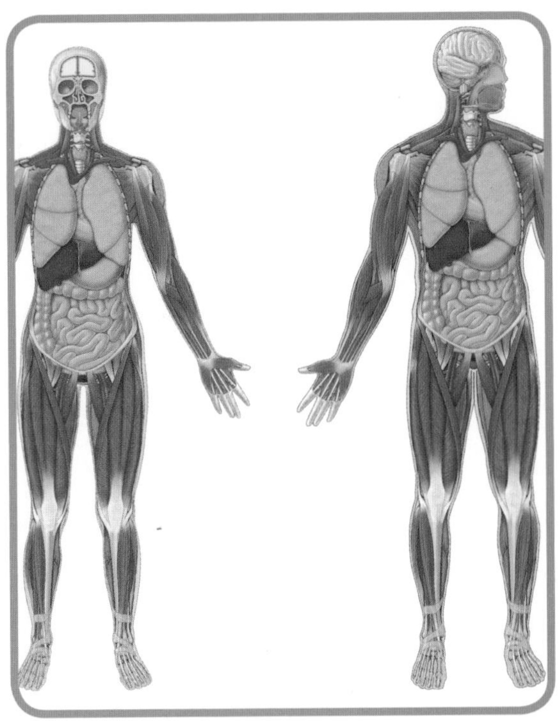

Clear View of the Human Body

Developed by
KEVIN PATTON and PAUL KRIEGER
Illustrated by
Dragonfly Media Group

Introduction

A complete understanding of human anatomy and physiology requires an appreciation for how structures within the body relate to one another. Such appreciation for anatomical structure has become especially important in the twenty-first century with the explosion in the use of diverse methods of medical imaging that rely on the ability to interpret sectional views of the human body.

The best way to develop your understanding of overall anatomical structure is to carefully dissect a large number of male and female human cadavers—then have those dissected specimens handy while reading and learning about each system of the body. Obviously, such multiple dissections and constant access to specimens are impractical for nearly everyone. However, the experience of a simple dissection can be approximated by layering several partially transparent, two-dimensional anatomical diagrams in a way that allows a student to "virtually" dissect the human body simply by paging through the layers.

This **Clear View of the Human Body** provides a handy tool for dissecting simulated male and female bodies. It also provides views of several different parts of the human body in a variety of cross sections. The many different anterior and posterior views also give you a perspective on body structure that is not available with ordinary anatomical diagrams. This Clear View is an always-available tool to help you learn the three-dimensional structure of the body in a way that allows you to see how they relate to each other in a complete body. It will always be right here in your textbook, so place a bookmark here and refer to the Clear View frequently as you study each of the systems of the human body.

Hints for Using the Clear View of the Body

1. Starting at the first page of the Clear View, slowly lift the page as you look at the anterior view of the male and female bodies. You will see deeper structures appear, as if you had dissected the body. As you lift each successive layer of images, you will be looking at deeper and deeper body structures. A key to the labels is found in the gray sidebar.
2. Starting with the second section of the Clear View, notice that you are looking at the posterior aspect of the male and female body. Lift each layer from the edge to reveal body structures in successive layers from the back to the front. This very unique view will help you understand structural relationships even better.
3. On each page of the Clear View, look at the transverse section represented in the sidebar. The section you are looking at on any one page is from the location shown in the larger diagram as a red line. In other words, if you cut the body at the red line and tilted the upper part of the body toward you, you would see what is shown in the section diagram. Notice that each section has its own labeling system that is separate from the labels used in the larger images.

KEY

1. Epicranius m.
2. Temporalis m.
3. Orbicularis oculi m.
4. Masseter m.
5. Orbicularis oris m.
6. Pectoralis major m.
7. Serratus anterior m.
8. Basilic vein
9. Brachial fascia
10. Cephalic vein
11. Rectus sheath
12. Linea alba
13. Rectus abdominis m.
14. Umbilicus
15. Abdominal oblique m., external
16. Abdominal oblique m., internal
17. Transverse abdominis m.
18. Inguinal ring, external
19. Fossa ovalis
20. Fascia of the thigh
21. Great saphenous vein
22. Parietal bone
23. Frontal bone
24. Temporal bone
25. Zygomatic bone
26. Maxilla
27. Mandible
28. Sternocleidomastoid m.
29. Sternohyoid muscle
30. Omohyoid muscle
31. Deltoid m.
32. Pectoralis minor m.
33. Sternum
34. Rib (costal) cartilage
35. Rib
36. Greater omentum
37. Frontal lobe
38. Parietal lobe
39. Temporal lobe
40. Cerebellum
41. Nasal septum
42. Brachiocephalic vein
43. Superior vena cava
44. Thymus gland
45. Right lung
46. Left lung
47. Pericardium
48. Liver
49. Gallbladder
50. Stomach
51. Transverse colon
52. Small intestines
53. Biceps brachii m.
54. Brachioradialis m.
55. Adductor longus m.
56. Sartorius m.
57. Quadriceps femoris m.
58. Patellar ligament
59. Tibialis anterior m.
60. Sup. extensor retinaculum
61. Inf. extensor retinaculum
62. Cerebrum of brain
63. Cerebellum
64. Brainstem
65. Maxillary sinus
66. Nasal cavity
67. Tongue
68. Thyroid gland
69. Heart
70. Hepatic veins
71. Esophagus
72. Spleen
73. Celiac artery
74. Portal vein
75. Duodenum
76. Pancreas
77. Mesenteric artery
78. Ascending colon
79. Transverse colon
80. Descending colon
81. Sigmoid colon
82. Mesentery
83. Appendix
84. Inguinal ligament
85. Pubic symphysis
86. Extensor carpi radialis m.
87. Pronator teres m.
88. Flexor carpi radialis m.
89. Flexor digitorum profundus m.
90. Quadriceps femoris m.
91. Extensor digitorum longus m.
92. Thyroid cartilage
93. Trachea
94. Aortic arch
95. Right lung
96. Left lung
97. Pulmonary artery
98. Right atrium
99. Right ventricle
100. Left atrium
101. Left ventricle
102. Coracobrachialis m.
103. Inferior vena cava
104. Descending aorta
105. Right kidney
106. Left kidney
107. Right ureter
108. Rectum
109. Urinary bladder
110. Prostate gland
111. Iliac artery and vein
112. Uterus
113. Parietal bone
114. Frontal sinus
115. Sphenoidal sinus
116. Occipital bone
117. Palatine process
118. Cervical vertebrae
119. Corpus callosum
120. Thalamus
121. Trapezius m.
122. Acromion process
123. Coracoid process
124. Humerus
125. Subscapularis m.
126. Deltoid m. (cut)
127. Triceps m.
128. Brachialis m.
129. Brachioradialis m.
130. Radius
131. Ulna
132. Diaphragm
133. Thoracic duct
134. Quadratus lumborum m.
135. Psoas m.
136. Lumbar vertebrae
137. Iliacus m.
138. Gluteus medius m.
139. Iliofemoral ligament
140. Sacral nerves
141. Sacrum
142. Coccyx
143. Femur
144. Vastus lateralis m.
145. Femoral artery and vein
146. Adductor magnus m.
147. Patella
148. Fibula
149. Tibia
150. Fibularis longus m.
151. Spinal cord
152. Nerve root
153. Platysma m.
154. Splenius capitis m.
155. Levator scapulae m.
156. Rhomboideus m.
157. Infraspinatus m.
158. Teres major m.
159. Lumbodorsal fascia
160. Erector spinae m.
161. Serratus post. inf. m.
162. Latissimus dorsi m.
163. Gluteus medius m.
164. Gluteus maximus m.
165. Iliotibial tract
166. Flexor carpi ulnaris m.
167. Extensor carpi ulnaris m.
168. Extensor digitorum m.
169. Carpal ligament, dorsal
170. Interosseous m.
171. Gluteus minimus m.
172. Piriformis m.
173. Gemellus sup. m.
174. Obturator internus m.
175. Gemellus inf. m.
176. Quadratus femoris m.
177. Biceps femoris m.
178. Gastrocnemius m.
179. Calcaneal (Achilles) tendon
180. Calcaneus bone
181. Subcutaneous fat
182. Corpus spongiosum
183. Corpora cavernosa
184. Umbilical ligaments
185. Epigastric artery and vein
186. Right testis
187. Transverse thoracic m.
188. Parietal pleura
189. Common bile duct
190. Lesser omentum
191. Flexor digitorum profundus
192. Epiglottis

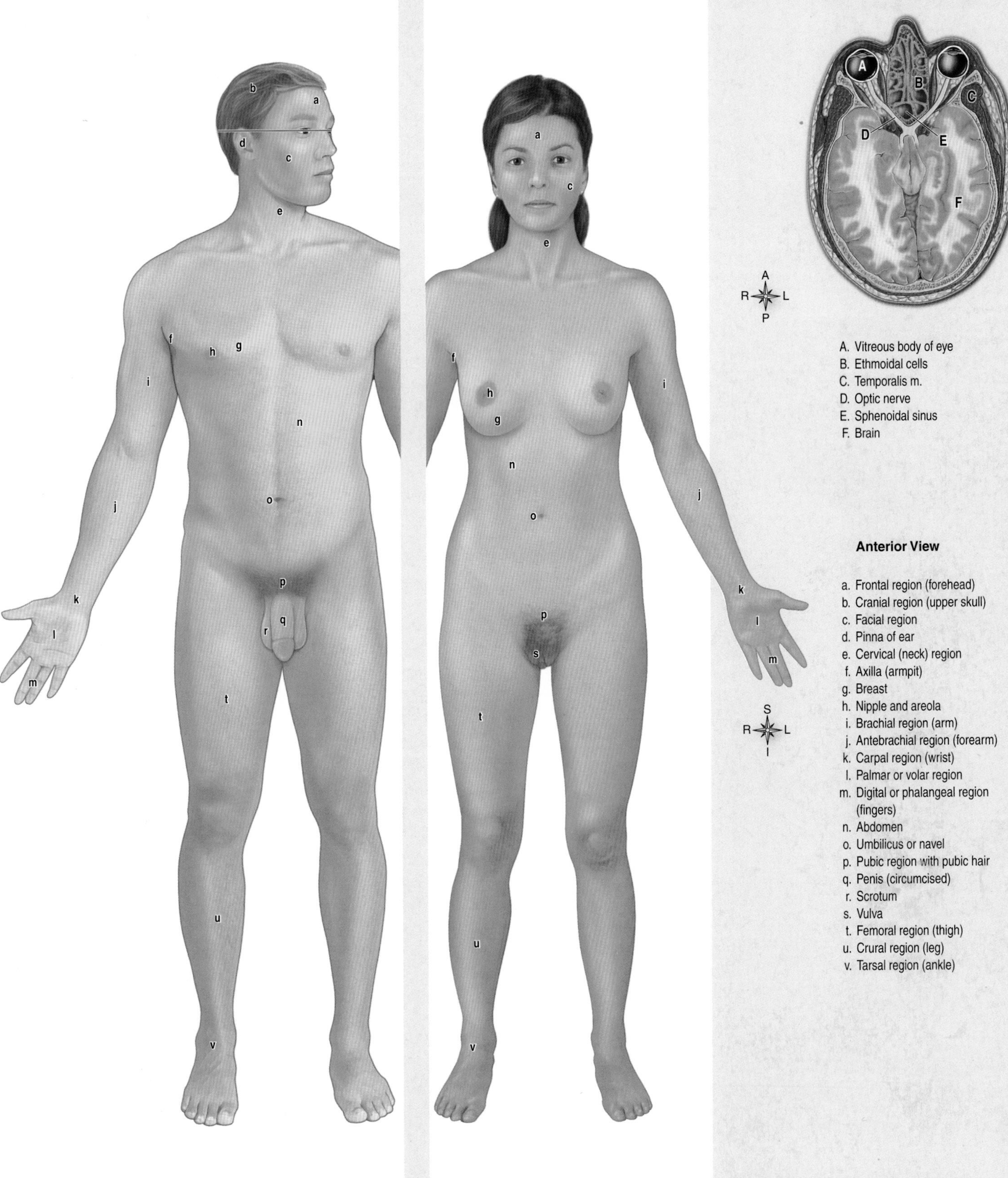

Head - Transverse Section
A
B
C
D
E
F
A
R
L
P
A. Vitreous body of eye
B. Ethmoidal cells
C. Temporalis m.
D. Optic nerve
E. Sphenoidal sinus
F. Brain
Anterior View
a. Frontal region (forehead)
b. Cranial region (upper skull)
c. Facial region
d. Pinna of ear
e. Cervical (neck) region
f. Axilla (armpit)
g. Breast
h. Nipple and areola
i. Brachial region (arm)
j. Antebrachial region (forearm)
k. Carpal region (wrist)
l. Palmar or volar region
m. Digital or phalangeal region (fingers)
n. Abdomen
o. Umbilicus or navel
p. Pubic region with pubic hair
q. Penis (circumcised)
r. Scrotum
s. Vulva
t. Femoral region (thigh)
u. Crural region (leg)
v. Tarsal region (ankle)
S
R
L
I

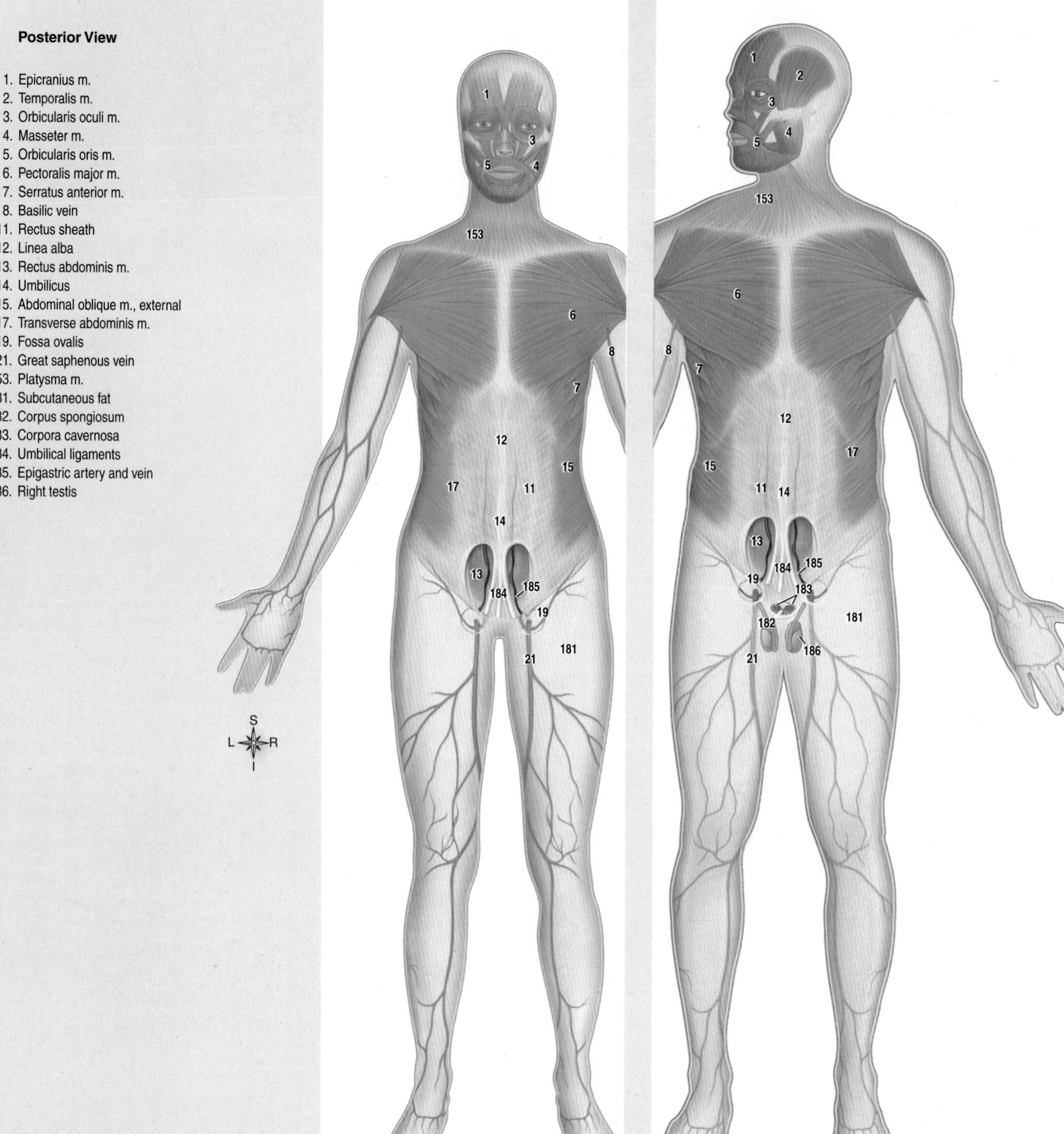
Posterior View
1. Epicranius m.
2. Temporalis m.
3. Orbicularis oculi m.
4. Masseter m.
5. Orbicularis oris m.
6. Pectoralis major m.
7. Serratus anterior m.
8. Basilic vein
11. Rectus sheath
12. Linea alba
13. Rectus abdominis m.
14. Umbilicus
15. Abdominal oblique m., external
17. Transverse abdominis m.
19. Fossa ovalis
21. Great saphenous vein
153. Platysma m.
181. Subcutaneous fat
182. Corpus spongiosum
183. Corpora cavernosa
184. Umbilical ligaments
185. Epigastric artery and vein
186. Right testis
S
L
R
I

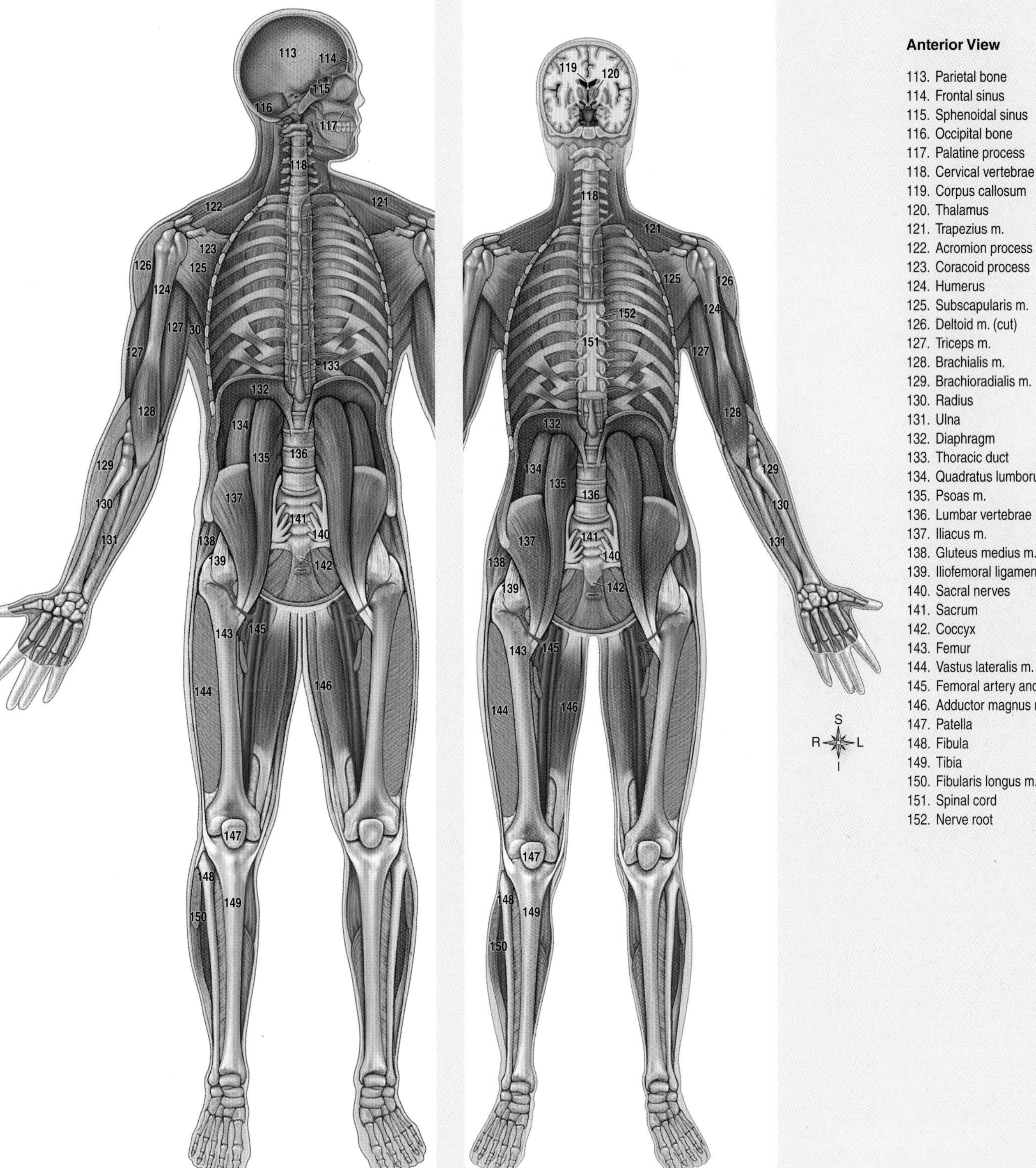

Anterior View

113. Parietal bone
114. Frontal sinus
115. Sphenoidal sinus
116. Occipital bone
117. Palatine process
118. Cervical vertebrae
119. Corpus callosum
120. Thalamus
121. Trapezius m.
122. Acromion process
123. Coracoid process
124. Humerus
125. Subscapularis m.
126. Deltoid m. (cut)
127. Triceps m.
128. Brachialis m.
129. Brachioradialis m.
130. Radius
131. Ulna
132. Diaphragm
133. Thoracic duct
134. Quadratus lumborum m.
135. Psoas m.
136. Lumbar vertebrae
137. Iliacus m.
138. Gluteus medius m.
139. Iliofemoral ligament
140. Sacral nerves
141. Sacrum
142. Coccyx
143. Femur
144. Vastus lateralis m.
145. Femoral artery and vein
146. Adductor magnus m.
147. Patella
148. Fibula
149. Tibia
150. Fibularis longus m.
151. Spinal cord
152. Nerve root

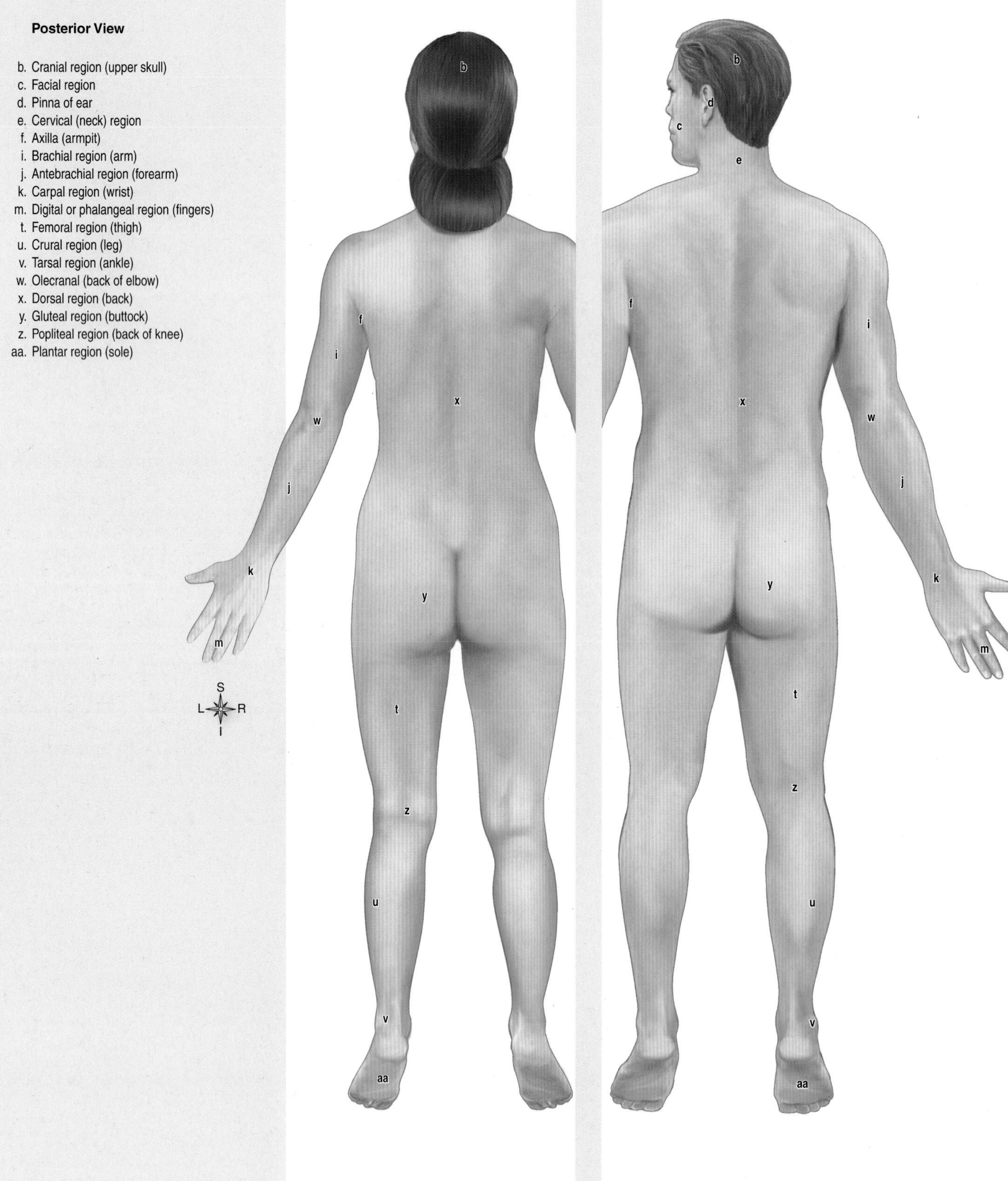

Posterior View

b. Cranial region (upper skull)
c. Facial region
d. Pinna of ear
e. Cervical (neck) region
f. Axilla (armpit)
i. Brachial region (arm)
j. Antebrachial region (forearm)
k. Carpal region (wrist)
m. Digital or phalangeal region (fingers)
t. Femoral region (thigh)
u. Crural region (leg)
v. Tarsal region (ankle)
w. Olecranal (back of elbow)
x. Dorsal region (back)
y. Gluteal region (buttock)
z. Popliteal region (back of knee)
aa. Plantar region (sole)

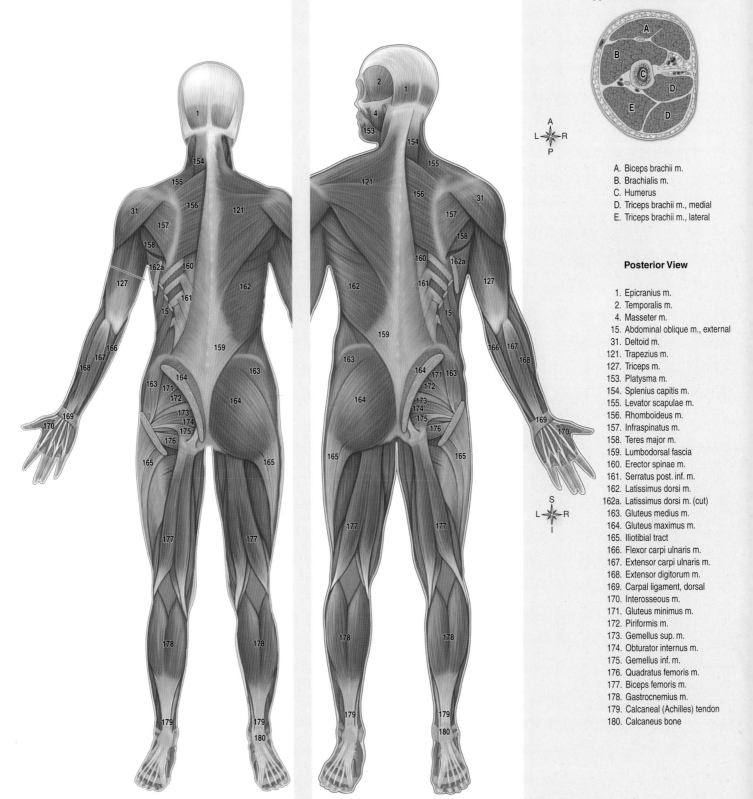

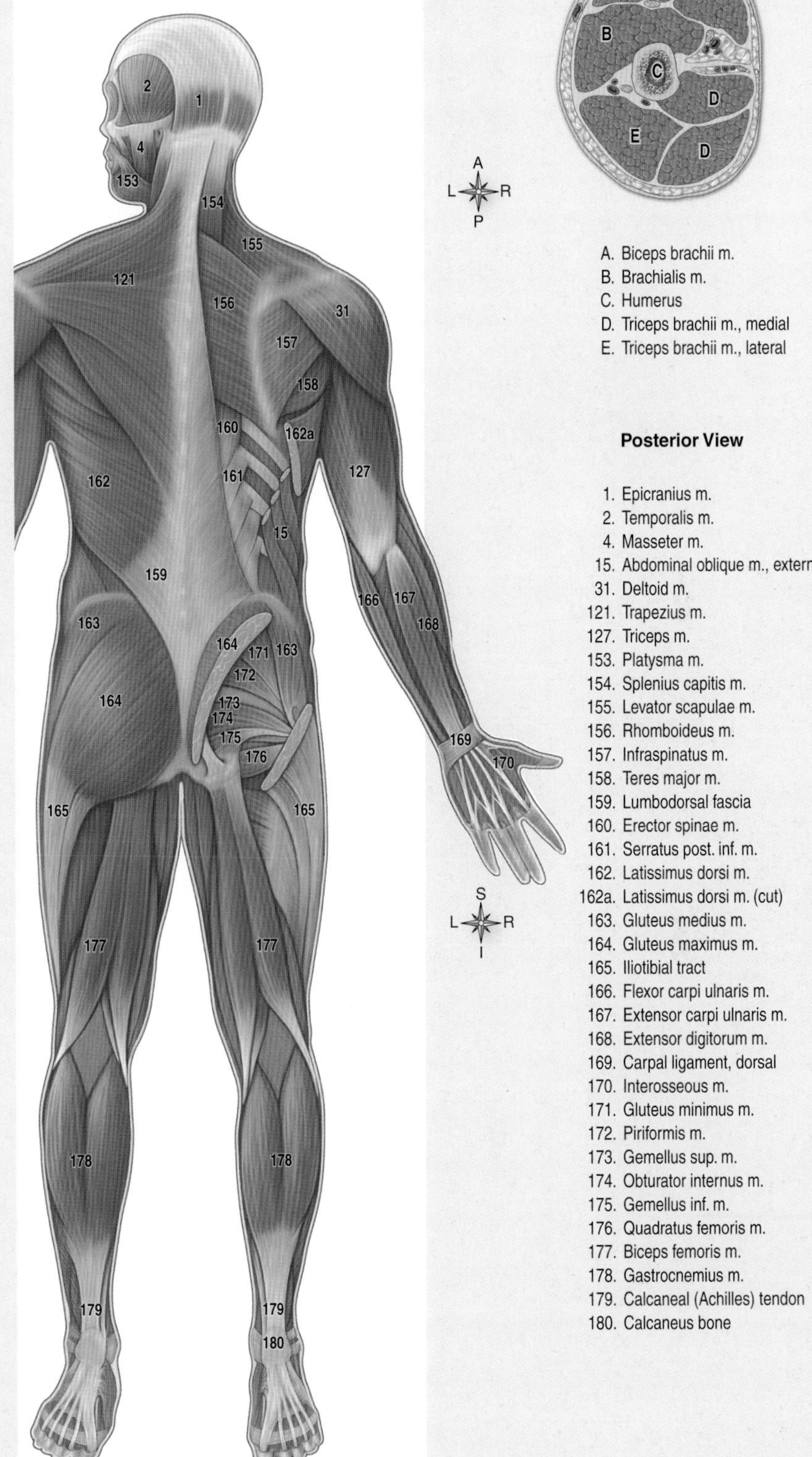

Upper Arm - Transverse Section

A. Biceps brachii m.
B. Brachialis m.
C. Humerus
D. Triceps brachii m., medial
E. Triceps brachii m., lateral

Posterior View

1. Epicranius m.
2. Temporalis m.
4. Masseter m.
15. Abdominal oblique m., external
31. Deltoid m.
121. Trapezius m.
127. Triceps m.
153. Platysma m.
154. Splenius capitis m.
155. Levator scapulae m.
156. Rhomboideus m.
157. Infraspinatus m.
158. Teres major m.
159. Lumbodorsal fascia
160. Erector spinae m.
161. Serratus post. inf. m.
162. Latissimus dorsi m.
162a. Latissimus dorsi m. (cut)
163. Gluteus medius m.
164. Gluteus maximus m.
165. Iliotibial tract
166. Flexor carpi ulnaris m.
167. Extensor carpi ulnaris m.
168. Extensor digitorum m.
169. Carpal ligament, dorsal
170. Interosseous m.
171. Gluteus minimus m.
172. Piriformis m.
173. Gemellus sup. m.
174. Obturator internus m.
175. Gemellus inf. m.
176. Quadratus femoris m.
177. Biceps femoris m.
178. Gastrocnemius m.
179. Calcaneal (Achilles) tendon
180. Calcaneus bone

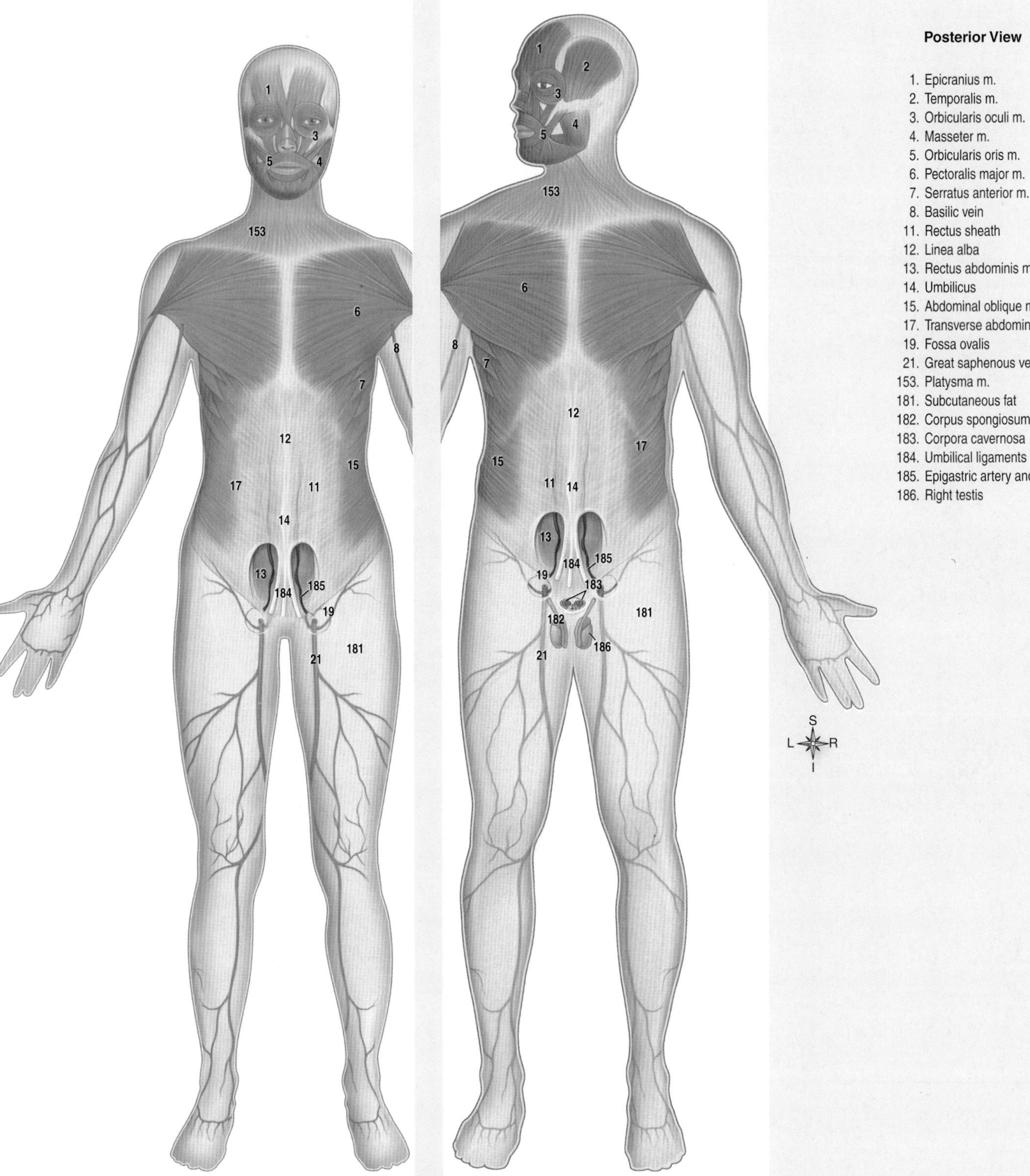

Posterior View

1. Epicranius m.
2. Temporalis m.
3. Orbicularis oculi m.
4. Masseter m.
5. Orbicularis oris m.
6. Pectoralis major m.
7. Serratus anterior m.
8. Basilic vein
11. Rectus sheath
12. Linea alba
13. Rectus abdominis m.
14. Umbilicus
15. Abdominal oblique m., external
17. Transverse abdominis m.
19. Fossa ovalis
21. Great saphenous vein
153. Platysma m.
181. Subcutaneous fat
182. Corpus spongiosum
183. Corpora cavernosa
184. Umbilical ligaments
185. Epigastric artery and vein
186. Right testis

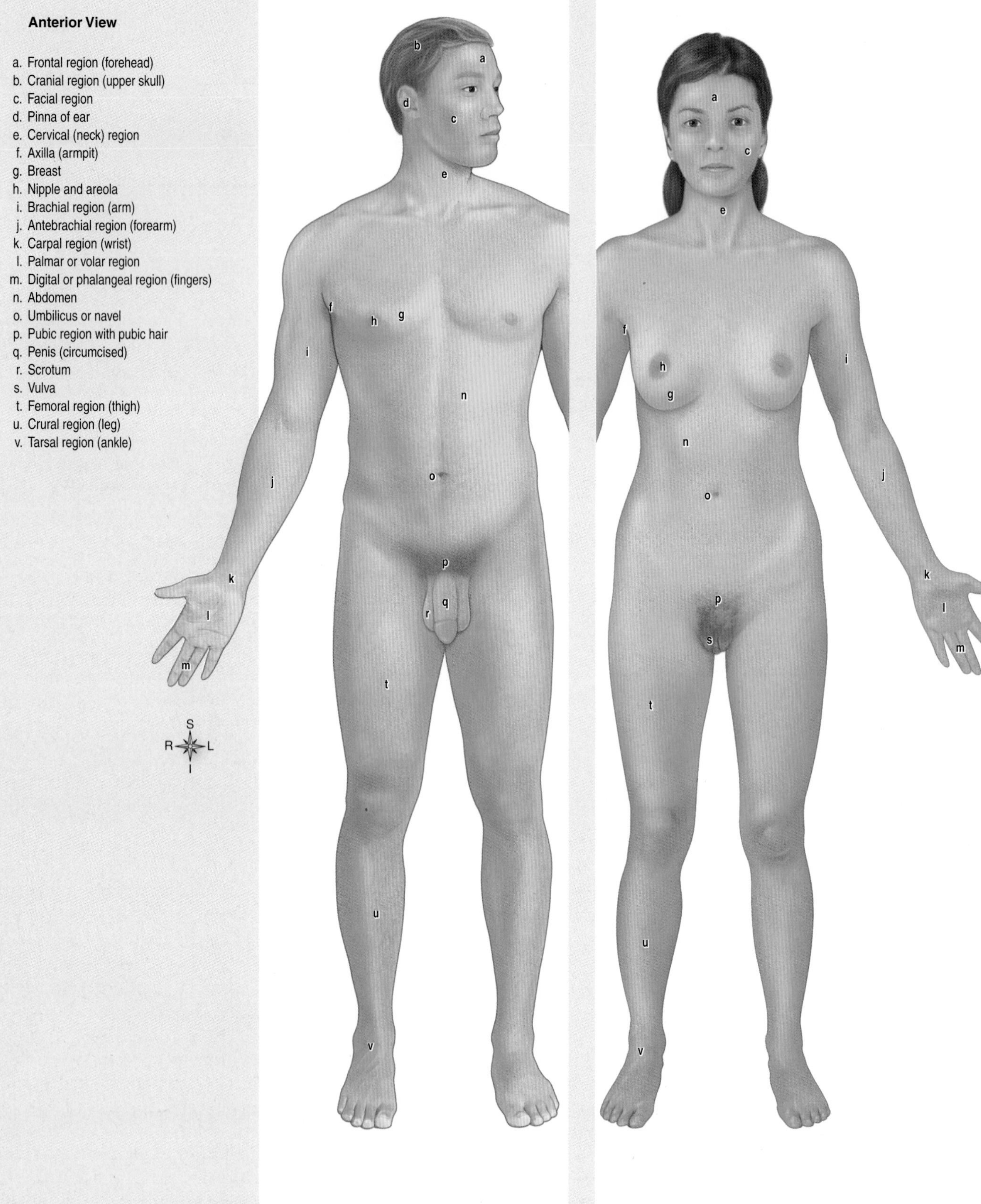

Anterior View
a. Frontal region (forehead)
b. Cranial region (upper skull)
c. Facial region
d. Pinna of ear
e. Cervical (neck) region
f. Axilla (armpit)
g. Breast
h. Nipple and areola
i. Brachial region (arm)
j. Antebrachial region (forearm)
k. Carpal region (wrist)
l. Palmar or volar region
m. Digital or phalangeal region (fingers)
n. Abdomen
o. Umbilicus or navel
p. Pubic region with pubic hair
q. Penis (circumcised)
r. Scrotum
s. Vulva
t. Femoral region (thigh)
u. Crural region (leg)
v. Tarsal region (ankle)
S
R
L
I

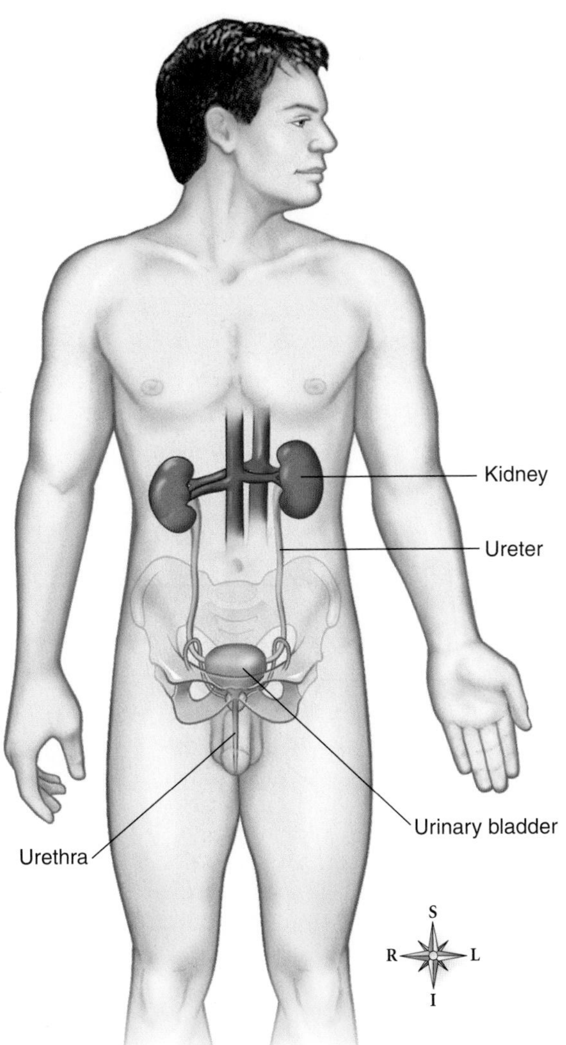

FIGURE 5-10 Urinary system.

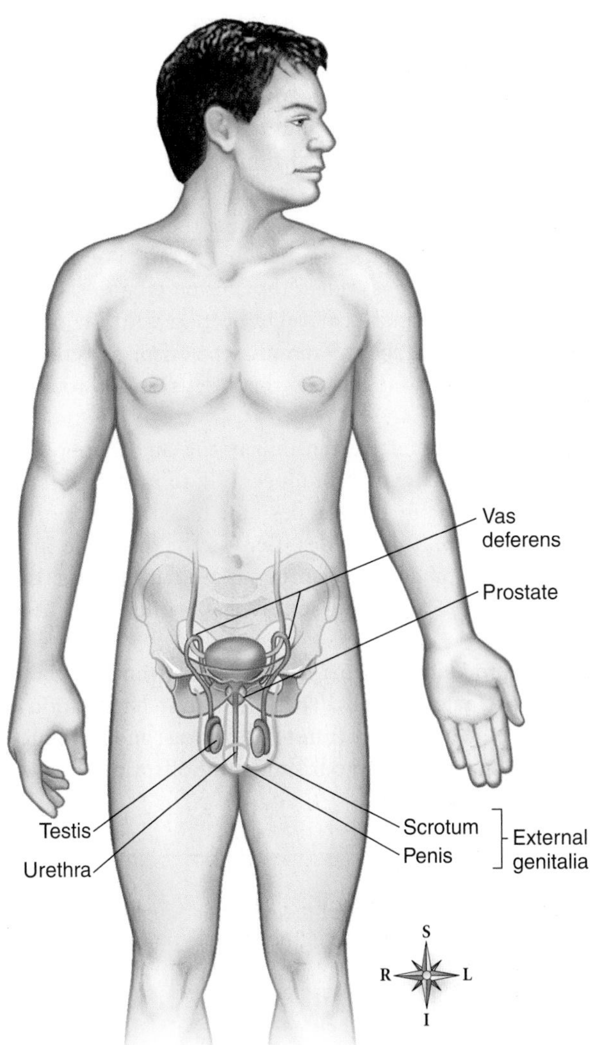

FIGURE 5-11 Male reproductive system.

Humans reproduce sexually (two-parent reproduction) and therefore we have two systems: the male reproductive system and the female reproductive system. An individual has either the male or the female system. Both systems have **gonads** that both produce sex cells for forming the offspring and produce hormones that regulate reproductive functions.

Male Reproductive System

The male reproductive structures shown in Figure 5-11 include the **testes,** which produce the sex cells and thus serve as the male gonads. The testes produce **sperm** and the male hormone *testosterone.* A tube called the **vas deferens** extends from each testis and leads to the urethra. Surrounding the upper urethra is the **prostate,** which is an exocrine gland.

The **penis** and **scrotum** are external structures and together are known as the external **genitalia.** The urethra, which is identified in Figure 5-10 as part of the urinary system, passes through the penis. It carries sperm to the exterior and acts as a passageway for the elimination of urine.

Functioning together, the male reproductive structures produce sperm and introduce them into the female reproductive tract, where fertilization can occur. Sperm produced by the testes travel through a number of ducts, including the vas deferens, to exit the body. The prostate and other accessory organs, which add fluid and nutrients to the sex cells as they pass through the ducts and the supporting structures (especially the penis), facilitate transfer of sex cells into the female reproductive tract.

Female Reproductive System

The female gonads are the **ovaries.** Other reproductive organs shown in Figure 5-12 include the **uterus, uterine tubes** or **fallopian tubes,** and the **vagina.** In the female the term **vulva** is used to describe the external genitalia.

Eggs, or **ova,** are sex cells produced by the ovaries. Ova travel through the uterine tubes, where they may be fertilized by sperm. As the offspring formed by the union of sperm and ovum matures, it moves down the uterine tube to the uterus, where it implants and forms a connection with the mother's blood vessels. After about 9 months, the offspring is delivered through the *cervix* (neck) of the uterus and through the vagina.

The breasts are fatty extensions of the skin that house the **mammary glands,** which produce milk to nurture offspring. They are present in both males and females, but normally only produce milk in females. Because of their role in supporting development of offspring, mammary glands usually are classified as accessory sex organs, rather than as skin glands.

The reproductive organs in the female produce the ova; receive the male sex cells (sperm); permit fertilization and transfer of the fertilized ovum to the uterus; and facilitate the development, birth, and nourishment of offspring.

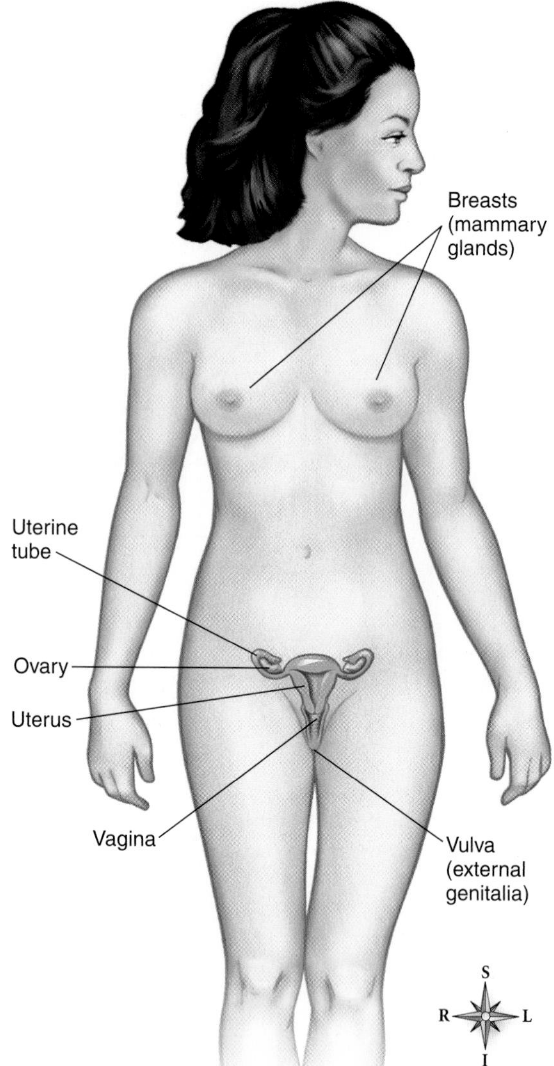

FIGURE 5-12 Female reproductive system.

QUICK CHECK

1. What are the functions of the lymphatic system?
2. What are three ways the immune system fights disease-causing microorganisms?
3. What functions besides gas exchange are performed by the respiratory system?
4. What are the primary organs of the digestive system?
5. What are the accessory organs of the digestive system?
6. What organ in males is shared by both the urinary system and the reproductive system?

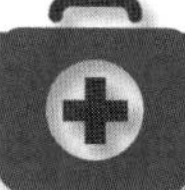

HEALTH AND WELL-BEING

CANCER SCREENING TESTS

Knowledge of the structure and function of the body organ systems is a critically important "first step" in understanding and using information that empowers us to become more sophisticated guardians of our own health and well-being. For example, a better understanding of the reproductive system helps individuals participate in a more direct and personal way in cancer prevention screening techniques.

Breast and testicular self-examinations to detect cancer are two important ways that women and men can participate directly in protecting their own health. In addition, regular examination of the skin surface to detect changes in moles or the appearance, or change in appearance, of other growths or pigmented areas can help in the early detection of skin cancer. Indeed, many other "danger signs of cancer," such as changes in bowel habits, persistent cough, or difficulty in swallowing, can be better understood and appropriate action steps can be initiated earlier with an understanding of the structure and function of the organ systems of the body. Information and specific instructions concerning cancer screening tests are available from the American Cancer Society and from most hospitals, clinics, and health-care providers.

The Body as a Whole

As you study the details of structure and function of the various organ systems in the chapters that follow, it is important that you focus on how each system and its component organs relate to other systems and to the body as a whole.

Table 5-1 lists major organs of each system and identifies the function of each system in the context of *homeostasis*. The concept of homeostasis, introduced in Chapter 1, explains how the body maintains or is able to restore relative constancy to its internal environment even when faced with changing external surroundings or internal needs.

For example, contraction of a muscle can produce a specific body movement only if it is attached appropriately to a bone in the skeletal system. In order for contraction to begin, muscles must first be stimulated by nervous impulses generated in

TABLE 5-1 Human Body Systems

BODY SYSTEM	MAJOR ORGANS		GENERAL FUNCTION
Integumentary	Skin (includes hair, nails, glands)		Separates internal environment from external environment
Skeletal	Bones Ligaments		Supports, protects, and moves body Stores minerals
Muscular	Muscles		Powers and directs skeletal movement Stabilizes the skeleton to maintain posture Generates heat
Nervous	Central Brain Spinal cord	Peripheral Cranial nerves and branches Peripheral nerves and branches Sense organs	Major regulatory systems of the internal environment Senses changes, integrates information, and sends signals to effectors (muscular organs, glands)
Endocrine	Pituitary gland Pineal gland Hypothalamus Thyroid gland Adrenal glands	Pancreatic islets Ovaries Testes Other glands	Regulates internal environment by secreting hormones that travel through bloodstream to target areas
Cardiovascular (circulatory)	Heart Arteries	Veins Capillaries	Transports nutrients, water, oxygen, hormones, wastes, and other materials within the internal environment
Lymphatic/Immune	Lymph nodes Lymph vessels Thymus	Spleen Tonsils Other lymphoid organs	Drains excess fluid from tissues, cleans it, and returns it to the blood Defends internal environment from injury by abnormal cells, foreign particles, and other irritants
Respiratory	Nose Pharynx Larynx	Trachea Bronchi Lungs	Exchanges O_2 and CO_2 between the internal and external environment
Digestive	Primary Mouth Pharynx Esophagus Stomach Small intestine Large intestine Rectum Anus	Accessory Teeth Salivary glands Tongue Liver Gallbladder Pancreas Appendix	Breaks apart nutrients from the external environment and absorbs them into the internal environment
Urinary	Kidneys Ureters	Urinary bladder Urethra	Adjusts internal environment by excreting excess water, salt, wastes, acids, and other substances
Reproductive	Male Testes Vas deferens Urethra Prostate Penis Scrotum	Female Ovaries Uterus Uterine (fallopian) tubes Vagina Vulva Mammary glands of breasts	Produces sex cells that form offspring, ensuring survival of genes Female system is also site of fertilization and early offspring development

the nervous system. Then, in order to continue contracting, they must receive both oxygen from the respiratory system and nutrients absorbed from the digestive system. Numerous waste products produced by contracting muscles must be eliminated by the urinary and respiratory systems. The cardiovascular system provides transportation for the respiratory gases, nutrients, and waste products of metabolism.

No one body system functions entirely independently of other systems. Instead, you will find that they are structurally and functionally interrelated and interdependent. Homeostasis can be maintained only by the coordinated and carefully regulated functioning of all body organ systems.

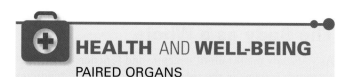

HEALTH AND WELL-BEING

PAIRED ORGANS

Have you ever wondered what advantage there might be in having two kidneys, two lungs, two eyes, and two of many other organs? Although the body could function well with only one of each, most of us are born with a pair of these organs. For paired organs that are vital to survival, such as the kidneys, this arrangement allows for the accidental loss of one organ without immediate threat to the survival of the individual. Athletes who have lost one vital organ through injury or disease are often counseled against participating in contact sports that carry the risk of damaging the remaining organ. If the second organ is damaged, total loss of a vital function, such as sight, or even death, may result.

LANGUAGE OF SCIENCE AND MEDICINE *(continued from p. 85)*

central nervous system (CNS)
(SEN-tral NER-vus SIS-tem)
[*centr-* **center,** *-al* **relating to,** *nerv-* **nerves,** *-ous* **relating to,** *system* **organized whole**]

circulatory system
(SER-kyoo-lah-tor-ee SIS-tem)
[*circulat-* **go around,** *-ory* **relating to,** *system* **organized whole**]

complement
(KOM-pleh-ment)
[*comple-* **complete,** *-ment* **result of action**]

digestive system
(dih-JES-tiv SIS-tem)
[*digest-* **break down,** *-ive* **pertaining to,** *system* **organized whole**]

endocrine system
(EN-doh-krin SIS-tem)
[*endo-* **inward or within,** *-crin-* **secrete,** *system* **organized whole**]

fallopian tube
(fal-LOH-pee-an toob)
[*Gabriele Fallopio* **Italian anatomist**]

feces
(FEE-seez)
[*feces* **waste**]

gastrointestinal (GI) tract
(gas-troh-in-TESS-tih-nul trakt)
[*gastr-* **stomach,** *-intestin-* **intestine,** *-al* **relating to,** *tract* **trail**]

genitalia
(jen-ih-TAIL-yah)
sing., genital
(JEN-ih-tul)
[*gen-* **produce,** *-al* **relating to**]

gonad
(GO-nad)
[*gon-* **offspring,** *-ad* **relating to**]

hormone
(HOR-mohn)
[*hormon-* **excite**]

hypothalamus
(hye-poh-THAL-ah-muss)
[*hypo-* **under or below,** *-thalamus* **inner chamber**]

immune system
(ih-MYOON SIS-tem)
[*immun-* **free (immunity),** *system* **organized whole**]

integument
(in-TEG-yoo-ment)
[*in-* **on,** *-teg-* **cover,** *-ment* **result of action**]

integumentary system
(in-teg-yoo-MEN-tar-ee SIS-tem)
[*in-* **on,** *-teg-* **cover,** *-ment* **result of action,** *-ary* **relating to,** *system* **organized whole**]

involuntary (smooth) muscle
(in-VOL-un-tair-ee MUSS-el)
[*in-* **not,** *volunt-* **will,** *mus-* **mouse,** *-cle* **little**]

joint
(joynt)
[*joint-* **to join**]

kidney
(KID-nee)
[*kidney-* **womb (shape)**]

larynx
(LAIR-inks)
[*larynx* **voice box**]

ligament
(LIG-ah-ment)
[*liga-* **bind,** *-ment* **result of action**]

lung
(lung)

lymph
(limf)
[*lymph* **water**]

lymph node
(limf nohd)
[*lymph* **water,** *nod-* **knot**]

lymphatic system
(lim-FAT-ik SIS-tem) duct
[*lymph-* **water,** *-atic* **relating to,** *system* **organized whole**]

lymphatic vessel
(lim-FAT-ik VES-el)
[*lymph-* **water,** *-atic* **relating to,** *vessel* **container**]

mammary gland
(MAM-mah-ree gland)
[*mamma-* **breast,** *-ry* **relating to,** *gland* **acorn**]

muscular system
(MUSS-kyoo-lar SIS-tem)
[*mus-* **mouse,** *-cul-* **little,** *-ar* **relating to,** *system* **organized whole**]

nerve impulse
(nerv IM-puls)
[*nervus* **nerve,** *impulse* **to drive**]

nervous system
(NER-vus SIS-tem)
[*nerv-* **nerves,** *-ous* **relating to,** *system* **organized whole**]

nose
(noz)
[*nose* **something obvious**]

organ
(OR-gan)
[*organ* **tool or instrument**]

ovary
(OH-var-ee)
[*ov-* **egg,** *-ar-* **relating to,** *-y* **location of process**]

ovum
(OH-vum)
pl., ova
(OH-vah)
[ovum **egg**]

pancreas
(PAN-kree-as)
[*pan-* **all,** *-creas* **flesh**]

parathyroid gland
(payr-ah-THYE-royd gland)
[*para-* **beside,** *-thyr-* **shield,** *-oid* **like,** *gland* **acorn**]

penis
(PEE-nis)
[*penis* **male sex organ**]

peripheral nervous system (PNS)
(peh-RIF-er-al NER-vus SIS-tem)
[*peri-* **around,** *-phera-* **boundary,** *-al* **relating to,** *nerv-* **nerves,** *-ous* **relating to,** *system* **organized whole**]

pharynx
(FAIR-inks)
[*pharynx* **throat**]

pineal gland
(PIN-ee-al gland)
[*pine-* **pine,** *-al* **relating to,** *gland* **acorn**]

pituitary gland
(pih-TOO-ih-tayr-ee gland)
[*pituit-* **phlegm,** *-ary* **relating to,** *gland* **acorn**]

prostate (gland)
(PROSS-tayt gland)
[*pro-* **before,** *-stat-* **set or place,** *gland* **acorn**]

radiography
(ray-dee-OG-rah-fee)
[*radi-* **ray, frequency,** *-graphy* **drawing**]

radiological technologist
(ray-dee-oh-LOJ-ih-kul tek-NOL-oh-jist)
[*radi(at)-* **emit rays,** *-log-* **words (study of),** *-ic* **relating to,** *-al* **relating to,** *techn-* **art or skill,** *-log-* **words (study of),** *-ist* **agent**]

radiologist
(ray-dee-AHL-oh-jist)
[*radi(at)-* **emit rays,** *-log-* **words (study of),** *-ist* **agent**]

reproductive system
(ree-proh-DUK-tiv SIS-tem)
[*re-* **again,** *-produce* **to bring forth,** *-tive* **relating to,** *system* **organized whole**]

respiratory system
(RES-pih-rah-tor-ee SIS-tem)
[*re-* **again,** *-spir-* **breathe,** *-tory* **relating to,** *system* **organized whole**]

scrotum
(SKROH-tum)
[*scrotum* **bag**]

sense organ
(sens OR-gan)
[*sense* **perception,** *organ-* **tool or instrument**]

skeletal system
(SKEL-eh-tal SIS-tem)
[*skeleto-* **dried body,** *-al* **relating to,** *system* **organized whole**]

smooth muscle
(smoothe MUSS-el)
[*smooth* **smooth,** *mus-* **mouse,** *-cle* **small**]

sperm
(spurm)
[*sperm* **seed**]

spleen
(spleen)

stimulus
(STIM-yoo-lus)
pl., stimuli
(STIM-yoo-lye)
[*stimulus* **incitement**]

system
(SIS-tem)
[*system* **organized whole**]

tendon
(TEN-don)
[*tend-* **pulled tight,** *-on* **unit**]

testis
(TES-tis)
pl., testes
(TES-teez)
[*testis* **witness (male gonad)**]

thoracic duct
(thoh-RASS-ik dukt)
[*thorac-* **chest (thorax),** *-ic* relating to, *duct* **to lead**]

thymus gland
(THY-mus gland)
[*thymus* **thyme flower,** *gland* **acorn**]

thyroid gland
(THY-royd gland)
[*thyro-* **shield,** *-oid* **like,** *gland* **acorn**]

tissue
(TISH-yoo)
[*tissue* **fabric**]

tonsil
(TAHN-sil)

trachea
(TRAY-kee-ah)
[*trachea* **rough duct**]

ureter
(YOOR-eh-ter)
[*ure-* **urine,** *-ter* **agent or channel**]

urethra
(yoo-REE-thrah)
[*ure-* **urine,** *-thr-* **agent or channel**]

urinary bladder
(YOOR-ih-nayr-ee BLAD-er)
[*urin-* **urine,** *-ary* **relating to,** *bladder* **blister, pimple**]

urinary system
(YOOR-ih-nayr-ee SIS-tem)
[*urin-* **urine,** *-ary* **relating to,** *system* **organized whole**]

urine
(YOOR-in)
[*ur-* **urine,** *-ine* **chemical**]

uterine tube
(YOO-ter-in toob)
[*uter-* **womb,** *-ine* **relating to,** *tube* **pipe**]

uterus
(YOO-ter-us)
[*uterus* **womb**]

vagina
(vah-JYE-nah)
[*vagina* **sheath**]

vas deferens
(vas DEF-er-enz)
pl. vasa deferentia
(VAS-ah def-er-EN-chah)
[*vas* **duct or vessel,** *deferens* **carrying away**]

vein
(vayn)
[*vena* **blood vessel**]

voluntary (skeletal) muscle
(VOL-un-tayr-ee MUSS-el)
[*volunt-* **will,** *mus-* **mouse,** *-cle* **little**]

vulva
(VUL-vah)
[*vulva* **wrapper**]

❑ OUTLINE SUMMARY

To download a digital audio version of the chapter summary for use with your device, access the ***Audio Chapter Summaries*** *online at evolve.elsevier.com.*

Hint *Scan this summary after reading the chapter to help you reinforce the key concepts. Later, use the summary as a quick review before your class or before a test.*

Definitions and Concepts

A. Organ — a structure made up of two or more kinds of tissues organized in such a way that they can together perform a more complex function than can any tissue alone
B. Organ system — a group of organs arranged in such a way that they can together perform a more complex function than can any organ alone
C. Knowledge of individual organs and how they are organized into groups makes the understanding of how a particular organ system functions as a whole more meaningful

Organ Systems

A. Integumentary system (see **Figure 5-1**)
  1. Structure
    a. Only one organ, the skin, but has many appendages (attached structures)
    b. Skin appendages
      (1) Hair
      (2) Nails
      (3) Microscopic sense receptors
      (4) Sweat glands
      (5) Oil glands
  2. Functions
    a. Protection — primary function
    b. Regulation of body temperature
    c. Synthesis of chemicals
    d. Sense organ
B. Skeletal system (see **Figure 5-2**)
  1. Structure
    a. Bones — organs of the skeletal system
      (1) 206 named bones in the skeleton
      (2) Additional variable bones occur in each individual
    b. Cartilage connects and cushions joined bones
    c. Ligaments — bands of fibrous tissue that hold bones together
    d. Joints — connections between bones that make movement possible
  2. Functions
    a. Supporting framework for entire body
    b. Protection of brain and internal organs
    c. Movement (with joints and muscles)
    d. Storage of minerals
    e. Formation of blood cells
C. Muscular system (see **Figure 5-3**)
  1. Structure
    a. Muscles are the primary organs
    b. Voluntary or striated skeletal muscle
    c. Involuntary or smooth muscle tissue in walls of some organs
    d. Cardiac muscle in wall of the heart
  2. Functions
    a. Movement
    b. Maintenance of body posture
    c. Production of heat
  3. Skeletomuscular system — combination of the skeletal and muscular systems
D. Nervous system (see **Figure 5-4**)
  1. Structure
    a. Central nervous system (CNS)
      (1) Brain
      (2) Spinal cord
    b. Peripheral nervous system (PNS)
      (1) Cranial nerves and their branches
      (2) Spinal nerves and their branches
      (3) Sense organs
  2. Functions
    a. Communication between body organs
    b. Integration of body functions
    c. Control of body functions
    d. Recognition of sensory stimuli
E. Endocrine system (see **Figure 5-5**)
  1. Structure — ductless glands that secrete signaling hormones directly into the blood
  2. Functions
    a. Same as nervous system — communication, integration, control
    b. Control is slow and of long duration
    c. Neuroendocrine system — combination of nervous and endocrine systems
    d. Examples of functions regulated by hormones:
      (1) Growth
      (2) Metabolism
      (3) Reproduction
      (4) Fluid and electrolyte balance
F. Cardiovascular system (also called *circulatory system*) (see **Figure 5-6**)
  1. Structure
    a. Heart
    b. Blood vessels
  2. Functions
    a. Transportation of substances throughout the body
    b. Regulation of body temperature
    c. Immunity (body defense)

G. Lymphatic and immune systems (see **Figure 5-7**)
  1. Lymphatic system
    a. Structure
      (1) Lymphatic vessels
      (2) Lymph nodes and tonsils
      (3) Thymus
      (4) Spleen
      (5) Red bone marrow
    b. Functions
      (1) Transportation of lymph
      (2) Immunity
  2. Immune system
    a. Structure
      (1) Unique cells
        (a) Phagocytes
        (b) Secretory cells
      (2) Defensive protein compounds
        (a) Antibodies
        (b) Complements
    b. Functions
      (1) Phagocytosis of bacteria
      (2) Chemical reactions that provide protection from harmful agents

H. Respiratory system (see **Figure 5-8**)
  1. Structure
    a. Nose
    b. Pharynx
    c. Larynx
    d. Trachea
    e. Bronchi
    f. Lungs
  2. Functions
    a. Exchange of waste gas (carbon dioxide) for oxygen in the alveoli of the lungs
    b. Filtration of irritants from inspired air
    c. Regulation of acid-base balance

I. Digestive system (see **Figure 5-9**)
  1. Structure
    a. Primary organs — form alimentary canal, or gastrointestinal (GI) tract
      (1) Mouth
      (2) Pharynx
      (3) Esophagus
      (4) Stomach
      (5) Small intestine
      (6) Large intestine
      (7) Rectum
      (8) Anal canal
    b. Accessory organs — assist the digestive process
      (1) Teeth
      (2) Salivary glands
      (3) Tongue
      (4) Liver
      (5) Gallbladder
      (6) Pancreas
      (7) Appendix
  2. Functions
    a. Mechanical and chemical breakdown (digestion) of food
    b. Absorption of nutrients
    c. Elimination of undigested waste product — referred to as *feces*
    d. Appendix holds bacteria that assist digestion

J. Urinary system (see **Figure 5-10**)
  1. Structure
    a. Kidneys
    b. Ureters
    c. Urinary bladder
    d. Urethra (part of both urinary and reproductive systems in males)
  2. Functions
    a. "Clearing," or cleaning, blood of waste products — excreted from the body as *urine*
    b. Electrolyte balance
    c. Water balance
    d. Acid-base balance

K. Reproductive systems
  1. Structure
    a. Male (see **Figure 5-11**)
      (1) Gonads — testes
      (2) Other structures — vas deferens, urethra, prostate, external genitalia (penis and scrotum)
    b. Female (see **Figure 5-12**)
      (1) Gonads — ovaries
      (2) Other structures — uterus, uterine (fallopian) tubes, vagina, external genitalia (vulva), mammary glands (breasts)
  2. Functions
    a. Survival of genes
    b. Production of sex cells (male: sperm; female: ova)
    c. Transfer and fertilization of sex cells
    d. Development and birth of offspring
    e. Nourishment of offspring
    f. Production of sex hormones

The Body as a Whole

A. No one body system functions entirely independently of other systems (see **Table 5-1**)

B. All body systems are structurally and functionally interrelated and interdependent

❑ ACTIVE LEARNING

STUDY TIPS

Hint *Use these tips to achieve success in meeting your learning goals.*

Chapter 5 is the perfect "big picture" or synopsis *chapter. It is a preview for most of the remaining chapters in the text.*

1. Put the name of the system on one side of a flash card and the function of that system and its organs on the other side. Notice how each organ contributes to the function of the system. Use **Table 5-1** as a resource.
2. In your study groups, go over the flash cards. Discuss how several systems need to be involved in accomplishing one function in the body, such as getting nutrients or oxygen to the cells.
3. Go over the questions in the back of the chapter and discuss possible test questions.
4. Consider starting some *running concept lists* for each of the systems and organs that you will encounter in this course. Each time you learn something new about each one, you can add your new knowledge to the appropriate concept list. See *my-ap.us/JlLFb6* to learn more about how to use running *concept lists*.
5. As you continue your studies, before you begin each chapter dealing with a particular system, it would be helpful to get an overview of that system by reviewing the synopsis of that system in this chapter.

Review Questions

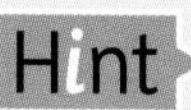

Write out the answers to these questions after reading the chapter and reviewing the Chapter Summary. If you simply think through the answer without writing it down, you won't retain much of your new learning.

Review the names of organ systems and individual organs in **Table 5-1**.

1. Define *organ* and *organ system.*
2. List examples of stimuli to which the skin sense receptors can respond.
3. Describe how the skin is able to assist in the body's ability to regulate temperature
4. List the function of tendons.
5. Describe some of the differences between the lymphatic and cardiovascular systems.
6. List the organs that help rid the body of waste and name the type of waste that each organ removes.
7. In addition to bone, name the other tissues included in the skeletal system.
8. List the 11 organ systems discussed in this chapter.
9. Most of the organ systems have more than one function. List two functions for the following systems: integumentary system, skeletal system, muscular system, lymphatic system, respiratory system, and urinary system.
10. Describe what is unique about the reproductive system.

Critical Thinking

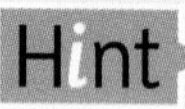

After finishing the Review Questions, write out the answers to these more in-depth questions to help you apply your new knowledge. Go back to sections of the chapter that relate to concepts that you find difficult.

11. Explain the differences between the nervous and endocrine systems. Include what types of functions are regulated and the "message carriers" for each system.
12. The term *balance* is used in this chapter. This is another term for *homeostasis.* Review the functions of the systems and list those functions that are homeostatic.
13. Jane's grandmother has a persistent cough. When Jane asked her grandmother about it, she shrugged it off by saying that she has had it for months and that it is nonproductive and just annoying. She further adds that it is probably just allergies. If you were Jane, how would you react to her grandmother's explanation?
14. Tom complained of pain in his abdomen one night and decided to go to the Emergency Department. His blood work was negative and a flat screen x-ray of his abdomen revealed nothing abnormal. The doctor, however, still suggested that Tom be admitted to the hospital. He advised Tom that he would be ordering some additional tests and x-rays. What are some x-ray options that the doctor might order and what are the individual advantages of these x-rays?

Chapter Test

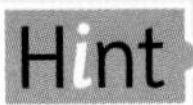

After studying the chapter, test your mastery by responding to these items. Try to answer them without looking up the answers. Then, verify the answers using the key in Appendix C at the back of this book.

1. The primary organs of the digestive system make a long tube called the __________.
2. __________ is another term for voluntary muscle.
3. Although it is part of the skeletal system, red bone marrow is often considered to also be a __________ structure.
4. The nervous system can generate special electrochemical signals called __________.
5. The __________, __________, __________, and __________ are called the accessory structures of the skin.
6. The __________ is part of both the lymphatic and endocrine systems.
7. The __________ is part of both the male reproductive and urinary systems.
8. The gonads for the male reproductive system are the __________. For the female reproductive system, the gonads are the __________.
9. The skeletal system is composed of bone tissue and these two related tissues: __________ and __________.

Match each function in Column B with the proper cell structure in Column A.

Column A	Column B
10. _____ Integumentary	a. Provides movement, body posture, and heat
11. _____ Skeletal	b. Uses hormones to regulate body functions
12. _____ Muscular	c. Transports fatty nutrients from the digestive system to the blood
13. _____ Nervous	d. Physical and chemical change in nutrients and absorption of them
14. _____ Endocrine	e. Cleans the blood of metabolic wastes and regulates electrolyte balance
15. _____ Cardiovascular	f. Protects underlying structures, sensory reception, and regulation of body temperature
16. _____ Lymphatic	g. Transports substances from one part of the body to another
17. _____ Respiratory	h. Ensures the survival of the species rather than the individual
18. _____ Digestive	i. Uses electrochemical signals to integrate and control body functions
19. _____ Urinary	j. Exchanges oxygen and carbon dioxide and regulates acid-base balance
20. _____ Reproductive	k. Provides a rigid framework for the body and stores minerals

Skin and Membranes

OUTLINE

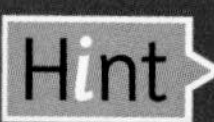

Scan this outline before you begin to read the chapter, as a preview of how the concepts are organized.

OBJECTIVES

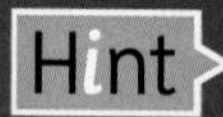

Before reading the chapter, review these goals for your learning.

After you have completed this chapter, you should be able to:

1. Classify, compare the structure of, and give examples of each type of body membrane.
2. Describe the structure and function of the epidermis and dermis.
3. List and briefly describe each accessory organ of the skin.
4. List and discuss the five primary functions of the integumentary system.
5. List and briefly describe the three most common types of skin cancer.
6. Classify burns and describe how to estimate the extent of a burn injury.

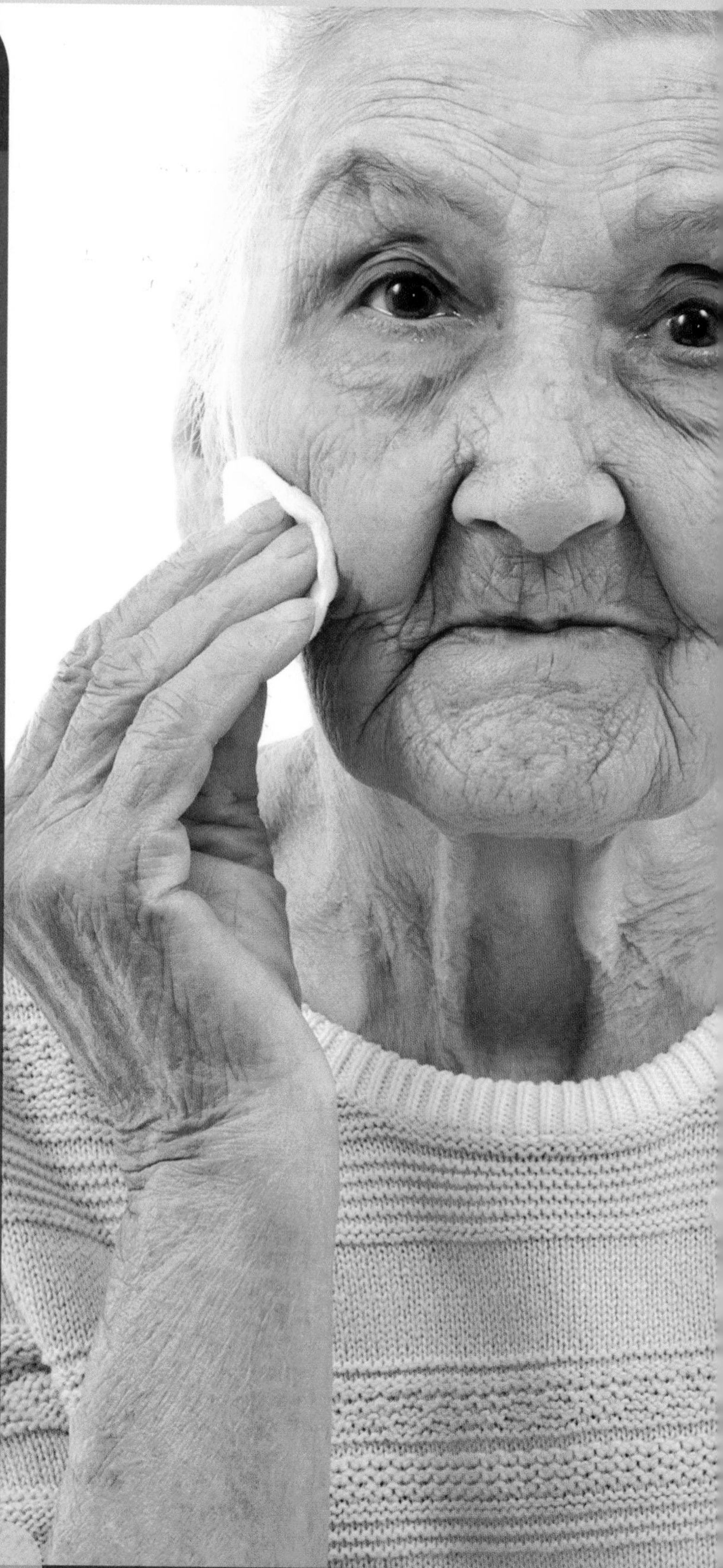

CHAPTER 6

In Chapter 1 the concept of progressive organization of body structures from simple to complex was established. Complexity in body structure and function progresses from cells to tissues and then to organs and organ systems. This chapter discusses the skin and its **appendages**—the hair, the nails, and the skin glands—as an organ system. This system is called the **integumentary system. Integument** is another name for the skin, and the skin itself is the principal organ of the integumentary system. The skin is one of a group of anatomically simple but functionally important sheet-like structures called *membranes.*

This chapter begins with classification and discussion of the important body membranes. Study of the integument follows—our first exploration of how the structure and function of a body system are interrelated.

Body Membranes

Classification of Membranes

The term **membrane** refers to a thin, sheetlike structure that may have many important functions in the body. Membranes cover and protect the body surface, line body cavities, and cover the inner surfaces of the hollow organs such as the digestive, reproductive, and respiratory passageways. Some membranes anchor organs to each other or to bones, and others cover the internal organs. In certain areas of the body, membranes secrete lubricating fluids that reduce friction during organ movements such as the beating of the heart or lung expansion and contraction.

LANGUAGE OF **SCIENCE** AND **MEDICINE**

Hint Before reading the chapter, say each of these terms out loud. This will help you to avoid stumbling over them as you read.

allergy
(AL-er-jee)
[*all-* **other,** *-erg-* **work,** *-y* **state**]

apocrine
(AP-oh-krin)
[*apo-* **from,** *crin-* **secrete**]

apocrine sweat gland
(AP-oh-krin swet gland)
[*apo-* **from,** *-crin* **secrete,** *gland* **acorn**]

appendage
(ah-PEN-dij)
[*append-* **hang upon,** *-age* **related to**]

arrector pili
(ah-REK-tor PYE-lye)
[*arrector* **raiser,** *pili* **of hair**]

basal cell carcinoma
(BAY-sal sel kar-sih-NOH-mah)
[*bas-* **base,** *-al* **relating to,** *cell* **storeroom,** *carcin-* **cancer,** *-oma* **tumor**]

basement membrane
(BAYS-ment MEM-brayn)
[*base-* **base,** *-ment* **thing,** *membrane* **thin skin**]

blackhead
(BLAK-hed)

blister
(BLIS-ter)

burn
(bern)

bursa
(BER-sah)
pl., bursae
(BER-see or BER-say)
[*bursa* **purse**]

comedo
(KOM-ee-doh)
[*comedo* **glutton (applied to secretions that resemble body-devouring worms)**]

Continued on p. 115

Membrane lubricants also decrease friction between bones in joints. There are two major categories or types of body membranes:

1. **Epithelial membranes** are composed of epithelial tissue and an underlying layer of fibrous connective tissue
2. **Connective tissue membranes** are composed exclusively of various types of connective tissue. No epithelial cells are present in this type of membrane

Epithelial Membranes

There are three types of epithelial tissue membranes in the body:

1. Cutaneous membrane
2. Serous membranes
3. Mucous membranes

Cutaneous Membrane

The **cutaneous membrane,** or skin, is the primary organ of the integumentary system. It is one of the most important and one of the largest and most visible organs of the body. In most individuals, the skin composes some 16% of the body weight. It fulfills the requirements necessary for an epithelial tissue membrane in that it has a superficial layer of epithelial cells and an underlying layer of supportive connective tissue. Its structure is uniquely suited to its many functions. The skin is discussed in depth later in the chapter.

Serous Membranes

As with all epithelial membranes, a **serous membrane** is composed of two distinct layers of tissue. The epithelial sheet is a thin layer of simple squamous epithelium. The connective tissue layer forms a very thin, gluelike **basement membrane** that holds and supports the epithelial cells.

The serous membrane that lines body cavities and covers the surfaces of organs in those cavities is in reality a single, continuous sheet of tissue covering two different surfaces. This arrangement results in two distinct layers of serous membranes. The first type of serous membrane layer lines body cavities, and the second type of serous layer covers the organs in those cavities.

The serous membrane that lines the walls of a body cavity much like wallpaper covers the walls of a room is called the **parietal** layer. The portion of the membrane that instead folds inward to cover the surface of organs within a body cavity is called the **visceral** layer.

Two serous membranes of the thoracic and abdominal cavities are identified in Figure 6-1. In the thoracic cavity the serous membrane around each lung is called the **pleura**. In the abdominal cavity, the serous membrane covering most of the organs is called the **peritoneum**. Look again at Figure 6-1 to note the placement of the *parietal pleura* and *visceral pleura* and the *parietal peritoneum* and *visceral peritoneum*. In both cases the parietal layer forms the lining of the body cavity, and the visceral layer covers the organs found in that cavity.

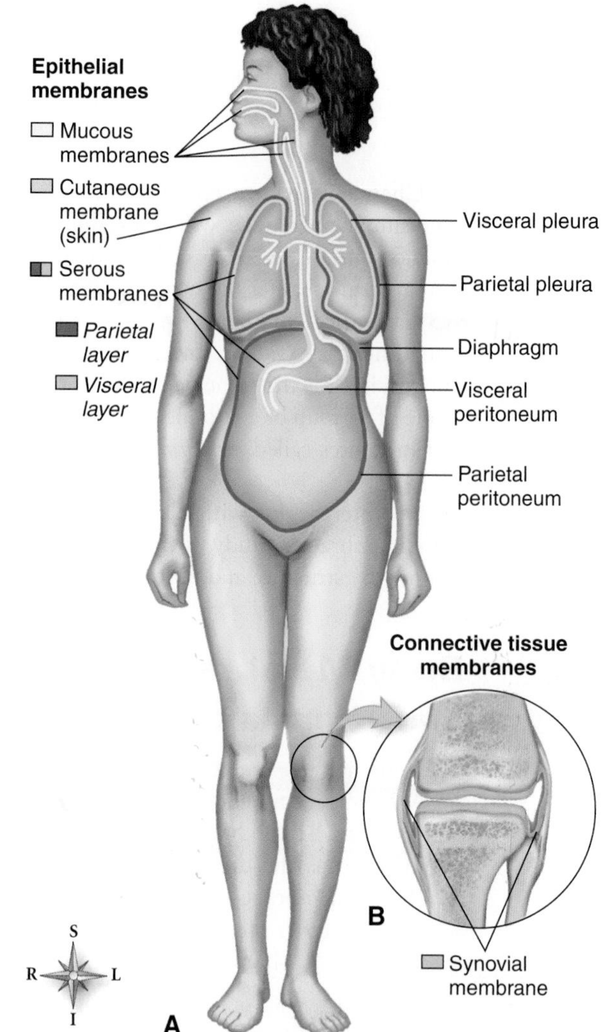

FIGURE 6-1 Types of body membranes. A, Epithelial membranes, including cutaneous membrane (skin), serous membranes (parietal and visceral pleura and peritoneum), and mucous membranes. **B,** Connective tissue membranes, including synovial membranes. See text for explanation.

Serous membranes secrete a thin, watery fluid that helps reduce friction and serves as a lubricant when organs rub against one another and against the walls of the cavities that contain them.

The heart is surrounded by a fibrous sac lined with a thin, slippery membrane that doubles back on itself to form a lubricating, fluid-filled pocket around the heart. Figure 6-2 shows how the serous membrane around the heart—the **pericardium**—resembles a water-filled balloon with a fist thrust into it.

Pleurisy is a very painful pathological condition characterized by inflammation of the serous membranes (pleura) that line the chest cavity and cover the lungs. Pain is caused by irritation and friction in the inflamed pleura as the lung rubs

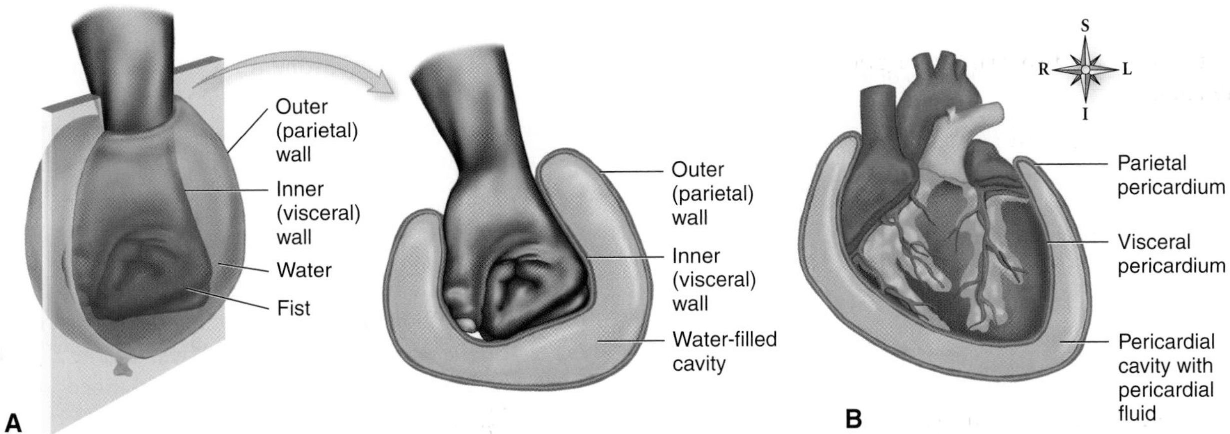

FIGURE 6-2 Serous membranes. A, The analogy of a fist thrust into a water-filled balloon demonstrates how a serous membrane forms a double-walled structure containing a thin pocket of fluid. **B,** The heart is surrounded by the serous pericardium, which forms a parietal and visceral layer filled with lubricating serous fluid called *pericardial fluid.*

against the wall of the chest cavity. In severe cases, the inflamed surfaces of the pleura fuse together and permanent damage may develop.

The term **peritonitis** is used to describe inflammation of the serous membranes in the abdominal cavity. Peritonitis can be a serious complication of an infected appendix.

To learn more about serous membranes, go to AnimationDirect at *evolve.elsevier.com.*

Mucous Membranes

Mucous membranes are epithelial membranes that contain both an epithelial layer and a fibrous connective tissue layer. These membranes line body surfaces opening directly to the exterior of the body. Examples of mucous membranes include those lining the respiratory, digestive, urinary, and reproductive tracts. The epithelial component of a mucous membrane varies, depending on its location and function. In most cases, the cell composition is either stratified squamous or simple columnar epithelia.

In the esophagus, for example, a tough, abrasion-resistant stratified squamous epithelium is found. This is a good example of the "structure fits function" principle. Without the protection of a tough epithelial lining, ingested food that is coarse, like popcorn, might cause injury to the esophageal wall when swallowed and may result in irritation or even infection and hemorrhage.

A thin layer of simple columnar epithelium lines the walls of the lower segments of the digestive tract. In the stomach and small intestine, ingested food undergoes digestion and is changed into a smooth, liquefied material that is no longer abrasive. The single layer of lining epithelial cells in these segments of the intestinal tract is well suited to a primary function: nutrient and water absorption.

The epithelial cells of most mucous membranes secrete a thick, slimy material called **mucus** that keeps the membranes moist and soft. The fibrous connective tissue underlying the epithelium in mucous membranes is called the **lamina propria.** Note that the term *mucous* identifies the type of membrane, whereas *mucus* refers to the secretion produced by that membrane.

The term **mucocutaneous junction** is used to describe the transitional area that serves as a point of "fusion" where skin and mucous membranes meet. Such junctions lack accessory organs such as hair or sweat glands that characterize skin. These transitional areas are generally moistened by mucous glands within the body orifices or openings where these junctions are located. The eyelids, lips, nasal openings, vulva, and anus have mucocutaneous junctions that may become sites of infection or irritation.

To learn more about mucous membranes, go to AnimationDirect at *evolve.elsevier.com.*

Connective Tissue Membranes

Unlike cutaneous, serous, and mucous membranes, connective tissue membranes do not contain epithelial components. The **synovial membranes** lining the joint capsules that surround and attach the ends of articulating bones in movable joints are classified as connective tissue membranes (see **Figure 6-1,** *B* and **Figure 7-25** on p. 144).

These membranes are smooth and slick and secrete a thick, colorless lubricating fluid called **synovial fluid.** The membrane itself, with its fluid that resembles egg white, helps reduce friction between the opposing surfaces of bones in movable joints. Synovial membranes also line the small, cushionlike sacs called **bursae** found between many moving body parts.

To learn more about connective tissue and synovial membrane, go to AnimationDirect at *evolve.elsevier.com.*

QUICK CHECK

1. What are the two main categories of membranes in the body?
2. Which of the body's membranes are types of epithelial membranes?
3. What fluid(s) is/are produced by serous, mucous, and synovial membranes? What is the function of each fluid?
4. What is the mucocutaneous junction?

The Skin

The brief description of the skin in Chapter 5 (see p. 86) identified it not only as the primary organ of the integumentary system but also as the largest and one of the most important organs of the body.

The skin is an architectural marvel. Consider the incredible number of structures fitting into 1 square inch of skin: 500 sweat glands; more than 1000 nerve endings; yards of tiny blood vessels; nearly 100 oil glands; 150 sensors for pressure, 75 for heat, and 10 for cold; and millions of skin cells.

Structure of the Skin

The skin, or cutaneous membrane, is a sheetlike organ composed of the following layers of distinct tissue (**Figure 6-3**):

1. The **epidermis** is the outermost layer of the skin. It is a relatively thin sheet of stratified squamous epithelium.
2. The **dermis** is the deeper of the two layers. It is thicker than the epidermis and is made up largely of connective tissue.

FIGURE 6-3 Microscopic view of the skin. The epidermis, shown in longitudinal section, is raised at one corner to reveal the ridges in the dermis.

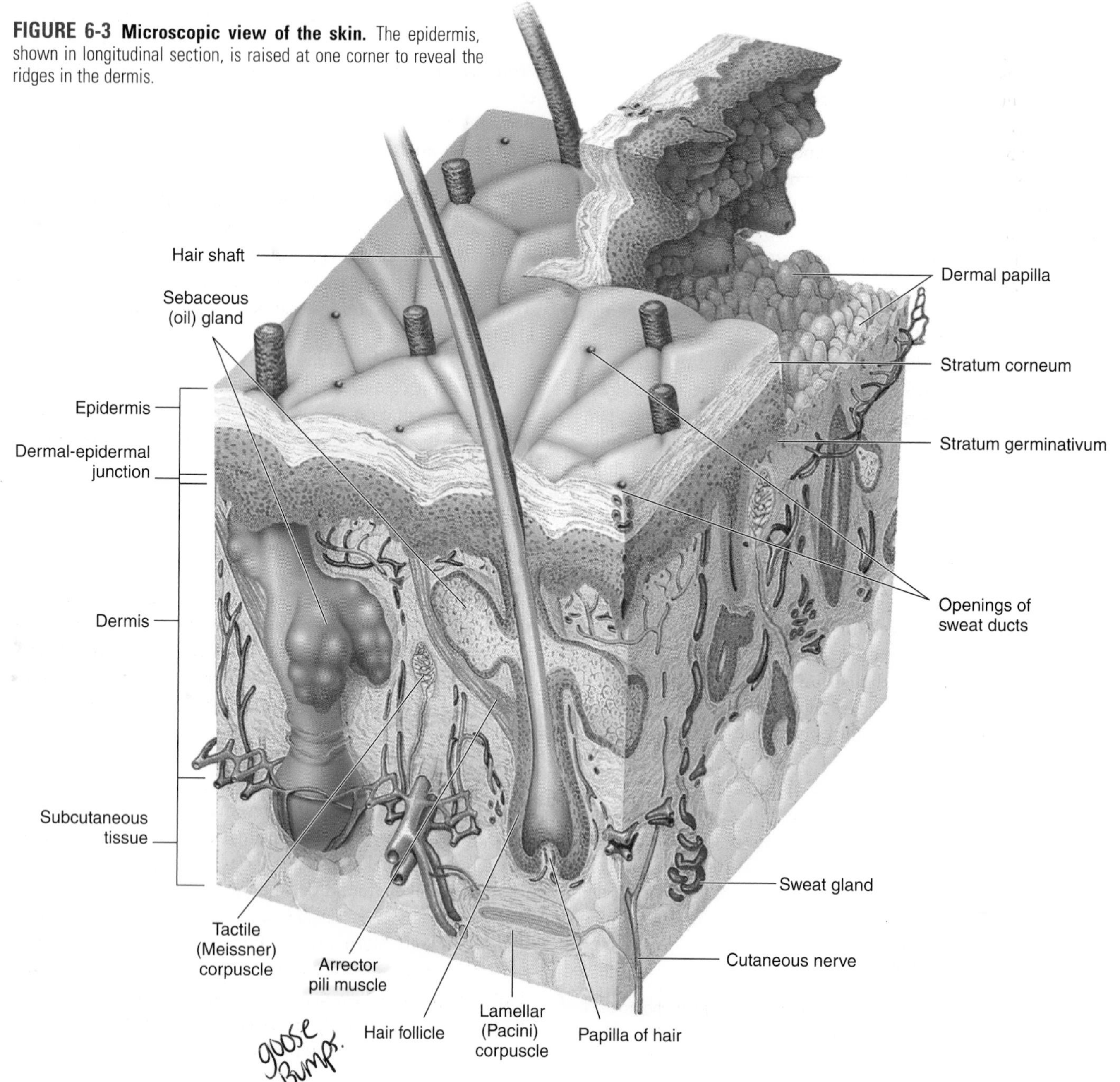

As you can see in Figure 6-3, the layers of the skin are supported by a thick layer of loose connective tissue and fat called **subcutaneous tissue,** or the **hypodermis**. Fat in the subcutaneous layer insulates the body from extremes of heat and cold. It also serves as a stored source of energy for the body and can be used as a food source if required. In addition, the subcutaneous tissue acts as a shock-absorbing pad and helps protect underlying tissues from injury caused by bumps and blows to the body surface.

Epidermis

The tightly packed epithelial cells of the epidermis are arranged in up to five distinct layers.

The basal cells of the innermost layer, called the **stratum germinativum**, undergo mitosis and reproduce themselves (see Figure 6-3). As new cells are produced in the deep layer of the epidermis, they are pushed upward through additional layers, or "strata" of cells.

As they approach the surface, the epithelial cells die and their cytoplasm is replaced by one of nature's most unique proteins, a substance called **keratin**. Keratin is a tough, waterproof material that provides cells in the outer layer of the skin with a horny, abrasion-resistant, and protective quality. The tough outermost layer of the epidermis is called the **stratum corneum**.

In the photomicrograph of the skin shown in Figure 6-4, many of the surface cells of the stratum corneum have been dislodged. These dry, dead cells filled with keratin "flake off" by the thousands onto our clothes, into our bath water, and onto things we handle. Millions of epithelial cells reproduce daily to replace the millions shed. This is just one example of the work our bodies do without our knowledge, continuing even when we seem to be resting.

Skin Pigment

The deepest cell layer of the stratum germinativum identified in Figure 6-3 is responsible for the production of a **pigment** that gives color to the skin. The term *pigment* comes from a Latin word meaning "paint." It is this epidermal layer that gives color to the skin.

The brown pigment **melanin** is produced by cells in this basal layer called **melanocytes**. Melanin produced and packaged in melanocytes is distributed to the surrounding epithelial cells, giving them a darker color. The higher the concentration of melanin distributed in the layers of epithelial cells, the deeper is the color of skin. The primary function of melanin is to absorb harmful ultraviolet (UV) radiation from sunlight before it reaches tissues below the outer layers of the epidermis.

The amount and type of melanin in your skin depends first on the skin color genes you have inherited. That is, heredity determines how dark or light your basic skin color is. However, other factors such as sunlight exposure can modify this hereditary effect. Prolonged exposure to sunlight in light-skinned people darkens the exposed area because it leads to increased melanin deposits in the epidermis—a protective mechanism that keeps deeper tissues safe from UV radiation.

If the skin contains little melanin, as under the nails where there is no melanin at all, a change in color can occur if the volume of blood in the skin changes significantly or if the amount of oxygen in the blood is increased or decreased. In these individuals, increased blood flow to the skin or increased blood oxygen levels can cause a pink flush to appear. However, if blood oxygen levels decrease or if actual blood flow is reduced dramatically, the skin turns a blue-gray color—a condition called **cyanosis**.

In general, the less abundant the melanin deposits in the skin are, the more visible will be the changes in color caused by the change in skin blood volume or oxygen level. Conversely, the richer the skin's pigmentation is, the less noticeable such changes will be.

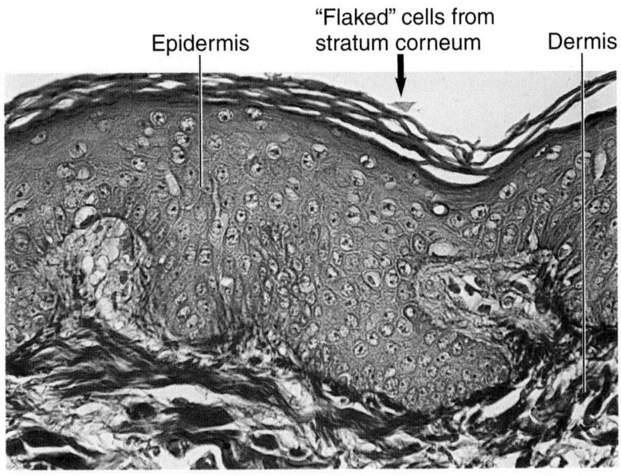

FIGURE 6-4 Photomicrograph of the skin. New cells of the epidermis are produced in stratum germinativum, where they are pushed upward and eventually die and flatten out to form stratum corneum (*arrow* shows dead cell falling away from skin). The deep region of the skin is the dermis, made up of connective tissue having few cells.

Dermal-Epidermal Junction

The junction that exists between the thin epidermal layer of skin above and the dermal layer below forms a type of basement membrane called the **dermal-epidermal junction.**

The deeper cells of the epidermis are packed tightly together. They are held firmly to one another and to the dermis below by cellular junctions between the membranes of adjacent cells, sometimes described as "spot welds," and by a unique type of gel that serves to "glue" the two layers of the skin together and provide support for the epidermis attached to its upper surface. Small nipplelike bumps that project upward from the dermis into the epidermis, called **dermal papillae**—which are discussed below—also play an important role in stabilizing the dermal-epidermal junction (see Figure 6-3).

If the junction is weakened or destroyed, the skin falls apart. When this occurs over a limited area because of burns, friction injuries, or exposure to irritants, **blisters** may result. Any widespread detachment of a large area of epidermis from the dermis is an extremely serious condition that may result in overwhelming infection and death.

Dermis

The dermis is the deeper of the two primary skin layers and is much thicker than the epidermis. The mechanical strength of the skin is in the dermis. It is composed largely of connective tissue. Instead of cells being crowded close together like the epithelial cells of the epidermis, they are scattered far apart, with many fibers in between. Some of the fibers are tough and strong (collagen or white fibers), and others are stretchable and elastic (elastic or yellow fibers).

Papillary Layer

The upper region, or *papillary layer,* of the dermis is characterized by parallel rows of tiny bumps called *dermal papillae,* which are visible in **Figure 6-3**. The papillary layer takes its name from the papillae on its surface. This layer of the dermis is composed essentially of loose connective tissue elements within a fine network of thin collagenous and elastic fibers (see Chapter 4, p. 74). The dermal papillae increase the surface area of the gluelike dermal-epidermal junction that helps bind the skin layers to each other. You may already know that glue holds rough surfaces together much more strongly than it binds smooth surfaces.

The ridges on the tips of the fingers and on the skin covering the palms of your hands result from the parallel arrangement of dermal papillae under the epidermis. The biological function of skin ridges is to improve our grip when making or using tools, for example, or walking barefooted on smooth surfaces. Friction ridges help us to walk upright without slipping and to make and hold tools. These ridges also help us sense textures on surfaces in our environment.

Friction ridges develop sometime before birth. Not only is their pattern unique in each individual but also it never changes except to grow larger—two facts that explain why our fingerprints or footprints can provide positive biological identification of who we are.

Reticular Layer

The deeper area, or *reticular layer,* of the dermis is filled with a dense network of interlacing fibers. Most of the fibers in this area are collagen that gives toughness to the skin. However, elastic fibers are also present. These make the skin stretchable and elastic (able to rebound). As we age, the number of elastic fibers in the dermis decreases, and the amount of fat stored in the subcutaneous tissue is reduced. Wrinkles develop as the skin loses elasticity. The skin sags and becomes less soft and pliant.

In addition to connective tissue elements, the dermis contains an extensive network of nerves and nerve endings to detect sensory information such as pain, pressure, touch, and temperature. At various levels of the dermis, there are muscle fibers, hair follicles, sweat and oil glands, and many blood vessels.

Subcutaneous Tissue

The **subcutaneous tissue** is often called the **superficial fascia** or *hypodermis* by anatomists. It is not a part or layer of the skin. Instead, it lies deep to the dermis and forms a connection between the skin and underlying structures of the body such as muscle and bone.

If you ever skin a piece of chicken before cooking, separation of the skin will occur in the "cleavage plane" that exists between the superficial fascia and the underlying structures. The spongy nature of subcutaneous tissue determines the relative mobility of the skin.

Loose fibrous and adipose tissue are prominent in subcutaneous tissue, and in obese individuals, fat content in this layer may exceed 10 cm or more in thickness. A surgical procedure called **liposuction** involves inserting a hollow tube into the subcutaneous tissue and removing fat with a vacuum aspirator.

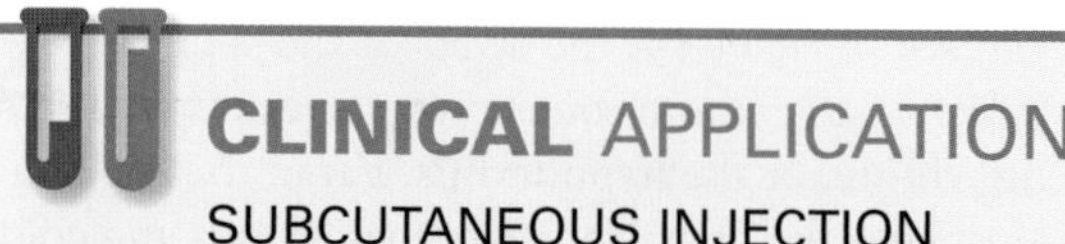

CLINICAL APPLICATION

SUBCUTANEOUS INJECTION

Although the subcutaneous layer is not part of the skin, it carries the major blood vessels and nerves that supply the skin superficial to it. The rich blood supply and loose, spongy texture of the subcutaneous layer make it an ideal site for the rapid and relatively pain-free absorption of injected material. Liquid medicines such as insulin and pelleted implant materials such as synthetic hormones are often administered by **subcutaneous injection** into this spongy and porous layer beneath the skin. Needles used to inject materials into the hypodermis are called *hypodermic needles.*

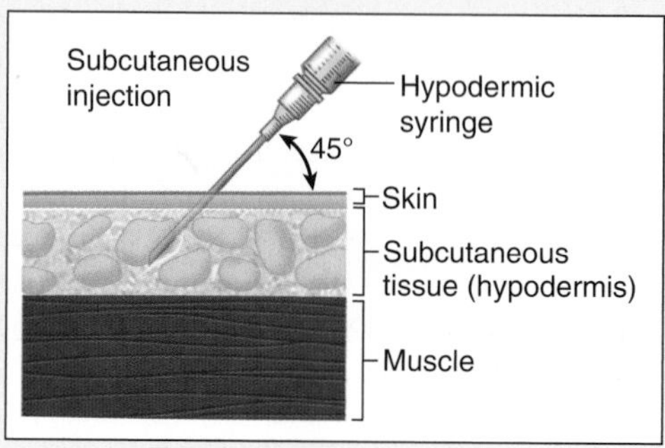

Hair, Nails, and Skin Receptors

Hair

Location of Hair

The human body is covered with millions of hairs. Indeed, at the time of birth most of the pocketlike **follicles** that are required for hair growth are already present. They develop early in fetal life and by birth are present in most parts of the skin. The hair of a newborn infant is extremely fine and soft. It is called **lanugo** from the Latin word meaning "down." In premature infants, lanugo may be noticeable over most of the body, but soon after birth the lanugo is lost and replaced by new hair that is stronger and more pigmented.

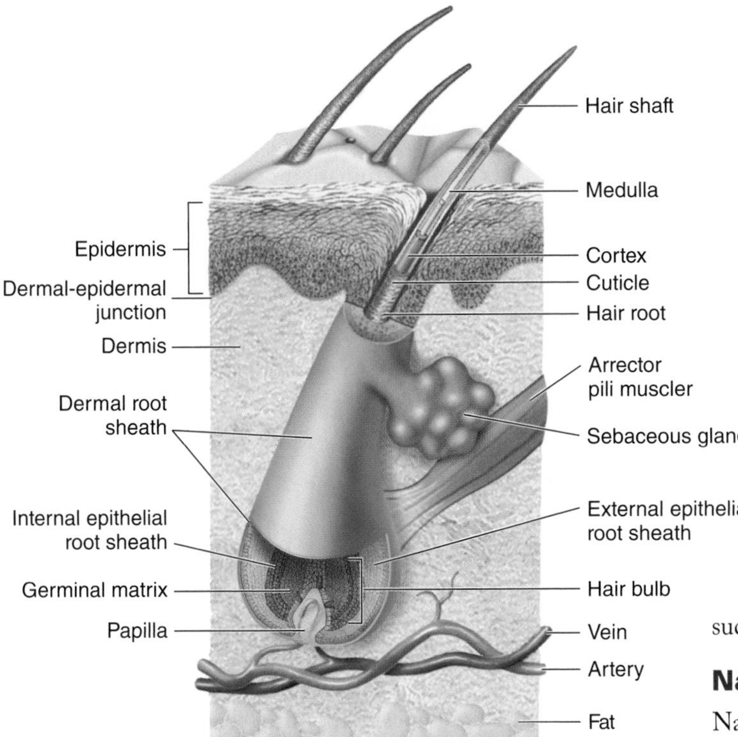

FIGURE 6-5 Hair follicle. Relationship of a hair follicle and related structures to the epidermal and dermal layers of the skin.

Although only a few areas of the skin are hairless—notably the lips, the palms of the hands, and the soles of the feet—most body hair remains almost invisible. Hair is most visible on the scalp, eyelids, and eyebrows. The coarse hair that first appears in the pubic and axillary regions at the time of puberty develops in response to the secretion of hormones.

Hair Growth

Hair growth begins when cells of the epidermal layer of the skin grow down into the dermis, forming a small tube called the **hair follicle.** The relationship of a hair follicle and its related structures to the epidermal and dermal layers of the skin is shown in **Figure 6-5**. Note in **Figure 6-5** that part of the hair, namely the *root*, lies hidden in the follicle. The visible part of a hair is called the *shaft.*

Hair growth begins from a small bump called the **hair papilla**, which is located at the base of the follicle. The papilla is nourished by dermal blood vessels and covered with a form of *stratum germinativum*—the epidermal growth layer. As in other areas of the skin, when new cells are formed, the older cells are pushed outward and become filled with keratin—producing a strong, keratinized cylinder of hair. The type of keratin in hair is a bit more rigid than the softer, more flexible keratin of stratum corneum.

As long as growth cells in the papilla of the hair follicle remain alive, new hair will replace any that is cut or plucked. Contrary to popular belief, frequent cutting or shaving does not make hair grow faster or become coarser. Why? It is because neither process affects the epithelial growth cells that form the hairs.

Arrector Pili Muscle

A tiny, smooth (involuntary) muscle can be seen at the follicle in **Figure 6-5** and **Figure 6-6**. It is called an **arrector pili** muscle. It is attached to the base of a dermal papilla above and to the side of a hair follicle below. Generally, these muscles contract only when we are frightened or cold.

When contraction occurs, each muscle simultaneously pulls on its two points of attachment (that is, up on a hair follicle but down on a part of the skin). This produces little raised places, commonly known as *goose bumps,* between the depressed points of the skin and at the same time pulls the hairs up until they are more or less straight. The name *arrector pili* describes the function of these muscles. It is Latin for "erectors of the hair."

We subconsciously recognize these facts in expressions such as "I was so frightened my hair stood on end."

Nails

Nails are classified as accessory organs of the skin and are produced by cells in the epidermis. They develop when epidermal cells over the terminal ends of the fingers and toes fill with keratin and become hard and platelike.

The components of a typical fingernail and its associated structures are shown in **Figure 6-7**. In this illustration the fingernail of the index finger is viewed from above and in sagittal section. (Recall that a sagittal section divides a body part into right and left portions.)

Look first at the posterior view of the nail in **Figure 6-7,** *A*. The visible part of the nail is called the **nail body.** The rest of the nail, namely the **root,** lies in a groove and is hidden by a fold of skin called the **cuticle**. In the sagittal section you can see the nail root from the side and note its relationship to the cuticle, which is folded back over its upper surface. The nail body nearest the root has a crescent-shaped white area known as the **lunula**, or "little moon." You should be able to identify

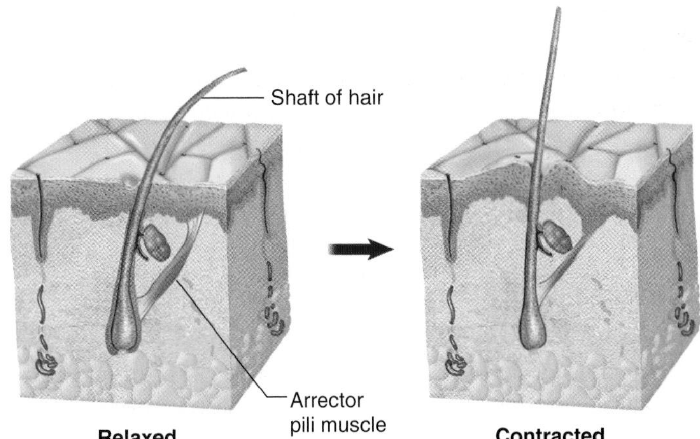

FIGURE 6-6 Arrector pili muscle. When the arrector pili muscle contracts, it pulls the follicle and hair into a more upright position, thus "fluffing up" the hair and pulling the surrounding skin into a "goose bump."

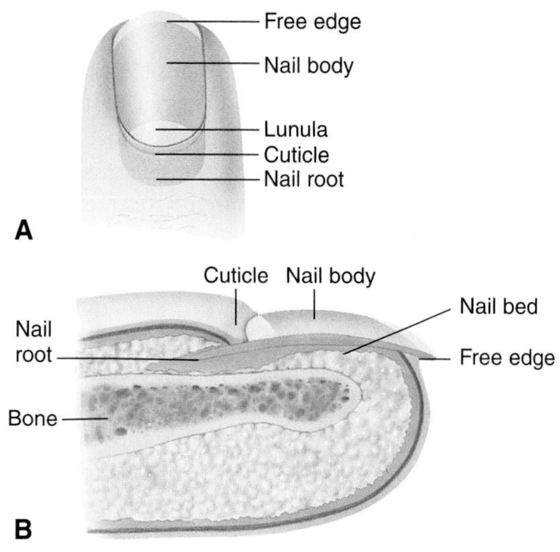

FIGURE 6-7 Structure of nails. A, Fingernail viewed from above. **B,** Sagittal section of fingernail and associated structures.

this area easily on your own nails. It is most noticeable on the thumbnail.

Now look at the sagittal section of the nail in Figure 6-7, *B*. Under the nail lies a layer of epithelium called the *nail bed.* Because it contains abundant blood vessels, it appears pink in color through the translucent nail bodies. If blood oxygen levels drop and cyanosis develops, the nail bed will turn blue.

Skin Receptors

Receptors in the skin make it possible for the body surface to act as a sense organ, relaying messages to the brain concerning sensations such as touch, pain, temperature, and pressure. Receptors, which differ in structure from the highly complex to the very simple, are discussed in detail in Chapter 10.

Two skin receptors are visible in Figure 6-3. One is a **lamellar corpuscle (Pacini corpuscle),** which detects pressure deep in the dermis. The other is the more superficial **tactile corpuscle (Meissner corpuscle),** which detects light touch. Other receptors mediate sensations such as crude touch, vibration, temperature, and pain.

Burn injuries, which are discussed later in the chapter, destroy skin receptors. By doing so, they also may destroy the ability of the burned skin to function as a sense organ.

Skin Glands

The skin glands include the two varieties of **sweat glands** and the tiny **sebaceous glands** (see Figure 6-3).

Sweat Glands

Also called **sudoriferous glands,** sweat glands are the most numerous of the skin glands. They can be classified into two groups—**eccrine** and **apocrine**—based on type of secretion and location.

Eccrine glands

Eccrine sweat glands are by far the more numerous, important, and widespread sweat glands in the body. They are quite small and, with few exceptions, are distributed over the total body surface. Throughout life they produce a transparent, watery liquid called **perspiration,** or *sweat.*

Sweat assists in the elimination of waste products such as ammonia and uric acid. In addition to elimination of waste, sweat plays a critical role in helping the body maintain a constant temperature. Anatomists estimate that a single square inch of skin on the palms of the hands contains about 3000 eccrine sweat glands.

With a magnifying glass you can locate the pinpoint-size openings on the skin that you probably call **pores.** The pores are outlets of small ducts from the eccrine sweat glands.

Apocrine glands

Apocrine sweat glands are found primarily in the skin in the axilla (armpit) and in the pigmented skin areas around the genitals. They are larger than the eccrine glands, and instead of watery sweat, they secrete a thicker secretion.

The odor associated with apocrine gland secretion is not caused by the secretion itself. Instead, it is caused by the contamination and decomposition of the secretion by skin bacteria. Apocrine glands enlarge and begin to function at puberty.

Sebaceous Glands

Sebaceous glands secrete oil for the hair and skin. Oil glands or sebaceous glands grow where hairs grow. Their tiny ducts open into hair follicles (see Figure 6-5) so that their secretion, called **sebum,** lubricates the hair and skin. Someone aptly described sebum as "nature's skin cream" because it prevents drying and cracking of the skin.

Sebum secretion increases during adolescence, stimulated by the increased blood levels of the sex hormones. Frequently sebum accumulates in and enlarges some of the ducts of the sebaceous glands, forming white pimples. This sebum often darkens when exposed to air, forming a **blackhead** or **comedo.** Sebum secretion decreases in late adulthood, contributing to increased wrinkling and cracking of the skin.

QUICK CHECK

1. What are the two major layers of the skin?
2. Where in the skin would you find layers of dead, keratinized cells?
3. How is hair formed?
4. Where in the skin would you find sensory nerve receptors?
5. Name five accessory structures of the skin.

Functions of the Skin

The skin, or cutaneous membrane, serves a number of important functions that contribute to survival. The most important functions are:

1. Protection
2. Temperature regulation
3. Sense organ activity
4. Excretion
5. Synthesis of vitamin D

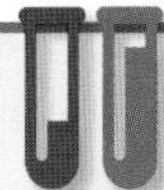

CLINICAL APPLICATION

REPAIR OF SKIN

Some of the most common skin lesions result from scrapes and cuts that our skin often endures in its role of protection. The illustration shows the way in which such injuries typically repair themselves. First, clotting of blood stops blood loss. Then cells of stratum germinativum produce more epithelial cells to rebuild the epidermis as the clot dissolves. At the same time, fiber-producing cells of the dermis replace torn collagen fibers. Often, the replaced fibrous tissue is denser than the original tissue—providing extra strength in the case of further injury but also sometimes producing a scar.

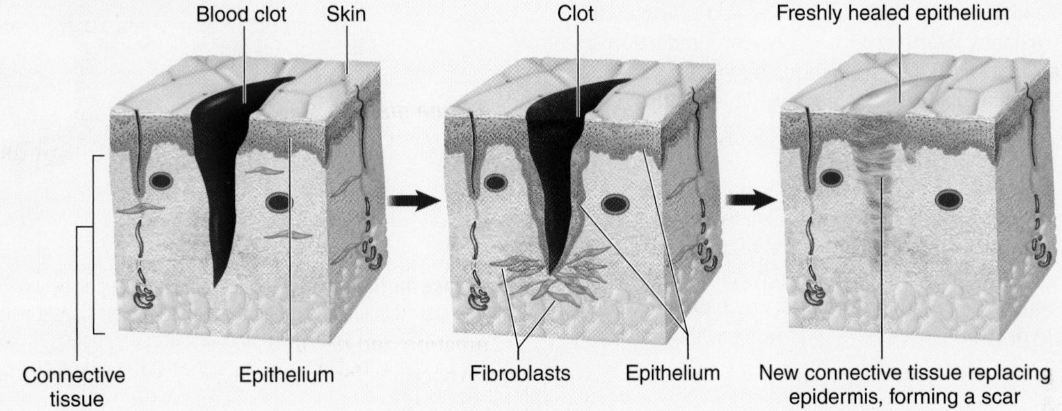

Skin Repair. A minor skin injury is followed by blood clotting and self-repair of the damaged epidermis and dermis. Thickened fibrous tissue produced during dermal repair may cause formation of a scar.

Protection

The skin as a whole is often described as our "first line of defense" against a multitude of hazards. It protects us against the daily invasion of deadly microbes. The tough, keratin-filled cells of the stratum corneum also resist the entry of harmful chemicals and protect against physical tears and cuts. Because it is waterproof, keratin also protects the body from excessive fluid loss. Melanin in the skin prevents the sun's harmful UV rays from penetrating the interior of the body.

Temperature Regulation

The skin plays a key role in regulating the body's temperature. Incredible as it seems, on a hot and humid day the skin can serve as a means for releasing almost 3000 calories of body heat—enough heat energy to boil more than 20 liters of water! It accomplishes this feat by regulating sweat secretion and by regulating the flow of blood close to the body surface. When sweat evaporates from the body surface, heat is also lost. The principle of heat loss through evaporation is basic to many cooling systems.

When increased quantities of blood are allowed to fill the vessels close to the skin, heat is also lost by radiation. Blood supply to the skin far exceeds the amount needed by the skin. The overabundant blood supply primarily enables the regulation of body temperature.

Changes in skin color noted in a hot or cold environment are related to the change in skin blood flow that helps regulate either heat loss or preservation of core body temperature—thus maintaining homeostasis of the body. Changes in skin blood flow, especially to the skin of the face and neck, can also occur as a result of certain skin diseases or sudden emotion. When blood supply increases, the skin reddens—a condition called *flushing* or *blushing*. Contraction of skin blood vessels reduces blood flow and causes the skin to take on a bluish color referred to as *cyanosis*.

Sense Organ Activity

The skin functions as an enormous sense organ. Its millions of nerve endings serve as antennas or receivers for the body, keeping it informed of changes in its environment. The two receptor types shown in **Figure 6-3** make it possible for the body to detect sensations of light touch (tactile corpuscles) and deep pressure (lamellar corpuscles). Other receptors make it possible for us to respond to sensations such as pain, heat, and cold.

Excretion

The term *excretion* refers to any process in which the body rids itself of waste or surplus substances. Excretion of substances in sweat can influence the amounts of certain ions (such as sodium) and waste products (such as uric acid, ammonia, and urea) that are present in the blood. Excess vitamins, drugs, and even hormones in the blood can also be excreted onto the skin by sweat.

HEALTH AND WELL BEING

EXERCISE AND THE SKIN

Excess heat produced by the skeletal muscles during exercise increases the core body temperature far beyond the normal range. Because blood in vessels near the skin's surface dissipates heat well, the body's control centers adjust blood flow so that more warm blood from the body's core is sent to the skin for cooling (see illustration). During exercise, blood flow in the skin can be so high that the skin takes on a redder coloration.

To help dissipate even more heat, sweat production increases to as high as 3 liters per hour during exercise. Although each sweat gland produces very little of this total, more than 3 million individual sweat glands are found throughout the skin.

Sweat evaporation is essential to keeping body temperature in balance, but excessive sweating can lead to a dangerous loss of fluid. Because normal amounts of drinking may not replace the water lost through sweating, it is important to increase fluid consumption during and after any type of exercise to avoid **dehydration**—excessive water loss that disrupts homeostasis.

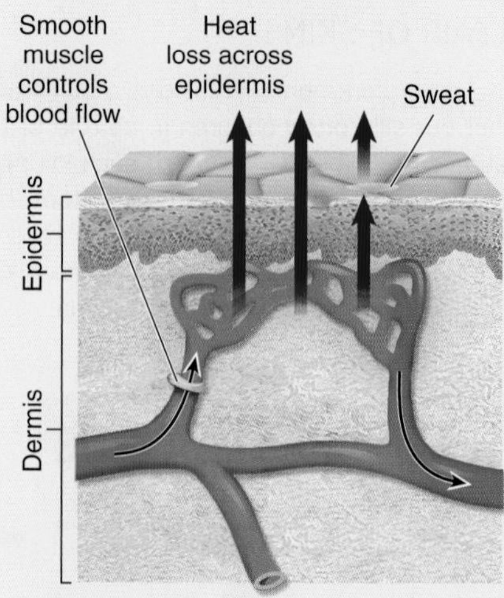

Heat loss during exercise Excess heat produced by working muscles can be lost from blood through the skin to the air. Sweat on the skin can also absorb some of the heat and evaporate—cooling the body further. These mechanisms help maintain homeostasis of body temperature.

Synthesis of Vitamin D

Synthesis of vitamin D is another important function of the skin. It occurs when the skin is exposed to UV light—usually from the sun. When this occurs, a precursor substance in skin cells is transported to the liver and kidneys where it is converted into an active form of vitamin D. Recent research has shown that vitamin D is critically important for good health, thus emphasizing the importance of this skin function.

Skin Cancer

The three most common types of skin cancer are **squamous cell carcinoma, basal cell carcinoma,** and **malignant melanoma.**

Although genetic predisposition plays a role, pathophysiologists believe that exposure to the sun's UV radiation is the most important factor in causing the common skin cancers. UV radiation damages the deoxyribonucleic acid (DNA) in skin cells, causing the mistakes in mitosis that produce cancer. Skin cells have a natural ability to repair UV damage to the DNA, but in some people, this inherent mechanism may not be able to deal with a massive amount of damage.

Kaposi Sarcoma

Kaposi sarcoma (KS) is caused by *Kaposi sarcoma–associated herpesvirus (KSHV),* also known as *human herpesvirus 8 (HHV8).* Once associated mainly with certain ethnic groups, a form of this cancer now also appears in many cases of immune deficiencies. Kaposi sarcoma, first appearing as purple papules (**Figure 6-8**, *A*), quickly spreads to the lymph nodes and internal organs.

Squamous Cell Carcinoma

A common type of skin cancer, squamous cell carcinoma, is a slow-growing malignant tumor of the epidermis. Lesions typical of this form of skin cancer begins as a hard, raised nodule that is usually painless (**Figure 6-8**, *B*). If not treated, squamous cell carcinomas will grow in size and eventually *metastasize*, or spread, invading other organs and areas of the body.

Basal Cell Carcinoma

Basal cell carcinoma, the most common type of skin cancer, usually appears on the upper face. Originating in cells at the base of the epidermis, this type of skin cancer is much less likely to metastasize than other types. It often appears first as a small, raised lesion that erodes in the center to form a bleeding, crusted crater (**Figure 6-8**, *C*).

Melanoma

Malignant melanoma is the most serious form of skin cancer. This type of cancer sometimes develops from a *benign* or noncancerous pigmented mole, and then transforms into a dark, spreading cancerous lesion (**Figure 6-8**, *D*). Benign moles should be checked regularly for warning signs of melanoma because early detection and removal are essential for successful treatment. The "ABCDE" rule of self-examination of moles is summarized in **Table 6-1**.

Unfortunately, the incidence of melanoma in the U.S. population is increasing. Epidemiological studies now show that adults who had more than two blistering sunburns before the age of 20 have a much greater risk of developing melanoma

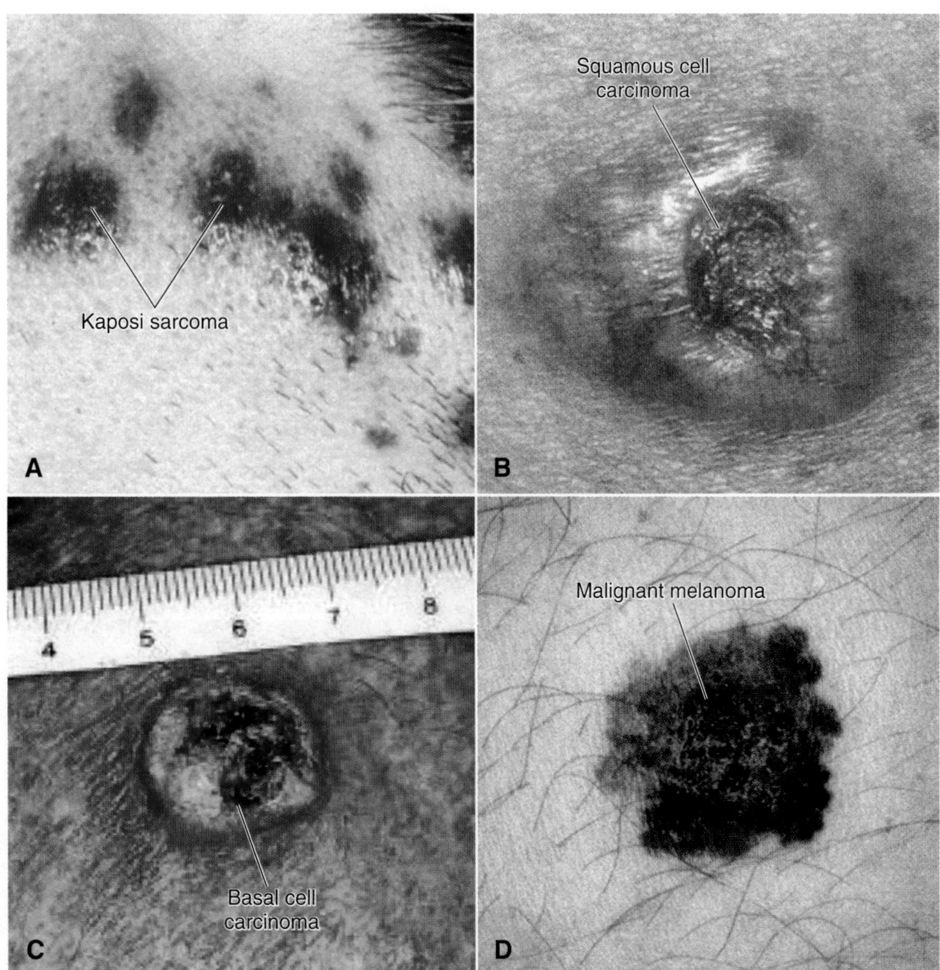

FIGURE 6-8 Examples of skin cancer lesions. **A,** Kaposi sarcoma. **B,** Squamous cell carcinoma. **C,** Basal cell carcinoma. **D,** Malignant melanoma.

than someone who experienced no such burns. Those who grew up in the 1970s and 1980s are now, as older adults, exhibiting melanoma at a much higher rate than those in previous generations.

Burns

Burns constitute one of the most serious and frequent problems that affect the skin. Typically, we think of a burn as an injury caused by fire or by contact of the skin with a hot surface. However, overexposure to UV light (sunburn) or contact of the skin with an electric current or a harmful chemical such as an acid can also cause burns.

The classification and seriousness of a burn injury, as well as appropriate treatment and the possibility for recovery, are determined by three major factors:

1. Depth and number of tissue layers involved
2. Total body surface area affected
3. Type of homeostatic mechanisms such as respiratory or blood pressure control and fluid and electrolyte balance that are damaged or destroyed

TABLE 6-1 Warning Signs of Malignant Melanoma

ABCDE	RULE
Asymmetry	Benign moles are usually symmetrical. Their halves are mirror images of each other. Melanoma lesions are asymmetrical or lopsided.
Border	Benign moles are outlined by a distinct border, but malignant melanomal lesions are often irregular or indistinct in shape.
Color	Benign moles may be any shade of brown but are relatively evenly colored. Melanoma lesions tend to be unevenly colored, exhibiting a mixture of shades or colors.
Diameter	By the time a melanoma lesion exhibits characteristics A, B, and C, it also is probably larger than 6 mm (¼ inch).
Evolving	Moles that continue to evolve, or change over time, may be cancerous. Besides the changes noted above, melanoma lesions may begin to itch, form an ulcer, or bleed.

The age and general state of health of the individual at the time of injury are also are important. A "moderately severe" burn in an otherwise healthy young adult may become a life-threatening "major" burn in an infant or an elderly individual with preexisting respiratory problems or heart disease.

Estimating Body Surface Area

When burns involve large areas of the skin, treatment and the possibility for recovery depend in large part on the *total area involved* and the *severity of the burn*. The severity of a burn is determined by the depth of the injury, as well as by the amount of body surface area affected.

The **"rule of nines"** is one of the most commonly used methods of determining the extent of a burn injury in adults. With this technique (Figure 6-9), the body is divided into 11 areas of 9% each, with the area around the genitals representing the additional 1% of body surface area.

As you can see in Figure 6-9, in the adult 9% of the skin covers the head and each upper extremity, including front and back surfaces. Twice as much, or 18%, of the total skin area covers the front and back of the trunk and each lower extremity, including front and back surfaces.

Classification of Burns

The classification system used to describe the severity of burns is based on the number of tissue layers involved (Figure 6-10). The most severe burns destroy not only layers of the skin and subcutaneous tissue but also underlying tissues.

First-Degree Burns

A **first-degree burn** (for example, a typical sunburn) causes minor discomfort and some reddening of the skin. Although the surface layers of the epidermis may peel in 1 to 3 days, no blistering occurs, and actual tissue destruction is minimal.

Second-Degree Burns

A **second-degree burn** involves the deep epidermal layers and always causes injury to the upper layers of the dermis. Although deep second-degree burns damage sweat glands, hair follicles, and sebaceous glands, complete destruction of the dermis does not occur. Blisters, severe pain, generalized swelling, and fluid loss characterize this type of burn. Scarring is common. First- and second-degree burns are called **partial-thickness burns.**

Third-Degree Burns

A **third-degree burn** is characterized by complete destruction of the epidermis and dermis. In addition, tissue death extends below the primary skin layers into the subcutaneous tissue.

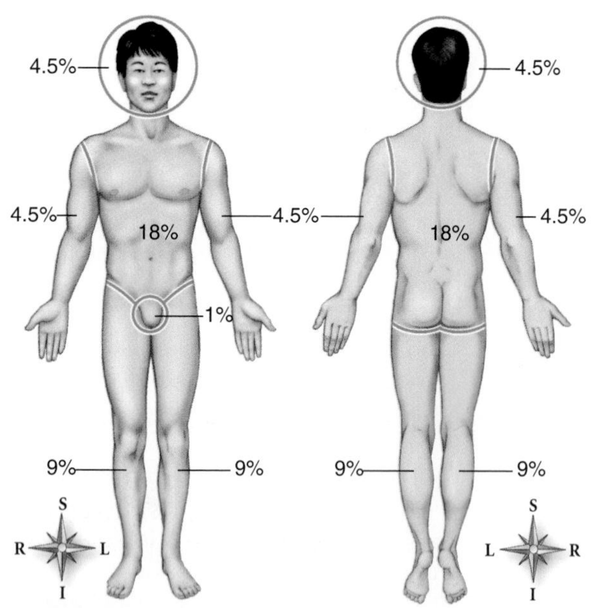

FIGURE 6-9 The "rule of nines." Dividing the body into 11 areas of 9% each helps to estimate the amount of skin surface burned in an adult.

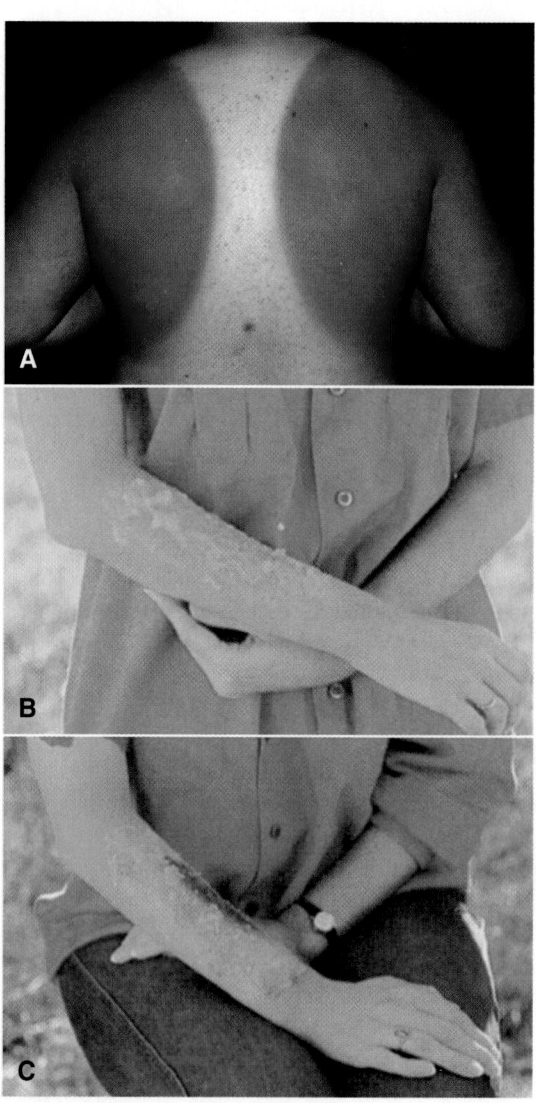

FIGURE 6-10 Classification of burns. Thickness of the damaged skin is one way to classify burns. **A,** First-degree, or partial-thickness, burn. **B,** Second-degree, or partial-thickness, burn. **C,** Third-degree, or full-thickness, burn.

Third-degree burns often involve underlying muscles and even bone. A third degree burn is a type of **full-thickness burn.**

One distinction between second- and third-degree burns is that third-degree lesions are insensitive to pain immediately after injury because of the destruction of nerve endings. However, intense pain occurs soon after the injury. The fluid loss that results from third-degree burns is a very serious problem. Another serious problem with third-degree burns is the great risk of infection because the protective functions of the skin are lost.

Fourth-Degree Burns

The term **fourth-degree burn** (not shown) is used to describe a full-thickness burn that extends below the subcutaneous tissue to reach muscle or bone. Such injuries may occur as a result of high-voltage electrical burns or from exposure to very intense heat over time. Treatment may require extensive skin grafting and even amputation of limbs.

To learn more about burns, go to AnimationDirect at *evolve.elsevier.com.*

QUICK CHECK

1. What are the five most important functions of the skin?
2. What sensory stimuli can be detected by the skin?
3. When referring to burns, what is meant by the "rule of nines"? How can the skin surface area covered by a burn be estimated?
4. How do first-degree, second-degree, third-degree, and fourth-degree burns differ?
5. How do basal cell carcinoma, squamous cell carcinoma, and melanoma differ?

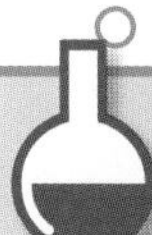

SCIENCE APPLICATIONS

SECRETS OF THE SKIN

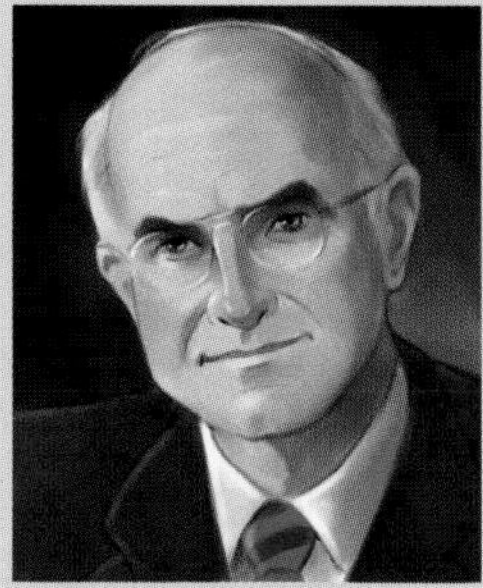

Dr. Joseph E. Murray (1919-2012)

The skin is our most visible organ, so it is no wonder that observing the structure and function of skin has generated sparks that have lit the fires of scientific discovery through the ages. The ancient Romans outlined the process of inflammation in detail after observing it first in the skin. In the twentieth century, Joseph Murray (see figure) noticed that skin he grafted onto burned soldiers he treated during World War II would eventually be rejected by the body. After the war, Murray tried to understand the body's immune reactions to transplanted tissues. His work led to the first successful kidney transplants. His breakthroughs in transplanting kidneys not only earned him a Nobel Prize in 1990, but also they paved the way for all the different types of tissue and organ transplantation that we see today.

Many scientists continue to study the secrets of the skin, and many physicians and other health care professionals also pioneer new methods of skin care and treatment in the fields of **dermatology, allergy, immunology,** *burn medicine,* **reconstructive surgery,** and **cosmetic surgery.** Additional practical applications of some of this skin science are practiced by people working with cosmetics and other skin treatments, nail treatments, and hair treatments. For example, *industrial researchers, product developers,* **cosmeticians,** *spa specialists,* and *hair stylists* all require some knowledge of current skin science to do their jobs effectively.

LANGUAGE OF SCIENCE AND MEDICINE *(continued from p. 103)*

connective tissue membrane
(kon-NEK-tiv TISH-yoo MEM-brayn)
[*con-* **together,** *-nect-* **bind,** *-ive* **relating to,** *tissu-* **fabric,** *membran-* **thin skin**]

cosmetic surgery
(koz-MET-ik SUR-jeh-ree)
[*cosmet-* **adorned,** *-ic* **relating to,** *surger-* **hand,** *-y* **activity**]

cosmetician
(koz-meh-TISH-un)
[*cosmet-* **adorned,** *-ic* **relating to**]

cutaneous membrane
(kyoo-TAYN-ee-us MEM-brayn)
[*cut-* **skin,** *-aneous* **relating to,** *membrane* **thin skin**]

cuticle
(KYOO-tih-kul)
[*cut-* **skin,** *-icle* **little**]

cyanosis
(sye-ah-NO-sis)
[*cyan-* **blue,** *-osis* **condition**]

dehydration
(dee-hye-DRAY-shun)
[*de-* **remove,** *-hydro* **water,** *-ation* **process**]

dermal papilla
(DER-mal pah-PIL-ah)
pl., papillae
(pah-PIL-ee)
[*derma-* **skin,** *-al* **relating to,** *papilla* **nipple**]

dermal-epidermal junction
(DER-mal EP-ih-der-mal JUNK-shun)
[*derma-* **skin,** *-al* **relating to,** *epi-* **on or upon,** *-derma-* **skin,** *-al* **relating to,** *junct-* **joined,** *-ion* **state**]

dermatology
(der-mah-TOL-uh-jee)
[*derma-* **skin,** *-log-* **words (study of),** *-y* **activity**]

dermis
(DER-mis)
[*dermis* **skin**]

eccrine
(EK-rin)
[*ec-* **out,** *-crin-* **secrete**]

eccrine sweat gland
(EK-rin swet gland)
[*ec-* **out,** *-crin-* **secrete,** *gland* **acorn**]

epidermis
(ep-ih-DER-mis)
[*epi-* **on or upon,** *-dermis* **skin**]

epithelial membrane
(ep-ih-THEE-lee-al)
[*epi-* **on or upon,** *-theli-* **nipple,** *-al* **relating to,** *membran-* **thin skin**]

first-degree burn
(furst dih-GREE bern)

follicle
(FOL-lih-kul)
[*foll-* **bag,** *-icle* **little**]

fourth-degree burn
(fohrth dih-GREE bern)

full-thickness burn
(ful THIK-nis bern)

hair follicle
(hair FOL-lih-kul)
[*foll-* **bag,** *-icle* **little**]

hair papilla
(hair pah-PIL-ah)
[*papilla* **nipple**]

hypodermis
(hye-poh-DER-mis)
[*hypo-* **under or below,** *-dermis* **skin**]

immunology
(im-yoo-NOL-uh-jee)
[*immuno-* **free (immunity),** *-logy* **study of**]

integument
(in-TEG-yoo-ment)
[*in-* **on,** *-teg-* **cover,** *-ment* **result of action**]

integumentary system
(in-teg-yoo-MEN-tar-ee SYS-tem)
[*in-* **on,** *-teg-* **cover,** *-ment-* **result of action,** *-ary* **relating to**]

Kaposi sarcoma (KS)
(KAH-poh-see sar-KOH-mah)
[*Moritz K. Kaposi* **Hungarian dermatologist,** *sarco-* **flesh,** *-oma* **tumor**]

keratin
(KER-ah-tin)
[*kera-* **horn,** *-in* **substance**]

lamellar corpuscle (Pacini corpuscle)
(lah-MEL-ar KOR-pus-ul)
[*lam-* **plate,** *-ella-* **little,** *-ar* **relating to,** *corpus-* **body,** *-cle* **little,** *Filippo Pacini* **Italian anatomist**]

lamina propria
(LAM-in-ah PROH-pree-ah)
[*lamina* **thin plate,** *propria* **proper**]

lanugo
(lah-NOO-go)
[*lanugo* **down**]

lunula
(LOO-nyoo-lah)
[*luna-* **moon,** *-ula* **small**]

liposuction
(LIP-oh-suk-shun or LYE-poh-suk-shun)
[*lipo-* **fat,** *-suct-* **sucked,** *-ion* **process**]

malignant
(mah-LIG-nant)
[*malign-* **bad,** *-ant* **state**]

melanin
(MEL-ah-nin)
[*melan-* **black,** *-in* **substance**]

melanocyte
(MEL-ah-noh-syte)
[*melan-* **black,** *-cyte* **cell**]

melanoma
(mel-ah-NO-mah)
[*melan-* **black,** *-oma* **tumor**]

membrane
(MEM-brayn)
[*membran-* **thin skin**]

mucocutaneous junction
(myoo-koh-kyoo-TAY-nee-us JUNK-shun)
[*muco-* **slime or mucus,** *-cut-* **skin,** *-aneous* **relating to,** *junct-* **joined,** *-ion* **state**]

mucous membrane
(MYOO-kus MEM-brayn)
[*muc-* **slime,** *-ous* **characterized by,** *membran-* **thin skin**]

mucus
(MYOO-kus)
[*mucus* **slime**]

nail body
(nayl BOD-ee)

parietal
(pah-RYE-ih-tal)
[*pariet-* **wall,** *-al* **relating to**]

partial-thickness burn
(PAR-shal THIK-nis bern)

pericardium
(pair-ih-KAR-dee-um)
pl., pericardia
(pair-ih-KAR-dee-ah)
[*peri-* **around,** *-cardi-* **heart,** *-um* **thing**]

peritoneum
(pair-ih-toh-NEE-um)
[*peri-* **around,** *-tone-* **stretched,** *-um* **thing**]

peritonitis
(pair-ih-toh-NYE-tis)
[*peri-* **around,** *-ton-* **stretch (peritoneum),** *-itis* **inflammation**]

perspiration (sweat)
(per-spih-RAY-shun)
[*per-* **through,** *-spire* **breathe,** *-ation* **process**]

pigment
(PIG-ment)
[*pigment* **paint**]

pleura
(PLOO-rah)
pl., pleurae
(PLOO-ree)
[*pleura* **side of body (rib)**]

pleurisy
(PLOOR-ih-see)
[*pleur-* **side of body (rib),** *-isy* **condition**]

pore
(por)

reconstructive surgery
(ree-kon-STRUK-tiv SUR-jeh-ree)
[*re-* **again,** *-con-* **with,** *-struct-* **build,** *-ive* **relating to,** *surger-* **hand,** *-y* **activity**]

rule of nines
(rool ov nahyns)

sebaceous gland
(seh-BAY-shus gland)
[*seb-* **tallow (hard animal fat),** *-ous* **relating to,** *gland* **acorn**]

sebum
(SEE-bum)
[*sebum* **grease**]

second-degree burn
(SEK-und dih-GREE bern)

serous membrane
(SEE-rus MEM-brayn)
[*sero-* **watery body fluid,** *-ous* **characterized by,** *membran-* **thin skin**]

squamous cell carcinoma
(SKWAY-mus sel kar-si-NOH-mah)
[*squam-* **scale,** *-ous* **characterized by,** *cell* **storeroom,** *carcin-* **cancer,** *-oma* **tumor**]

stratum corneum
(STRAH-tum KOR-nee-um)
[*stratum* **layer,** *corneum* **horn**]

stratum germinativum
(STRAH-tum jer-min-ah-TYE-vum)
[*stratum* **layer,** *germinativum* **something that sprouts**]

subcutaneous injection
(sub-kyoo-TAY-nee-us in-JEK-shun)
[*sub-* **under,** *cut-* **skin,** *-aneous* **relating to,** *in-* **in,** *-ject-* **throw,** *-tion* **process**]

subcutaneous tissue
(sub-kyoo-TAY-nee-us TISH-yoo)
[*sub-* **beneath,** *-cut-* **skin,** *-ous* **relating to,** *tissu-* **fabric**]

sudoriferous (sweat) gland
(soo-doh-RIF-er-us gland)
[*sudo-* **sweat,** *-fer-* **bear or carry,** *-ous* **relating to,** *gland* **acorn**]

superficial fascia
(soo-per-FISH-al FAH-shah)
[*super-* **over or above,** *-fici-* **face,** *-al* **relating to,** *fascia* **band**]

sweat gland
(swet gland)
[*gland* **acorn**]

synovial fluid
(sih-NO-vee-al FLOO-id)
[*syn-* **together,** *-ovi-* **egg (white),** *-al* **relating to**]

synovial membrane
(sih-NO-vee-al MEM-brayn)
[*syn-* **together,** *-ovi-* **egg (white),** *-al* **relating to,** *membran-* **thin skin**]

tactile corpuscle (Meissner corpuscle)
(TAK-tyle KOR-pus-ul [MYZ-ner KOR-pus-ul])
[*tact-* **touch,** *-ile* **relating to,** *corpus-* **body,** *-cle* **little** (*George Meissner* **German physiologist**)]

third-degree burn
(third dih-GREE bern)

visceral
(VIS-er-al)
[*viscer-* **internal organ,** *-al* **relating to**]

❑ OUTLINE SUMMARY

To download a digital audio version of the chapter summary for use with your device, access the ***Audio Chapter Summaries*** *online at evolve.elsevier.com.*

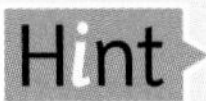

Scan this summary after reading the chapter to help you reinforce the key concepts. Later, use the summary as a quick review before your class or before a test.

Body Membranes

A. Classification of body membranes (see **Figure 6-1**)
  1. Epithelial membranes — composed of epithelial tissue and an underlying layer of connective tissue
  2. Connective tissue membranes — composed largely of various types of connective tissue
B. Epithelial membranes
  1. Cutaneous membrane — the skin
  2. Serous membranes — simple squamous epithelium on a connective tissue basement membrane (see **Figure 6-1**)
    a. Layers (see **Figure 6-2**)
      (1) Parietal — lines wall of body cavity
      (2) Visceral — covers organs within body cavity
    b. Examples
      (1) Pericardium—parietal and visceral layers line a fibrous sac around the heart and a visceral layer covers the heart wall
      (2) Pleura — parietal and visceral layers line walls of thoracic cavity and cover the lungs
      (3) Peritoneum — parietal and visceral layers line walls of abdominal cavity and cover the organs in that cavity
    c. Diseases
      (1) Pleurisy — inflammation of the serous membranes that line the chest cavity and cover the lungs
      (2) Peritonitis — inflammation of the serous membranes in the abdominal cavity that line the walls and cover the abdominal organs
  3. Mucous membranes
    a. Line body surfaces that open directly to the exterior
    b. Produce mucus, a thick secretion that keeps the membranes soft and moist
C. Connective tissue membranes
  1. Do not contain epithelial components
  2. Produce a lubricant called *synovial fluid*
  3. Examples are the synovial membranes lining the joint capsules that surround and attach the ends of articulating bones in movable joints and in the lining of bursal sacs

The Skin

A. Structure (see **Figure 6-3**) — two primary layers called *epidermis* and *dermis*
  1. Epidermis
    a. Outermost and thinnest primary layer of skin
    b. Composed of several layers of stratified squamous epithelium
    c. Stratum germinativum — innermost (deepest) layer of cells that continually reproduce, and new cells move toward the surface
    d. As cells approach the surface, they are filled with a tough, waterproof protein called *keratin* and eventually flake off (see **Figure 6-4**)
    e. Stratum corneum — outermost layer of keratin-filled cells
  2. Skin pigment
    a. Basal layer of stratum germinativum has pigment-producing melanocyte cells
      (1) The brown pigment melanin produced by melanocytes is distributed to other epithelial cells, giving skin a darker color
      (2) Amount and type of melanin, determined by genes, helps determine basic skin color
    b. Skin color changes
      (1) Sunlight promotes additional pigmentation
      (2) Pink flush indicates increased blood volume or increased blood oxygen
      (3) Cyanosis—bluish color of skin indicates decreased blood oxygen level

3. Dermal-epidermal junction
   a. Gluelike layer between the dermis and epidermis
   b. Small bumps called dermal papillae help stabilize the junction
   c. Blisters — caused by breakdown of union between cells or primary layers of skin
4. Dermis
   a. Deeper and thicker of the two primary skin layers and composed largely of connective tissue
   b. Upper papillary layer of dermis characterized by parallel rows of tiny bumps called *dermal papillae*
   c. Ridges and grooves in dermis form pattern unique to each individual
      (1) Basis of fingerprinting
      (2) Improves grip for tool use and walking
   d. Deeper reticular layer of dermis filled with network of tough, interlacing, collagenous, and stretchable elastic fibers
      (1) Number of elastic fibers decreases with age and contributes to wrinkle formation
      (2) Dermis also contains nerve endings, muscle fibers, hair follicles, sweat and sebaceous glands, and many blood vessels
5. Subcutaneous tissue
   a. Also called the *superficial fascia* or hypodermis
   b. Located deep to the dermis, but is not part of the skin
   c. Loose fibrous and adipose tissue are prominent in this layer

B. Hair, nails, and skin receptors
1. Hair (see **Figure 6-5**)
   a. Soft hair of fetus and newborn is called *lanugo*
   b. Hair growth requires epidermal tubelike structure called *hair follicle*
   c. Hair growth begins from hair papilla
   d. Hair root lies hidden in follicle and visible part of hair called *shaft*
   e. Arrector pili — smooth muscle of the skin that produces "goose bumps" and causes hair to stand up straight (see **Figure 6-6**)
2. Nails (see **Figure 6-7**)
   a. Produced by epidermal cells over terminal ends of fingers and toes
   b. Visible part is called *nail body*
   c. Root lies in a groove and is hidden by cuticle
   d. Crescent-shaped area nearest root is called *lunula*
   e. Nail bed may change color with change in blood flow
3. Skin receptors (see **Figure 6-3**)
   a. Sensory nerve endings — make it possible for skin to act as a sense organ
   b. Tactile (Meissner) corpuscle — capable of detecting light touch
   c. Lamellar (Pacini) corpuscle — capable of detecting pressure

C. Skin glands
1. Sweat, or sudoriferous, glands
   a. Eccrine sweat glands
      (1) Most numerous, important, and widespread of the sweat glands
      (2) Produce perspiration or sweat, which flows out through pores on skin surface
      (3) Function throughout life and assist in body heat regulation
   b. Apocrine glands
      (1) Found primarily in axilla and around genitalia
      (2) Secrete a thicker secretion quite different from eccrine perspiration
      (3) Breakdown of secretion by skin bacteria produces odor
   c. Sebaceous glands
      (1) Secrete oil or sebum for hair and skin
      (2) Level of secretion increases during adolescence
      (3) Amount of secretion is regulated by sex hormones
      (4) Sebum in sebaceous gland ducts may darken to form a blackhead

D. Functions of the skin
1. Protection — first line of defense against
   a. Infection by microbes
   b. UV rays from sun
   c. Harmful chemicals
   d. Cuts and tears
2. Temperature regulation
   a. Skin can release almost 3000 calories of body heat per day
      (1) Mechanisms of temperature regulation
         (a) Regulation of sweat secretion
         (b) Regulation of flow of blood close to the body surface
3. Sense organ activity
   a. Skin functions as an enormous sense organ
   b. Receptors serve as receivers for the body, keeping it informed of changes in its environment
4. Excretion—sweat can rid the body of ions and wastes
5. Synthesis of vitamin D

Skin Cancer

A. Types (see **Figure 6-8**)
1. Squamous cell carcinoma
2. Basal cell carcinoma
3. Malignant melanoma
4. Kaposi sarcoma

B. Causes
1. Genetic predisposition
2. Sun's UV radiation damages skin cell DNA, causing mistakes during mitosis
3. Viral infection

C. Kaposi sarcoma (KS)
   1. Caused by Kaposi sarcoma–associated herpes virus (KSHV)
   2. Purple papules on skin surface, which quickly metastasize internally
D. Squamous cell carcinoma
   1. Common type of skin cancer
   2. Slow growing
   3. Lesions begin as painless, hard, raised nodules
   4. Will metastasize
E. Basal cell carcinoma (most common type of skin cancer)
   1. Originates in cells at base of epidermis — often on upper face
   2. Lesions begin as small raised areas that erode in center, bleed, and crust over
   3. Less likely to metastasize than other skin cancer types
F. Malignant melanoma
   1. Most serious form of skin cancer
   2. May develop from benign, pigmented moles or excess UV radiation
   3. Incidence in the United States is increasing
   4. ABCDE rule of self-examination (see **Table 6-1**)

Burns

A. Treatment and recovery or survival depend on total area involved and severity or depth of the burn
B. Body surface area is estimated using the "rule of nines" (see **Figure 6-9**) in adults
   1. Body is divided into 11 areas of 9% each
   2. Additional 1% of body surface area is around the genitals
C. Classification of burns (see **Figure 6-10**)
   1. First-degree (partial-thickness) burns — only the surface layers of epidermis involved
   2. Second-degree (partial-thickness) burns — involve the deep epidermal layers and always cause injury to the upper layers of the dermis
   3. Third-degree (full-thickness) burns — characterized by complete destruction of the epidermis and dermis
      a. Lesion is insensitive to pain because of destruction of nerve endings immediately after injury — intense pain is soon experienced after the initial injury
      b. Risk of infection is increased
   4. Fourth-degree burns—full-thickness burns that extend to muscle or bone

❑ ACTIVE LEARNING

STUDY TIPS

Hint *Use these tips to achieve success in meeting your learning goals.*

1. Before studying Chapter 6, go back and review the discussion of the integumentary system in Chapters 4 and 5. Keep in mind that the principle of "structure fits function" will help explain many of the anatomical and functional characteristics of the skin.
2. The body membranes are either epithelial or connective. The epithelial membranes cover or protect. The difference between mucous and serous membranes is their location in the body. If the membrane is exposed to the environment, it is a mucous membrane. Connective tissue membranes cover joints.
3. The skin is divided into two major layers: epidermis and dermis. *Epi* means "on," so the epidermis is *on* the dermis and serves a protective function. The dermis contains most of the skin structures, including the nails, sense receptors, hair, glands, blood vessels, and muscles.
4. The functions of the skin—protection, sensation, and heat regulation, for example—are related to its location and anatomical components.
5. Burns are classified by how much damage has been done to the layers of the skin and how much, if any, damage has occurred to deeper structures such as muscle and bone.
6. In your study groups, make a photocopy or use your mobile device to take a photo of illustrations of the membranes, the microscopic view of the skin, the hair, and the nails. Cover the labels and quiz each other on the location and function of various structures.
7. In your study group, go over the questions in the back of the chapter, and discuss possible test questions. Use online resources that provide tutorials and diagrams. One example is *studyblue.com.* This is a free online site that allows you to create flash cards, and download apps for all academic disciplines. Other flash card sites and tips are found at *my-ap.us/LzuowE.*
8. Review the Language of Science and Medicine terms and their word origins to help you better understand the meaning of the terms in this chapter.
9. Review the outline at the end of this chapter. This outline provides an overview of the material and would help you understand the general concepts of the chapter.

Review Questions

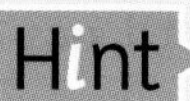

Write out the answers to these questions after reading the chapter and reviewing the Chapter Summary. If you simply think through the answer without writing it down, you won't retain much of your new learning.

1. Define *membrane* and name the two major categories of body membranes.
2. Describe the structure and function of cutaneous membrane.
3. Explain the structure and function of serous membrane. Identify the difference between the parietal and visceral layers and the difference between the pleura and pericardium.
4. Explain the structure and function of mucous membrane and include an explanation of the mucocutaneous junction.
5. Explain the structure of synovial membrane. What is the function of synovial fluid?
6. Name and briefly describe the layers of the epidermis.
7. Explain the structure of the dermis.
8. Differentiate between the *hair papilla*, the *hair root*, and the *hair shaft*.
9. Explain what occurs when the arrector pili contract.
10. Name the four receptors of the skin. To what type of stimuli does each respond?
11. Give the location of the eccrine glands and their function, and describe the type of fluid they produce.
12. Give the location of the apocrine glands and their function, and describe the type of fluid they produce.
13. Give the location of the sebaceous glands and their function, and describe the type of fluid they produce.
14. What are five primary functions of skin?
15. Explain the difference between second-degree and third-degree burns. Which is considered a "full-thickness" burn?

Critical Thinking

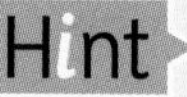

After finishing the Review Questions, write out the answers to these more in-depth questions to help you apply your new knowledge. Go back to sections of the chapter that relate to concepts that you find difficult.

16. Explain the protective function of melanin.
17. Explain fully the role of the skin in temperature regulation.
18. If a person burned all of his back, the back of his right arm, and the back of his right thigh, approximately what percent of his body surface area would be involved? How did you determine this?
19. Jimmy recently had a carcinoma removed from his face. His doctor performed a biopsy and the report came back with the following information: small lesion with center erosion; no metastasis noted. What type of skin cancer does this description suggest?

Chapter Test

Hint *After studying the chapter, test your mastery by responding to these items. Try to answer them without looking up the answers. Then, verify the answers using the key in Appendix C at the back of this book.*

1. The ________, ________, and ________ are the three types of epithelial membranes.
2. Epithelial membranes are usually composed of two distinct layers: the epithelial layer and a supportive connective tissue layer called the ________
3. The membrane lining the interior of the chest wall is called the ________
4. The membrane covering the organs of the abdomen is called the ________
5. The connective tissue membrane that lines the space between the bone and joints is called the ________
6. The two main layers of the epidermis of the skin are the ________ and the ________
7. As new skin cells approach the surface of the skin, their cytoplasm is replaced by a unique waterproof protein called ________
8. The upper region of the dermis forms projections called ________ that form unique fingerprints.
9. The ________ are sweat glands that can be found all over the body and produce a transparent watery liquid.
10. The ________ are sweat glands that can be found in the armpits and produce a thicker secretion.
11. The sebaceous glands secrete an oil called ________
12. ________, ________, and ________ are the three functions of the skin.
13. The receptors in the skin that respond to pressure deep in the dermis are the:
    a. tactile (Meissner) corpuscles
    b. lamellar (Pacini) corpuscles
    c. pili
    d. dermal papillae
14. Which of the following is not a warning sign of melanoma?
    a. Asymmetry
    b. Color
    c. Density
    d. Evolving
15. The receptors in the skin that respond to light touch are the:
    a. tactile (Meissner) corpuscles
    b. lamellar (Pacini) corpuscles
    c. pili
    d. dermal papillae
16. Which burn extends below the subcutaneous tissue to reach muscle or bone? It is a full-thickness burn that is also known as a:
    a. First-degree burn
    b. Second-degree burn
    c. Third-degree burn
    d. Fourth-degree burn

Match each description of a part of the hair in Column B with the name of the structure in Column A.

Column A	Column B
17. ________ Hair follicle	a. The part of the hair hidden in the follicle
18. ________ Hair papilla	b. The growth of the epidermal cells into the dermis forming a small tube
19. ________ Hair root	c. The part of the hair that is visible and extends from the follicle
20. ________ Hair shaft	d. A cuplike cluster of cells where hair growth begins

Skeletal System

OUTLINE

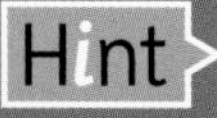

Scan this outline before you begin to read the chapter, as a preview of how the concepts are organized.

OBJECTIVES

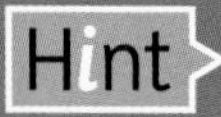

Before reading the chapter, review these goals for your learning.

After you have completed this chapter, you should be able to:

1. List and discuss the generalized functions of the skeletal system.
2. Identify the major anatomical structures found in a typical long bone.
3. Discuss the microscopic structure of bone and cartilage, including the identification of specific cell types and structural features.
4. Explain how bones are formed, how they grow, and how they are remodeled.
5. Identify the two major divisions of the skeleton and list the bones found in each area.
6. Explain why individual human skeletons can vary from each other.
7. List and compare the major types of joints in the body and give an example of each.

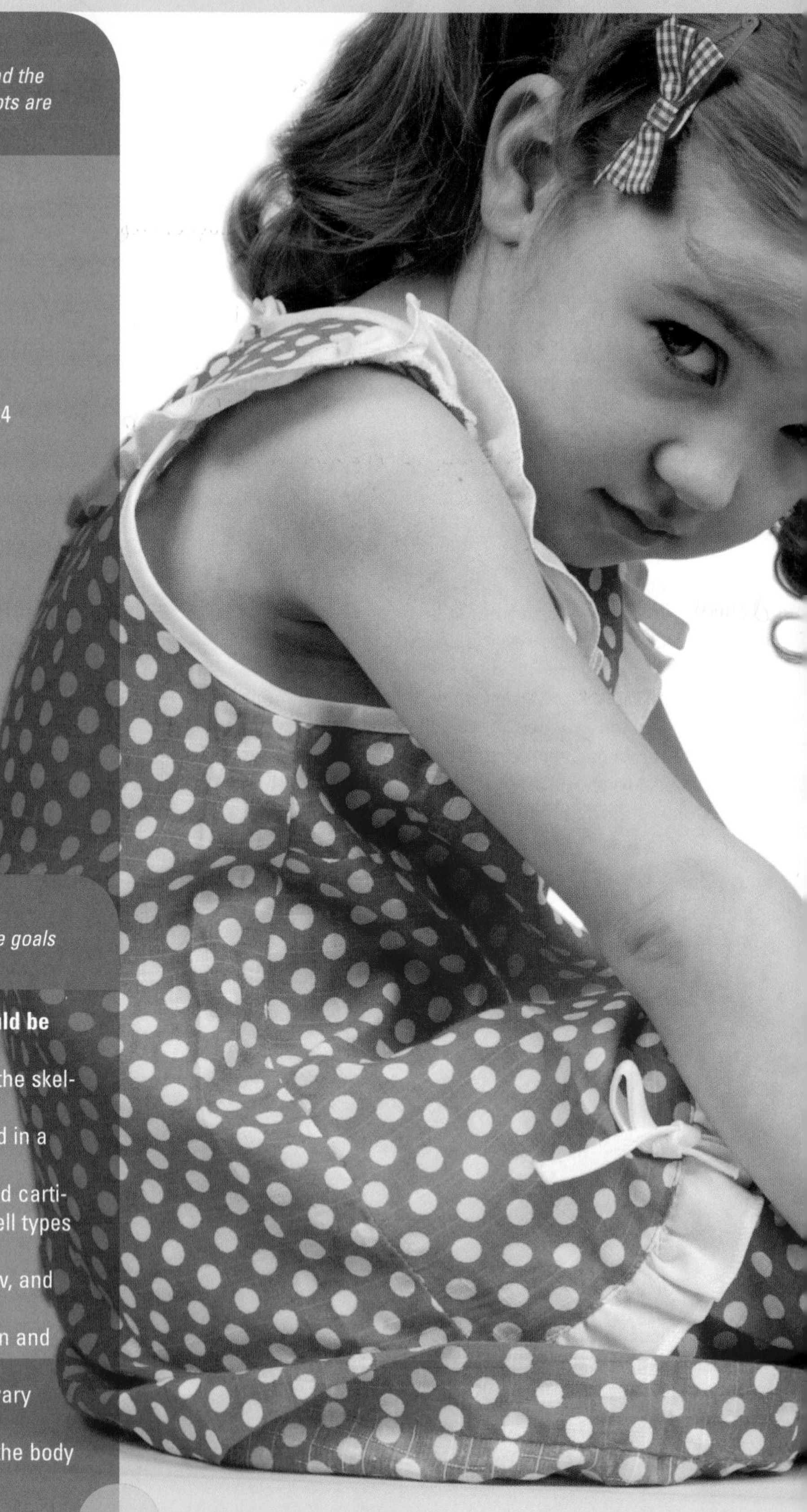

CHAPTER 7

The primary organs of the skeletal system—bones—lie buried beneath the muscles and other soft tissues, providing a rigid framework and support structure for the whole body. In this respect the skeletal system functions like steel girders in a building. However, unlike steel girders, bones can be moved. Bones are also living organs. They can remodel themselves and help the body respond to a changing environment. This ability of bones to change allows our bodies to grow and adapt to new situations.

Our study of the skeletal system begins with an overview of its function. We then classify bones by their structure and describe the characteristics of a typical bone. After discussing the microscopic structure of skeletal tissues, we briefly outline bone growth and formation. Having this information, the study of specific bones and the way they are assembled in the skeleton will be more meaningful. The chapter ends with a discussion of skeletal variations and an overview of joints between bones.

An understanding of how bones articulate with one another in joints and how they relate to other body structures provides a basis for understanding the functions of many other organ systems. Coordinated movement, for example, is possible only because of the way bones are joined to one another and because of the way muscles are attached to those bones. In addition, knowing where specific bones are in the body will assist you in locating other body structures that are discussed in later chapters.

Functions of the Skeletal System

Support

The skeleton provides the internal framework of the body much like tent poles help maintain the structure of a tent. Skeletal muscles are attached to the

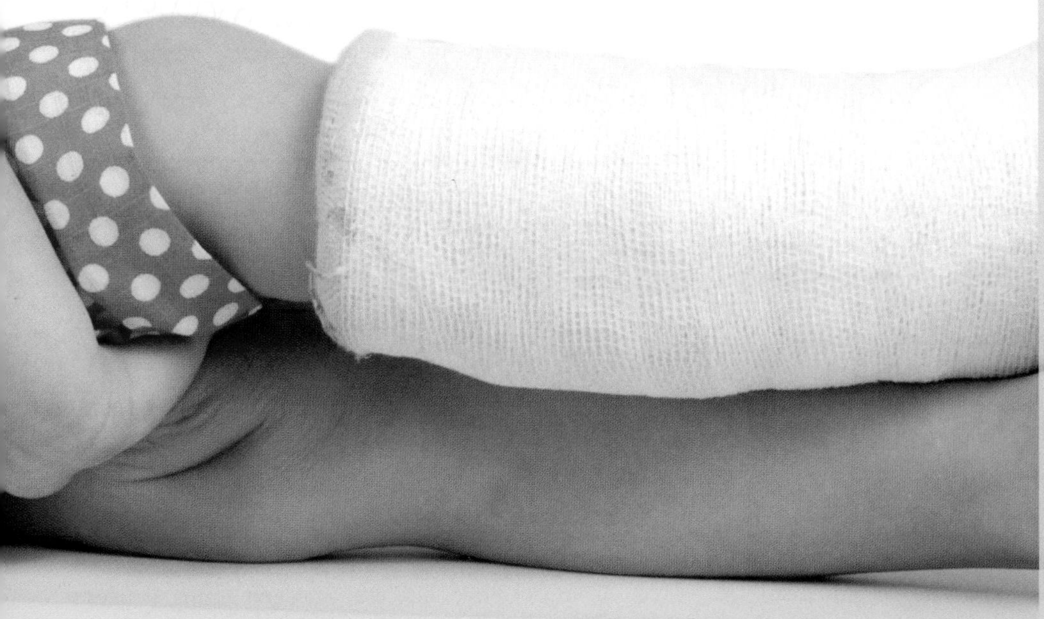

LANGUAGE OF SCIENCE AND MEDICINE

Hint Before reading the chapter, say each of these terms out loud. This will help you to avoid stumbling over them as you read.

abduct
(ab-DUKT)
[*ab-* **away,** *-duct-* **lead**]

abduction
(ab-DUK-shun)
[*ab-* **away,** *-duct-* **lead,** *-tion* **process**]

acetabulum
(as-eh-TAB-yoo-lum)
[*acetabulum* **vinegar cup**]

adduct
(ad-DUKT)
[*ad-* **toward,** *-duct-* **lead**]

adduction
(ad-DUK-shun)
[*ad-* **toward,** *-duct-* **lead,** *-tion* **process**]

amphiarthrosis
(am-fee-ar-THROH-sis)
pl., amphiarthroses
(am-fee-ar-THROH-seez)
[*amphi-* **both sides,** *-arthr-* **joint,** *-osis* **condition**]

appendicular skeleton
(ah-pen-DIK-yoo-lar SKEL-eh-ton)
[*append-* **hang upon,** *-ic-* **relating to,** *-ul-* **little,** *-ar* **relating to,** *skeleton* **dried body**]

arch

articular cartilage
(ar-TIK-yoo-lar KAR-tih-lij)
[*artic-* **joint,** *-ul-* **little,** *-ar* **relating to,** *cartilage* **gristle**]

articulation
(ar-tik-yoo-LAY-shun)
[*artic-* **joint,** *-ul-* **little,** *-ation* **state**]

athletic trainer
(ath-LET-ik TRAY-ner)
[*athlet-* **prize contender,** *-ic* **relating to**]

Continued on p. 148

bones, and internal organs are found in the cavities surrounded by the bones and skeletal muscles. The skeletal system can provide this support only when the composition of the bone is strong enough to hold the weight and yet flexible enough to withstand twisting forces.

Protection

The skeletal system protects the soft tissues that are located inside of bony cavities. The skull protects the brain, and the ribs and breastbone protect vital organs in the chest (heart and lungs). Bone also contains a vital tissue (*red bone marrow*, the blood cell–forming tissue) that produces red blood cells and several types of white blood cells that protect the body from disease.

Movement

Muscles are anchored firmly to bones. As muscles contract and shorten, they pull on bones and thereby move them. Movable joints in the skeleton make such movement possible.

Storage

Bones play an important part in maintaining homeostasis of blood calcium, a vital substance required for normal nerve and muscle function. They serve as a safety deposit box for calcium. When the amount of calcium in blood increases to an above-normal level, calcium moves out of the blood and into the bones for storage. Conversely, when blood calcium decreases to a below-normal level, calcium moves in the opposite direction. It comes out of storage in bones and enters the blood.

The balance of calcium deposits and withdrawals to and from the skeleton is regulated by a balance of hormones. For example, **calcitonin (CT)** from the *thyroid gland* increases mineralization of bone and thus reduces blood calcium. **Parathyroid hormone (PTH)** from the *parathyroid glands* counterbalances the effects of calcitonin by decreasing calcium in the bone and thus increasing blood calcium.

The cavities inside some bones also store fat.

Hematopoiesis

The term **hematopoiesis** is used to describe the process of blood cell formation. It is a combination of two Greek word parts: *hemato-* meaning "blood" and *-poiesis* meaning "a making." Blood cell formation is a vital process carried on in **red bone marrow.** Red bone marrow is soft connective tissue inside the hard walls of some bones that produces both red and white blood cells.

Gross Structure of Bones

Bone Types

There are four major types of bones, classified according to overall structure. Their names suggest their shapes:

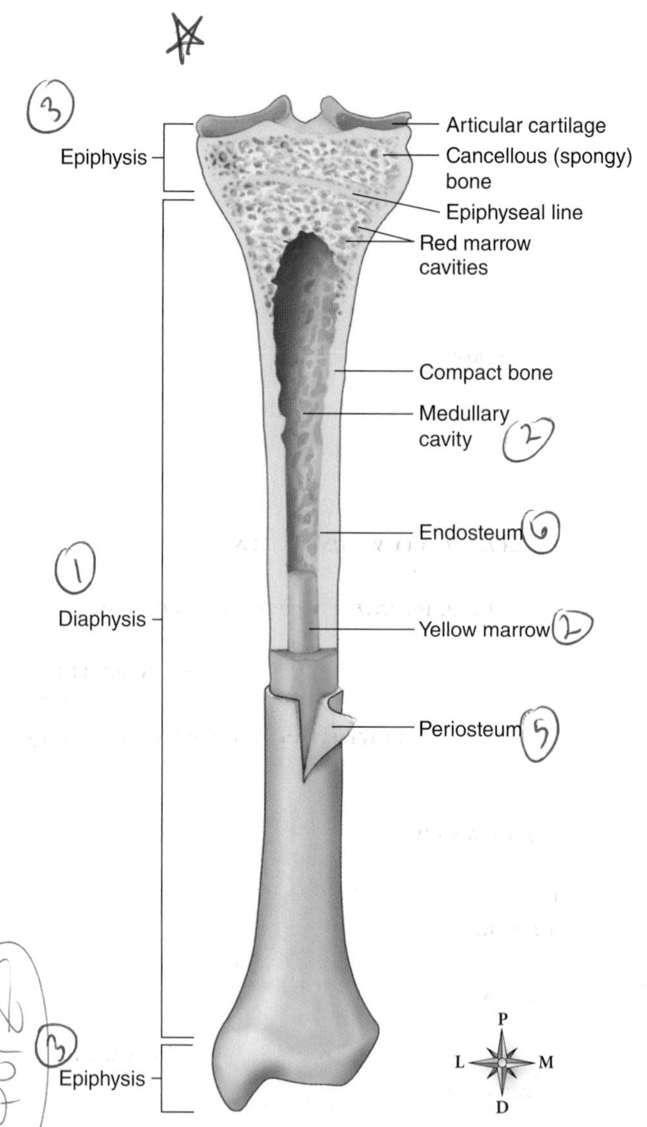

FIGURE 7-1 Long bone. Frontal section of the right tibia (long bone of the leg) showing the typical structures of a long bone.

- *Long bones*—for example, humerus or arm bone
- *Short bones*—for example, carpals or wrist bones
- *Flat bones*—for example, frontal or skull bone
- *Irregular bones*—for example, vertebrae or spinal bones

Some scientists recognize an additional category called *sesamoid* ("like a sesame seed") or *round,* which may develop within a tendon. An example of sesamoid bone is the kneecap (patella), which develops within the patellar tendon.

Many important bones in the skeleton are classified as long bones, and all bones of the body have several common characteristics. By studying a typical long bone, you can become familiar with the structural features of the entire group of human bones.

Structure of Long Bones

Figure 7-1 will help you learn the names of the main parts of a long bone. Identify each of the following:

1. **Diaphysis** or *shaft*—a hollow tube made of hard, compact bone, hence a rigid and strong structure light enough in weight to permit easy movement

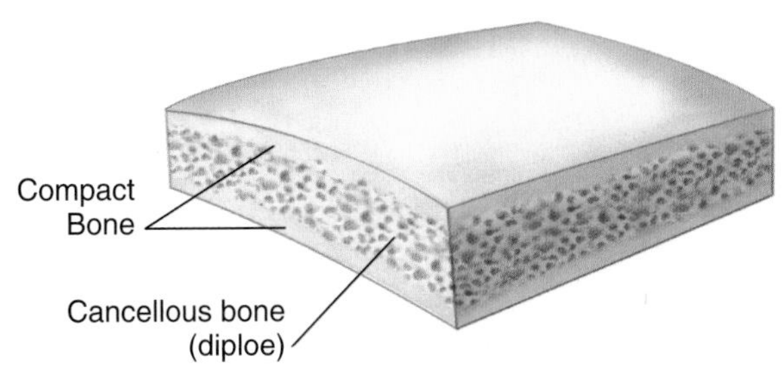

FIGURE 7-2 Flat bone. The diploe is a cancellous (spongy) bone layer sandwiched between two compact bone layers.

2. **Medullary cavity**—the hollow area inside the diaphysis of a bone; contains soft **yellow bone marrow,** an inactive, fatty form of marrow found in the adult skeleton
3. **Epiphyses** or the ends of the bone—red bone marrow fills in small spaces in the spongy bone composing the epiphyses; some yellow marrow may appear as a person ages
4. **Articular cartilage**—a thin layer of cartilage covering each epiphysis; functions like a small rubber cushion would if it were placed over the ends of bones where they form a joint
5. **Periosteum**—a strong membrane of dense fibrous tissue covering a long bone everywhere except at joint surfaces, where it is covered by articular cartilage
6. **Endosteum**—a thin membrane that lines the medullary cavity

Structure of Flat Bones

Flat bones, such as the sternum (breastbone), the ribs, and many of the skull bones have a simpler structure than most long bones. As Figure 7-2 shows, flat bones have a layer of cancellous bone between outer layers of compact bone. The cancellous bone layer is called the **diploe.**

QUICK CHECK

1. What are the organs of the skeletal system?
2. What are the five major functions of the skeletal system?
3. What are the four categories of bones in the skeleton?
4. What are the major features of a long bone? How does the typical flat bone differ?

Microscopic Structure of Bones

The bones of the skeletal system contain two major types of connective tissue: *bone* and *cartilage.*

Bone Tissue Structure

Bone tissue has different microscopic structures, depending on its location and function. In Figure 7-3, *A,* the outer layer of bone is hard and dense. Bone of this type is called **compact bone.** Compact bone appears solid to the naked eye. The porous bone tissue on the inside of individual bones is called **cancellous bone** or **spongy bone.**

Cancellous Bone (Spongy Bone)

As the name implies, spongy bone contains many spaces—like a bath sponge. The cavities are filled with red or yellow marrow. The beams that form the lattice of spongy bone are called **trabeculae.** Figure 7-3, *B,* shows the microscopic appearance of cancellous bone.

Compact Bone

As you can see in Figure 7-3 and Figure 7-4, compact bone does not contain a network of open spaces. Instead, the extracellular matrix is organized into numerous structural units called **osteons** or *haversian systems.* Each circular and tubelike osteon is composed of calcified matrix arranged in multiple layers that resemble the rings of an onion. Each ring is called a **concentric lamella.**

The circular lamellae surround the **central canal,** or *haversian canal,* which contains blood vessels. The central canals are connected to each other by **transverse canals,** sometimes called *Volkmann canals.*

Bones are not lifeless structures. Within their hard, seemingly lifeless matrix are many living bone cells called **osteocytes.** Osteocytes are mature bone cells that were formerly active bone-making osteoblast cells, but which have now become dormant. These osteocytes lie between the hard layers of the lamellae in little spaces called **lacunae.**

In Figure 7-3, *B,* and Figure 7-4, note that tiny passageways, or canals, called **canaliculi** connect the lacunae with one another and with the central canal in each osteon. Nutrients pass along cell extensions of the osteocytes from the blood vessel in the central canal through the canaliculi and are distributed to all osteocytes of the osteon.

Note also in Figure 7-3, *B,* that numerous blood vessels from the outer **periosteum** enter the bone and eventually pass through transverse canals—and eventually to central canals.

Cartilage Tissue Structure

Cartilage both resembles and differs from bone. As with bone, it consists more of intercellular substance than of cells. Innumerable collagenous fibers reinforce the matrix of both tissues. However, in cartilage the fibers are embedded in a firm gel instead of in a calcified cement substance like they are in bone. As a result, cartilage has the flexibility of a firm plastic rather than the rigidity of bone.

Cartilage cells, called **chondrocytes,** as with the osteocytes of bone, are located in lacunae (Figure 7-5). In cartilage, lacunae are suspended in the cartilage matrix much like air bubbles in a block of Swiss cheese. Because there are no blood vessels in cartilage, nutrients must diffuse through the matrix to reach the cells. Because of this lack of blood vessels, cartilage rebuilds itself very slowly after an injury.

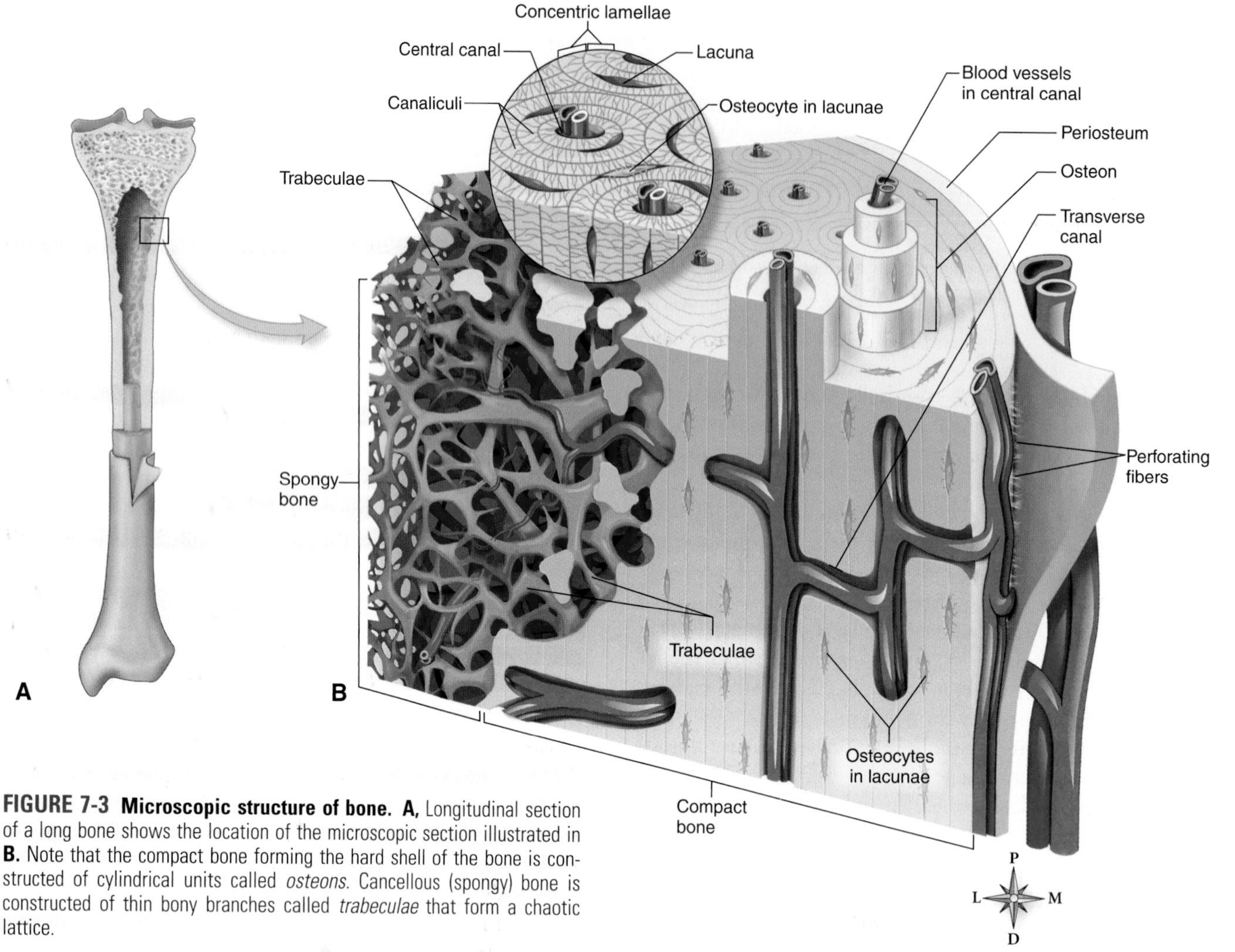

FIGURE 7-3 Microscopic structure of bone. A, Longitudinal section of a long bone shows the location of the microscopic section illustrated in **B.** Note that the compact bone forming the hard shell of the bone is constructed of cylindrical units called *osteons.* Cancellous (spongy) bone is constructed of thin bony branches called *trabeculae* that form a chaotic lattice.

Ossification: the process of bone formation

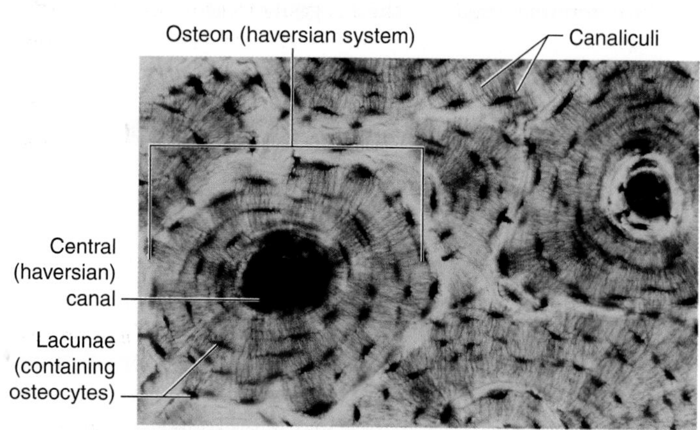

FIGURE 7-4 Compact bone. Photomicrograph shows circular cross section of a cylindrical osteon.

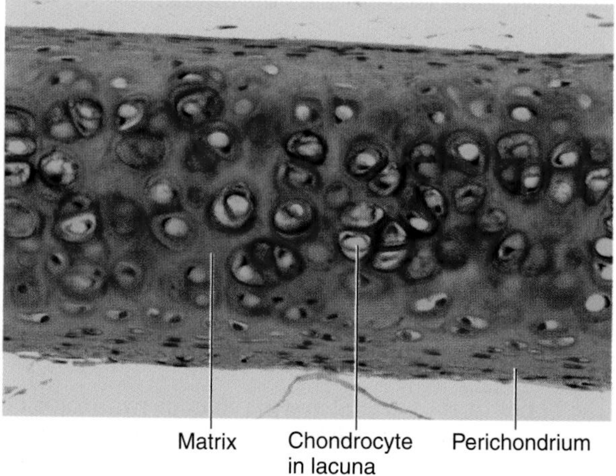

FIGURE 7-5 Cartilage tissue. Photomicrograph shows chondrocytes scattered around the tissue matrix in spaces called lacunae.

Bone Development

Making and Remodeling Bone

When the skeleton begins to form in a baby before its birth, it consists not of bones but of cartilage and fibrous structures shaped like bones. Gradually these cartilage "models" become transformed into real bones when the cartilage is replaced with calcified bone matrix. This process of constantly "remodeling" a growing bone as it changes from a small cartilage model to the characteristic shape and proportion of the adult bone requires continuous activity by bone-forming cells called **osteoblasts** and bone-reabsorbing cells called **osteoclasts,** both seen in Figure 7-6.

The laying down of bone matrix is an ongoing process. Osteoblasts first lay down organic collagen fibers if needed. They also release a solution of inorganic calcium salts that crystallize on the fibers. The fibers reinforce the matrix to withstand twisting forces and the mineral crystals calcify the bone to make it as "hard as bone."

When an osteoblast becomes "trapped" between lamellae of hard bone matrix, they stop forming bone and are called osteocytes. Osteocytes resume their bone-making activity when osteoclasts (or an injury) remove the surrounding bone. Osteoclasts release acids that dissolve the calcium crystals. This has two effects: the hard bone matrix is removed, and the calcium ions are released from bone tissue to diffuse into the bloodstream.

The combined breaking-building actions of the osteoblasts and osteoclasts remodels bones into their adult shapes (Figure 7-7). The process of "sculpting" by the bone-forming and bone-reabsorbing cells allows bones to respond to stress or injury by changing size, shape, and density.

When a bone is mechanically stressed from the pull of a muscle, the osteoblasts are stimulated to strengthen the bone at that location to resist the stress of pulling muscle. For this reason, athletes or dancers may have denser, stronger bones than less active people.

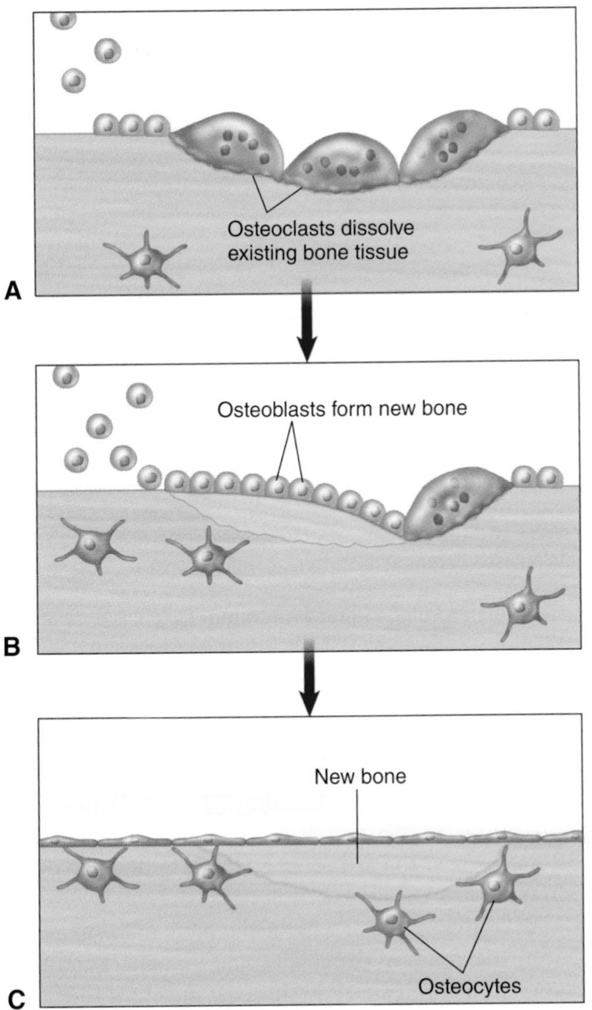

FIGURE 7-6 Bone remodeling. During remodeling of bone, bone-dissolving osteoclasts remove the hard calcium salts in bone matrix (**A**). Osteoblasts then form new bone matrix in the area (**B**) until they eventually become surrounded and "trapped" by hard bone and are then called osteocytes (**C**).

Endochondral Ossification

Many bones of the body are formed from cartilage models, as illustrated in Figure 7-7 and Figure 7-8. This process is called **endochondral ossification,** meaning "formed in cartilage."

As you can see in Figure 7-7, a long bone grows and ultimately becomes "ossified" from small centers within a developing bone. These centers of ossification are located in the *epiphyses* at the ends of a long bone and from a larger center located in the *diaphysis* (**shaft**) of the bone. An area of cartilage called an **epiphyseal plate** remains between the epiphyses and the diaphysis as long as growth continues. Growth ceases when all epiphyseal cartilage is transformed into bone. All that remains is an *epiphyseal line* that marks the location where the two centers of ossification have fused together.

Physicians sometimes use concepts of bone development to determine whether a child is going to grow any more. They have an x-ray study performed on the child's wrist. If it shows a layer of epiphyseal cartilage, they know that additional growth will occur. However, if it shows no epiphyseal cartilage, they know that growth has stopped and that the individual has attained adult height.

Intramembranous Ossification

Some bones, such as the skull bones illustrated in Figure 7-8, are formed by calcification of fibrous membranes in a process called **intramembranous ossification**.

The soft spots, or **fontanels,** on a newborn baby's skull are areas of fibrous membrane that have not yet fully ossified (see Figure 7-8). As intramembranous ossification progresses, a hard bone plate forms a complete flat bone.

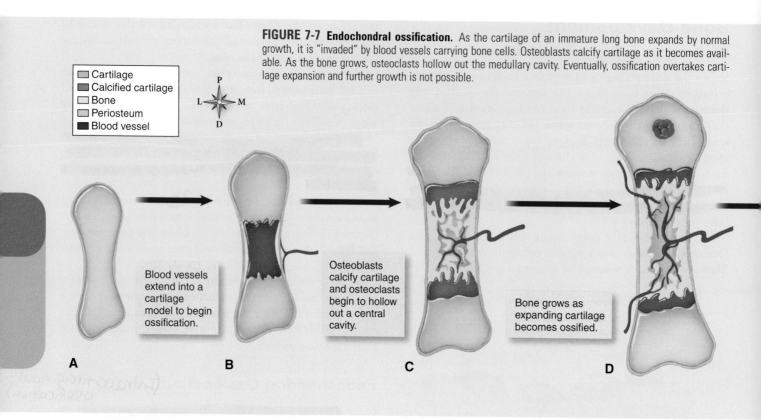

FIGURE 7-7 Endochondral ossification. As the cartilage of an immature long bone expands by normal growth, it is "invaded" by blood vessels carrying bone cells. Osteoblasts calcify cartilage as it becomes available. As the bone grows, osteoclasts hollow out the medullary cavity. Eventually, ossification overtakes cartilage expansion and further growth is not possible.

Cartilage
Calcified cartilage
Bone
Periosteum
Blood vessel

P
L M
D

A Blood vessels extend into a cartilage model to begin ossification.

B Osteoblasts calcify cartilage and osteoclasts begin to hollow out a central cavity.

C Bone grows as expanding cartilage becomes ossified.

D

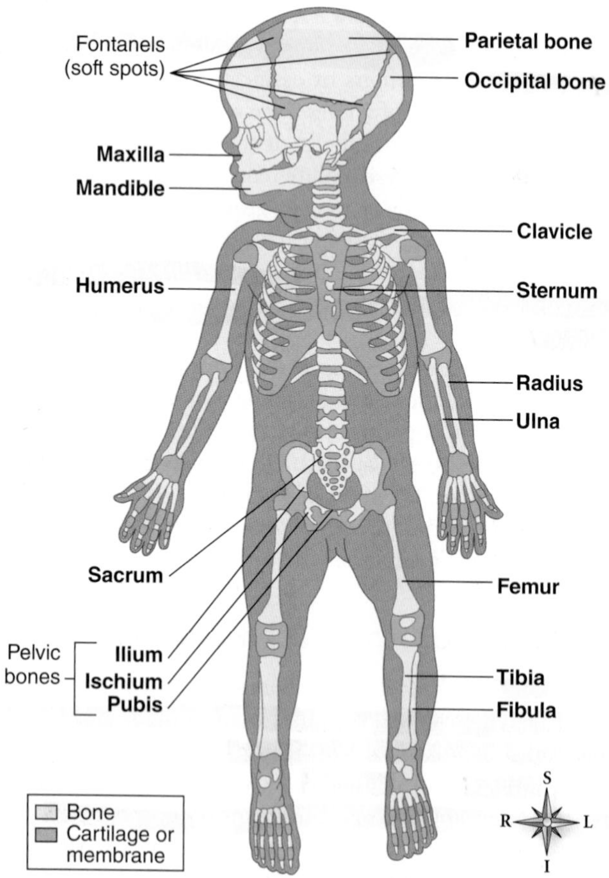

FIGURE 7-8 Bone development in a newborn. An infant's skeleton has many bones that are not yet completely ossified.

To learn more about bone formation and growth, go to AnimationDirect at *evolve.elsevier.com*.

QUICK CHECK

1. What is the basic structural unit of compact bone tissue called?
2. What are the primary structures of a long bone?
3. What are osteocytes? Where would you find them in bone tissue?
4. How does cartilage differ from bone?
5. What is ossification? What is the role of the osteoblast?

Axial Skeleton

The human skeleton has two divisions: the **axial skeleton** and the **appendicular skeleton.** Go back to **Figure 1-9** on p. 12 to review the axial-appendicular division of body regions.

Bones of the center, or axis, of the body make up the axial skeleton. The bones of the skull, spine, and chest and the hyoid bone in the neck are all in the axial skeleton. The bones of the upper and lower extremities or appendages make up the appendicular skeleton. The appendicular skeleton consists of the bones of the upper extremities (shoulder, pectoral girdles, arms, wrists, and hands) and the lower extremities (hip, pelvic girdles, legs, ankles, and feet) (**Table 7-1**).

Locate the various parts of the axial skeleton and the appendicular skeleton in **Figure 7-9**.

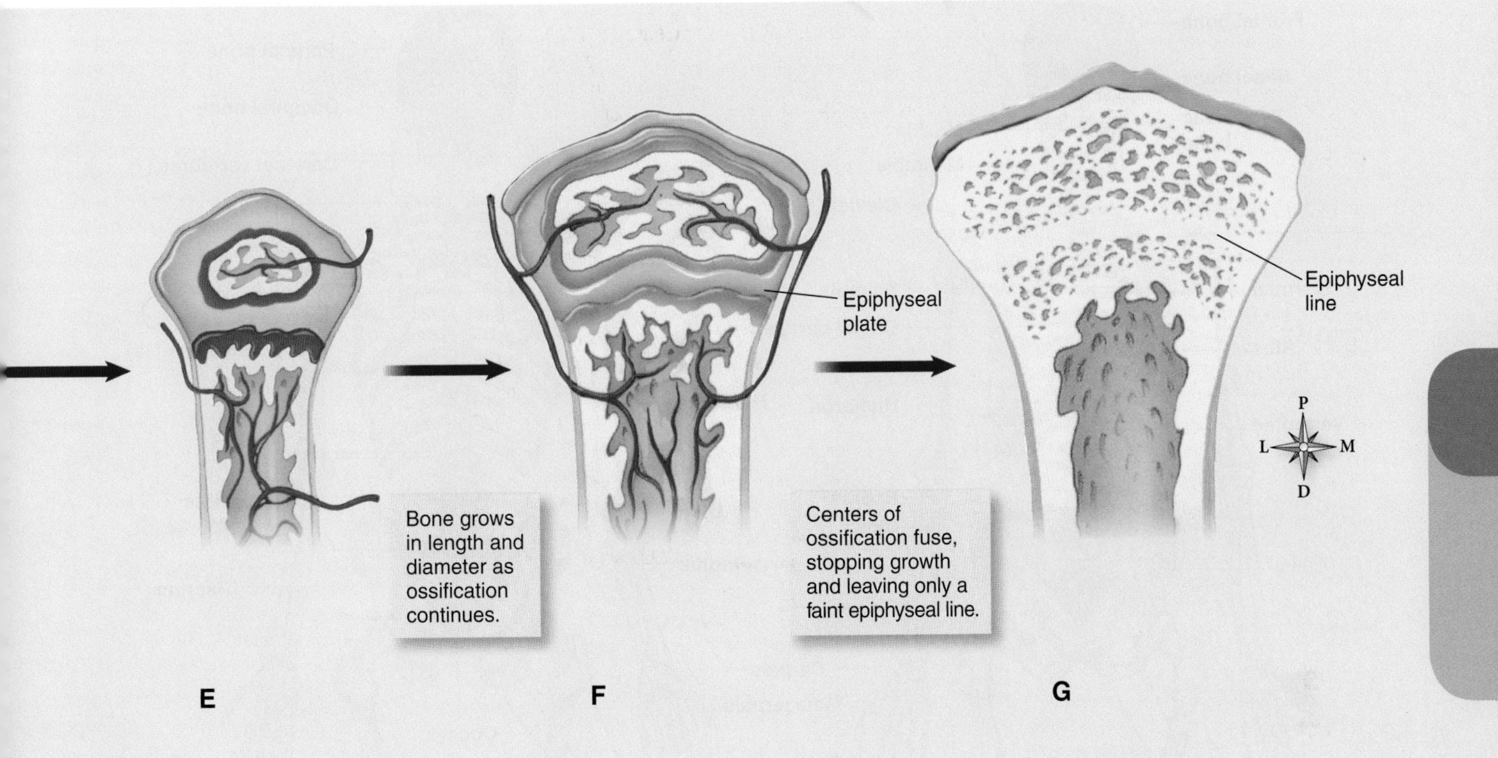
Epiphyseal plate
Epiphyseal line
Bone grows in length and diameter as ossification continues.
Centers of ossification fuse, stopping growth and leaving only a faint epiphyseal line.
P
L
M
D
E
F
G

TABLE 7-1 Main Parts of the Skeleton*

AXIAL SKELETON†	APPENDICULAR SKELETON‡
Skull	Upper extremities
Cranial bones	Pectoral (shoulder) girdle
Ear bones	Arm and forearm bones
Face bones	Wrist bones
Spine	Hand bones
Vertebrae	Lower extremities
Thorax	Pelvic (hip) girdle
Ribs	Thigh and leg bones
Sternum	Ankle bones
Hyoid bone	Foot bones

*Total bones = 206.
†Total = 80 bones.
‡Total = 126 bones.

Skull

The skull consists of 8 bones that form the **cranium,** 14 bones that form the **face,** and 6 tiny bones in the **middle ear.** You can learn the names and locations of these bones by studying **Table 7-2**. Find as many of them as you can on **Figure 7-10**. Feel their outlines in your own body where possible. Examine them on a skeleton if you have access to one.

"My sinuses give me so much trouble." Have you ever heard this complaint or perhaps uttered it yourself? **Sinuses**

HEALTH AND WELL-BEING

OSTEOPOROSIS

Osteoporosis is one of the most common and serious of all bone diseases. It is characterized by excessive loss of calcified matrix and collagenous fibers from bone. Osteoporosis occurs most often in elderly white females. Although white and black males are also susceptible, black women are seldom affected by it.

Because sex hormones play important roles in stimulating osteoblast activity after puberty, decreasing levels of these hormones in the blood of elderly persons reduce new bone growth and the maintenance of existing bone mass. Therefore some reabsorption of bone and subsequent loss of bone mass are accepted consequences of advancing years. However, bone loss in osteoporosis goes far beyond the modest decrease normally seen in old age. The result is a dangerous pathological condition resulting in bone degeneration, increased susceptibility to "spontaneous fractures," and pathological curvature of the spine.

Treatment may include drug therapy and dietary supplements of calcium and vitamin D to replace deficiencies or to offset intestinal malabsorption. Some of the effects of osteoporosis can be prevented by starting exercise while still a young adult, which strengthens bone, and maintaining a diet sufficient in calcium throughout life.

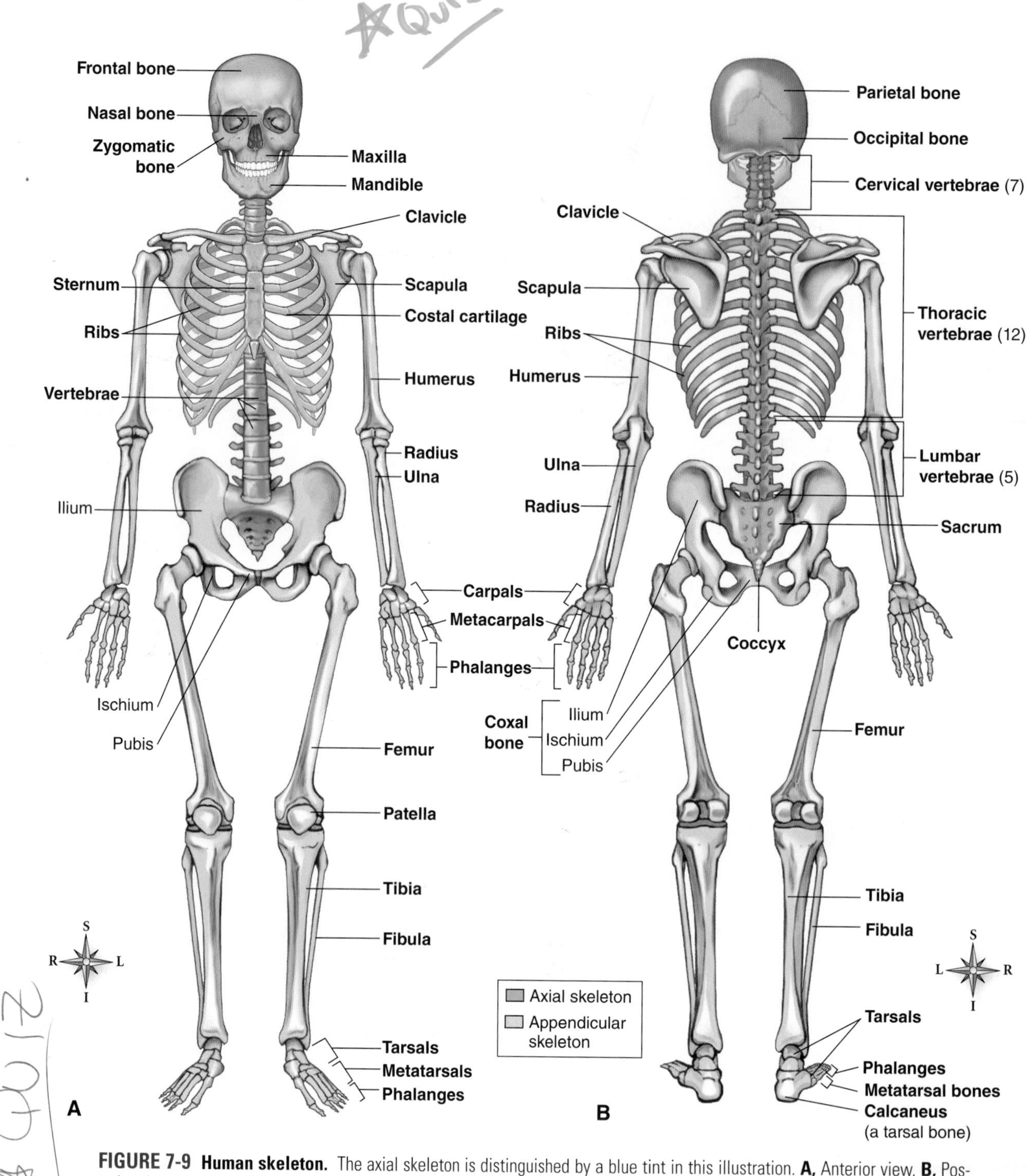

FIGURE 7-9 Human skeleton. The axial skeleton is distinguished by a blue tint in this illustration. **A,** Anterior view. **B,** Posterior view.

are spaces or cavities within some of the cranial bones (**Figure 7-11**). Four pairs of them (those within the frontal, maxillary, sphenoid, and ethmoid bones) have openings into the nose and thus are referred to as **paranasal sinuses.**

Air-filled sinuses are necessary to make the skull light enough for the neck to hold the head upright. But sinuses can give trouble when the mucous membrane that lines them becomes inflamed, swollen, and painful. For example, inflammation in the frontal sinus *(frontal sinusitis)* often starts from a nasal infection. (The suffix *-itis* added to a word means "inflammation of.")

Note in **Figure 7-10** that the two parietal bones, which give shape to the bulging topside of the skull, form immovable joints called **sutures** with several bones: the *lambdoidal suture*

TABLE 7-2 Bones of the Skull

NAME	NUMBER	DESCRIPTION
Cranial Bones		
Frontal	1	Forehead bone; also forms front part of floor of cranium and most of upper part of eye sockets; cavity inside bone above upper margins of eye sockets (orbits) called *frontal sinus;* lined with mucous membrane
Parietal	2	Form bulging topsides of cranium
Temporal	2	Form lower sides of cranium; contain *middle* and *inner ear structures; mastoid sinuses* are mucosa-lined spaces in *mastoid process,* the protuberance behind ear; *external auditory canal* is tube leading into temporal bone; muscles attach to *styloid process*
Occipital	1	Forms back of skull; spinal cord enters cranium through large hole *(foramen magnum)* in occipital bone
Sphenoid	1	Forms central part of floor of cranium; pituitary gland located in small depression in sphenoid called *sella turcica (Turkish saddle);* muscles attach to *pterygoid process*
Ethmoid	1	Uniquely shaped bone that helps form floor of cranium; side walls, roof of nose, and part of its middle partition (nasal septum—made up of the *vomer* bone and the *perpendicular plate* of the ethmoid bone); and part of orbit. Contains honeycomblike spaces, the *ethmoid sinuses; superior* and *middle conchae* are projections of ethmoid bone that form "ledges" along side wall of each nasal cavity
Face Bones		
Nasal	2	Small bones that form upper part of bridge of nose
Maxilla	2	Upper jawbones; also help form roof of mouth, floor, and side walls of nose and floor of orbit; large cavity in maxillary bone is *maxillary sinus*
Zygomatic	2	Cheek bones; also help form orbit
Mandible	1	Lower jawbone articulates with temporal bone at *condyloid process;* only bone of skull that moves freely; *mental foramen* is hole for blood vessels and nerves
Lacrimal	2	Small bones; help form medial wall of eye socket and side wall of nasal cavity
Palatine	2	Form back part of roof of mouth and floor and side walls of nose and part of floor of orbit
Inferior nasal concha	2	Form curved "ledge" along inside of side wall of nose, below middle concha
Vomer	1	Forms lower, back part of nasal septum
Ear Bones		
Malleus	2	Malleus, incus, and stapes are tiny bones in middle ear cavity in temporal bone; *malleus* means "hammer"—shape of bone
Incus	2	*Incus* means "anvil"—shape of bone
Stapes	2	*Stapes* means "stirrup"—shape of bone
Hyoid Bone		
Hyoid bone	1	U-shaped bone in neck; not joined to any other bone (not part of skull); between mandible and upper edge of larynx

with the occipital bone, the *squamous suture* with the temporal bone and part of the sphenoid, and the *coronal suture* with the frontal bone.

You may be familiar with the "soft spots" on a baby's skull. These are six *fontanels,* or areas where intramembranous ossification is incomplete at birth. You can see them in **Figure 7-8**. Fontanels allow some compression of the skull during birth without much risk of breaking the skull bones. They may also be important in determining the position of the baby's head before delivery. The soft membranes of the fontanels also allow additional bone to form around the margins of the skull bones, thus permitting early rapid growth of an infant's skull.

The fontanels eventually fuse to form the immovable joints called *sutures* before a baby is 2 years old.

Hyoid Bone

The odd little **hyoid bone** resembles the Greek letter upsilon (Y or υ). Unlike other bones, it does not form a joint with any other bone of the skeleton. As you can see in **Figure 7-12**, the

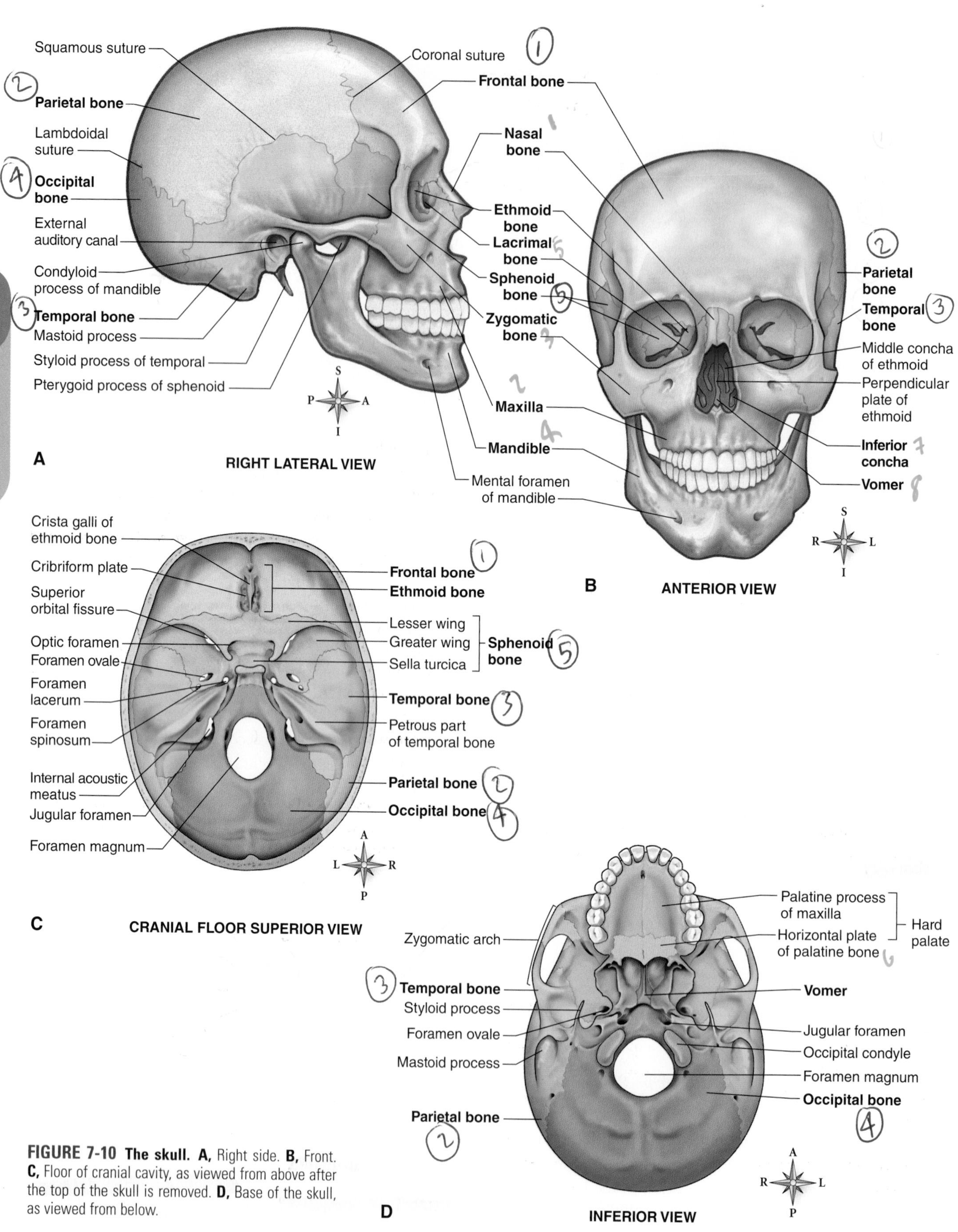

FIGURE 7-10 The skull. **A,** Right side. **B,** Front. **C,** Floor of cranial cavity, as viewed from above after the top of the skull is removed. **D,** Base of the skull, as viewed from below.

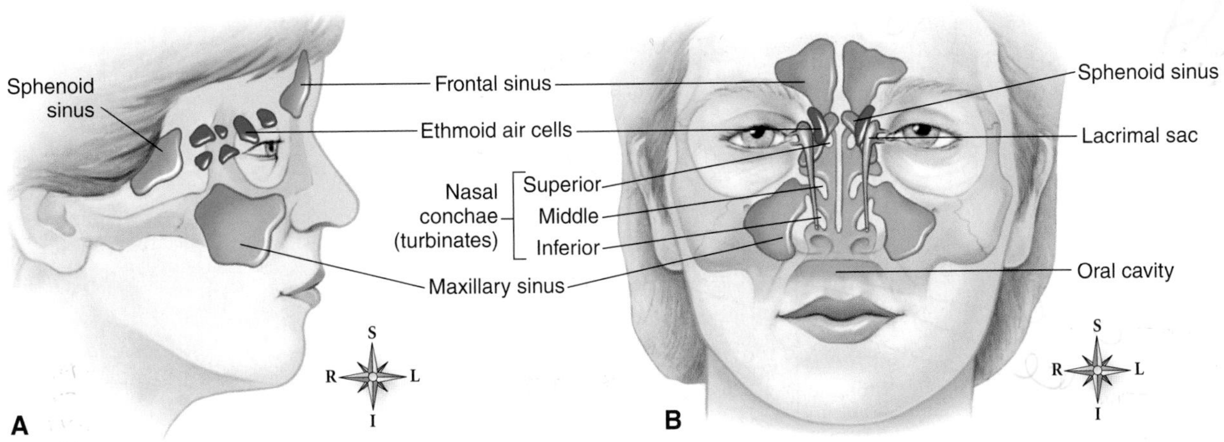

FIGURE 7-11 Paranasal sinuses. A, Lateral view of the head, showing location of sinuses. **B,** Anterior view, showing sinuses and their relationship to the nasal cavity.

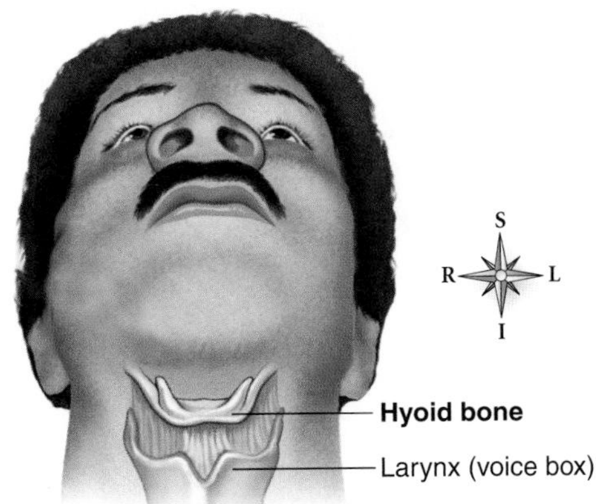

FIGURE 7-12 Hyoid bone. The U-shaped hyoid bone is unique because it does not attach to any other bone of the skeleton.

hyoid bone is located in the neck, where it serves as an anchor for tongue muscles and helps support the larynx (voice box).

Vertebral Column (Spine)

Vertebrae

The term *vertebral column* may conjure up a mental picture of the spine as a single long bone shaped like a column in a building, but this is far from true. The vertebral column consists of a series of 24 separate bones, or **vertebrae,** connected in such a way that they form a flexible curved rod (**Figure 7-13**). Different sections of the vertebral column have different names: *cervical* region, *thoracic* region, and *lumbar* region.

Two additional bones—modified vertebrae—are found at the inferior end of the vertebral column. These are the **sacrum** and **coccyx**.

All 26 bones of the vertebral column are illustrated in **Figure 7-13** and described in **Table 7-3**.

Although individual vertebrae are small bones that are irregular in shape, they have several well-defined parts. Note, for example, in **Figure 7-14**, the body of the lumbar vertebra, its *spinous process* (or spine), its two *transverse processes,* and the hole in its center, called the *vertebral foramen*. The *superior* and *inferior articular processes* permit limited and controlled movement between adjacent vertebrae.

To feel the tip of the spinous process of one of your vertebrae, simply bend your head forward and run your fingers down the back of your neck until you feel a projection of bone at shoulder level. This is the tip of the seventh cervical vertebra's long, forked spinous process. The seven cervical vertebrae form the supporting framework of the neck.

At the top of **Figure 7-13**, *C*, you can see that the first two cervical vertebrae have an unusual structure compared to the rest of the vertebrae. **Figure 7-15** shows that the first cervical vertebra—called the **atlas**—is a ring made up of an *anterior arch* and *posterior arch*. The superior articular processes join with the processes called *occipital condyles* on the base of the

TABLE 7-3 Bones of the Vertebral Column

NAME	NUMBER	DESCRIPTION
Cervical	7	Upper seven vertebrae, in neck region; first cervical vertebra called *atlas;* second, *axis*
Thoracic vertebrae	12	Next 12 vertebrae; ribs attach to these
Lumbar vertebrae	5	Next five vertebrae; located in small of back
Sacrum	1	In child, five separate vertebrae; in adult, fused into one
Coccyx	1	In child, three to five separate vertebrae; in adult, fused into one

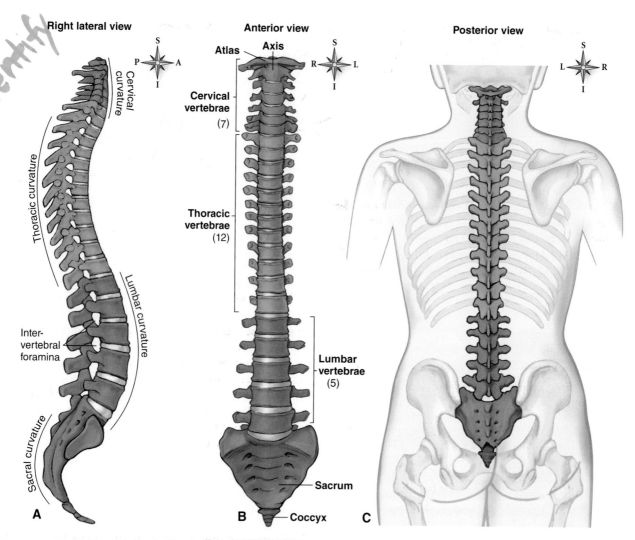

Right lateral view

Cervical curvature
Thoracic curvature
Lumbar curvature
Sacral curvature
Inter-vertebral foramina
A

Anterior view

Atlas
Axis
Cervical vertebrae (7)
Thoracic vertebrae (12)
Lumbar vertebrae (5)
Sacrum
Coccyx
B

Posterior view

C

FIGURE 7-13 **The vertebral column.**

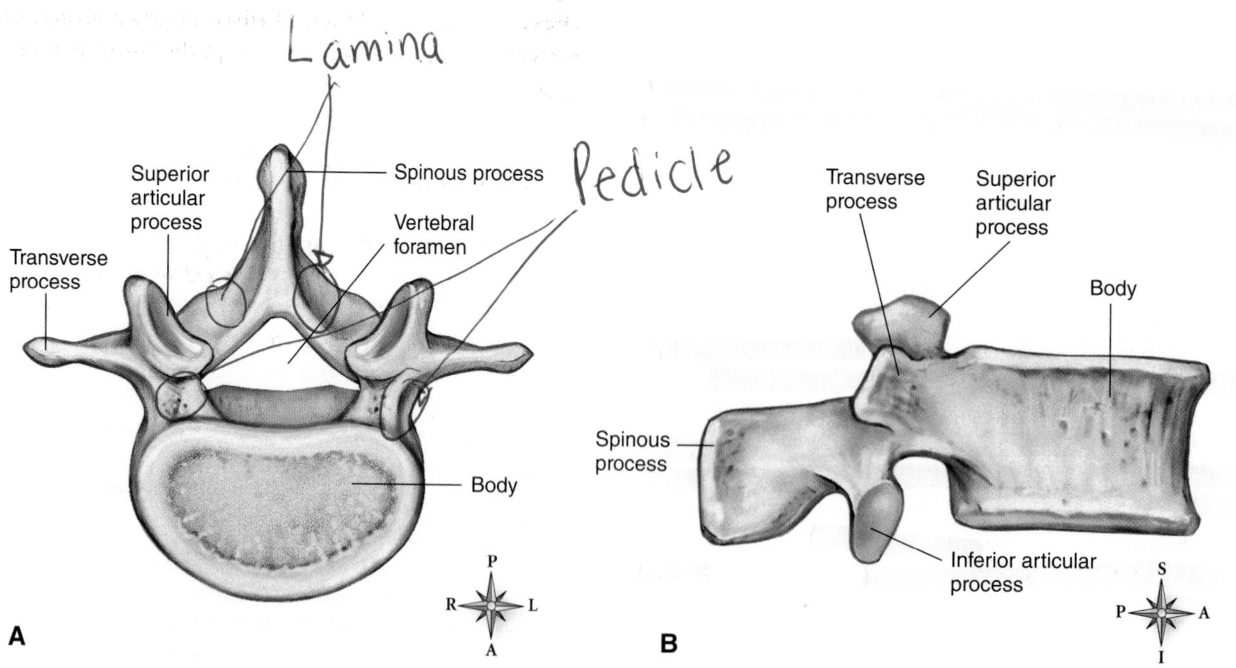

FIGURE 7-14 **The third lumbar vertebra.** **A,** From above. **B,** From the side.

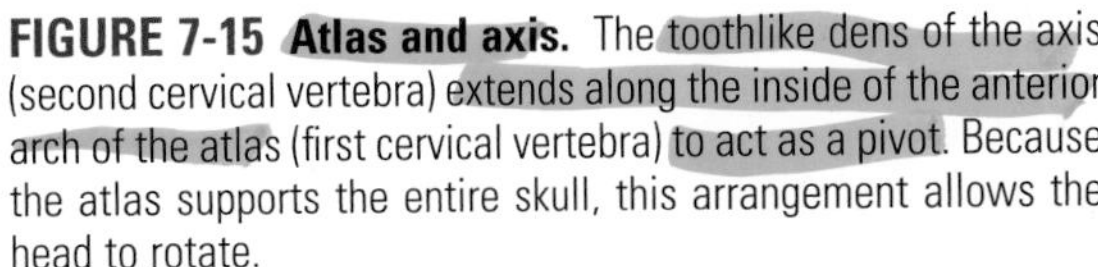

FIGURE 7-15 Atlas and axis. The toothlike dens of the axis (second cervical vertebra) extends along the inside of the anterior arch of the atlas (first cervical vertebra) to act as a pivot. Because the atlas supports the entire skull, this arrangement allows the head to rotate.

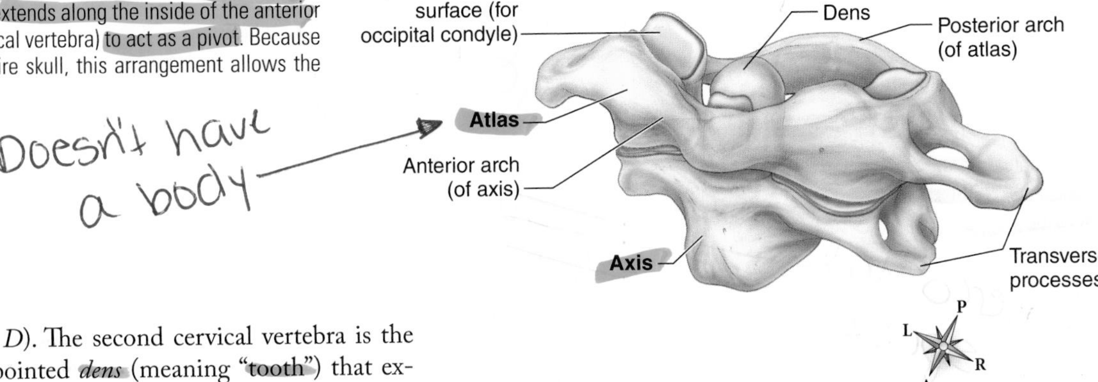

skull (see Figure 7-10, *D*). The second cervical vertebra is the **axis.** The axis has a pointed *dens* (meaning "tooth") that extends up into the curve of the atlas's anterior arch to act as pivot around which the atlas (and the skull) can swivel left and right. This is yet another example of *structure fits function* because rotation of the neck would be very limited without this unique structure.

Spinal Curvatures

Have you ever noticed the four curves in your spine? Your neck and the small of your back curve slightly inward or forward, whereas the chest region of the spine and the lowermost portion curve in the opposite direction (see Figure 7-13).

When you look at the spine from the rear, you will see the cervical and lumbar curves of the spine, called *concave curvatures,* and the thoracic and sacral curves, called *convex curvatures.*

This is not true, however, of a newborn baby's spine. It forms a continuous convex curve from top to bottom (Figure 7-16). Gradually, as the baby learns to hold up his or her head, a reverse or concave curve develops in the neck (cervical region). Later, as the baby learns to stand, the lumbar region of his or her spine also becomes concave.

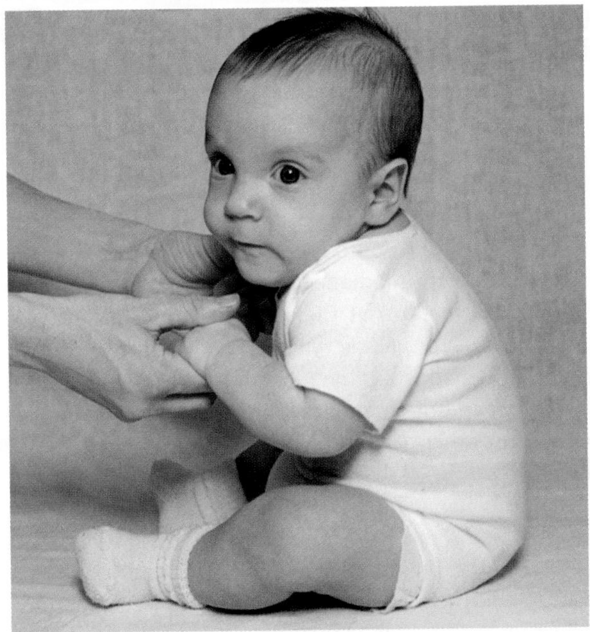

FIGURE 7-16 Spinal curvature of an infant. The spine of the newborn baby forms a continuous convex curve.

The normal curves of the spine have important functions. They give it enough strength to support the weight of the rest of the body. These curves also make it possible to balance the weight of the body, which is necessary for us to stand and walk on two feet instead of having to crawl on all fours. A curved structure has more strength than a straight one of the same size and materials. (The next time you pass a bridge, look to see whether or not its supports form a curve.)

Clearly the spine needs to be a strong structure. It supports the head that is balanced on top of it, the ribs and internal organs that are suspended from it in front, and the hips and legs that are attached to it below.

Thorax

Twelve pairs of ribs, the sternum (breastbone), and the thoracic vertebrae form the bony cage known as the **thorax** or **chest.** Each of the 12 pairs of **ribs** is attached posteriorly to a vertebra. Also, all of the ribs, except the lower two pairs, are also attached to the **sternum** and so have anterior and posterior anchors.

Look closely at Figure 7-17 and you can see that the first seven pairs of ribs (sometimes referred to as the *true ribs*) are attached to the sternum by costal cartilage. The eighth, ninth, and tenth pairs of ribs are attached to the cartilage of the seventh ribs and are sometimes called *false ribs.* The last two pairs of ribs, in contrast, are not attached to any costal cartilage and consequently seem to float free in front, hence their descriptive name, *floating ribs* (Table 7-4).

QUICK CHECK

1. What is the difference between the axial skeleton and the appendicular skeleton?
2. What is a suture? A fontanel? A sinus?
3. What are the three major categories of vertebrae? How many bones are in each section?
4. How is a false rib different from a true rib?
5. Name the spinal curves in the concave curvature and the spinal curves in the convex curvatures of the body.

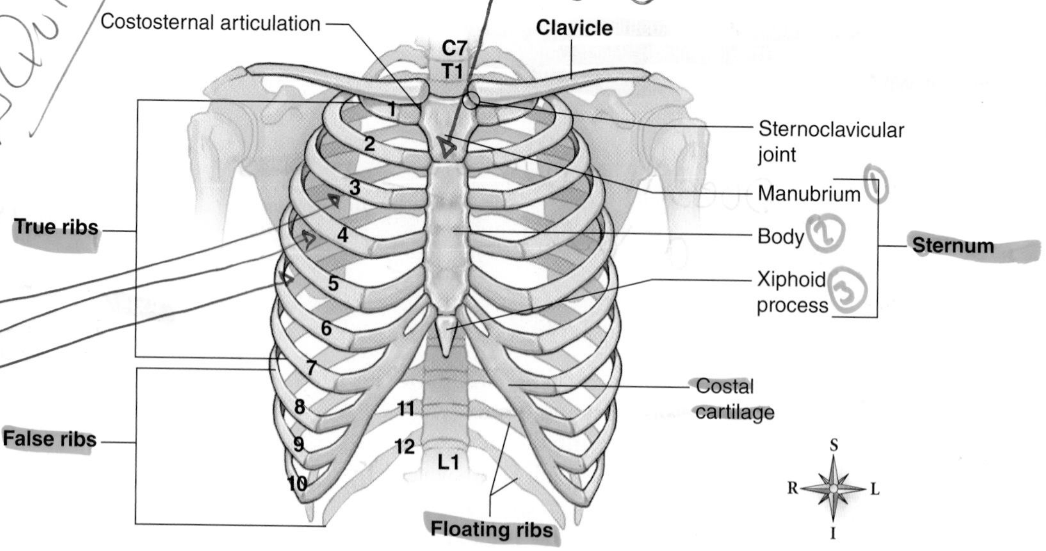

FIGURE 7-17 Bones of the thorax. Rib pairs 1 through 7, the true ribs, are attached by cartilage to the sternum. Rib pairs 8 through 10, the false ribs, are attached to the cartilage of the seventh pair. Rib pairs 11 and 12 are called floating ribs because they have no anterior cartilage attachments.

TABLE 7-4 Bones of the Thorax

NAME	NUMBER	DESCRIPTION
True ribs	14	Upper seven pairs; attached to sternum by *costal cartilages*
False ribs	10	Lower five pairs; first three pairs attached to sternum by costal cartilage of seventh ribs; lowest two pairs do not attach to sternum, therefore called *floating ribs*
Sternum	1	Breastbone; shaped like a dagger; piece of cartilage at lower end of bone called *xiphoid process;* superior portion called the *manubrium*

Appendicular Skeleton

Of the 206 bones that form the skeleton as a whole, 126 are found in the appendicular subdivision.

Look again at **Figure 7-9** to identify the appendicular components of the skeleton. Note that the bones in the shoulder or pectoral girdle connect the bones of the arm, forearm, wrist, and hands to the axial skeleton of the thorax, and the hip or pelvic girdle connects the bones of the thigh, leg, ankle, and foot to the axial skeleton of the pelvis.

Upper Extremity

The **scapula,** or shoulder blade, and the **clavicle,** or collarbone, compose the *shoulder girdle,* or **pectoral girdle.** This structure connects the upper extremity to the axial skeleton. The only direct point of attachment between these bones occurs at the **sternoclavicular joint** between the clavicle and the sternum or breastbone. As you can see in **Figure 7-9** and **Figure 7-17**, this joint is very small. Because the upper extremity is capable of a wide range of motion, great pressures can occur at or near the joint. As a result, fractures of the clavicle are very common.

The **humerus** is the long bone of the arm and the second longest bone in the body. It is attached at the concave glenoid cavity of the scapula at its proximal end, where it is held in place and permitted to move by a group of muscles that are together called the *rotator cuff.*

The distal end of the humerus articulates with the two bones of the forearm at the elbow joint. The bones of the forearm are the **radius** and the **ulna.**

The anatomy of the elbow is a good example of how structure is related to function. Note in **Figure 7-18** that the rounded *trochlea* of the humerus fits into the *trochlear notch* of the ulna to form a hingelike structure that allows the elbow to bend or *flex.* Notice also that the large bony process of the ulna, called the **olecranon,** fits nicely into a large depression on the posterior surface of the humerus, called the **olecranon fossa.** This arrangement prevents the "hinge" of the elbow to extend beyond a straight-arm position—a stability needed to hold objects efficiently.

The radius and the ulna of the forearm articulate with each other and with the distal end of the humerus at the elbow joint. In addition, they also touch each another distally where they articulate with the bones of the wrist. In the anatomical position, with the arm at the side and the palm facing forward, the radius runs along the lateral side of the forearm, and the ulna is located along the medial side of the forearm.

The wrist and the hand have more bones in them for their size than any other part of the body—8 **carpal** or wrist bones, 5 **metacarpal** bones that form the support structure for the palm of the hand, and 14 **phalanges,** or finger, bones—27 bones in all (**Table 7-5**). This composition is very important structurally. The presence of many small bones in the hand and wrist and the many movable joints between them makes the human hand highly maneuverable—allowing us to easily make and use tools.

Figure 7-19 shows the relationships between the bones of the wrist and hand.

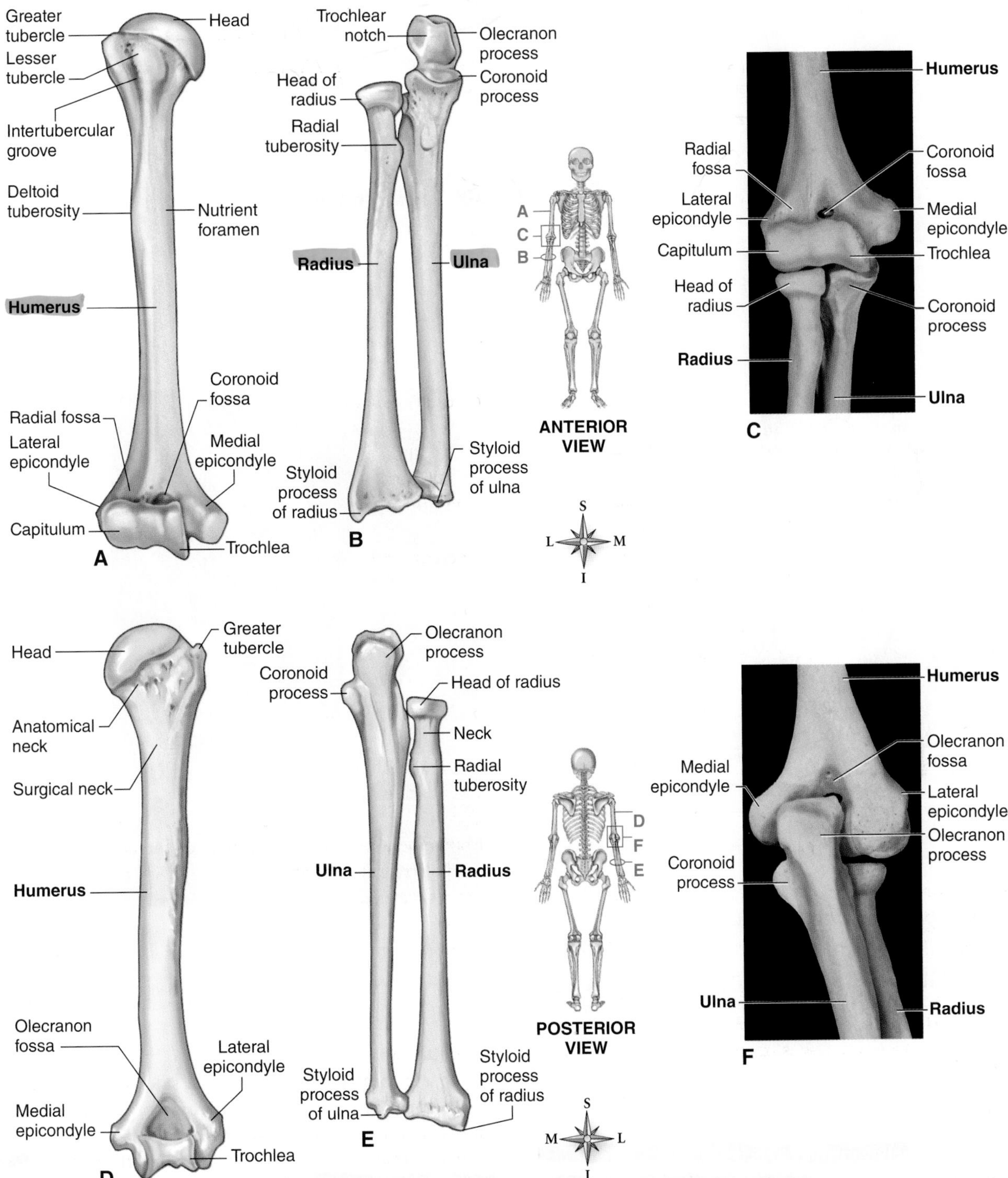

FIGURE 7-18 Bones of the right arm, elbow, and forearm.

TABLE 7-5 Bones of the Upper Extremities

NAME	NUMBER	DESCRIPTION
Clavicle	2	Collarbones; only joints between pectoral (shoulder) and axial skeleton are those between each clavicle and sternum *(sternoclavicular joints)*
Scapula	2	Shoulder blades; scapula plus clavicle forms *pectoral (shoulder); acromion process*—tip of shoulder that forms joint with clavicle; *glenoid cavity*—arm socket
Humerus	2	Arm bone (Muscles are attached to the *greater tubercle* and to the *medial* and *lateral epicondyles;* the *trochlea* articulates with the ulna; the *surgical neck* is a common fracture site.)
Radius	2	Bone on thumb (lateral) side of forearm (Muscles are attached to the *radial tuberosity* and to the *styloid process.*)
Ulna	2	Bone on little finger (medial) side of forearm; *olecranon*—process of ulna known as *elbow* or "funny bone" (Muscles are attached to the *coronoid process* and to the *styloid process.*)
Carpal bones	16	Short bones at upper end of hand; anatomical wrist
Metacarpals	10	Form framework of palm of hand
Phalanges	28	Finger bones; three in each finger, two in each thumb

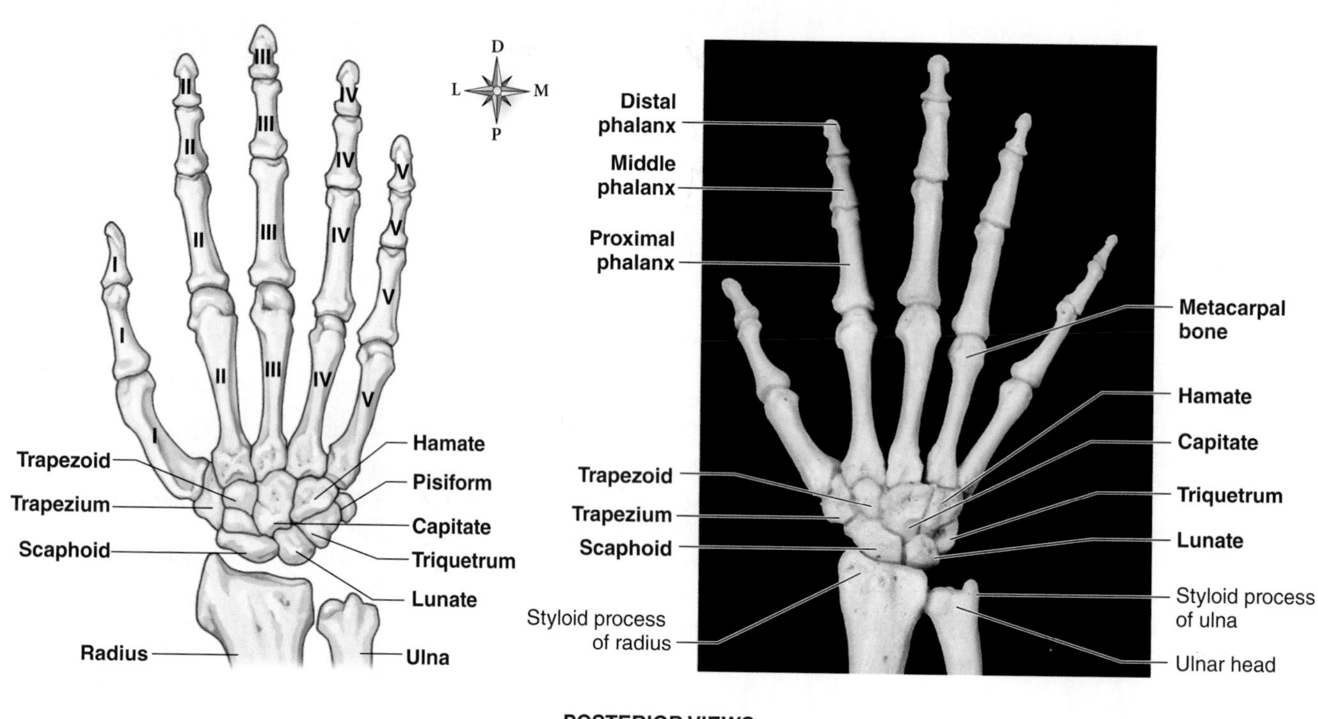

FIGURE 7-19 Bones of the right hand and wrist. Posterior view (back of hand and wrist). There are 14 phalanges in each hand. Each of these bones is called a *phalanx* (dorsal view).

Lower Extremity

The *hip girdle,* or **pelvic girdle,** connects the legs to the trunk. The pelvic girdle as a whole consists of two large **coxal bones,** one located on each side of the pelvis, attached inferiorly to the *sacrum* of the vertebral column. This ringlike arrangement of bones provides a strong base of support for the torso and connects the lower extremities to the axial skeleton. In an infant's body, each coxal bone consists of three separate bones—the **ilium,** the **ischium,** and the **pubis** (see Figure 7-8). These bones grow together to become one coxal bone in an adult (see Figure 7-9 and Figure 7-23).

Just as the humerus is the only bone in the arm, the **femur** is the only bone in the thigh (Figure 7-20). It is the longest bone in the body and articulates proximally at the hip with the coxal bone in a deep, cup-shaped socket called the **acetabulum.** The articulation of the head of the femur in the acetabulum is more stable than the articulation of the head of the humerus with the scapula in the upper extremity. As a result, dislocation of the hip occurs less often than does

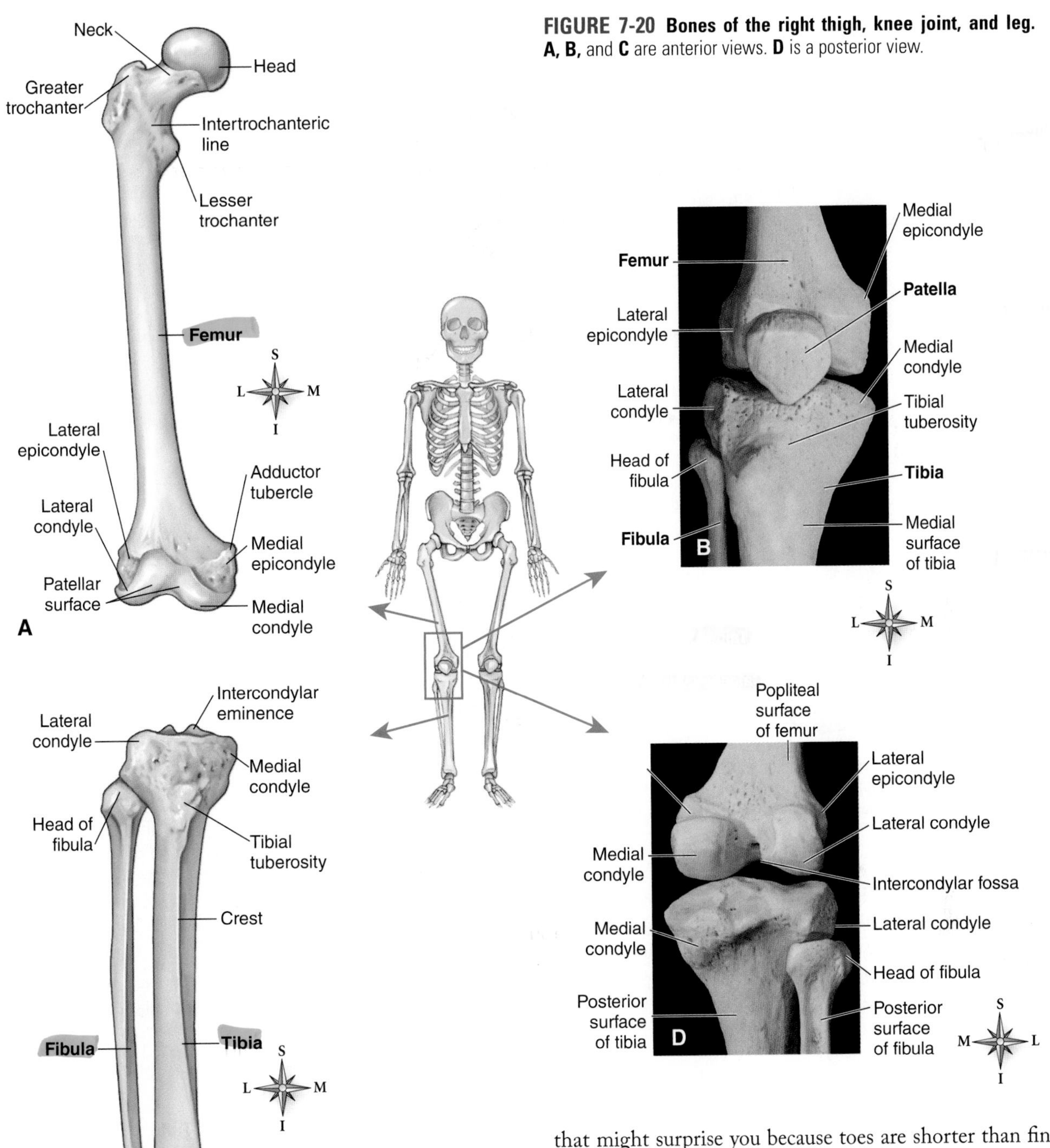

FIGURE 7-20 Bones of the right thigh, knee joint, and leg. **A, B,** and **C** are anterior views. **D** is a posterior view.

disarticulation of the shoulder. Distally, the femur articulates with the knee cap, or **patella,** and the **tibia,** or "shinbone." The tibia forms a rather sharp edge or crest along the front of your leg. A slender, non–weight-bearing, and rather fragile bone named the **fibula** lies along the outer or lateral border of the leg.

Toe bones have the same name as finger bones—**phalanges.** There is the same number of toe bones as finger bones, a fact that might surprise you because toes are shorter than fingers. Foot bones comparable to the metacarpals and carpals of the hand have slightly different names. They are called **metatarsals** and **tarsals** in the foot (Figure 7-21). Just as each hand contains five metacarpal bones, each foot contains five metatarsal bones. However, the foot has only seven tarsal bones, in contrast to the hand's eight carpals. The largest tarsal bone is the **calcaneus,** or heel bone. The bones of the lower extremities are summarized in Table 7-6.

You stand on your feet, so certain features of their structure make them able to support the body's weight. The great toe, for example, is considerably more solid and less mobile than the thumb. The foot bones are held together in such a way as to form springy lengthwise and crosswise arches. These provide great supporting strength and a highly stable base.

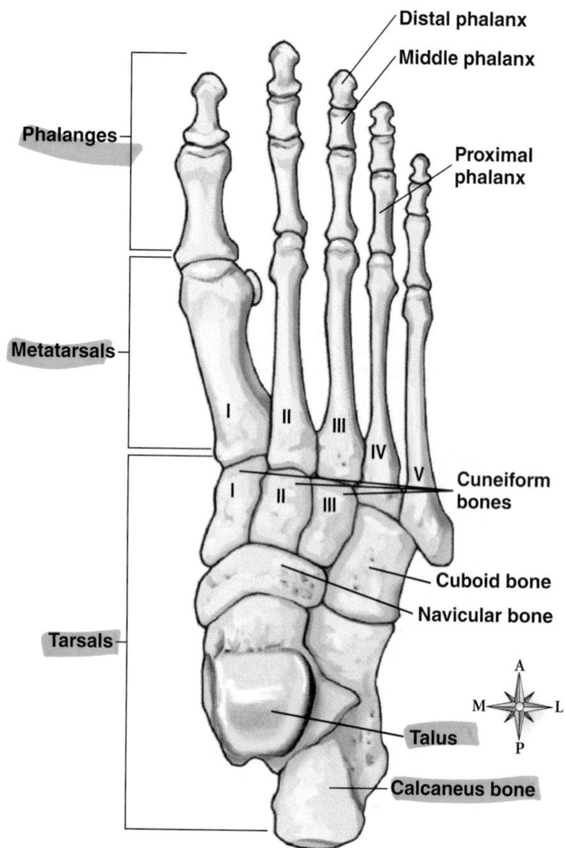

FIGURE 7-21 Bones of the right foot. Compare the names and numbers of foot bones (viewed here from above) with those of the hand bones shown in **Figure 7-19**.

Strong ligaments and leg muscle tendons normally hold the foot bones firmly in their arched positions. Frequently, however, the foot ligaments and tendons weaken. The arches then flatten, a condition appropriately called *fallen arches* or *flatfeet* (**Figure 7-22**, *B*).

TABLE 7-6 Bones of the Lower Extremities

NAME	NUMBER	DESCRIPTION
Coxal bone	2	Hip bone; *ilium*—upper flaring part of pelvic bone; *ischium*—lower back part; *pubic bone*—lower front part; *acetabulum*—hip socket; *symphysis pubis*—cartilaginous joint in midline between two pubic bones; *pelvic inlet*—opening into *true pelvis* or pelvic cavity; if pelvic inlet is misshapen or too small, infant skull cannot enter true pelvis for natural birth
Femur	2	Thigh bones; *head of femur*—ball-shaped upper end of bone; fits into acetabulum (Muscles are attached to the *greater* and *lesser trochanters* and to the *lateral* and *medial epicondyles;* the *lateral* and *medial condyles* form articulations at the knee.)
Patella	2	Kneecap
Tibia	2	Shinbone; *medial malleolus*—rounded projection at lower end of tibia commonly called *inner anklebone;* muscles are attached to the *tibial tuberosity*
Fibula	2	Long slender bone of lateral side of leg; *lateral malleolus*—rounded projection at lower end of fibula commonly called *outer anklebone*
Tarsal bones	14	Form heel and back part of foot; anatomical ankle; largest is the *calcaneus*
Metatarsals	10	Form part of foot to which toes are attached; tarsal and metatarsal bones arranged so that they form three arches in foot; *inner longitudinal arch* and *outer longitudinal arch,* which extend from front to back of foot, and *transverse* or *metatarsal arch,* which extends across foot
Phalanges	28	Toe bones; three in each of the smaller toes, two in each great toe

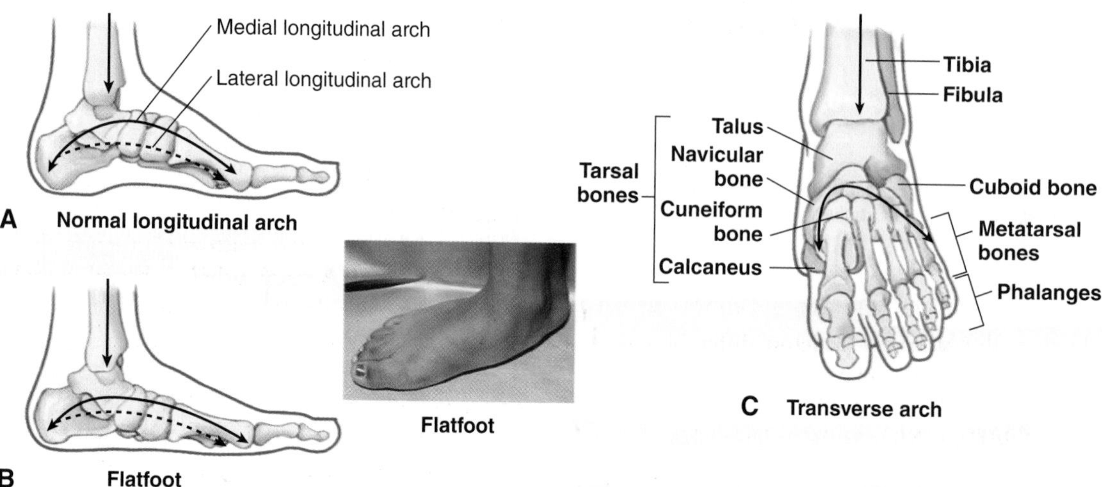

FIGURE 7-22 Arches of the foot. A, Medial and lateral longitudinal arches. (*Arrows* show direction of force.) **B,** "Flatfoot" occurs when tendons and ligaments weaken and the arches fall. **C,** Transverse arch.

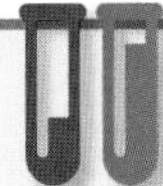

CLINICAL APPLICATION

PALPABLE BONY LANDMARKS

Health professionals often identify externally palpable bony landmarks when dealing with the sick and injured. **Palpable** bony landmarks are bones that can be touched and identified through the skin. They serve as reference points in identifying other body structures.

There are externally palpable bony landmarks throughout the body. Many skull bones, such as the zygomatic bone, can be palpated. The medial and lateral epicondyles of the humerus, the olecranon of the ulna, and the styloid process of the ulna and the radius at the wrist can be palpated on the upper extremity. The highest corner of the shoulder is the acromion process of the scapula.

When you put your hands on your hips, you can feel the superior edge of the ilium called the *iliac crest.* The anterior end of the crest, called the *anterior superior iliac spine,* is a prominent landmark used often as a clinical reference. The medial malleolus of the tibia and the lateral malleolus of the fibula are prominent at the ankle. The calcaneus or heel bone is easily palpated on the posterior aspect of the foot. On the anterior aspect of the lower extremity, examples of palpable bony landmarks include the patella, or knee cap; the anterior border of the tibia, or shinbone; and the metatarsals and phalanges of the toes. Try to identify as many of the externally palpable bones of the skeleton as possible on your own body. Using these as points of reference will make it easier for you to visualize the placement of other bones that cannot be touched or palpated through the skin.

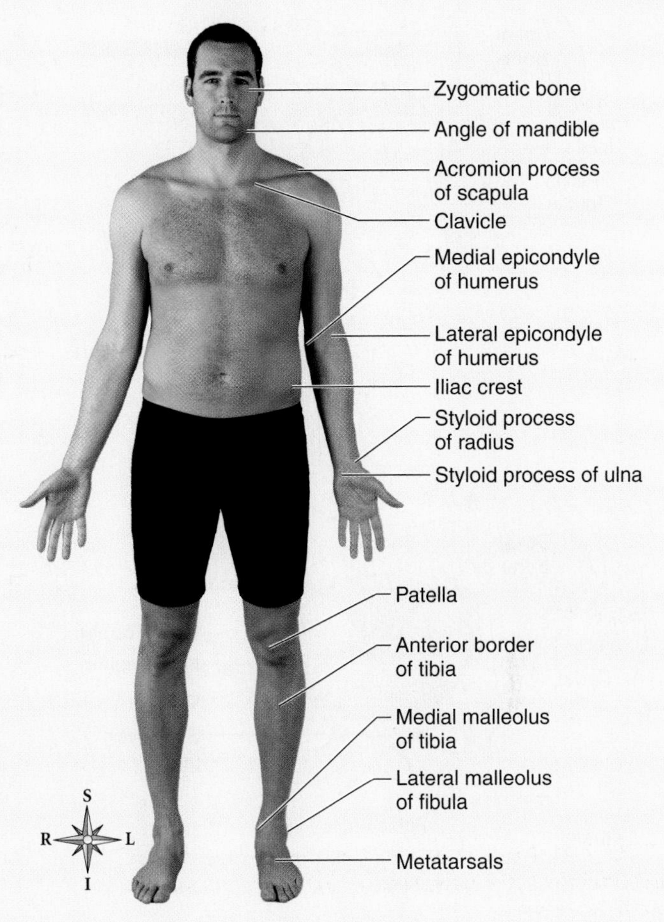

Two arches extend in a lengthwise direction in the foot (**Figure 7-22**, *A*). One lies on the inside part of the foot and is called the **medial longitudinal arch.** The other lies along the outer edge of the foot and is named the **lateral longitudinal arch.** Another arch extends across the ball of the foot. This arch is called the **transverse,** or **metatarsal, arch** (**Figure 7-22**, *C*).

Skeletal Variations

Many different factors cause each individual's skeleton to vary from all other human skeletons. In this section, we explore a few of those factors.

Male and Female Skeletal Differences

A man's skeleton and a woman's skeleton differ in several ways. If you were to examine a male skeleton and a female skeleton placed side by side, you would probably first notice the difference in their sizes. Most male skeletons have bones that are larger, with more distinct bumps and other markings, than most female skeletons. This difference results partly from the difference in muscle tension on bones—the more tension on bone, the bigger and denser the bone gets at the points of muscle attachment. These male-female distinctions are visible in nearly every bone of the body, so it is no wonder that forensic scientists can often accurately determine the sex of human remains using just a few bones.

Perhaps the most obvious of the many structural differences between the male and female skeletons are in the *pelvic girdle* or **pelvis**—the ring formed by the two pelvic (coxal) bones and sacrum. The word *pelvis* means "basin." The wide structure of the female pelvis allows the body of a fetus to be cradled in it before birth, and its wide opening allows the baby to pass through it during birth.

Although the individual male coxal bones are generally larger than the individual female coxal bones, together the male coxal bones form a narrower structure than do the female coxal bones. A man's pelvis is shaped more like a funnel than the broad, shallow basin of the female pelvis (**Figure 7-23**).

You can also see in **Figure 7-23** that the openings from the abdomen into and through the pelvis—the pelvic inlet and pelvic outlet—are both normally much wider in the female than in the male. This effect is partly because the angle at the front of the female pelvis where the two pubic bones join is wider than in the male. Such an arrangement allows more room for a fetus's head to move through during childbirth.

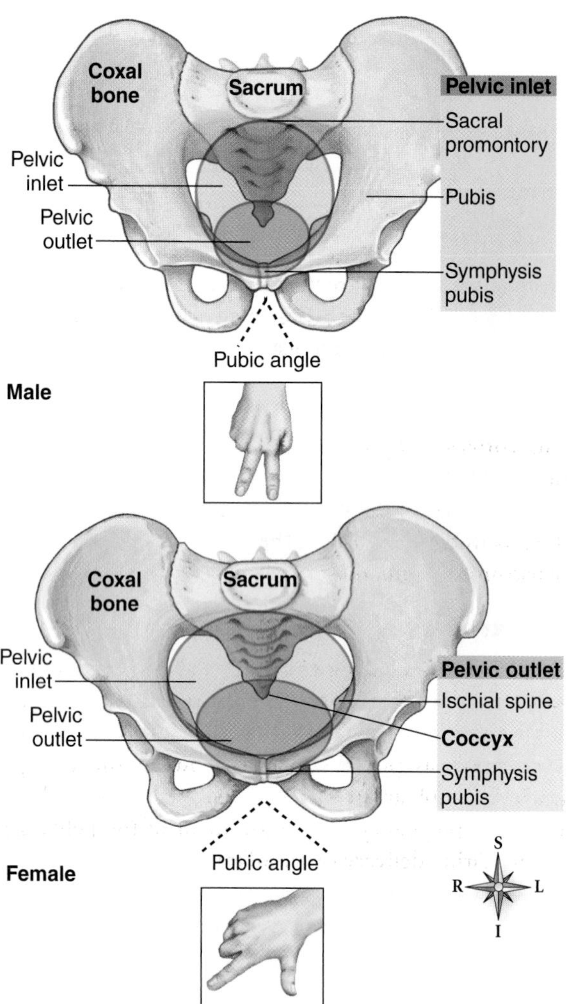

FIGURE 7-23 Comparison of the male pelvis and female pelvis. Notice the narrower width of the male pelvis, giving it a more funnel-like shape than the female pelvis. The insets show how the hand can be used to show how the pubic angles differ.

Age Differences

As we learned earlier in the chapter, during childhood and adolescence the bones of the skeleton enlarge and become more ossified. The human skeleton is considered to reach its mature state around age 25. From then until about age 50 or so, the skeleton is in a state of active maintenance, continually remodeling—dissolving and rebuilding—bone tissue.

After age 50, the density of bone often decreases slowly because of a shift in the remodeling activity. An elderly person's skeleton often weighs much less than it did when they were in their 30s.

Environmental Factors

Among the many factors that can cause variations in one's skeleton is nutrition. Without enough calcium and vitamin D, especially during the developmental years, the skeleton may not reach its full potential of growth or it may show signs of early degeneration.

Load-bearing, or mechanical stress, of using the skeleton affects how bone tissue is remodeled. Exercise has a profound effect on the skeleton. An active older person can reverse much or all of the bone loss associated with aging. Scientists can sometimes tell a person's occupation by which bones—or which parts of bones—are more developed. For example, a person who works with heavy loads on their right arm every day will have denser bones in the right arm and shoulder than in the left arm. Breaks and repairs similarly cause individual variations in the skeleton.

QUICK CHECK

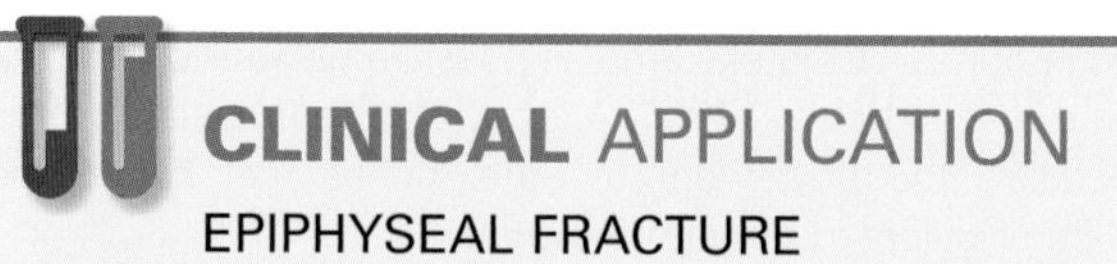

1. How many bones are in the appendicular skeleton?
2. Name 8 bones of the upper extremities and 8 bones of the lower extremities.
3. What are the phalanges? Why are there two different sets of phalanges?
4. What are metacarpal bones? How do they differ from metatarsal bones?
5. How does the female pelvis differ from the male pelvis?

CLINICAL APPLICATION

EPIPHYSEAL FRACTURE

The point of articulation between the epiphysis and diaphysis of a growing long bone is susceptible to injury if overstressed, especially in the young child or preadolescent athlete. In these individuals the epiphyseal plate can be separated from the diaphysis or epiphysis, causing an epiphyseal fracture. This x-ray study shows such a fracture in a young boy. Without successful treatment, an epiphyseal fracture may inhibit normal growth. Stunted bone growth, in turn, may cause the affected limb to be shorter than the unaffected limb.

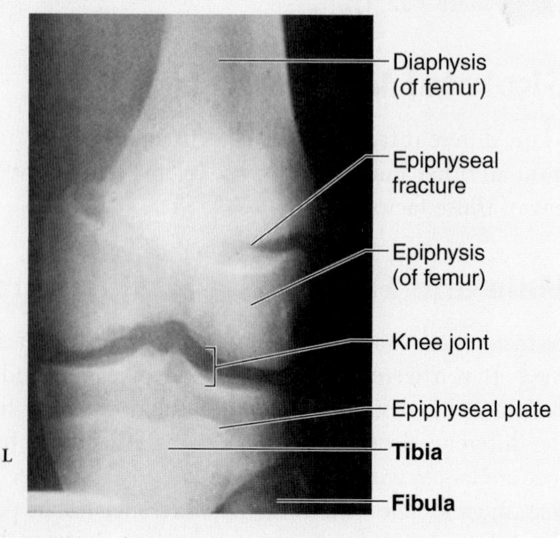

Joints

Articulation of Bones

The term *joint* is borrowed from carpentry, where it refers to the structure formed when pieces of wood are joined together. In anatomy, a joint is the structure formed when bones join together. Joints are also called **articulations**—a term based on the word part *arthro*, which means "joint."

Every bone in the body, except one, connects to at least one other bone. In other words, every bone but one forms a joint with some other bone. The exception is the hyoid bone in the neck, to which the tongue anchors. Most of us probably never think much about our joints unless something goes wrong with them and they do not function properly. Then their tremendous importance becomes painfully clear.

Joints hold our bones together securely and at the same time make it possible for movement to occur between the bones—between most of them, that is. Without joints we could not move our arms, legs, or many other of our body parts. Our bodies would, in short, be rigid, immobile hulks.

Try, for example, to move your arm at your shoulder joint in as many directions as you can. Try to do the same thing at your elbow joint. Now examine the shape of the bones at each of these joints on a skeleton or in **Figure 7-9**. Looking at the anatomy, do you understand why you cannot move your arm at your elbow in nearly as many directions as you can at your shoulder?

Kinds of Joints

One method classifies joints into three types according to the degree of movement they allow:

1. Synarthroses — no movement
2. Amphiarthroses — slight movement
3. Diarthroses — free movement

Differences in joint structure account for differences in the degree of movement that is possible—yet another example of the structure-function relationship in the body.

Synarthroses

A **synarthrosis** is a joint in which no significant movement occurs. This functional characteristic is produced by the fibrous connective tissue between the articulating (joining) bones, holding them tightly together. The joints between cranial bones are synarthroses, commonly called *sutures* (**Figure 7-24**, *A*).

Amphiarthroses

An **amphiarthrosis** is a joint in which only slight movement is possible. Amphiarthroses are usually made up of cartilage, which joins the bones tightly—but often with slight flexibility.

The symphysis pubis, the joint between the two pubic bones, is an amphiarthrosis (**Figure 7-24**, *B*). It normally only flexes late in pregnancy when movement of the pelvic girdle is helpful during delivery of an infant.

Joints between the bodies of the vertebrae are also amphiarthroses. These joints make it possible to flex the trunk

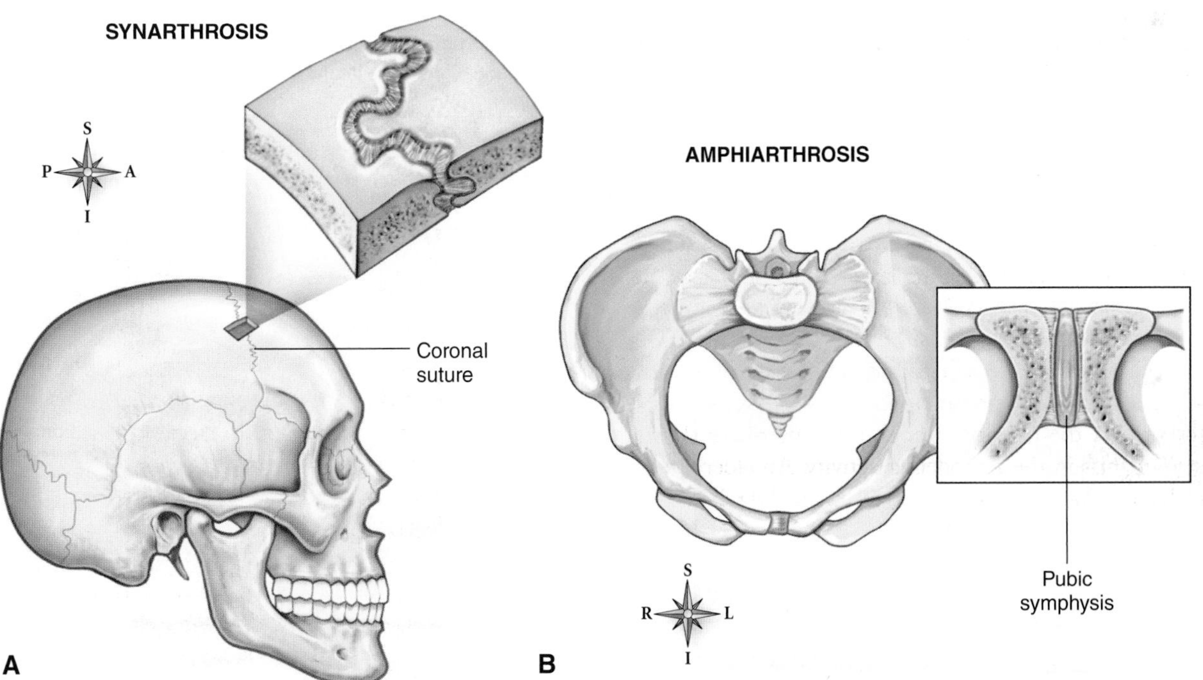

FIGURE 7-24 Joints of the skeleton. A, Synarthrotic joint. **B,** Amphiarthrotic joint.

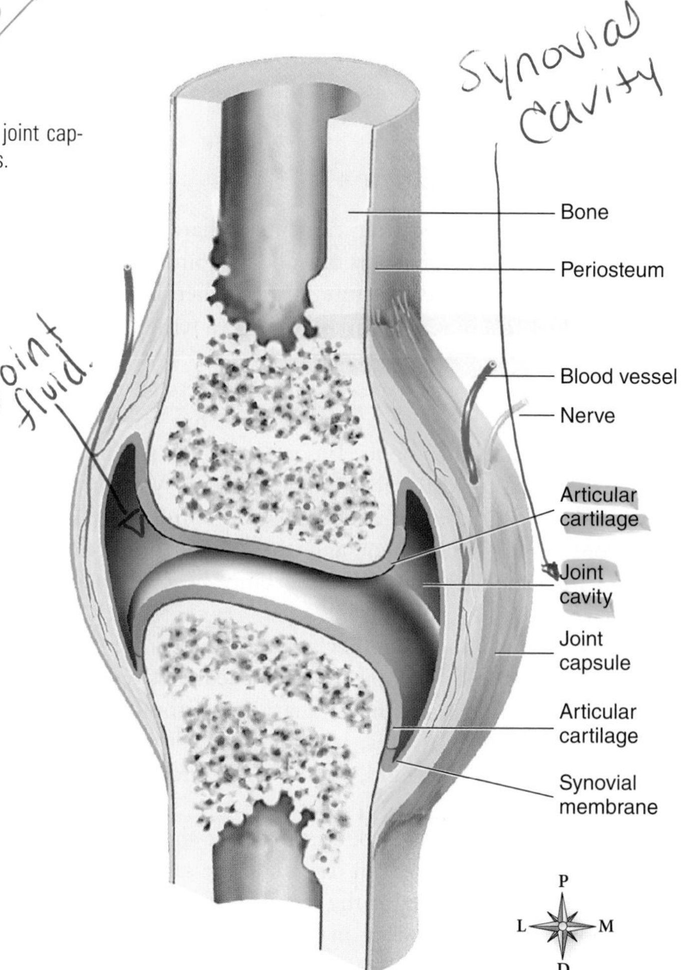

FIGURE 7-25 Structure of a diarthrotic joint. Each diarthrosis has a joint capsule, a joint cavity, and a layer of cartilage over the ends of the joined bones.

forward or sideways and even to circumduct and rotate it. Strong ligaments connect the bodies of the vertebrae, and fibrous disks lie between them. The central core of these intervertebral disks consists of a pulpy, elastic substance that loses some of its resiliency with age.

Diarthroses

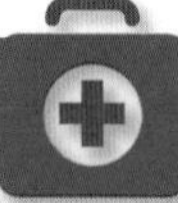

Fortunately most of our joints are **diarthroses.** Such joints allow considerable movement, sometimes in many directions and sometimes in only one or two directions.

Structure of Diarthroses

Diarthroses (freely movable joints) are made alike in certain ways. All have a joint capsule, a joint cavity, and a layer of cartilage over the ends of two joining bones (**Figure 7-25**). The **joint capsule** is made of the body's strongest and toughest material—fibrous connective tissue—and is lined with a smooth, slippery synovial membrane. The capsule fits over the ends of the two bones somewhat like a sleeve. Because it attaches firmly to the shaft of each bone to form its covering (called the *periosteum, peri* means "around," and *osteum* means "bone"), the joint capsule holds the bones securely together but at the same time permits movement at the joint. The

HEALTH AND WELL-BEING

THE KNEE JOINT

The knee is the largest and most vulnerable joint. Because the knee is often subjected to sudden, strong forces during athletic activity, knee injuries are among the most common type of athletic injury. Sometimes, the concave disks of articular cartilage called **menisci** on the tibia tear when the knee twists while bearing weight. The ligaments holding the tibia and femur together can also be injured in this way.

The figure shows tears in the lateral and medial ligaments outside the joint cavity, as well as tears in the crossed **cruciate ligaments** inside the joint. Knee injuries may also occur when a weight-bearing knee is hit by another person or a moving object.

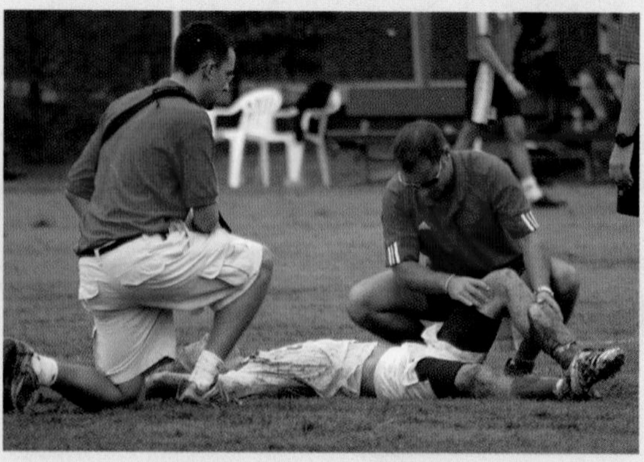

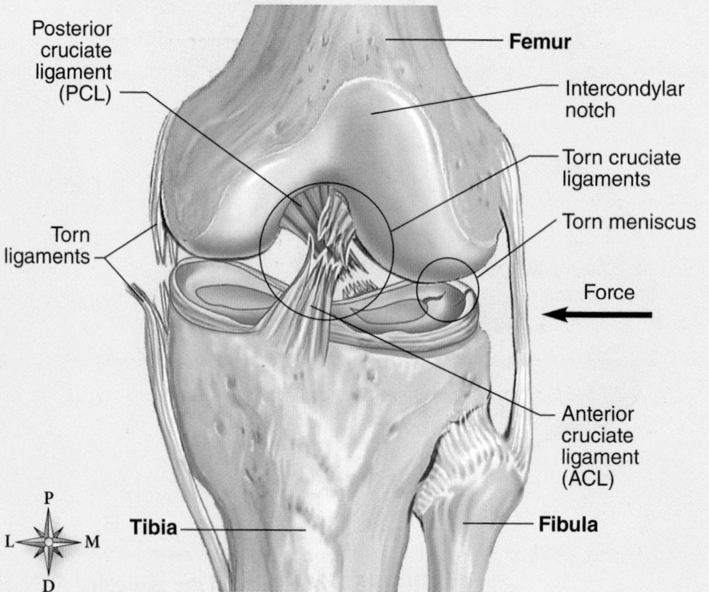

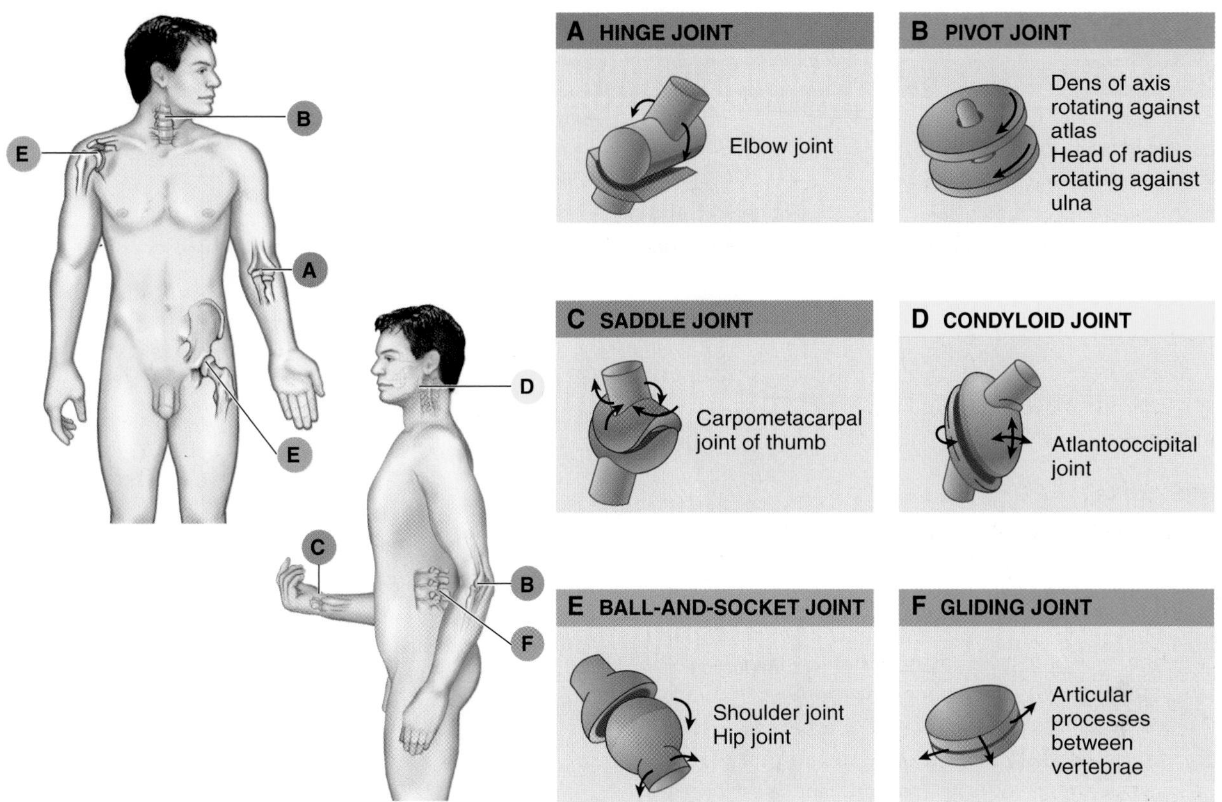

FIGURE 7-26 Types of diarthrotic joints. Notice that the structure of each type dictates its function (movement). The mechanical diagrams represent the type of action at the highlighted anatomical joints.

structure of the joint capsule, in other words, helps make possible the joint's function.

Ligaments (cords or bands made of the same strong fibrous connective tissue as the joint capsule) also grow out of the periosteum and lash the two bones together even more firmly.

The layer of **articular cartilage** over the joint ends of bones acts like a rubber heel on a shoe—it absorbs jolts. The articular cartilage also provides a smooth surface so the bones of the joint can move with little friction.

A joint cavity where the bones join together is lined with **synovial membrane,** which secretes a lubricating fluid *(synovial fluid)* that allows easier movement with less friction. In some joints, the synovial membrane forms a pocketlike extension or a pouch filled alongside a joint. Called a **bursa,** this pocket of fluid acts as a shock-absorbing cushion around the bones of the joint. Irritation, injury, or infection of a bursa can cause inflammation—a condition called *bursitis.*

Function of Diarthroses

There are several types of diarthroses: *ball-and-socket, hinge, pivot, saddle, gliding,* and *condyloid* joints (Figure 7-26). Because they differ in structure, they differ also in their possible range of movement.

Ball-and-socket Joints

In a **ball-and-socket joint,** a ball-shaped head of one bone fits into a concave socket of another bone. Shoulder and hip joints, for example, are ball-and-socket joints.

Of all the joints in our bodies, these permit the widest range of movements. Think for a moment about how many ways you can move your arms. You can move them forward, you can move them backward, you can move them away from the sides of your body, and you can move them back down to your sides. You can also move them around so your hands make a circle.

Hinge Joints

Hinge joints, like the hinges on a door, allow movements in only two directions, namely, *flexion* and *extension.* **Flexion** is bending a joint and **extension** is straightening it out (Table 7-7). Elbow and knee joints and the joints in the fingers are hinge joints.

Pivot Joints

Pivot joints are those in which a small projection of one bone pivots in an arch of another bone. For example, recall that a projection of the *axis* (second cervical vertebra) is a point around which an arch of the *atlas* (first cervical vertebra) can pivot (see Figure 7-15). This permits **rotation** of the head, which rests on the atlas.

Saddle Joints

Only one pair of **saddle joints** exists in the body—between the metacarpal bone of each thumb and a carpal bone of the wrist (the name of this carpal bone is the *trapezium*). Because the articulating surfaces of these bones are saddle-shaped,

TABLE 7-7 Types of Joint Movements

MOVEMENT	EXAMPLE	MOVEMENT	EXAMPLE
Flexion (to *flex* a joint) Reduces the angle of the joint, as in bending the elbow	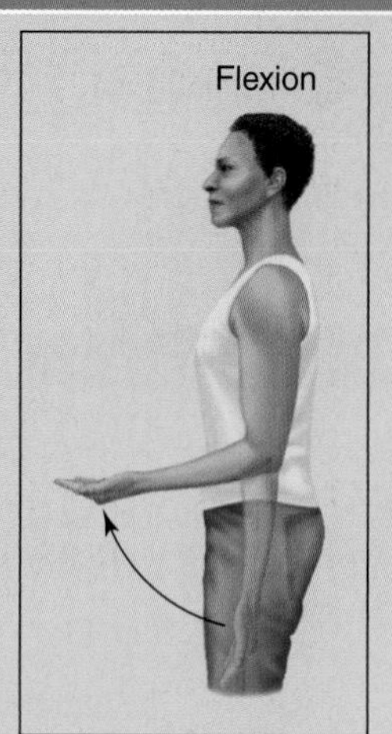	**Extension** (to *extend* a joint) Increases the angle of a joint, as in straightening a bent elbow	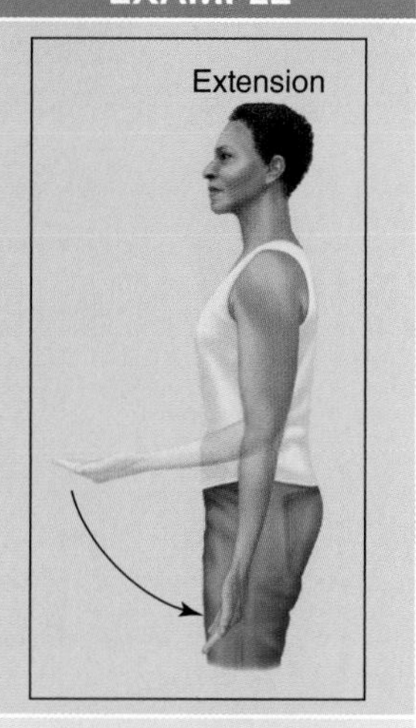
Abduction (to *abduct* a joint) Increases the angle of a joint to move a part away from the midline, as in moving the arm to the side and away from the body	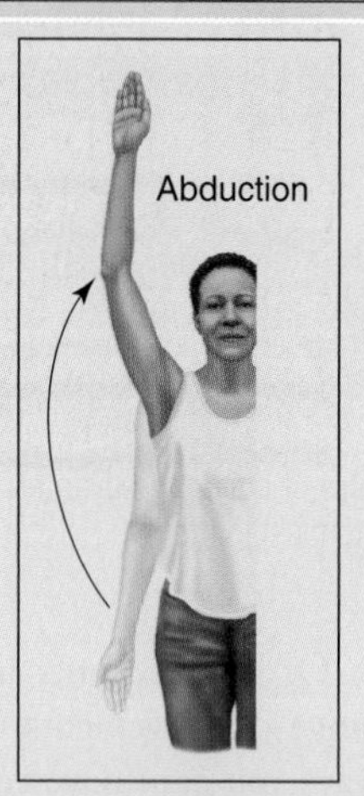	**Adduction** (to *adduct* a joint) Decreases the angle of a joint to move a part toward the midline, as in moving the arm in and down from the side	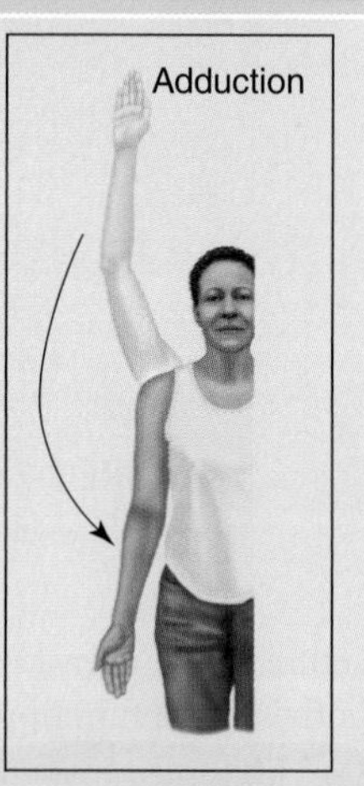
Rotation (to *rotate* a joint) Spins one bone relative to another, as in rotating the head at the neck joint	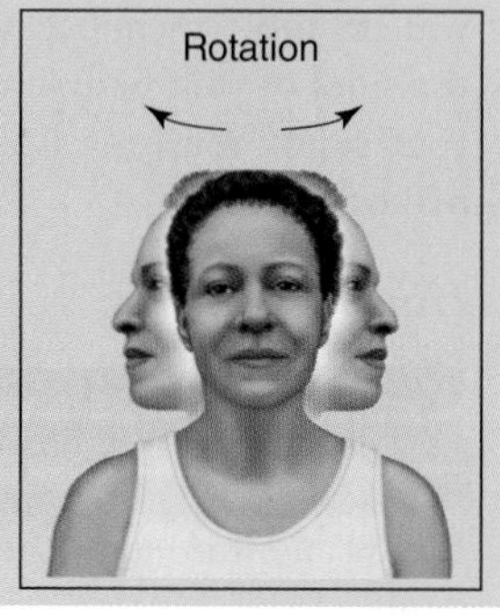	**Circumduction** (to *circumduct* a joint) Moves the distal end of a bone in a circle, while circumducting a joint, keeping the proximal end relatively stable, as in moving the arm in a circle and thus circumducting the shoulder joint 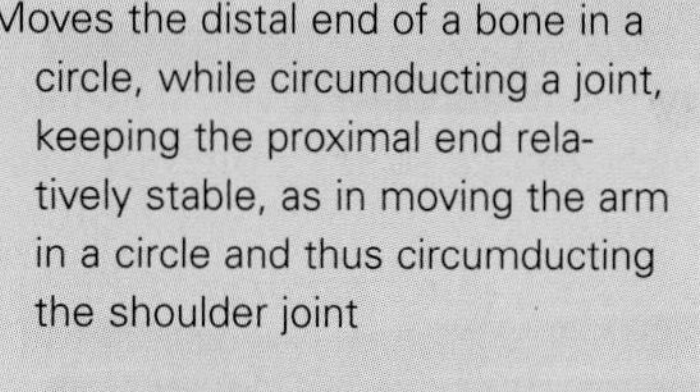	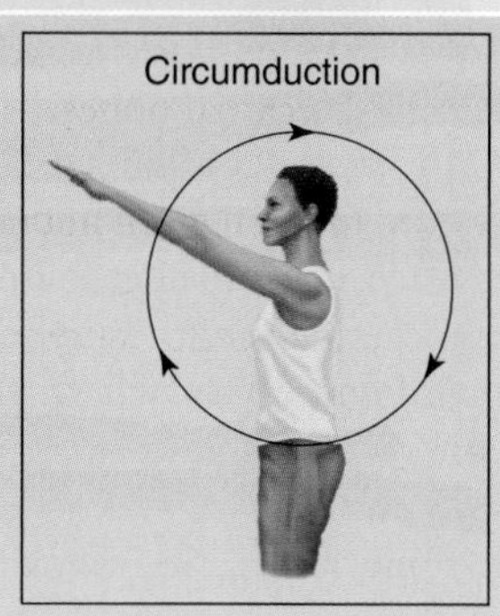

Your study of these movements continues in Chapter 8, beginning on p. 164.

they make possible the human thumb's great mobility, a mobility no animal's thumb possesses. We can **flex, extend, abduct, adduct,** and **circumduct** our thumbs, and most important of all, we can move our thumbs to touch the tip of any one of our fingers. (This movement is called *opposing the thumb to the fingers.*)

Without the saddle joints at the base of each of our thumbs, we could not do such a simple act as picking up a pin or grasping a pencil between thumb and forefinger.

Gliding Joints

Gliding joints are the least movable diarthrotic joints. Their flat articulating surfaces allow limited gliding movements, such as that at the superior and inferior articulating processes between successive vertebrae.

Condyloid joints

Condyloid joints are those in which a condyle (an oval projection) fits into an elliptical socket. An example is the fit

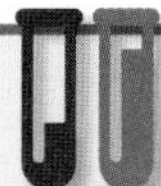

CLINICAL APPLICATION

TOTAL HIP REPLACEMENT

Because *total hip replacement (THR)* is the most common orthopedic operation performed on older persons (more than 300,000 procedures per year in the United States), home health care professionals often work with patients recovering from THR surgery.

The THR procedure involves replacement of the femoral head by a metal prosthesis and the acetabular socket by a polyethylene cup. The prostheses are usually coated with a porous material that allows natural growth of bone to mesh with the artificial material. Such meshing of tissue and prostheses ensures stability of the parts without the loosening that the use of glues in the past often allowed. First introduced in 1953, THR technique has advanced to the state that the procedure has very high success rates in older adults.

Patients at home after THR surgery should progress through proper surgical healing and recovery, including stabilization of the prostheses as new tissue grows into their porous surfaces. THR patients should also expect some improvement in regained use of the affected hip, including weight-bearing and walking movements.

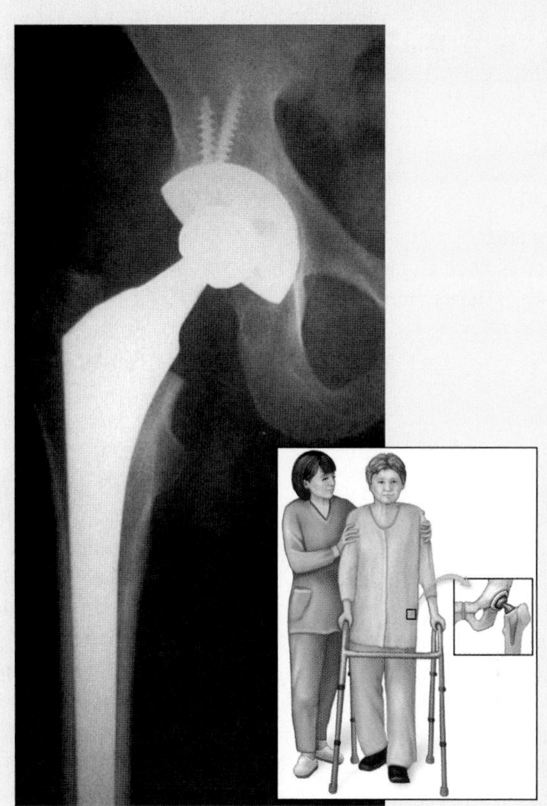

of the distal end of the radius into depressions in the carpal bones.

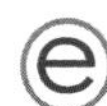

To learn more about types of joint movement, go to AnimationDirect at *evolve.elsevier.com*.

QUICK CHECK

1. What are the three major types of joints in the skeleton? Give an example of each.
2. What is the degree of movement for each of the three major types of joints in the skeleton?
3. What membrane in a diarthrotic joint provides lubrication for movement?
4. What is a ligament?
5. What is meant by "flexing" the elbow? Extending the elbow?

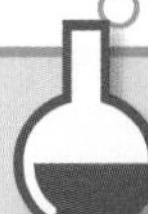

SCIENCE APPLICATIONS

BONES AND JOINTS

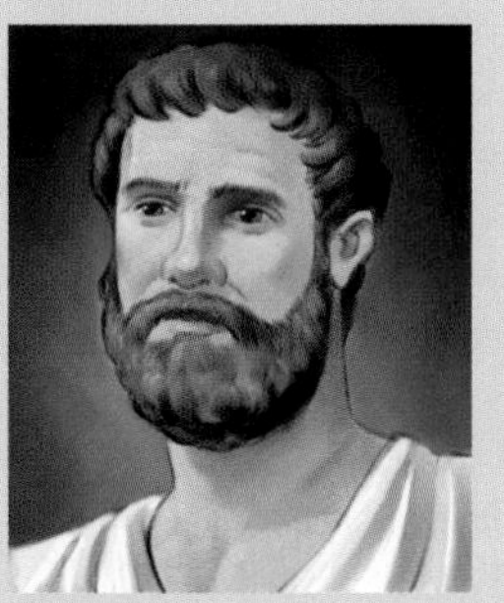

Hippocrates
(ca. 460-377 B.C.E.)

Ever since 400 B.C.E., when Hippocrates (the Greek physician often regarded as a founder of the medical profession) first described treatments of human bone and joint disorders and injuries, many approaches to treating the human skeleton have been taken. **Physical therapists** and **occupational therapists** help patients regain movement in joints through physical exercises and **orthopedic surgeons** help their patients by means of surgical operations. Because the skeleton, with its many bones and joints, is the framework of the entire body, it is not surprising to learn that many different health professionals work directly with the skeleton. **Podiatrists** work with the bones and joints of the foot and ankle, **athletic trainers** and **sports physicians** work with many parts of the skeleton, and **chiropractors** often work to align the vertebral column. *Radiographic technologists* and *radiologists* are often called upon to make medical images of the bones and joints and interpret the meaning of these images.

LANGUAGE OF **SCIENCE** AND **MEDICINE** *(continued from p. 123)*

atlas
(AT-lis)
[*Atlas,* **Greek mythical figure who supports the world**]

axial skeleton
(AK-see-al SKEL-eh-ton)
[*axi-* **axis,** *-al* **relating to,** *skeleton* **dried body**]

axis
(AK-sis)
pl., axes
(AK-seez)

ball-and-socket joint

bursa
(BER-sah)
pl., bursae
(BER-see or BER-say)
[*bursa* **purse**]

calcaneus
(kal-KAY-nee-us)
[*calcane-* **heel,** *-ous* **having to do with**]

calcitonin (CT)
(kal-sih-TOH-nin)
[*calci-* **lime (calcium),** *-ton-* **tone,** *-in* **substance**]

canaliculus
(kan-ah-LIK-yoo-lus)
pl., canaliculi
(kan-ah-LIK-yoo-lye)
[*canal-* **channel,** *-uculus* **little**]

cancellous bone
(KAN-seh-lus bohn)
[*cancel-* **lattice,** *-ous* **characterized by**]

carpal
(KAR-pul)
[*carp-* **wrist,** *-al* **relating to**]

cartilage
(KAR-tih-lij)
[*cartilage* **gristle**]

central canal
(SEN-tral kah-NAL)
[*centr-* **center,** *-al* **relating to,** *canal* **channel**]

chest

chiropractor
(KYE-roh-prak-ter)
[*chiro-* **hand,** *-practic-* **practical,** *-or* **agent**]

chondrocyte
(KON-droh-syte)
[*chondro-* **cartilage,** *-cyte* **cell**]

circumduct
(ser-kum-DUKT)
[*circum-* **around,** *-duct-* **lead**]

circumduction
(ser-kum-DUK-shun)
[*circum-* **around,** *-duct-* **lead,** *-tion* **process**]

clavicle
(KLAV-ih-kul)
[*clavi-* **key,** *-cle* **little**]

coccyx
(KOK-sis)
[*coccyx* **cuckoo (beak)**]

compact bone
(kom-PAKT bohn)

concentric lamella
(kon-SEN-trik lah-MEL-ah)
pl., lamellae
(lah-MEL-ee)
[*con-* **together,** *-centr-* **center,** *-ic* **relating to,** *lam-* **plate,** *-ella* **little**]

condyloid joint
(KON-dih-loyd joynt)
[*condylo-* **knuckle,** *-oid* **like**]

coxal bone
(kok-SAL bohn)
[*coxa-* **hip,** *-al* **relating to**]

cranium
(KRAY-nee-um)
[*cranium* **skull**]

cruciate ligament
(KRU-shee-ayt)
[*cruci-* **cross,** *-ate* **of or like**]

diaphysis
(dye-AF-ih-sis)
pl., diaphyses
(dye-AF-ih-seez)
[*dia-* **through or apart,** *-physis* **growth**]

diarthrosis
(dye-ar-THROH-sis)
pl., diarthroses
(dye-ar-THROH-seez)
[*dia-* **between,** *-arthr-* **joint,** *-osis* **condition**]

diploe
(DIP-loh-EE)
[*diploe* **folded over (doubled)**]

endochondral ossification
(en-doh-KON-dral os-ih-fih-KAY-shun)
[*endo-* **inward or within,** *-chondr-* **cartilage,** *-al* **relating to,** *oss-* **bone,** *-fication* **to make**]

endosteum
(en-DOS-tee-um)
[*endo-* **within,** *-osteum* **bone**]

epiphyseal plate
(ep-ih-FEEZ-ee-al playt)
[*epi-* **on,** *-phys-* **growth,** *-al* **relating to,** *plate* **flat**]

epiphysis
(eh-PIF-ih-sis)
pl., epiphyses
(eh-PIF-ih-seez)
[*epi-* **upon,** *-physis* **growth**]

extend
(ek-STEND)
[*ex-* **outward,** *-tens-* **stretch**]

extension
(ek-STEN-shun)
[*ex-* **outward,** *-tens-* **stretch,** *-sion* **process**]

face
(fays)

femur
(FEE-mur)
[*femur* **thigh**]

fibula
(FIB-yoo-lah)
[*fibula* **clasp**]

flex
(FLEKS)
[*flex* **bend**]

flexion
(FLEK-shun)
[*flex-* **bend,** *-ion* **process**]

fontanel
(FON-tah-nel)
[*fontan-* **fountain or source,** *-el* **little**]

gliding joint
(GLY-ding joynt)

hematopoiesis
(hee-mat-oh-poy-EE-sis)
[*hemo-* **blood,** *-poiesis* **making**]

hinge joint
(hinj joynt)

humerus
(HYOO-mer-us)
[humerus **arm**]

hyoid bone
(HYE-oyd bohn)
[*hy-* **Greek letter upsilon (Υ or υ),** *-oid* **like**]

ilium
(IL-ee-um)
[*ilium* **flank**]

intramembranous ossification
(in-trah-MEM-brah-nus os-ih-fih-KAY-shun)
[*intra-* **within,** *-membran-* **thin skin,** *-ous* **characterized by,** *os-* **bone,** *-fic-* **make,** *-ation* **process**]

ischium
(IS-kee-um)
[*ischium* **hip joint**]

joint capsule
(joynt CAP-sool)

lacuna
(lah-KOO-nah)
pl., lacunae
(lah-KOO-nee)
[*lacuna* **pit**]

lateral longitudinal arch
(LAT-er-all lawnj-ih-TOOD-in-al)
[*later-* **side,** *-al* **relating to,** *longitud-* **length,** *-al* **relating to**]

ligament
(LIG-ah-ment)
[*liga-* **bind,** *-ment* **result of action]**

medial longitudinal arch
(MEE-dee-al lon-jih-TOO-dih-nal arch)
[*medi-* **middle,** *-al* **relating to,** *longitud-* **length,** *-al* **relating to]**

medullary cavity
(MED-oo-layr-ee KAV-ih-tee)
[*medulla-* **marrow,** *-y* **related to,** *cav-* **hollow,** *-ity* **state]**

meniscus
(meh-NIS-kus)
pl., menisci
(meh-NIS-eye or meh-NIS-kye)
[*meniscus* **crescent]**

metacarpal
(met-ah-KAR-pal)
[*meta-* **beyond,** *-carp-* **wrist,** *-al* **relating to]**

metatarsal
(met-ah-TAR-sal)
[*meta-* **beyond,** *-tars-* **ankle,** *-al* **relating to]**

middle ear
(MID-ul eer)

occupational therapist
(ak-yoo-PAY-shun-al THAYR-ah-pist)
[*occup-* **occupy,** *-tion-* **process,** *-al* **relating to,** *therap-* **treatment,** *-ist* **agent]**

olecranon
(oh-LEK-rah-nohn)
[*ole-* **elbow,** *-cran-* **head,** *-on* **unit]**

olecranon fossa
(oh-LEK-rah-non FOSS-ah)
[*ole-* **elbow,** *-cran-* **head,** *-on* **unit,** *fossa* **ditch]**

orthopedic surgeon
(or-thoh-PEE-dik SUR-jen)
[*ortho-* **straight or normal,** *-ped-* **feet,** *-ic* **relating to,** *surg-* **hand,** *-eon* **practitioner]**

osteoblast
(OS-tee-oh-blast)
[*osteo-* **bone,** *-blast* **bud or sprout]**

osteoclast
(OS-tee-oh-klast)
[*osteo-* **bone,** *-clast* **break]**

osteocyte
(OS-tee-oh-syte)
[*osteo-* **bone,** *-cyte* **cell]**

osteon (haversian system)
(AHS-tee-on [hah-VER-zhun or HAV-er-zhun SIS-tem])
[*osteo-* **bone,** *-on* **unit,** *Clopton Havers,* **English physician]**

osteoporosis
(os-tee-oh-poh-ROH-sis)
[*osteo-* **bone,** *-poro-* **pore,** *-osis* **condition]**

palpable
(PAL-pah-bul)
[*palp-* **touch gently,** *-able* **capable]**

paranasal sinus
(payr-ah-NAY-zal SYE-nus)
[*para-* **beside,** *-nas-* **nose,** *-al* **relating to,** *sinus* **hollow]**

parathyroid hormone (PTH)
(pair-ah-THYE-royd HOR-mohn)
[*para-* **besides,** *-thyr-* **shield,** *-oid* **like,** *hormon-* **excite]**

patella
(pah-TEL-ah)
[*pat-* **dish,** *-ella* **small]**

pectoral girdle
(PEK-toh-ral GIRD-el)
[*pector-* **breast,** *-al* **relating to,** *girdle* **belt]**

pelvic girdle
(PEL-vic GER-dul)
[*pelvi-* **basin,** *-ic* **relating to,** *girdle* **belt]**

pelvis
(PEL-vis)
pl., pelves or pelvises
(PEL-veez or PEL-vis-ez)
[*pelvis* **basin]**

periosteum
(pair-ee-OS-tee-um)
[*peri-* **around,** *-osteum* **bone]**

phalanges
(fah-LAN-jeez)
sing., phalanx
(fah-LANKS)
[*phalanx* **formation of soldiers in rows]**

physical therapist
(FIS-ik-al THAYR-ah-pist)
[*physic-* **medicine,** *-al* **relating to,** *therap-* **treatment,** *-ist* **agent]**

pivot joint
(PIV-it joynt)

podiatrist
(poh-DYE-ah-trist)
[*pod-* **foot,** *-iatr-* **treatment,** *-ist* **agent]**

pubis
(PYOO-bis)
[*pubis* **groin]**

radius
(RAY-dee-us)
[*radius* **ray]**

red bone marrow
(red bohn MAR-oh)

rib

rotation
(roh-TAY-shun)
[*rot-* **turn,** *-ation* **process]**

sacrum
(SAY-krum)
[*sacr-* **holy,** *-um* **thing]**

saddle joint
(SAD-el joynt)

scapula
(SKAP-yoo-lah)
[*scapula* **shoulder blade]**

shaft

sinus
(SYE-nus)
[*sinus* **hollow]**

spongy bone
(SPUN-jee bohn)
[*spong-* **sponge,** *-y* **characterized by]**

sports physician
(sports fih-ZISH-un)
[*physic-* **medicine,** *-ian* **practitioner]**

sternoclavicular joint
(ster-no-klah-VIK-yoo-lar joynt)
[*sterno-* **breastbone (sternum),** *-clavi-* **key,** *-ular* **relating to]**

sternum
(STER-num)
pl., sterna or sternums
(STER-nah or STER-numz)
[*sternum* **breastbone]**

suture
(SOO-chur)
[*suture* **seam]**

synarthrosis
(sin-ar-THROH-sis)
pl., synarthroses
(sin-ar-THROH-seez)
[*syn-* **together,** *-arthr-* **joint,** *-osis* **condition]**

synovial membrane
(sih-NO-vee-all MEM-brayne)
[*syn-* **together,** *-ovi-* **egg (white),** *-al* **relating to,** *membran-* **thin skin]**

tarsal
(TAR-sal)
[*tars-* **ankle,** *-al* **relating to]**

thorax (chest)
(THOH-raks)
[*thorax* **chest]**

tibia
(TIB-ee-ah)
[*tibia* **shin bone]**

trabecula
(trah-BEK-yoo-lah)
pl., trabeculae
(trah-BEK-yoo-lee)
[*trab-* **beam,** *-ula* **little]**

transverse canal (Volkmann canal)
(tranz-VERS kah-NAL [VOLK-man])
[*trans-* **across,** *-vers-* **turn,** *Richard von Volkmann,* **German surgeon]**

ulna
(UHL-nah)
[*ulna* **elbow]**

vertebra
(VER-teh-bra)
pl., vertebrae
(VER-teh-bree or VER-teh-bray)
[*vertebra* **joint or turning part]**

yellow bone marrow
(YEL-oh bohn MAR-oh)

❑ OUTLINE SUMMARY

To download a digital audio version of the chapter summary for use with your device, access the ***Audio Chapter Summaries*** *online at evolve.elsevier.com.*

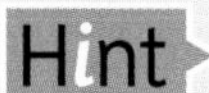

Scan this summary after reading the chapter to help you reinforce the key concepts. Later, use the summary as a quick review before your class or before a test.

Functions of the Skeletal System

A. Supports and gives shape to the body
B. Protects internal organs
C. Helps make movements possible when bones at moveable joints are pulled by muscles
D. Storage of vital substances
   1. Calcium — hormones regulate calcium storage: calcitonin (CT) increases storage and parathyroid hormone (PTH) reduces stores of calcium
   2. Fat — stored in cavities of some bones
E. Hematopoiesis — blood cell formation in red bone marrow

Gross Structure of Bones

A. Four major types, according to overall shape of the bone
   1. Long — Example: humerus (arm)
   2. Short — Example: carpals (wrist)
   3. Flat — Example: frontal (skull)
   4. Irregular — Example: vertebrae (spinal cord)
   5. Some also recognize a sesamoid (round) bone category — Example: patella (kneecap)
B. Structure of long bones (see **Figure 7-1**)
   1. Diaphysis or shaft — hollow tube of hard compact bone
   2. Medullary cavity — hollow area inside diaphysis that contains yellow marrow
   3. Epiphyses, or ends of the bone — spongy bone that contains red bone marrow
   4. Articular cartilage — covers epiphyses and functions as a cushion
   5. Periosteum — strong membrane covering bone everywhere except at joint surfaces
   6. Endosteum — thin membrane lining medullary cavity
C. Structure of flat bones (see **Figure 7-2**)
   1. Spongy bone layer sandwiched between two compact bone layers
   2. Diploe — spongy bone layer of a flat bone

Microscopic Structure of Bones

A. Bone tissue structure (see **Figure 7-3**)
   1. Cancellous (spongy) bone
      a. Texture results from needlelike threads of bone called *trabeculae* surrounded by a network of open spaces
      b. Found in epiphyses of bones
      c. Spaces contain red bone marrow
   2. Compact bone
      a. Structural unit is an osteon — calcified matrix arranged in multiple layers or rings called concentric lamella (see **Figure 7-4**)
      b. Bone cells are called *osteocytes* and are found inside spaces called *lacunae,* which are connected by tiny tubes called *canaliculi*
B. Cartilage (see **Figure 7-5**)
   1. Cell type called *chondrocyte*
   2. Matrix is gel-like and lacks blood vessels

Bone Development

A. Making and remodeling bone tissue (see **Figure 7-6**)
   1. Early bone development (before birth) consists of cartilage and fibrous structures
   2. Osteoblasts
      a. Form new bone matrix by encrusting collagen fibers with calcium crystals
      b. Osteocytes are inactive osteoblasts
   3. Osteoclasts dissolve bone, releasing calcium ions for reabsorption into the bloodstream
   4. Remodeling is a combined action of making and dissolving bone matrix that eventually sculpts bone into the adult shape
B. Endochondral ossification — cartilage models gradually replaced by calcified bone (see **Figure 7-7** and **Figure 7-8**)
C. Intramembranous ossification — fibrous membranes are ossified into hard bone plates; fontanels are soft, not-yet-ossified regions

Axial Skeleton

A. Skeleton can be divided into central *axial* and peripheral *appendicular* regions (see **Figure 7-9** and **Table 7-1**)
B. Axial skeleton includes 80 bones:
   1. Skull (see **Figure 7-10** and **Table 7-2**)
      a. Bones of the cranium (8), face (14), and middle ear (6)
      b. Includes spaces called paranasal sinuses (see **Figure 7-11**)
   2. Hyoid bone (see **Figure 7-12**)
   3. Vertebral column (spine) — vertebrae (24 total: cervical [7], thoracic [12], lumbar [5]), sacrum, coccyx (see **Figure 7-13** through **Figure 7-16** and **Table 7-3**)
   4. Thorax — ribs (24), sternum (see **Figure 7-17** and **Table 7-4**)

Appendicular Skeleton

A. Bones of the upper and lower extremities (126)
B. Upper extremity (64) (**Table 7-5**)
   1. Pectoral (shoulder) girdle — scapula (2), clavicle (2)
   2. Arm and forearm — humerus (2), radius (2), ulna (2) (see **Figure 7-18**)

3. Wrist and hand — carpal bones (16), metacarpal bones (10), phalanges (28) (see **Figure 7-19**)

C. Lower extremity (62) (see **Table 7-6**)
1. Pelvic (hip) girdle — coxal bone (2)
2. Thigh and leg — femur (2), patella (2), tibia (2), fibula (2) (see **Figure 7-20**)
3. Ankle and foot — tarsal bones (14), metatarsal bones (10), phalanges (28) (see **Figure 7-21** and **Figure 7-22**)
4. Arched structure of foot provides dynamic support for entire skeleton

Skeletal Variations

A. Male and female skeletal differences
1. Size — male skeleton generally larger
2. Shape of pelvis — male pelvis deep and narrow, female pelvis shallow and broad
3. Size of pelvic inlet — female pelvic inlet generally wider, normally large enough for baby's head to pass through it (see **Figure 7-23**)
4. Pubic angle — angle between pubic bones of female generally wider

B. Age differences
1. Bones enlarge and become more ossified until maturity at age 25
2. Bones actively remodel (dissolve and rebuild) in middle adulthood
3. Bones become less dense during elderly years

C. Environmental factors
1. Nutrition affects growth and maintenance of bone tissue
2. Mechanical stress, including exercise, affects bone remodeling

Joints

A. Articulation — a joint between two or more bones

B. Every bone except the hyoid (which anchors the tongue) connects to at least one other bone.

C. Kinds of joints
1. Synarthroses (no movement) — fibrous connective tissue grows between articulating bones; for example, sutures of skull (see **Figure 7-24**)
2. Amphiarthroses (slight movement) — cartilage connects articulating bones; for example, symphysis pubis (see **Figure 7-24**)
3. Diarthroses (free movement) — most joints belong to this class
   a. Structure (see **Figure 7-25**)
      (1) Structures of freely movable joints — joint capsule and ligaments hold adjoining bones together but permit movement at joint
      (2) Articular cartilage — covers joint ends of bones where they form joints with other bones
      (3) Synovial membrane — lines joint capsule and secretes lubricating fluid
      (4) Joint cavity — space between joint ends of bones
      (5) Bursa — fluid-filled pouch that absorbs shock; inflammation of bursa is called *bursitis*
   b. Functions of freely movable joints — ball-and-socket, hinge, pivot, saddle, gliding, and condyloid — allow different kinds of movements determined by the structure of each joint (see **Figure 7-26** and **Table 7-7**)

❑ ACTIVE LEARNING

STUDY TIPS

Hint *Use these tips to achieve success in meeting your learning goals.*

To make the study of the skeletal system more efficient, we suggest these tips:

1. Before studying Chapter 7, go back to Chapter 5 and review the synopsis of the skeletal system.
2. There are several terms in this chapter that use prefixes or suffixes that help explain their meaning. The prefixes *epi-* (upon) and *endo-* (within) were discussed earlier. *Peri-* means "around," *osteo-* or *os-* refers to bone, *chondro-* refers to cartilage, *-cyte* means "cell," *-blast* means "young cell" or "building cell," and *-clast* means "to destroy." Knowing the meaning of these prefixes or suffixes makes most of the terms self-explanatory. Start a section in your notebook listing these common word parts and terms that use them—then add to your list as you continue through the rest of this book.
3. When studying the microscopic structure of the skeletal system, remember that bone tissue heals fairly well, whereas cartilage doesn't. This is because there are many blood vessels throughout the bone, but not in cartilage. The cells must have a way of receiving food and oxygen and a way to get rid of waste products. The structure of the osteon allows this to occur.
4. Reviewing the figures of the full skeleton and the skull may be the best way to learn the bones of the skeleton. Use flash cards or online resources to supplement the text material. One such online resource is: *getbodysmart.com*. This site has excellent illustrations, tutorials, and quizzes. Additional online tips are found at *my-ap.us/JJEEMF*.
5. The joints are named based on the amount of movement they allow (*arthro* means "joint"). The joint capsule is an example of a synovial membrane discussed in Chapter 6.
6. In your study group you can use flash cards to learn the terms in the bone structure and joints. Discuss the formation and structure of the osteon. A photocopy or a cell phone picture of the skeleton figures with the labels blackened out will help you learn the names and characteristics of the bones. There is no real shortcut to learning the names and locations of the bones; it's simply a memorization task, but quizzing each other will help you learn them faster.
7. Review the Language of Science terms and their word origins to help you better understand the meaning of the names of the bones.
8. In your study group, go over the questions at the end of the chapter and discuss possible test questions.

Review Questions

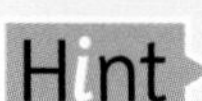

Write out the answers to these questions after reading the chapter and reviewing the Chapter Summary. If you simply think through the answer without writing it down, you won't retain much of your new learning.

1. List and briefly explain the five functions of the skeletal system.
2. List the main structures found in a typical long bone.
3. Describe the structure of the osteon.
4. Describe the structure of cartilage.
5. Explain briefly the process of endochondral ossification and include the function of osteoblasts and osteoclasts.
6. Explain the importance of the epiphyseal plate.
7. List the bones that are included in the axial skeleton and the bones included in the appendicular skeleton.
8. The vertebral column is divided into five sections based on location. Name the sections and give the number of vertebrae in each section.
9. Distinguish between true, false, and floating ribs and list how many ribs are in each category.
10. Describe and give an example of a synarthrotic joint.
11. Describe and give an example of an amphiarthrotic joint.
12. Describe and give an example of four types of diarthrotic joints.
13. Briefly describe a joint capsule.

Critical Thinking

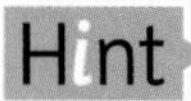

After finishing the Review Questions, write out the answers to these more in-depth questions to help you apply your new knowledge. Go back to sections of the chapter that relate to concepts that you find difficult.

14. When a patient receives a bone marrow transplant, what vital process is being restored?
15. Explain how the canaliculi allow bone to heal more efficiently than cartilage.
16. What effect does the task of childbearing have on the differences between the male and female skeleton?
17. Explain how the anatomy of the elbow is a good example of how "structure fits function."

Chapter Test

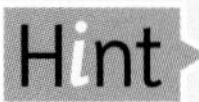

After studying the chapter, test your mastery by responding to these items. Try to answer them without looking up the answers. Then, verify the answers using the key in Appendix C at the back of this book.

1. The thin layer of cartilage on the end of bones where they form joints is called the articular cartilage.
2. The hollow area in the shaft of long bones where marrow is located is called the medulary cavity.
3. The needlelike threads of spongy bone are called trabeculae.
4. The structural units of compact bone are called haversian system.
5. Osteocytes and chondrocytes live in small spaces in the matrix called lacunae.
6. The haversian canal is synonymous with central canal.
7. Bone-forming cells are called osteoblasts.
8. The process of forming bone from cartilage is called endochondral ossification.
9. If a(n) epiphiseal plate remains between the epiphysis and diaphysis, bone growth can continue.
10. The two major divisions of the human skeleton are the axial skeleton and the appendicular skeleton.
11. The three types of joints named based on the amount of movement they allow are synathroses, amphiarthroses, and diarthroses.
12. The ligaments are cords or bands made of strong connective tissue that holds two bones together.
13. Which of the following is not a function of the skeletal system?
    a. mineral storage
    b. blood formation
    (c.) heat regulation
    d. protection
14. The strong fibrous membrane covering a long bone everywhere except for the joint is called the:
    a. endosteum
    (b.) periosteum
    c. diaphysis
    d. epiphysis
15. The fibrous inner lining of the hollow tube in a long bone is called the:
    (a.) endosteum
    b. periosteum
    c. diaphysis
    d. epiphysis
16. The end of a long bone is called the:
    a. endosteum
    b. periosteum
    c. diaphysis
    (d.) epiphysis
17. The shaft of a long bone is called the:
    a. endosteum
    b. periosteum
    (c.) diaphysis
    d. epiphysis

Match the bones in Column A with their locations in Column B.

Column A		Column B
18. B	ulna	a. skull
19. A	mandible	b. upper extremity
20. B	humerus	c. trunk
21. B	metatarsals	d. lower extremity
22. D	tibia	
23. C	rib	
24. D	fibula	
25. c	sternum	
26. B	scapula	
27. D	femur	
28. B	metacarpals	
29. a	frontal bone	
30. D	patella	
31. a	zygomatic bone	
32. b	clavicle	
33. A	occipital bone	
34. B	carpals	
35. A	maxilla	

Muscular System

OUTLINE

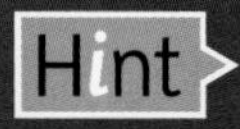

Scan this outline before you begin to read the chapter, as a preview of how the concepts are organized.

OBJECTIVES

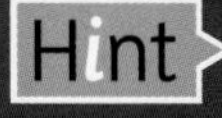

Before reading the chapter, review these goals for your learning.

After you have completed this chapter, you should be able to:

1. List, locate in the body, and compare the structure and function of the three major types of muscle tissue.
2. Discuss the microscopic structure and function of a skeletal muscle, including sarcomere and motor unit.
3. Discuss how a muscle is stimulated and compare the major types of skeletal muscle contractions.
4. List and explain the primary effects of exercise on the structure and function of skeletal muscles.
5. List and explain the most common types of movement produced by skeletal muscles.
6. Name, identify on a model or diagram, and give the function of the major muscles of the body discussed in this chapter.

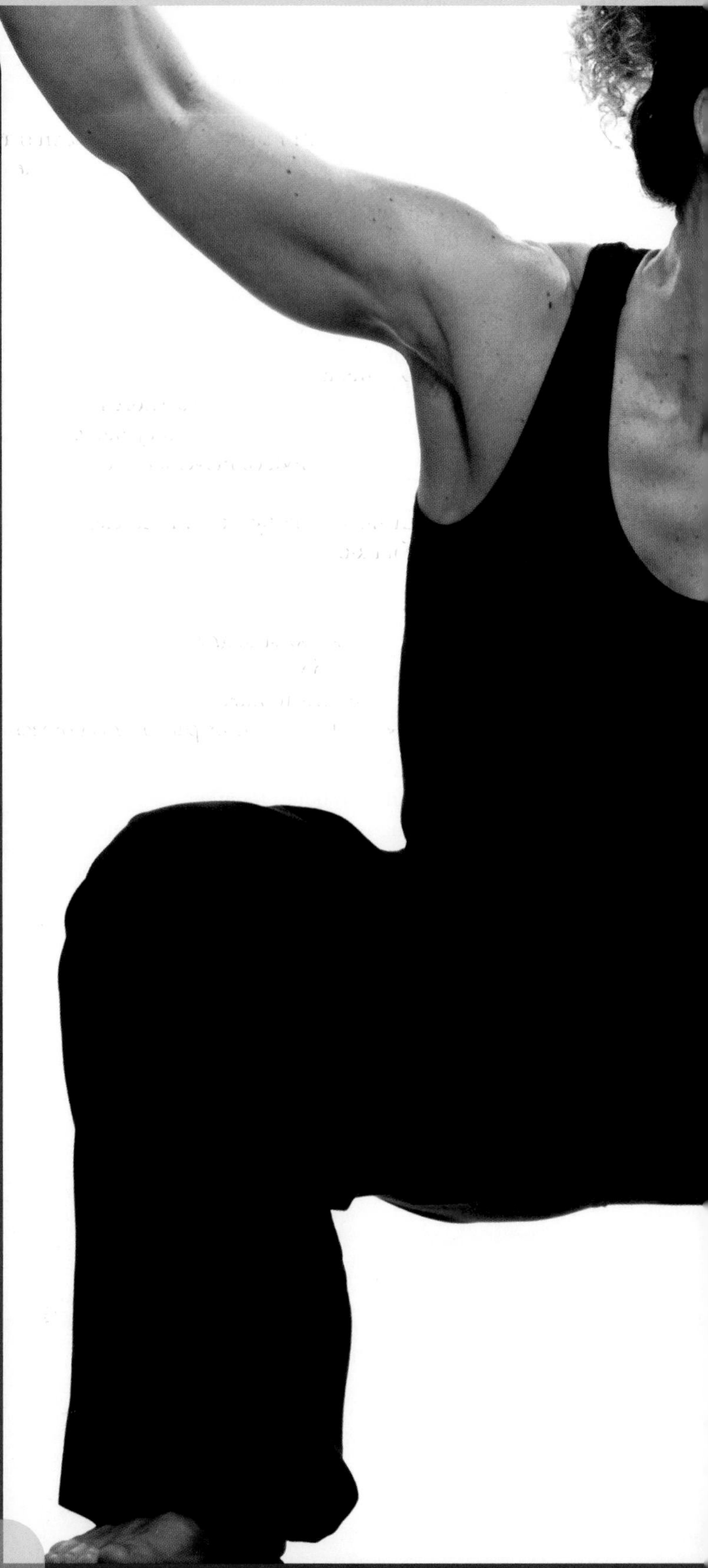

CHAPTER 8

We initially review the three types of muscle tissue introduced earlier (see Chapter 4), but the plan for this chapter is to focus on skeletal or voluntary muscle—those muscle masses that attach to bones and actually move them about when contraction or shortening of muscle cells, or muscle fibers, occurs.

If you weigh 120 pounds, about 50 pounds of your weight comes from your skeletal muscles, the "red meat" of the body that is attached to your bones.

Muscular movement occurs when chemical energy from nutrient molecules is transferred to protein filaments in each muscle fiber and then converted to mechanical energy that attempts to shorten (contract) the muscle. As the muscle fibers in a muscle contract, they pull on the bones to which they are attached and thus produce movement of the body.

Movements caused by skeletal muscle contraction vary in complexity from blinking an eye to the coordinated and fluid movements of a gifted athlete. Not many of our body structures can claim as great an importance for happy, active living as can our voluntary muscles, and only a few can boast of greater importance for life itself. Our ability to survive often depends on our ability to adjust to the changing conditions of our environment to maintain homeostasis. Movements frequently constitute a major part of this homeostatic adjustment.

LANGUAGE OF SCIENCE AND MEDICINE

Hint Before reading the chapter, say each of these terms out loud. This will help you to avoid stumbling over them as you read.

abduction
(ab-DUK-shun)
[*ab-* **away,** *-duct-* **lead,** *-tion* **process**]

acetylcholine (ACh)
(as-ee-til-KOH-leen)
[*acetyl-* **vinegar,** *-chole-* **bile,** *-ine* **made of**]

actin
(AK-tin)
[*act-* **act or do,** *-in* **substance**]

adduction
(ad-DUK-shun)
[*ad-* **toward,** *-duct-* **lead,** *-tion* **process**]

adductor muscle
(ad-DUK-tor MUS-el)
[*ad-* **toward,** *-duct-* **lead,** *-or* **condition,** *mus-* **mouse,** *-cle* **small**]

aerobic training
(air-OH-bik TRAYN-ing)
[*aer-* **air,** *-bi-* **life,** *-ic* **relating to**]

all or none
(all or nun)

antagonist
(an-TAG-oh-nist)
[*ant-* **against,** *-agon-* **struggle,** *-ist* **agent**]

biceps brachii
(BYE-seps BRAY-kee-eye)
[*bi-* **two,** *-cep* **head,** *brachii* **related to the arm**]

biomechanical engineering
(bye-oh-meh-KAN-ik-al en-juh-NEER-ing)
[*bio-* **life,** *-mechan-* **machine,** *-ic-* **relating to,** *-al* **relating to,** *engin-* **devise or design,** *-eer* **practitioner**]

Continued on p. 171

Muscle Tissue

Skeletal Muscle

Under the microscope, threadlike and cylindrical **skeletal muscle** cells appear in bundles. They are characterized by many crosswise stripes and multiple nuclei (**Figure 8-1**, *A*). Each fine thread is a muscle cell—usually called a **muscle fiber.**

This type of muscle tissue has three names: *skeletal muscle,* because it attaches to bone; *striated muscle,* because of its cross stripes or striations; and *voluntary muscle,* because its contractions can be controlled voluntarily.

Cardiac Muscle

In addition to **skeletal muscle,** the body also contains two other types of muscle tissue: cardiac muscle and smooth muscle. **Cardiac muscle** composes the bulk of the heart. Fibers in this type of muscle tissue are also cylindrical, branch frequently (**Figure 8-1**, *B*), and then recombine into a continuous mass of interconnected tissue. As with skeletal muscle fibers, the cardiac muscle fibers have cross striations. They also have unique dark bands called **intercalated disks,** where the plasma membranes of adjacent cardiac fibers come in contact with each other.

Cardiac muscle tissue demonstrates the principle that "structure fits function." The interconnected nature of cardiac muscle fibers helps the tissue to contract as a unit and increases the efficiency of the heart muscle in pumping blood.

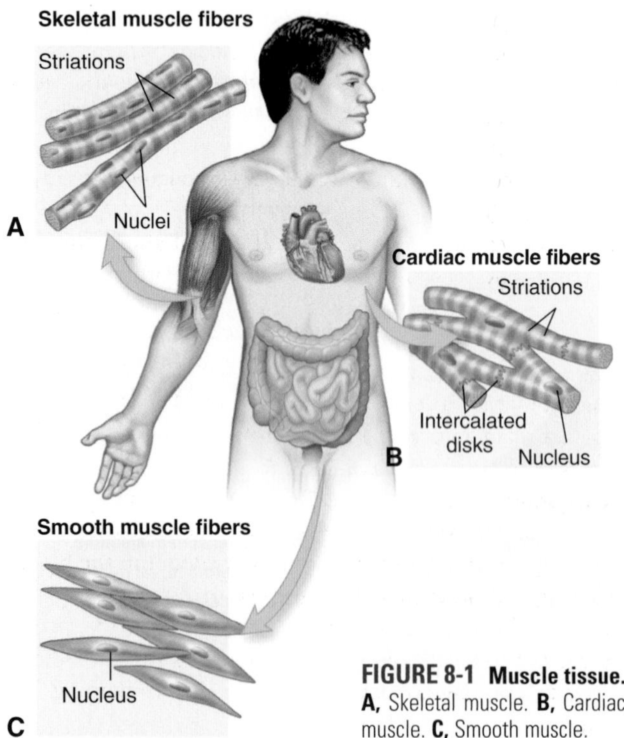

FIGURE 8-1 Muscle tissue. **A,** Skeletal muscle. **B,** Cardiac muscle. **C,** Smooth muscle.

Smooth Muscle

Smooth muscle fibers are tapered at each end and have a single nucleus (**Figure 8-1**, *C*). Because they lack cross stripes or striations, they are sometimes called *nonstriated* muscle fibers. They have a smooth, even appearance when viewed through a microscope. They are called *involuntary* because we normally do not have control over their contractions.

Smooth or involuntary muscle forms an important part of blood vessel walls and of many hollow internal organs (viscera) such as the gut, urethra, and ureters. Because of its location in many visceral structures, it is sometimes also called *visceral muscle.*

Although we cannot willfully control the action of smooth muscle, its contractions are highly regulated, which promotes efficient food passage through the digestive tract or urine through the ureters into the bladder.

All three muscle fiber types—skeletal, cardiac, and smooth—specialize in contraction or shortening. Every movement we make is produced by contractions of skeletal muscle fibers. Contractions of cardiac muscle fibers pump the blood through the heart, and smooth muscle contractions help pump blood and other substances through our other hollow organs.

Structure of Skeletal Muscle

Muscle Organs

A skeletal muscle is an organ composed mainly of skeletal muscle fibers and connective tissue. Fibrous connective tissue wraps around each individual muscle fiber, then continues as it wraps around groups of muscle fibers called *fascicles,* and then forms a "wrapper" around the entire muscle organ. *Fascia* is the loose connective tissue outside the muscle organs that forms a flexible, sticky "packing material" between muscles, bones, and the skin.

Most skeletal muscles attach to two bones that have a movable joint between them. In other words, most muscles extend from one bone across a joint to another bone. Also, one of the two bones is usually more stationary during a given movement than the other. The muscle's attachment to this more stationary bone is called its **origin.** Its attachment to the more movable bone is called the muscle's **insertion.** The rest of the muscle (all of it except its two ends) is called the *body* of the muscle (**Figure 8-2**).

Tendons anchor muscles firmly to bones and are made of dense, fibrous connective tissue that extends from the muscle "wrappers" described earlier. In the shape of heavy cords or broad sheets, tendons have great strength. They do not tear or pull away from bone easily. Yet any emergency room nurse or physician sees many tendon injuries—severed tendons and tendons torn loose from bones.

Small fluid-filled sacs called **bursae** lie between some tendons and the bones beneath them. Recall from Chapter 7 that these small connective tissue sacs are lined with **synovial**

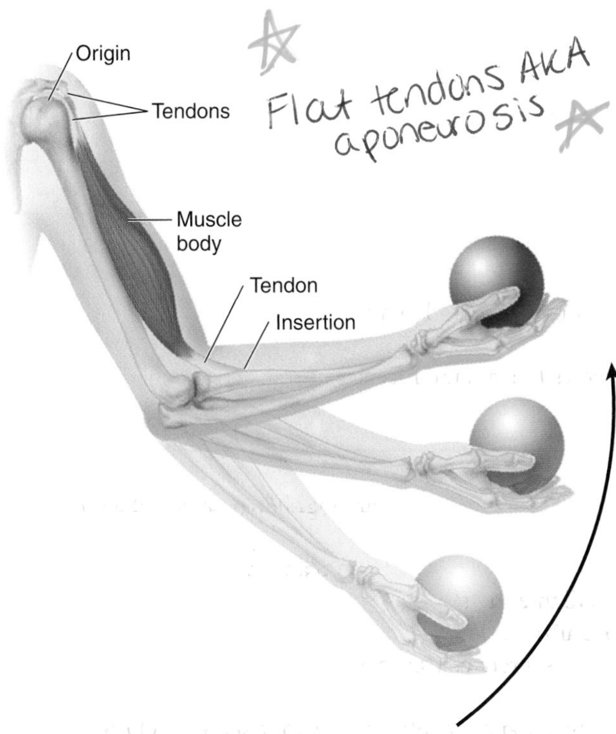

FIGURE 8-2 Attachments of a skeletal muscle. A muscle originates at a relatively stable part of the skeleton (origin) and inserts at the skeletal part that is moved when the muscle contracts (insertion).

membrane. The synovial membrane secretes a slippery lubricating fluid *(synovial fluid)* that fills the bursa. Like a small, flexible cushion, a bursa makes it easier for a tendon to slide over a bone when the tendon's muscle shortens.

Tendon sheaths enclose some tendons. Because these tube-shaped structures are also lined with synovial membrane and are moistened with synovial fluid, they, like the bursae, facilitate body movement.

Muscle Fibers

Structure of Muscle Fibers

Skeletal muscle tissue consists of elongated contractile cells, or *muscle fibers,* that look like long, tapered cylinders. Their flexible connective tissue wrappings hold them together in parallel groups, allowing the muscle fibers to all pull together in the same direction—as a team.

Each skeletal muscle fiber has a unique cytoskeleton structure. The fiber's internal framework is organized into many long cylinders, each made up of two kinds of threadlike microfilaments called **thick** and **thin myofilaments.** The thick myofilaments are formed from a protein called **myosin,** and the thin myofilaments are composed mainly of the protein **actin.**

Each shaftlike myosin molecule has a "head" that sticks out toward the actin molecules. At rest, the actin is blocked from connecting with the myosin heads by small proteins attached to the actin. During contraction, however, the blocking proteins release actin and the myosin heads connect to form *crossbridges* between the thick and thin filaments.

Find the label **sarcomere** in Figure 8-3. Think of the sarcomere as the basic functional or *contractile unit* of skeletal muscle. The submicroscopic structure of a sarcomere consists of numerous thick and thin myofilaments arranged so that, when viewed under a microscope, dark and light stripes, or cross striations, are seen. The repeating units, or sarcomeres, are separated from each other by dark bands called *Z lines* or *Z disks.*

Although the sarcomeres in the upper portions (Figure 8-3, *A*) and in the electron micrograph (EM) of Figure 8-3, *C,* are in a relaxed state, the thick and thin myofilaments, which are lying parallel to each other, still overlap. Now look at the diagrams in the middle portion of Figure 8-3, *B.* Note that contraction of the muscle causes the two types of myofilaments to slide toward each other and shorten the sarcomere and thus the entire muscle. When the muscle relaxes, the sarcomeres can return to resting length, and the filaments resume their resting positions.

Contraction of Muscle Fibers

An explanation of how a skeletal muscle contracts is provided by the **sliding filament model.** According to this model, during contraction, the thick and thin myofilaments in a muscle fiber first attach to one another by forming crossbridges that then act as levers to ratchet or pull the myofilaments past each other.

The connecting bridges between the myofilaments form only if calcium is present. During the relaxed state, calcium ions (Ca^{++}) are stored within the smooth endoplasmic reticulum (ER) in the muscle cell. When a nerve signal stimulates the muscle fiber, the ER releases Ca^{++} into the cytoplasm. There, the Ca^{++} ions bind to the blocking proteins in thin filaments and permit actin to react with myosin. The myosin heads connect to actin, pull, release, and then pull again. This ratcheting of myosin heads thus pulls the thin filaments toward the center of the sarcomere—producing the muscle contraction (Figure 8-4).

The contraction process of a muscle cell also requires energy. This energy is supplied by glucose and other nutrients.

The energy must be transferred to myosin heads by adenosine triphosphate (ATP) molecules, the energy-transfer molecules of the cell. Oxygen is required to transfer energy to ATP and make it available to the myosin heads, so it is not surprising that many muscles have high oxygen requirements.

To supplement the oxygen carried to muscle fibers by the hemoglobin of blood, muscle fibers contain **myoglobin**—a red, oxygen-storing pigment similar to hemoglobin. During rest, oxygen carried to muscles by hemoglobin in the blood is taken up by myoglobin within muscle fibers. As oxygen is used up quickly during muscle contractions, oxygen from myoglobin adds to the oxygen from hemoglobin—thereby allowing maximum "recharging" of energy-containing ATP molecules.

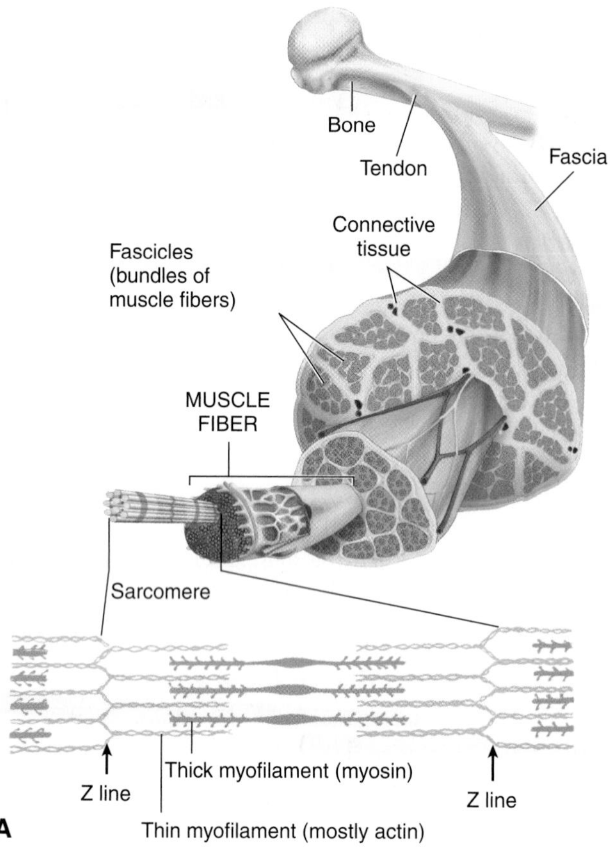

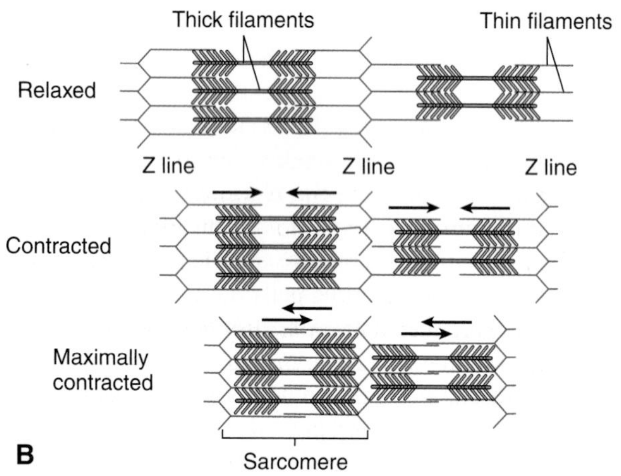

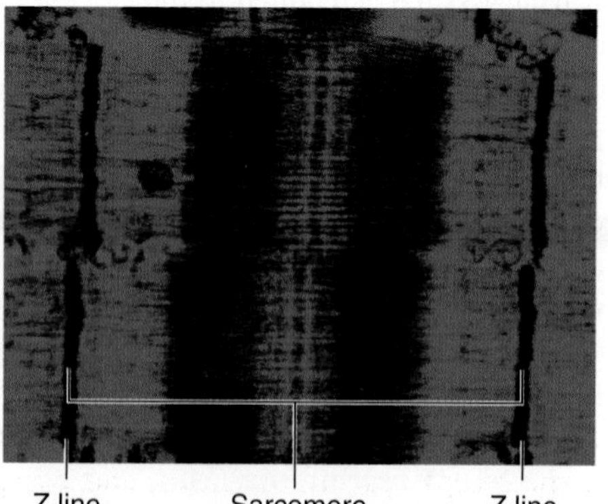

FIGURE 8-3 Structure of skeletal muscle. A, Each muscle organ has many muscle fibers, each containing many bundles of thick and thin filaments. The expanded diagram shows the overlapping thick and thin filaments arranged to form adjacent segments called *sarcomeres.* **B,** During contraction, the thin filaments are pulled toward the center of each sarcomere, shortening the whole muscle. **C,** This electron micrograph shows that the overlapping thick and thin filaments within each sarcomere create a pattern of dark striations in the muscle. The extreme magnification allowed by electron microscopy has revolutionized our concept of the structure and function of skeletal muscle and other tissues.

We discuss the processes of transferring energy to ATP to cellular processes in Chapter 17.

QUICK CHECK

1. What are the three main types of muscle tissue? How do they differ?
2. What is the origin and insertion of a muscle? What is a tendon?
3. How do a muscle's myofilaments provide the mechanism for movement?

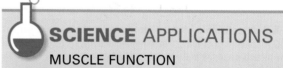

SCIENCE APPLICATIONS

MUSCLE FUNCTION

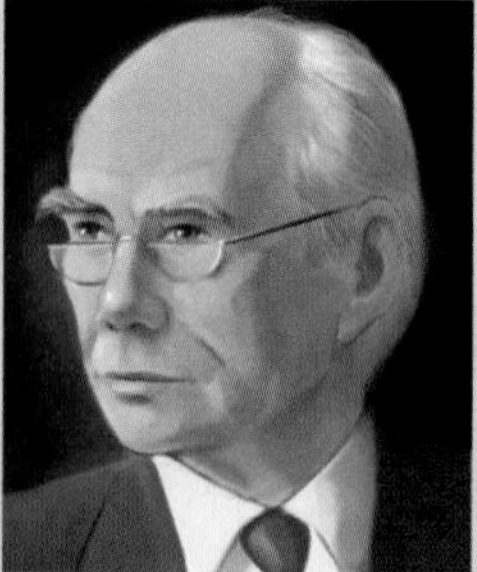

Andrew F. Huxley (1917-2012)

The British physiologist Andrew F. Huxley is largely responsible for explaining how muscle fibers contract. After making pioneering discoveries in how nerves conduct impulses, a feat for which he shared the 1963 Nobel Prize in Medicine or Physiology, Huxley turned his attention to muscle fibers. It was he who, in the 1950s, proposed the sliding filament model along with its mechanical explanation of muscle contraction.

Today, research physiologists continue to find out more about how muscle fibers work. These discoveries are being applied in many different professions. For example, **nutritionists** use this information in advising athletes and others concerning what and when to eat to maximize muscular strength and endurance. *Athletes* themselves, along with their *coaches* and *athletic trainers,* use current concepts of muscle science in helping them improve their performance.

Health professionals such as **physicians, nurses,** *physical therapists,* and *occupational therapists* use information about muscular problems such as myasthenia gravis and muscular dystrophy to help clients improve their mobility and quality of life. Many other professions such as **massage therapy; ergonomics; physical education;** and *fitness, dance, art,* and **biomechanical engineering** also rely on up-to-date information on muscle structure and function for optimal performance.

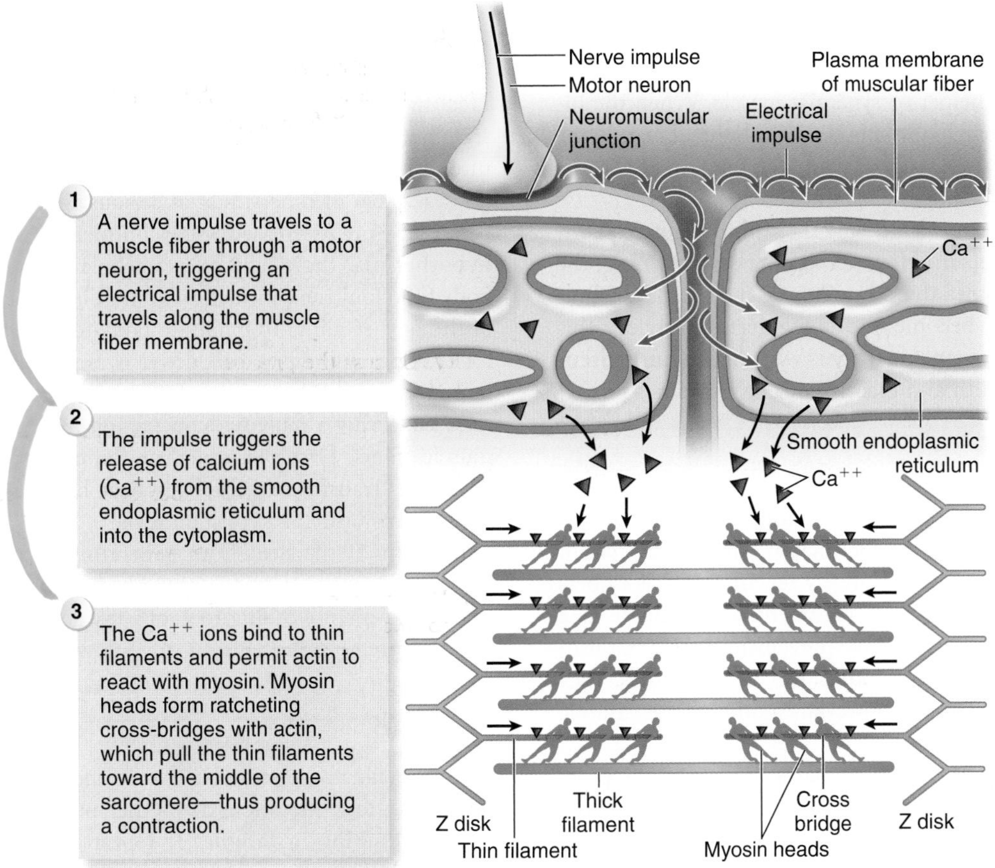

1
A nerve impulse travels to a muscle fiber through a motor neuron, triggering an electrical impulse that travels along the muscle fiber membrane.
2
The impulse triggers the release of calcium ions (Ca^{++}) from the smooth endoplasmic reticulum and into the cytoplasm.
3
The Ca^{++} ions bind to thin filaments and permit actin to react with myosin. Myosin heads form ratcheting cross-bridges with actin, which pull the thin filaments toward the middle of the sarcomere—thus producing a contraction.
Nerve impulse
Motor neuron
Neuromuscular junction
Electrical impulse
Plasma membrane of muscular fiber
Ca^{++}
Smooth endoplasmic reticulum
Ca^{++}
Z disk
Thin filament
Thick filament
Cross bridge
Myosin heads
Z disk

FIGURE 8-4 Muscle contraction mechanism.

Functions of Skeletal Muscle

The functions of the muscular system are many. Most obviously, this system *produces movement* of the skeleton and permits us to move our whole body, as well as our individual limbs. By producing continuous tension on the skeleton—**muscle tone**—this system also helps maintain a stable body position, or *posture*. As discussed in Chapter 1, skeletal muscles also *produce heat* and thus help us maintain homeostatic balance of body temperature.

Movement

One tremendously important function of skeletal muscle contractions therefore is to produce body movements.

Muscles move bones by pulling on them. Because the length of a skeletal muscle becomes shorter as its fibers contract, the bones to which the muscle attaches move closer together. As a rule, only the insertion bone moves. Look again at Figure 8-2. As the ball is lifted, the shortening of the muscle body pulls the insertion bone toward the origin bone. The origin bone stays put, holding firm, while the insertion bone moves toward it. Remember this simple rule: a muscle's insertion bone moves toward its origin bone. It can help you understand most muscle actions.

Shortening of a muscle is the primary example of muscle action in this chapter, but it is important to remember that muscles can also produce tension as they extend. This occurs when muscles lengthen under tension, as the muscle insertion is pulled by a load away from the origin. For example, when you lower a heavy bowling ball from your shoulder the muscles in your arm produce tension as they lengthen and allow you to gently lower it—otherwise the ball would suddenly fall and possibly cause injury. Tension during muscle lengthening is often called *eccentric contraction*.

Voluntary muscular movement is normally smooth and free of jerks and tremors because skeletal muscles generally work in coordinated teams, not individually. Several muscles contract while others relax to produce almost any movement that you can imagine. Of all the muscles contracting simultaneously, the one that is mainly responsible for producing a particular movement is called the **prime mover** for that movement. The other muscles that help in producing the movement are called **synergist muscles.**

As prime movers and synergist muscles at a joint contract, other muscles, called **antagonist muscles,** relax. When antagonist muscles contract, they produce a movement opposite to that of the prime movers and their synergist muscles.

Locate the biceps brachii, brachialis, and triceps brachii muscles in Figure 8-7. All of these muscles are involved in bending and straightening the forearm at the elbow joint. The biceps brachii is the prime mover during bending, and the brachialis is its helper or synergist muscle. When the biceps brachii and brachialis muscles bend the forearm, the triceps brachii relaxes. Therefore while the forearm bends, the triceps brachii is the antagonistic muscle.

While the forearm straightens, these three muscles continue to work as a team. However, during straightening, the triceps brachii becomes the prime mover and the biceps brachii and brachialis become the antagonistic muscles. This combined and coordinated activity is what makes our muscular movements smooth and graceful.

Posture

We are able to maintain our body position because of a continuous, low-strength muscle contraction called *muscle tone* or **tonic contraction.** Because relatively few of a muscle's fibers shorten at one time in a tonic contraction, the muscle as a whole does not shorten, and no movement occurs. Consequently, tonic contractions do not move any body parts. They do hold muscles in position, however. In other words, muscle tone maintains **posture.**

Good posture means that body parts are held in the positions that favor best function. These positions balance the distribution of weight and therefore put the least strain on muscles, tendons, ligaments, and bones.

Skeletal muscle tone maintains posture by counteracting the pull of gravity. Gravity tends to pull the head and trunk down and forward, but the tone in certain back and neck muscles pulls just hard enough in the opposite direction to overcome the force of gravity and hold the head and trunk erect.

Heat Production

Healthy survival depends on our ability to maintain a constant body temperature. A fever or elevation in body temperature of only a degree or two above 37° C (98.6° F) is almost always a sign of illness. Just as serious is a fall in body temperature. Any decrease below normal, a condition called **hypothermia,** drastically affects cellular activity and normal body function. The contraction of muscle fibers produces most of the heat required to maintain body temperature.

Energy required to produce a muscle contraction is obtained from ATP. Some of the energy transferred to ATP and released during a muscular contraction is used to shorten the muscle fibers. However, much of the energy is lost as heat during its transfer to ATP. This heat helps us maintain our body temperature at a constant level.

Sometimes the heat from generating ATP during heavy muscle use can produce too much heat, and we have to sweat or shed layers of clothing to cool back down to our set point temperature.

Fatigue

If muscle fibers are stimulated repeatedly without adequate periods of rest, the strength of the muscle contraction decreases, resulting in **fatigue.** If repeated stimulation occurs, the strength of the contraction continues to decrease, and eventually the muscle loses its ability to contract.

During exercise, the stored ATP required for muscle contraction becomes depleted. Formation of more ATP results in a rapid consumption of oxygen and nutrients, often outstripping the ability of the muscle's blood supply to replenish

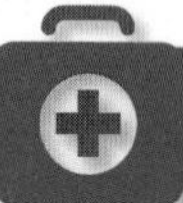

HEALTH AND WELL-BEING

SLOW AND FAST MUSCLE FIBERS

Sports physiologists know there are three basic skeletal muscle fiber types in the body: slow, fast, and intermediate fibers. Each type is best suited to a particular style of muscular contraction—a fact that is useful when considering how different muscles are used in various athletic activities.

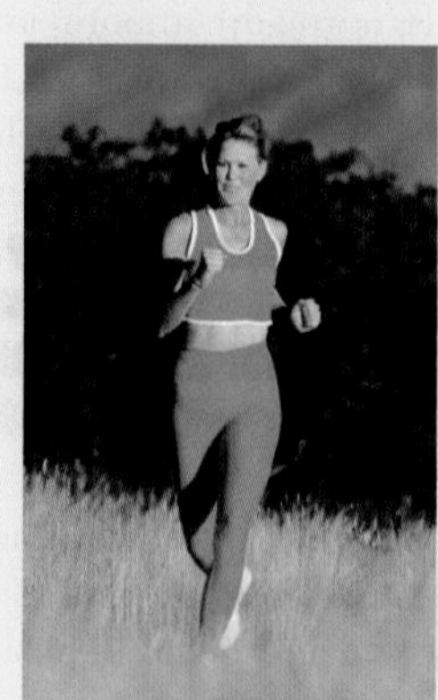

Slow fibers are also called "red fibers" because they have a high content of oxygen-storing myoglobin (a red pigment similar to hemoglobin). Slow fibers are best suited to endurance activities such as long-distance running (pictured) because they do not fatigue easily. Muscles that maintain body position—posture—have a proportion of slow fibers.

Fast fibers are also called "white fibers" because they have a low red myoglobin content. Fast fibers are best suited for quick, powerful contractions because even though they fatigue quickly, they can produce a great amount of ATP very quickly. Fast fibers are well suited to sprinting and weightlifting events. Muscles that move the fingers have a high proportion of fast fibers—a big help when playing computer games or musical instruments.

Intermediate fibers have characteristics between the extremes of slow and fast fibers. This muscle type is found in muscles such as the calf muscle (gastrocnemius), which is used both for posture and occasional brief, powerful contractions such as jumping.

Each muscle of the body is a mixture of varying proportions of slow, fast, and intermediate fibers.

them. When oxygen supplies run low, the muscle fibers switch to a type of energy conversion that does not require oxygen. This process produces lactic acid that may contribute to a burning sensation in muscle during exercise.

The simple term **oxygen debt** describes the continued increased metabolism that must occur in a cell to remove excess lactic acid that accumulates during prolonged exercise. Thus the depleted energy reserves are replaced. Labored breathing after the cessation of exercise is required to "pay the debt" of oxygen required for the metabolic effort.

The technical name for oxygen debt used by exercise physiologists is *excess post-exercise oxygen consumption (EPOC),* a term that more directly describes what happens after exercise.

The oxygen debt mechanism is a good example of homeostasis at work. The body returns the cells' energy and oxygen reserves to normal, resting levels.

Role of Other Body Systems in Movement

Remember that muscles do not function alone. Other structures, such as bones and joints, must function along with them. Most skeletal muscles cause movements by pulling on bones across movable joints.

However, the respiratory, circulatory, nervous, muscular, and skeletal systems all play essential roles in producing normal movements. This fact has great practical importance. For example, a person might have perfectly normal muscles and still not be able to move normally. He or she might have a nervous system disorder that shuts off impulses to certain skeletal muscles, which results in **paralysis.** *Multiple sclerosis (MS)* acts in this way, but so do some other conditions such as a brain hemorrhage, a brain tumor, or a spinal cord injury.

Skeletal system disorders, especially arthritis, have disabling effects on body movement.

Muscle functioning, then, depends on the functioning of many other parts of the body. This fact illustrates a principle that is repeated often in this book. It can be simply stated: Each part of the body is one of many components in a large, interactive system that maintains homeostasis. The normal function of one part depends on the normal function of the other parts.

QUICK CHECK

1. What are the three primary functions of the muscular system?
2. When a prime mover muscle contracts, what does its antagonist do?
3. How would you define the term *posture?*
4. How does muscle function affect body temperature?
5. What is *oxygen debt?*
6. What roles do the respiratory, circulatory, nervous, and skeletal systems play in producing normal movements?

Motor Unit

Before a skeletal muscle can contract and pull on a bone to move it, the muscle must first be stimulated by nerve impulses. Muscle fibers are stimulated by a nerve fiber called a **motor neuron** (**Figure 8-5**). The point of contact between the nerve ending and the muscle fiber is called a **neuromuscular junction** (NMJ).

Signal chemicals called neurotransmitters are released by the motor neuron in response to a nervous impulse. The type of neurotransmitter operating in each NMJ is called **acetylcholine (ACh)**. The released ACh moves across the NMJ and triggers events within the muscle fiber that result in contraction or shortening of the muscle fiber. A single motor neuron, with the muscle fibers it innervates, is called a **motor unit** (see **Figure 8-5**).

Muscle Stimulus

In a laboratory setting, a single muscle fiber can be isolated and subjected to stimuli of varying intensities so that it can be studied. Such experiments show that a muscle fiber does not contract until an applied stimulus reaches a certain level of intensity. The minimal level of stimulation required to cause a fiber to contract is called the **threshold stimulus.**

When a muscle fiber is subjected to a threshold stimulus, it contracts completely. Because of this, muscle fibers are said to respond **"all or none."** However, a muscle is composed of many muscle fibers that are controlled by different motor units and that have different threshold-stimulus levels. Although each fiber in a muscle such as the biceps brachii responds all or none when subjected to a threshold stimulus, the muscle as a whole does not.

This fact has tremendous importance in everyday life. It allows you to pick up a 2-liter bottle of soda or a 20-kg weight because different numbers of motor units can be activated for different loads. Once activated, however, each fiber always responds all or none.

Types of Skeletal Muscle Contraction

In addition to the tonic contraction of muscle that maintains muscle tone and posture, other types of contraction also occur. These additional types of muscle contraction include the following:

1. Twitch contraction
2. Tetanic contraction
3. Isotonic contraction
4. Isometric contraction

Twitch and Tetanic Contractions

A **twitch** is a quick, jerky response to a stimulus. Twitch contractions can be seen in isolated muscles during research, but they play a minimal role in normal muscle activity. To

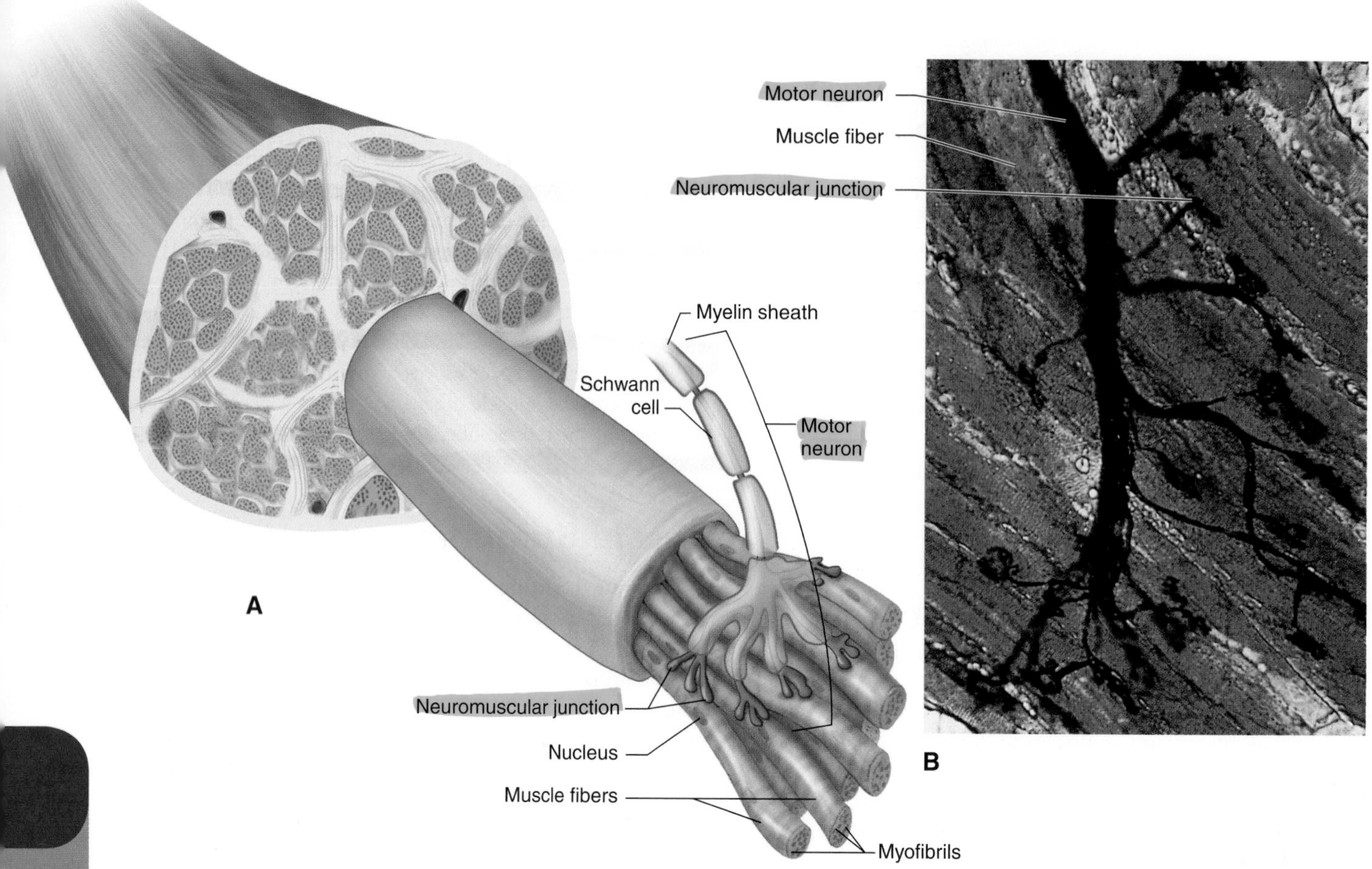

FIGURE 8-5 Motor unit. A, A motor unit consists of one motor neuron and the muscle fibers supplied by its branches. **B,** Micrograph of a motor unit. **C,** Diagram of several motor units, each controlled by its own motor neuron.

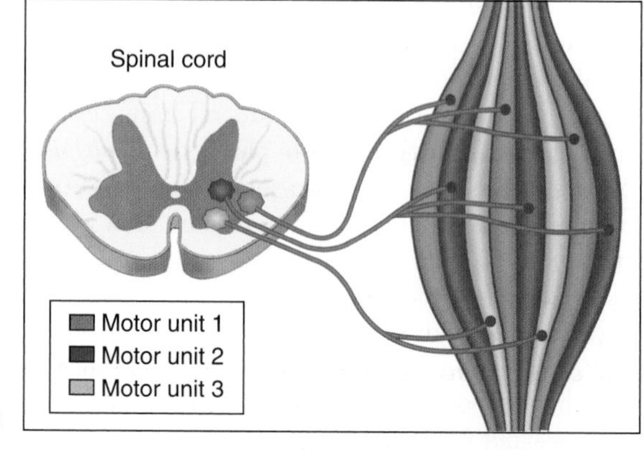

accomplish the coordinated and fluid muscular movements needed for most daily tasks, muscles must contract not in a jerky but in a smooth and sustained way.

A **tetanic contraction** is a more sustained and steady response than a twitch. It is produced by a series of stimuli bombarding the muscle in rapid succession. Contractions "melt" together to produce a sustained contraction, or **tetanus.** About 30 stimuli per second, for example, evoke a tetanic contraction in certain types of skeletal muscle. Tetanic contraction is not necessarily a maximal contraction in which each muscle fiber responds at the same time. In most cases, only a few groups of muscle fibers undergo contractions at any one time.

Isotonic Contraction

In most cases, **isotonic contraction** of muscle produces movement at a joint. With this type of contraction, the muscle changes length, and the insertion end moves relative to the point of origin (**Figure 8-6,** *A*).

There are two types of isotonic contraction. One is **concentric contraction,** in which the muscle shortens. The other is **eccentric contraction,** in which the muscle lengthens but still provides work. For example lifting this book requires concentric contraction of the biceps muscle that flexes your elbow. Lowering the book slowly and safely requires eccentric contraction of the biceps muscle. Thus what we call muscle "contraction" really means any pulling of the muscle whether it shortens or not.

Walking, running, breathing, lifting, twisting, and most body movements are examples of isotonic contraction.

Isometric Contraction

Contraction of a skeletal muscle does not always produce movement. Sometimes it increases the tension within a muscle but does not change the length of the muscle. When the muscle contracts and no movement results, it is called an **isometric contraction.** The word *isometric* comes from Greek

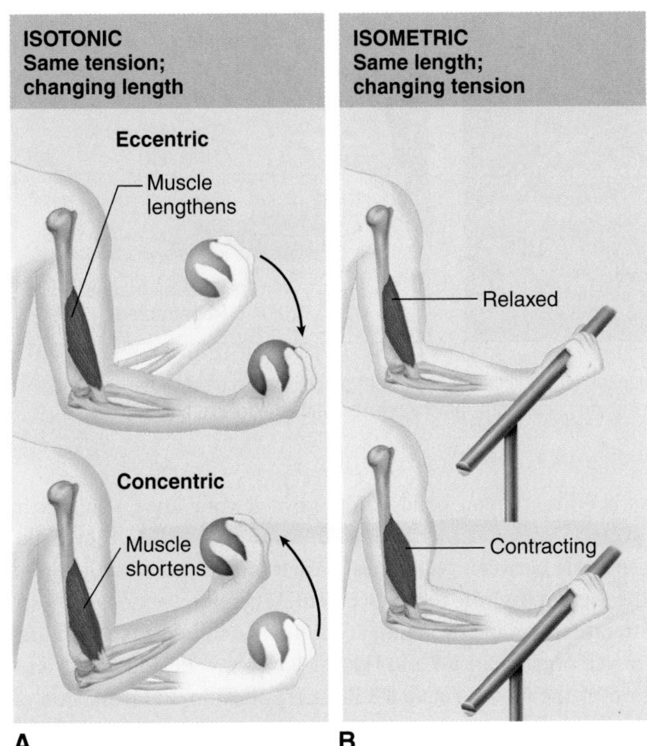

FIGURE 8-6 Types of muscle contraction. A, In isotonic contraction the muscle changes length, producing movement. **B,** In isometric contraction the muscle pulls forcefully against a load but does not shorten.

words that mean "equal measure." In other words, a muscle's length during an isometric contraction and during relaxation is about equal.

Although muscles do not shorten (and thus produce no movement) during isometric contractions, tension within them increases (Figure 8-6, *B*). Because of this, repeated isometric contractions make muscles grow larger and stronger. Pushing against a wall or other immovable object is a good example of isometric exercise. Although no movement occurs and the muscle does not shorten, its internal tension increases dramatically.

Effects of Exercise on Skeletal Muscle

We know that exercise is good for us. Some of the benefits of regular, properly practiced exercise are greatly improved muscle tone, better posture, more efficient heart and lung function, less fatigue, and looking and feeling better.

Skeletal muscles undergo changes that correspond to the amount of work that they normally do. During prolonged inactivity, muscles usually shrink in mass, a condition called **disuse atrophy.** Exercise, on the other hand, may cause an increase in muscle size called **hypertrophy.**

RESEARCH, ISSUES, AND TRENDS

ENHANCING MUSCLE STRENGTH

The most obvious and effective way of increasing skeletal muscle strength is by strength training; that is, regularly pulling against heavy resistance. The maximal amount of muscular strength one can achieve is determined mainly by genetics. However, there are a number of chemical enhancements athletes have tried over the centuries to improve strength.

An early fad among athletes in the twentieth century was the overuse of vitamin supplements. Although moderate vitamin supplementation will ensure adequate intake of vitamins necessary for good muscle function, overuse may lead to *hypervitaminosis* and possibly serious consequences.

Another type of chemical often abused by athletes is *anabolic steroids.* Anabolic steroids are usually synthetic derivatives of the male hormone *testosterone.* As with naturally produced testosterone, they do in fact stimulate an increase in muscle size and strength, making them attractive to coaches and athletes wanting to win their events. However, prolonged use of these hormones can cause serious, even life-threatening, hormonal imbalances. For this reason, anabolic steroids are banned from most organized sports.

Sports physiologists are now investigating a whole variety of chemicals, such as *creatine phosphate* and various coenzymes that are reported to enhance strength or endurance. Always carefully review the latest research findings on these substances with the help of a health or exercise professional before using them yourself, or you may suffer serious health consequences.

Muscle hypertrophy can be enhanced by **strength training,** which involves contracting muscles against heavy resistance. Isometric exercises and weight lifting are common strength-training activities. This type of training results in increased numbers of myofilaments in each muscle fiber. Although the number of muscle fibers stays the same, the increased number of myofilaments greatly increases the mass of the muscle.

Endurance training, often called **aerobic training,** does not usually result in muscle hypertrophy. Instead, this type of exercise program increases a muscle's ability to sustain moderate exercise over a long period. Aerobic activities such as running, bicycling, or other primarily isotonic movements increase the number of blood vessels in a muscle without significantly increasing its size. The increased blood flow allows a more efficient delivery of oxygen and glucose to muscle fibers during exercise. Aerobic training also causes an increase in the number of mitochondria in muscle fibers. This allows production of more ATP as a rapid energy source.

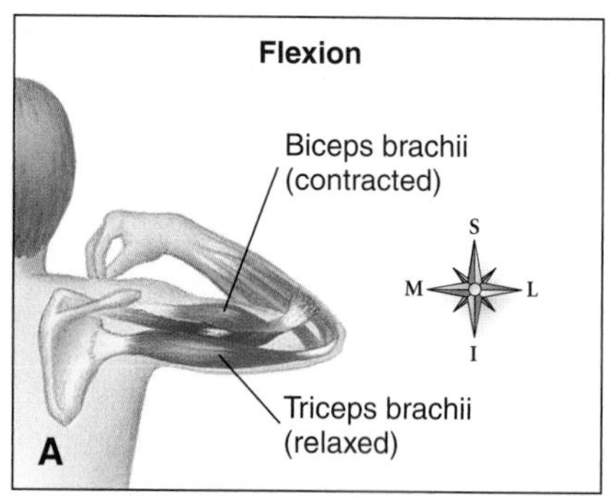

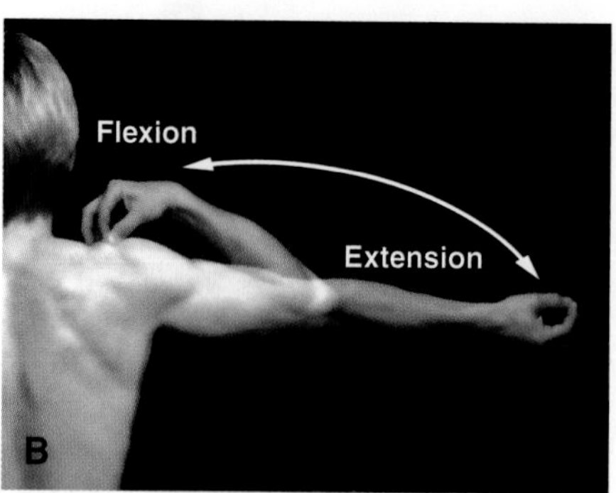

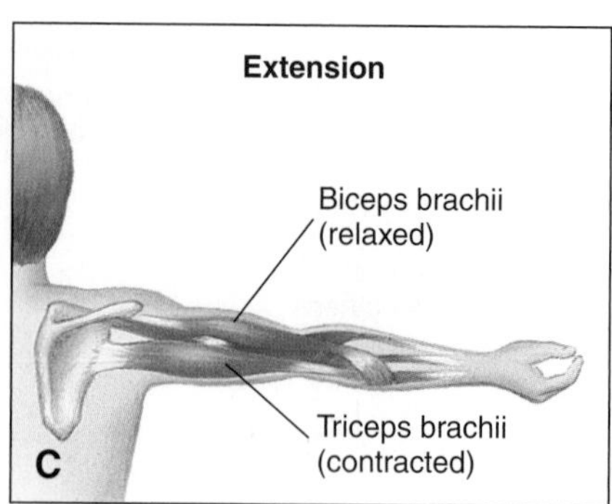

FIGURE 8-7 Flexion and extension of the elbow. A and **B,** When the elbow is flexed, the biceps brachii contracts while its antagonist, the triceps brachii, relaxes. **B** and **C,** When the elbow is extended, the biceps brachii relaxes while the triceps brachii contracts.

QUICK CHECK

1. What is a *motor unit?*
2. How does a muscle produce different levels of strength?
3. What is the difference between *isotonic* and *isometric* muscle contractions?
4. How does strength training affect a person's muscles?
5. What role does acetylcholine play in muscle contraction?

Movements Produced by Skeletal Muscle Contractions

The particular type of movement that occurs at any joint depends on the muscles acting at that joint, on their origin and insertion points, on the shapes of the bones involved, and the joint type (see Chapter 7). Muscles acting on some joints produce movement in several directions, whereas only limited movement is possible at other joints. The terms most often used to describe body movements are described in the following sections.

Angular Movements

Flexion is a movement that makes the angle between two bones at their joint smaller than it was at the beginning of the movement. Most flexions are movements commonly described as bending. If you bend your elbow or your knee, you flex it. **Extension** movements are the opposite of flexions. They make the angle between two bones at their joint larger than it was at the beginning of the movement. Therefore, extensions are straightening or stretching movements rather than bending movements. **Figure 8-7** and **Figure 8-9**, *A*, show flexion and extension of the elbow. **Figure 8-8** illustrates flexion and extension of the knee.

Abduction means moving a part away from the midline of the body, such as moving your arm out to the side. **Adduction** means moving a part toward the midline, such as bringing your arms down to your sides from an elevated position. **Figure 8-9**, *B*, shows abduction and adduction.

Circular Movements

Rotation is movement around a longitudinal axis. You rotate your head and neck by moving your skull from side to side as in shaking your head "no" (**Figure 8-9**, *C*). **Circumduction** moves a part so that its distal end moves in a circle. When a pitcher winds up to throw a ball, she circumducts her arm (**Figure 8-9**, *D*).

Supination and **pronation** refer to hand positions that result from rotation of the forearm. (The term *prone* refers to the body as a whole lying face down. *Supine* means lying face up.) Supination results in a hand position with the palm

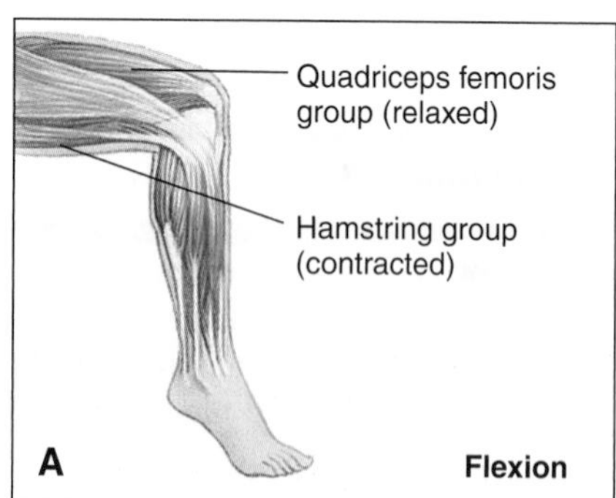

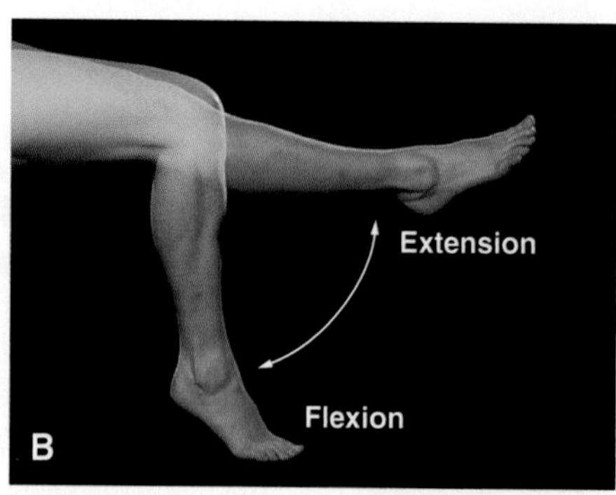

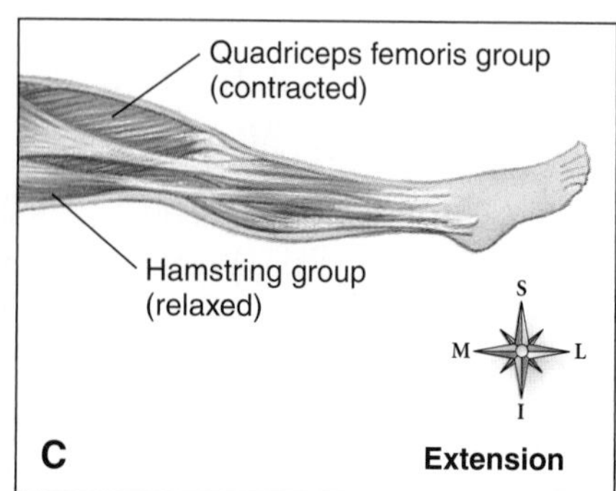

FIGURE 8-8 Flexion and extension of the knee. A and **B,** When the knee flexes, muscles of the hamstring group contract while their antagonists in the quadriceps femoris group relax. **B** and **C,** When the knee extends, the hamstring muscles relax while the quadriceps femoris muscle contracts.

turned to the anterior position (as in the anatomical position), and pronation occurs when you turn the palm of your hand so that it faces posteriorly (**Figure 8-9**, *E*).

Special Movements

Some body parts, such as the foot, are difficult to describe with ordinary terms, so special terms are often used to describe their unique movements.

Dorsiflexion and **plantar flexion** refer to ankle movements. In dorsiflexion the dorsum, or top, of the foot is elevated with the toes pointing upward. In plantar flexion the bottom of the foot is directed downward so that you are in effect standing on your toes (**Figure 8-9**, *F*).

Inversion and **eversion** are also ankle movements. Inversion turns the ankle so that the bottom of the foot faces toward the midline of the body (**Figure 8-9**, *G*). Eversion turns the ankle in the opposite direction, so that the bottom of the foot faces toward the side of the body (**Figure 8-9**, *H*).

ANGULAR

A

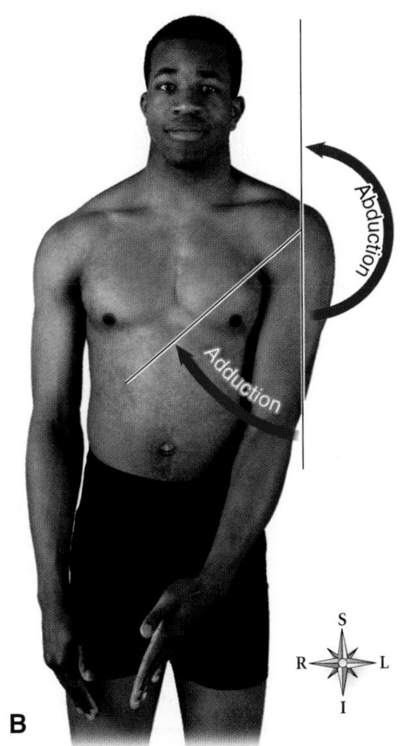

CIRCULAR

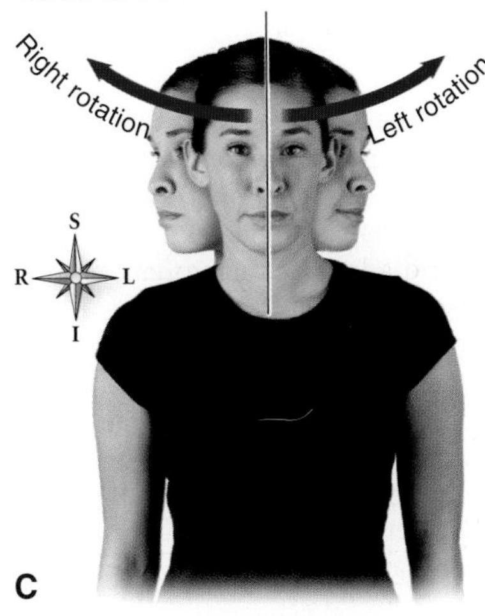

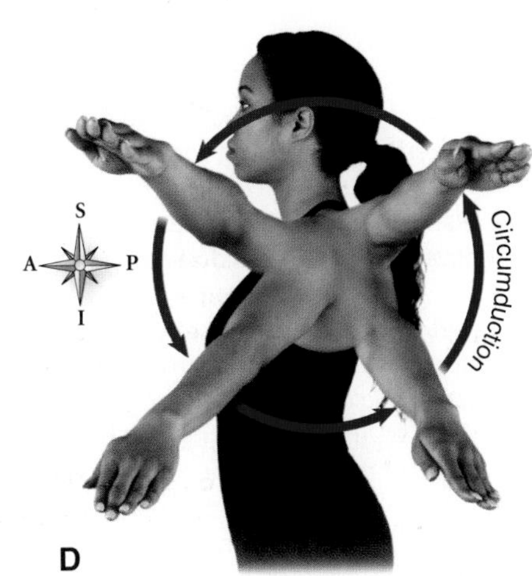

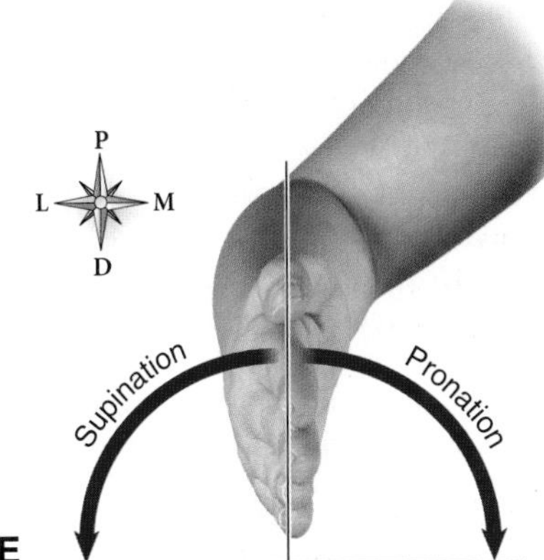

SPECIAL

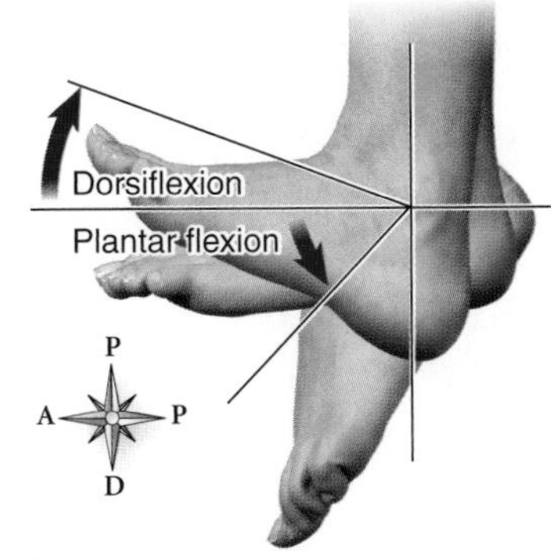

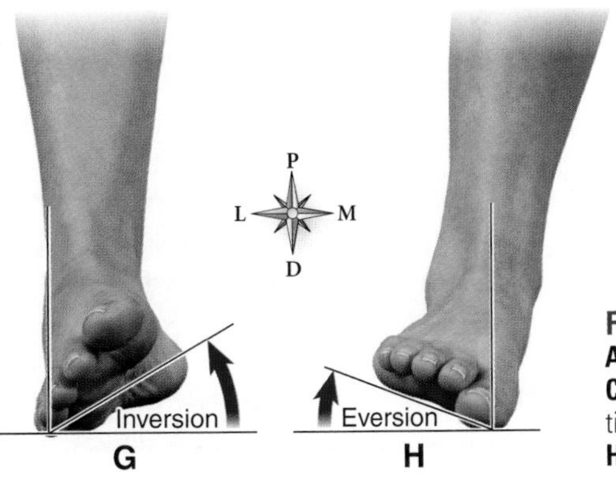

FIGURE 8-9 Examples of body movements. A, Flexion and extension. **B,** Adduction and abduction. **C,** Rotation. **D,** Circumduction. **E,** Pronation and supination. **F,** Dorsiflexion and plantar flexion. **G,** Inversion. **H,** Eversion.

TABLE 8-1 Muscles Grouped According to Function

PART MOVED	FLEXORS	EXTENSORS	ABDUCTORS	ADDUCTORS
Arm	Pectoralis major	Latissimus dorsi	Deltoid	Pectoralis major and latissimus dorsi contracting together
Forearm	Biceps brachii	Triceps brachii	None	None
Thigh	Iliopsoas Sartorius Rectus femoris	Gluteus maximus Hamstring group	Gluteus medius	Adductor group
Leg	Hamstrings	Quadriceps group	None	None
Foot	Tibialis anterior	Gastrocnemius Soleus	Fibularis longus Fibularis brevis	Tibialis anterior Fibularis tertius

As you study the illustrations and learn to recognize the muscles discussed in this chapter, you should attempt to group them according to function, as in **Table 8-1**. You will note, for example, that flexors produce many of the movements used for walking, sitting, swimming, typing, and many other activities. Extensors also function in these activities but perhaps play their most important role in maintaining an upright posture.

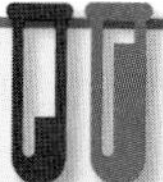

CLINICAL APPLICATION

CARPAL TUNNEL SYNDROME

Some physicians specialize in the field of occupational health, the study of health matters related to work or the workplace. Many problems seen by occupational health experts are caused by repetitive motions of the wrists or other joints. Word processors (typists) and meat cutters, for example, are at risk of developing conditions caused by repetitive motion injuries.

One common problem often caused by such repetitive motion is **tenosynovitis**—inflammation of the tendon sheath. Tenosynovitis can be painful, and the swelling characteristic of this condition can limit movement in affected parts of the body. For example, swelling of the tendon sheath around tendons in an area of the wrist known as the *carpal tunnel* can limit movement of the wrist, hand, and fingers.

The figure shows the relative positions of the tendon sheath and medial nerve within the carpal tunnel. If this swelling, or any other lesion in the carpal tunnel, presses on the *median nerve,* a condition called **carpal tunnel syndrome** may result. Because the median nerve connects to the palm and radial side (thumb side) of the hand, carpal tunnel syndrome is characterized by weakness, pain, and tingling in that part of the hand. The pain and tingling may also radiate to the forearm and shoulder.

Prolonged and severe cases of carpal tunnel syndrome may be relieved by injection of anti-inflammatory agents. A permanent cure is sometimes accomplished by surgically cutting the fibrous band called the *flexor retinaculum* enclosing the carpal tunnel—thus relieving pressure on the median nerve.

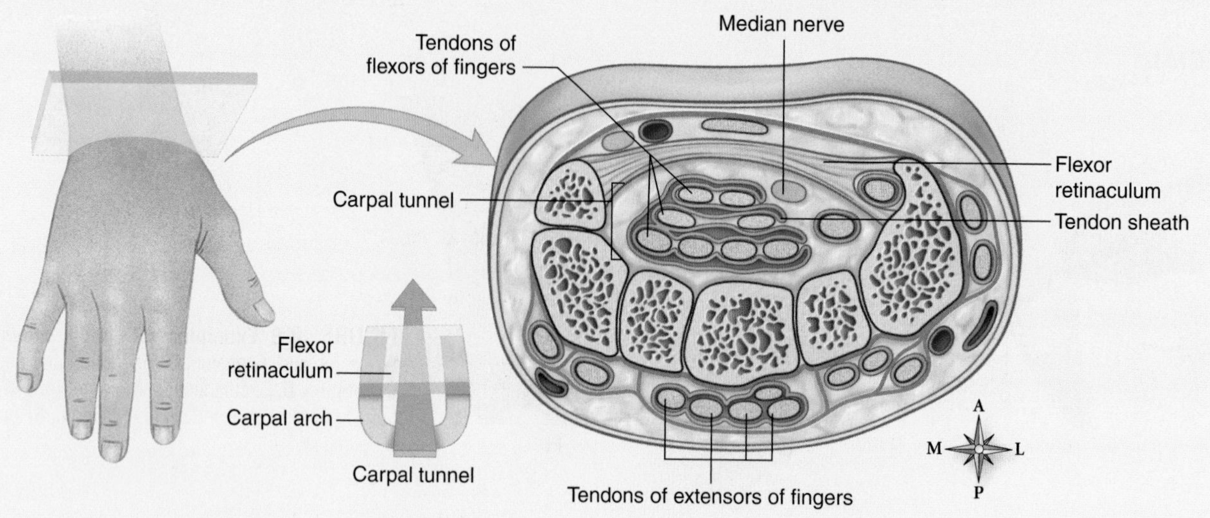

QUICK CHECK

1. When a person flexes the knee, what movement is this?
2. What happens when a person abducts his or her arm?
3. How is dorsiflexion of the foot performed?

Skeletal Muscle Groups

In the paragraphs that follow, representative muscles from the most important skeletal muscle groups are discussed. Refer to **Figure 8-10** often so that you will be able to see a muscle as you read about its placement on the body and its function. **Table 8-2** identifies and groups muscles according to function and provides information about muscle action and points of origin and insertion. Keep in mind that muscles move bones, and the bones that they move are their insertion bones.

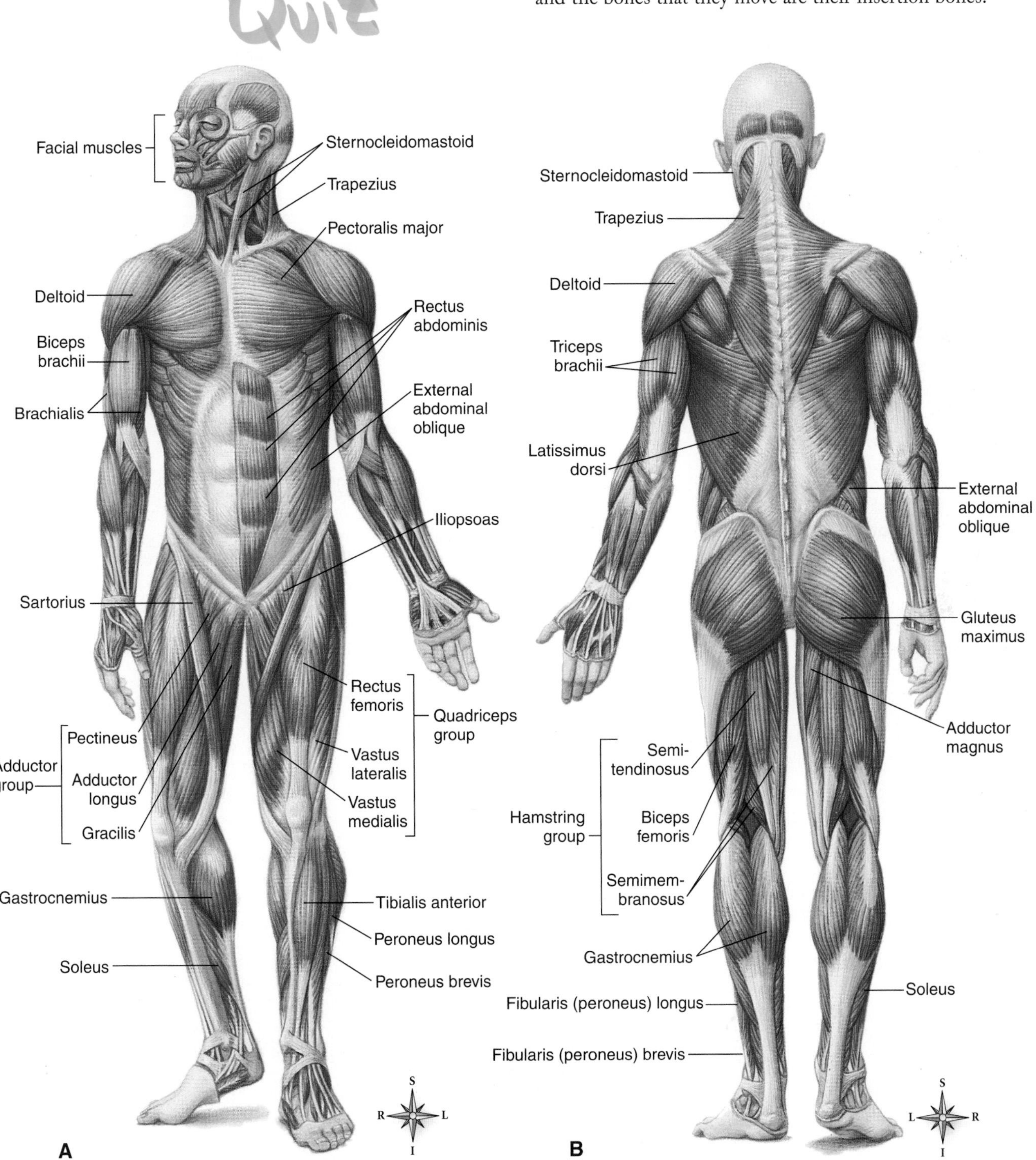

FIGURE 8-10 General overview of the body musculature. A, Anterior view. **B,** Posterior view.

TABLE 8-2 Principal Muscles of the Body

MUSCLE	FUNCTION	INSERTION	ORIGIN
Muscles of the Head and Neck			
Frontal	Raises eyebrow	Skin of eyebrow	Occipital bone
Orbicularis oculi	Closes eye	Maxilla and frontal bone	Maxilla and frontal bone (encircles eye)
Orbicularis oris	Draws lips together	Encircles lips	Encircles lips
Zygomaticus	Elevates corners of mouth and lips	Angle of mouth and upper lip	Zygomatic
Masseter	Closes jaw	Mandible	Zygomatic arch
Temporal	Closes jaw	Mandible	Temporal region of the skull
Sternocleidomastoid	Rotates and flexes head and neck	Mastoid process	Sternum and clavicle
Trapezius	Extends head and neck Moves or stabilizes scapula	Scapula	Skull and upper vertebrae
Muscles That Move the Upper Extremities			
Pectoralis major	Flexes and helps adduct arm	Humerus	Sternum, clavicle, and upper rib cartilages
Latissimus dorsi	Extends and helps adduct arm	Humerus	Vertebrae and ilium
Deltoid	Abducts arm	Humerus	Clavicle and scapula
Biceps brachii	Flexes elbow	Radius	Scapula
Triceps brachii	Extends elbow	Ulna	Scapula and humerus
Muscles of the Trunk			
External oblique	Compresses abdomen	Midline of abdomen	Lower thoracic cage
Internal oblique	Compresses abdomen	Midline of abdomen	Pelvis
Transversus abdominis	Compresses abdomen	Midline of abdomen	Ribs, vertebrae, and pelvis
Rectus abdominis	Flexes trunk	Lower rib cage	Pubis
Diaphragm	Expands thoracic cavity during inspiration	Circumference of lower rib cage	Fibrous tissue (central tendon) at center of diaphragm
Muscles That Move the Lower Extremities			
Iliopsoas	Flexes thigh or trunk	Femur	Ilium and vertebrae
Sartorius	Flexes thigh and rotates leg	Tibia	Ilium
Gluteus maximus	Extends thigh	Femur	Ilium, sacrum, coccyx
Adductor Group			
Adductor longus	Adducts thigh	Femur	Pubis
Gracilis	Adducts thigh	Tibia	Pubis
Pectineus	Adducts thigh	Femur	Pubis
Hamstring Group			
Semimembranosus	Flexes knee	Tibia	Ischium
Semitendinosus	Flexes knee	Tibia	Ischium
Biceps femoris	Flexes knee	Fibula	Ischium and femur
Quadriceps Group			
Rectus femoris	Extends knee	Tibia	Ilium
Vastus lateralis Vastus intermedius Vastus medialis	Extend knee	Tibia	Femur
Fibularis Group			
Fibularis longus Fibularis brevis Fibularis tertius	Evert and plantar flex ankle (tertius dorsiflexes ankle)	Tarsal and metatarsals (ankle and foot)	Tibia and fibula
Tibialis anterior	Dorsiflexes ankle	Metatarsals (foot)	Tibia
Gastrocnemius	Plantar flexes ankle	Calcaneus (heel)	Femur
Soleus	Plantar flexes ankle	Calcaneus (heel)	Tibia and fibula

Muscles of the Head and Neck

The *muscles of facial expression* (**Figure 8-11**) allow us to communicate many different emotions nonverbally. Contraction of the **frontal muscle,** for example, allows you to raise your eyebrows in surprise and furrow the skin of your forehead into a frown. The **orbicularis oris,** called the *kissing muscle,* puckers the lips. The **zygomaticus** elevates the corners of the mouth and lips and has been called the *smiling muscle.*

The *muscles of mastication* are responsible for closing the mouth and producing chewing movements. The term **mastication** refers to chewing. As a group, they are among the strongest muscles in the body. The two largest muscles of the group, identified in **Figure 8-11**, are the **masseter,** which elevates the mandible, and the **temporal,** which assists the masseter in closing the jaw.

The **sternocleidomastoid** and **trapezius** muscles are easily identified in **Figure 8-10** and **Figure 8-11**. The two sternocleidomastoid muscles are located on the anterior surface of the neck. They originate on the sternum and then pass up and cross the neck to insert on the mastoid process of the skull. Working together, they flex the head on the chest. If only one contracts, the head is both flexed and tilted to the opposite side.

The triangular-shaped trapezius muscles form the line from each shoulder to the neck on its posterior surface. They have a wide line of origin extending from the base of the skull down the spinal column to the last thoracic vertebra. When contracted, the trapezius muscles help elevate the shoulders and extend the head backward.

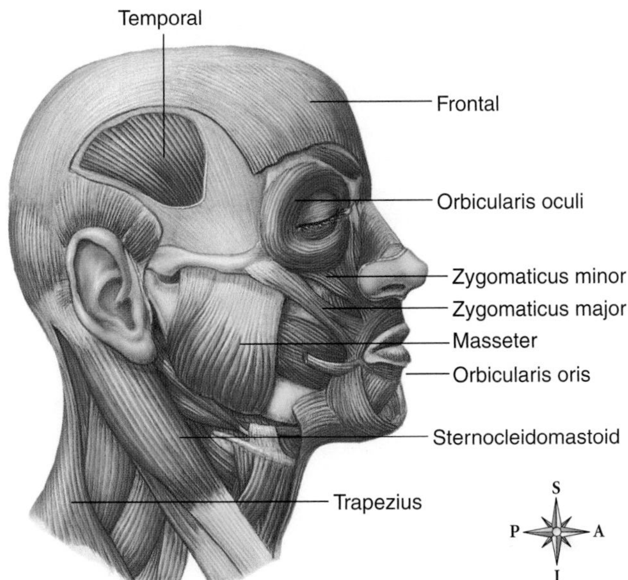

FIGURE 8-11 Muscles of the head and neck. Muscles that produce most facial expressions surround the eyes, nose, and mouth. Large muscles of mastication stretch from the upper skull to the lower jaw. These powerful muscles produce chewing movements. The neck muscles connect the skull to the trunk of the body, rotating the head or bending the neck.

Muscles That Move the Upper Extremities

The upper extremity is attached to the thorax by the fan-shaped **pectoralis major** muscle, which covers the upper chest, and by the **latissimus dorsi** muscle, which originates from structures over the lower back (see **Figure 8-10** and **Figure 8-12**). Both muscles insert on the humerus. The pectoralis major is a flexor, and the latissimus dorsi is an extensor of the arm.

The **deltoid** muscle forms the thick, rounded prominence over the shoulder and arm (see **Figure 8-10**). The muscle takes its origin from the scapula and clavicle and inserts on the humerus. It is a powerful abductor of the arm.

As the name implies, the **biceps brachii** is a two-headed muscle that serves as a primary flexor of the forearm (see **Figure 8-10**). It originates from the bones of the shoulder girdle and inserts on the radius in the forearm.

The **triceps brachii** is on the posterior or back surface of the arm. It has three heads of origin from the shoulder girdle and inserts into the olecranon process of the ulna. The triceps is an extensor of the elbow and thus performs a straightening function. Because this muscle is responsible for delivering blows during fights, it is often called the *boxer's muscle.*

Muscles of the Trunk

The muscles of the anterior or front side of the abdomen are arranged in three layers, with the fibers in each layer running in different directions much like the layers of wood in a sheet of plywood (see **Figure 8-12**). The result is a very strong "girdle" of muscle that covers and supports the abdominal cavity and its internal organs.

The three layers of muscle in the anterolateral (side) abdominal walls are arranged as follows: the outermost layer or **external oblique;** a middle layer or **internal oblique;** and the innermost layer or **transversus abdominis.**

In addition to these sheetlike muscles, the band- or strap-shaped **rectus abdominis** muscle runs down the midline of the abdomen from the thorax to the pubis. The rectus abdominis and external oblique muscles can be seen in **Figure 8-12**. In addition to protecting the abdominal viscera, the rectus abdominis flexes the vertebral column.

The *respiratory muscles* are discussed in Chapter 15. **Intercostal muscles,** located between the ribs, and the sheet-like **diaphragm** separating the thoracic and abdominal cavities change the size and shape of the chest during breathing. As a result, air is moved into or out of the lungs.

Muscles That Move the Lower Extremities

The **iliopsoas** originates from deep within the pelvis and the lower vertebrae to insert on the lesser trochanter of the femur and capsule of the hip joint. It is generally classified as a flexor of the thigh and an important postural muscle that stabilizes and keeps the trunk from falling over backward when you

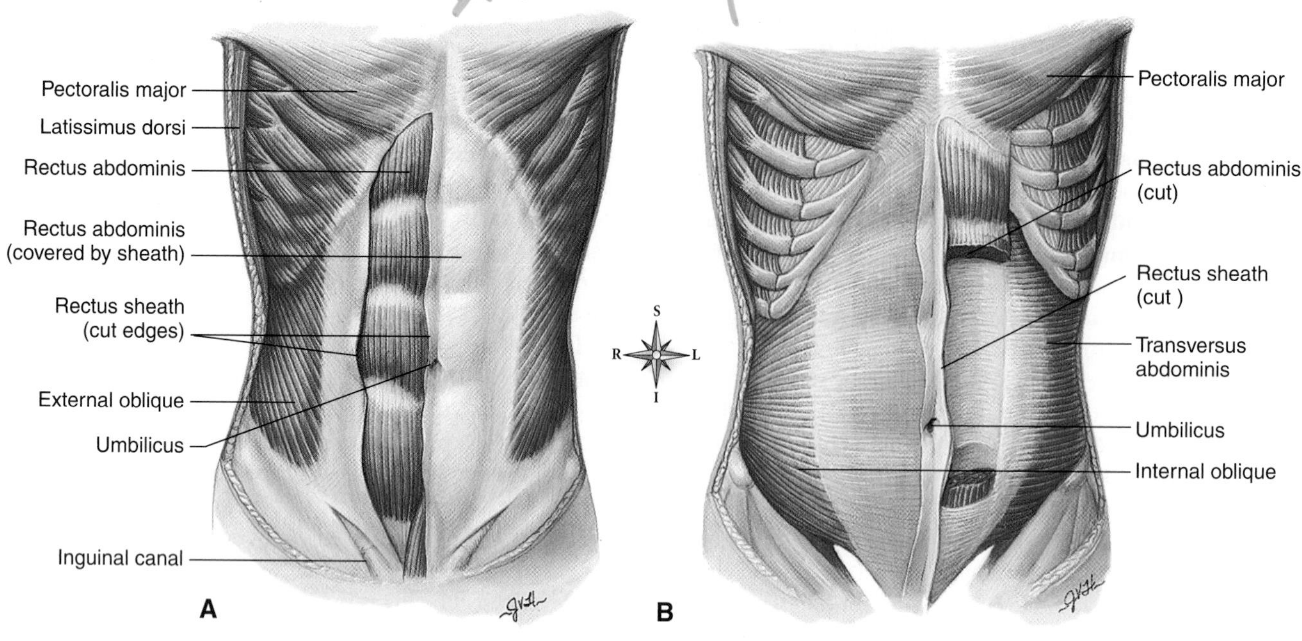

FIGURE 8-12 Muscles of the trunk. A, Anterior view showing superficial muscles. **B,** Anterior view showing deeper muscles.

CLINICAL APPLICATION

MUSCLE INJURY

Injuries to skeletal muscles resulting from overexertion or trauma usually result in a **muscle strain.** Muscle strains are characterized by muscle pain, or *myalgia,* and involve overstretching or tearing of muscle fibers. If an injury occurs in the area of a joint and a ligament is damaged, the injury may be called a *sprain.*

Any muscle inflammation, including that caused by a muscle strain, is termed *myositis.* If tendon inflammation occurs with myositis, as when one experiences a *charley horse,* the condition is termed *fibromyositis.* Although inflammation may subside in a few hours or days, it usually takes several weeks for damaged muscle fibers to repair themselves. Some damaged muscle cells may be replaced by fibrous tissue, forming scars. Occasionally, hard calcium is deposited in the scar tissue.

Cramps are painful muscle spasms (involuntary twitches). Cramps often result from mild myositis or fibromyositis, but they also can be a symptom of any irritation or of an ion and water imbalance.

Minor trauma to the body, especially a limb, may cause a muscle *bruise* or *contusion.* Muscle contusions involve local internal bleeding and inflammation. Severe trauma to a skeletal muscle may cause a *crush injury.* Crush injuries not only greatly damage the affected muscle tissue but also cause the release of muscle fiber contents into the bloodstream, which can be life threatening. For example, the reddish muscle pigment *myoglobin* can accumulate in the blood and cause kidney failure.

Stress-induced muscle tension can result in myalgia and stiffness in the neck and back and is thought to be one cause of "stress headaches." Headache and back pain clinics use a variety of strategies to treat stress-induced muscle tension. These treatments include massage, biofeedback, and relaxation training.

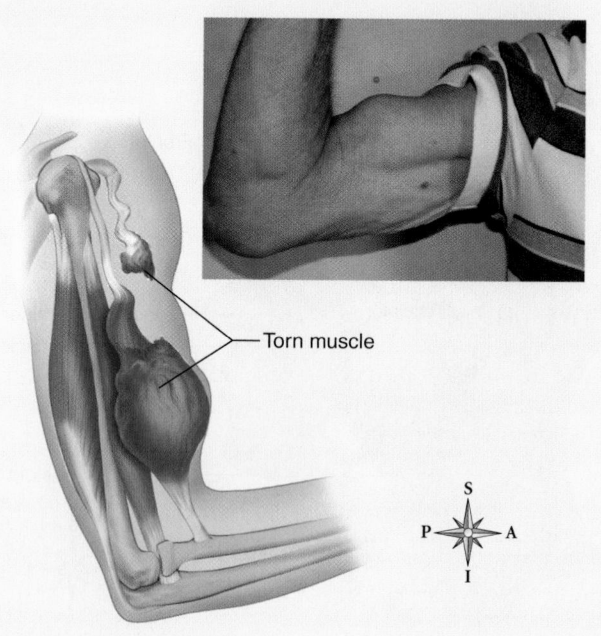

Muscle strain. Severe strain of the biceps brachii muscle. When a muscle is severely strained, it may break in two pieces, causing a visible gap in muscle tissue under the skin. Notice how the broken ends of the muscle reflexively contract (spasm) to form a knot of tissue.

stand. However, if the thigh is fixed so that it cannot move, the iliopsoas flexes the *trunk.* An example would be doing sit-ups.

The **gluteus maximus** forms the outer contour and much of the substance of the buttock. It is an important extensor of the thigh (see Figure 8-10) and supports the torso in the erect position.

The **adductor muscles** originate on the bony pelvis and insert on the femur. They are located on the inner or medial side of the thighs. These muscles adduct, or press, the thighs together.

The three **hamstring muscles** are called the *semimembranosus, semitendinosus,* and *biceps femoris.* Acting together, they serve as powerful flexors of the leg (see Figure 8-10). They originate on the ischium and insert on the tibia or fibula.

The **quadriceps femoris** muscle group covers the upper thigh. The four thigh muscles—the *rectus femoris* and three *vastus* muscles—extend the leg (see Figure 8-10 and Table 8-2). One component of the quadriceps group has its origin on the pelvis, and the remaining three originate on the femur. All four insert on the tibia. Only two of the vastus muscles are visible in Figure 8-10. The vastus intermedius is covered by the rectus femoris and is not visible.

The **tibialis anterior** muscle (see Figure 8-10) is located on the anterior or front surface of the leg. It dorsiflexes the foot. The **gastrocnemius** is the primary calf muscle. Note in Figure 8-10 that it has two fleshy components arising from both sides of the femur. It inserts through the calcaneal (Achilles) tendon into the heel bone or calcaneus. The gastrocnemius is responsible for plantar flexion of the foot. Since it is used to stand on tiptoe, it is sometimes called the *toe dancer's muscle.*

A group of three muscles called the **fibularis group** or **peroneus group** (see Figure 8-10) is found along the sides of the leg. As a group, these muscles evert and plantar flex the foot. A long tendon from one component of the group—the *fibularis longus* muscle tendon—forms a support arch for the foot (see Figure 7-22).

QUICK CHECK

1. What are the functions of the *muscles of mastication*?
2. Why is the triceps brachii muscle sometimes called the "boxer's muscle"?
3. What action do the hamstring muscles perform?
4. What are the two primary respiratory muscles?

LANGUAGE OF SCIENCE AND MEDICINE *(continued from p. 155)*

bursa
(BER-sah)
pl., bursae
(BER-see or BER-say)
[*bursa* **purse**]

cardiac muscle
(KAR-dee-ak MUS-el)
[*cardi-* **heart**, *-ac* **relating to**, *mus-* **mouse**, *-cle* **small**]

carpal tunnel syndrome
(KAR-pul TUN-el SIN-drohm)
[*carp-* **wrist**, *-al* **relating to**, *syn-* **together**, *-drome* **running or (race) course**]

circumduction
(ser-kum-DUK-shun)
[*circum-* **around**, *-duct-* **lead**, *-tion* **process**]

concentric contraction
(kon-SEN-trik kon-TRAK-shun)
[*con-* **together**, *-centr-* **center**, *-ic* **relating to**, *con-* **together**, *-tract-* **drag or draw**, *-tion* **process**]

deltoid
(DEL-toyd)
[*delta-* **triangle**, *-oid* **like**]

diaphragm
(DYE-ah-fram)
[*dia-* **across**, *-phrag-* **enclose**, *-(u)m* **thing**]

disuse atrophy
(DIS-yoos AT-roh-fee)
[*dis-* **absence of**, *a-* **without**, *-troph-* **nourishment**, *-y* **state**]

dorsiflexion
(dor-sih-FLEK-shun)
[*dorsi-* **back**, *-flex-* **bend**, *-ion* **process**]

eccentric contraction
(ek-SENT-rik kon-TRAK-shun)
[*ec-* **out of**, *-centr-* **center**, *-ic* **relating to**, *con-* **together**, *-tract-* **drag or draw**, *-tion* **process**]

endurance training
(en-DOOR-ents TRAYN-ing)

ergonomics
(er-go-NOM-iks)
[*ergo-* **work**, *-nom-* **arrangement**, *-ic* **relating to**]

eversion
(ee-VER-zhun)
[*e(x)-* **outward**, *-ver-* **turn**, *-sion* **process**]

extension
(ek-STEN-shun)
[*ex-* **outward**, *-tens-* **stretch**, *-sion* **process**]

external oblique
(eks-TER-nal oh-BLEEK)
[*extern-* **outside**, *-al* **relating to**, *obliq-* **slanted**]

fatigue
(fah-TEEG)

fibularis group
(fib-YOO-lay-ris groop)
[*fibula-* **clasp (fibula bone)**, *-aris* **relating to**]

flexion
(FLEK-shun)
[*flex-* **bend**, *-ion* **process**]

frontal muscle
(FRUN-tal MUS-el)
[*front-* **forehead**, *-al* **relating to**, *mus-* **mouse**, *-cle* **small**]

gastrocnemius
(GAS-trok-NEE-mee-us)
[*gastro-* **belly**, *-cnemius* **leg**]

gluteus maximus
(GLOO-tee-us MAX-ih-mus)
[*gluteus* **buttocks**, *maximus* **greatest**]

hamstring muscle
(HAM-string MUS-el)
[*ham-* **hollow of knee**, *-string* **(tendon)**, *mus-* **mouse**, *-cle* **small**]

hypertrophy
(hye-PER-troh-fee)
[*hyper-* **excessive**, *-troph-* **nourishment**, *-y* **state**]

hypothermia
(hye-poh-THER-mee-ah)
[*hypo-* **under or below**, *-therm-* **heat**, *-ia* **abnormal condition**]

iliopsoas
(il-ee-oh-SO-as)
[*ilio-* **loin or gut**, *-psoas* **loin muscle**]

insertion
(in-SER-shun)
[*in-* **in**, *-ser-* **join**, *-tion* **process**]

intercalated disk
(in-TER-kah-lay-ted disk)
[*inter-* **between**, *-cala-* **calendar**, *-ate* **act of**]

intercostal muscle
(in-ter-KOS-tal MUS-el)
[*inter-* **between,** *-costa-* **rib,** *-al* **relating to,** *mus-* **mouse,** *-cle* **small**]

internal oblique
(in-TER-nal oh-BLEEK)
[*intern-* **inside,** *-al* **relating to,** *obliq-* **slanted,** *mus-* **mouse,** *-cle* **little**]

inversion
(in-VER-zhun)
[*in-* **in,** *-ver-* **turn,** *-sion* **process**]

isometric contraction
(eye-soh-MET-rik kon-TRAK-shun)
[*iso-* **equal,** *metric* **relating to measure,** *con-* **together,** *-tract-* **drag or draw,** *-tion* **process**]

isotonic contraction
(eye-soh-TON-ik kon-TRAK-shun)
[*iso-* **equal,** *-ton-* **tension,** *-ic* **relating to,** *con-* **together,** *-tract-* **drag or draw,** *-tion* **process**]

latissimus dorsi
(lah-TIS-ih-mus DOR-sye)
[*latissimus* **broadest,** *dorsi* **relating to back**]

massage therapy
(mah-SAHJ THAYR-ah-pee)
[*mass-* **handle,** *-age* **process,** *therap-* **treatment,** *-y* **activity**]

masseter
(mah-SEE-ter)
[*masseter* **chewer**]

mastication
(mass-tih-KAY-shun)
[*mastica-* **chew,** *-ation* **process**]

motor neuron
(MOH-ter NOO-ron)
[*mot-* **movement,** *-or* **agent,** *neuron* **nerve**]

motor unit
(MOH-ter YOO-nit)
[*mot-* **movement,** *-or* **agent,** *unit* **single**]

muscle fiber
(MUS-el FYE-ber)
[*mus-* **mouse,** *-cle* **little,** *fibr-* **thread**]

muscle strain
(MUS-el strayn)
[*mus-* **mouse,** *-cle* **little,** *str(a)n* **overstretch**]

muscle tone
(MUS-el tohn)
[*mus-* **mouse,** *-cle* **little,** *tone* **stretching**]

myofilament
(my-oh-FIL-ah-ment)
[*myo-* **muscle,** *-fila-* **thread,** *-ment* **thing**]

myoglobin
(my-oh-GLO-bin)
[*myo-* **muscle,** *-glob-* **ball,** *-in* **substance**]

myosin
(MY-oh-sin)
[*myos-* **muscle,** *-in* **substance**]

neuromuscular junction (NMJ)
(noo-roh-MUS-kyoo-lar JUNG-shun)
[*neuro-* **nerve,** *-mus-* **mouse,** *-cul-* **little,** *-ar* **relating to,** *-junc* **join,** *-tion* **condition**]

nurse
(nurs)
[*nurs-* **nourish or nurture**]

nutritionist
(noo-TRISH-en-ist)
[*nutri-* **nourish,** *-tion* **process,** *-ist* **agent**]

orbicularis oris
(or-bik-yoo-LAR-is OR-is)
[*orbi-* **circle,** *-cul-* **little,** *-aris* **relating to,** *oris* **relating to mouth**]

origin
(OR-ih-jin)
[*origin* **source**]

oxygen debt
(AHK-sih-jen det)
[*oxy-* **sharp,** *-gen* **produce,** *debt* **thing owed**]

paralysis
(pah-RAL-ih-sis)
[*para-* **beside,** *-lysis* **loosening**]

pectoralis major
(pek-teh-RAH-lis MAY-jor)
[*pector-* **breast,** *-alis* **relating to,** *major* **greater**]

peroneus group
(per-ohn-EE-us groop)
[*pero-* **boot,** *-us* **thing**]

physical education
(FIS-ik-al ed-yoo-KAY-shun)
[*physic-* **medicine,** *-al* **relating to**]

physician
(fih-ZISH-en)
[*physic-* **medicine,** *-ian* **practitioner**]

plantar flexion
(PLAN-tar FLEK-shun)
[*planta-* **sole,** *-ar* **relating to,** *flex-* **bend,** *-ion* **process**]

posture
(POS-chur)
[*postur-* **position**]

prime mover
(pryme MOO-ver)
[*prime* **first order**]

pronation
(proh-NAY- shun)
[*prona-* **bend forward,** *-ation* **process**]

quadriceps femoris
(KWOD-reh-seps feh-MOR-is)
[*quadri-* **four,** *-ceps* **head,** *femoris* **related to the thigh (femur)**]

rectus abdominis
(REK-tus ab-DOM-ih-nus)
[*rectus* **straight,** *abdominis* **related to the abdomen**]

rotation
(roh-TAY-shun)
[*rot-* **turn,** *-ation* **process**]

sarcomere
(SAR-koh-meer)
[*sarco-* **flesh,** *-mere* **part**]

skeletal muscle
(SKEL-et-al)
[*skelet-* **dried body,** *-al* **relating to,** *mus-* **mouse,** *-cle* **small**]

sliding filament model
(SLY-ding FIL-ah-ment MAH-del)
[*slide-* **glide,** *-ing* **action,** *fila-* **thread,** *-ment* **thing,** *model* **standard**]

smooth muscle
(smoothe MUS-el)
[*smooth* **smooth,** *mus-* **mouse,** *-cle* **small**]

sternocleidomastoid
(STERN-oh-KLYE-doh-MAS-toyd)
[*sterno-* **breastbone (sternum),** *-cleid-* **key (clavicle),** *-masto-* **breast (mastoid process),** *-oid* **like**]

strength training
(STRENG-th TRAYN-ing)
[*strength-* **power,** *train-* **instruct,** *-ing* **action**]

supination
(soo-pih-NAY-shun)
[*supin-* **turned backward (belly up),** *-ation* **process**]

synergist
(SIN-er-jist)
[*syn-* **together,** *-erg-* **to work,** *-ist* **agent**]

synovial membrane
(sih-NOH-vee-al MEM-brayn)
[*syn-* **together,** *-ovi-* **egg (white),** *-al* **relating to,** *membran-* **thin skin**]

temporal
(TEM-poh-ral)
[*tempora-* **temple (of head),** *-al* **relating to**]

tendon
(TEN-don)
[*tend-* **pulled tight,** *-on* **unit**]

tendon sheath
(TEN-don sheeth)
[*tend-* **pulled tight,** *-on* **unit**]

tenosynovitis
(ten-oh-sin-oh-VYE-tis)
[*teno-* **pulled tight (tendon),** *-syn-* **together,** *-ovi-* **egg white (joint fluid),** *-itis* **inflammation**]

tetanic contraction
(teh-TAN-ik kon-TRAK-shun)
[*tetanus* **tension,** *-ic* **pertaining to,** *con-* **together,** *-tract-* **drag or draw,** *-tion* **process**]

tetanus
(TET-ah-nus)
[*tetanus* **tension**]

threshold stimulus
(THRESH-hold STIM-yoo-lus)
[*stimul-* **to excite,** *-us* **thing**]

tibialis anterior
(tib-ee-AL-is an-TEER-ee-or)
[*tibia-* **shinbone,** *-alis* **relating to,** *ante-* **front,** *-er-* **more,** *-or* **quality**]

tonic contraction
(TAHN-ik kon-TRAK-shun)
[*ton-* **stretch,** *-ic* **relating to,** *con-* **together,** *-tract-* **drag or draw,** *-tion* **process**]

transversus abdominis
(tranz-VERS-us ab-DAH-min-us)
[*trans-* **across,** *-vers-* **turn,** *abdomin-* **belly**]

trapezius
(trah-PEE-zee-us)
[*trapezius* **small table (irregular 4-sided shape)**]

triceps brachii
(TRY-seps BRAY-kee-eye)
[*tri-* **three,** *-ceps* **head,** *brachii* **related to the arm**]

twitch
(twich)
[*twitch* **quick jerk**]

zygomaticus
(zye-goh-MAT-ik-us)
[*zygo-* **union or yoke,** *-ic-* **relating to,** *-us* **thing**]

❑ OUTLINE SUMMARY

To download a digital audio version of the chapter summary for use with your device, access the ***Audio Chapter Summaries*** *online at evolve.elsevier.com.*

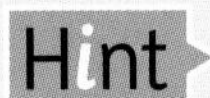

Scan this summary after reading the chapter to help you reinforce the key concepts. Later, use the summary as a quick review before your class or before a test.

Introduction

A. Muscular tissue enables the body and its parts to move
   1. Three types of muscle tissue exist in body (see Chapter 4)
   2. Movement caused by muscle cells (called *fibers*) either shortening or contracting
   3. Muscle movement occurs when chemical energy (obtained from food) is converted into mechanical energy

Muscle Tissue

A. Types of muscle tissue (see **Figure 8-1**)
   1. Skeletal muscle — also called *striated* or *voluntary muscle*
      a. Microscope reveals crosswise stripes or striations
      b. Contractions can be voluntarily controlled
   2. Cardiac muscle — composes bulk of heart
      a. Cardiac muscle fibers are branched
      b. Has dark bands called *intercalated disks*
      c. Cardiac muscle fiber interconnections allow heart to contract efficiently as a unit
   3. Nonstriated muscle, or involuntary muscle — also called *smooth* or *visceral muscle*
      a. Lacks striations when seen under a microscope; appears smooth
      b. Found in walls of hollow structures such as digestive tract, blood vessels, etc.
      c. Contractions not under voluntary control

B. Function — all muscle fibers specialize in contraction (shortening)

Structure of Skeletal Muscle

A. Muscle organs — mainly striated muscle fibers and connective tissue
   1. Connective tissue forms "wrappers" around each muscle fiber, around fascicles (groups) of muscle fibers, and around the entire muscle; fascia surrounds muscle organs and nearby structures
   2. Most skeletal muscles extend from one bone across a joint to another bone
   3. Regions of a skeletal muscle (see **Figure 8-2**)
      a. Origin — attachment to the bone that remains relatively stationary or fixed when movement at the joint occurs
      b. Insertion — point of attachment to the bone that moves when a muscle contracts
      c. Body — main part of the muscle
   4. Muscles attach to bone by tendons — strong cords or sheets of fibrous connective tissue that extend from the muscle organ; some tendons enclosed in synovial-lined tubes (tendon sheaths) and lubricated by synovial fluid
   5. Bursae — small synovial-lined sacs containing a small amount of synovial fluid; located between some tendons and underlying bones

B. Muscle fibers (see **Figure 8-3**)
   1. Contractile cells are called *muscle fibers;* connective tissue holds muscle fibers in parallel groupings
   2. Fibers of the cytoskeleton form cylinders made up of myofilaments
      a. Thick myofilaments contain myosin
      b. Thin myofilaments contain mainly actin
      c. Basic functional (contractile) units called *sarcomeres* are separated from each other by dark bands called *Z lines*

3. Muscle fiber contraction explained by sliding filament model
   a. Thick and thin myofilaments slide past each other to contract
   b. Contraction requires calcium and energy-rich ATP molecules (see **Figure 8-4**)

Functions of Skeletal Muscle

A. Movement
   1. Muscles produce movement by pulling on bones as a muscle contracts
      a. The insertion bone is pulled closer to the origin bone
      b. Movement occurs at the joint between the origin and the insertion
   2. Groups of muscles usually contract to produce a single movement
      a. Prime mover — mainly responsible for producing a given movement
      b. Synergist — helps the prime mover produce a given movement
      c. Antagonist — opposes the action of a prime mover in any given movement

B. Posture
   1. A continuous, low-strength muscle contraction called *tonic contraction* (muscle tone) enables us to maintain body position
      a. Only a few of a muscle's fibers shorten at one time
      b. Produces no movement of body parts
      c. Maintains muscle tone called *posture*
   2. Good posture favors best body functioning
   3. Skeletal muscle tone maintains good posture by counteracting the pull of gravity

C. Heat production
   1. Survival depends on the body's ability to maintain a constant body temperature
      a. Fever — an elevated body temperature — often a sign of illness
      b. Hypothermia — a body temperature below normal
   2. Contraction of muscle fibers produces most of the heat required to maintain normal body temperature

D. Fatigue
   1. Reduced strength of muscle contraction
   2. Caused by repeated muscle stimulation without adequate periods of rest
   3. Repeated muscular contraction depletes cellular ATP stores and outstrips the ability of the blood supply to replenish oxygen and nutrients
   4. Contraction in the absence of adequate oxygen produces lactic acid, which contributes to muscle soreness
   5. *Oxygen debt* — term used to describe the metabolic effort required to burn excess lactic acid that may accumulate during prolonged periods of exercise
      a. Labored breathing after strenuous exercise is required to "pay the debt"
      b. This increased metabolism helps restore energy and oxygen reserves to pre-exercise levels

Role of Other Body Systems in Movement

A. Muscle functioning depends on the functioning of many other parts of the body
B. Most muscles cause movements by pulling on bones across movable joints
C. Respiratory, circulatory, nervous, muscular, and skeletal systems play essential roles in producing normal movements
D. Multiple sclerosis, brain hemorrhage, and spinal cord injury are examples of how pathological conditions in other body organ systems can dramatically affect movement

Motor Unit

A. Stimulation of a muscle by a nerve impulse is required before a muscle can shorten and produce movement
B. Motor neuron — nerve cell that transmits an impulse to a muscle, causing contraction
C. Neuromuscular junction (NMJ)
   1. Point of contact between a nerve ending and a muscle fiber
   2. Chemicals called neurotransmitters cross the NMJ to trigger contraction in muscle
   3. Acetylcholine (ACh) is the neurotransmitter operating at each NMJ
D. Motor unit — combination of a motor neuron with the muscle fibers it controls (see **Figure 8-5**)

Muscle Stimulus

A. A muscle will contract only if an applied stimulus reaches a certain level of intensity
   1. Threshold stimulus — minimal level of stimulation required to cause a muscle fiber to contract
B. Once stimulated by a threshold stimulus, a muscle fiber will contract completely, a response called *all or none*
C. Different muscle fibers in a muscle are controlled by different motor units having different threshold-stimulus levels
   1. Although individual muscle fibers always respond all or none to a threshold stimulus, the muscle as a whole does not
   2. Different motor units responding to different threshold stimuli permit a muscle as a whole to execute contractions of graded force

Types of Skeletal Muscle Contraction

A. Twitch and tetanic contractions
   1. Twitch contractions are laboratory phenomena, not normal muscle activity; they are a single contraction of muscle fibers caused by a single threshold stimulus
   2. Tetanic contractions are sustained muscular contractions caused by stimuli hitting a muscle in rapid succession

B. Isotonic contractions (see **Figure 8-6**)
   1. Contractions that produce movement at a joint because the muscle changes length
   2. Concentric contractions — the muscle shortens insertion end of the muscle to move toward the point of origin
   3. Eccentric contractions — the muscle lengthens under tension, thus moving the insertion away from the origin
   4. Most types of body movements (walking, running, etc.) are produced by isotonic contractions

C. Isometric contractions (see **Figure 8-6**)
   1. Contractions that do not produce movement; the muscle as a whole does not shorten
   2. Although no movement occurs, tension within the muscle increases

Effects of Exercise on Skeletal Muscle

A. Exercise, if regular and properly practiced, improves muscle tone and posture, results in more efficient heart and lung functioning, and reduces fatigue

B. Muscles change in relation to the amount of work they normally do
   1. Prolonged inactivity causes disuse atrophy
   2. Regular exercise increases muscle size, called *hypertrophy*

C. Strength training is exercise involving contraction of muscles against heavy resistance
   1. Strength training increases the numbers of myofilaments in each muscle fiber, and as a result, the total mass of the muscle increases
   2. Strength training does not increase the number of muscle fibers

D. Endurance training is exercise that increases a muscle's ability to sustain moderate exercise over a long period; it is sometimes called *aerobic training*
   1. Endurance training allows more efficient delivery of oxygen and nutrients to a muscle via increased blood flow
   2. Endurance training does not usually result in muscle hypertrophy

Movements Produced by Skeletal Muscle Contractions

(see **Figure 8-7** through **Figure 8-9**)

A. Angular movements
   1. Flexion — decreases an angle
   2. Extension — increases an angle
   3. Abduction — away from the midline
   4. Adduction — toward the midline

B. Circular movements
   1. Rotation — around an axis
   2. Circumduction — move distal end of a part in a circle
   3. Supination and pronation — hand positions that result from twisting of the forearm

C. Special movements—those not easily described with general terms
   1. Dorsiflexion and plantar flexion — foot movements (upward and downward ankle movement)
   2. Inversion and eversion — foot movements (sideways)

Skeletal Muscle Groups (see **Table 8-2**)

A. Muscles of the head and neck (see **Figure 8-10** and **Figure 8-11**)
   1. Facial muscles
      a. Orbicularis oculi
      b. Orbicularis oris
      c. Zygomaticus
   2. Muscles of mastication
      a. Masseter
      b. Temporal
   3. Sternocleidomastoid — flexes head
   4. Trapezius — elevates shoulders and extends head

B. Muscles that move the upper extremities
   1. Pectoralis major — flexes arm
   2. Latissimus dorsi — extends arm
   3. Deltoid — abducts arm
   4. Biceps brachii — flexes forearm
   5. Triceps brachii — extends forearm

C. Muscles of the trunk (see **Figure 8-12**)
   1. Abdominal muscles
      a. Rectus abdominis
      b. External oblique
      c. Internal oblique
      d. Transversus abdominis
   2. Respiratory muscles
      a. Intercostal muscles
      b. Diaphragm

D. Muscles that move the lower extremities (see **Figure 8-10**)
   1. Iliopsoas — flexes thigh
   2. Gluteus maximus — extends thigh
   3. Adductor muscles — adduct thighs
   4. Hamstring muscles — flex leg
      a. Semimembranosus
      b. Semitendinosus
      c. Biceps femoris

5. Quadriceps femoris group — extends leg
   a. Rectus femoris
   b. Vastus muscles
6. Tibialis anterior — dorsiflexes foot
7. Gastrocnemius — plantar flexes foot
8. Peroneus group — flexes foot

❑ ACTIVE LEARNING

STUDY TIPS

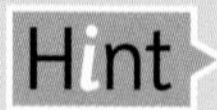

Use these tips to achieve success in meeting your learning goals.

To make the study of the muscular system more efficient, we suggest these tips:

1. Before studying Chapter 8, go back to Chapter 5 and review the synopsis of the muscular system. Also review the three types of muscle tissue covered in Chapter 4.
2. There are two prefixes that refer to muscle: *myo-* and *sarco-*. Several terms in the chapter have these prefixes.
3. It is important that you understand the terms *origin* and *insertion* when they are first presented. They will be used repeatedly in this chapter.
4. Movement is one of the functions of the muscle system. To create movement, muscle cells (muscle fibers) must get shorter. It is important to understand the mechanisms that make muscle fibers shorter and supply the energy to do so.
5. To create movement, muscle fibers usually get shorter. The sarcomere is the structure in the muscle that actually shortens or pulls. The sliding filament model explains how this shortening occurs. The shortening of the sarcomere requires energy. ATP supplies this energy and is most efficiently formed when oxygen is supplied to the muscle. When you can't supply the muscle with enough oxygen, your muscle "borrows" energy, using a process that creates lactic acid and develops an "oxygen debt."
6. The names of the muscles are probably less familiar to you than the names of the bones. But muscle names can give you information about the muscle. Muscles are named for their shape: *deltoid, trapezius.* They are named for the number of origins they have: *triceps* brachii, their points of attachment: *sternocleidomastoid,* their size: gluteus *maximus,* and the direction of the muscle fibers: *rectus* abdominis (*rectus* means the muscle has fibers running parallel to the midline of the body). When you are learning the muscles, try to look for meaning in the muscle names. Review the Language of Science and Medicine terms and their word origins to help you better understand the meaning of the muscle names. Check out tips online at *my-ap.us/LnDZ2U.*
7. Most of the terms for muscle movement are fairly straightforward. One way to remember the difference between supination and pronation is that when your hand is supinated, you can hold a bowl of soup. And in *add*uction, you *add* to your body; you pull the appendage into the trunk (silly, but effective).
8. Prepare flash cards and refer to online resources to help you learn the terms in this chapter. Review them in your study group. Also discuss the process of contraction and fatigue, and be sure you understand the movement terms. If you are asked to learn the names and locations of the muscles, a photocopy of the muscle figures with the labels blackened out can be used to quiz each other. There are many online labeling exercises *(getbodysmart.com)* that you can use as tutorials. If you are asked to learn the function, origin, and insertion of the muscles, prepare and use flash cards along with the figures.
9. Answer the questions at the end of the chapter and discuss possible test questions in your study group. Review the outline at the end of this chapter. This outline provides an overview of the material and will help you understand the general concepts of the chapter.

Review Questions

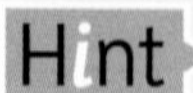

Write out the answers to these questions after reading the chapter and reviewing the Chapter Summary. If you simply think through the answer without writing it down, you won't retain much of your new learning.

1. Briefly describe the structure of skeletal muscle.
2. Describe the microscopic structure of a skeletal muscle sarcomere and motor unit
3. Briefly describe the structure of cardiac muscle.
4. Briefly describe the structure of smooth muscle.
5. Briefly describe the structure and give the functions of tendons, bursae, and synovial membranes.
6. Explain how tonic contractions help maintain posture.
7. Give an example of how two body systems other than the muscular system contribute to the movement of the body.
8. Describe how a muscle is stimulated.
9. Explain twitch and tetanic contractions.
10. Explain isotonic contractions.
11. Explain isometric contractions.
12. Describe "strength training" and explain the expected results.
13. Describe "endurance training" and explain the expected results.
14. Describe the following movements: flexion, extension, abduction, adduction, and rotation.

15. Name two muscles of the trunk and give their origin, insertion, and function.
16. Name two muscles of the head or neck and give their origin, insertion, and function.
17. Name two muscles that move the upper extremity and give their origin, insertion, and function.
18. Name three muscles that move the lower extremity and give their origin, insertion, and function.

Critical Thinking

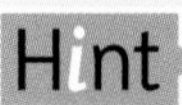

After finishing the Review Questions, write out the answers to these more in-depth questions to help you apply your new knowledge. Go back to sections of the chapter that relate to concepts that you find difficult.

19. Draw and label a relaxed sarcomere, and include actin, myosin, and Z lines. Explain the process that causes the sarcomere to contract.
20. Explain the interaction of the prime mover, the synergist, and the antagonist in efficient movement.
21. Describe the conditions that cause a muscle to develop an "oxygen debt." How is the oxygen debt "paid off"?
22. How does cardiac muscle tissue demonstrate the principle "structure fits function"?

Chapter Test

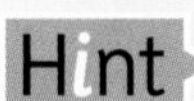

After studying the chapter, test your mastery by responding to these items. Try to answer them without looking up the answers. Then, verify the answers using the key in Appendix C at the back of this book.

1. __muscle fiber__ is another name for muscle cell.
2. Cardiac muscle makes up the bulk of the tissue of the __Heart__.
3. The muscle attachment to the more movable bone is called the __insertiom__
4. The muscle attachment to the more stationary bone is called the __origin__.
5. __Actin__ is the protein that makes up the thin myofilaments.
6. __Myosin__ is the protein that makes up the thick myofilaments.
7. The __sarcomere__ is the basic functional unit of contraction in a skeletal muscle.
8. The three functions of the muscular system are __posture__, __movement__ and __Heat__.
9. The molecule __ATP__ supplies energy for muscle contraction.
10. __lactic Acid__ is the waste product produced when the muscle must switch to an energy supplying process that does not require oxygen.
11. A single motor neuron with all the muscle fibers it innervates is called a __motor__. unit
12. ________ is the minimal level of stimulation required to cause a muscle fiber to contract. threshold stimulus
13. __isotonic__ is a type of muscle contraction that produces movement in a joint and allows the muscle to shorten.
14. __isometric__ is a type of muscle contraction that does not produce movement and does not allow the muscle to shorten but does increase muscle tension.
15. __abduction__ is a term describing movement of a body part away from the midline of the body.
16. __extension__ is a term used to describe the movement that is the opposite of flexion
17. __Supination__ describes the hand position when the body is in anatomical position.
18. Skeletal muscles can also be called:
    a. visceral muscles
    b. voluntary muscles
    c. cardiac muscles
    d. all of the above
19. Smooth muscles can also be called:
    a. visceral muscles
    b. involuntary muscles
    c. nonstriated muscles
    d. all of the above

Match the muscles in Column A with the locations in Column B.

Column A		Column B
20. __A__	temporal muscle	a. muscles of the head or neck
21. __B__	biceps brachii	b. muscles that move the upper extremity
22. __D__	sartorius	c. muscles of the trunk
23. __D__	gastrocnemius	d. muscles that move the lower extremity
24. __a__	masseter	
25. __C__	pectoralis major	
26. __C__	external oblique	
27. __d__	gluteus maximus	
28. __A__	sternocleidomastoid	
29. __C__	rectus abdominis	
30. __D__	rectus femoris	
31. __B__	triceps brachii	

Nervous System

OUTLINE

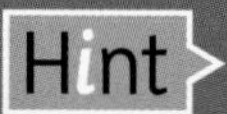

Scan this outline before you begin to read the chapter, as a preview of how the concepts are organized.

OBJECTIVES

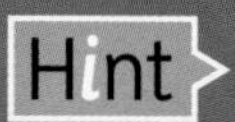

Before reading the chapter, review these goals for your learning.

After you have completed this chapter, you should be able to:

1. List the organs and divisions of the nervous system and describe the generalized functions of the system as a whole.
2. Identify the major types of cells in the nervous system and discuss the functions of each.
3. Identify the anatomical components of a reflex arc and explain its function.
4. Explain the mechanisms of transmission of a nerve impulse along a nerve fiber and across a synapse.
5. Identify the major anatomical components of the brain and spinal cord and briefly comment on the functions of each.
6. Compare and contrast cranial and spinal nerves.
7. Discuss the anatomical and functional characteristics of the two divisions of the autonomic nervous system.

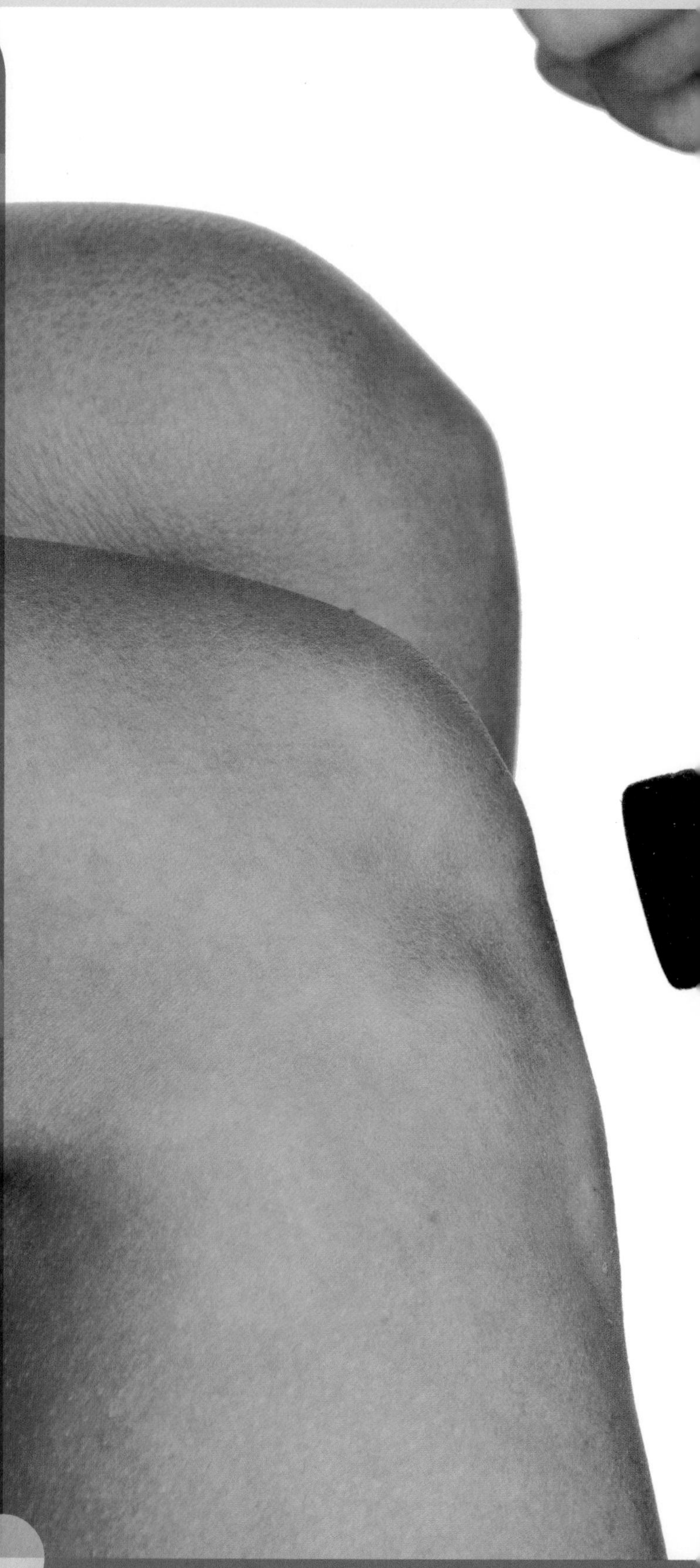

CHAPTER 9

The human body must accomplish a gigantic and enormously complex job—keeping itself alive and healthy. Each one of its billions of cells performs some activity that is a part of this function. Control of the body's billions of cells is accomplished in part by two body-wide communication systems: the nervous system and the endocrine system. Both systems transmit information from one part of the body to another, but they do it in different ways. The nervous system transmits information very rapidly by nerve impulses conducted from one body area to another. The endocrine system transmits information more slowly by chemicals secreted by ductless glands into the bloodstream and then circulated to other parts of the body.

Nerve impulses and hormones send signals to body structures, increasing or decreasing their activities as needed for healthy survival. In other words, the communication systems of the body are also its control and integrating systems. They combine the body's hundreds of functions into its one overall function of keeping itself alive and healthy.

Recall that homeostasis is the balanced and controlled internal environment of the body that is basic to life itself. Homeostasis is possible only if our physiological control and integration systems function properly. Our plan for this chapter is to name the cells, organs, and divisions of the nervous system and then explain how nerve impulses move between one area of the body and another.

We not only discuss the major structures of the nervous system, such as the brain, spinal cord, and nerves, but also learn how they function to maintain and regulate homeostasis. In Chapter 10, we consider the senses.

Organization of the Nervous System

The organs of the nervous system as a whole include the brain and spinal cord, the numerous nerves of the body, the special sense organs such as the eyes and ears, and the microscopic sense organs such as those found in the skin. The system as a whole consists of two principal divisions called the *central nervous system* and the *peripheral nervous system* (**Figure 9-1**).

Because the brain and spinal cord occupy a midline or central location in the body, together they are called the **central nervous system,** or **CNS.** Similarly, the usual designation for the nerves of the body is the **peripheral nervous system,** or **PNS.** The term *peripheral* is appropriate because nerves extend to outlying or peripheral parts of the body.

A subdivision of the peripheral nervous system, called the **autonomic nervous system,** or **ANS,** consists of structures that regulate the body's automatic or involuntary functions (for example, heart rate, contractions of the stomach and intestines, and secretion of chemical compounds by glands).

To learn more about the divisions of the nervous system, go to AnimationDirect at *evolve.elsevier.com*.

LANGUAGE OF **SCIENCE** AND **MEDICINE**

Hint Before reading the chapter, say each of these terms out loud. This will help you to avoid stumbling over them as you read.

acetylcholine (ACh)
(as-ee-til-KOH-leen)
[*acetyl-* **vinegar,** *-chole-* **bile,** *-ine* **made of**]

action potential
(AK-shun poh-TEN-shal)
[*act-* **moving,** *-ion* **condition,** *poten-* **power,** *-ial* **relating to**]

adrenergic fiber
(ad-ren-ER-jik FYE-ber)
[*ad-* **toward,** *-ren-* **kidney,** *-erg-* **work,** *-ic* **relating to,** *fibr-* **thread**]

afferent neuron
(AF-fer-ent NOO-ron)
[*a[d]-* **toward,** *-fer-* **carry,** *-ent* **relating to,** *neuron* **string or nerve**]

anesthesia
(an-es-THEE-zhah)
[*an-* **absence,** *-esthesia* **feeling**]

antidiuretic hormone (ADH)
(an-tee-dye-yoo-RET-ik HOR-mohn)
[*anti-* **against,** *-dia-* **through,** *-uret-* **urination,** *-ic* **relating to,** *hormon-* **excite**]

arachnoid mater
(ah-RAK-noyd MAH-ter)
[*arachn-* **spider(web),** *-oid* **like,** *mater* **mother**]

astrocyte
(ASS-troh-syte)
[*astro-* **star shaped,** *-cyte* **cell**]

autonomic effector
(aw-toh-NOM-ik ef-FEK-tor)
[*auto-* **self,** *-nom-* **rule,** *-ic* **relating to,** *effect-* **accomplish,** *-or* **agent**]

autonomic nervous system (ANS)
(aw-toh-NAHM-ik NER-vus SIS-tem)
[*auto-* **self,** *-nom-* **rule,** *-ic* **relating to,** *nerv-* **nerve,** *-ous,* **relating to**]

Continued on p. 204

Cells of the Nervous System

In Chapter 4, we learned that nervous tissue is the major component of the nervous system. And we learned two major types of cells are found in nervous tissue: **neurons** or nerve cells and **glia,** which are support cells (see **Figure 4-19** on p. 79). Neurons conduct impulses, whereas glia support neurons.

Neurons

Neuron Structure

Each neuron consists of three parts: a main part called the neuron **cell body,** one or more branching projections called **dendrites,** and one elongated projection known as an **axon.**

The axon shown in **Figure 9-2**, *B,* is surrounded by a segmented wrapping of a material called **myelin.** Myelin is a white, fatty substance formed by *Schwann cells* that wrap around some axons outside the central nervous system. Such fibers are called **myelinated fibers.** In **Figure 9-2**, *B,* one such axon has been enlarged to show additional detail. **Nodes of Ranvier** are gaps between adjacent Schwann cells.

The outer wrapped layer of a Schwann cell is called the **neurilemma.** It is clinically significant that axons in the brain and spinal cord have no neurilemma, because neurilemma plays an essential part in the regeneration of cut and injured axons. Therefore the potential for regeneration in the brain

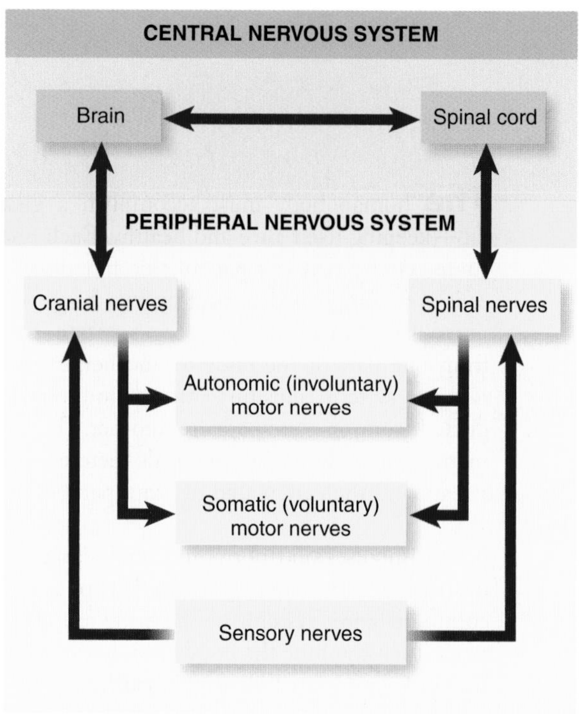

FIGURE 9-1 Divisions of the nervous system.

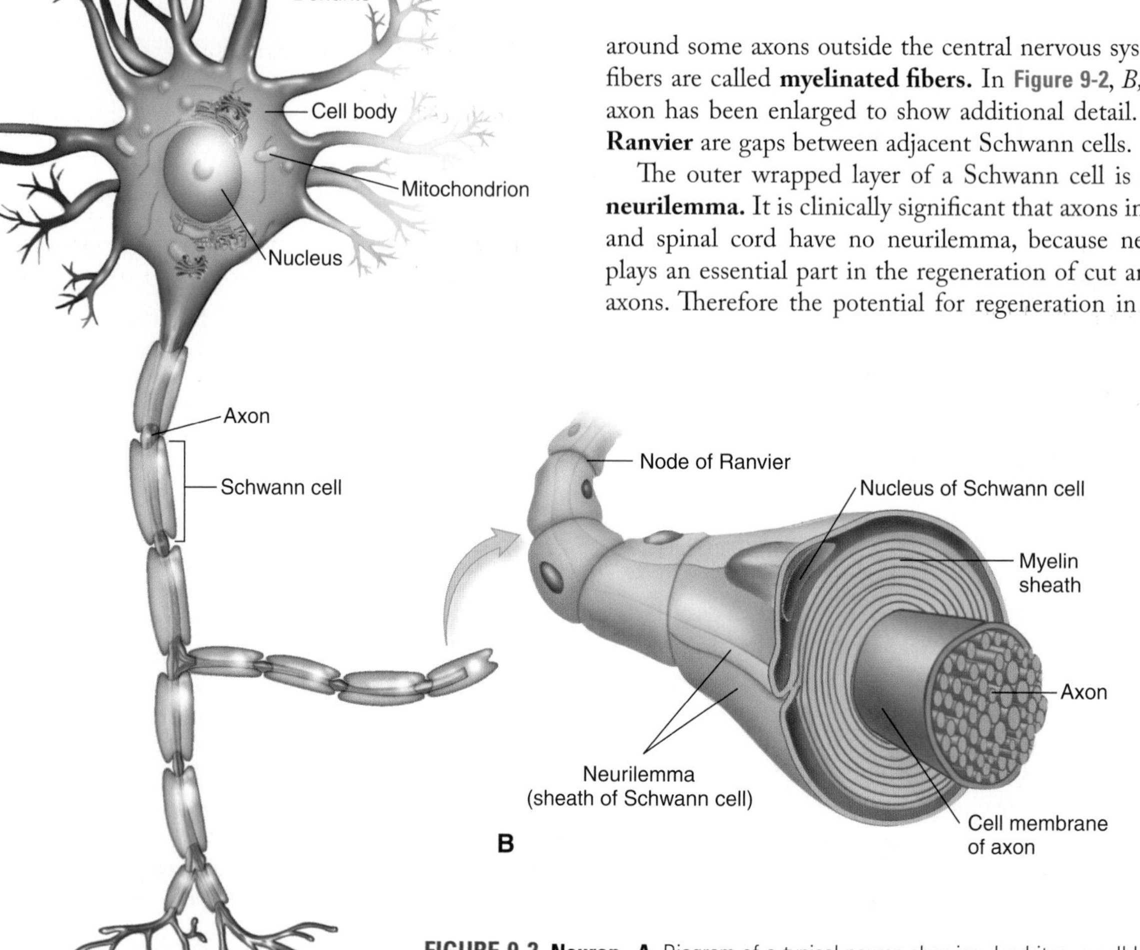

FIGURE 9-2 Neuron. A, Diagram of a typical neuron showing dendrites, a cell body, and an axon. **B,** Segment of a myelinated axon cut to show detail of the concentric layers of the Schwann cell filled with myelin.

and spinal cord is far less than it is in the peripheral nervous system.

Identify each part on the neuron shown in Figure 9-2. Dendrites are the processes or projections that carry impulses to the neuron cell bodies, and axons are the processes that carry impulses away from the neuron cell bodies.

Types of Neurons

There are three major types of neurons classified according to the direction in which they carry impulses.

Sensory Neurons

Sensory neurons carry impulses to the spinal cord and brain from all parts of the body. Sensory neurons are also called **afferent neurons.**

Motor Neurons

Motor neurons carry impulses in the opposite direction—away from the brain and spinal cord. They do not conduct impulses to all parts of the body—only to two kinds of tissue—muscle and glandular epithelial tissue. Motor neurons are also called **efferent neurons.**

Interneurons

Interneurons conduct impulses from sensory neurons to motor neurons. They also often connect with each other to form complex, central networks of nerve fibers. Interneurons are sometimes called *central* or *connecting* neurons.

Glia

Function of Glia

Glia—or **neuroglia**—do not specialize in transmitting impulses. Instead, they are special types of supporting cells. Their name is appropriate because it is derived from the Greek word *glia* meaning "glue." One function of glial cells is to hold the functioning neurons together and protect them.

We now know that glia perform many different functions, including the regulation of neuron function. Therefore, they not only act as "glue" in the physical sense but also help bring the various functions of nervous tissue together into a coordinated whole.

An important reason for discussing glia is that one of the most common types of brain tumor—called **glioma**—develops from them.

Central Glia

Glia vary in size and shape (Figure 9-3). Some are relatively large cells that look somewhat like stars because of the threadlike extensions that jut out from their surfaces. These glial cells are called **astrocytes,** a word that means "star cells" (see Figure 9-3, *A*). Their threadlike branches attach to neurons and to small blood vessels, holding these structures close to each other.

Along with the walls of the blood vessels, astrocyte branches form a two-layer structure called the **blood-brain barrier (BBB)**. As its name implies, the BBB separates the blood tissue and nervous tissue to protect vital brain tissue from harmful chemicals that might be in the blood.

Microglia are smaller than astrocytes (see Figure 9-3, *B*). They usually remain stationary, but in inflamed or degenerating brain tissue, they enlarge, move about, and act as microbe-eating scavengers. They surround the microbes, draw them into their cytoplasm, and digest them. They likewise help clean up cell damage resulting from injury or disease. Recall from Chapter 3 that phagocytosis is the scientific name for this important cellular process.

The **oligodendrocytes** help hold nerve fibers together and also serve another and probably more important function: they produce the fatty myelin sheath that envelops nerve fibers located in the brain and spinal cord.

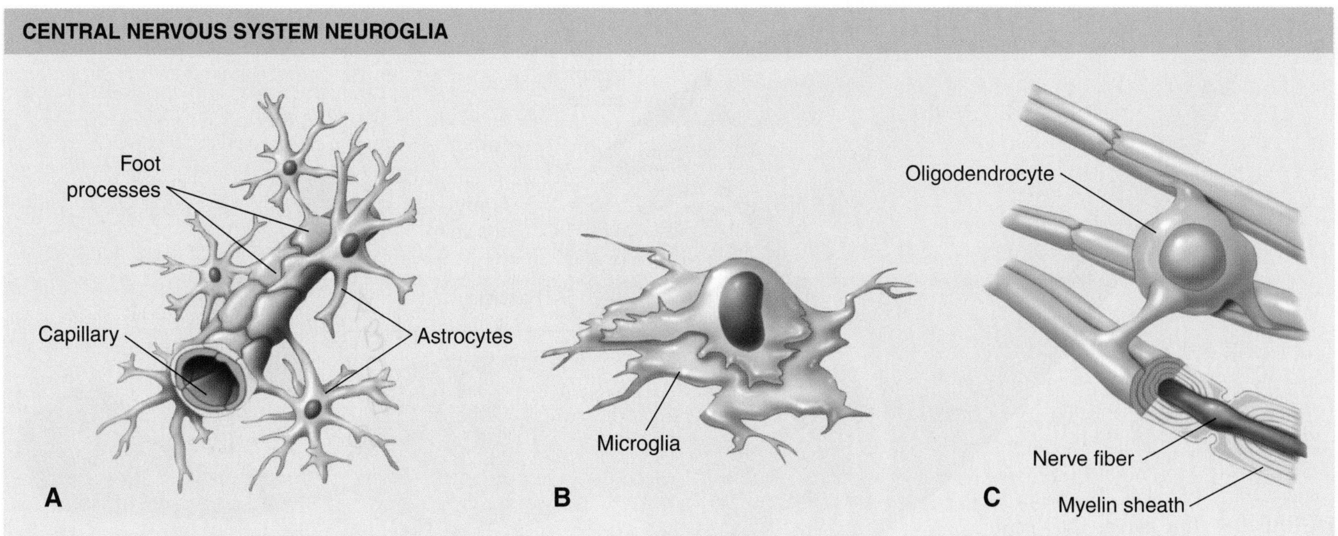

FIGURE 9-3 Central glia. A, Astrocytes have extensions attached to blood vessels in the brain. **B,** Microglia within the central nervous system can enlarge and consume microbes by phagocytosis. **C,** Oligodendrocytes have extensions that form myelin sheaths around axons in the central nervous system.

Peripheral Glia

Schwann cells are glial cells that also form myelin sheaths but do so only in the peripheral nervous system. Notice in Figure 9-3, *C*, that each oligodendrocyte can form part of the myelin sheath around several axons but Schwann cells wrap entirely around only one axon.

QUICK CHECK

1. What is the difference between the central nervous system and the peripheral nervous system?
2. What are the major features of a neuron?
3. How are glia different from neurons?
4. What are three types of central glia cells? Give an example of a peripheral glia cell.
5. What are the three major types of neurons? Classify them according to the direction in which they transmit impulses.

Nerves and Tracts

A **nerve** is a group of peripheral nerve fibers (axons) bundled together like the strands of a cable. Peripheral nerve fibers usually have a myelin sheath. Because myelin is white, peripheral nerves often look white.

Figure 9-4 shows that each axon in a nerve is surrounded by a thin wrapping of fibrous connective tissue called the **endoneurium.** Groups of these wrapped axons are called **fascicles.** Each fascicle is surrounded by a thin, fibrous **perineurium.** A tough, fibrous sheath called the **epineurium** covers the whole nerve.

Bundles of axons in the CNS, called **tracts,** also are myelinated and thus form the **white matter** of the brain and spinal cord. Brain and spinal cord tissue composed of cell bodies and unmyelinated axons and dendrites is called **gray matter** because of its characteristic gray appearance.

Nerve Signals

Reflex Arcs

Neuron Pathways

During every moment of our lives, nerve impulses speed over neurons to and from our spinal cords and brains. If all impulse conduction ceases, life itself ceases. Only neurons can provide the rapid communication between cells that is necessary for maintaining life. Hormones are the only other kind of signal the body can send, and they travel much more slowly than nerve signals. Hormones can move from one part of the body to another only via circulating blood. Compared with nerve impulse conduction, circulation is a very slow process.

Nerve impulses, also called **action potentials,** can travel over trillions of routes—routes made up of neurons because they are the cells that conduct impulses. Hence the routes traveled by nerve impulses are sometimes spoken of as *neuron pathways.*

A basic type of neuron pathway, called a **reflex arc,** is important to nervous system functioning. The simplest kind of reflex arc is a two-neuron arc, so-called because it consists of only two types of neurons: sensory neurons and motor neurons. Three-neuron arcs are the next simplest kind. They, of course, consist of all three kinds of neurons: sensory neurons, interneurons, and motor neurons.

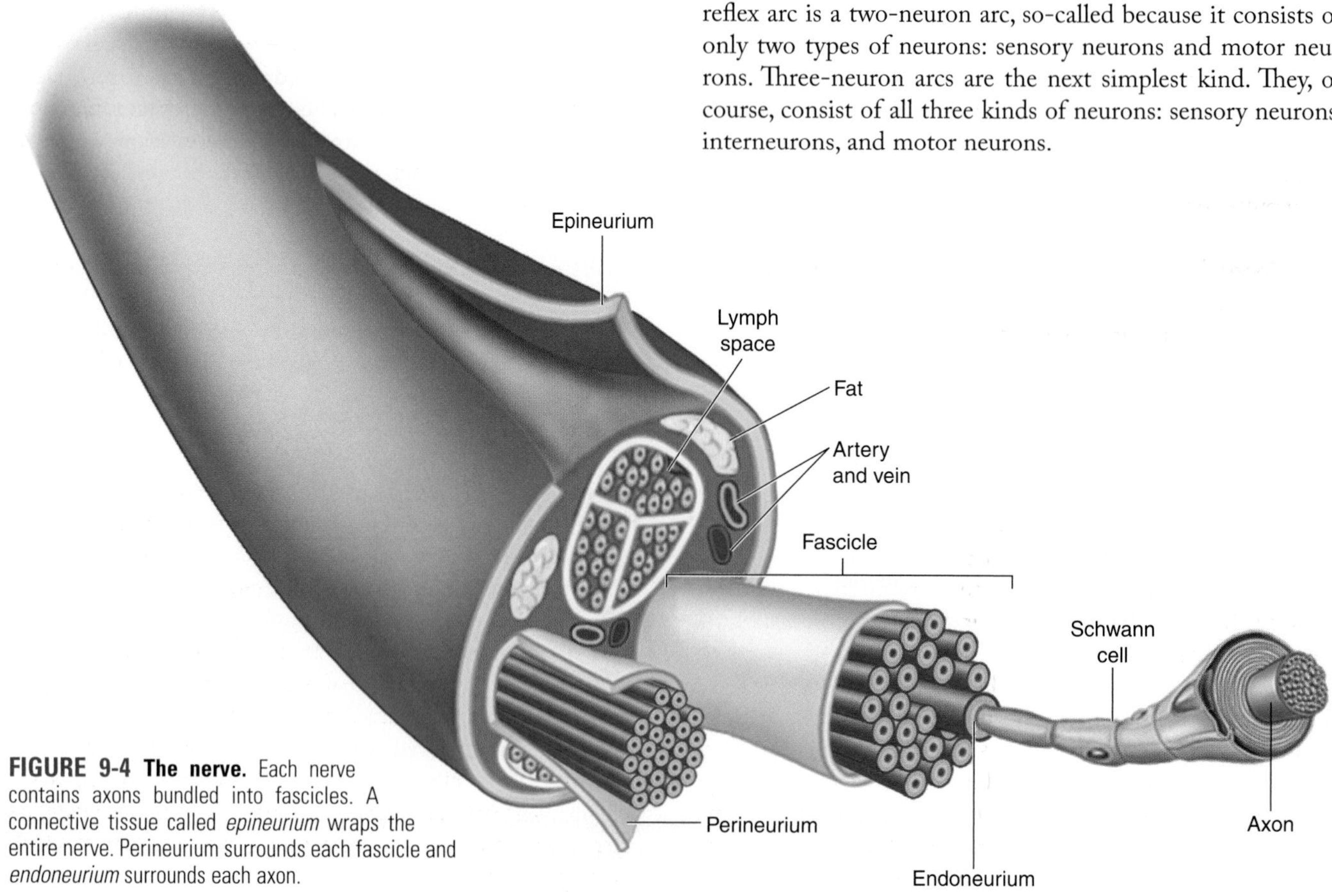

FIGURE 9-4 The nerve. Each nerve contains axons bundled into fascicles. A connective tissue called *epineurium* wraps the entire nerve. Perineurium surrounds each fascicle and *endoneurium* surrounds each axon.

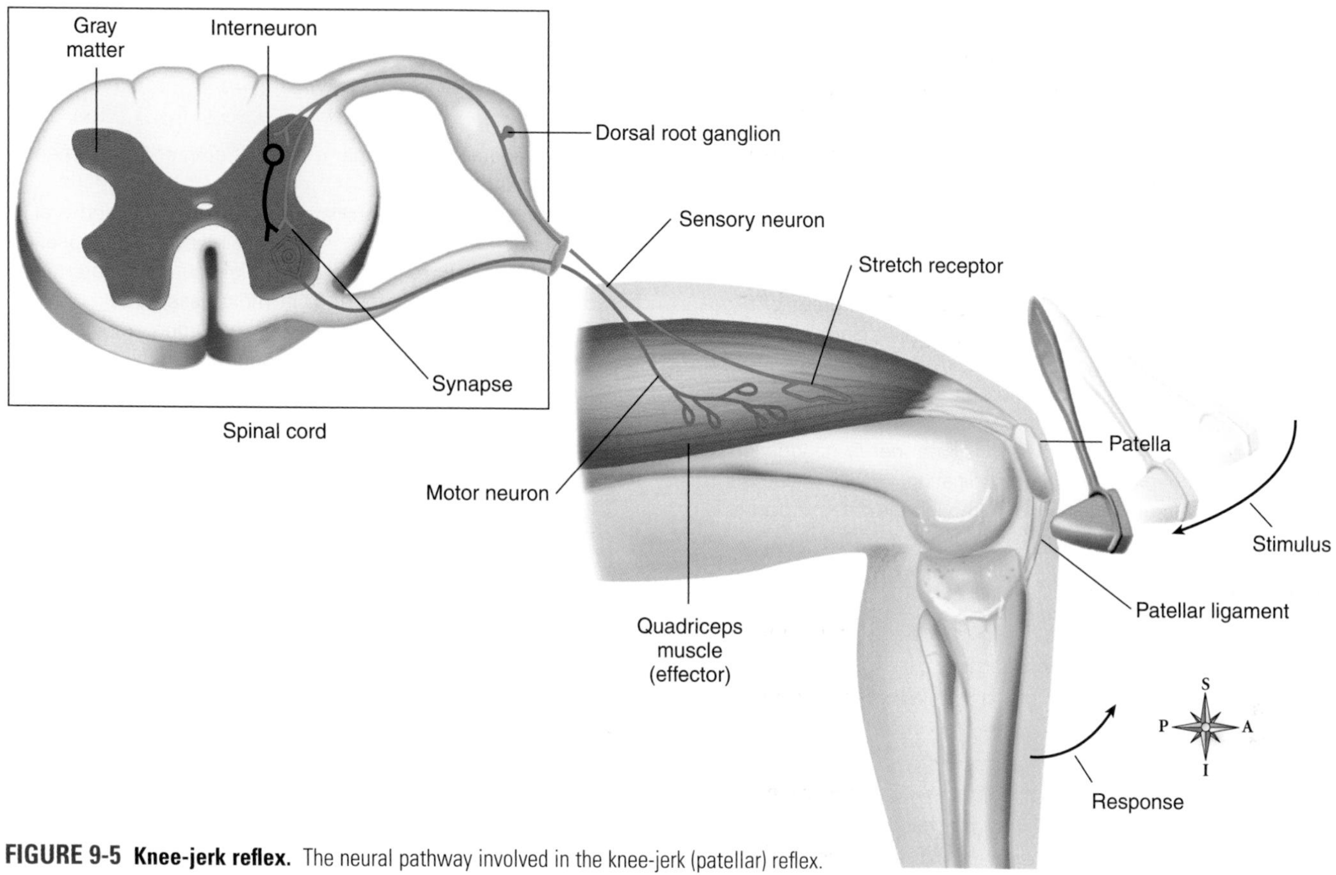

FIGURE 9-5 Knee-jerk reflex. The neural pathway involved in the knee-jerk (patellar) reflex.

Structure of Reflex Arcs

Reflex arcs are like one-way streets: they allow impulse conduction in only one direction. The next paragraph describes this direction in detail. Look frequently at Figure 9-5 as you read it.

Impulse conduction normally starts in receptors. **Receptors** are the beginnings of dendrites of sensory neurons. They are often located far from the spinal cord (in tendons, skin, or mucous membranes, for example).

In Figure 9-5 the sensory receptors are located in the quadriceps muscle group. In the reflex that is illustrated there, stretch receptors are stimulated when muscles are stretched as a result of a tap on the patellar ligament from a rubber hammer used by a physician to elicit a reflex during a physical examination. The nerve impulse that is generated, its neurological pathway, and its ultimate "knee-jerk" effect are an example of the simplest form of a two-neuron reflex arc.

In the knee-jerk reflex, only sensory and motor neurons are involved. The nerve impulse that is generated by stimulation of the stretch receptors travels along the length of the sensory neuron's dendrite to its cell body located in the *dorsal root ganglion (posterior root ganglion).* A **ganglion** is a group of nerve-cell bodies located in the PNS. This ganglion is located near the spinal cord. Each dorsal root ganglion contains not one sensory neuron cell body, as shown in Figure 9-5, but hundreds of them.

The axon of the sensory neuron travels from the cell body in the dorsal root ganglion and ends near the dendrites of another neuron located in the gray matter of the spinal cord. A microscopic space separates the axon ending of one neuron from the dendrites of another neuron. This gap serves as a junction between nerve cells called a **synapse.** The nerve impulse stops at the synapse, chemical signals are sent across the gap, and then a new impulse continues along the dendrites, cell body, and axon of the motor neuron.

The motor neuron axon forms a synapse with a structure called an **effector,** an organ that puts nerve signals "into effect." Effectors are usually muscles or glands, and muscle contractions and gland secretion are the kinds of reflexes operated by these effectors.

Reflex Responses

The response to impulse conduction over a reflex arc is called a **reflex.** In short, impulse conduction by a reflex arc causes a reflex to occur. In our example reflex, the nerve impulses that reach the quadriceps muscle (the effector) result in the "knee-jerk" response.

Now turn your attention to the *interneuron* shown in Figure 9-5. Some reflexes involve three rather than two neurons. In these more complex types of responses, an interneuron, in addition to a sensory and a motor neuron, is involved. In three-neuron reflexes, the end of the sensory neuron's axon synapses first with an interneuron before chemical signals are sent across a second synapse, resulting in conduction through the motor neuron.

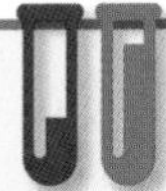

CLINICAL APPLICATION

MULTIPLE SCLEROSIS (MS)

Many diseases are associated with disorders of the oligodendrocytes. Because these glial cells are involved in myelin formation, these diseases are called **myelin disorders.** The most common primary disease of the CNS is a myelin disorder called **multiple sclerosis,** or **MS.** It is characterized by myelin loss and destruction accompanied by varying degrees of oligodendrocyte cell injury and death. The result is demyelination of the white matter of the CNS. Hard, plaquelike lesions replace the destroyed myelin, and affected areas are invaded by inflammatory cells.

As the myelin around axons is lost, nerve conduction is impaired, and weakness, incoordination, visual impairment, and speech disturbances occur. Although the disease occurs in both sexes and all age groups, it is most common in women between 20 and 40 years.

The cause of MS may be related to autoimmunity and viral infections in some individuals. MS typically involves relapses and is chronic in nature, but some cases of acute and unremitting disease have been reported. In most cases, MS is prolonged, with remissions and relapses occurring over many years. Television personality and author Montel Williams reports that he lived with recurring episodes of MS for 20 years before he realized that he has the condition.

Although there is not yet a cure for MS, early diagnosis and treatment can slow or stop its progression.

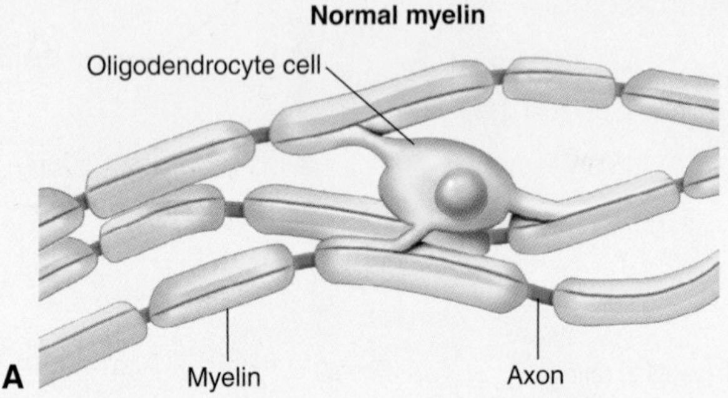

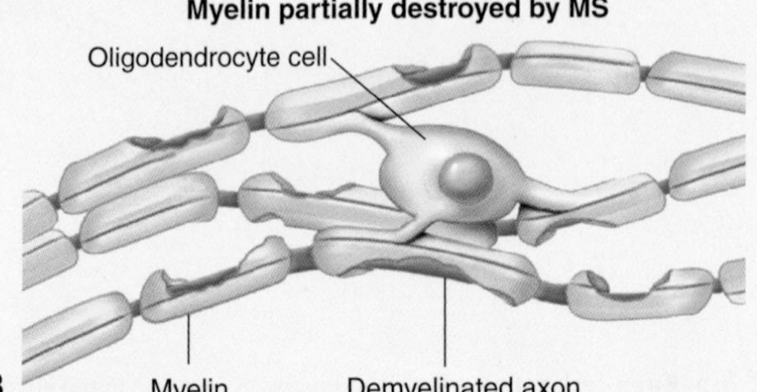

Effects of multiple sclerosis (MS). A, A normal myelin sheath allows rapid conduction. **B,** In MS, the myelin sheath is damaged, disrupting nerve conduction.

For example, application of an irritating stimulus to the skin of the thigh initiates a three-neuron reflex response that causes contraction of muscles to pull the leg away from the irritant—a three-neuron arc reaction called the **withdrawal reflex.**

All interneurons lie entirely within the gray matter of the brain or spinal cord. Gray matter forms the H-shaped inner core of the spinal cord. Because of the presence of an interneuron, three-neuron reflex arcs have two synapses. A two-neuron reflex arc, however, has only a sensory neuron and a motor neuron with one synapse between them.

Identify the motor neuron in **Figure 9-5**. Observe that its dendrites and cell body, like those of an interneuron, are located in the spinal cord's gray matter. The axon of this motor neuron, however, runs through the ventral root (anterior root) of the spinal nerve and terminates in a muscle.

QUICK CHECK

1. How is white matter different from gray matter?
2. What is the function of a reflex arc?
3. What is a sensory receptor? How does it relate to the reflex arc?
4. What is an effector? How does it relate to the reflex arc?

Nerve Impulses

Definition of a Nerve Impulse

What are nerve impulses? Here is one widely accepted definition: a nerve impulse is a self-propagating wave of electrical disturbance that travels along the surface of a neuron's plasma membrane. You might visualize this as a tiny spark sizzling its way along a fuse.

Nerve impulses do not continually race along every nerve cell's surface. First they have to be initiated by a stimulus, a change in the neuron's environment. Pressure, temperature, and chemical changes are the usual stimuli.

Mechanism of a Nerve Impulse

Figure 9-6 depicts a simplified summary of the mechanism of a nerve impulse.

The membrane of each resting neuron has a slight positive charge on the outside and a negative charge on the inside, a state called *polarization.* This occurs because there is normally an excess of sodium ions (Na^+) on the outside of the membrane.

When a section of the membrane is stimulated, its Na^+ channels suddenly open, and Na^+ ions rush inward. The inside

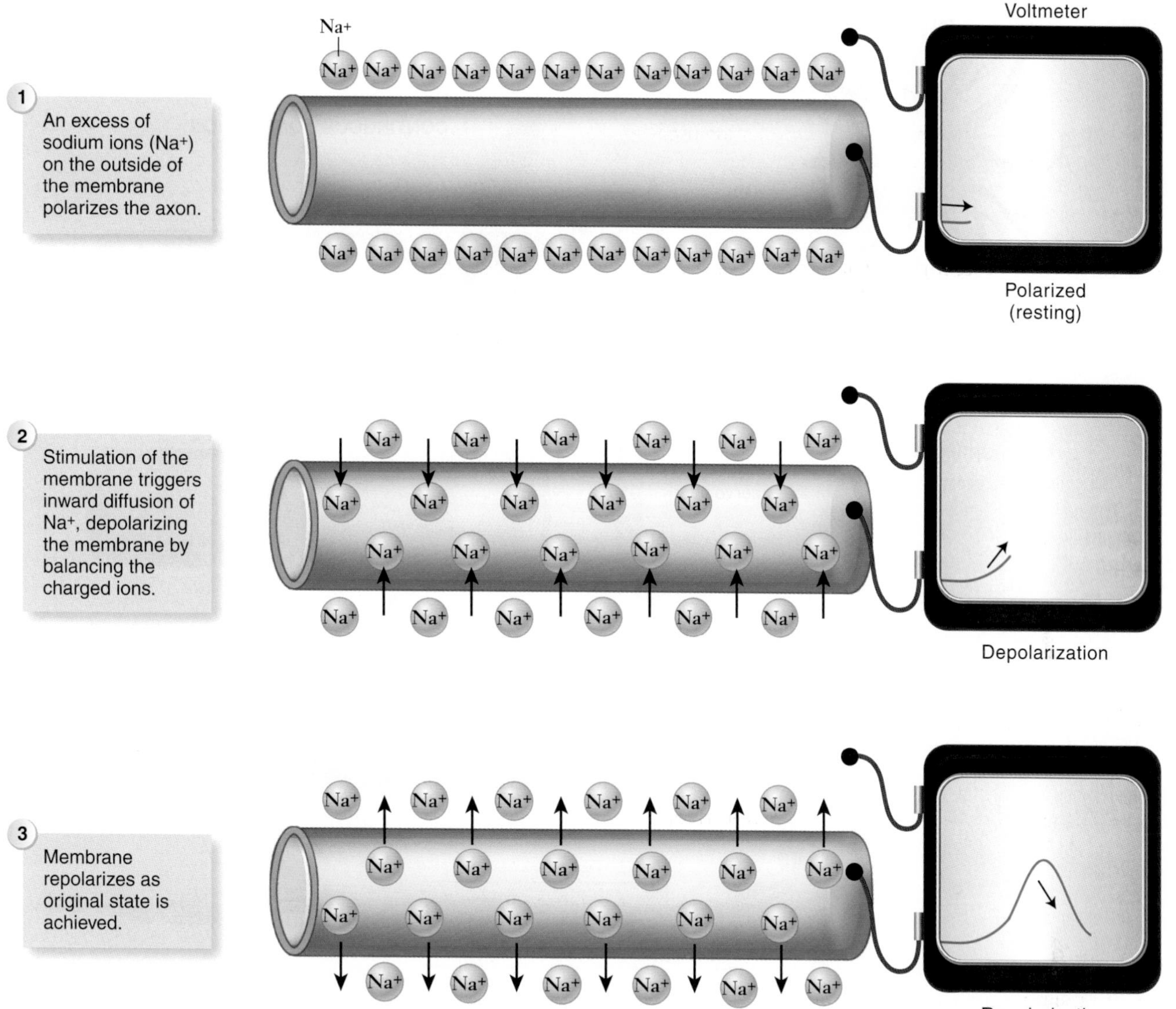
Voltmeter
Na+
1
An excess of sodium ions (Na+) on the outside of the membrane polarizes the axon.
Polarized (resting)
2
Stimulation of the membrane triggers inward diffusion of Na+, depolarizing the membrane by balancing the charged ions.
Depolarization
3
Membrane repolarizes as original state is achieved.
Repolarization

FIGURE 9-6 Mechanism of the nerve impulse. A voltmeter *(right)* shows how the charge difference across the membrane fluctuates as the balance of positive ions (Na^+) changes.

of the membrane temporarily becomes positive, and the outside becomes negative—a process called *depolarization.*

The depolarized section of the membrane then immediately recovers—a process called *repolarization.* However, the depolarization has already stimulated Na^+ channels in the next section of the membrane to open.

Conduction of Nerve Impulses

The impulse—or *action potential*—cannot go backwards during the brief moment of repolarization and recovery of the previous section of membrane. Thus a self-propagating wave of electrical disturbance—a nerve impulse—travels continuously in one direction across the neuron's surface (**Figure 9-7**, *A*).

Nerve impulses are also called *action potentials* because each one is a difference in charge (called "electrical potential") that usually triggers an action by the cell—in this case, transmission of the impulse itself.

If the traveling impulse encounters a section of membrane covered with insulating myelin, it simply "jumps" around the myelin to the next gap in the myelin sheath. Called **saltatory conduction,** this type of impulse travel is much faster than is possible in nonmyelinated sections. Saltatory conduction is illustrated in **Figure 9-7**, *B*.

To learn more about nerve impulses, go to AnimationDirect at *evolve.elsevier.com.*

The Synapse

Structure and Function of a Synapse

Transmission of signals from one neuron to the next—across the synapse—is an important part of the nerve conduction process. By definition, a synapse is the place where impulses

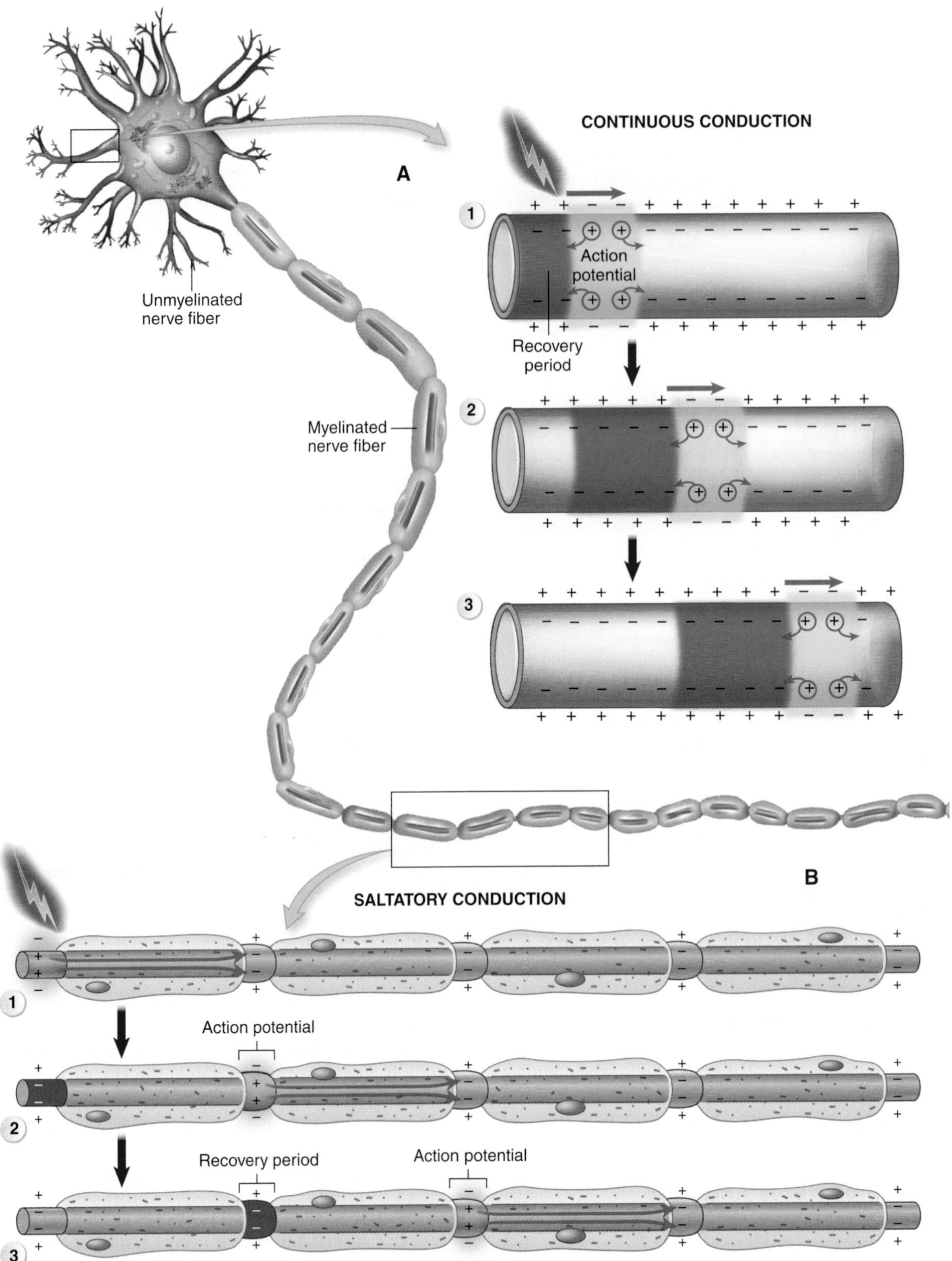

FIGURE 9-7 Conduction of nerve impulses. A, In an unmyelinated fiber, a nerve impulse (action potential, shown with yellow glow) is a *continuous,* self-propagating wave of electrical disturbance. The dark blue area of "recovery" during repolarization cannot be restimulated, preventing backward conduction. **B,** In a myelinated fiber, the action potential "jumps" around the insulating myelin in a rapid type of conduction called *saltatory conduction.*

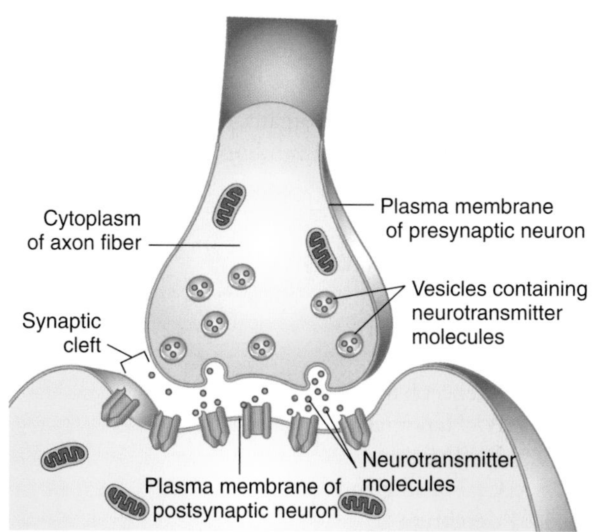

FIGURE 9-8 Components of a synapse. Diagram shows synaptic knob or axon terminal of presynaptic neuron, the plasma membrane of a postsynaptic neuron, and a synaptic cleft. On the arrival of an action potential at a synaptic knob, neurotransmitter molecules are released from vesicles in the knob into the synaptic cleft. Binding of neurotransmitter molecules to their receptor molecules in the plasma membrane of the postsynaptic neuron triggers the opening of ion channels—thereby initiating impulse conduction in the postsynaptic neuron.

are transmitted from one neuron, called the **presynaptic neuron,** to another neuron, called the **postsynaptic neuron.**

Three structures make up a typical synapse: a synaptic knob, a synaptic cleft, and the plasma membrane of a postsynaptic neuron.

A **synaptic knob** is a tiny bulge at the end of a terminal branch of a presynaptic neuron's axon (Figure 9-8). Each synaptic knob contains many small sacs or vesicles. Each vesicle contains a very small quantity of a chemical compound called a *neurotransmitter.* When a nerve impulse arrives at the synaptic knob, neurotransmitter molecules are released from the vesicles into the **synaptic cleft.**

The synaptic cleft is the space between a synaptic knob and the plasma membrane of a *postsynaptic neuron.* It is an incredibly narrow space—only about two millionths of a centimeter in width. The synaptic cleft is filled with extracellular matrix that holds the synaptic structure in place. Identify the synaptic cleft in Figure 9-8.

The plasma membrane of a postsynaptic neuron has protein molecules embedded in it opposite each synaptic knob. These serve as receptors to which neurotransmitter molecules bind. This binding can initiate an impulse in the postsynaptic neuron by opening ion channels in the postsynaptic membrane.

After impulse conduction by postsynaptic neurons is initiated, neurotransmitter activity is rapidly terminated. Either one or both of two mechanisms cause this. Some neurotransmitter molecules are transported out of the synaptic cleft back into synaptic knobs. Other neurotransmitter molecules are broken apart into inactive compounds by specific enzymes in the extracellular matrix of the synaptic cleft.

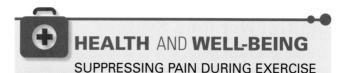

HEALTH AND WELL-BEING

SUPPRESSING PAIN DURING EXERCISE

Research shows that the release of endorphins increases during heavy exercise. Endorphins inhibit pain, so it is no wonder that pain associated with muscle fatigue decreases when endorphins are present. Normally, pain is a warning signal that calls attention to injuries or dangerous circumstances. However, it is better to inhibit severe pain if it would stop us from continuing an activity that may be necessary for survival. Athletes and others who exercise heavily have even reported a unique feeling of well-being or euphoria associated with elevated endorphin levels.

Neurotransmitters

Neurotransmitters are chemicals by which neurons communicate. As previously noted, at trillions of synapses in the CNS, presynaptic neurons release neurotransmitters that assist, stimulate, or inhibit postsynaptic neurons. At least 30 different compounds have been identified as neurotransmitters. They are not distributed randomly through the spinal cord and brain. Instead, specific neurotransmitters are localized in discrete groups of neurons and released in specific pathways.

For example, the substance named **acetylcholine** (**ACh**) is released at some of the synapses in the spinal cord and at neuromuscular (nerve-muscle) junctions. Other well-known neurotransmitters include **norepinephrine, dopamine,** and **serotonin.** They belong to a group of compounds called **catecholamines,** which may play a role in sleep, motor function, mood, and pleasure recognition.

Two morphinelike neurotransmitters called **endorphins** and **enkephalins** are released at various spinal cord and brain synapses in the pain conduction pathway. These neurotransmitters inhibit conduction of pain impulses. They are natural pain killers.

Very small molecules such as **nitric oxide** (**NO**) also have an important role as neurotransmitters. Unlike most other neurotransmitters, NO diffuses directly across the plasma membrane of neurons rather than being released from vesicles.

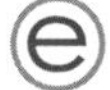
To learn more about the synapse, go to AnimationDirect at *evolve.elsevier.com.*

QUICK CHECK

1. How does myelin increase the speed of nerve impulse conduction?
2. What is the structure and function of a synapse?
3. How do neurotransmitters transmit signals across the synapse?
4. What is a postsynaptic neuron?

Central Nervous System

The central nervous system (CNS), as its name implies, is centrally located. Its two major structures, the brain and spinal cord, are found along the midline of the body (**Figure 9-9**).

The brain is protected in the cranial cavity of the skull, and the spinal cord is surrounded in the spinal cavity by the vertebral column. In addition, the brain and spinal cord are also protected by three membranes called *meninges,* which are discussed in a later section of this chapter.

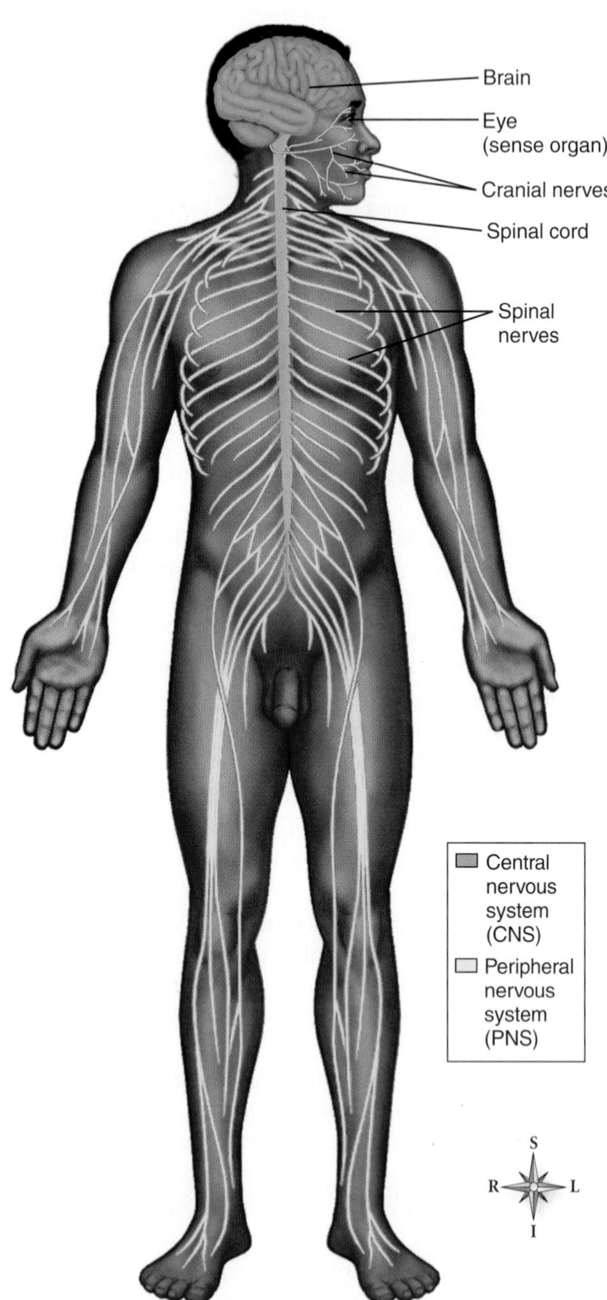

FIGURE 9-9 The nervous system. The brain and spinal cord (highlighted green) constitute the central nervous system (CNS) and the nerves make up the peripheral nervous system (PNS) shown in yellow.

Brain

Divisions of the Brain

The brain, one of our largest organs, consists of the following major divisions, named in ascending order, beginning with most inferior part:

I. Brainstem
   A. Medulla oblongata
   B. Pons
   C. Midbrain
II. Cerebellum
III. Diencephalon
   A. Hypothalamus
   B. Thalamus
   C. Pineal gland
IV. Cerebrum

Observe in **Figure 9-10** the location and relative sizes of the different divisions of the brain

Brainstem

The lowest part of the brainstem is the medulla oblongata. Immediately above the medulla lies the pons and above that the midbrain. Together these three structures are called the *brainstem* (see **Figure 9-10**).

The **medulla oblongata** is an enlarged, upward extension of the spinal cord. It lies just inside the cranial cavity above the large hole in the occipital bone called the *foramen magnum.* The **pons** bulges out a bit more than medulla, forming a bridge to the narrower **midbrain.**

In the brainstem, small bits of gray matter mix closely and intricately with white matter to form the **reticular formation** (*reticular* means "netlike"). In the spinal cord, gray and white matter do not intermingle. Gray matter forms the interior core of the spinal cord, and white matter surrounds it.

All three parts of the brainstem function as two-way conduction paths. Sensory fibers conduct impulses up from the spinal cord to other parts of the brain, and motor fibers conduct impulses down from the brain to the spinal cord.

In addition, many important reflex centers lie in the brainstem. The cardiac, respiratory, and vasomotor centers (collectively called the *vital centers*), for example, are located in the medulla. Impulses from these centers control heartbeat, respiration, and blood vessel diameter (which is important in regulating blood pressure).

Cerebellum

Structure

Look at **Figure 9-10** to find the location, appearance, and size of the cerebellum. The **cerebellum** is the second largest part of the human brain. It lies under the occipital lobe of the cerebrum. In the cerebellum, folded gray matter composes the thin outer layer and forms a large surface area of nervous connections that allow for a huge amount of information processing. White matter tracts form most of the interior. Notice that these tracts branch in a treelike pattern called the *arbor vitae* (literally, "living tree").

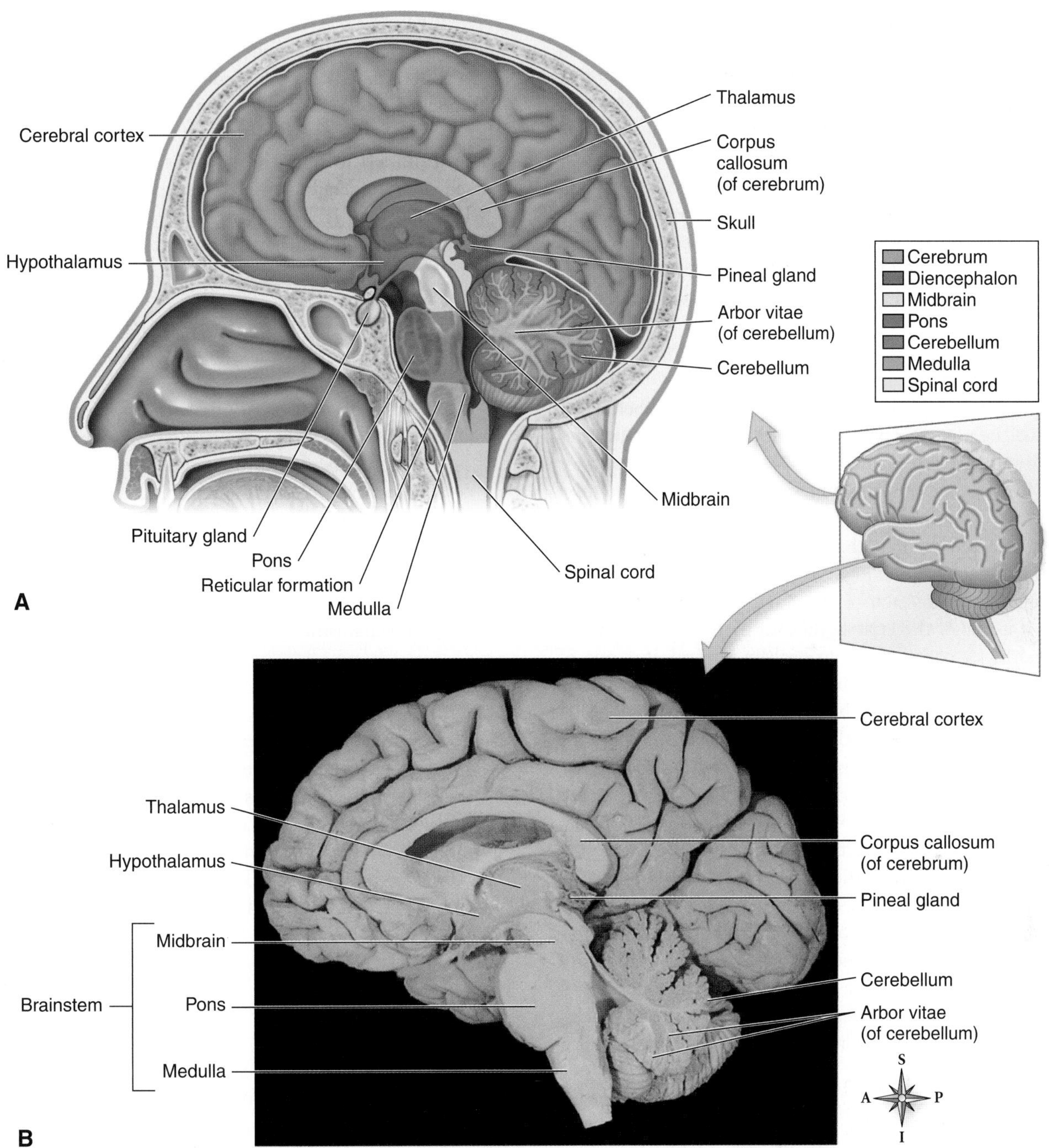

FIGURE 9-10 Major regions of the central nervous system. A, Sagittal sections of the brain and spinal cord. **B,** Section of preserved brain.

Functions

Most of our previous knowledge about cerebellar functions has come from observing patients who have some sort of disease of the cerebellum and from animals that have had the cerebellum removed. From such observations, we know that the cerebellum plays an essential part in the production of normal movements.

Perhaps a few examples will make this clear. A patient who has a tumor of the cerebellum frequently loses his balance and topples over; he may feel like a drunken man when he walks. He cannot coordinate his muscles normally. He may complain, for instance, that he is clumsy about everything he does—that he cannot even drive a nail or draw a straight line. With the loss of normal cerebellar functioning, he has lost the ability to make precise movements.

The most obvious functions of the cerebellum, then, are to produce smooth coordinated movements, maintain equilibrium, and sustain normal postures.

Recent studies using new brain imaging methods show that the cerebellum may have far more functions than earlier observed. The cerebellum may assist the cerebrum and other parts of the brain, perhaps having an overall coordinating function for the whole brain.

Diencephalon

The **diencephalon** is a small but important part of the brain located between the midbrain below and the cerebrum above. It consists of three major structures: hypothalamus, thalamus, and pineal gland. Find these structures in **Figure 9-10** before reading further.

Hypothalamus

The **hypothalamus,** as its name suggests, is located below the thalamus. The posterior pituitary gland, the stalk that attaches it to the undersurface of the brain, and areas of gray matter located in the side walls of a fluid-filled space called the *third ventricle* are extensions of the hypothalamus. Identify the pituitary gland and the hypothalamus in **Figure 9-10**.

The old adage, "Don't judge by appearances," applies well to appraising the importance of the hypothalamus. Measured by size, it is one of the least significant parts of the brain, but measured by its contribution to healthy survival, it is one of the most important brain structures.

Impulses from neurons whose dendrites and cell bodies lie in the hypothalamus are conducted by their axons to neurons located in the spinal cord, and many of these impulses are then relayed to muscles and glands all over the body. Thus the hypothalamus exerts major control over virtually all internal organs. Among the vital functions that it helps control are the heartbeat, constriction and dilation of blood vessels, and contractions of the stomach and intestines.

Some neurons in the hypothalamus function in a surprising way; they make the hormones that the posterior pituitary gland secretes into the blood. Because one of these hormones (called **antidiuretic hormone,** or **ADH**) affects the volume of urine excreted, the hypothalamus plays an essential role in maintaining the body's water balance.

Some of the neurons in the hypothalamus function as endocrine (ductless) glands. Their axons secrete chemicals called *releasing hormones* into the blood, which then carries them to the anterior pituitary gland. Releasing hormones, as their name suggests, control the release of certain anterior pituitary hormones. These in turn influence the hormone secretion of other endocrine glands. Thus the hypothalamus indirectly helps control the functioning of every cell in the body.

The hypothalamus is a crucial part of the mechanism for maintaining body temperature. Therefore marked elevation in body temperature in the absence of disease frequently characterizes injuries or other abnormalities of the hypothalamus. In addition, this important center is involved in functions such as the regulation of water balance, sleep cycles, and the control of appetite and many emotions involved in pleasure, fear, anger, sexual arousal, and pain.

Thalamus

Just above the hypothalamus is a dumbbell-shaped section of gray matter called the **thalamus.** Each enlarged end of the dumbbell lies in a lateral wall of a fluid-filled chamber called the *third ventricle.* The thin center section of the thalamus passes from left to right through this ventricle, which is discussed in more detail later in this chapter.

The thalamus is composed chiefly of dendrites and cell bodies of neurons that have axons extending up toward the sensory areas of the cerebrum. The thalamus performs the following functions:

1. It helps produce sensations. Its neurons relay impulses to the cerebral cortex from the sense organs of the body.
2. It associates sensations with emotions. Almost all sensations are accompanied by a feeling of some degree of pleasantness or unpleasantness. The way that these pleasant and unpleasant feelings are produced is unknown except that they seem to be associated with the arrival of sensory impulses in the thalamus.
3. It plays a part in the so-called *arousal* or alerting mechanism.

Pineal Gland

Posterior to the thalamus is a tiny mass protruding from the back of the diencephalon called the **pineal gland** or *pineal body.* It resembles a small pine nut or kernel of corn.

The pineal gland receives sensory information about the strength of light seen by the eyes and adjusts its output of the hormone *melatonin.* Melatonin is known as "the timekeeping hormone" because it helps keep the body's clock "on time" with the daily, monthly, and seasonal cycles of sunlight and moonlight. We will return to this amazing little organ in Chapter 11 (p. 253).

Cerebrum

Structure

The **cerebrum** is the largest and uppermost part of the brain. If you were to look at the outer surface of the cerebrum, the first features you might notice are its many ridges and grooves. The ridges are called *convolutions* or **gyri,** and the grooves are called **sulci.**

The deepest sulci are called *fissures.* The longitudinal fissure divides the cerebrum into right and left halves or hemispheres. These halves are almost separate structures except for an inferior central band called the **corpus callosum,** which is made up of white matter tracts (see **Figure 9-10**).

Two deep sulci subdivide each cerebral hemisphere into four major lobes and each lobe into numerous convolutions. The lobes are named for the bones that lie over them: the frontal lobe, the parietal lobe, the temporal lobe, and the occipital lobe. Identify these in **Figure 9-11,** *A.*

A thin layer of gray matter called the **cerebral cortex,** made up of neuron dendrites and cell bodies, forms the surface of the cerebrum.

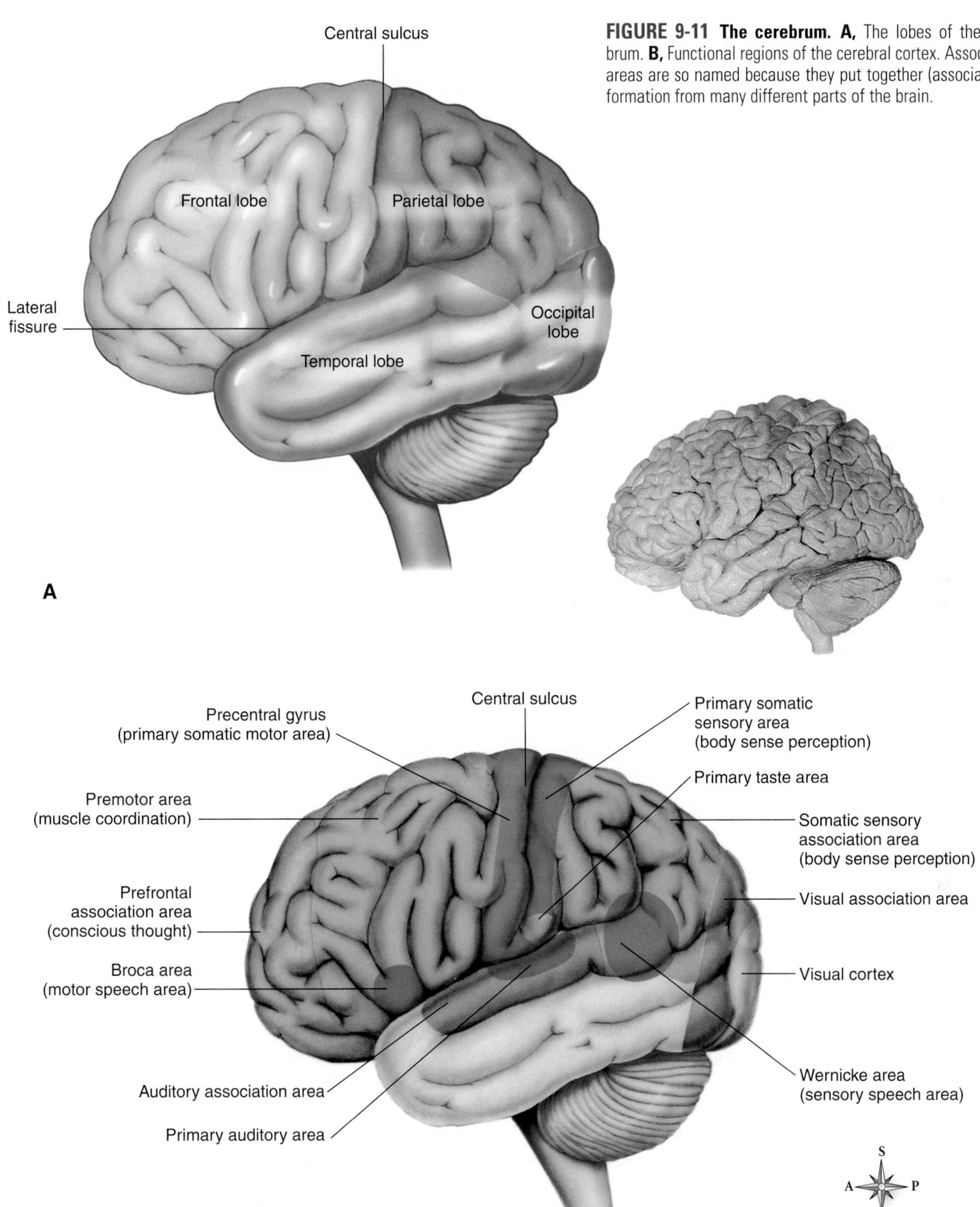

FIGURE 9-11 The cerebrum. A, The lobes of the cerebrum. **B,** Functional regions of the cerebral cortex. Association areas are so named because they put together (associate) information from many different parts of the brain.

White matter, made up of bundles of nerve fibers (tracts), composes most of the interior of the cerebrum. Within this white matter, however, are a few islands of gray matter known as the **basal nuclei** or **basal ganglia,** whose functioning is essential for producing automatic movements and postures.

Functions

What functions does the cerebrum perform? This is a hard question to answer briefly because the neurons of the cerebrum do not function alone. They function with many other neurons in many other parts of the brain and in the spinal

RESEARCH, ISSUES, AND TRENDS

PARKINSON DISEASE

Parkinson disease (**PD**) is a chronic nervous disorder resulting from a deficiency of the neurotransmitter dopamine in the basal nuclei of the cerebrum. The group of signs associated with this disorder is a syndrome called *parkinsonism.* Parkinsonism is characterized by rigidity and trembling of the head and extremities, a forward tilt of the trunk, and shuffling manner of walking, as you can see in the figure. You may have noticed these characteristics in former boxing champion Muhammad Ali, the actor Michael J. Fox, or others you may know with PD. All of these characteristics result from a lack of dopamine, leading to misinformation in the part of the brain that normally prevents the skeletal muscles from being overstimulated.

Dopamine injection into the blood and dopamine pills are not effective treatments because dopamine cannot cross the blood-brain barrier. A breakthrough in the treatment of PD came when the drug *levodopa* or *L-dopa* was found to increase the dopamine levels in afflicted patients. Neurons use L-dopa, which can cross the blood-brain barrier, to make dopamine. For some reason, L-dopa does not always have the desired effects in individual patients, so a number of alternatives have been developed. One option that has had some success is the surgical grafting of normal dopamine-secreting cells into the brains of individuals with PD. Another experimental option is an artificial implant that gives electrical stimulation to the basal nuclei, causing them to produce more dopamine.

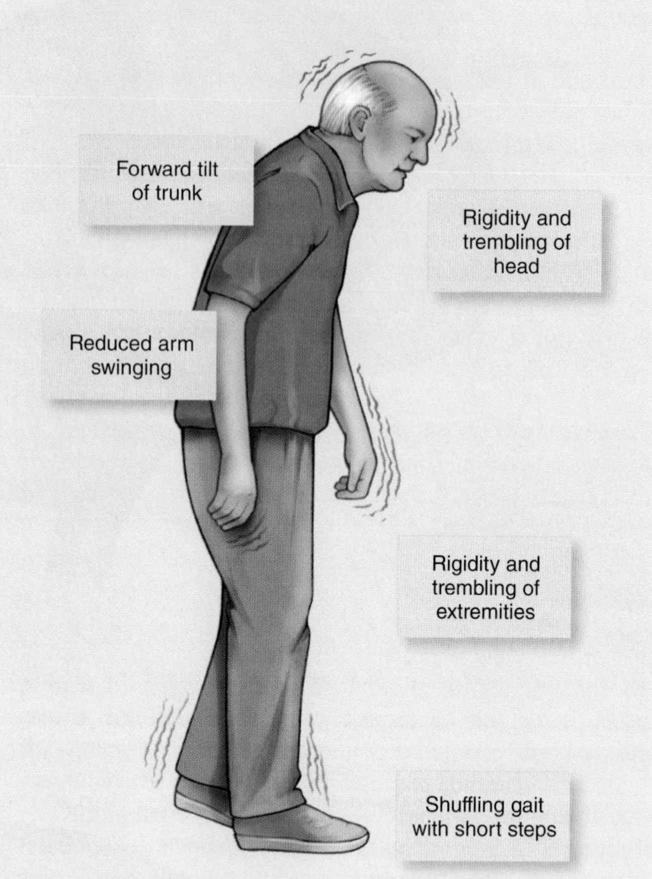

cord. Neurons of these various structures continually bring impulses to cerebral neurons and also continually carry impulses away from them.

If all other neurons were functioning normally and only cerebral neurons were not functioning, here are some of the things that you could not do. You could not think or use your will. You could not remember anything that has ever happened to you. You could not decide to make the smallest movement, nor could you make it. You would neither see nor hear. You could not experience any of the sensations that make life so rich and varied. Nothing would anger or frighten you, and nothing would bring you joy or sorrow. You would, in short, be unconscious.

These terms sum up the major cerebral functions: consciousness, thinking, memory, sensations, emotions, and willed movements. **Figure 9-11**, *B,* shows the areas of the cerebral cortex essential for willed movements, general sensations, vision, hearing, and normal speech.

Injury or disease can destroy neurons. A common example is the destruction of neurons of the motor area of the cerebrum that results from a **cerebrovascular accident** (**CVA**), which is a hemorrhage from or cessation of blood flow through cerebral blood vessels. When this happens, the victim can no longer voluntarily move the parts of the body on the side opposite to the side on which the CVA occurred. In nontechnical language, we say that he or she has suffered a stroke. Note in **Figure 9-11**, *B,* the location of the *primary somatic motor area* in the frontal lobe of the cerebrum.

It is important to understand that specific areas of the cortex have specific functions, as shown in **Figure 9-11**, *B.* For example, the temporal lobe's auditory areas interpret incoming nervous signals from the ear as very specific sounds. The visual area of the cortex in the occipital lobe helps you identify and understand specific images.

This *localization* of function explains the specific symptoms associated with an injury to localized areas of the cerebral cortex after a stroke or traumatic injury to the head. **Table 9-1** summarizes the major components of the brain and their main functions.

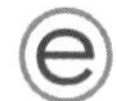
To learn more about areas of the brain that control body functions, go to AnimationDirect at *evolve.elsevier.com.*

TABLE 9-1 Functions of Major Divisions of the Brain

BRAIN AREA	FUNCTION
Brainstem	
Medulla oblongata	Two-way conduction pathway between the spinal cord and higher brain centers; cardiac, respiratory, and vasomotor control center
Pons	Two-way conduction pathway between areas of the brain and other regions of the body; influences respiration
Midbrain	Two-way conduction pathway; relay for visual and auditory impulses
Cerebellum	Muscle coordination; maintenance of equilibrium and posture
Diencephalon	
Hypothalamus	Regulation of body temperature, water balance, sleep-cycle control, appetite, and sexual arousal
Thalamus	Sensory relay station from various body areas to cerebral cortex; emotions and alerting or arousal mechanisms
Pineal gland	Adjusts output of melatonin in response to changes in external light, to keep the body's internal clock on time
Cerebrum	Sensory perception, emotions, willed movements, consciousness, and memory

QUICK CHECK

1. What are the four main divisions of the brain? What is the function of each division?
2. What regions make up the brainstem? What is the function of each region of the brainstem?
3. Why is the hypothalamus said to be a link between the nervous system and endocrine system?
4. In which part of your brain does thinking and memory occur?

Spinal Cord

Structure

If you are of average height, your spinal cord is about 17 or 18 inches long (**Figure 9-12**). It lies inside the spinal column in the spinal cavity and extends from the occipital bone down to the bottom of the first lumbar vertebra. Place your hands on your hips, and they will line up with your fourth lumbar vertebra. Your spinal cord ends just above this level.

Look now at **Figure 9-13**. Notice the H-shaped core of the spinal cord. It consists of gray matter and thus is composed mainly of dendrites and cell bodies of neurons. Columns of white matter form the outer portion of the spinal cord, and bundles of myelinated nerve fibers—the **spinal tracts**—make up the white columns.

Spinal cord tracts provide two-way conduction paths to and from the brain. *Ascending tracts* conduct impulses up the spinal cord to the brain. *Descending tracts* conduct impulses down the spinal cord from the brain. Tracts are functional organizations in that all axons composing one tract serve one general function. For instance, fibers of the spinothalamic tracts serve a sensory function. They carry impulses that produce sensations of crude touch, pain, and temperature. Other ascending tracts shown in **Figure 9-13** include the gracilis and cuneatus tracts, which transmit sensations of touch and pressure up to the brain, and the anterior and posterior spinocerebellar tracts, which transmit information about muscle length to the cerebellum. Descending tracts include the lateral and ventral corticospinal tracts, which carry impulses controlling many voluntary movements.

Functions

To try to understand spinal cord functions, think about a hotel telephone switching system. Suppose a guest in Room 108 calls the switching system and keys in the extension number for Room 520, and in a second or so, someone in that room answers. Very briefly, three events took place: a message traveled into the switching system, the system routed the message along the proper path, and the message traveled out from the switching system toward Room 520. The telephone switching system provided the network of connections that made possible the completion of the call. We might say that the switching system transferred the incoming call to an outgoing line.

The spinal cord functions similarly. It contains the centers for thousands and thousands of reflex arcs. Look back at **Figure 9-5**. The interneuron shown there is an example of a spinal cord reflex center. It switches or transfers incoming sensory impulses to outgoing motor impulses, thereby making it possible for a reflex to occur.

Reflexes that result from conduction over arcs whose centers lie in the spinal cord are called *spinal cord reflexes.* Two common kinds of spinal cord reflexes are withdrawal and jerk reflexes. An example of a withdrawal reflex is pulling one's hand away from a hot surface. The familiar knee jerk is an example of a jerk reflex.

In addition to functioning as the primary reflex center of the body, the spinal cord tracts, as previously noted, carry impulses to and from the brain. Sensory impulses travel up to the brain in ascending tracts, and motor impulses travel down from the brain in descending tracts.

If an injury cuts the spinal cord all the way across, impulses can no longer travel to the brain from any part of the body located below the injury, nor can they travel from the brain down to these parts. In short, this kind of spinal cord injury produces a loss of sensation, which is called **anesthesia,** and a loss of the ability to make voluntary movements, which is called **paralysis.**

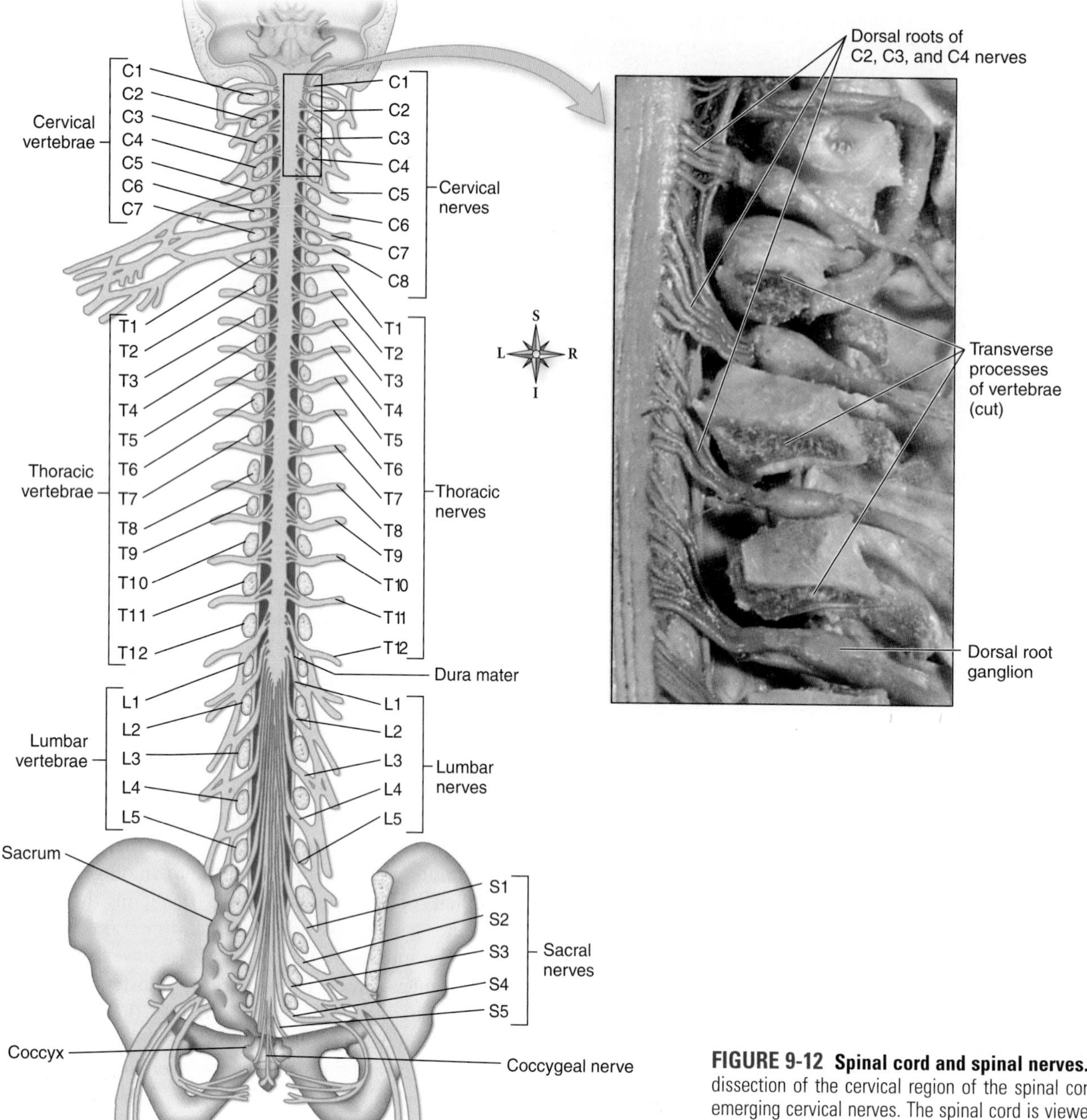

FIGURE 9-12 Spinal cord and spinal nerves. Inset is a dissection of the cervical region of the spinal cord showing emerging cervical nerves. The spinal cord is viewed from behind (posterior aspect).

Coverings and Fluid Spaces

Meninges and Bone

Nervous tissue is not a sturdy tissue. Even moderate pressure can kill nerve cells, so nature safeguards the chief organs made of this tissue—the spinal cord and the brain—by surrounding them with a tough, fluid-cushioned set of membranes called the **meninges.**

The spinal meninges form a tubelike covering around the spinal cord and line the bony vertebral foramen of the vertebrae that surround the spinal cord. Look at **Figure 9-14**, and you can identify the three layers of the spinal meninges. They are the **dura mater,** which is the tough outer layer that lines the vertebral canal, the **pia mater,** which is the innermost membrane covering the spinal cord itself, and the **arachnoid mater,** which is the membrane between the dura and the pia mater. The arachnoid mater resembles a cobweb with fluid in its spaces. The word *arachnoid* means "like a spider web." It comes from *arachne,* the Greek word for spider.

The meninges that form the protective covering around the spinal cord also extend up and around the brain to enclose it completely.

The meninges are inner, soft coverings of the CNS. They are, in turn, surrounded by the hard bone of the skull and vertebrae—forming a highly protective shield from injury.

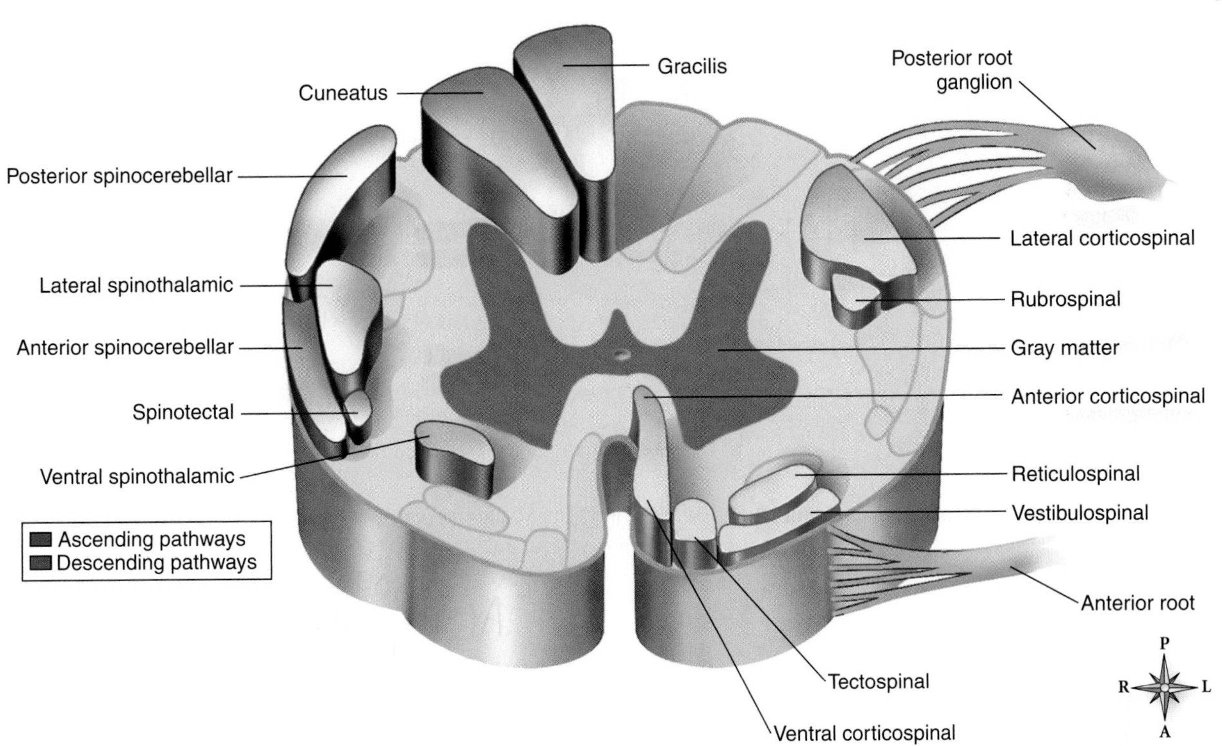

FIGURE 9-13 Spinal cord cross section. Cross section of the spinal cord showing some of the major pathways. The ascending tracts are shown in blue and the descending tracts are shown in red. You can also see the gray matter in the center of the spinal cord (brown) and the nerve roots (yellow) attached to the spinal cord.

Cerebrospinal Fluid Spaces

Fluid fills the subarachnoid spaces between the pia mater and arachnoid in the brain and spinal cord. This fluid is called **cerebrospinal fluid (CSF)**.

CSF also fills spaces in the brain called cerebral **ventricles.** In Figure 9-15, you can see the irregular shapes of the ventricles of the brain. These illustrations can also help you visualize the location of the ventricles if you remember that these large spaces lie deep inside the brain and that there are two lateral ventricles. One lies inside the right half of the cerebrum (the largest part of the human brain), and the other lies inside the left half.

CSF forms continually from fluid filtering out of the blood in a network of brain capillaries known as the **choroid plexus** and into the ventricles.

CSF is one of the body's circulating fluids. CSF seeps from the lateral ventricles into the third ventricle and flows down through the cerebral aqueduct (find this in Figure 9-15 and Figure 9-16) into the fourth ventricle. Most of the CSF moves through tiny openings from the fourth ventricle into the subarachnoid space near the cerebellum. Some of it moves into the small, tubelike central canal of the spinal cord and then out into the subarachnoid spaces. Then CSF moves leisurely down and around the spinal cord and up and around the brain (in the subarachnoid spaces of their meninges) and returns to the blood (in the veins of the brain).

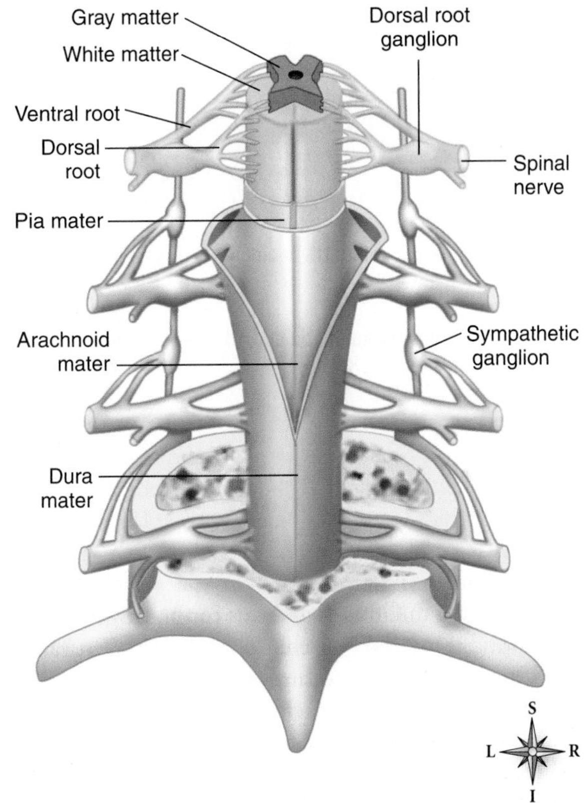

FIGURE 9-14 Spinal cord and its coverings. The meninges, spinal nerves, and sympathetic trunk are visible.

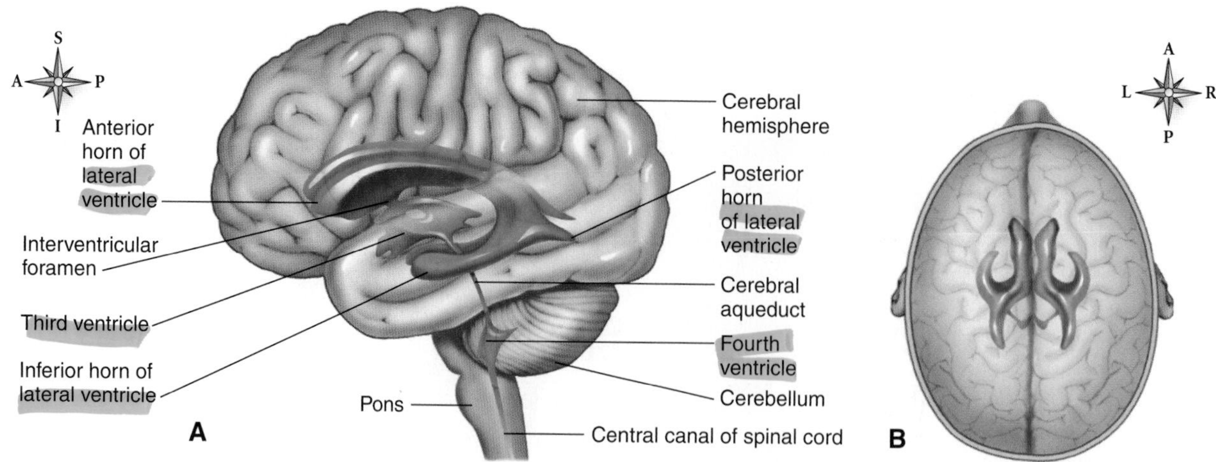

FIGURE 9-15 Fluid spaces of the brain. A, The ventricles highlighted within the brain in a left lateral view. **B,** The ventricles as seen from above.

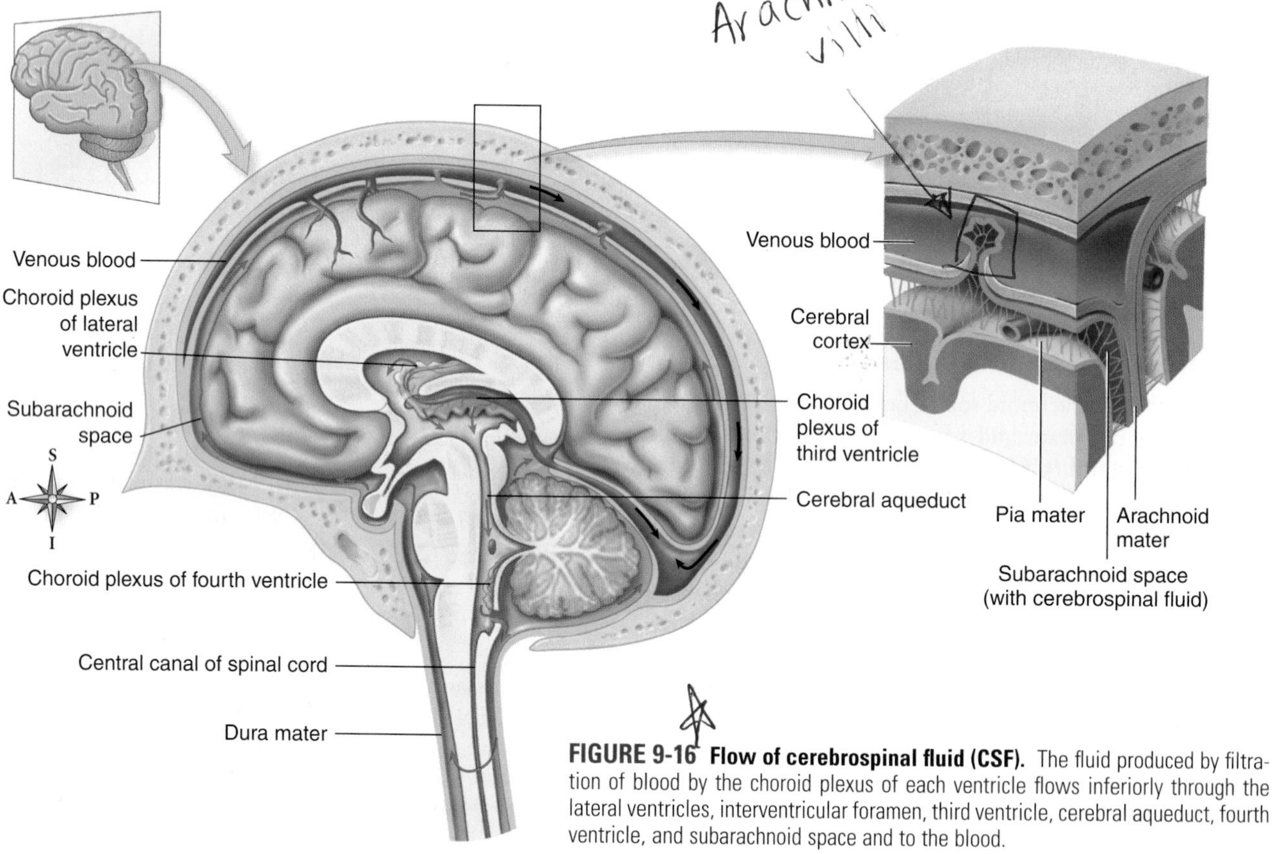

FIGURE 9-16 Flow of cerebrospinal fluid (CSF). The fluid produced by filtration of blood by the choroid plexus of each ventricle flows inferiorly through the lateral ventricles, interventricular foramen, third ventricle, cerebral aqueduct, fourth ventricle, and subarachnoid space and to the blood.

Remembering that this fluid forms continually from blood, circulates, and is resorbed into blood can be useful. It can help you understand certain abnormalities. Suppose a person has a brain tumor that presses on the cerebral aqueduct. This blocks the way for the return of CSF to the blood. Because the fluid continues to form but cannot drain away, it accumulates in the ventricles or in the meninges, creating enough pressure to damage or deform the nearby soft nervous tissue.

Other conditions can cause an accumulation of CSF in the ventricles. An example is **hydrocephalus** or "water on the brain." One form of treatment involves surgical placement of a hollow tube or catheter through the blocked channel so that CSF can drain into another location in the body.

QUICK CHECK

1. What are the major functions of the spinal cord?
2. What are spinal tracts?
3. What is the name, location, and function of each of the three meninges?
4. What is cerebrospinal fluid?

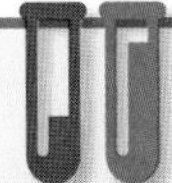

CLINICAL APPLICATION

LUMBAR PUNCTURE

The meninges, the fluid-containing membranes surrounding the brain and spinal cord, extend beyond the spinal cord, an anatomical fact that allows physicians to perform lumbar punctures without putting the spinal cord at risk of injury. A **lumbar puncture,** or "spinal tap," is the withdrawal of some cerebrospinal fluid (CSF) from the subarachnoid space in the lumbar region of the spinal cord.

The physician inserts a needle just above or below the fourth lumbar vertebra, knowing that the spinal cord ends an inch or more above this level. The fourth lumbar vertebra can be easily located because it lies on a line with the iliac crest. Placing an adult patient on his side and having him arch his back by drawing the knees and chest together separates the vertebrae sufficiently to introduce the needle.

Lumbar punctures are often performed when CSF is needed for analysis or when it is necessary to reduce pressure caused by swelling of the brain or spinal cord after injury or disease. The normal sample of CSF from a lumbar puncture shown here is slightly yellowish and clear, but the red color in the abnormal sample indicates bleeding (in this case, a hemorrhage in the subarachnoid space).

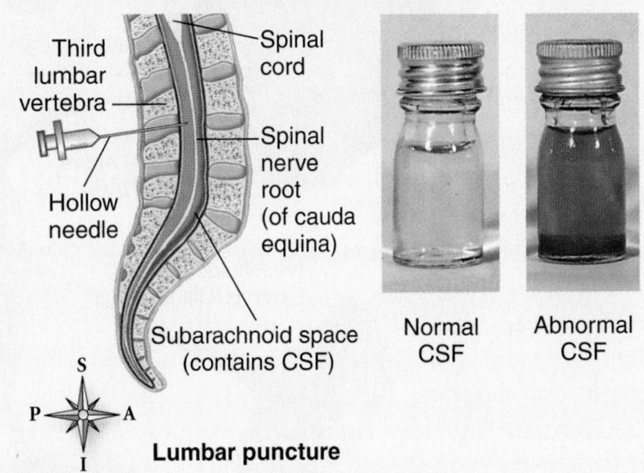

Lumbar puncture

Peripheral Nervous System

The nerves connecting the brain and spinal cord to other parts of the body constitute the peripheral nervous system (PNS). This system includes **cranial** and **spinal nerves** that connect the brain and spinal cord, respectively, to peripheral structures such as the skin surface and the skeletal muscles. In addition, other structures in the autonomic nervous system (ANS) are considered part of the PNS. These connect the brain and spinal cord to various glands in the body and to the cardiac and smooth muscles in the thorax and abdomen.

Cranial Nerves

Twelve pairs of cranial nerves are attached to the undersurface of the brain. **Figure 9-17** shows the attachments of these nerves to the brainstem and diencephalon. Their fibers conduct impulses between the brain and structures in the head and neck and in the thoracic and abdominal cavities.

For example, the second cranial nerve (optic nerve) conducts impulses from the eye to the brain, where these impulses produce vision. The third cranial nerve (oculomotor nerve) conducts impulses from the brain to muscles in the eye, where they cause contractions that move the eye. The tenth cranial nerve (vagus nerve) conducts impulses between the medulla oblongata and structures in the neck and thoracic and abdominal cavities. The names of each cranial nerve and a brief description of their functions are listed in **Table 9-2**.

To learn more about cranial nerves, go to AnimationDirect at *evolve.elsevier.com*.

Spinal Nerves

Structure

Thirty-one pairs of nerves are attached to the spinal cord in the following order: 8 pairs are attached to the cervical segments, 12 pairs are attached to the thoracic segments, 5 pairs are attached to the lumbar segments, 5 pairs are attached to the sacral segments, and 1 pair is attached to the coccygeal segment (see **Figure 9-12**).

Unlike cranial nerves, spinal nerves have no special names; instead, a letter and number identify each one. C1, for example, indicates the pair of spinal nerves attached to the first segment of the cervical part of the spinal cord, and T8 indicates nerves attached to the eighth segment of the thoracic part of the spinal cord.

In **Figure 9-12** the cervical area of the spine has been dissected to show the emerging spinal nerves in that area. After spinal nerves exit from the spinal cord, they branch to form the many peripheral nerves of the trunk and limbs. Sometimes, nerve fibers from several spinal nerves are reorganized to form a single peripheral nerve. This reorganization can be seen as a network of intersecting or "braided" branches called a **plexus. Figure 9-12** shows several plexuses.

Functions

Spinal nerves conduct impulses between the spinal cord and the parts of the body not supplied by cranial nerves. The spinal nerves shown in **Figure 9-12** contain, as do all spinal nerves, sensory and motor fibers. Spinal nerves therefore function to make possible sensations and movements. A disease or injury that prevents conduction by a spinal nerve thus results in a loss of feeling and a loss of movement in the part supplied by that nerve.

Detailed mapping of the skin's surface reveals a close relationship between the source on the spinal cord of each spinal

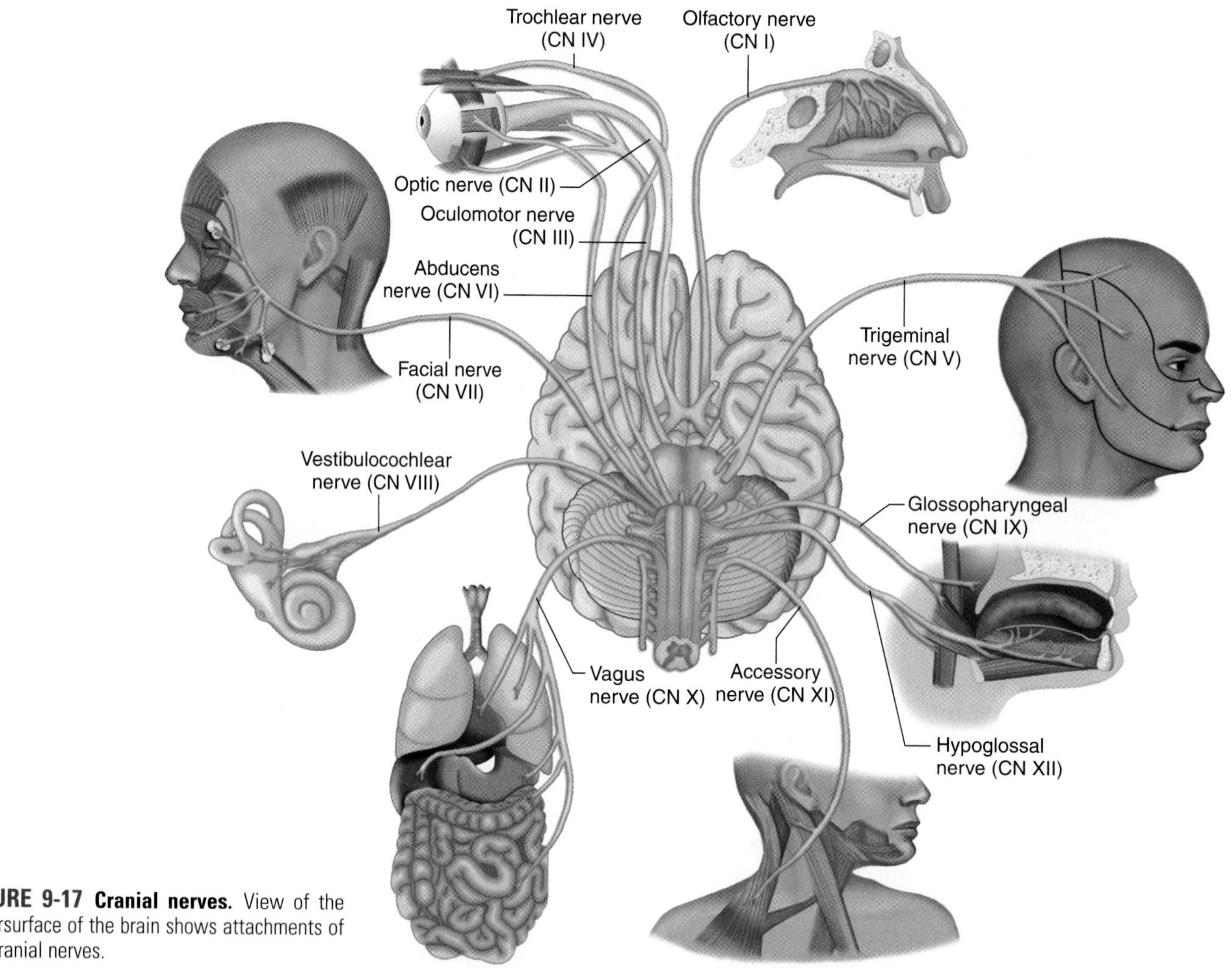

FIGURE 9-17 Cranial nerves. View of the undersurface of the brain shows attachments of the cranial nerves.

TABLE 9-2 Cranial Nerves

NERVE*		CONDUCT IMPULSES	MAIN FUNCTIONS
I	Olfactory	From nose to brain	Sense of smell
II	Optic	From eye to brain	Vision
III	Oculomotor	From brain to eye muscles	Eye movements
IV	Trochlear	From brain to external eye muscles	Eye movements
V	Trigeminal	From skin and mucous membrane of head and from teeth to brain; also from brain to chewing muscles	Sensations of face, scalp, and teeth; chewing movements
VI	Abducens	From brain to external eye muscles	Eye movements
VII	Facial	From taste buds of tongue to brain; from brain to face muscles	Sense of taste; contraction of muscles of facial expression
VIII	Vestibulocochlear	From ear to brain	Hearing; sense of balance
IX	Glossopharyngeal	From throat and taste buds of tongue to brain; also from brain to throat muscles and salivary glands	Sensations of throat, taste, swallowing movements, secretion of saliva
X	Vagus	From throat, larynx, and organs in thoracic and abdominal cavities to brain; also from brain to muscles of throat and to organs in thoracic and abdominal cavities	Sensations of throat and larynx and of thoracic and abdominal organs; swallowing, voice production, slowing of heartbeat, acceleration of peristalsis (gut movements)
XI	Accessory	From brain to certain shoulder and neck muscles	Shoulder movements; turning movements of head
XII	Hypoglossal	From brain to muscles of tongue	Tongue movements

*The first letters of the words in the following sentence are the first letters of the names of the cranial nerves, in the correct order. Many anatomy students find that using this sentence, or one like it, helps in memorizing the names and numbers of the cranial nerves. It is "**O**n **O**ld **O**lympus' **T**iny **T**ops, **A** **F**riendly **V**iking **G**rew **V**ines **A**nd **H**ops."

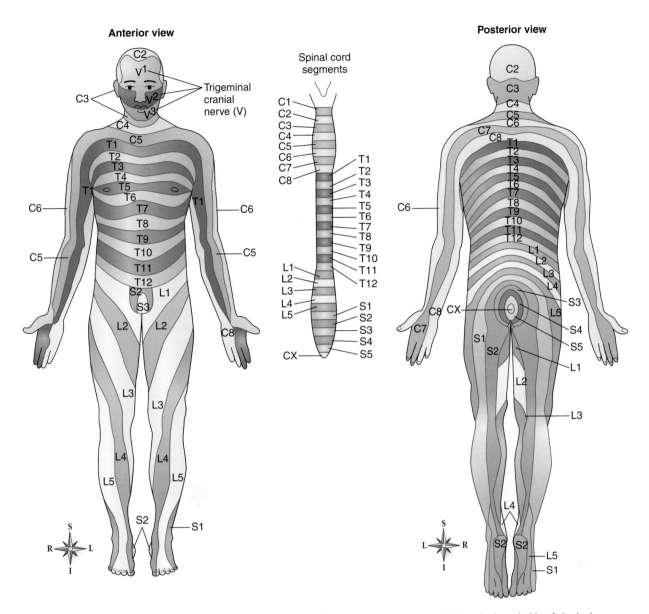

FIGURE 9-18 Dermatomes. Segmental dermatome distribution of spinal nerves to the front, back, and side of the body. *C*, Cervical segments; *T*, thoracic segments; *L*, lumbar segments; *S*, sacral segments; *CX*, coccygeal segment.

nerve and the part of the body that it innervates. Knowledge of the segmental arrangement of spinal nerves is useful to physicians. For instance, a neurologist can identify the site of a spinal cord or nerve abnormality by noting the area of the body that is insensitive to a pinprick. Skin surface areas that are supplied by a single spinal nerve are called **dermatomes.** A dermatome "map" of the body is shown in Figure 9-18.

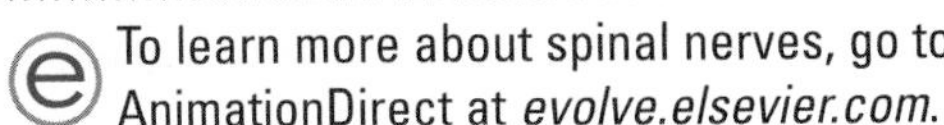

To learn more about spinal nerves, go to AnimationDirect at *evolve.elsevier.com*.

QUICK CHECK

1. How many cranial nerves are located in the peripheral nervous system? How many spinal nerves?
2. What is a spinal nerve *plexus?*
3. What are *dermatomes?*

Autonomic Nervous System

The autonomic nervous system (ANS) consists of certain motor neurons that conduct impulses from the spinal cord or brainstem to the following kinds of tissues:

1. Cardiac muscle tissue
2. Smooth muscle tissue
3. Glandular epithelial tissue

The ANS includes the parts of the nervous system that regulate involuntary functions (for example, the heartbeat, contractions of the stomach and intestines, and secretions by glands). On the other hand, motor nerves that control the voluntary actions of skeletal muscles are sometimes called the *somatic nervous system.*

The ANS consists of two divisions called the **sympathetic division** and the **parasympathetic division** (Figure 9-19).

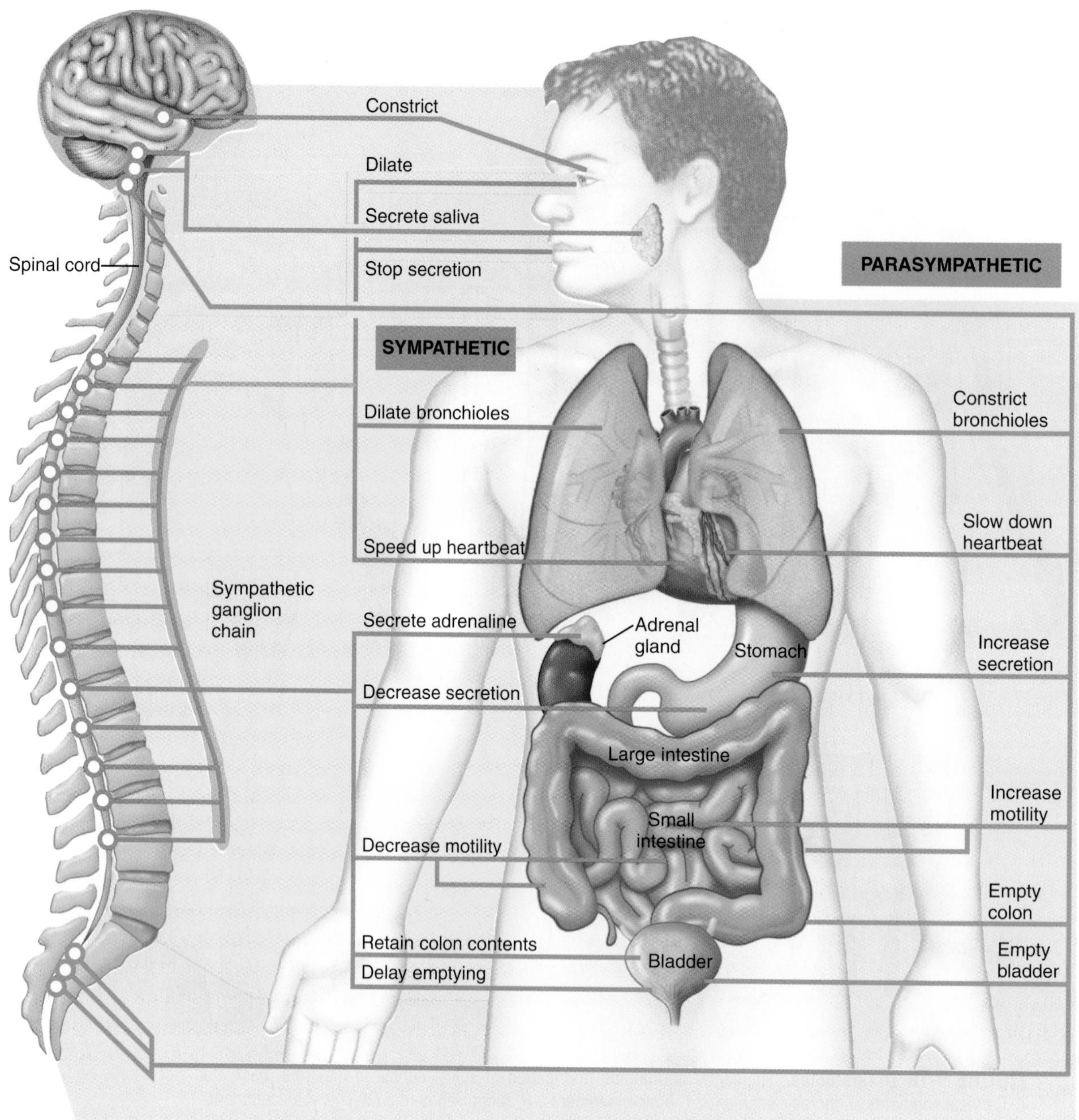

FIGURE 9-19 Innervation of major target organs by the autonomic nervous system. The sympathetic pathways are highlighted with orange, and the parasympathetic pathways are highlighted with green.

Functional Anatomy

Autonomic neurons are the motor neurons that make up the ANS. The dendrites and cell bodies of some autonomic neurons are located in the gray matter of the spinal cord or brainstem. Their axons extend from these structures and terminate in peripheral "junction boxes" called **ganglia.** These autonomic neurons are called **preganglionic neurons** because they conduct impulses between the spinal cord and a ganglion.

In the autonomic ganglia, the axon endings of preganglionic neurons synapse with the dendrites or cell bodies of postganglionic neurons. **Postganglionic neurons,** as their name suggests, conduct impulses from a ganglion to cardiac muscle, smooth muscle, or glandular epithelial tissue.

Autonomic or **visceral effectors** are the tissues to which autonomic neurons conduct impulses. Specifically, visceral effectors are cardiac muscle that makes up the wall of the heart, smooth muscle that partially makes up the walls of blood vessels and other hollow internal organs, and glandular epithelial tissue that makes up the secreting part of a gland.

Autonomic Conduction Paths

Conduction paths to visceral and somatic effectors from the CNS (spinal cord or brainstem) differ somewhat. Autonomic paths to visceral effectors, as the right side of **Figure 9-20** shows, consist of two-neuron relays. Impulses travel over preganglionic neurons from the spinal cord or brainstem to autonomic

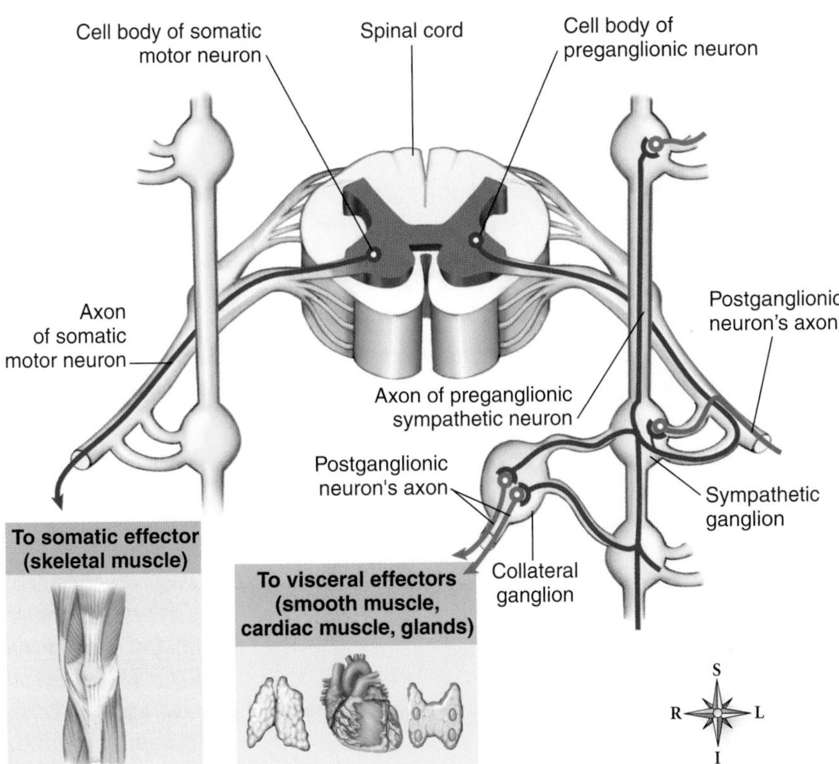

FIGURE 9-20 Autonomic conduction paths. The left side of the diagram shows that one somatic motor neuron conducts impulses all the way from the spinal cord to a somatic effector. Conduction from the spinal cord to any visceral effector, however, requires a relay of at least two autonomic motor neurons—a preganglionic and a postganglionic neuron, shown on the right side of the diagram. Both types of pathways occur on left and right sides.

ganglia. There, they are relayed across synapses to postganglionic neurons, which then conduct the impulses from the ganglia to visceral effectors.

Compare the autonomic conduction path with the somatic conduction path illustrated on the left side of **Figure 9-20**. A single somatic motor neuron, like the ones shown here, conducts impulses all the way from the spinal cord or brainstem to somatic effectors with no intervening synapses.

Sympathetic Division

Structure

Sympathetic preganglionic neurons have dendrites and cell bodies in the gray matter of the thoracic and upper lumbar segments of the spinal cord. For this reason, the sympathetic system has also been referred to as the *thoracolumbar system.*

Look now at the right side of **Figure 9-20**. Follow the course of the axon of the sympathetic preganglionic neuron shown there. It leaves the spinal cord in the anterior (ventral) root of a spinal nerve. It next enters the spinal nerve but soon leaves it to extend to and through a sympathetic ganglion and terminate in a collateral ganglion. There, it synapses with several postganglionic neurons whose axons extend to terminate in visceral effectors.

Also shown in **Figure 9-20**, branches of the preganglionic axon may ascend or descend to terminate in ganglia above and below their point of origin. All sympathetic preganglionic axons therefore synapse with many postganglionic neurons, and these frequently terminate in widely separated organs. Hence sympathetic responses are usually widespread, involving many organs rather than just one.

Sympathetic postganglionic neurons have dendrites and cell bodies in sympathetic ganglia. Sympathetic ganglia are located in front of and at each side of the spinal column. Because short fibers extend between the sympathetic ganglia, they look a little like two chains of beads and are often referred to as the *sympathetic chain ganglia.*

Axons of sympathetic postganglionic neurons travel in spinal nerves to blood vessels, sweat glands, and arrector pili hair muscles all over the body. Separate autonomic nerves distribute many sympathetic postganglionic axons to various internal organs.

Functions

The sympathetic division functions as an emergency system. Impulses over sympathetic fibers take control of many internal organs when we exercise strenuously and when strong emotions—anger, fear, hate, anxiety—are elicited. In short, when we must cope with stress of any kind, sympathetic impulses increase to many visceral effectors and rapidly produce widespread changes within our bodies.

The middle column of **Table 9-3** indicates many sympathetic responses. The heart beats faster. Most blood vessels constrict, causing blood pressure to increase. Blood vessels in skeletal muscles dilate, supplying the muscles with more blood. Sweat glands and adrenal glands secrete more abundantly. Salivary and other digestive glands secrete more sparingly. Digestive tract contractions (peristalsis) become sluggish, hampering digestion.

Together, all these varied sympathetic responses make us ready for strenuous muscular work. We need such physiological preparation when facing a threat—we must be ready to either resist (fight) the threat or to avoid (fly from) the threat. Therefore, this group of changes induced by sympathetic control is known as the **fight-or-flight response.**

Parasympathetic Division

Structure

The dendrites and cell bodies of **parasympathetic preganglionic neurons** are located in the gray matter of the brainstem and the sacral segments of the spinal cord. For this reason, the parasympathetic system has also been referred to as the *craniosacral system.*

The parasympathetic preganglionic axons extend some distance before terminating in the parasympathetic ganglia located in the head and in the thoracic and abdominal cavities close to the visceral effectors that they control. The dendrites and cell bodies of **parasympathetic postganglionic neurons**

TABLE 9-3 Autonomic Functions

VISCERAL EFFECTORS	SYMPATHETIC CONTROL	PARASYMPATHETIC CONTROL
Heart muscle	Accelerates heartbeat	Slows heartbeat
Smooth muscle		
Of most blood vessels	Constricts blood vessels	None
Of blood vessels in skeletal muscles	Dilates blood vessels	None
Of the digestive tract	Decreases peristalsis; inhibits defecation	Increases peristalsis
Of the anal sphincter	Stimulates—closes sphincter	Inhibits—opens sphincter for defecation
Of the urinary bladder	Inhibits—relaxes bladder	Stimulates—contracts bladder
Of the urinary sphincters	Stimulates—closes sphincter	Inhibits—opens sphincter for urination
Of the eye		
Iris	Stimulates radial fibers—dilation of pupil	Stimulates circular fibers—contraction of pupil
Ciliary	Inhibits—accommodation for far vision (flattening of lens)	Stimulates—accommodation for near vision (bulging of lens)
Of hairs (arrector pili)	Stimulates—"goose pimples"	No parasympathetic fibers
Glands		
Adrenal medulla	Increases epinephrine secretion	None
Sweat glands	Increases sweat secretion	None
Digestive glands	Decreases secretion of digestive juices	Increases secretion of digestive juices

lie in these outlying parasympathetic ganglia, and their short axons extend into the nearby structures. Therefore each parasympathetic preganglionic neuron synapses only with postganglionic neurons to a single effector.

For this reason, parasympathetic stimulation frequently involves response by only one organ. This is in stark contrast to sympathetic responses, which involve numerous organs.

Functions

The parasympathetic system dominates control of many visceral effectors under normal, everyday conditions. Impulses carried by parasympathetic fibers, for example, tend to slow heartbeat, increase peristalsis, and increase secretion of digestive juices and insulin (see **Table 9-3**). Thus we can think of parasympathetic function as counterbalancing sympathetic function.

Autonomic Neurotransmitters

Turn your attention now to **Figure 9-21**. It reveals information about autonomic neurotransmitters, the chemical compounds released from the axon terminals of autonomic neurons.

Observe that three of the axons shown in **Figure 9-21**—the sympathetic preganglionic axon, the parasympathetic preganglionic axon, and the parasympathetic postganglionic axon—release acetylcholine. These axons are therefore classified as **cholinergic fibers.**

Only one type of autonomic axon releases the neurotransmitter norepinephrine (noradrenaline). This is the axon of a sympathetic postganglionic neuron, and such neurons are classified as **adrenergic fibers.**

That each division of the ANS signals its effectors with a different neurotransmitter explains how an organ can tell which division is stimulating it. The heart, for example, responds to acetylcholine from the parasympathetic division by slowing down. The presence of norepinephrine at the heart, on the other hand, is a signal from the sympathetic division, and the response is an increase in heart activity.

Autonomic Nervous System as a Whole

The function of the autonomic nervous system is to regulate the body's automatic, involuntary functions in ways that maintain or quickly restore homeostasis.

Many internal organs are *dually innervated* by the ANS. In other words, they receive fibers from parasympathetic and sympathetic divisions. Parasympathetic and sympathetic impulses continually bombard them and, as **Table 9-3** indicates, influence their function in opposite or antagonistic ways.

For example, the heart continually receives sympathetic impulses that make it beat faster and parasympathetic impulses that slow it down. The ratio between these two antagonistic forces, determined by the ratio between the two different autonomic neurotransmitters, determines the actual heart rate.

The term *autonomic nervous system* is something of a misnomer. It seems to imply that this part of the nervous system is independent from other parts. But this is not true. Dendrites and cell bodies of preganglionic neurons are located, as observed in **Figure 9-20** and **Figure 9-21**, in the spinal cord and brainstem. They are continually influenced directly or indirectly by impulses from neurons located above them, notably by some in the hypothalamus and in the parts of the cerebral cortex called the **limbic system** or *emotional brain.* Through

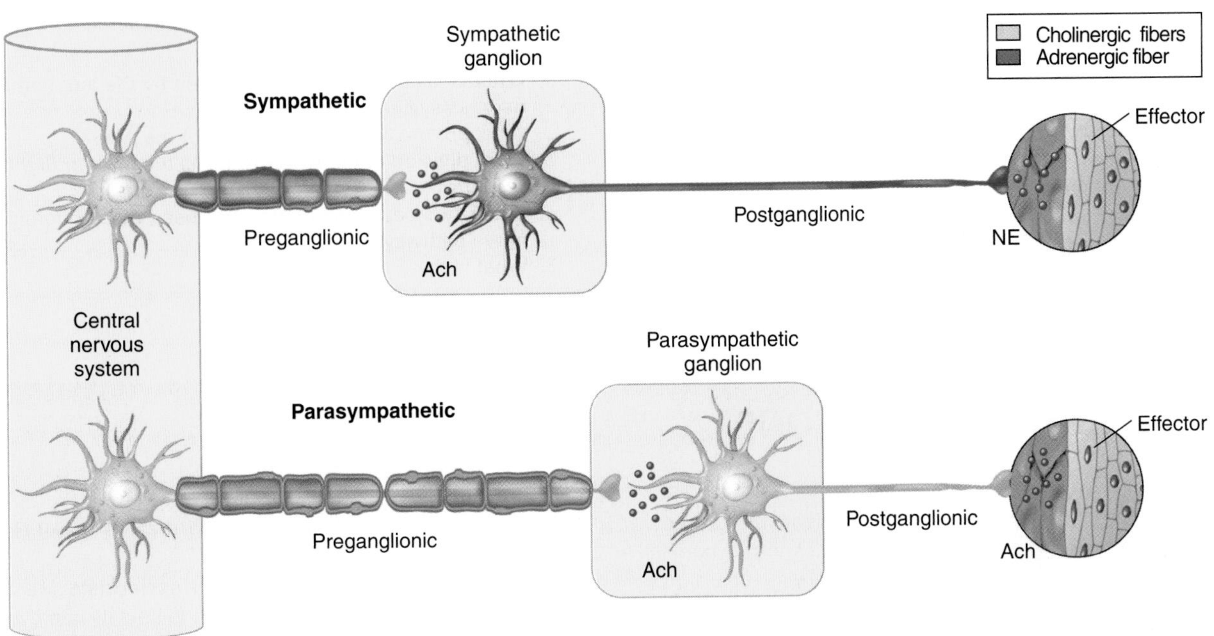

FIGURE 9-21 Autonomic neurotransmitters. Three of the four fiber types are cholinergic, secreting the neurotransmitter acetylcholine *(Ach)* into a synapse. Only the sympathetic postganglionic fiber is adrenergic, secreting norepinephrine *(NE)* into a synapse.

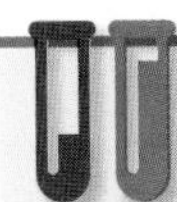

CLINICAL APPLICATION

HERPES ZOSTER, OR SHINGLES

Herpes zoster, or **shingles,** is a unique viral infection that almost always affects the skin of a single dermatome. It is caused by a varicella zoster virus (VZV) of chickenpox. Nearly 15% of the population will suffer from shingles at least once by the time they reach the age of 80.

In most cases the disease results from reactivation of the varicella virus. The virus probably traveled through a cutaneous nerve and remained dormant in a dorsal root ganglion for years after an episode of chickenpox. If the body's immunological protective mechanism becomes diminished in the elderly after stress, or in individuals undergoing cancer therapy or taking immunosuppressive drugs, the virus may reactivate. If this occurs, the virus travels over the sensory nerve to the skin of a single dermatome. The result is a painful eruption of red, swollen plaques or vesicles that eventually rupture and crust before clearing in 2 to 3 weeks.

In severe cases, extensive inflammation, hemorrhagic blisters, and secondary bacterial infection may lead to permanent scarring. In most cases, the eruption of vesicles is preceded by 4 to 5 days of preeruptive pain, burning, and itching in the affected dermatome. Although an attack of herpes zoster does not confer lasting immunity, only 5% of cases are recurrences.

Some health officials are concerned about a possible shingles epidemic among adults caused by widespread use of chickenpox vaccines in children. Apparently, adults who have not had occasional immune-boosting exposures to children with chickenpox have an increased risk of developing shingles. A shingles vaccine is available for use in people 50 and older who have had chickenpox.

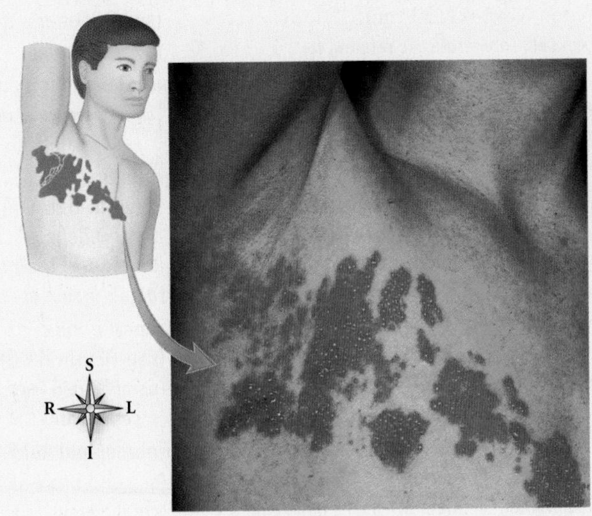

conduction paths from these areas, emotions can produce widespread changes in the automatic functions of our bodies, in cardiac and smooth muscle contractions, and in secretion by glands. Anger and fear, for example, lead to increased sympathetic activity and the fight-or-flight response.

According to some physiologists, the slightly altered state of consciousness known as *meditation* leads to decreased sympathetic activity and a group of changes opposite to those of the fight-or-flight response.

QUICK CHECK

1. What kinds of tissues are controlled by the autonomic nervous system (ANS)?
2. What are the two main divisions of the ANS?
3. What division of the ANS produces the *fight-or-flight response?*
4. Which two neurotransmitters are used by autonomic nerve pathways?
5. What is the limbic system?

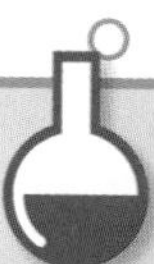

SCIENCE APPLICATIONS

NEUROSCIENCE

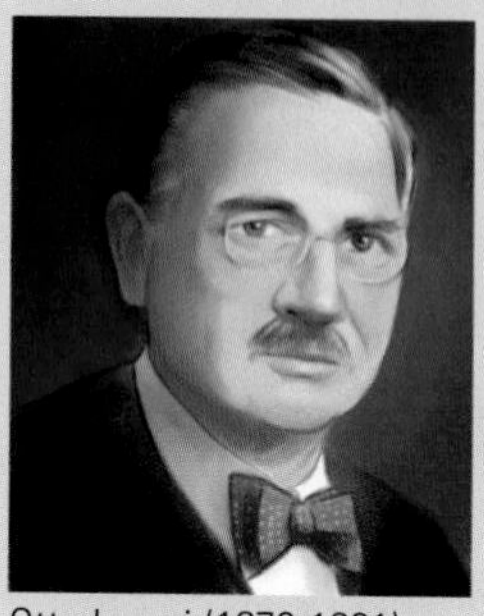

Otto Loewi (1873-1961)

The Austrian scientist Otto Loewi started his studies in the humanities, not science. When he did begin university studies in medicine, he often skipped his science classes to attend lectures in philosophy. But after Dr. Loewi turned his attention to human biology, he was brilliant. In 1921, when trying to design an experiment to find out how neurons communicate with other cells, he had a dream in which the answer came to him. He rushed to his lab and performed a famous experiment in which he discovered what we know as acetylcholine. For his work that showed that it is neurotransmitters that carry signals from neurons, Loewi shared a Nobel Prize in 1936. And, not surprisingly, Loewi later spent some of his time studying how dreams may help us understand subconscious thoughts.

Many professions depend on **neuroscientists** like Otto Loewi to provide information they need to help us improve our lives. For example, **neurologists, psychiatrists,** and other medical professionals use this information to treat disorders of the nervous system. **Pharmacologists** use these ideas to develop drug treatments that affect the nervous system—and **pharmacists** and **pharmacy technicians** supply these treatments. Mental health professionals such as **psychologists** and *counselors* use concepts derived from neuroscience to better understand human emotions and behavior. Even people who specialize in *business* and *marketing* use some of the neuroscience discoveries—their focus is learning how to entice buyers to buy certain products or, perhaps, to predict the behavior of crowds.

LANGUAGE OF SCIENCE AND MEDICINE *(continued from p. 179)*

autonomic neuron
(aw-toh-NOM-ik NOO-ron)
[*auto-* **self,** *-nom-* **rule,** *-ic* **relating to,** *neuron* **nerve**]

axon
(AK-son)
[*axon* **axle**]

basal nuclei (basal ganglia)
(BAY-sal NOO-klee-eye [GANG-glee-ah])
sing., basal nucleus or ganglion
(BAY-sal NOO-klee-us [GANG-glee-un])
[*bas-* **foundation,** *-al* **relating to,** *nucle-* **nut or kernel** (*ganglion* **knot**)]

blood-brain barrier (BBB)
(blud brayn BAYR-ee-er)

catecholamine
(kat-eh-KOHL-ah-meen)
[*catech-* **melt,** *-ol-* **alcohol,** *-amine* **ammonia compound**]

cell body
(sell BOD-ee)
[*cell* **storeroom**]

central nervous system (CNS)
[*centr-* **center,** *-al* **relating to,** *nerv-* **nerve,** *-ous* **relating to**]

cerebellum
(sayr-eh-BEL-um)
pl., cerebella or cerebellums
(sayr-eh-BEL-ah or sayr-eh-BEL-umz)
[*cereb-* **brain,** *-ell-* **small,** *-um* **thing**]

cerebral cortex
(seh-REE-bral KOR-teks)
[*cerebr-* **brain (cerebrum),** *-al* **relating to,** *cortex* **bark**]

cerebrospinal fluid
(seh-ree-broh-SPY-nal FLOO-id)
[*cerebr-* **brain,** *-spin-* **backbone,** *-al* **relating to**]

cerebrovascular accident (CVA)
(SAYR-eh-broh-VAS-kyoo-lar)
[*cerebr-* **brain,** *-vas-* **vessel,** *-cul-* **little,** *-ar* **relating to**]

cerebrum
(seh-REE-brum)
[*cerebrum* **brain**]

cholinergic fiber
(koh-lin-ER-jik FYE-ber)
[*chole-* **bile,** *-erg-* **work,** *-ic* **relating to,** *fibr-* **thread**]

choroid plexus
(KOH-royd PLEK-sus)
pl., choroid plexuses
(KOH-royd PLEK-sus-ez)
[*chorio-* **skin,** *-oid* **like,** *plexus* **braid or network**]

corpus callosum
(KOHR-pus kah-LOH-sum)
pl., corpora callosa
(KOHR-por-ah kah-LOH-sah)
[*corpus* **body,** *callosum* **callous or tough**]

cranial nerve
(KRAY-nee-al nerv)
[*crani-* **skull,** *-al* **relating to**]

dendrite
(DEN-dryte)
[*dendr-* **tree,** *-ite* **part (branch)**]

dermatome
(DER-mah-tohm)
[*derma-* **skin,** *-tome* **cut (segment)**]

diencephalon
(dye-en-SEF-ah-lon)
[*di-* **between,** *-en-* **within,** *-cephalon* **head**]

dopamine
(DOH-pah-meen)
[*dopa-* **amino acid,** *-amine* **ammonia**]

dura mater
(DOO-rah MAH-ter)
[*dura* **hard,** *mater* **mother**]

effector
(ef-FEK-tor)
[*effect-* **accomplish,** *-or* **agent**]

efferent neuron
(EF-fer-ent NOO-ron)
[*e-* **away,** *-fer-* **carry,** *-ent* **relating to,** *neuron* **string or nerve**]

endoneurium
(en-doh-NOO-ree-um)
[*endo-* **inward,** *-neuri-* **nerve,** *-um* **thing**]

endorphin
(en-DOR-fin)
[*endo-* **within,** *-(m)orph-* **Morpheus (Roman god of dreams),** *-in* **substance**]

enkephalin
(en-KEF-ah-lin)
[*en-* **within,** *-kephalo-* **head,** *-in* **substance**]

epineurium
(ep-ih-NOO-ree-um)
[*epi-* **upon,** *-neuri-* **nerve,** *-um* **thing**]

fascicle
(FAS-ih-kul)
[*fasci-* **band or bundle,** *-cle* **small**]

fight-or-flight response
(fyte or flyte ree-SPAHNS)

ganglion
(GANG-lee-on)
pl., ganglia
(GANG-lee-ah)
[*gangli-* **knot,** *-on* **unit**]

glia
(GLEE-ah)
sing., glial cell
(GLEE-al sel)
[*glia* **glue**]

glioma
(glee-OH-mah)
[*glio-* **neuroglia,** *-oma* **tumor**]

gray matter
(gray MAT-ter)

gyri
(JYE-rye)
sing., gyrus
(JYE-rus)
[*gyrus* **circle**]

herpes zoster
(HER-peez ZOS-ter)
[*herpe* **creep,** *zoster* **girdle**]

hydrocephalus
(hye-droh-SEF-ah-lus
[*hydro-* **water,** *-cephalus* **head**]

hypothalamus
(hye-poh-THAL-ah-mus)
[*hypo-* **under or below,** *-thalamus* **inner chamber**]

interneuron
(in-ter-NOO-ron)
[*inter-* **between,** *-neuron* **nerve**]

limbic system
(LIM-bik SIS-tem)
[*limb-* **edge,** *-ic* **relating to**]

lumbar puncture
(LUM-bar)
[*lumb-* **loin,** *-ar* **relating to**]

medulla oblongata
(meh-DUL-ah ob-long-GAH-tah)
[*medulla* **marrow or pith,** *oblongata* **oblong**]

meninges
(meh-NIN-jeez)
sing., meninx
(meh-NINKS)
[*meninx* **membrane**]

microglia
(my-KROG-lee-ah)
sing., microglial cell
(my-KROG-lee-al sel)
[*micro-* **small,** *-glia* **glue**]

midbrain
(MID-brayn)
[*mid-* **middle,** *-brain* **skull**]

motor neuron
(MOH-ter NOO-ron)
[*mot-* **movement,** *-or* **agent,** *neuron* **nerve**]

multiple sclerosis (MS)
(MULT-ih-pul skleh-ROH-sis)
[*multi-* **many,** *-pl-* **fold,** *sclera-* **hard,** *-osis* **condition**]

myelin
(MY-eh-lin)
[*myel-* **marrow,** *-in* **substance**]

myelin disorder
(MY-eh-lin)
[*myel-* **marrow,** *-in* **substance**]

myelinated fiber
(MY-eh-lih-nay-ted FYE-ber)
[*myel-* **marrow,** *-in-* **substance,** *-ate* **act of,** *fibr-* **thread**]

nerve
(nerv)

neurilemma
(noo-rih-LEM-mah)
[*neuri-* **neuron,** *-lemma* **sheath**]

neuroglia
(noo-ROH-glee-ah or noo-roh-GLEE-ah)
sing., neuroglial cell
(noo-ROH-glee-al sel)
[*neur-* **nerve,** *-glia* **glue**]

neurologist
(noo-ROL-uh-jist)
[*neuro-* **nerve,** *-log-* **words (study of),** *-ist* **agent**]

neuron
(NOO-ron)
[*neuron* **string or nerve**]

neuroscientist
(noo-roh-SYE-en-tist)
[*neuro-* **nerve,** *-scien-* **knowledge,** *-ist* **agent**]

neurotransmitter
(noo-roh-tranz-MIT-ter)
[*neuro-* **nerve,** *-trans-* **across,** *-mitt-* **send,** *-er* **agent**]

nitric oxide (NO)
(NYE-trik AWK-syde)
[*nitr-* **nitrogen,** *-ic* **relating to,** *ox-* **oxygen,** *-ide* **chemical**]

nodes of Ranvier
(nohd of rahn-vee-AY)
[*nod-* **knot,** *Louis A. Ranvier,* **French pathologist**]

norepinephrine
(nor-ep-ih-NEF-rin)
[*nor-* **chemical prefix (unbranched C chain),** *-epi-* **upon,** *-nephr-* **kidney,** *-ine* **substance**]

oligodendrocyte
(ohl-ih-goh-DEN-droh-syte)
[*oligo-* **few,** *-dendr-* **part (branch) of,** *-cyte* **cell**]

paralysis
(pah-RAL-ih-sis)
[*para-* **beside,** *-lysis* **loosening**]

parasympathetic division
(payr-ah-sim-pah-THET-ik dih-VIZH-un)
[*para-* **beside,** *-sym-* **together,** *-pathe-* **feel,** *-ic* **relating to**]

parasympathetic postganglionic neuron
(payr-ah-sim-pah-THET-ik post-gang-glee-ON-ik NOO-ron)
[*para-* **beside,** *-sym-* **together,** *-pathe-* **feel,** *-ic* **relating to,** *post-* **after,** *-ganglion-* **knot,** *-ic* **relating to,** *neuron* **string or nerve**]

parasympathetic preganglionic neuron
(payr-ah-sim-pah-THET-ik pree-gang-glee-ON-ik NOO-ron)
[*para-* **beside,** *-sym-* **together,** *-pathe-* **feel,** *-ic* **relating to,** *pre-* **before,** *-ganglion-* **knot,** *-ic* **relating to,** *neuron* **string or nerve**]

Parkinson disease (PD)
(PARK-in-son)
[*James Parkinson* **English physician**]

perineurium
(payr-ih-NOO-ree-um)
[*peri-* **around,** *-neur-* **nerve,** *-um* **thing**]

peripheral nervous system (PNS)
(peh-RIF-er-al NER-vus SIS-tem)
[*peri-* **around,** *-phera-* **boundary,** *-al* **relating to,** *nerv-* **nerve,** *-ous* **relating to,** *system* **organized whole**]

pharmacist
(FAR-mah-sist)
[*pharmac-* **drug,** *-ist* **agent**]

pharmacologist
(far-mah-KAHL-oh-jist)
[*pharmaco-* **drug,** *-log-* **words (study of),** *-ist* **agent**]

pharmacy technician
(FAR-mah-see tek-NISH-en)
[*pharmac-* **drug,** *-y* **location of activity,** *techn-* **art or skill,** *-ic* **relating to,** *-ian* **practitioner**]

pia mater
(PEE-ah MAH-ter)
[*pia* **tender,** *mater* **mother**]

pineal gland
(PIN-ee-al gland)
[*pine-* **pine,** *-al* **relating to,** *gland* **acorn**]

plexus
(PLEK-sus)
[*plexus* **braid or network**]
pl., plexuses
(PLEK-sus-ez)

pons
(ponz)
[*pons* **bridge**]

postganglionic neuron
(post-gang-glee-ON-ik NOO-ron)
[*post-* **after,** *-ganglion-* **knot,** *-ic* **relating to,** *neuron* **nerve**]

postsynaptic neuron
(post-sih-NAP-tik NOO-ron)
[*post-* **after,** *-syn-* **together,** *-apt-* **join,** *-ic* **relating to,** *neuron* **nerve**]

preganglionic neuron
(pree-gang-glee-ON-ik NOO-ron)
[*pre-* **before,** *-ganglion-* **knot,** *-ic* **relating to,** *neuron* **nerve**]

presynaptic neuron
(pree-sih-NAP-tik NOO-ron)
[*pre-* **before,** *-syn-* **together,** *-apt-* **join,** *-ic* **relating to,** *neuron* **nerve**]

psychiatrist
(sye-KYE-ah-trist)
[*psych-* **mind,** *-iatr-* **treatment,** *-ist* **agent**]

psychologist
(sye-KOL-uh-jist)
[*psych-* **mind,** *-log-* **words (study of),** *-ist* **agent**]

receptor
(ree-SEP-tor)
[*recept-* **receive,** *-or* **agent**]

reflex
(REE-fleks)
[*re-* **again,** *-flex* **bend**]

reflex arc
(REE-fleks ark)
[*re-* **back or again,** *-flex* **bend,** *arc* **curve**]

reticular formation
(reh-TIK-yoo-lar)
[*ret-* **net,** *-ic-* **relating to,** *-ul-* **little,** *-ar* **characterized by**]

saltatory conduction
(SAL-tah-tor-ee kon-DUK-shun)
[*salta-* **leap,** *-ory* **relating to,** *con-* **with,** *-duct-* **lead,** *-ion* **process**]

Schwann cell
(shwon *or* shvon sel)
[*Theodor Schwann* **German anatomist,** *cell* **storeroom**]

sensory neuron
(SEN-sor-ee NOO-ron)
[*sens-* **feel,** *-ory* **relating to,** *neuron* **string or nerve**]

serotonin
(sair-oh-TOH-nin)
[*sero-* **watery body fluid,** *-ton-* **tension,** *-in* **substance**]

shingles
(SHING-gulz)
[from *cingulum* **girdle (inflammation often extends around the middle of the body, like a girdle)**]

spinal nerve
(SPY-nal nerv)
[*spin-* **backbone,** *-al* **relating to**]

spinal tract
(SPY-nal trakt)
[*spin-* **backbone,** *-al* **relating to,** *trac* **course or trail**]

sulci
(SUL-kye or SUL-kee)
sing., sulcus
[*sulcus* **furrow**]

sympathetic division
(sim-pah-THET-ik dih-VIZH-un)
[*sym-* **together,** *-pathe-* **feel,** *-ic* **relating to**]

sympathetic postganglionic neuron
(sim-pah-THET-ik post-gang-glee-ON-ik NOO-ron)
[*sym-* **together,** *-pathe-* **feel,** *-ic* **relating to,** *post-* **after,** *-ganglion-* **knot,** *-ic* **relating to,** *neuron* **string or nerve**]

sympathetic preganglionic neuron
(sim-pah-THET-ik pree-gang-glee-ON-ik NOO-ron)
[*sym-* **together,** *-pathe-* **feel,** *-ic* **relating to,** *pre-* **before,** *-ganglion-* **knot,** *-ic* **relating to,** *neuron* **string or nerve**]

synapse
(SIN-aps)
[*syn-* **together,** *-aps-* **join**]

synaptic cleft
(sin-AP-tik kleft)
[*syn-* **together,** *-apt-* **join,** *-ic* **relating to**]

synaptic knob
(sin-AP-tik nob)
[*syn-* **together,** *-apt-* **join,** *-ic* **relating to**]

thalamus
(THAL-ah-mus)
[*thalamus* **inner chamber**]

tract
(trakt)
[*trac-* **course or trail**]

ventricle
(VEN-trih-kul)
[*ventr-* **belly,** *-icle* **little**]

visceral effector
(VISS-er-al ee-FEK-tor)
[*viscer-* **internal organ,** *-al* **relating to,** *effect-* **accomplish,** *-or* **agent**]

white matter
(wyte MAT-ter)

withdrawal reflex
(with-DRAW-ul REE-fleks)
[*with-* **away,** *-draw-* **draw,** *-al* **relating to,** *re-* **again,** *-flex* **bend**]

❑ OUTLINE SUMMARY

*To download a digital audio version of the chapter summary for use with your device, access the **Audio Chapter Summaries** online at evolve.elsevier.com.*

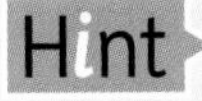

Scan this summary after reading the chapter to help you reinforce the key concepts. Later, use the summary as a quick review before your class or before a test.

Organization of the Nervous System (See Figure 9-1)

A. Central nervous system (CNS) — brain and spinal cord
B. Peripheral nervous system (PNS) — all nerves
C. Autonomic nervous system (ANS)

Cells of the Nervous System

A. Neurons
  1. Neuron structure
    a. Consist of three main parts — dendrites, cell body of neuron, and axon (see **Figure 9-2**)
      (1) Dendrites — branching projections that conduct impulses to cell body of neuron
      (2) Axon — elongated projection that conducts impulses *away* from cell body of neuron
        (a) Myelin — white, fatty substance formed by glia, surrounding some axons as a sheath
        (b) Nodes of Ranvier — gaps in the myelin sheath
        (c) Neurilemma — outer layer of myelin sheath needed for repair of damaged axons
  2. Neuron types are classified according to function
    a. Sensory (afferent) neurons — conduct impulses to the spinal cord and brain
    b. Motor (efferent) neurons — conduct impulses away from brain and spinal cord to muscles and glands
    c. Interneurons — conduct impulses from sensory neurons to motor neurons or among a network of interneurons; also known as *central* or *connecting neurons*
B. Glia (neuroglia)
  1. Function—support cells, bringing the cells of nervous tissue together structurally and functionally
  2. Central glia — three main types of glial cells of the CNS (see **Figure 9-3**)
    a. Astrocytes — star-shaped cells that anchor small blood vessels to neurons
    b. Microglia — small cells that move in inflamed brain tissue carrying on phagocytosis
    c. Oligodendrocytes — form myelin sheaths on axons in the CNS
  3. Peripheral glia—Schwann cells form myelin sheaths on axons of the PNS (see **Figure 9-2**)

Nerves and Tracts

A. Nerve — bundle of peripheral axons (see **Figure 9-4**)
B. Nerve coverings — fibrous connective tissue
  1. Endoneurium — surrounds individual fibers within a nerve
  2. Perineurium — surrounds a group (fascicle) of nerve fibers
  3. Epineurium — surrounds the entire nerve
C. Tract — bundle of central axons
  1. White matter — tissue composed primarily of myelinated axons (nerves or tracts)
  2. Gray matter — tissue composed primarily of cell bodies and unmyelinated fibers

Nerve Signals

A. Reflex arcs
  1. Nerve impulses are conducted from receptors to effectors over neuron pathways or reflex arcs; conduction by a reflex arc results in a reflex (that is, contraction by a muscle or secretion by a gland)
  2. The simplest reflex arcs are two-neuron arcs — consisting of sensory neurons synapsing in the spinal cord with motor neurons
  3. Three-neuron arcs consist of sensory neurons synapsing in the spinal cord with interneurons that synapse with motor neurons (see **Figure 9-5**)
B. Nerve impulses
  1. Definition — self-propagating wave of electrical disturbance that travels along the surface of a neuron membrane (also called *action potential*)
  2. Mechanism (see **Figure 9-6**)
    a. At rest, the neuron's membrane is slightly positive on the outside — polarized — from a slight excess of Na^+ on the outside
    b. A stimulus triggers the opening of Na^+ channels in the plasma membrane of the neuron
    c. Inward movement of Na^+ depolarizes the membrane by making the inside more positive than the outside at the stimulated point; this depolarization is a nerve impulse (action potential)
  3. Conduction of nerve impulses (see **Figure 9-7**)
    a. Continuous conduction—the stimulated section of membrane immediately repolarizes, but by that time the depolarization has already triggered the next section of membrane to depolarize, thus propagating a wave of electrical disturbances (depolarizations) all the way down the membrane
    b. Saltatory conduction—in myelinated fibers, conduction can "jump" from gap to gap and thus greatly speed up the rate of conduction
C. The synapse
  1. Definition — the place where impulses are transmitted from one neuron to another (the postsynaptic neuron) (see **Figure 9-8**)

2. Synapse made of three structures — synaptic knob, synaptic cleft, and plasma membrane
3. Neurotransmitters bind to specific receptor molecules in the membrane of a postsynaptic neuron, opening ion channels and thereby stimulating impulse conduction by the membrane
4. Names of neurotransmitters — acetylcholine, catecholamines (norepinephrine, dopamine, and serotonin), endorphins, enkephalins, nitric oxide (NO), and other compounds

Central Nervous System

A. Divisions of the brain (see **Figure 9-9**, **Figure 9-10**, and **Table 9-1**)
   1. Brainstem
      a. Consists of three parts of brain, named in ascending order: the medulla oblongata, pons, and midbrain
      b. Structure — white matter with bits of gray matter scattered through it
      c. Functions
         (1) All three parts of brainstem are two-way conduction paths
            (a) Sensory tracts in the brainstem conduct impulses to the higher parts of the brain
            (b) Motor tracts conduct from the higher parts of the brain to the spinal cord
         (2) Gray matter areas in the brainstem function as important reflex centers
   2. Cerebellum
      a. Structure
         (1) Second largest part of the human brain
         (2) Gray matter outer layer is thin but highly folded, forming a large surface area for processing information
         (3) *Arbor vitae* — internal, treelike network of white matter tracts
      b. Function
         (1) Helps control muscle contractions to produce coordinated movements so that we can maintain balance, move smoothly, and sustain normal postures
         (2) Variety of additional coordinating effects, assisting the cerebrum and other regions of the brain
   3. Diencephalon
      a. Hypothalamus
         (1) Consists mainly of the posterior pituitary gland, pituitary stalk, and gray matter
         (2) Acts as the major center for controlling the ANS; therefore, it helps control the functioning of most internal organs
         (3) Controls hormone secretion by anterior and posterior pituitary glands; therefore, it indirectly helps control hormone secretion by most other endocrine glands
         (4) Contains centers for controlling body temperature, appetite, wakefulness, and pleasure
      b. Thalamus
         (1) Dumbbell-shaped mass of gray matter extending toward each cerebral hemisphere
         (2) Relays sensory impulses to cerebral cortex sensory areas
         (3) In some way produces the emotions of pleasantness or unpleasantness associated with sensations
      c. Pineal gland (pineal body)
         (1) Small body resembling a pine nut behind the thalamus
         (2) Adjusts output of "timekeeping hormone" melatonin in response to changing levels of external light (sunlight and moonlight)
   4. Cerebrum (see **Figure 9-11**)
      a. Largest part of the human brain
      b. Outer layer of gray matter is the cerebral cortex; made up of lobes; composed mainly of dendrites and cell bodies of neurons
      c. Interior of the cerebrum composed mainly of white matter
         (1) Tracts — nerve fibers arranged in bundles
         (2) Basal nuclei — islands of gray matter regulate automatic movements and posture
      d. Functions of the cerebrum — mental processes of all types, including sensations, consciousness, memory, and voluntary control of movements

B. Spinal cord (see **Figure 9-12**)
   1. Columns of white matter, composed of bundles of myelinated nerve fibers, form the outer portion of the H-shaped core of the spinal cord; bundles of axons called *tracts* (see **Figure 9-13**)
   2. Interior composed of gray matter made up mainly of neuron dendrites and cell bodies
   3. Spinal cord tracts provide two-way conduction paths — ascending and descending
   4. Spinal cord functions as the primary center for all spinal cord reflexes; sensory tracts conduct impulses to the brain, and motor tracts conduct impulses from the brain

C. Coverings and fluid spaces of the brain and spinal cord
   1. Meninges and bone (see **Figure 9-14** and **Figure 9-16**)
      a. Cerebral and spinal meninges
         (1) Dura mater—tough outer membrane
         (2) Arachnoid mater—cobweblike middle layer
         (3) Pia mater—delicate inner layer adhering to brain and spinal cord
      b. Cranial bones and vertebrae form hard outer covering
   2. Cerebrospinal fluid spaces (see **Figure 9-15** and **Figure 9-16**)
      a. Subarachnoid spaces of meninges
      b. Central canal inside cord
      c. Ventricles in brain

Peripheral Nervous System

A. Cranial nerves (see **Figure 9-17** and **Table 9-2**)
   1. Twelve pairs — attached to undersurface of the brain
   2. Connect brain with the neck and structures in the thorax and abdomen
B. Spinal nerves
   1. Thirty-one pairs — contain dendrites of sensory neurons and axons of motor neurons
   2. Conduct impulses necessary for sensations and voluntary movements
C. Dermatome — skin surface area supplied by a single cranial or spinal nerve (see **Figure 9-18**)

Autonomic Nervous System

A. Functional anatomy
   1. Autonomic nervous system — motor neurons that conduct impulses from the CNS to cardiac muscle, smooth muscle, and glandular epithelial tissue; regulates the body's automatic or involuntary functions (see **Figure 9-19**)
   2. Autonomic neurons — preganglionic autonomic neurons conduct from spinal cord or brainstem to an autonomic ganglion; postganglionic neurons conduct from autonomic ganglia to cardiac muscle, smooth muscle, and glandular epithelial tissue
   3. Autonomic or visceral effectors — tissues to which autonomic neurons conduct impulses (that is, cardiac and smooth muscle and glandular epithelial tissue)
   4. Composed of two divisions — the sympathetic system and the parasympathetic system
B. Autonomic conduction paths (see **Figure 9-20**)
   1. Consist of two-neuron relays (that is, preganglionic neurons from the CNS to autonomic ganglia, synapses, postganglionic neurons from ganglia to visceral effectors)
   2. In contrast, somatic motor neurons conduct all the way from the CNS to somatic effectors with no intervening synapses
C. Sympathetic division
   1. Dendrites and cell bodies of sympathetic preganglionic neurons are located in the gray matter of the thoracic and upper lumbar segments of the spinal cord
   2. Axons leave the spinal cord in the anterior roots of spinal nerves, extend to sympathetic or collateral ganglia, and synapse with several postganglionic neurons whose axons extend to spinal or autonomic nerves to terminate in visceral effectors
   3. A chain of sympathetic ganglia is in front of and at each side of the spinal column
   4. Functions of the sympathetic division
      a. Serves as the emergency or stress system, controlling visceral effectors during strenuous exercise and when strong emotions (anger, fear, hate, or anxiety) are triggered
      b. Group of changes induced by sympathetic control is called the *fight-or-flight response*
D. Parasympathetic division
   1. Structure
      a. Parasympathetic preganglionic neurons have dendrites and cell bodies in the gray matter of the brainstem and the sacral segments of the spinal cord
      b. Parasympathetic preganglionic neurons terminate in parasympathetic ganglia located in the head and the thoracic and abdominal cavities close to visceral effectors
      c. Each parasympathetic preganglionic neuron synapses with postganglionic neurons to only one effector
   2. Function—dominates control of many visceral effectors under normal, everyday conditions; counterbalances sympathetic function
E. Autonomic neurotransmitters (see **Figure 9-21**)
   1. Cholinergic fibers — preganglionic axons of parasympathetic and sympathetic systems and parasympathetic postganglionic axons release acetylcholine
   2. Adrenergic fibers — axons of sympathetic postganglionic neurons release norepinephrine (noradrenaline)
F. Autonomic nervous system as a whole (see **Table 9-3**)
   1. Regulates the body's automatic functions in ways that maintain or quickly restore homeostasis
   2. Many visceral effectors are doubly innervated (that is, they receive fibers from parasympathetic and sympathetic divisions and are influenced in opposite ways by the two divisions)

❑ ACTIVE LEARNING

STUDY TIPS

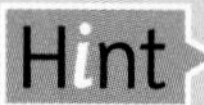

Use these tips to achieve success in meeting your learning goals.

To make the study of the nervous system more efficient, we suggest these tips:

1. Before studying Chapter 9, review the synopsis of the nervous system in Chapter 5.
2. Keep in mind that the nervous system functions as one organized system. The function of the nervous system involves two major processes: conduction of nerve impulses and passing of the nerve impulse across a synapse. Nerve impulses are an exchange of ions between the interior and exterior of the neuron.
3. The synapse requires the production, release, and deactivation of neurotransmitters. Neurotransmitters function by stimulating receptors in the neuron on the other side of the synapse.
4. The material on the central nervous system can be learned best by using flash cards that match up structure and function. Use online resources that provide tutorials and animations (for example, *getbodysmart.com*).
5. Use mnemonics (memory aids) to help you remember cranial nerves and other structures or functions. See *my-ap.us/12WL7BI* for tips.
6. In your study group, you should go over the terms presented in the first part of the chapter. Review the Language of Science and Medicine terms and their word origins to help you better understand the meaning of the nervous system terms. Discuss the processes of nerve impulse transmission and what occurs at the synapse. Review the flash cards with the names and functions of the parts of the central nervous system. Remember that most of the structures in the central nervous system have more than one function. If you learn the general functions of the sympathetic and parasympathetic divisions now, the specific effects you will see in later chapters will be easier to remember.

Review Questions

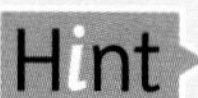

Write out the answers to these questions after reading the chapter and reviewing the Chapter Summary. If you simply think through the answer without writing it down, you won't retain much of your new learning.

1. Draw and label the three parts of the neuron and explain the function of the dendrite and axon.
2. Name the three types of neurons classified according to the direction in which the impulse is transmitted. Define and explain each of them.
3. Define or explain the following terms: *myelin*, *node of Ranvier*, and *neurilemma*.
4. Provide the name and list the function of the three types of central glia cells.
5. Provide the name and list the function of the peripheral glia cells.
6. Define or explain the following terms: *epineurium*, *perineurium*, and *endoneurium*.
7. Explain the difference between gray matter and white matter.
8. Explain how a reflex arc functions. Name two types of reflex arc.
9. Explain what occurs during a nerve impulse. Describe what occurs during *saltatory conduction*.
10. Explain fully what occurs at a synapse. Explain the two ways in which neurotransmitter activity is terminated.
11. Describe and list the functions of the medulla oblongata.
12. Describe and list the functions of the hypothalamus.
13. Describe and list the functions of the thalamus.
14. Describe and list the functions of the cerebellum.
15. Name the general functions of the cerebrum. List the specific functions of the occipital and temporal lobes.
16. Describe and list the functions of the spinal cord.
17. Name and describe the three layers of the meninges.
18. Describe the function of cerebrospinal fluid and where it is produced.
19. Provide the number of nerve pairs that are generated from each section of the spinal cord and explain how they are named. Describe a plexus.
20. Explain the structure and function of the sympathetic nervous system.
21. Explain the structure and function of the parasympathetic nervous system.
22. Explain the "emotional brain."

Critical Thinking

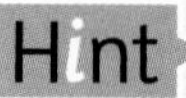

After finishing the Review Questions, write out the answers to these more in-depth questions to help you apply your new knowledge. Go back to sections of the chapter that relate to concepts that you find difficult.

23. Compare the functional regions of the frontal, parietal, occipital, and temporal lobes.
24. Which of the cranial nerves deals primarily with motor function? Which deal primarily with sensory function?

25. There is a type of medication that inhibits the functioning of acetylcholinesterase (the enzyme that deactivates acetylcholine). Explain the side effects the medication would have on the visceral effectors.
26. Olivia was speaking at a luncheon. She had her regular breakfast of toast, juice and coffee. She admits to being slightly nervous and she has no appetite for lunch. She is also slightly nauseated. Be specific and cite some possible reason for Olivia's symptoms from your knowledge of the nervous system.

Chapter Test

Hint *After studying the chapter, test your mastery by responding to these items. Try to answer them without looking up the answers. Then, verify the answers using the key in Appendix C at the back of this book.*

1. _____ is the name of the nervous system division that includes the nerves that extend to the outlying parts of the body.
2. _____ is the name of the nervous system division that includes the brain and spinal cord.
3. A group of peripheral axons bundled together in an epineurium is called a _____.
4. The two types of cells found in the nervous system are _____ and _____.
5. The knee jerk is of a type of neural pathway called a _____
6. _____ is a self-propagating wave of electrical disturbance that travels along the surface of a neuron's plasma membrane.
7. The exterior of a resting neuron has a slight _____ charge, whereas the interior has a slight _____ charge.
8. During a nerve impulse, _____ is the ion that rushes into the neuron.
9. The _____ is the place where impulses are passed from one neuron to another.
10. Acetylcholine and dopamine are examples of _____, which are chemicals used by neurons to communicate.
11. _____, _____, and _____ are the three membranes that make up the meninges.
12. There are _____ pairs of cranial nerves and _____ pairs of nerves that come from the spinal cord.
13. _____ are skin surface areas supplied by a single spinal nerve.
14. _____ is the part of the autonomic nervous system that regulates effectors during nonstress conditions.
15. _____ is the part of the autonomic nervous system that regulates the "fight-or-flight" response.
16. The preganglionic axons of the sympathetic nervous system release the neurotransmitter _____. The postganglionic axons release _____
17. The preganglionic axons of the parasympathetic nervous system release the neurotransmitter _____. The postganglionic axons release _____.
18. The autonomic nervous system consists of neurons that conduct impulses from the brain or spinal cord to _____ tissue, _____ tissue, and _____ tissue.

Match each function or description in Column B with the correct term in Column A.

Column A

19. _____ dendrite
20. _____ axon
21. _____ myelin
22. _____ Schwann cells
23. _____ astrocytes
24. _____ microglia
25. _____ oligodendrocyte
26. _____ medulla oblongata
27. _____ pons
28. _____ midbrain
29. _____ hypothalamus
30. _____ thalamus
31. _____ cerebellum
32. _____ cerebrum
33. _____ spinal cord

Column B

a. cells that make myelin for axons outside the CNS
b. glia cells that help form the blood-brain barrier
c. a single projection that carries nerve impulses away from the cell body
d. cells that make myelin for axons inside the CNS
e. a white fatty substance that surrounds and insulates the axon
f. cells that act as microbe-eating scavengers in the CNS
g. a highly branched part of the neuron that carries impulses toward the cell body
h. part of the brainstem that is a conduction pathway between areas of the brain and body; influences respiration
i. sensory relay station from various body areas to the cerebral cortex; also involved with emotions and alerting and arousal mechanisms
j. carries messages to and from the brain to the rest of the body; also mediates reflexes
k. part of the brainstem that contains cardiac, respiratory, and vasomotor centers
l. sensory perception, willed movements, consciousness, and memory are mediated here
m. regulates body temperature, water balance, sleep-wake cycles, appetite, and sexual arousal
n. regulates muscle coordination, maintenance of equilibrium, and posture
o. part of the brainstem that contains relays for visual and auditory impulses

Senses

OUTLINE

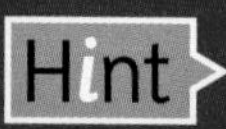

Scan this outline before you begin to read the chapter, as a preview of how the concepts are organized.

OBJECTIVES

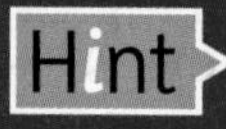

Before reading the chapter, review these goals for your learning.

After you have completed this chapter, you should be able to:

1. Classify sense organs as general or special and explain the basic differences between the two groups.
2. Discuss how a stimulus is converted into a sensation.
3. Discuss the general sense organs and their functions.
4. Describe the structure of the eye and the functions of its components.
5. Discuss the anatomy of the ear and its sensory function in hearing and equilibrium.
6. Describe the anatomy of the tongue and its sensory function in taste.
7. Describe the anatomy of the nasal cavity and its sensory function in smell.
8. Discuss how senses are integrated.

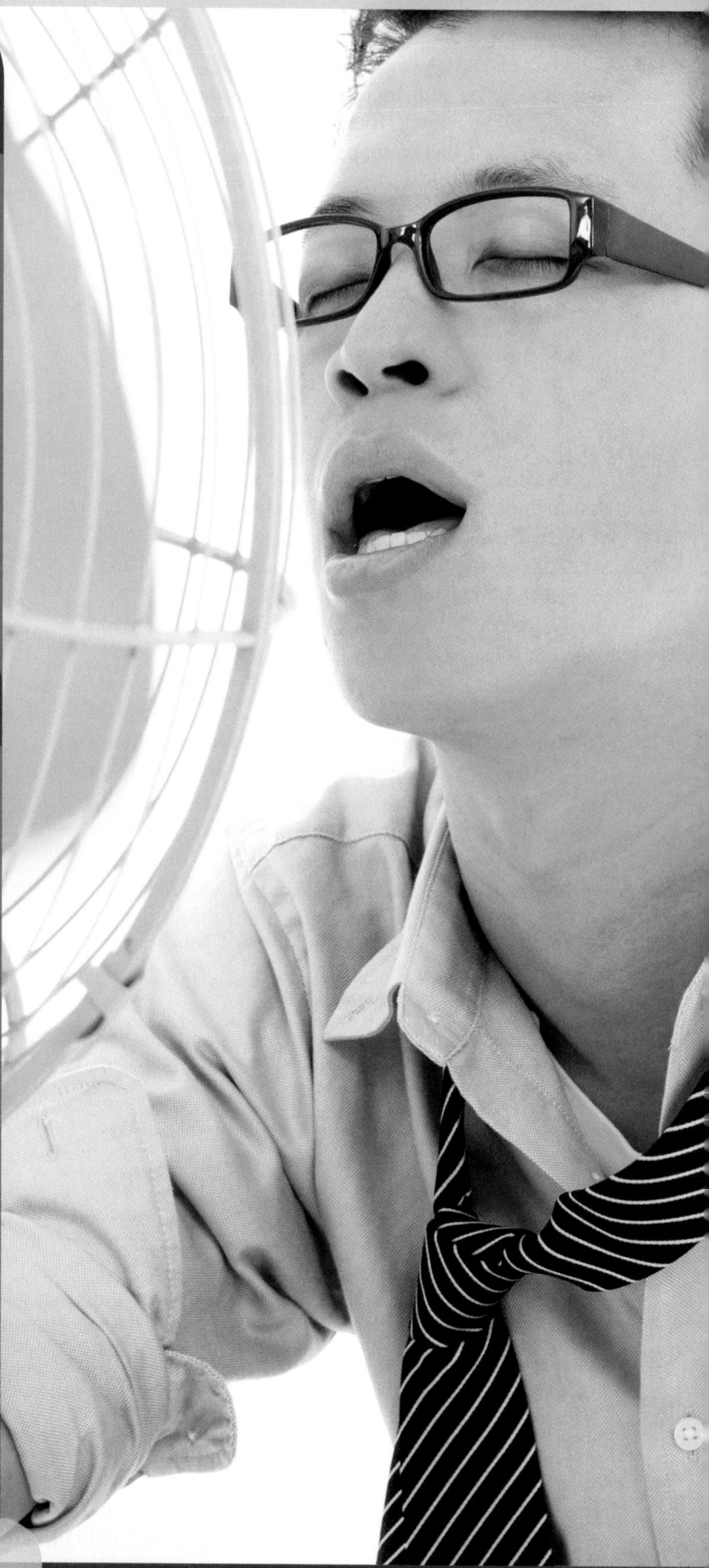

CHAPTER 10

If you were asked to name the sense organs, what organs would you name? Can you think of any besides the eyes, ears, nose, and taste buds? Actually there are millions of other sense organs throughout the body in our skin, internal organs, and muscles. They constitute the many *sensory receptors* that allow us to respond to stimuli such as touch, pressure, temperature, and pain. These microscopic receptors are located at the tips of dendrites of sensory neurons.

Our ability to detect changes in our external and internal environments is a requirement for maintaining homeostasis and for survival itself. We can initiate protective reflexes important to homeostasis only if we can *sense* a change or danger.

External dangers may be detected by sight or hearing. If the danger is internal, such as overstretching a muscle, detecting an increase in body temperature (fever), or sensing the pain caused by an ulcer, other receptors make us aware of the problem and permit us to take appropriate action to maintain homeostasis.

Classification of Senses

The senses are often classified as either **general senses** or **special senses.**

LANGUAGE OF **SCIENCE** AND **MEDICINE**

Hint Before reading the chapter, say each of these terms out loud. This will help you to avoid stumbling over them as you read.

adaptation
(ad-ap-TAY-shun)
[*adapt-* **fit to,** *-tion* **process**]

aqueous humor
(AY-kwee-us HYOO-mer)
[*aqu-* **water,** *-ous* **relating to,** *humor* **body fluid**]

audiologist
(aw-dee-OL-oh-jist)
[*audio-* **hear,** *-log-* **words (study of),** *-ist* **agent**]

auditory tube (eustachian tube)
(AW-dih-toh-ree toob [yoo-STAY-shun toob])
[*audit-* **hear,** *-ory* **relating to,** (*Bartolomeo Eustachio* **Italian anatomist**), *-an* **relating to**]

auricle
(AW-rih-kul)
[*auri-* **ear,** *-icle* **little**]

bony labyrinth
(BOHN-ee LAB-eh-rinth)
[*labyrinth* **maze**]

cataract
(KAT-ah-rakt)
[*cataract* **waterfall**]

cerumen
(seh-ROO-men)
[*cer(a)-* **wax,** *-men* **formed of**]

ceruminous gland
(seh-ROO-mih-nus gland)
[*cer(a)-* **wax,** *-min-* **formed of,** *-ous* **relating to,** *gland*]

chemoreceptor
(kee-moh-ree-SEP-tor)
[*chemo-* **chemical,** *-recept-* **receive,** *-or* **agent**]

choroid
(KOH-royd)
[*chor-* **skin,** *-oid* **like**]

Continued on p. 229

General Senses

The *general senses* are those detected by rather simple, microscopic receptors that are widely distributed throughout the body in the skin, muscles, tendons, joints, and other internal organs of the body. They are responsible for such sensations as pain, temperature, touch, pressure, and body position.

Special Senses

The special senses are those detected by receptors that are grouped in specific areas and associated with complex structures that facilitate these senses. The senses of smell, taste, vision, hearing, and equilibrium are considered special senses because their receptors are grouped within distinct structures that enhance their function.

Sensory Receptor Types

Individual receptor cells are often identified structurally according to whether they are *encapsulated* or *unencapsulated*, that is, whether they are covered by some sort of capsule or are "free" or "naked" of any such covering.

Sensory receptor cells are also classified functionally by the types, or *modes*, of stimuli that activate them:

1. **Photoreceptors**—sensitive to change in intensity or color of light, as in vision
2. **Chemoreceptors**—sensitive to presence of certain chemicals, as in taste or smell
3. **Pain receptors**—sensitive to physical injury
4. **Thermoreceptors**—sensitive to changes in temperature
5. **Mechanoreceptors**—sensitive to mechanical stimuli that change their position or shape

TABLE 10-1 General Sense Organs

TYPE	MAIN LOCATION	GENERAL SENSES
Free Nerve Endings (Naked Nerve Endings)		
	Skin and mucosa (epithelial layers)	Pain, crude touch, temperature, itch, tickle
Encapsulated Nerve Endings		
Tactile corpuscle (Meissner corpuscle)	Skin (in papillae of dermis) and fingertips and lips (numerous)	Fine or light touch and low-frequency vibration
Ruffini corpuscle (bulbous corpuscle)	Skin (dermal layer) and subcutaneous tissue of fingers	Persistent touch and pressure
Lamellar corpuscle (Pacini corpuscle)	Subcutaneous, submucous, and subserous tissues; around joints, in mammary glands, and external genitals of both sexes	Deep pressure and high-frequency vibration
Bulboid corpuscle (Krause end bulb)	Skin (dermal layer), subcutaneous tissue, mucosa of lips and eyelids, and external genitals	Touch
Golgi tendon organ	Near junction of tendons and muscles	Proprioception (sense of muscle tension)
Muscle spindle	Skeletal muscles	Proprioception (sense of muscle length)

Table 10-1 identifies the general sense organs as either free nerve endings or one of the six types of encapsulated nerve endings, whereas Table 10-2 identifies the type of receptor cells in the special sense organs that are stimulated by specific types of stimuli.

Sensory Pathways

All sense organs, regardless of size, type, or location, have in common some important functional characteristics. First, they must be able to sense or detect a stimulus or a change in the quality or intensity of a particular stimulus in their environment. Next, detection of a stimulus must be converted into a nerve impulse. This signal is then conducted over a nervous system "pathway" to the brain, where the incoming information is filtered and sorted—often comparing it to information coming in along other sensory pathways. Only after all of this processing of information is the sensation actually perceived in the brain.

The sensory pathway for the general senses typically involves conduction of action potentials generated in the receptors through the spinal cord to the thalamus (cutaneous or skin receptors) or cerebellum (proprioceptors) where they synapse, and impulses are then relayed to specific areas of the cerebral cortex for conscious sensory interpretation.

The sensory pathways for the special senses are varied, but also ultimately end in specific sensory areas of the cerebral cortex.

General Senses

Distribution of General Sense Receptors

Microscopic general sense organ receptors are found in almost every part of the body but they are most concentrated in the skin (Figure 10-1). However, these receptors are not evenly distributed over the body surface or in the internal organs. Also, they do not all respond to the same type of stimulus. To demonstrate this, try touching any point of your skin on a fingertip with the tip of a toothpick. You can hardly miss stimulating at least one receptor and almost instantaneously experiencing a sensation of touch.

The ability to distinguish one touch stimulus from two is called *two-point discrimination.* A neurological test that measures this function involves simultaneously touching two points on the skin over one area of the body to determine whether the ability to feel the two separate stimuli is present. The skin over different parts of the body will respond differently because of the differing numbers of touch receptors that are present.

Touch receptors are distributed closely together over the fingertips (2 to 8 mm apart), relatively close together over the palms (8 to 12 mm), and quite far apart over the back of the torso (40 to 60 mm). Lesions to the parietal lobe of the brain will impair two-point discrimination.

TABLE 10-2 Special Sense Organs

SENSE ORGAN	SPECIFIC RECEPTOR	TYPE OF RECEPTOR	SENSE
Eye	Rods and cones	Photoreceptor	Vision
Ear	Organ of Corti (spiral organ)	Mechanoreceptor	Hearing
	Cristae ampullares	Mechanoreceptor	Dynamic equilibrium
	Maculae	Mechanoreceptor	Static equilibrium
Nose	Olfactory cells	Chemoreceptor	Smell
Taste buds	Gustatory cells	Chemoreceptor	Taste

Modes of Sensation

Stimulation of general sensory receptors can lead to a variety of sensations. The difference in what kind of stimuli is detected is called the **mode** of the sensation. Different general sensory receptors can detect vibration, deep pressure, light pressure, pain, stretch, or temperature.

Examples of general sensory receptors of various modes are listed in Table 10-1 and illustrated in Figure 10-1.

Some general sensory receptors found near the point of junction between tendons and muscles and others found deep within skeletal muscle tissue are called **proprioceptors.** When stimulated by stretch, these mechanoreceptors provide us with information concerning the position or movement of the different parts of the body as well as the length and the extent of contraction of our muscles.

The Golgi tendon receptors and muscle spindles identified in Table 10-1 are important proprioceptors.

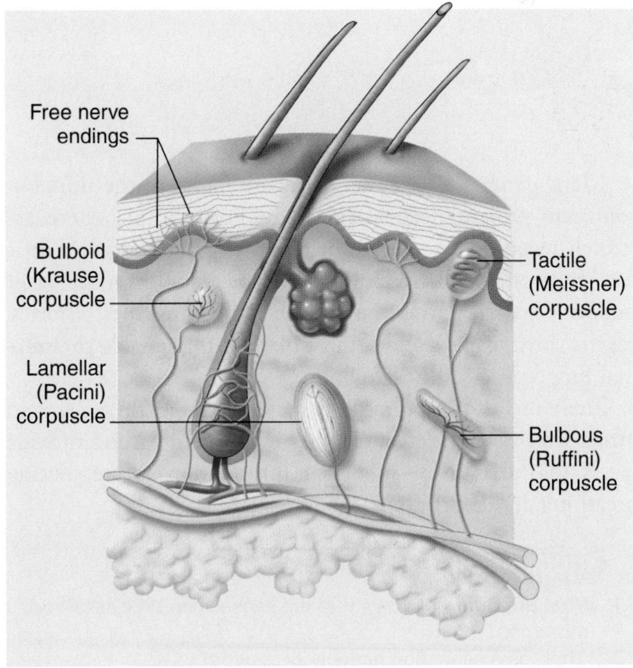

FIGURE 10-1 General sense receptors. This section of skin shows the placement of some of the receptors described in Table 10-1.

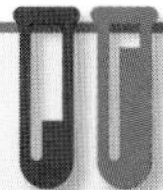

CLINICAL APPLICATION

REFERRED PAIN

The stimulation of pain receptors in deep structures may be felt as pain in the skin that lies over the affected organ or in an area of skin on the body surface far removed from the site of disease or injury. **Referred pain** is the term for this phenomenon.

The cause of referred pain is related to a convergence of sensory nerve impulses from both the diseased organ and the skin in the area of referred pain. For example, pain originating in an organ deep in the abdominal cavity is often interpreted as coming from an area of skin whose sensory fibers enter the same segment of the spinal cord as the sensory fibers from the deep structure.

A classic example is the referred pain often associated with a heart attack. Sensory fibers from the skin on the chest over the heart and from the tissue of the heart itself enter the first to the fifth thoracic spinal cord segments and so do sensory fibers from the skin areas over the left shoulder and inner surface of the left arm. Part *A* of the figure shows the primary sensory fibers from both the skin and heart converging in the spinal cord. Sensory impulses from both these areas travel to the brain over a common pathway—the secondary sensory fiber. Thus the brain may locate the pain of a heart attack in the shoulder or arm (part *B* of the figure).

Misinterpretation in the brain in regard to the true location of sensory neurons being stimulated causes referred pain. In clinical medicine, an understanding of referred pain can be an important determinant in whether the correct diagnosis of disease is made (see figure).

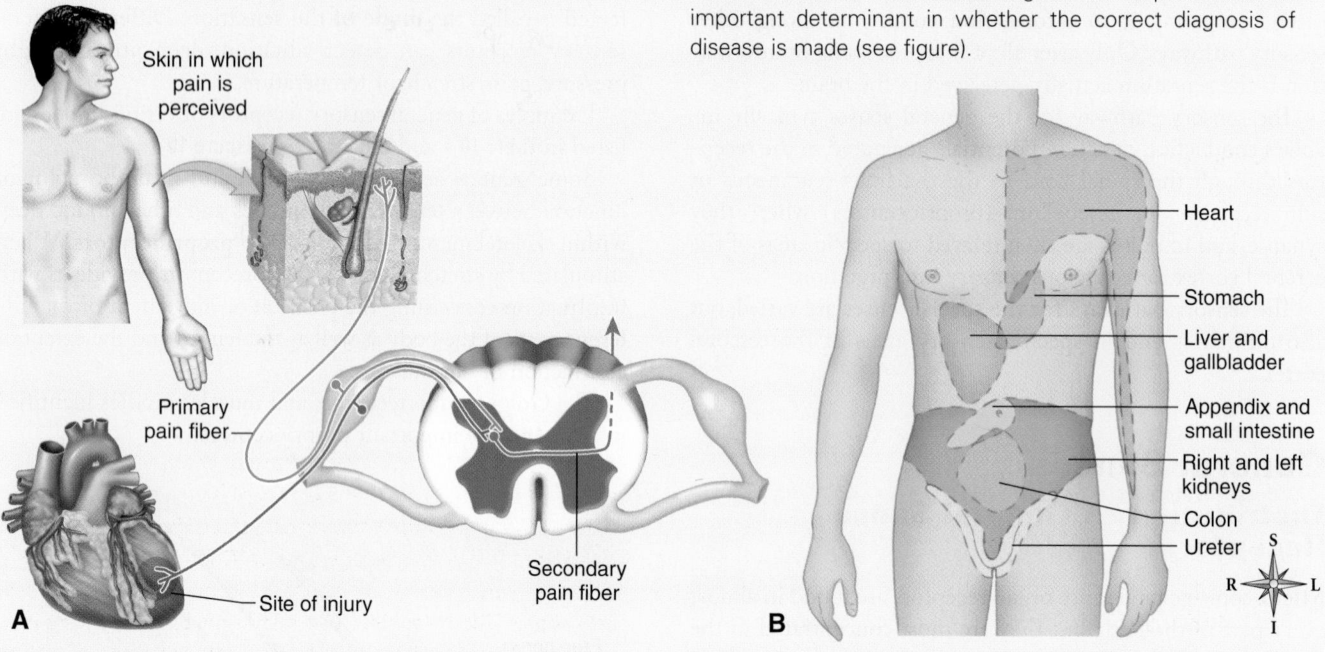

Many general sensory receptors are found in the skin, but some are present deep in the body. For example, there are stretch receptors in your stomach that signal you when it is full. There are also stretch (pressure) receptors in most other hollow organs such as the stomach and intestines, arteries, vagina (birth canal), and urinary bladder that enable the normal functioning of those organs.

There are also important chemoreceptors in the aorta and other arteries that detect changes in pH and carbon dioxide levels in the blood—important information for regulating breathing and heart rate.

QUICK CHECK

1. What are different ways that the senses can be classified into types?
2. Where is a sensation actually perceived?
3. What is the function of a *proprioceptor?*
4. What is *two-point discrimination?*

Special Senses

Vision

Vision detects the color and intensity of light in our external environment. But when focused by the eyes and processed by the brain, it can do much more. For example, we can recognize the outlines and depth of objects, analyze movement, and determine distances. In this section, we discuss that complex and amazing tool of vision—the eye.

Structure and Function of the Eye

When you look at a person's eye, you see only a small part of the whole eye. As you can see in **Figure 10-2**, the eyeball is a fluid-filled sphere having a wall of three layers:

1. Fibrous layer
   - Sclera
   - Cornea

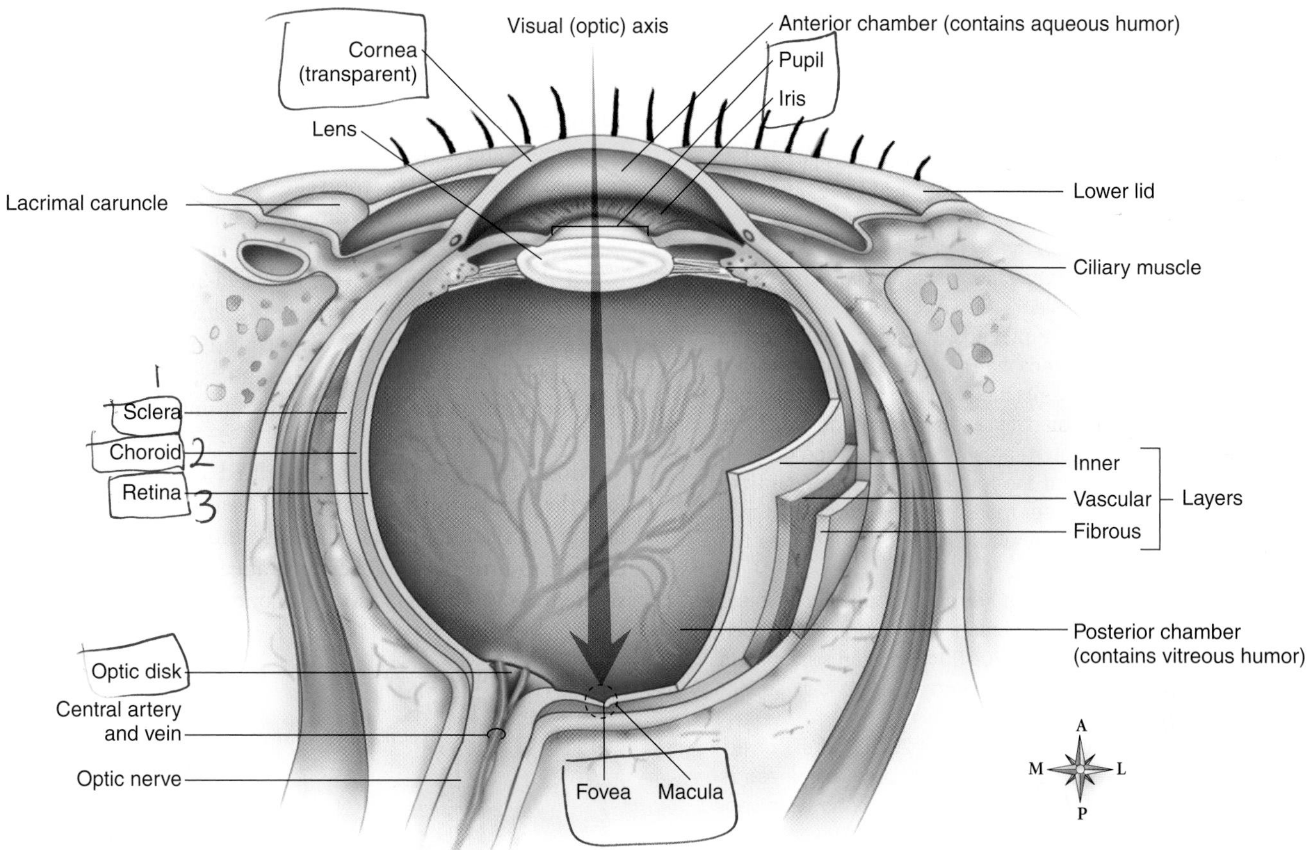

FIGURE 10-2 Eye. This transverse (horizontal) section through the left eyeball is shown as if viewed from above.

2. Vascular layer
   - Choroid
   - Ciliary muscle
   - Iris
   - Lens
3. Inner layer
   - Retina
   - Optic nerve
   - Retinal blood vessels

Fibrous Layer

The *fibrous layer* of the eyeball consists of tough fibrous tissue.

The "white" of the eye is part of the fibrous layer called the **sclera.** The sclera, made white by its dense bundles of collagen fibers, forms most of the fibrous layer.

The transparent circle on the anterior of the fibrous layer is called the **cornea.** The cornea is sometimes spoken of as the window of the eye because of its transparency.

Inflammation of the cornea is called *keratitis.* In addition to possible loss of transparency that may result from inflammation, any change in the shape of the cornea can dramatically change the ability of the eye to focus an image on the retina.

The fact that the shape of the cornea affects the eye's focus explains the popularity of surgical procedures that use lasers or other specialty instruments to "sculpt" and change the shape of the cornea. The result is improvement of many visual problems without the use of eyeglasses or contact lenses.

A mucous membrane known as the **conjunctiva** lines the eyelids and covers the fibrous layer in front. The blood vessels you see on the surface of the sclera actually belong to the conjunctiva. Inflammation of this important membrane is called *conjunctivitis* and is most often caused by bacterial or viral infection, allergy, or environmental factors. The conjunctiva is kept moist by tears secreted by the **lacrimal gland.**

Vascular Layer

The middle layer of the eyeball is called the *vascular layer* because it has a dense network of blood vessels.

Most of the vascular layer is made up of the **choroid,** which contains a large amount of the dark pigment *melanin.* This almost-black layer helps prevent the scattering of incoming light rays, which could make it hard for the eye to focus an image.

Several involuntary muscles make up the anterior part of the choroid. Some are in the **iris,** the colored structure seen through the cornea. The iris may appear blue, green, brown, gray, or some combination of these colors when seen through the transparent cornea because of the pigments in this layer of the eyeball.

The black center of the iris is really a hole in this doughnut-shaped muscle—it is the **pupil** of the eye. Some of the fibers

CLINICAL APPLICATION

VISUAL ACUITY

Visual acuity is the clearness or sharpness of visual perception. Acuity is affected by our focusing ability, the efficiency of the retina, and the proper function of the visual pathway and processing centers in the brain.

One common way to measure visual acuity is to use the familiar test chart on which letters or other objects of various sizes and shapes are printed. The subject is asked to identify the smallest object that he or she can see from a distance of 20 feet (6.1 m). The resulting determination of visual acuity is expressed as a double number such as "20-20." The first number represents the distance (in feet) between the subject and the test chart—the standard being 20. The second number represents the number of feet a person with normal acuity would have to stand to see the same objects clearly.

Thus a finding of 20-20 is normal because the subject can see at 20 feet what a person with normal acuity can see at 20 feet. A person with 20-100 vision can see objects at 20 feet that a person with normal vision can see at 100 feet.

People whose acuity is worse than 20-200 after correction are considered to be legally blind. Legal blindness is the designation used to identify the severity of a wide variety of visual disorders so that laws that involve visual acuity can be enforced. For example, laws that govern the awarding of driving licenses often require that drivers have a minimum level of visual acuity.

Smaller charts, such as the one shown in the figure, can be used to test near vision acuity.

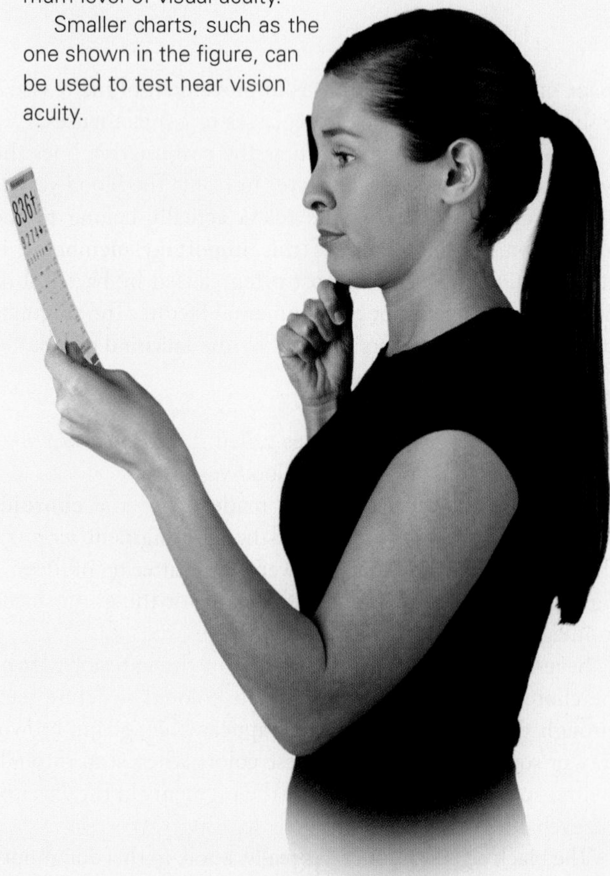

of the iris are arranged like spokes in a wheel. When they contract, the pupils dilate, letting in more light rays. Other fibers are circular. When they contract, the pupils constrict, letting in fewer light rays. Normally, the pupils constrict in bright light and dilate in dim light. **Figure 10-3** shows how these muscles work under the control of autonomic nerves.

The **lens** of the eye lies directly behind the pupil. It is held in place by a ligament attached to an involuntary muscle called the **ciliary muscle** (see **Figure 10-2**). When we look at distant objects, the ciliary muscle is relaxed, and the lens has only a slightly curved shape. To focus on near objects, the ciliary muscle must contract. As it contracts, it pulls the choroid coat forward toward the lens, thus causing the lens to bulge and curve even more.

Most of us become more farsighted as we grow older and lose the ability to focus on close objects because our lenses lose at least some of their elasticity and can no longer bulge enough to bring near objects into focus. **Presbyopia** or "oldsightedness" is the name for this condition.

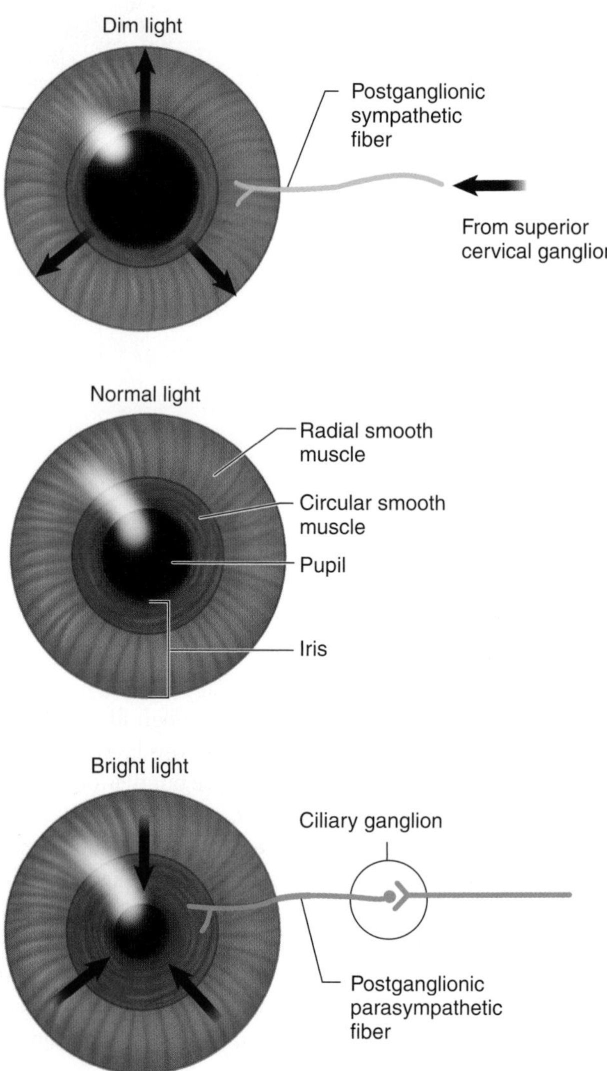

FIGURE 10-3 Control of pupil. This diagram of the muscular parts of the iris shows autonomic nerves stimulating radial muscles to dilate the pupil *(top)* and stimulating circular muscle to constrict the pupil *(bottom)*.

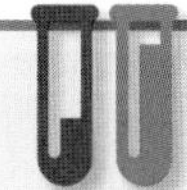

FIGURE 10-4 Cells of the retina. Photoreceptors called *rods* and *cones* (notice their shapes) detect changes in light and relay the information to bipolar neurons. The bipolar cells, in turn, conduct the information to ganglion cells. The information leaves the eye by way of the optic nerve.

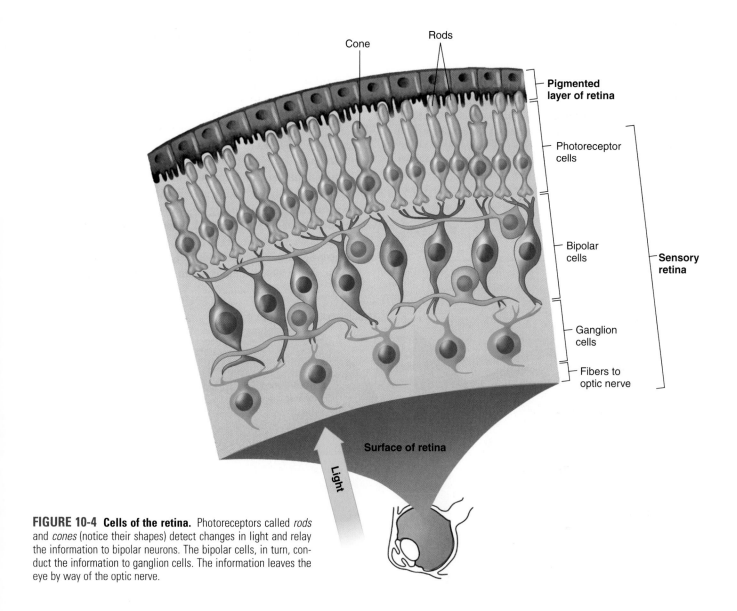

In most young people, the lens is both transparent and somewhat elastic so that it is capable of changing shape. Unfortunately, in some individuals, long-time exposure to ultraviolet (UV) radiation in sunlight may cause the lens to become hard, lose its transparency, and become "milky" in appearance. This condition is called a **cataract.** Cataract formation may occur in one or both eyes. Once it begins, cataract formation tends to be progressive and may result in blindness. Cataracts can be removed surgically and the defective lens replaced with an artificial implant.

Inner Layer

The **retina** makes up most of the *inner layer* of the eyeball. It contains microscopic photoreceptor cells to detect light (**Figure 10-4**). Most of these receptor cells are called *rods* and *cones* because of their shapes. Dim light of various wavelengths—or colors—can stimulate the rods, giving us monochrome (colorless) vision when lighting is low. However, fairly bright light is necessary to stimulate the cones. In other

CLINICAL APPLICATION

MACULAR DEGENERATION

A serious and widespread visual problem affecting more than 1.5 million Americans over age 65 is called *age-related macular degeneration,* or *AMD.* The most common type of AMD (about 85% of cases) is called "dry" AMD. In these individuals, as the macular area of the retina degenerates and the disease progresses over time, the central visual field is gradually lost and the ability to distinguish fine detail diminishes. Although total blindness seldom occurs and varying amounts of peripheral vision remain, AMD patients are unable to read or drive and other daily activities are severely restricted because of the loss of clear "straight-ahead" sight. A less common (10% to 15% of cases) but more severe type of AMD is called "wet" AMD. In these patients, fragile and leaking blood vessels damage the retina over the macula lutea, and rapid loss of central vision may occur.

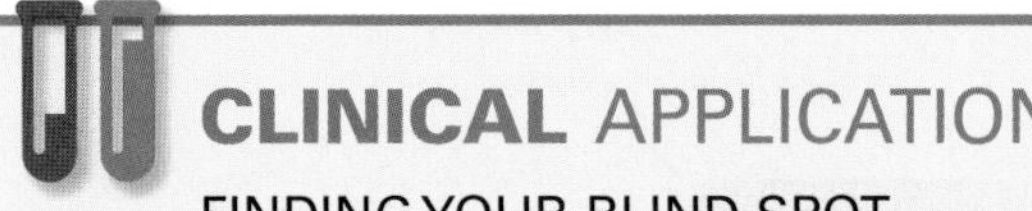

CLINICAL APPLICATION

FINDING YOUR BLIND SPOT

Demonstrate the location of the blind spot in your visual field by covering your left eye and looking at the objects below. While staring at the block, begin about 35 cm (12 inches) from objects and slowly bring the figures closer to your eye. At one point, the circle will seem to disappear because its image has fallen on the blind spot.

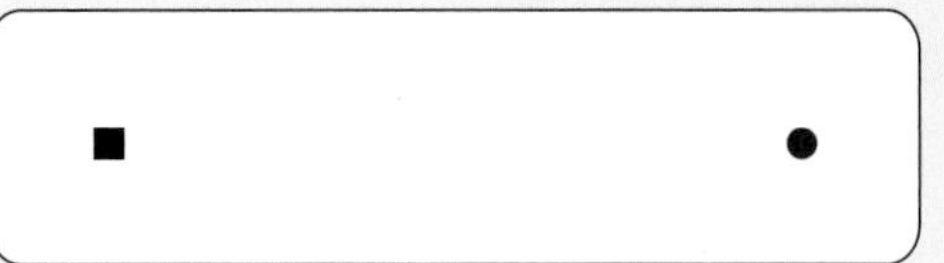

words, **rods** are the receptors for night vision and **cones** are the receptors for daytime vision.

There are three kinds of cones; each is sensitive to a different color: red, green, or blue. Scattered throughout the central portion of the retina, these three types of cones allow us to distinguish between different colors—but only in bright light.

There is a yellowish area near the center of the retina called the **macula lutea**—a term that means "yellow spot." It surrounds a small depression, called the **fovea centralis,** which contains the greatest concentration of cones of any area of the retina. These structures are identified in **Figure 10-2** but can also be seen using a common medical device called an **ophthalmoscope,** shown in **Figure 10-5**.

In good light, greater visual acuity, or sharpness of visual perception, can be obtained if we look directly at an object and focus the image on the fovea. But in dim light or darkness, we

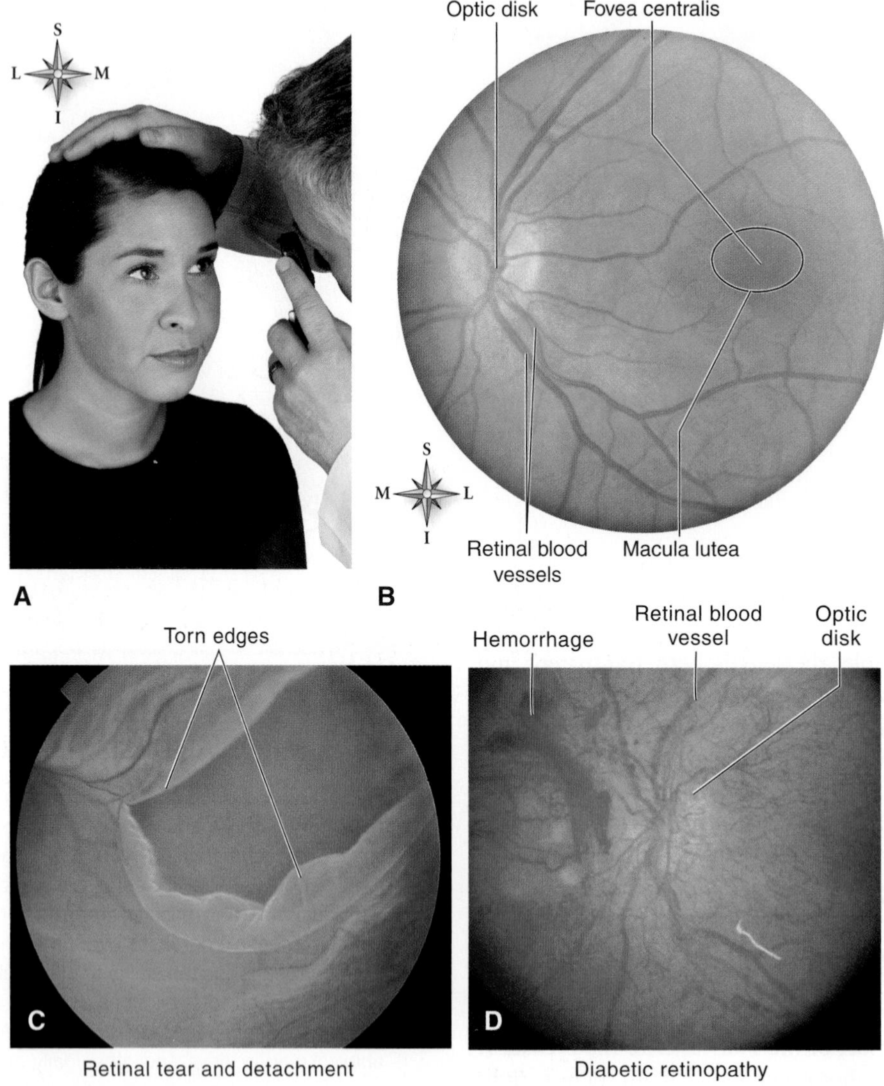

FIGURE 10-5 Examining the eye. A, Using an opthalmoscope to view the retina. **B,** Ophthalmoscopic view of the retina, as seen through the pupil. **C,** A case of retinal tear and detachment. **D,** Diabetes can produce abnormal blood vessels and bleeding of the retina.

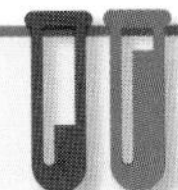

CLINICAL APPLICATION

FOCUSING PROBLEMS

Focusing a clear image on the retina is essential for good vision. In the normal eye *(A)*, light rays enter the eye and are focused into a clear, upside-down image on the retina. The brain can easily right the upside-down image in our conscious perception but cannot fix an image that is not sharply focused. If our eyes are elongated *(B)*, the image focuses in front of the retina rather than on it. The retina receives only a fuzzy image. This condition, called **myopia,** or *nearsightedness,* can be corrected by using contact lenses, glasses *(C)*, or refractive eye surgery. If our eyes are shorter than normal *(D)*, the image focuses behind the retina, also producing a fuzzy image. This condition, called **hyperopia,** or *farsightedness,* can also be corrected by lenses *(E)* or refractive surgery. *Astigmatism* is an abnormal eye condition resulting in blurred vision. It is caused by an irregular curvature of the lens.

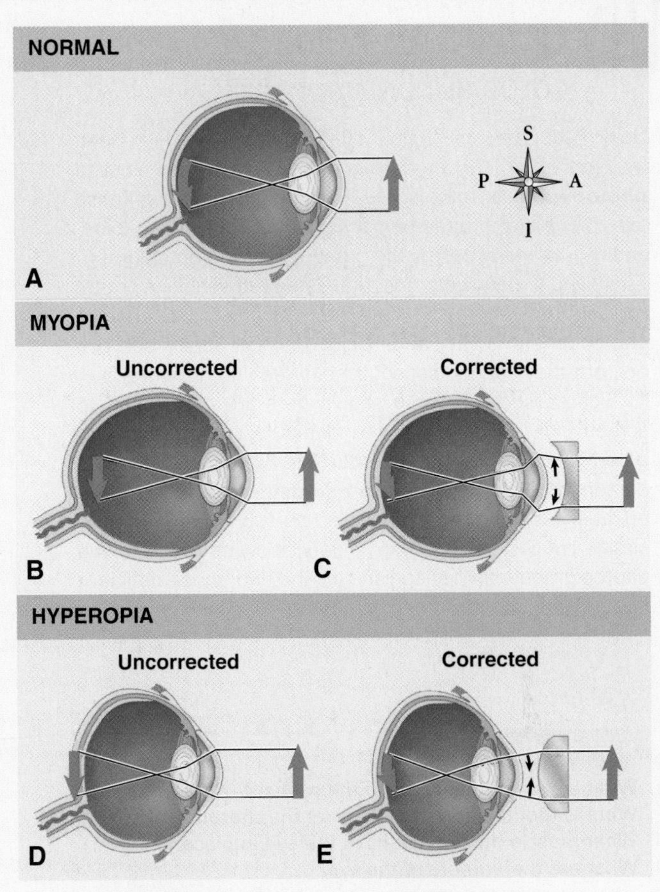

see an object better if we look slightly to the side of it, thereby focusing the image nearer the periphery of the retina, where the rods are more plentiful.

Figure 10-4 also shows **ganglion cells**, which are also sensitive to light. Ganglion cells, like rods, are sensitive to various wavelengths (colors) of light, but they are not used to form visual images. Instead, information from ganglion cells helps the body determine whether it is day or night, as well as the level of moonlight (monthly phases). This helps our body's *internal clock* mechanisms synchronize themselves to the daily, monthly, and seasonal rhythms of our external environment.

Fluids of the Eyeball

Fluids fill the hollow spaces inside the eyeball. They maintain the normal shape of the eyeball and help refract light rays; that is, the fluids bend light rays to bring them to focus on the retina.

Aqueous humor is the name of the watery fluid in front of the lens (in the anterior chamber of the eye), and **vitreous humor** is the name of the jellylike fluid behind the lens (in the posterior chamber). Aqueous humor is constantly being formed, drained, and replaced in the anterior chamber. If drainage is blocked for any reason, the internal pressure within the eye will increase, and damage that could lead to blindness will occur. This condition is called **glaucoma.**

Visual Pathway

Light is the stimulus that results in vision (that is, our ability to see objects as they exist in our environment). Besides detecting intensity (brightness) and wavelength (color) of light, we can also perceive images and their movements.

Light enters the eye through the pupil and is *refracted,* or bent, so that it is focused on the retina. **Refraction** occurs as light passes through the cornea, the aqueous humor, the lens, and the vitreous humor on its way to the retina.

The innermost layer of the retina contains the rods and cones, which are the **photoreceptor cells** of the eye (see Figure 10-4). They respond to a light stimulus by producing a nervous impulse. The rod and cone photoreceptor cells synapse with neurons in the bipolar and ganglionic layers of the retina.

Nervous signals eventually leave the retina and exit the eye through the optic nerve on the posterior surface of the eyeball. No rods or cones are present in the area of the retina where the optic nerve fibers exit. The result is a "blind spot" known as the **optic disk** (see Figure 10-2).

After leaving the eye, the optic nerves enter the brain and travel to the visual cortex of the occipital lobe. Eventually, *visual interpretation* of the nervous impulses generated by light striking the retina results in "seeing."

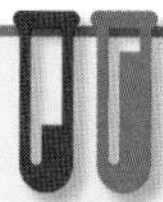

CLINICAL APPLICATION

COLOR BLINDNESS

Color blindness, usually an inherited condition, is caused by mistakes in producing three chemicals called **photopigments** in the cones. Each photopigment is sensitive to one of the three primary colors of light: green, blue, and red. In many cases, the green-sensitive photopigment is missing or deficient; other times, the red-sensitive photopigment is abnormal. (Deficiency of the blue-sensitive photopigment is very rare.) Color-blind individuals see colors, but they cannot distinguish between them normally.

Figures such as those shown here are often used to screen individuals for color blindness. A person with red-green blindness cannot see the 74 in Figure *A,* whereas a person with normal vision can. To determine which photopigment is deficient, a color-blind person may try a figure similar to *B.* Persons with a deficiency of red-sensitive photopigment can distinguish only the two; those deficient in green-sensitive photopigment can only see the four.

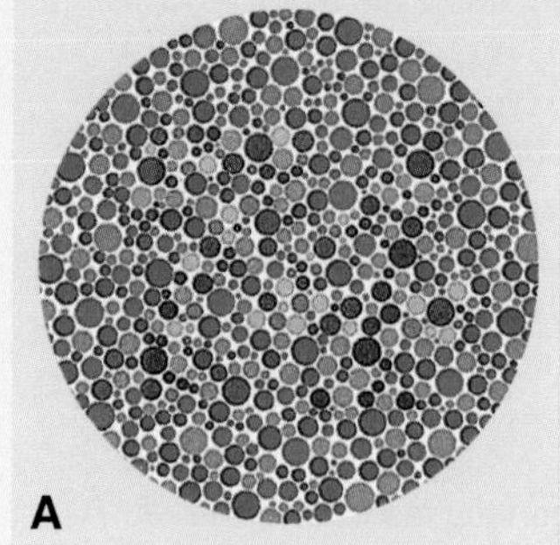

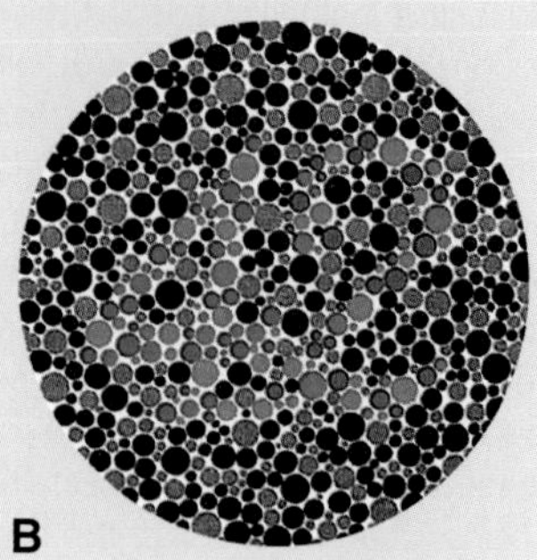

QUICK CHECK

1. What are the three layers of the eyeball?
2. What is the function of melanin in the choroid?
3. What muscle holds the lens of the eye in place?
4. What are the *humors* of the eye?
5. How are rods and cones used in vision? How are they alike? How are they different?
6. What is the function of the ganglia cells of the eye?

Hearing and Equilibrium

In addition to its role in hearing, the ear also functions as the sense organ of balance, or *equilibrium.* The stimulation or "trigger" that activates receptors involved with hearing and equilibrium is mechanical, and the receptors themselves are called **mechanoreceptors.** In hearing, sound vibrations trigger nervous impulses that are eventually perceived in the brain as sound. In equilibrium, changes in position or movement of the body trigger impulses that lead to the sensations of balance.

Structure and Function of the Ear

The ear is more than an appendage on the side of the head. A large part of the ear and its most important functional part lie hidden from view deep inside the temporal bone. The ear is divided into the following anatomical areas (**Figure 10-6**):

1. External ear
2. Middle ear
3. Inner ear

External Ear

The external ear has two parts: the **auricle,** or pinna, and the **external acoustic canal.** The auricle is the appendage on the side of the head surrounding the opening of the external acoustic canal. The canal itself is a curving tube about 2.5 cm (1 inch) in length. It extends into the temporal bone and ends at the **tympanic membrane,** or **eardrum,** which is a partition between the external and middle ear. Sound waves traveling through the external acoustic canal strike the tympanic membrane and cause it to vibrate.

The skin of the auditory canal, especially in its outer one third, contains many short hairs and **ceruminous glands** that produce a waxy substance called **cerumen** that may collect in the canal and impair hearing by absorbing or blocking the passage of sound waves.

A medical device called an **otoscope** can be used to view the external acoustic canal and eardrum (**Figure 10-7**).

Middle Ear

The middle ear is a tiny and very thin epithelium-lined cavity hollowed out of the temporal bone. It is an air-filled space housing three very small bones. The names of these ear bones, called **ossicles,** describe their shapes: **malleus** (hammer), **incus** (anvil), and **stapes** (stirrup).

The "handle" of the malleus attaches to the inside of the tympanic membrane, and the "head" attaches to the incus. The incus attaches to the stapes, and the stapes presses against a membrane that covers a small opening, the *oval window.* The oval window separates the middle ear from the inner ear. When sound waves cause the eardrum to vibrate, that movement is transmitted and amplified by the ear ossicles as it passes through the middle ear. Movement of the stapes against the oval window causes movement of fluid in the inner ear.

A point worth mentioning, because it explains the frequent spread of infection from the throat to the ear, is the fact that a tube—the **auditory tube** or **eustachian tube**—connects the throat with the middle ear. The epithelial lining of the middle

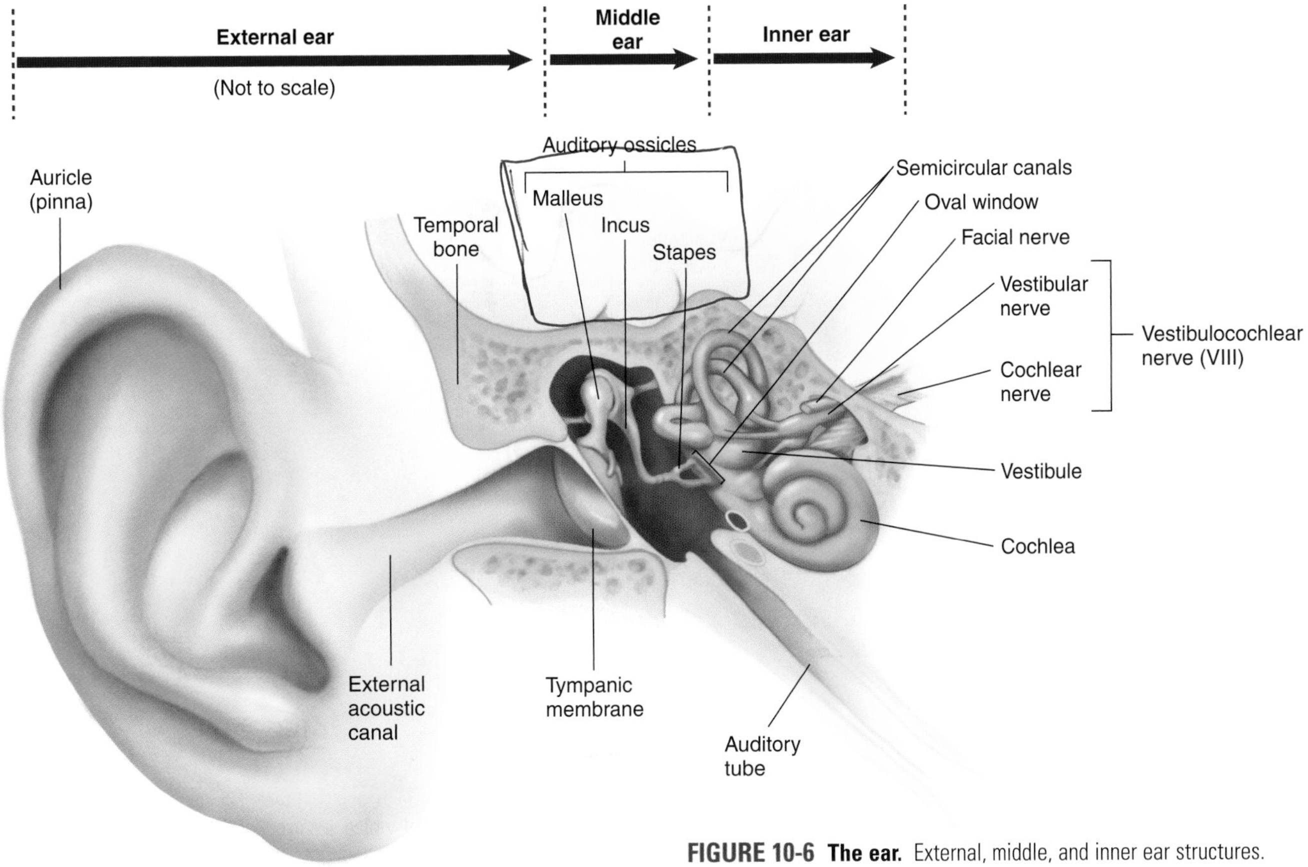

FIGURE 10-6 The ear. External, middle, and inner ear structures.

ears, auditory tubes, and throat are extensions of one continuous membrane. A sore throat may thus spread to produce a middle ear infection called **otitis media** (Figure 10-7, *C*).

The function of a healthy auditory tube is to equalize air pressure between the middle ear and the outside environment. When air pressures are unequal, the tympanic membrane may remain stretched—sometimes becoming quite painful and reducing its ability to vibrate.

Inner Ear

Anatomically, the inner ear consists of three spaces in the temporal bone, assembled in a complex maze called the **bony labyrinth.** This odd-shaped bony space is filled with a watery fluid called **perilymph** and is divided into the following parts: **vestibule, semicircular canals,** and **cochlea.** The vestibule is adjacent to the oval window between the semicircular canals and the cochlea (Figure 10-8).

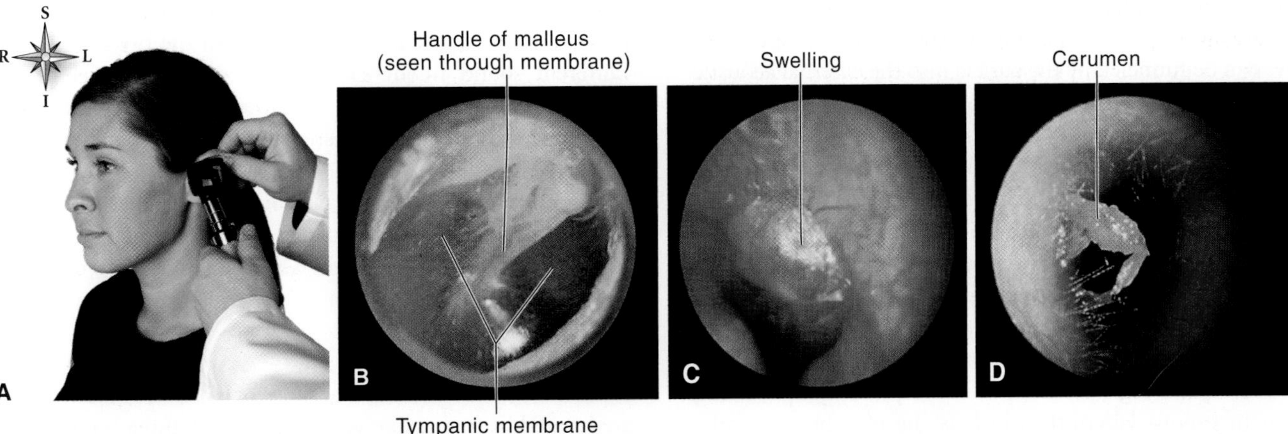

FIGURE 10-7 Examining the external ear. A, Using a lighted otoscope to view the external ear canal and tympanic membrane. **B,** Note the translucent, pearly-gray appearance of a normal tympanic membrane (with a bit of white glare from the otoscope light in the lower right). The "handle" of the malleus can be seen attaching near the center of the inner surface of the membrane. **C,** Acute otitis media. Note the red, thickened, and bulging tympanic membrane. **D,** Cerumen (earwax) in ear canal.

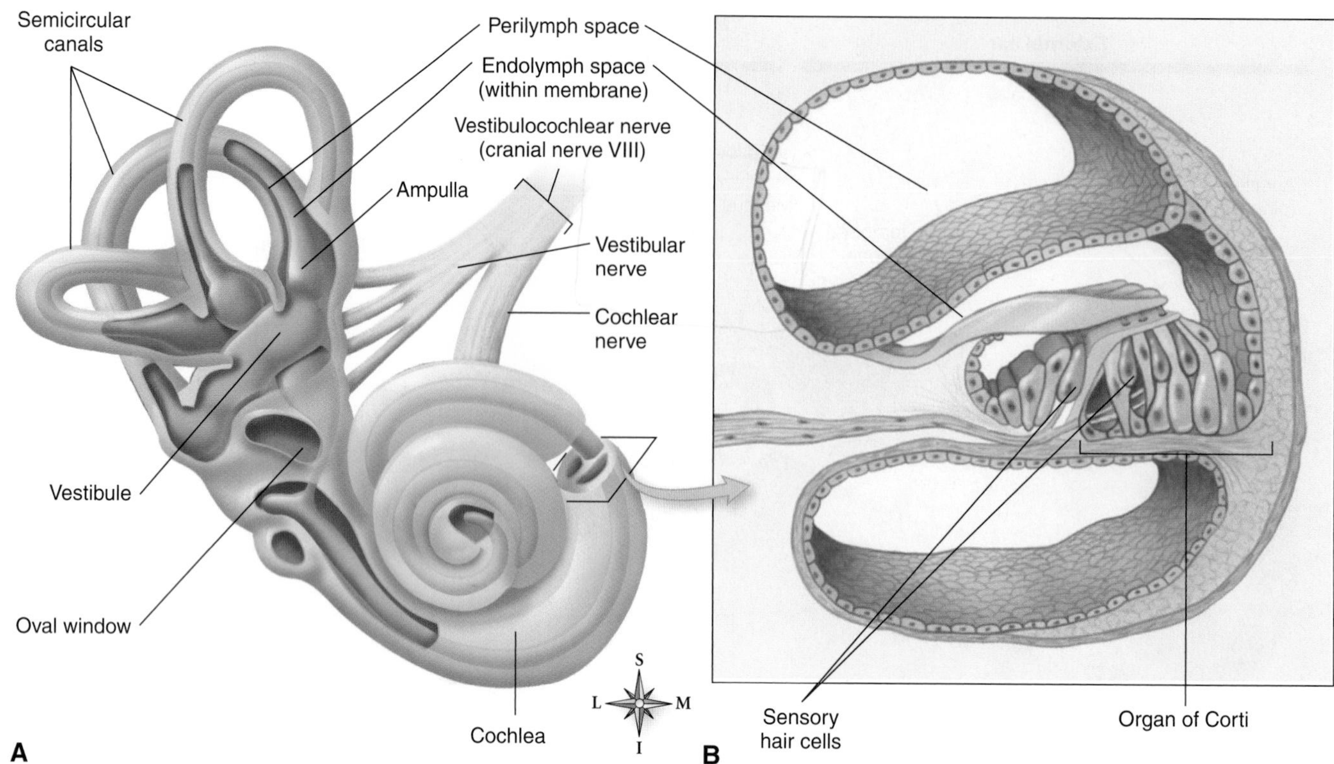

FIGURE 10-8 The inner ear. A, The bony labyrinth is the hard outer wall of the entire inner ear and includes semicircular canals, vestibule, and cochlea. Within the bony labyrinth is the membranous labyrinth *(purple)*, which is surrounded by perilymph and filled with endolymph. Each ampulla in the vestibule contains a crista ampullaris that detects changes in head position and sends sensory impulses through the vestibular nerve to the brain. **B,** The inset shows a section of the membranous cochlea. Hair cells in the organ of Corti detect sound and send the information through the cochlear nerve. The vestibular and cochlear nerves join to form the vestibulocochlear nerve, or cranial nerve VIII.

Note in **Figure 10-8** that a balloonlike membranous sac is suspended in the perilymph and follows the shape of the bony labyrinth much like a "tube within a tube." This is the **membranous labyrinth,** and it is filled with a thicker fluid called **endolymph.**

Hearing

Hearing is the sensation of the intensity and *frequency* (tone) of sounds in our environment.

Sound waves are simply pressure waves in the air. Such waves can be funneled by the auricle into the external acoustic canal and strike the tympanic membrane. Sound waves cause the eardrum to vibrate, and that movement is then transmitted and amplified by the ear ossicles as it passes through the middle ear. Movement of the stapes against the oval window causes movement of perilymph fluid in the inner ear, which in turn triggers vibrations of the endolymph.

The vibration waves now travel through the fluid of the inner ear to the organ of hearing—the **organ of Corti**—which lies within the curling, snail-shaped cochlea. Also called the **spiral organ,** it is surrounded by endolymph, filling the membranous labyrinth, which is the membranous tube within the bony cochlea. Ciliated "hair cells" on the organ of Corti generate nerve impulses when they are bent by the movement of endolymph set in motion by sound waves (see **Figure 10-8** and **Figure 10-9**).

This activation of mechanoreceptors in the organ of Corti inside the cochlea of the inner ear generates nervous impulses that travel through the **cochlear nerve** to the brain and results in hearing.

Hearing loss caused by nerve impairment is common in the elderly. Called **presbycusis,** this progressive hearing loss associated with aging results from degeneration of sensory nerve tissue in the ear and the vestibulocochlear nerve.

A similar type of hearing loss occurs after chronic exposure to loud noises that damages receptors in the organ of Corti. Different sound frequencies (tones) stimulate different regions of the organ of Corti; therefore, hearing impairment is limited to only frequencies associated with the damaged portion of the organ of Corti.

The portion of the organ of Corti that degenerates first in presbycusis is normally stimulated by high-frequency sounds. Thus the inability to hear high-pitched sounds is common among the elderly.

Equilibrium

The mechanoreceptors for our sense of balance, or *equilibrium,* are located in the saclike vestibule and the three semicircular canals of the inner ear.

Within the vestibule are two structures, each made up of a patch of sensory hairs coated with a thick glob of heavy gel. Each of these structures is called a **macula.** When you bend

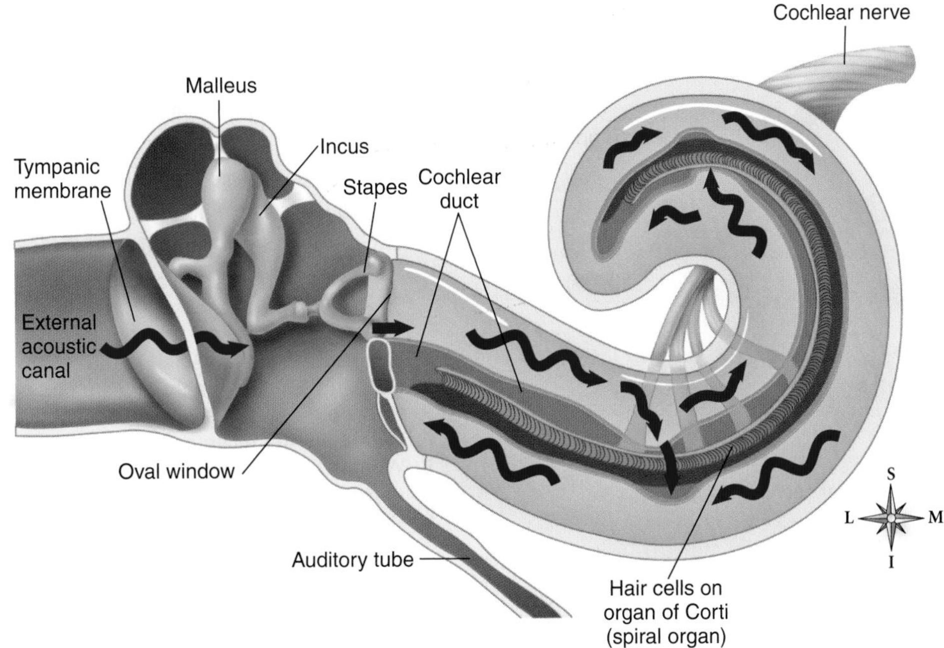

FIGURE 10-9 Effect of sound waves in the ear. Sound waves strike the tympanic membrane and cause it to vibrate. This vibration causes the membrane of the oval window to vibrate. This vibration causes the perilymph in the bony labyrinth of the cochlea to move, which causes the endolymph in the membranous labyrinth of the cochlea or cochlear duct to move. This movement of endolymph stimulates hair cells on the organ of Corti to generate a nerve impulse. The nerve impulse travels over the cochlear nerve, which becomes a part of the eighth cranial nerve. Eventually, nerve impulses reach the auditory cortex and are interpreted as sound.

your head, gravity acts on the heavy gel to pull it one way or the other (**Figure 10-10**). This, in turn, bends the cilia of the hair cells and thus produces a nerve signal. This signal is interpreted by the brain as our "sense of gravity" or **static equilibrium.**

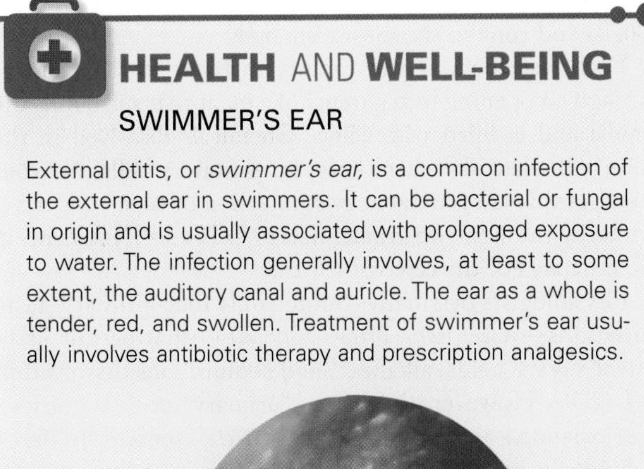

HEALTH AND WELL-BEING

SWIMMER'S EAR

External otitis, or *swimmer's ear,* is a common infection of the external ear in swimmers. It can be bacterial or fungal in origin and is usually associated with prolonged exposure to water. The infection generally involves, at least to some extent, the auditory canal and auricle. The ear as a whole is tender, red, and swollen. Treatment of swimmer's ear usually involves antibiotic therapy and prescription analgesics.

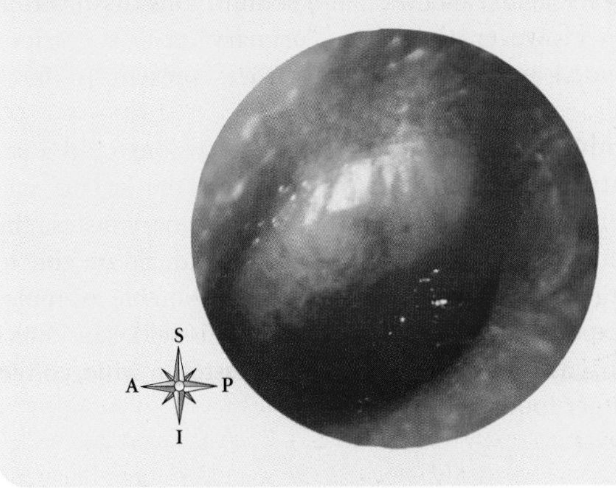

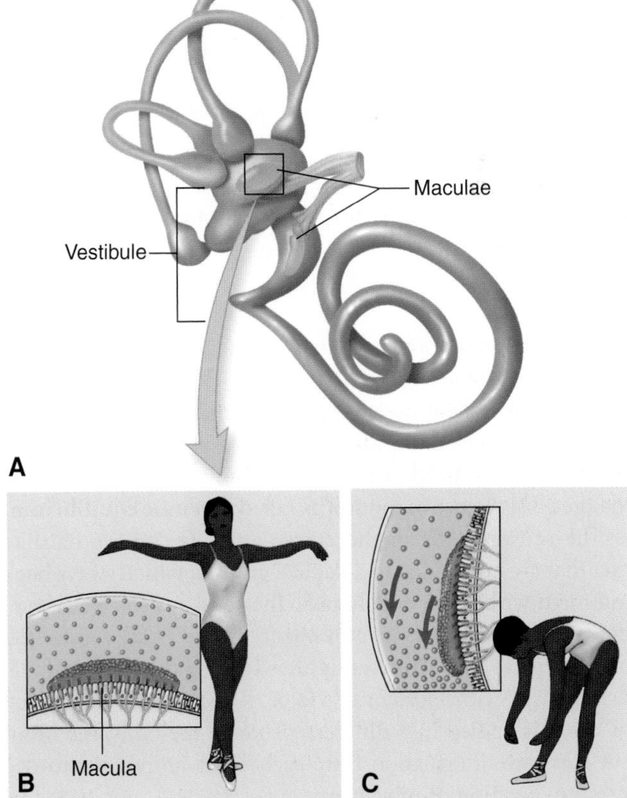

FIGURE 10-10 Static equilibrium. A, Structure of vestibule showing placement of the maculae, which have mechanoreceptors that detect our "sense of gravity" or *static equilibrium.* **B,** Macula stationary in upright position. **C,** Macula displaced by gravity as person bends over.

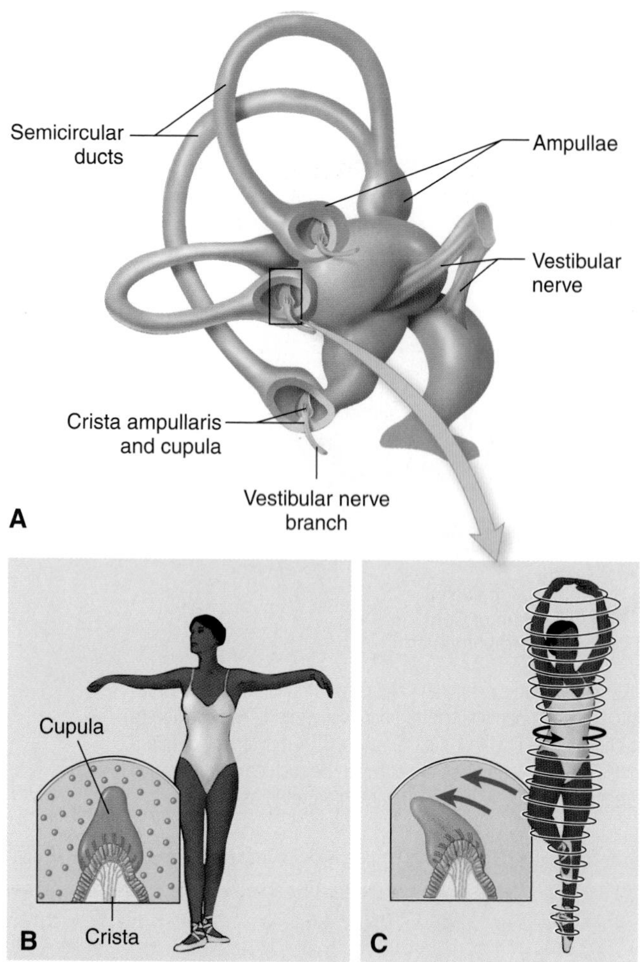

FIGURE 10-11 Dynamic equilibrium. A, Semicircular ducts showing location of the crista ampullaris and cupula in ampullae. **B,** When a person is at rest, the crista ampullaris and cupula do not move. **C,** As a person begins to spin, the cupula bends and the crista ampullaris is displaced by the endolymph in a direction opposite to the direction of spin. This produces the sensation of dynamic equilibrium.

The three semicircular canals are half-circles oriented at right angles to one another (**Figure 10-11**). Within each canal is a dilated area called the *ampulla* that contains a sensory structure called a **crista ampullaris,** which generates a nerve impulse when the speed or direction of movement of your head changes. This "sense of motion" is called **dynamic equilibrium.**

The sensory cells in the cristae ampullares have hairlike cilia that are embedded in a flaplike **cupula,** which sways back and forth within the endolymph. The sensory cells are stimulated when a change in movement of the head causes the endolymph to move differently, thus causing the crista ampullaris to sway with more or less force. Because each semicircular canal is angled in a different plane of the body, the brain can compare information from each crista ampullaris to determine direction of movement.

Nerves from mechanoreceptors in the vestibule join those from the semicircular canals to form the **vestibular nerve.** The vestibular nerve then joins with the cochlear nerve to form the *vestibulocochlear nerve (cranial nerve VIII)* (see **Figure 10-8**). Eventually, nervous impulses passing through this nerve reach the cerebellum and medulla—ultimately reaching the cerebral cortex.

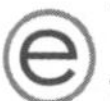
To learn more about the pathway of sound waves, go to AnimationDirect at *evolve.elsevier.com*.

QUICK CHECK

1. What senses are detected in the ear?
2. Can you describe the three main parts of the ear?
3. How do the ossicles work in helping a person to hear?
4. Where are the receptor cells for hearing?
5. What is the function of the *spiral organ?* What is another name for this organ?
6. What is the difference between *static equilibrium* and *dynamic equilibrium?*

Taste

Our sense of taste—or **gustation**—allows us to chemically analyze food before we bite or swallow it.

The **taste buds** are the sense organs of taste. They contain both supporting cells and chemoreceptors called **gustatory cells.** These cells generate the nervous impulses ultimately interpreted by the brain as taste (**Figure 10-12**).

Although a few taste buds are located in the lining of the mouth and on the soft palate, most are located on the sides of much larger and differing shaped bumps scattered across the tongue called **papillae.** About 10 to 15 large **circumvallate papillae** form an inverted "V" pattern at the back of the tongue and contain the most taste buds.

Each taste bud, as you can see in **Figure 10-12**, *C,* opens through an opening into a trenchlike moat that surrounds the papilla and is filled with saliva. Chemicals dissolved in the saliva stimulate the chemoreceptor gustatory cells. Nervous impulses that are generated by stimulation of taste buds travel primarily through two cranial nerves (VII and IX) to end in the taste area of the cerebral cortex.

Physiologists originally counted only four "primary" taste sensations—*sweet, sour, bitter,* and *salty*—that permit us to detect sugars, acids, alkalines, and sodium ions dissolved in our saliva. However, the list of "primary" taste sensations has expanded to include several others present in most individuals.

Currently, **metallic** taste (to detect metal ions) and a savory, meaty taste called **umami** (to detect the amino acid glutamate) have been added to the list of primary tastes. The list continues to grow. Of course, some individuals are able to sense a larger number of tastes than others. Notable examples include "experts" and "supertasters" who, it is said, can detect literally dozens of discrete and different tastes in wine, coffee, tea, and other foods and beverages.

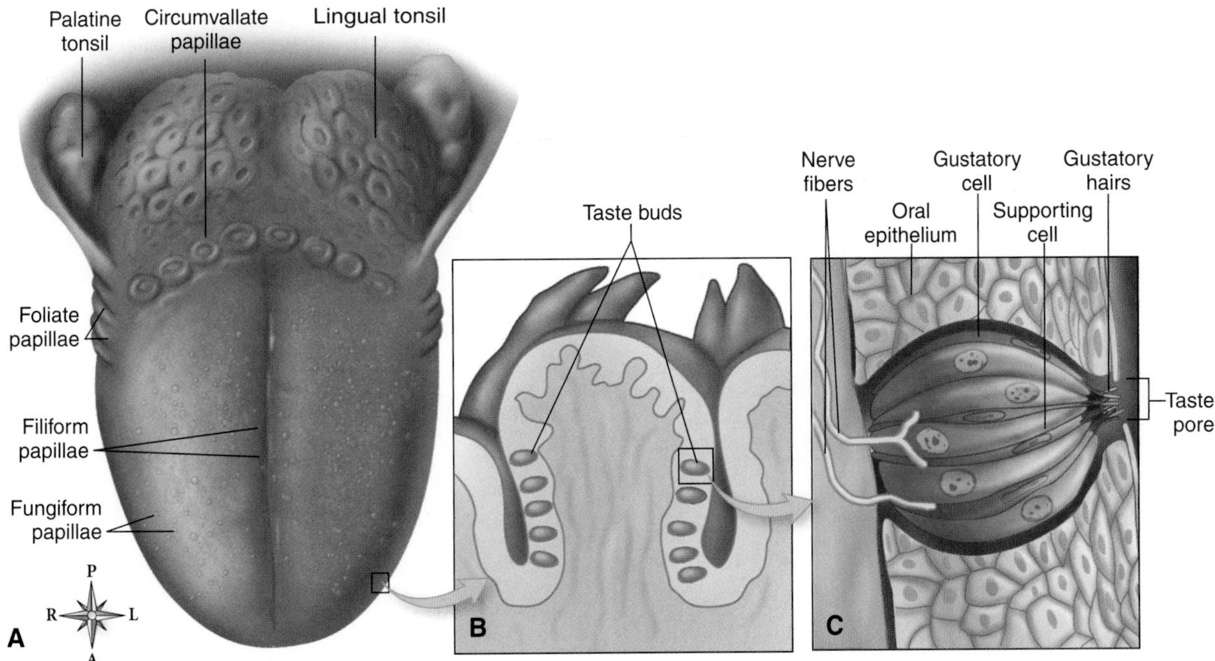

FIGURE 10-12 The tongue. A, Dorsal surface of tongue showing circumvallate papillae. **B,** Section through a papilla with taste buds on the side. **C,** Enlarged view of a section through a taste bud.

Smell

The sense of smell, or **olfaction**, helps us detect certain chemicals in our environment.

The chemoreceptors responsible for olfaction are located in a small area of epithelial tissue in the upper part of the nasal cavity (**Figure 10-13**). The location of the **olfactory receptors** is somewhat hidden, and we must often forcefully sniff the air to smell delicate odors.

Each olfactory cell has a number of sensory cilia that detect different chemicals and cause the cell to respond by generating a nervous impulse. To be detected by olfactory receptors, chemicals must be dissolved in the watery mucus that lines the nasal cavity.

The olfactory receptors are extremely sensitive and respond quickly to even very slight odors. However, after a short time they develop a kind of fatigue and lose their ability to respond. This decrease in receptor sensitivity is called **adaptation** and explains why odors that are at first very noticeable are soon not sensed at all.

After the olfactory cells are stimulated by odor-causing chemicals, the resulting nerve impulse travels through the olfactory nerves in the olfactory bulb and tract and then enters the thalamus for relay to the olfactory centers in the cortex of the brain, where the nervous impulses are interpreted as specific odors.

The pathways taken by olfactory nerve impulses and the areas where these impulses are interpreted are closely associated with the *limbic system* of the brain important in memory and emotion (see Chapter 9, p. 202). For this reason, we may retain vivid and long-lasting memories of particular smells and odors. The pleasant smell of bread or cookies baking in a grandmother's kitchen may be part of a childhood memory that lasts a lifetime.

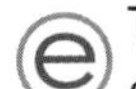
To learn more about how the brain interprets odors, go to AnimationDirect at *evolve.elsevier.com*.

Integration of Senses

Looking at the "big picture" of sensation, we should remind ourselves that sensations are all perceived in the brain—not at the individual receptors scattered throughout the body. Some sensory signals never get to the brain, others are amplified or muffled in the brain. All incoming signals are integrated with other sensory signals and even memories to produce our perceptions, which are really a combined sensation of our world at that moment.

For example, most of what we think of as flavor sensations result from a combination of sensory stimuli detected by gustatory cells, olfactory receptors, and even touch and pain receptors. In other words, the myriad unique flavors we recognize are not just tastes alone but are a combined sensation based on tastes, odors, touch, temperature, and pain.

For this reason, severe nasal congestion can interfere with the stimulation of the olfactory receptors by odors from foods in the mouth, which can markedly dull flavor sensations (see **Figure 10-13**). Some foods seem to have a different flavor if they are crispy or warm or cold. And some spicy foods stimulate

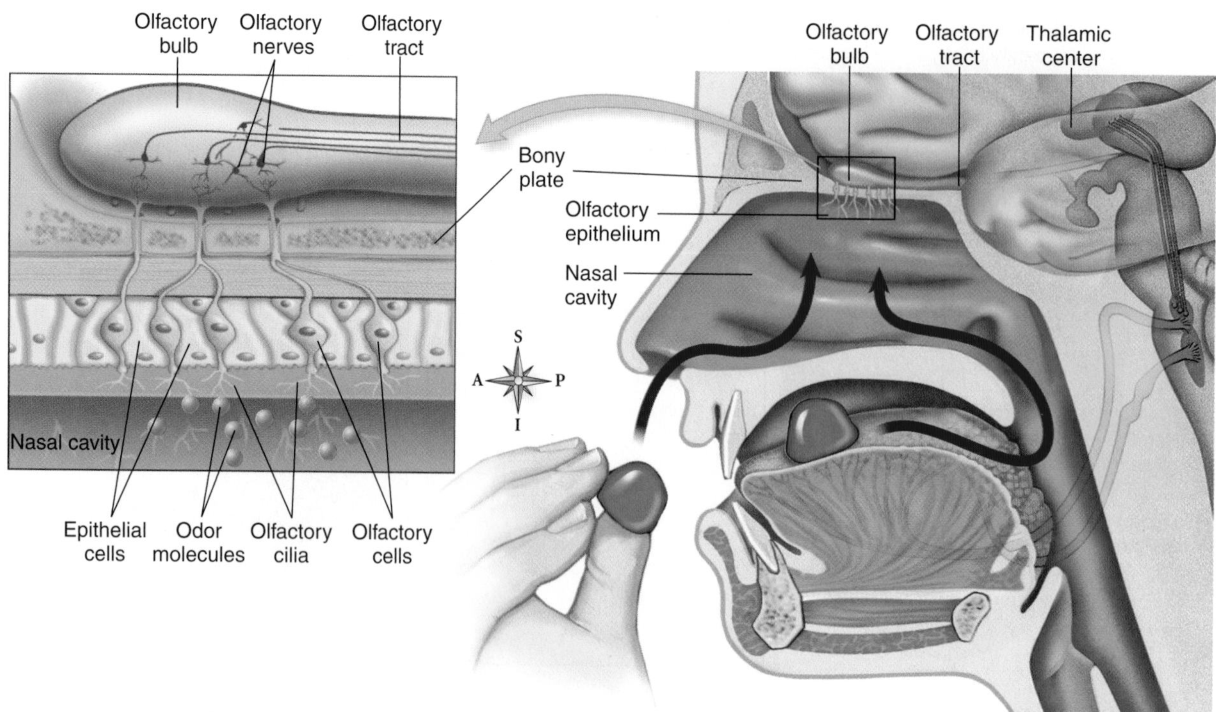

FIGURE 10-13 Olfactory structures. Gas molecules stimulate olfactory cells in the nasal epithelium. Sensory information is then conducted along nerves in the olfactory bulb and olfactory tract to sensory processing centers in the brain.

pain or temperature receptors to produce a "hot" flavor. Some mints can produce a sensation of coolness that adds to our experience of flavor.

Smell sensations, even more than other modes of sensation, are often powerful triggers of memory. Yet all sensations are compared to our learned memories, which help us accurately interpret what we are sensing at any one moment.

We often combine the senses of equilibrium with vision and proprioception to maintain our posture and balance—thus maintaining a safe body position under changing circumstances.

We should also remind ourselves that some sensory information is processed and perceived subconsciously. You cannot "feel" your blood pH go up or down, but your brain is

SCIENCE APPLICATIONS

SENSES

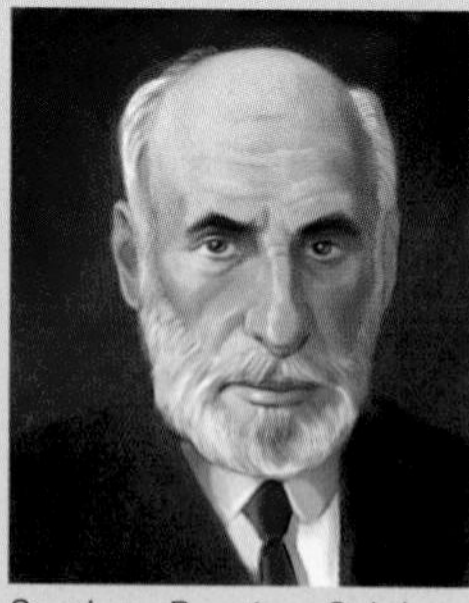

Santiago Ramón y Cajal (1852-1934)

Santiago Ramón y Cajal is considered by many to be the originator of the modern view of the nervous system's organization. He not only uncovered much about sensory centers of the cortex and the structure of the retina but also made important discoveries about nearly every part of the nervous system. Most of this Spanish researcher's ideas about the nervous system are intact today. Although Santiago wanted to be an artist, his father convinced him to follow in his footsteps and become an anatomist—a choice that led to his receiving a Nobel Prize in 1906.

The study of the sensory aspect of the nervous system and its relationships with the rest of the body is useful in many different fields. For example, the ideas used by **optometrists** and **ophthalmologists, otologists** and **audiologists,** and other professionals who assess and treat sensory disorders are based on neuroscience.

Many other fields make indirect use of neuroscience as well. For example, *artists* use what we know of visual perception in creating their works, *musicians* and *architects* make use of our knowledge of sound perception when performing in or designing concert halls, and *aerospace professionals* can use what we know of equilibrium and how it is perceived in the brain to understand motion sickness.

constantly aware of such changes. Likewise, you cannot state your current blood oxygen saturation—but your subconscious mind is aware of the precise level.

Lastly, we should not forget that senses do eventually start to fail us as we age. Mechanoreceptors in our ears become less sensitive, our lenses become less able to adjust our visual focus, and we slowly lose taste and smell function. This may explain why some foods "just don't taste the same" as they did when we were younger.

QUICK CHECK

1. Where are taste receptors located?
2. Can you name the primary tastes that humans can perceive?
3. What is the job of olfactory receptors?
4. In what organ are all senses experienced?

LANGUAGE OF SCIENCE AND MEDICINE *(continued from p. 213)*

ciliary muscle
(SIL-ee-ayr-ee)
[*ciliary* **eyelids or eyelashes,** *mus-* **mouse,** *-cle* **little**]

circumvallate papilla
(ser-kum-VAL-ayt pah-PIL-ah)
pl., papillae
(pah-PIL-ee)
[*circum-* **around,** *-vall-* **post or stake,** *-ate* **relating to,** *papilla* **nipple**]

cochlea
(KOHK-lee-ah)
[*cochlea* **snail shell**]

cochlear nerve
(KOHK-lee-ar nerv)
[*cochlea-* **snail shell,** *-ar* **relating to**]

cone
(cohn)

conjunctiva
(kon-junk-TYE-vah)
[*con-* **together,** *-junct* **join**]

cornea
(KOR-nee-ah)
[*corn-* **horn,** *-a* **thing**]

crista ampullaris
(KRIS-tah am-pyoo-LAYR-is)
[*crista* **ridge,** *ampu-* **flask,** *-ulla-* **little,** *-aris* **relating to**]

cupula
(KYOO-pyoo-lah)
pl., cupulae
(KYOO-pyoo-lee)
[*cup-* **tub,** *-ula* **little**]

dynamic equilibrium
(dye-NAM-ik ee-kwi-LIB-ree-um)
[*dynam-* **moving force,** *-ic* **relating to,** *equi-* **equal,** *-libr-* **balance**]

eardrum
(EAR-drum)

endolymph
(EN-doh-limf)
[*endo-* **within,** *-lymph* **water**]

eustachian tube
(yoo-STAY-shun)
[*Bartolomeo Eustachio* **Italian anatomist,** *-an* **relating to**]

external acoustic canal
(eks-TER-nal ah-KOO-stik kah-NAL)
[*extern-* **outside,** *-al* **relating to,** *acoust-* **hearing,** *-ic* **relating to**]

fovea centralis
(FOH-vee-ah sen-TRAL-is)
[*fovea* **pit,** *centralis* **in the center**]

ganglion cell
(GANG-lee-on sel)
[*gangli-* **knot,** *-on* **unit,** *cell* **storeroom**]

general senses
(JEN-er-al SEN-sez)

glaucoma
(glaw-KOH-mah)
[*glauco-* **gray or silver,** *-oma* **tumor (growth)**]

gustation
(GUS-tay-shun)
[*gusta-* **taste,** *-tion* **process**]

gustatory cell
(GUS-tah-tor-ee sel)
[*gusta-* **taste,** *-ory* **relating to,** *cell* **storeroom**]

hyperopia
(hye-per-OH-pee-ah)
[*hyper-* **excessive or above,** *-op-* **vision,** *-ia* **condition**]

incus
(IN-kus)
[*incus* **anvil**]

iris
(EYE-ris)
[*iris* **rainbow**]

lacrimal gland
(LAK-rih-mal gland)
[*lacrima-* **tear,** *-al* **relating to,** *gland* **acorn**]

lens
(lenz)
[*lens* **lentil**]

macula
(MAK-yoo-lah)
pl., maculae or maculas
(MAK-yoo-lee or MAK-yoo-lahz)
[*macula* **spot**]

macula lutea
(MAK-yoo-lah LOO-tee-ah)
[*macula* **spot,** *lutea* **yellow**]

malleus
(MAL-ee-us)
[*malleus* **hammer**]

mechanoreceptor
(mek-an-oh-ree-SEP-tor)
[*mechano-* **machine (mechanical),** *-recept-* **receive,** *-or* **agent**]

membranous labyrinth
(MEM-brah-nus LAB-eh-rinth)
[*membran-* **thin skin,** *-ous* **characterized by,** *labyrinth* **maze**]

metallic
(meh-TAL-ik)
[*metal-* **metal,** *-ic* **relating to**]

mode
(mohd)

myopia
(my-OH-pee-ah)
[*myops-* **nearsighted,** *-op-* **vision,** *-ia* **condition**]

olfaction
(ohl-FAK-shun)
[*olfact-* **smell,** *-ion* **process**]

olfactory receptor
(ohl-FAK-tor-ee ree-SEP-tor)
[*olfact-* **smell,** *-ory* **relating to,** *recept-* **receive,** *-or* **agent**]

ophthalmologist
(off-thal-MOL-eh-jist)
[*oph-* **eye or vision,** *-thalm-* **inner chamber,** *-o-* **combining vowel,** *-log-* **words (study of),** *-ist* **agent**]

ophthalmoscope
(off-THAL-mah-skohp)
[*oph-* **eye or vision,** *-thalmo-* **inner chamber,** *-scop-* **see**]

optic disk
(OP-tic disk)
[*opti-* **vision,** *-ic* **relating to**]

optometrist
(op-TOM-eh-trist)
[*opti-* **vision,** *-metr-* **measure,** *-ist* **agent**]

organ of Corti
(OR-gan KOR-tee)
[*organ-* **tool or instrument,** *Alfonso Corti* **Italian anatomist**]

ossicle
(OS-sih-kul)
[*os-* **bone,** *-icle* **little**]

otitis media
(oh-TYE-tis MEE-dee-ah)
[*ot-* **ear,** *-itis* **inflammation,** *medi-* **middle,** *-ia* **condition**]

otologist
(oh-TOL-o-jist)
[*oto-* **ear,** *-log-* **words (study of),** *-ist* **agent**]

otoscope
(OH-toh-skohp)
[*oto-* **ear,** *-scop-* **see**]

pain receptor
(payn ree-SEP-tor)
[*recept-* **receive,** *-or* **agent**]

papilla
(pah-PIL-ah)
pl., papillae
(pah-PIL-ee)
[*papilla* **nipple**]

perilymph
(PAYR-ih-limf)
[*peri-* **around,** *-lymph* **water**]

photopigment
(foh-toh-PIG-ment)
[*photo-* **light,** *-pigment* **paint**]

photoreceptor
(FOH-toh-ree-sep-tor)
[*photo-* **light,** *-recept-* **receive,** *-or* **agent**]

presbycusis
(pres-bih-KYOO-sis)
[*presby-* **elderly,** *-cusis* **hearing**]

presbyopia
(pres-bee-OH-pee-ah)
[*presby-* **aging,** *-op-* **vision,** *-ia* **condition**]

proprioceptor
(proh-pree-oh-SEP-tor)
[*propri-* **one's own,** *-(re)cept-* **receive,** *-or* **agent**]

pupil
(PYOO-pil)
[*pup-* **doll,** *-il* **little**]

referred pain
(re-FERD payn)

refraction
(ree-FRAK-shun)
[*re-* **back or again,** *-fract-* **break,** *-tion* **process**]

retina
(RET-ih-nah)
[*ret-* **net,** *-ina* **relating to**]

rod
(rod)

sclera
(SKLEH-rah)
[*sclera* **hard**]

semicircular canal
(sem-ih-SIR-kyoo-lar kah-nal)
[*semi-* **half,** *-circul-* **circle,** *-ar* **relating to**]

special senses
(SPESH-ul SEN-sez)

spiral organ
(SPY-rel OR-gun)
[*spir-* **coiled,** *-al* **relating to,** *organ* **tool or instrument**]

stapes
(STAY-peez)
[*stapes* **stirrup**]

static equilibrium
(ee-kwih-LIB-ree-um)
[*stat-* **stand,** *-ic* **relating to,** *equi-* **equal,** *-libr-* **balance**]

taste bud
(tayst bud)

thermoreceptor
(ther-moh-ree-SEP-tor)
[*thermo-* **heat,** *-cept-* **receive,** *-or* **agent**]

tympanic membrane
(tim-PAN-ik MEM-brayn)
[*tympan-* **drum,** *-ic* **relating to,** *membran-* **thin skin**]

umami
(oo-MAH-mee)
[*umami* **savory**]

vestibular nerve
(ves-TIB-yoo-lar nerv)
[*vestibul-* **entrance hall,** *-ar* **relating to**]

vestibule
(VES-tih-byool)
[*vestibul-* **entrance hall**]

vitreous humor
(VIT-ree-us HYOO-mer)
[*vitre-* **glassy,** *-ous* **of or like,** *humor* **fluid**]

❑ OUTLINE SUMMARY

To download a digital audio version of the chapter summary for use with your device, access the ***Audio Chapter Summaries*** *online at evolve.elsevier.com.*

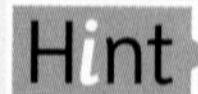

Scan this summary after reading the chapter to help you reinforce the key concepts. Later, use the summary as a quick review before your class or before a test.

Classification of Senses

A. General senses
 1. Detected by sensory organs that exist as individual cells or receptor units (see **Table 10-1**)
 2. Widely distributed throughout the body

B. Special senses (see **Table 10-2**)
 1. Detected by large and complex organs, or localized grouping of sensory receptors

C. Sensory receptor types
   1. Classified by presence or absence of covering capsule
      a. Encapsulated
      b. Unencapsulated ("free" or "naked")
   2. Classified by type of stimuli (mode) required to activate receptors
      a. Photoreceptors (light)
      b. Chemoreceptors (chemicals)
      c. Pain receptors (injury)
      d. Thermoreceptors (temperature change)
      e. Mechanoreceptors (movement or shape change)

Sensory Pathways

A. All sense organs have common functional characteristics
   1. All are able to detect a particular stimulus
   2. A stimulus results in generation of a nerve impulse
   3. A nerve impulse is processed and perceived as a sensation in the central nervous system

General Senses

A. Distribution is widespread; single-cell receptors are common
B. Mode—the kind of stimulus or change a receptor or sense is able to detect
   1. Examples of general sensory receptors and their modes (see **Figure 10-1**, **Table 10-1**)
      a. Free nerve ending — pain, temperature, and crude touch
      b. Tactile corpuscle (Meissner corpuscle) — fine touch and vibration
      c. Bulbous corpuscle (Ruffini corpuscle) — touch and pressure
      d. Lamellar corpuscle (Pacini corpuscle) — pressure and vibration
      e. Bulboid corpuscle (Krause end bulb) — touch
      f. Golgi tendon organ — proprioception
      g. Muscle spindle — proprioception
   2. General sense organs are also found in deep organs of the body

Special Senses

A. Vision
   1. Eye (see **Figure 10-2**)
      a. Layers of eyeball
         (1) Fibrous layer — tough outer coat
            (a) Sclera — "white" of eye
            (b) Cornea — transparent part over iris
            (c) Conjunctiva — mucous membrane that covers front of fibrous layer and extends to inside of eyelids
            (d) Lacrimal gland — secretes tears that moisten conjunctiva
         (2) Vascular layer — has dense network of blood vessels
            (a) Choroid — pigmented, melanin-rich layer prevents scattering of light
            (b) Iris — the colored part of the eye; the pupil is the hole in the center of the iris; contraction of smooth muscle dilates or constricts pupil (see **Figure 10-3**)
            (c) Lens — transparent body behind the pupil; focuses or refracts light rays on the retina
            (d) Ciliary muscle — near front of vascular layer, just outside the edge of the iris; contraction affects shape of lens just behind the iris, thus altering focus for near objects
         (3) Inner layer — innermost sensory layer
            (a) Retina — contains various kinds of photoreceptors (see **Figure 10-4** and **Figure 10-5**)
               i. Rods — receptors for night vision and peripheral vision
               ii. Cones — receptors for day vision and color vision
               iii. Ganglion cells — receptors for changing light patterns of days, months, seasons
      b. Eye fluids
         (1) Aqueous humor — in the anterior chamber in front of the lens
         (2) Vitreous humor — in the posterior chamber behind the lens
   2. Visual pathway
      a. Vision detects intensity (brightness) and wavelength (color) of light, as well as images and motion
      b. Light must be refracted (focused) by the eye to form a detectable image
      c. Innermost layer of retina contains rods and cones
      d. Impulse travels from the rods and cones through the bipolar and ganglionic layers of retina (see **Figure 10-4**)
      e. Nerve impulse leaves the eye through the optic nerve; the point of exit is free of receptors and is therefore called a *blind spot*
      f. Visual interpretation occurs in the visual cortex of the cerebrum

B. Hearing and equilibrium
  1. The ear functions in hearing and in equilibrium using receptors called *mechanoreceptors*
  2. Ear (see **Figure 10-6**)
     a. External ear
        (1) Auricle (pinna)
        (2) External acoustic canal (see **Figure 10-7**)
           (a) Curving canal 2.5 cm (1 inch) in length
           (b) Contains ceruminous glands
           (c) Ends at the tympanic membrane
     b. Middle ear
        (1) Houses ear ossicles — malleus, incus, and stapes
        (2) Ends in the oval window
        (3) The auditory (eustachian) tube connects the middle ear to the throat
        (4) Inflammation called *otitis media*
     c. Inner ear (see **Figure 10-8**)
        (1) Bony labyrinth filled with perilymph
        (2) Subdivided into the vestibule, semicircular canals, and cochlea
        (3) Membranous labyrinth filled with endolymph
  3. Hearing (see **Figure 10-9**)
     a. Hearing detects changes in intensity and frequency (tone) of sound waves, which are pressure waves
     b. Sound waves funneled by auricle into external acoustic canal and vibrate the tympanic membrane
     c. Vibrations of tympanic membrane are amplified by auditory ossicles and transmitted to the oval window
     d. Vibrations of the oval window trigger vibrations of perilymph, which in turn vibrates the endolymph
     e. Sensory hair cells on the organ of Corti (spiral organ) respond when bent by the movement of surrounding endolymph set in motion by sound waves; can become damaged by chronic exposure to loud noise
  4. Equilibrium — two types of balance: static and dynamic
     a. Static equilibrium — sense of gravity (see **Figure 10-10**)
        (1) Detected by ciliated hair cells (mechanoreceptors) of the two maculae in the vestibule
        (2) When the head tilts, gravity pulls the heavy gel of each macula, bending the sensory cilia and producing a nerve signal
     b. Dynamic equilibrium — sense of speed and direction of movement (see **Figure 10-11**)
        (1) Detected by ciliated hair cells (mechanoreceptors) of the crista ampullaris (with flaplike cupula) in the ampulla of each semicircular canal
        (2) When speed or direction of movement of head changes, the flow of endolymph in semicircular canals is altered, which causes change in bending of sensory cilia (producing a nerve signal)
     c. Vestibular nerve carries nerve impulses from the equilibrium receptors of the vestibule; joins with cochlear nerve to form vestibulocochlear nerve (cranial nerve VIII)

C. Taste
  1. Sense of taste is also called gustation
  2. Receptors are chemoreceptors called gustatory cells, located in *taste buds* (see **Figure 10-12**)
  3. Cranial nerves VII and IX carry gustatory impulses
  4. Primary taste modes
     a. Sweet — detects sugars
     b. Sour — detects acids
     c. Bitter — detects alkaline solutions
     d. Salty — detects sodium ions
     e. Metallic — detects metal ions
     f. Umami (savory) — detects glutamate (an amino acid)

D. Smell
  1. Olfactory receptors — sensory fibers of olfactory or cranial nerve I lie in olfactory mucosa of nasal cavity (see **Figure 10-13**)
  2. Olfactory receptors are extremely sensitive but easily adapt (become fatigued)
  3. Odor-causing chemicals initiate a nervous signal that is interpreted as a specific odor by the brain
  4. Olfaction has a strong relationship with emotions and memory

E. Integration of senses
  1. All senses are processed and finally perceived in the brain (not receptors)
  2. Sensory information is combined to form an overall sensory perception of our world
     a. Flavor
        (1) Combination of gustatory and olfactory senses; can be affected by other senses, such as touch, pain, or temperature
        (2) Nasal congestion interferes with stimulation of olfactory receptors and thereby dulls flavor sensations
     b. Posture and balance — both senses of equilibrium with vision and proprioception — combine to help us maintain a safe body position
  3. Some sensory information is processed subconsciously
  4. Our senses may decline as we age

❑ ACTIVE LEARNING

STUDY TIPS

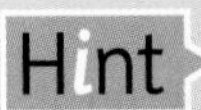

Use these tips to achieve success in meeting your learning goals.

1. Each of the body's senses must go through the following processes to perform its function: (1) detect the physical stimulus to which it responds and (2) convert that stimulus into a nerve impulse. For example, the eye must let light in and focus it on a specific point; the receptors convert that stimulus into a nerve impulse and send it to the brain.
2. When you study structures and their specific function in a sensory system, focus on how they contribute to one of these two processes. Use flash cards and other online resources to learn the specific structures and their functions in each sensory system.
3. In your study group, discuss how each of the sensory systems detect and respond to a stimulus. Copy the figures of the sense organs, block out the labels, and quiz each other on the name, location, and function of each structure. Use online labeling exercises *(www.getbodysmart.com)* as a resource.
4. Review the Language of Science terms. Review the questions and outline summary at the end of the chapter and discuss possible test questions in your study group.

Review Questions

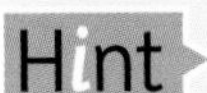

Write out the answers to these questions after reading the chapter and reviewing the Chapter Summary. If you simply think through the answer without writing it down, you won't retain much of your new learning.

1. Name the general senses found in the skin or subcutaneous tissue and list the type of stimuli to which each of them respond. Identify which of these general senses are unencapsulated.
2. Name the two general senses of proprioception and give the location of each.
3. Describe the type of information that proprioceptors provide.
4. Explain how the iris changes the size of the pupil.
5. Explain how the ciliary muscle allows the eye to focus on near and far objects.
6. Define *presbyopia,* and describe the common cause of this condition.
7. Name the two types of receptor cells in the retina. Explain the difference between these two receptors.
8. Define *glaucoma,* and describe its cause.
9. Describe *cataracts,* how they are caused, and what can be done to prevent them.
10. Explain what is meant by the visual pathway. Include in your description of the visual pathway the blind spot, and what causes it.
11. Briefly explain the structure of the external ear.
12. Explain how sound waves are transmitted through the middle ear.
13. Describe how sound waves are converted to an auditory impulse.
14. Explain how the structures in the inner ear help maintain balance or equilibrium.
15. Identify where the gustatory cells are located, and name the "primary" tastes to which they respond.
16. Explain how the sense of smell is stimulated.

Critical Thinking

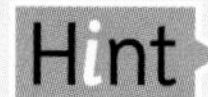

After finishing the Review Questions, write out the answers to these more in-depth questions to help you apply your new knowledge. Go back to sections of the chapter that relate to concepts that you find difficult.

17. Explain why food loses some of its taste when you have a bad cold with a stuffy nose.
18. Explain why the longer you are in a newly painted room, the less able you are to smell the paint.
19. Where in the eye is light sensed? Where is it perceived? (Be specific.)
20. Explain why the smell of a "doctor's office" or the smell of a turkey cooking on Thanksgiving can easily generate an emotional response.

Chapter Test

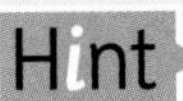

After studying the chapter, test your mastery by responding to these items. Try to answer them without looking up the answers. Then, verify the answers using the key in Appendix C at the back of this book.

1. The eye can be classified as a photoreceptor. Taste and smell can be classified as Chemo-receptors and Golgi tendon organs and muscle spindles can be classified as proprioceptors
2. The specific mechanoreceptor for hearing is the Spiral organ
3. The specific mechanoreceptor for balance is the crista ampullaris
4. The gustatory cells are involved with the sense of taste.
5. Six "primary" kinds of taste sensations that result from the stimulation of the taste buds are sour, sweet, salty, metallic, Bitter, and umami
6. Taste buds can be found on much larger structures on the tongue called papillae.
7. The chemoreceptors responsible for the sense of smell are the olfactory receptors

Match each function or description in Column B with the corresponding structure of the eye in Column A.

Column A	Column B
8. e sclera	a. tears are formed in this gland
9. i cornea	b. hole in the eye that lets light in
10. j iris	c. receptors for night or dim light vision
11. B pupil	d. thick jellylike fluid or humor of the eye
12. A lacrimal	e. tough, white outer layer of the eye
13. g lens	f. receptors for red, blue, and green color vision
14. C rods	g. ciliary muscles pull on this to help the eye focus
15. f cones	h. dark pigmented middle layer of the eye that prevents the scattering of incoming light
16. H choroid coat	i. transparent part of the sclera, the window of the eye
17. D vitreous	j. colored part of the front of the eye
18. K aqueous	k. thin, watery humor of the eye

Match each function or description in Column B with the corresponding structure of the ear in Column A.

Column A	Column B
19. f tympanic membrane	a. tube connecting the middle ear and the throat
20. g ossicles	b. watery fluid that fills the bony labyrinth
21. a auditory tube	c. snail-shaped structure in the inner ear
22. b perilymph	d. the organ of hearing
23. e endolymph	e. thick fluid in the membranous labyrinth
24. c cochlea	f. another term for eardrum
25. d spiral organ	g. collective name for incus, malleus, and stapes

Endocrine System

OUTLINE

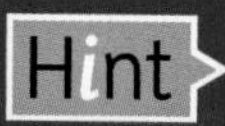

Scan this outline before you begin to read the chapter, as a preview of how the concepts are organized.

OBJECTIVES

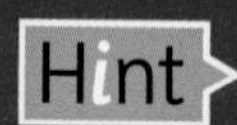

Before reading the chapter, review these goals for your learning.

After you have completed this chapter, you should be able to:

1. Distinguish between endocrine and exocrine glands and define the terms *hormone, hypersecretion,* and *hyposecretion.*
2. Identify and locate the primary endocrine glands and list the major hormones produced by each gland.
3. Describe the mechanisms of nonsteroid and steroid hormone action.
4. Explain how negative and positive feedback mechanisms regulate the secretion of endocrine hormones.
5. Define and explain the importance of prostaglandins (PGs).
6. Identify the principal functions of each major endocrine gland and the hormones that each releases.
7. Describe the conditions that may result from hyposecretion or hypersecretion of endocrine hormones, including gigantism, diabetes insipidus, goiter, cretinism, *diabetes mellitus,* and glycosuria.

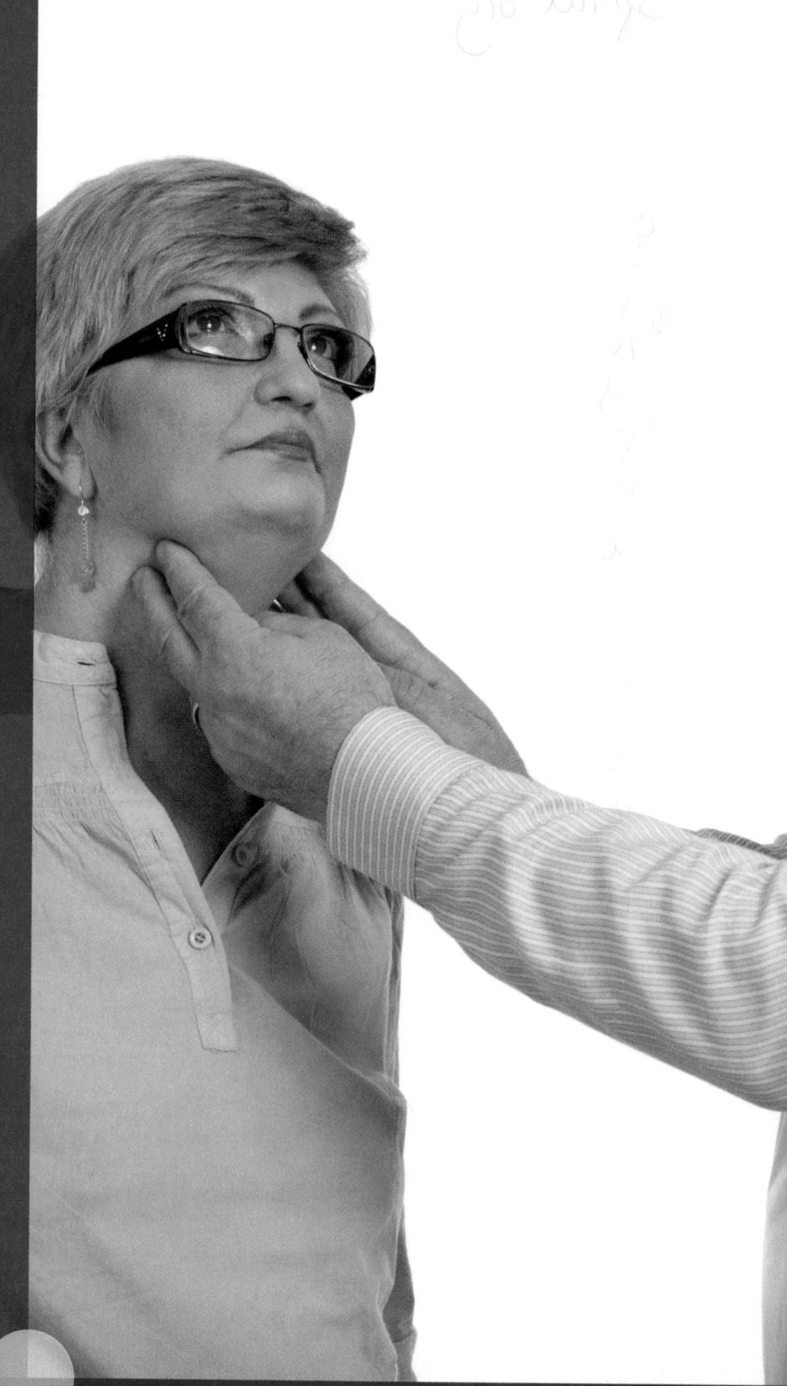

CHAPTER 11

Have you ever known anyone with thyroid problems or diabetes? Surely you have seen the dramatic changes that happen to a person's body as he or she goes through puberty. These are all proof of the importance of the endocrine system in normal development and health.

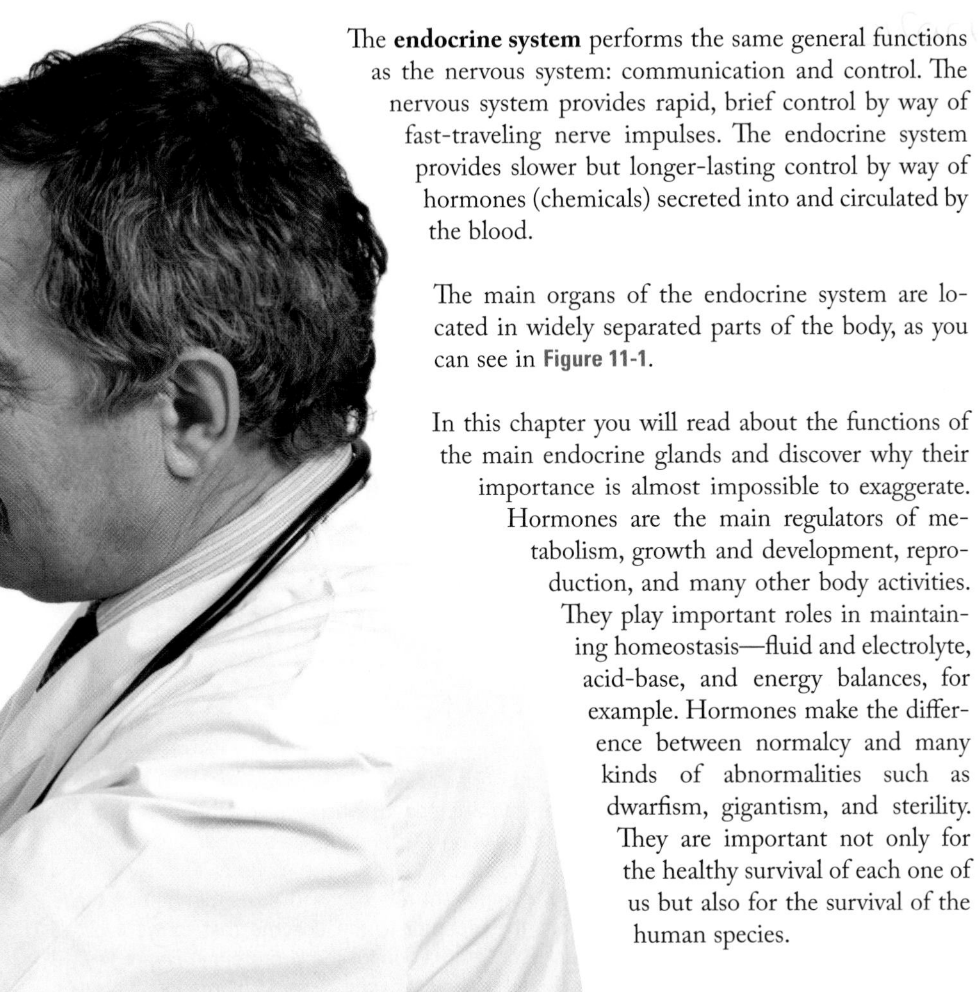

The **endocrine system** performs the same general functions as the nervous system: communication and control. The nervous system provides rapid, brief control by way of fast-traveling nerve impulses. The endocrine system provides slower but longer-lasting control by way of hormones (chemicals) secreted into and circulated by the blood.

The main organs of the endocrine system are located in widely separated parts of the body, as you can see in **Figure 11-1**.

In this chapter you will read about the functions of the main endocrine glands and discover why their importance is almost impossible to exaggerate. Hormones are the main regulators of metabolism, growth and development, reproduction, and many other body activities. They play important roles in maintaining homeostasis—fluid and electrolyte, acid-base, and energy balances, for example. Hormones make the difference between normalcy and many kinds of abnormalities such as dwarfism, gigantism, and sterility. They are important not only for the healthy survival of each one of us but also for the survival of the human species.

Endocrine Glands

All organs of the endocrine system are glands, but not all glands are organs of the endocrine system. Of the two types of glands in the body—**exocrine glands** and **endocrine glands**—only endocrine glands belong to this system.

LANGUAGE OF SCIENCE AND MEDICINE

Hint Before reading the chapter, say each of these terms out loud. This will help you to avoid stumbling over them as you read.

acromegaly
(ak-roh-MEG-ah-lee)
[*acro-* **extremities,** *-mega-* **great,** *-aly* **state**]

Addison disease
(AD-ih-son dih-ZEEZ)
[*Thomas Addison* **English physician,** *dis-* **opposite of,** *-ease* **comfort**]

adenohypophysis
(ad-eh-no-hye-POF-ih-sis)
[*adeno-* **gland,** *-hypo-* **under or below,** *-physis* **growth**]

adrenal cortex
(ah-DREE-nal KOR-teks)
[*ad-* **toward,** *-ren-* **kidney,** *-al* **relating to,** *cortex* **bark**]

adrenal medulla
(ah-DREE-nal meh-DUL-ah)
[*ad-* **toward,** *-ren-* **kidney,** *-al* **relating to,** *medulla* **marrow or pith**]

adrenocorticotropic hormone (ACTH)
(ah-dree-noh-kor-teh-koh-TROH-pic HOR-mohn)
[*adreno-* **gland,** *-cortic-* **bark,** *-trop-* **nourish,** *-ic* **relating to,** *hormon-* **excite**]

aldosterone
(AL-doh-steh-rohn *or* al-DAH-stair-ohn)
[*aldo-* **aldehyde,** *-stero-* **solid or steroid derivative,** *-one* **chemical**]

anabolism
(ah-NAB-oh-liz-em)
[*anabol-* **build up,** *-ism* **action**]

androgen
(AN-droh-jen)
[*andro-* **male,** *-gen* **produce**]

Continued on p. 254

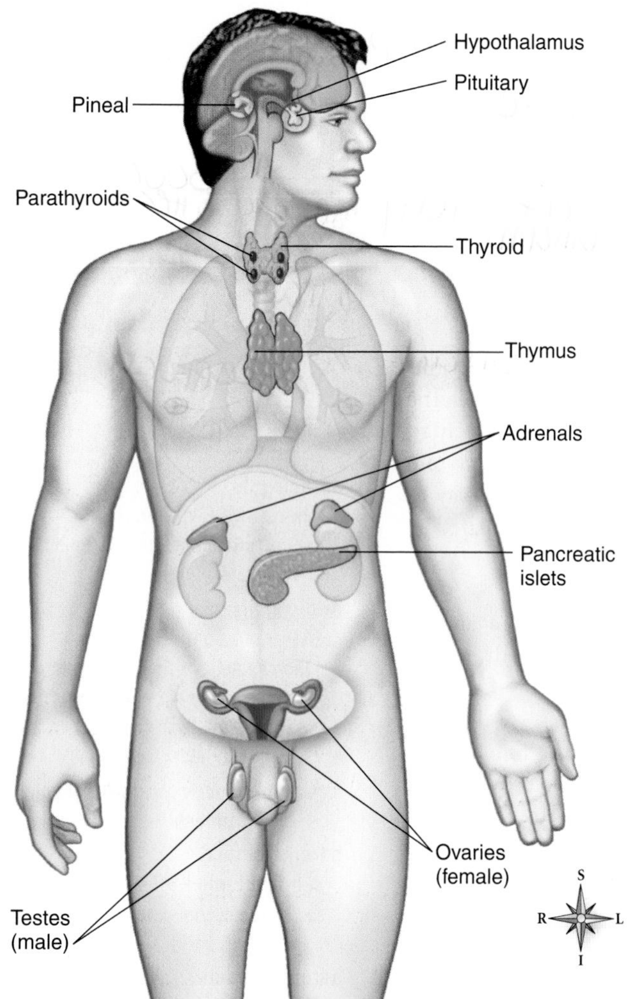

FIGURE 11-1 Location of the endocrine glands. Thymus gland is shown at maximum size at puberty.

You may recall from Chapters 4 and 5 that exocrine glands secrete their products into ducts that empty onto a surface or into a cavity. For example, sweat glands produce a watery secretion that empties onto the surface of the skin. Salivary glands are also exocrine glands, secreting saliva that flows into the mouth.

Endocrine glands, on the other hand, are ductless glands. They secrete chemicals known as **hormones** into intercellular spaces. From there, the hormones diffuse directly into the blood and are carried throughout the body. Each hormone molecule may then bind to a cell that has specific receptors for that hormone, triggering a reaction in the cell. Such a cell is called a **target cell.**

The list of endocrine glands and the organs in which their target cells are found *(target organs)* continues to grow. The names, locations, and functions of the well-known endocrine glands are given in **Figure 11-1** and **Table 11-1**.

Diseases of the endocrine glands are numerous, varied, and sometimes spectacular. Tumors or other abnormalities often cause a gland to secrete too much or too little hormone. Production of too much hormone by a diseased gland is called **hypersecretion.** If too little hormone is produced, the condition is called **hyposecretion.**

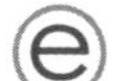
To learn more about the endocrine system, go to AnimationDirect at *evolve.elsevier.com.*

Mechanisms of Hormone Action

A hormone causes its target cells to respond in particular ways; this has been the subject of intense interest and research. The two major classes of hormones—**nonsteroid hormones** and **steroid hormones**—differ in the mechanisms by which they influence target cells.

Nonsteroid Hormones

Nonsteroid hormones are whole proteins, shorter chains of amino acids, or simply versions of single amino acids. Nonsteroid hormones typically work according to the *second messenger mechanism.* According to this concept, a nonsteroid protein hormone, such as thyroid-stimulating hormone, acts as a "first messenger" (that is, it delivers its chemical message from the cells of an endocrine gland to highly specific membrane receptor sites on the target cells).

This interaction between a hormone and its specific receptor site on the target cell's plasma membrane is often compared with the fitting of a unique key into a lock. (This idea is the *lock-and-key model* of chemical activity.)

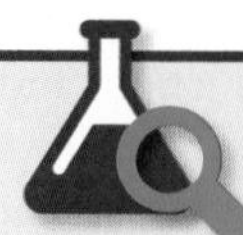

RESEARCH, ISSUES, AND TRENDS

SECOND MESSENGER SYSTEMS

Rapid and revolutionary discoveries about how nonsteroid hormones act on their target cells began with the pioneering work of Earl Sutherland, who received the 1971 Nobel Prize for formulating the second messenger hypothesis, and new discoveries continue to be made to this day.

Later, the important role of the *G protein* in getting the signal from the receptor to the enzyme that forms cyclic AMP was discovered. Look for the G protein in **Figure 11-2**. More recently, the role of nitric oxide (NO) in second messenger systems has been worked out. All of these discoveries resulted in Nobel Prizes, which shows the importance the scientific community has placed on them. Why? By working out the details of how hormones work, we can more clearly understand how and why things can go wrong that affect endocrine disorders. Perhaps we may even gain new knowledge about disorders that we previously did not even know involved hormone mechanisms.

Once the processes of disease mechanisms are figured out, we hope scientists will be able to design tests that can screen for such problems. Or perhaps they can develop drugs that will "fix" the broken mechanisms and cure the disease. Although this complex subject may seem like more than you want to learn right now, you will discover that understanding how hormones act on target cells—the concept of **signal transduction**—will prepare you for the revolution in medicine that is now upon us.

After the hormone attaches to its specific receptor site, a number of chemical reactions occur. These reactions activate molecules within the cell called **second messengers.**

One example of this mechanism occurs when the hormone-receptor interaction changes energy-rich ATP molecules inside the cell into **cyclic AMP (adenosine monophosphate).** Cyclic AMP serves as the second messenger, delivering information inside the cell that regulates the cell's activity. For example, cyclic AMP causes thyroid cells to respond to thyroid-stimulating hormone by secreting a thyroid hormone such as thyroxine. Cyclic AMP is only one of several second messengers that have been discovered.

In summary, nonsteroid hormones serve as first messengers, providing communication between endocrine glands and target organs. Another molecule, such as cyclic AMP, then acts as the second messenger, providing communication within a hormone's target cells. Figure 11-2 summarizes the mechanism of nonsteroid hormone action as explained by the second messenger hypothesis.

Steroid Hormones

The primary actions of small, lipid-soluble steroid hormones such as estrogen do not occur by the second messenger system. Because they are lipid soluble, steroid hormones can pass intact directly through the plasma membrane of the target cell.

Once inside the cell, steroid hormones pass through the cytoplasm and enter the nucleus where they bind with a receptor (according to the lock-and-key model) to form a hormone-receptor complex. This complex acts on DNA, which ultimately causes the formation of a new protein in the cytoplasm that then produces specific effects in the target cell. In the case of estrogen, for example, that effect might be breast development in the female adolescent.

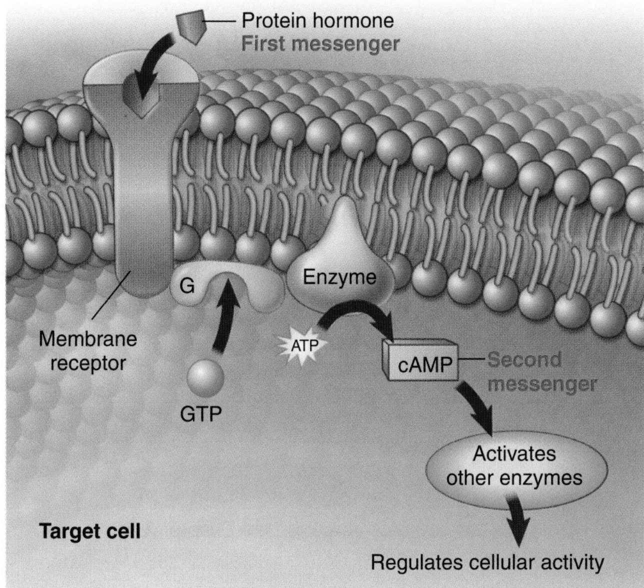

FIGURE 11-2 Mechanism of nonsteroid hormone action. The hormone acts as a "first messenger," delivering its message via the bloodstream to a membrane receptor in the target cell much like a key fits into a lock. The "second messenger" is cyclic AMP (cAMP), which forms in response to the first messenger's actions. cAMP causes the cell to respond and perform its specialized function. Variations of this mechanism also exist.

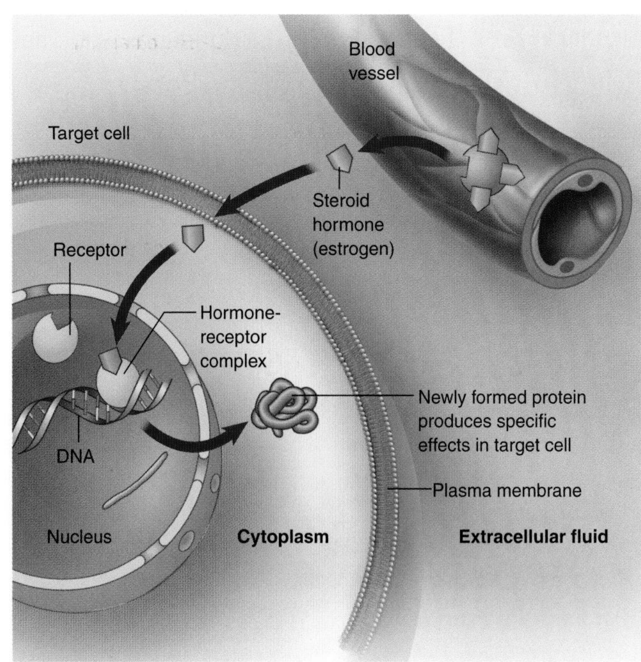

FIGURE 11-3 Mechanism of steroid hormone action. Steroid hormones pass through the plasma membrane and enter the nucleus to form a hormone receptor complex that acts on DNA. As a result, a new protein is formed in the cytoplasm that produces specific effects in the target cell.

Figure 11-3 summarizes this mechanism of steroid hormone action. Because it takes some time to accomplish all of the steps illustrated in the diagram, steroid hormone responses typically are slow compared with responses triggered by nonsteroid hormones.

Besides the primary effects of steroids produced by the DNA-triggering mechanism just described, steroid hormones may also trigger membrane receptors to produce a variety of secondary effects. These secondary effects usually appear much more rapidly than do the primary steroid effects.

QUICK CHECK

1. What is the chemical messenger used by the endocrine system?
2. How do nonsteroid hormones and steroid hormones differ? How are they alike?
3. What is a *second messenger* system?
4. How does the *lock-and-key model* of chemical activity affect nonsteroid hormones?

Regulation of Hormone Secretion

Negative Feedback

The regulation of hormone levels in the blood depends primarily on the homeostatic mechanism called *negative feedback* (see Chapter 1, p. 15).

TABLE 11-1 Endocrine Glands, Hormones, and Their Functions

GLAND/HORMONE	FUNCTION
Anterior Pituitary	
Thyroid-stimulating hormone (TSH)	Tropic hormone Stimulates secretion of thyroid hormones
Adrenocorticotropic hormone (ACTH)	Tropic hormone Stimulates secretion of adrenal cortex hormones
Follicle-stimulating hormone (FSH)	Tropic hormone *Female:* stimulates development of ovarian follicles and secretion of estrogens *Male:* stimulates seminiferous tubules of testes to grow and produce sperm
Luteinizing hormone (LH)	Tropic hormone *Female:* stimulates maturation of ovarian follicle and ovum; stimulates secretion of estrogen; triggers ovulation; stimulates development of corpus luteum (luteinization) *Male:* stimulates interstitial cells of the testes to secrete testosterone
Growth hormone (GH)	Stimulates growth in all organs; mobilizes nutrient molecules, causing an increase in blood glucose concentration
Prolactin (PRL) (lactogenic hormone)	Stimulates breast development during pregnancy and milk secretion (milk let-down) after pregnancy
Posterior Pituitary*	
Antidiuretic hormone (ADH)	Stimulates retention of water by the kidneys
Oxytocin (OT)	Stimulates uterine contractions at the end of pregnancy; Stimulates the release of milk into the breast ducts
Hypothalamus	
Releasing hormones (RHs) (several)	Stimulate the anterior pituitary to release hormones
Inhibiting hormones (IHs) (several)	Inhibit the anterior pituitary's secretion of hormones
Thyroid	
Thyroxine (T_4) and triiodothyronine (T_3)	Stimulate the energy metabolism of all cells
Calcitonin (CT)	Inhibits the breakdown of bone; causes a decrease in blood calcium concentration
Parathyroid	
Parathyroid hormone (PTH)	Stimulates the breakdown of bone; causes an increase in blood calcium concentration
Adrenal Cortex	
Mineralocorticoids (MCs): aldosterone	Regulate electrolyte and fluid homeostasis
Glucocorticoids (GCs): cortisol (hydrocortisone)	Stimulate gluconeogenesis, causing an increase in blood glucose concentration; also have anti-inflammatory, anti-immunity, and antiallergy effects
Sex hormones (androgens)	Stimulate sexual drive in the female but have negligible effects in the male
Adrenal Medulla	
Epinephrine (Epi) (adrenaline) and norepinephrine (NR)	Prolong and intensify the sympathetic nervous response during stress
Pancreatic Islets	
Glucagon	Stimulates liver glycogenolysis, causing an increase in blood glucose concentration
Insulin	Promotes glucose entry into all cells, causing a decrease in blood glucose concentration
Ovary	
Estrogens	Promote development and maintenance of female sexual characteristics (see Chapter 21)
Progesterone	Promotes conditions required for pregnancy (see Chapter 21)
Testis	
Testosterone	Promotes development and maintenance of male sexual characteristics (see Chapter 21)
Thymus	
Thymosins	Promote development of immune-system cells
Placenta	
Chorionic gonadotropin, estrogens, progesterone	Promote conditions required during early pregnancy

*Posterior pituitary hormones are synthesized in the hypothalamus but released from axon terminals in the posterior pituitary.

TABLE 11-1 Endocrine Glands, Hormones, and Their Functions—cont'd

GLAND/HORMONE	FUNCTION
Pineal Gland	
Melatonin	Inhibits tropic hormones that affect the ovaries; helps regulate the body's internal clock and sleep cycles
Heart (Atria)	
Atrial natriuretic hormone (ANH)	Regulates fluid and electrolyte homeostasis
Gastrointestinal (GI) Tract	
Ghrelin	Affects energy balance (metabolism)
Fat-Storing Cells	
Leptin	Controls how hungry or full we feel

The principle of **negative feedback** can be illustrated by using the hormone insulin as an example. When released from endocrine cells in the pancreas, insulin lowers "blood sugar levels" or glucose concentration in the blood. Normally, elevated blood sugar levels occur after a meal, after the absorption of sugars from the digestive tract takes place. The elevated blood sugar stimulates the release of insulin from the pancreas. Insulin then assists in the transfer of sugar from the blood into cells, causing blood sugar levels to drop back toward the normal set point.

As blood sugar levels drop, the endocrine cells in the pancreas slow their production and release of insulin. These responses are *negative because they reverse the direction of a disturbance to the stability of the internal environment of the body.* Therefore this homeostatic mechanism is called a *negative feedback control mechanism* because it reverses the change in blood sugar level (**Figure 11-4**).

Positive Feedback

Positive feedback mechanisms, which are uncommon, amplify changes rather than reverse them. Usually, such amplification threatens homeostasis, but in some situations it can help the body maintain its stability.

For example, during labor, the muscle contractions that push the baby through the birth canal become stronger and stronger by means of a positive feedback mechanism that regulates secretion of the hormone oxytocin (see **Figure 1-12** on p. 15).

Levels of Regulation

The endocrine system provides a good example of the concept of different levels of homeostatic regulation. Regulating the secretion of a particular hormone is one level of control, but that in turn regulates specific functions in the target cells, which in turn changes some particular function of the body.

Typically, additional levels of control are involved in maintaining homeostasis. For example, feedback may trigger the secretion of a "releasing" hormone that targets another gland and triggers the secretion of that second gland's hormone.

Feedback may instead trigger autonomic nervous stimulation of a gland, which then secretes a releasing hormone. In turn, the releasing hormone triggers the release of another hormone that regulates its target cells, which change their functions to produce an effect that changes a variable to move back toward its set point.

Often, *all* the levels of control are receiving and reacting to feedback—thus providing extra efficiency and precision to the homeostatic control of body function.

Prostaglandins

Prostaglandins (PGs), or tissue hormones, are important and extremely powerful lipid substances found in a wide variety of tissues. PGs are modified versions of fatty acids. PGs play an important role in communication and in the control of many body functions but do not meet the definition of a typical hormone.

The term *tissue hormone* is appropriate because in many instances a prostaglandin is produced in a tissue and then diffuses only a short distance to act on cells within that tissue. Typical hormones influence and control activities of widely separated organs; typical PGs influence activities of neighboring cells.

PGs, along with several other tissue hormones such as *leukotrienes* and *thromboxane,* are sometimes called **paracrine** agents. The term *paracrine* literally means "secrete beside"—an apt description for a regulatory agent released right next to its target cell.

The prostaglandins in the body can be divided into several groups. Three classes of prostaglandins—prostaglandin A (PGA), prostaglandin E (PGE), and prostaglandin F (PGF)—are among the best known.

PGs have profound effects on many body functions. They influence respiration, blood pressure, gastrointestinal secretions, inflammation, and the reproductive system. Researchers believe that most PGs regulate cells by influencing the production of cyclic AMP.

Although much research is yet to be done, PGs are already playing an important role in the treatment of conditions such as high blood pressure, asthma, and ulcers. In fact, many common treatments such as aspirin cause their effects by altering the functions of PGs in the body.

QUICK CHECK

1. How does negative feedback affect hormone levels in the blood?
2. Why are prostaglandins called *tissue hormones?*
3. What are paracrine agents? Name an example of a paracrine agent.

Pituitary Gland

Structure of the Pituitary Gland

The **pituitary gland** is a small but mighty structure. Although no larger than a pea, it is really two glands—each a different type. One is called the *anterior pituitary gland* or **adenohypophysis,** and the other is called the *posterior pituitary gland* or **neurohypophysis.**

Differences between the two glands are indicated by their names—*adeno* means "gland," and *neuro* means "nervous." The adenohypophysis has the epithelial structure of an endocrine gland, whereas the neurohypophysis has the cellular structure of nervous tissue. Hormones secreted by the adenohypophysis serve very different functions from those released from the neurohypophysis.

The protected location of this dual gland suggests its importance. The pituitary gland lies buried deep in the cranial cavity, in a well-protected location. It sits securely within a "seat" called the **sella turcica** formed by two bony projections at the top of the sphenoid bone (see Figure 7-10, *C,* on p. 132).

A stem-like structure, the *pituitary stalk,* attaches the gland to the undersurface of the

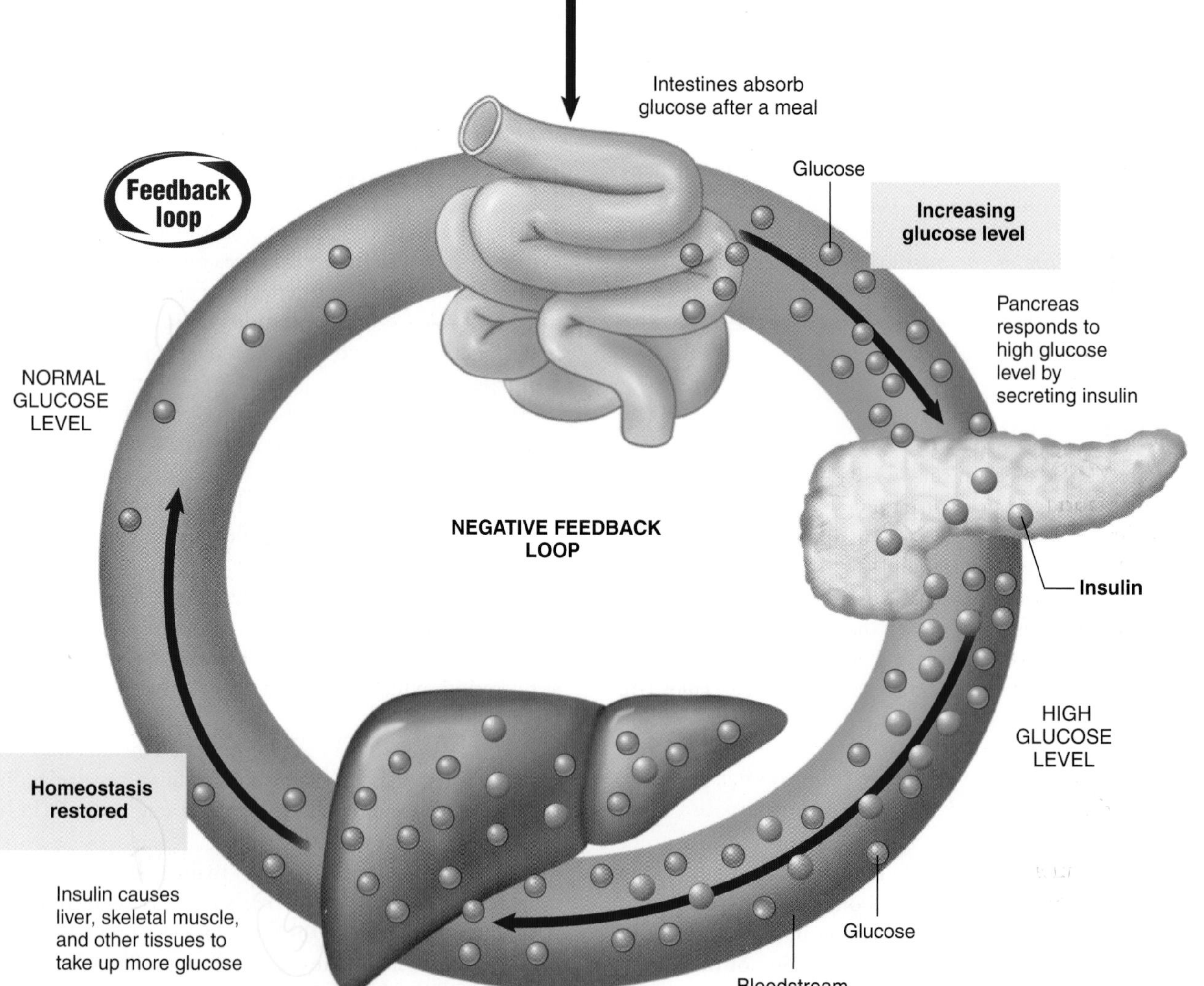

FIGURE 11-4 Negative feedback. The secretion of most hormones is regulated by negative feedback mechanisms that tend to reverse any deviations from normal. In this example, an increase in blood glucose triggers secretion of insulin. Because insulin promotes glucose uptake by cells, the blood glucose level is restored to its lower, normal level.

brain. More specifically, the stalk attaches the pituitary body to the hypothalamus.

Anterior Pituitary Gland Hormones

The anterior pituitary gland (adenohypophysis) secretes several major hormones. Each of the four hormones listed as a **tropic hormone** in Table 11-1 stimulates another endocrine gland to grow and secrete its hormones.

Because the anterior pituitary gland exerts tropic control over the structure and function of the thyroid gland, the adrenal cortex, the ovarian follicles, and the corpus luteum, it was sometimes called the *master gland.* However, because its secretions are in turn controlled by the hypothalamus and other mechanisms, the anterior pituitary is hardly the master of body function it was once thought to be.

Thyroid-stimulating Hormone

Thyroid-stimulating hormone (TSH) acts on the thyroid gland. As its name suggests, it stimulates the thyroid gland to increase secretion of thyroid hormone.

Adrenocorticotropic Hormone

The **adrenocorticotropic hormone (ACTH)** acts on the adrenal cortex. It stimulates the adrenal cortex to increase in size and to secrete larger amounts of its hormones, especially larger amounts of cortisol (hydrocortisone).

Follicle-stimulating Hormone

Follicle-stimulating hormone (FSH) stimulates the primary ovarian follicles in an ovary to start growing and to continue developing to maturity (that is, to the point of ovulation). FSH also stimulates follicle cells to secrete estrogens. In the male, FSH stimulates the seminiferous tubules to grow and form sperm.

Luteinizing Hormone

Luteinizing hormone (LH) acts with FSH to perform several functions. It stimulates a follicle and ovum to complete their growth to maturity, it stimulates follicle cells to secrete estrogens, and it causes ovulation (rupturing of the mature follicle with expulsion of its ripe ovum). Because of this function, LH is sometimes called the *ovulating hormone.*

LH also stimulates the formation of a golden body, the corpus luteum, from the ruptured follicle. This process—called **luteinization**—is the one that earned LH its title of *luteinizing hormone.* As it promotes luteinization, LH stimulates the corpus luteum to produce the hormone progesterone.

The male pituitary gland also secretes LH. In males, LH stimulates interstitial cells in the testes to develop and secrete testosterone, the male sex hormone.

Growth Hormone

Another important hormone secreted by the anterior pituitary gland is **growth hormone (GH).** GH speeds up the movement of digested proteins (amino acids) out of the blood and

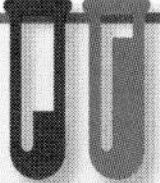

CLINICAL APPLICATION

GROWTH HORMONE ABNORMALITIES

Hypersecretion of growth hormone during the early years of life produces a condition called **gigantism.** The photo in Figure *A* shows a 22-year-old man on the left with gigantism next to his normal identical twin on the right. The name *gigantism* suggests the obvious characteristics of this condition. The child grows to giant size.

Hyposecretion of the growth hormone may produce pituitary **dwarfism,** *which is characterized by abnormally short stature.*

If the anterior pituitary gland secretes too much growth hormone after the normal growth years, then the disease called **acromegaly** develops. Characteristics of this disease are enlargement of the bones of the hands, feet, jaws, and face (Figure *B*). The facial appearance typical of acromegaly results from the combination of bone and soft tissue overgrowth. A prominent forehead and large nose are characteristic. In addition, the skin is characterized by large, widened pores, and the mandible grows in length so that the lower jaw protrudes and separation of the lower teeth commonly occurs.

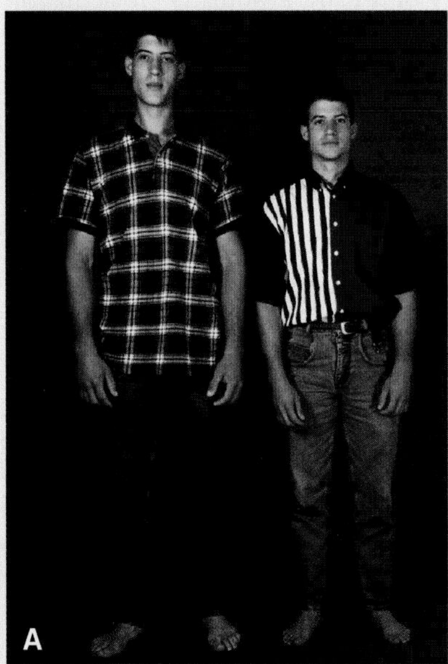

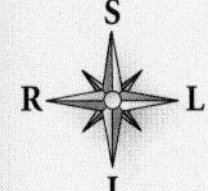

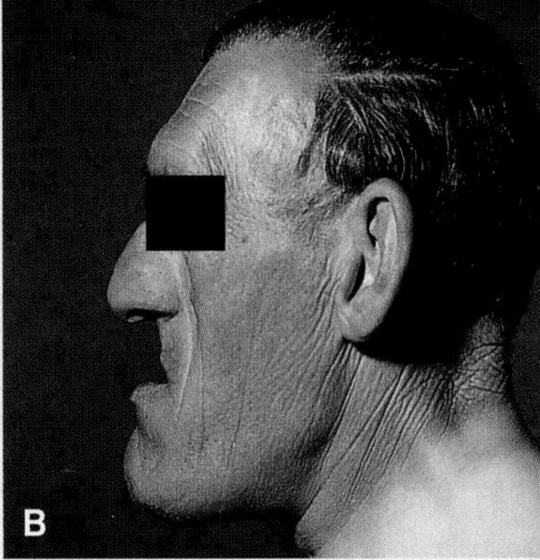

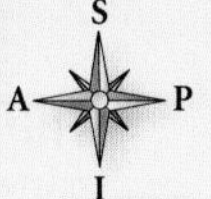

into the cells, and this accelerates the cells' **anabolism** (building-up) of amino acids to form tissue proteins (see Chapter 17). This anabolic action promotes normal growth.

Growth hormone also affects fat and carbohydrate metabolism. It accelerates fat catabolism (breakdown) but slows glucose catabolism. This means that less glucose leaves the blood to enter cells, and therefore the amount of glucose in the blood increases. Thus growth hormone and insulin have opposite effects on blood glucose. Insulin decreases blood glucose, and growth hormone increases it.

Too much insulin in the blood produces **hypoglycemia** (lower than normal blood glucose concentration). Too much growth hormone produces **hyperglycemia** (higher than normal blood glucose concentration).

Also called *human growth hormone (hGH),* this hormone is used by some people to keep themselves youthful or to boost athletic performance. These unapproved uses can have dangerous side effects by disrupting normal hormone balances in the body.

Prolactin

The anterior pituitary gland also secretes **prolactin (PRL)**. During pregnancy, prolactin stimulates the breast development necessary for eventual lactation (milk secretion). Also, soon after delivery of a baby, a woman's prolactin stimulates the breasts to start secreting milk, a function suggested by prolactin's other name, *lactogenic hormone.*

Figure 11-5 provides a summary of anterior pituitary hormone target organs and functions.

Posterior Pituitary Gland Hormones

The posterior pituitary gland (neurohypophysis) releases two hormones—*antidiuretic hormone* and *oxytocin.* Both hormones are produced in cell bodies that are located in the hypothalamus but are released from the ends of axons that are located in the posterior pituitary gland.

Antidiuretic Hormone

Antidiuretic hormone (ADH) is a major regulator of fluid balance in the human body. ADH accelerates the reabsorption of water from urine in kidney tubules back into the blood. With more water moving out of the tubules into the blood, less water remains in the tubules, and therefore less urine leaves the body.

The term *antidiuretic* is appropriate because *anti-* means "against" and *diuretic* means "increasing the volume of urine excreted." Therefore *antidiuretic* means "acting against an increase in urine volume"—in other words, ADH acts to decrease urine volume and thus prevent dehydration.

Hyposecretion of ADH results in **diabetes insipidus**, a condition in which large volumes of urine are formed. Dehydration and electrolyte imbalances may cause serious problems. Although increased water intake can relieve mild symptoms, many cases also require administering a synthetic form of ADH.

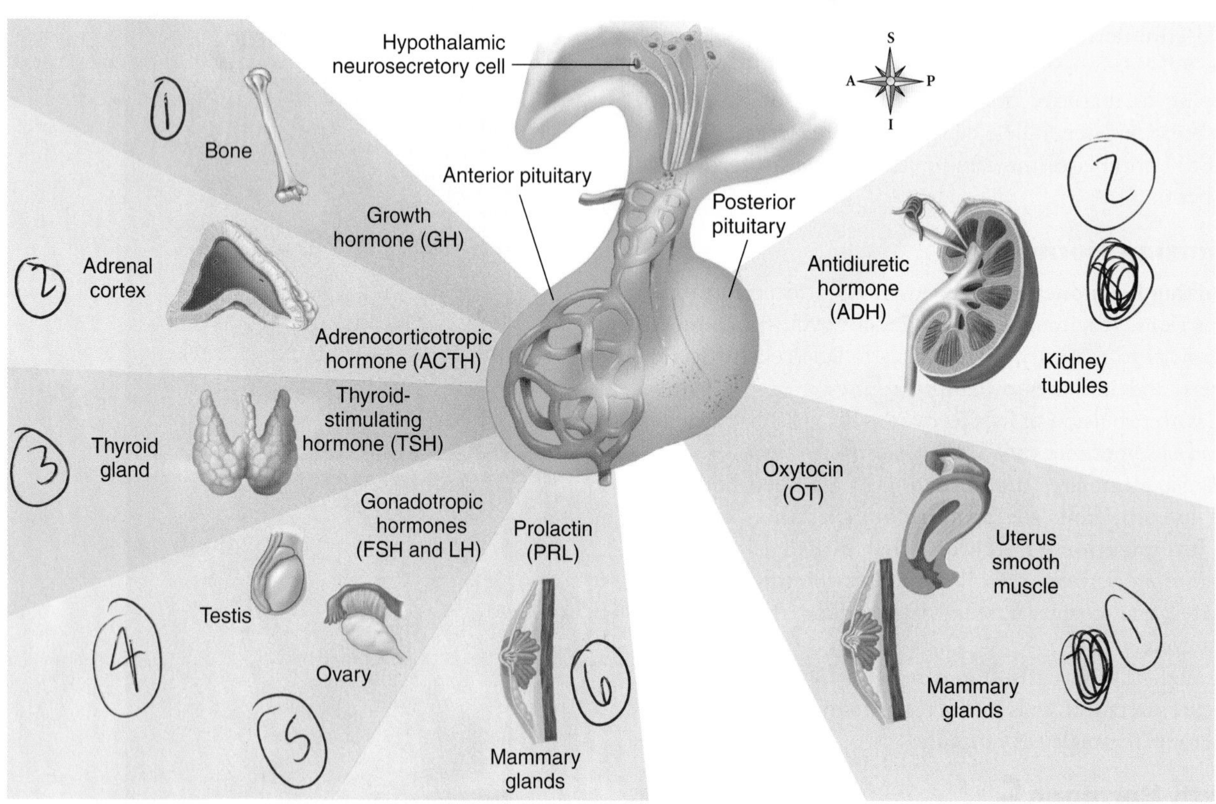

FIGURE 11-5 Pituitary hormones. Principal anterior pituitary hormones and their major target organs *(shaded purple)* and posterior pituitary hormones and some major target organs *(shaded blue).*

Oxytocin

The posterior pituitary hormone **oxytocin (OT)** is secreted at high levels by a woman's body before and after she has a baby. Oxytocin stimulates contraction of the smooth muscle of the pregnant uterus and is believed to initiate and maintain labor. This is why physicians sometimes prescribe oxytocin injections to induce or increase labor.

Oxytocin also performs a function important to a newborn baby. It causes the glandular cells of the breast to release milk into ducts from which a baby can easily obtain it by sucking. In short, oxytocin stimulates "milk let-down."

Oxytocin is also thought to enhance social bonding—a function helpful in supporting the mother-infant bond.

The right side of **Figure 11-5** summarizes posterior pituitary functions.

Hypothalamus

In discussing ADH and oxytocin, we noted that these hormones were *released* from the posterior lobe of the pituitary. Actual production of these two hormones occurs in the hypothalamus. Two groups of secretory neurons in the hypothalamus synthesize the posterior pituitary hormones, which then pass down along axons into the pituitary gland. Release of ADH and oxytocin into the blood is controlled by nervous stimulation.

In addition to oxytocin and ADH, the hypothalamus also produces substances called **releasing hormones (RHs)** and **inhibiting hormones (IHs).** These substances are produced in the hypothalamus and then released directly into a unique blood capillary system. This system carries the hormones to the anterior pituitary gland, where they stimulate or inhibit the release of anterior pituitary hormones into the general circulation.

The combined nervous and endocrine functions of the hypothalamus allow the nervous system to influence many endocrine functions. Therefore the hypothalamus plays a dominant role in the regulation of many body functions related to homeostasis. Examples include the regulation of body temperature, appetite, and thirst.

QUICK CHECK

1. How are the anterior pituitary and posterior pituitary different? How are they alike?
2. What makes a hormone a *tropic* hormone?
3. Name the hormones produced by the pituitary gland.
4. How does the hypothalamus control the pituitary gland?
5. What hormone is being used by some people to keep youthful or to boost athletic performance? Why is this not approved for safe use?

Thyroid Gland

The thyroid gland lies in the neck just below the larynx (**Figure 11-6**).

As **Figure 11-7** shows, thyroid tissue is organized into many chambers called **thyroid follicles.** Each thyroid follicle is filled with a thick fluid having many fine, suspended particles called *colloid.*

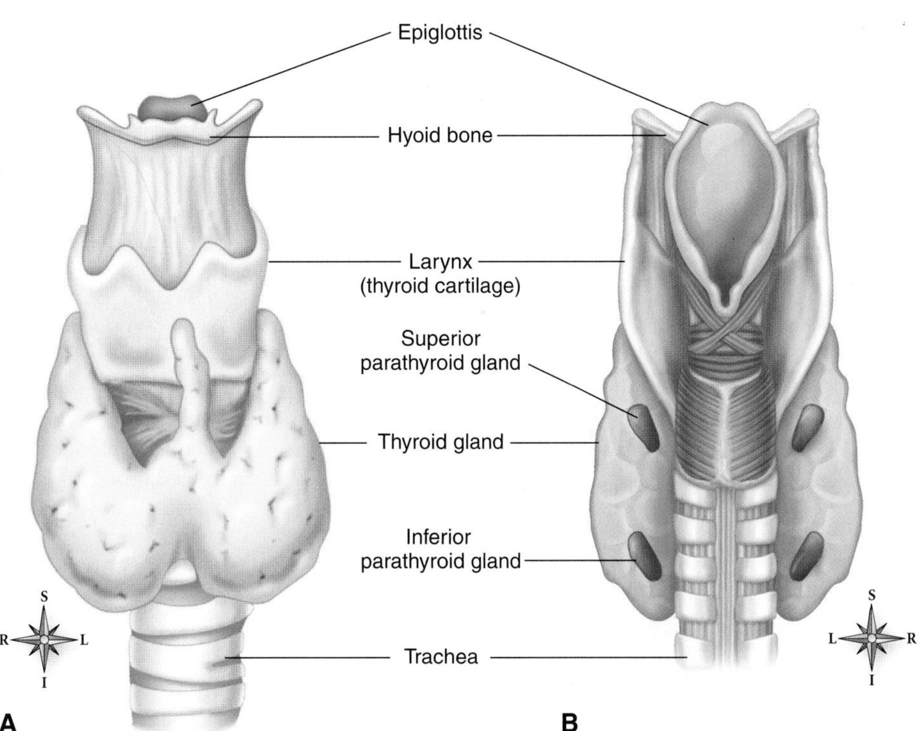

FIGURE 11-6 Thyroid and parathyroid glands. Note their relationship to each other and to the larynx (voice box) and trachea.

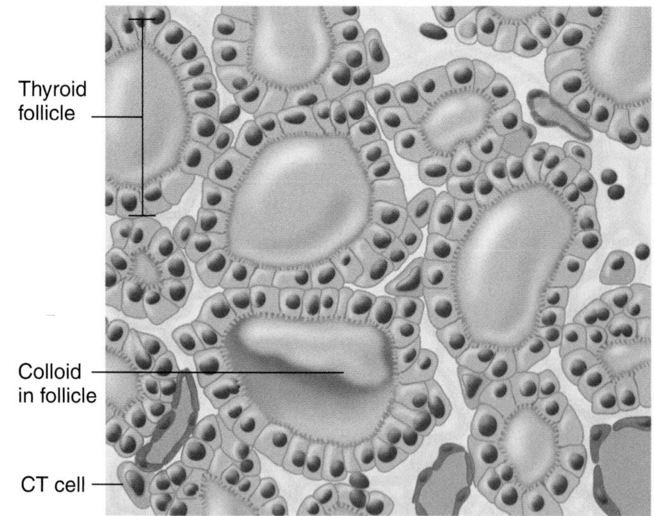

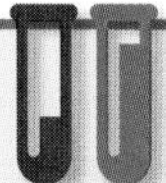

FIGURE 11-7 Thyroid gland tissue. Thyroid hormone is produced by follicular cells in the walls of the thyroid follicles. Note that each of the follicles is filled with colloid—a fluid with fine, suspended particles. The colloid serves as a storage medium for the thyroid hormones. Another type of thyroid gland cells, called CT cells, are outside the follicles and secrete calcitonin (CT).

The thyroid gland secretes two thyroid hormones and the hormone **calcitonin (CT).**

Thyroid Hormone

What was once thought of as a single thyroid hormone is actually two similar hormones: **triiodothyronine (T_3)** and **thyroxine (T_4)**.

Of the two thyroid hormones, T_4 is the more abundant. However, T_3 is the more potent and is considered by physiologists to be the principal thyroid hormone. One molecule of T_4 contains four atoms of iodine, and one molecule of T_3, as its name suggests, contains three iodine atoms. For thyroid hormones to be produced in adequate amounts, the diet must contain sufficient iodine.

Most endocrine glands do not store their hormones but instead secrete them directly into the blood as they are produced. The thyroid gland is different in that it stores considerable amounts of the thyroid hormones in the form of molecules suspended in fluid as a colloid, as seen in Figure 11-7. The colloid material is stored in the follicles of the gland, and when the thyroid hormones are needed, they are released from the colloid and secreted into the blood.

CLINICAL APPLICATION

THYROID HORMONE ABNORMALITIES

Hyperthyroidism, or oversecretion of the thyroid hormones, dramatically increases the metabolic rate. Nutrients are metabolized by the cells at an excessive rate, and individuals who suffer from this condition lose weight, are irritable, have an increased appetite, and often show protrusion of the eyeballs due in part to edema of tissue at the back of the eye socket (see Figure *A*).

Hypothyroidism, or undersecretion of thyroid hormones, can be caused by and result in a number of different medical conditions. Low dietary intake of iodine causes a painless enlargement of the thyroid gland called **simple goiter,** shown in Figure *B*. This condition was once common in areas of the United States where the iodine content of the soil and water is inadequate. The use of iodized salt has dramatically reduced the incidence of simple goiter caused by low iodine intake. In simple goiter the gland enlarges to compensate for the lack of iodine in the diet necessary for the synthesis of thyroid hormones.

Hyposecretion of thyroid hormones during the formative years leads to a condition called **cretinism.** It is characterized by a low metabolic rate; retarded growth and sexual development; and, often, mental retardation. Fortunately, health screening for low thyroid function can lead to treatment before cretinism develops.

Later in life, deficient thyroid hormone secretion produces the disease called **myxedema.** The low metabolic rate that characterizes myxedema leads to lessened mental and physical vigor, weight gain, loss of hair, and swelling of tissues.

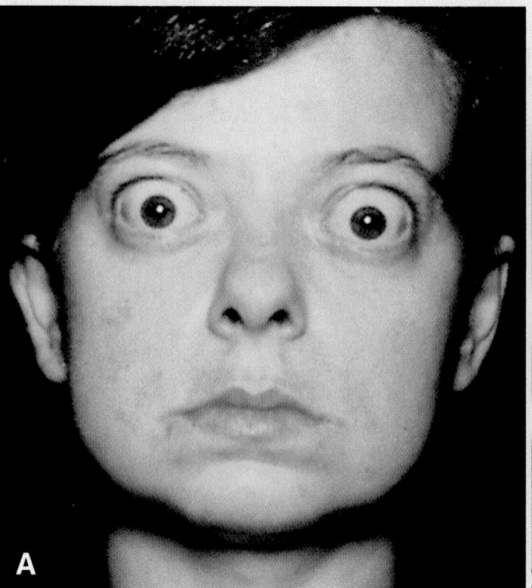

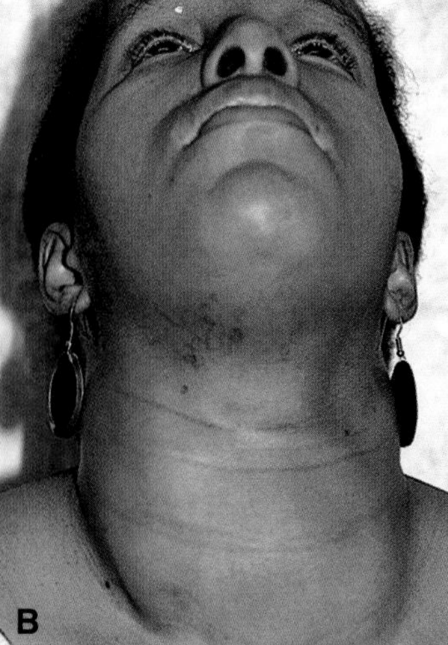

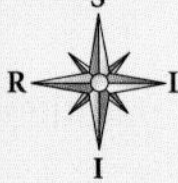

T_4 and T_3 are small, nonsteroid hormones that are able to enter their target cell to find their receptors. This is an exception to the general model of nonsteroid action requiring an internal second messenger.

T_4 and T_3 influence every one of the trillions of cells in our bodies. They make them speed up their release of energy from nutrients. In other words, these thyroid hormones stimulate cellular metabolism. This has far-reaching effects. Because all body functions depend on a normal supply of energy, they all depend on normal thyroid secretion. Even normal mental and physical growth and development depend on normal thyroid functioning.

Calcitonin

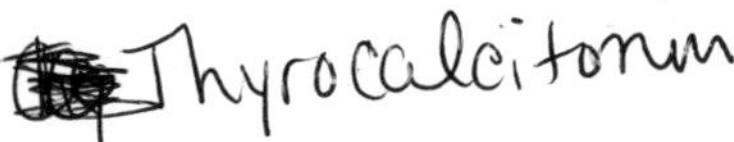

Calcitonin (CT) is secreted by thyroid gland cells—sometimes called *CT cells*—that lie outside the thyroid follicles.

Calcitonin decreases the concentration of calcium in the blood by first acting on bone to inhibit its breakdown. With less bone being resorbed, less calcium moves out of bone into blood, and, as a result, the concentration of calcium in blood decreases.

An increase in calcitonin secretion quickly follows any increase in blood calcium concentration, even if it is a slight one. This causes blood calcium concentration to decrease to its normal level. Calcitonin thus helps maintain homeostasis of blood calcium. It prevents a harmful excess of calcium in the blood, a condition called **hypercalcemia**, from developing.

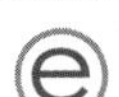

To learn more about thyroid secretion, go to AnimationDirect at *evolve.elsevier.com*.

Parathyroid Glands

The **parathyroid glands** are small lumps of glandular epithelium. There are usually four of them, and they are found on the posterior surfaces of the thyroid gland (see **Figure 11-6**).

The parathyroid glands secrete **parathyroid hormone (PTH).**

PTH increases the concentration of calcium in the blood—the opposite effect of the thyroid gland's calcitonin. Whereas calcitonin acts to decrease the amount of calcium being dissolved and reabsorbed from bone, PTH acts to increase it.

PTH stimulates mineral-dissolving osteoclast cells in bone tissue to increase their breakdown of bone's hard matrix, a process that frees the calcium stored in the matrix. The released calcium then moves out of bone into blood, and this in turn increases the blood's calcium concentration.

Figure 11-8 provides a summary of the antagonistic effects of calcitonin and parathyroid hormone. This is a matter of life-and-death importance because our cells are extremely sensitive to changing amounts of blood calcium. They cannot function normally with too much or too little calcium.

For example, with too much blood calcium, brain cells and heart cells soon cease to function normally; a person becomes mentally disturbed, and the heart may stop. However, with too little blood calcium, nerve cells become overactive, sometimes to such a degree that they bombard muscles with so many impulses that the muscles go into spasms.

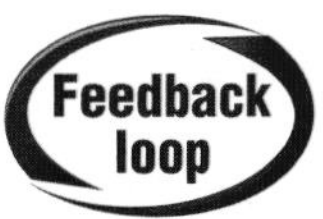

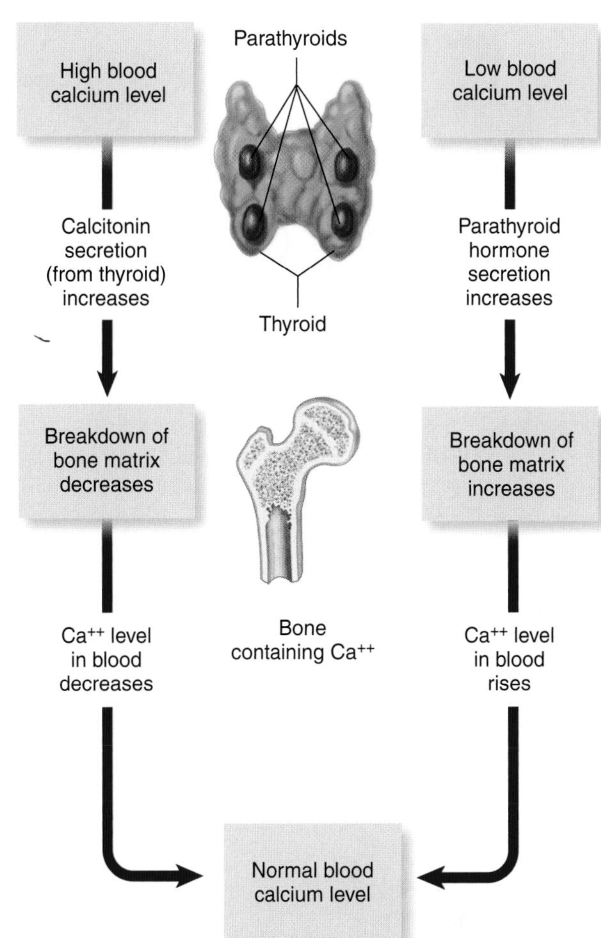

FIGURE 11-8 Regulation of blood calcium levels. Calcitonin and parathyroid hormones have antagonistic (opposite) effects on calcium concentration in the blood.

QUICK CHECK

1. Where are the thyroid and parathyroid glands located?
2. What gland stores its hormones for later use?
3. Calcitonin and parathyroid hormone both regulate the blood concentration of what important ion?
4. What hormones are exceptions to the general model of nonsteroid action requiring an internal second messenger?

Adrenal Glands

As you can see in **Figure 11-1** and **Figure 11-9**, an adrenal gland curves over the superior surface of each kidney.

From the surface an adrenal gland appears to be only one organ, but it is actually two separate endocrine glands: the

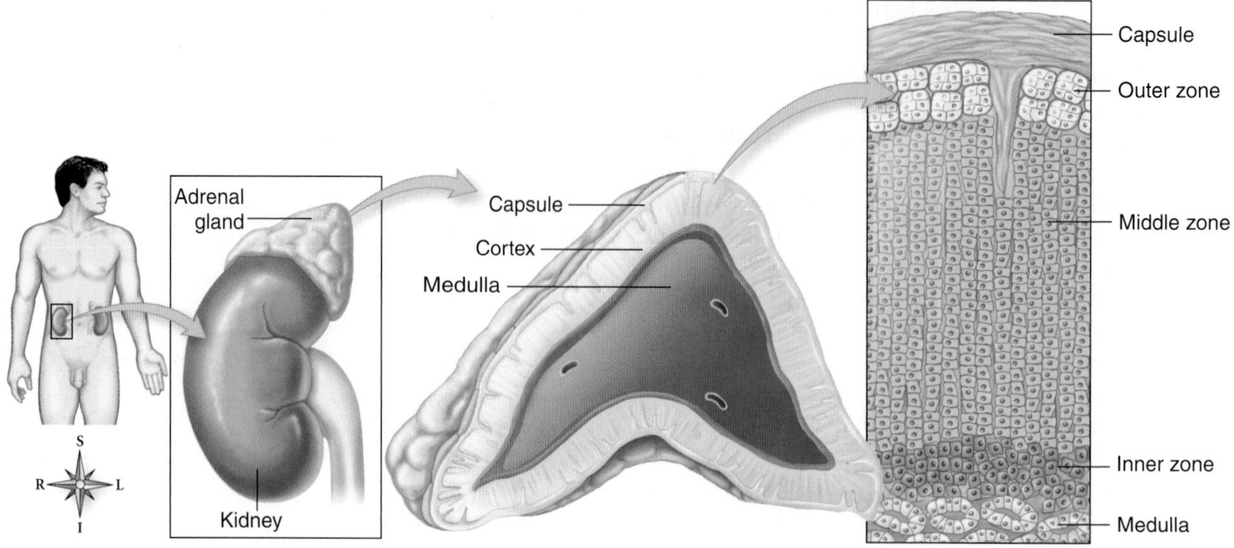

FIGURE 11-9 The adrenal gland. The three cell layers of the adrenal cortex are easily seen here. The outer zone cells secrete mineralocorticoids (aldosterone). The middle zone cells secrete glucocorticoids (hydrocortisone). The inner zone cells secrete sex hormones (androgens).

adrenal cortex and the *adrenal medulla.* Does this two-glands-in-one structure remind you of another endocrine organ? (See p. 242.)

The adrenal cortex is the outer part of an adrenal gland and is made up of glandular epithelium. The adrenal medulla is the inner part and it is made up of secretory nervous tissue—much like the secretory nervous tissue of the posterior pituitary. Each part releases a different set of hormones, as you might expect.

Adrenal Cortex

Three different zones or layers of cells make up the **adrenal cortex** as you can see in Figure 11-9. Follow this diagram carefully as you read the following paragraph and you will easily see the special function of each layer of the adrenal cortex.

Zones of the Adrenal Cortex

Hormones secreted by the three cell layers or zones of the adrenal cortex are called **corticoids**, all of which are steroid hormones.

The outer zone of adrenal cortex cells secretes hormones called **mineralocorticoids (MCs).** The main mineralocorticoid is the hormone *aldosterone.*

The middle zone secretes **glucocorticoids (GCs).** *Cortisol* is the chief glucocorticoid.

The innermost or deepest zone of the cortex secretes small amounts of *sex hormones.* Sex hormones secreted by the adrenal cortex resemble testosterone.

A brief discussion of the functions of the main corticoid hormones follows.

Aldosterone

As their name suggests, *mineralocorticoids* help control the amount of certain mineral salts (mainly sodium chloride) in the blood.

Aldosterone is the chief mineralocorticoid. Remember its main functions—to increase the amount of sodium and decrease the amount of potassium in the blood—because these changes lead to other profound changes.

Aldosterone increases blood sodium and decreases blood potassium by influencing the kidney tubules. It causes them to speed up their reabsorption of sodium back into the blood so that less of it will be lost in the urine. At the same time, aldosterone causes the tubules to increase their secretion of potassium so that more of this mineral will be lost in the urine. The effects of aldosterone speed up kidney reabsorption of water.

Cortisol

An important role of glucocorticoids is to help maintain normal blood glucose concentration. **Cortisol,** or **hydrocortisone,** is the chief glucocorticoid produced by the adrenal cortex.

Cortisol and other glucocorticoids increase **gluconeogenesis,** a process in liver cells that converts amino acids or glycerol to glucose. Glucocorticoids act in several ways to increase gluconeogenesis. They promote the breakdown of tissue proteins to amino acids, especially in muscle cells. Amino acids thus formed move out of the tissue cells into blood and circulate to the liver. Liver cells then change them to glucose by the process of gluconeogenesis. The newly formed glucose leaves the liver cells and enters the blood. This action increases blood glucose concentration.

In addition to performing these functions—which are necessary for maintaining normal blood glucose concentration—glucocorticoids such as cortisol also play an essential part in maintaining normal blood pressure. They act in a complicated way to make it possible for two other hormones secreted by the adrenal medulla to partially constrict blood vessels, a condition necessary for maintaining normal blood pressure.

Also, glucocorticoids act with these hormones from the adrenal medulla to produce an anti-inflammatory effect. They bring about a normal recovery from inflammations produced by many kinds of agents. The use of hydrocortisone to relieve skin rashes, for example, is based on the anti-inflammatory effect of glucocorticoids.

Another effect produced by glucocorticoids is called their *anti-immunity, antiallergy effect.* Glucocorticoids bring about a decrease in the number of certain cells that produce antibodies, substances that make us immune to some factors and allergic to others.

When extreme stimuli act on the body, they produce an internal state or condition known as **stress**. Surgery, hemorrhage, infections, severe burns, and intense emotions are examples of extreme stimuli that bring on stress. The normal adrenal cortex responds to the condition of stress by quickly increasing its secretion of glucocorticoids. This fact is well established. What is still not known, however, is whether the increased amount of glucocorticoids helps the body cope successfully with stress.

Increased glucocorticoid secretion is only one of many ways in which the body responds to stress, but it is one of the first stress responses, and it brings about many of the other stress responses. Examine **Figure 11-10** to discover what stress responses are produced by a high concentration of glucocorticoids in the blood.

When resisting (or avoiding) a threat, the increased blood glucose can help improve our skeletal muscle function. Reduced inflammation may help keep us less swollen—and thus more mobile—while we deal with the threat. Decreased immunity may help us focus all our resources on the more immediate threat. Immunity resumes after a threatening encounter to deal with any damage.

Frequent or prolonged stress responses could cause metabolic problems by disturbing normal mechanisms keeping blood glucose and stored fats in balance. Chronic stress may also increase our susceptibility to cancer and infections by reducing our immunity. Prolonging the anti-inflammatory effects may cause constriction of blood vessels—possibly raising our blood pressure.

Sex Hormones

The **sex hormones** that are secreted by the inner zone are male hormones **(androgens)** similar to testosterone. These hormones are secreted in small amounts in both adult males and females, but they play an early role in the development of reproductive organs.

In women, these androgens may stimulate the female sexual drive. In men, so much testosterone is secreted by the testes that adrenal androgens are physiologically insignificant.

Adrenal Medulla

The **adrenal medulla,** or inner portion of the adrenal gland shown in **Figure 11-9**, secretes the hormones **epinephrine (Epi)** and **norepinephrine (NR).** Epinephrine is also known as *adrenaline.*

Our bodies have many ways to defend themselves against enemies that threaten their well-being. A physiologist might say that the body resists stress by making many stress

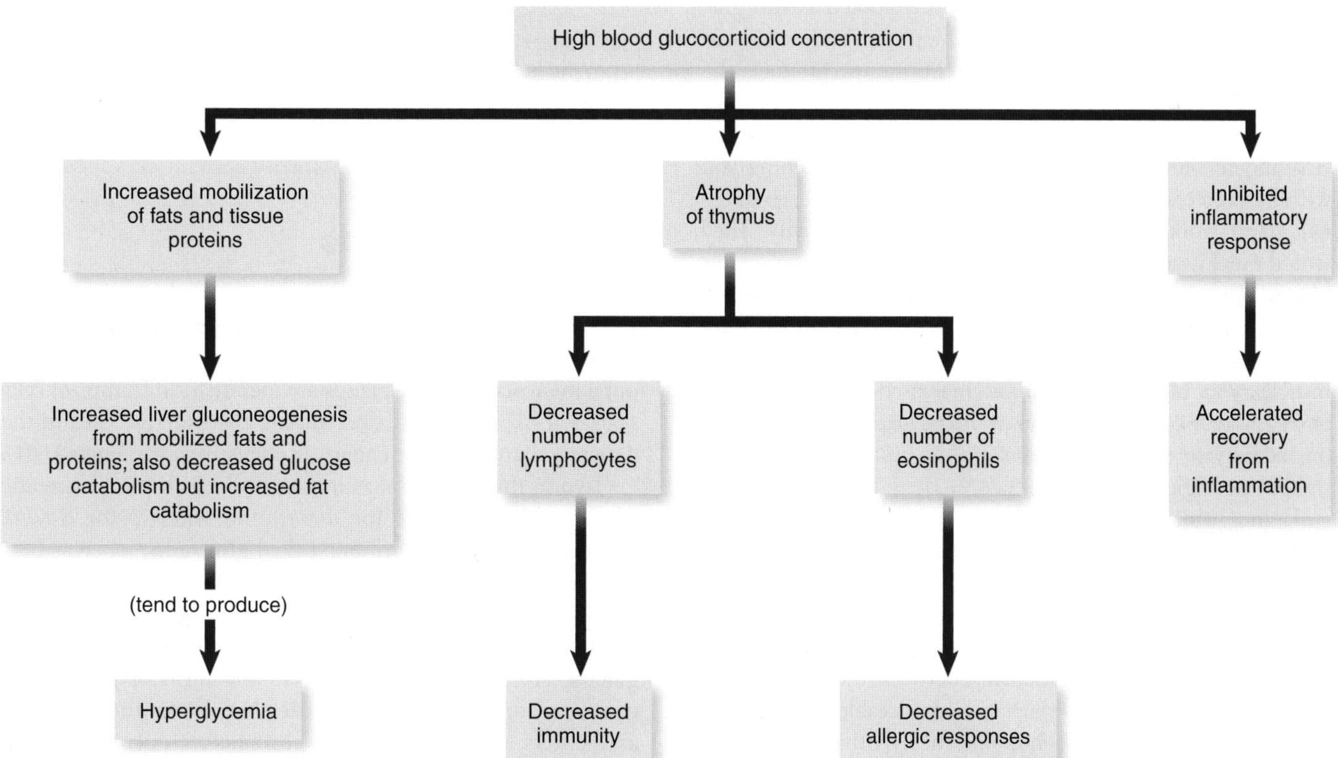

FIGURE 11-10 Stress responses. Stress may trigger elevated secretion of glucocorticoids (GCs) into the blood. This flow chart shows the possible effects induced by high blood GC concentration.

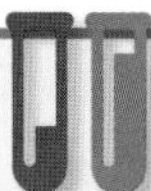

CLINICAL APPLICATION

ADRENAL HORMONE ABNORMALITIES

Injury, disease states, or malfunction of the adrenal glands can result in hypersecretion or hyposecretion of several different hormones.

Tumors of the adrenal cortex located in the middle zone of the cortex often result in the production of abnormally large amounts of glucocorticoids. The medical name for this condition is **Cushing syndrome.** Figure *A* shows a boy just diagnosed with Cushing syndrome. Figure *B* shows the same boy 4 months later, after treatment.

For some reason, many more women than men develop Cushing syndrome. Its most noticeable features are the so-called moon face and the buffalo hump on the upper back that develop because of redistribution of body fat. These individuals also have elevated blood sugar levels and suffer frequent infections. Surgical removal of a glucocorticoid-producing tumor may result in dramatic improvement of the moon-face symptom within 6 months.

Deficiency, or hyposecretion, of adrenal cortex hormones results in a condition called **Addison disease.** President John F. Kennedy suffered from Addison disease, which causes reduced cortical hormone levels resulting in muscle weakness, reduced blood sugar, nausea, loss of appetite, and weight loss.

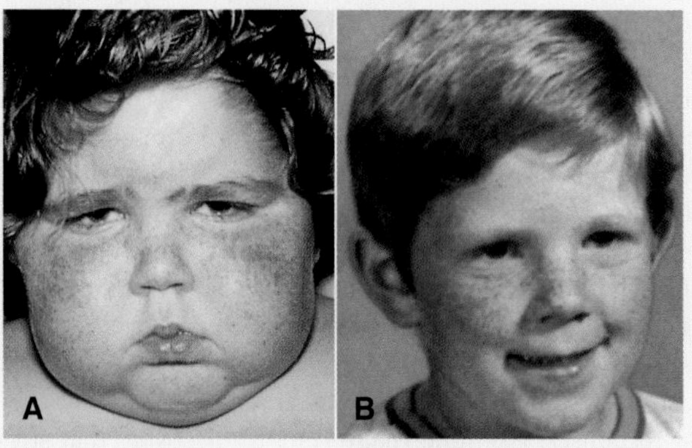

responses. We have just discussed increased glucocorticoid secretion. An even faster-acting stress response is increased hormone secretion by the adrenal medulla.

The adrenal medulla responds very rapidly to stress because nerve impulses conducted by sympathetic nerve fibers stimulate the adrenal medulla. When stimulated, it literally squirts epinephrine and norepinephrine into the blood. As with glucocorticoids, these hormones may help the body resist or avoid stress. In other words, these hormones produce the body's "fight-or-flight" response to danger (stress).

Suppose you suddenly faced some threatening situation. Imagine encountering a large animal that is threatening you with bared teeth. Almost instantly, the medulla of each adrenal gland would be galvanized into feverish activity. They would quickly secrete large amounts of epinephrine into your blood. Many of your body functions would seem to be supercharged. Your heart would beat faster, your blood pressure would rise, more blood would be pumped to your skeletal muscles, your blood would contain increased glucose for more energy, and so on. In short, you would be geared up for strenuous activity to either *resist* or *avoid* the animal attack—thus the phrase "fight or flight."

Epinephrine prolongs and intensifies changes in body function brought about by the stimulation of the sympathetic subdivision of the autonomic nervous system. Recall from Chapter 9 that sympathetic or adrenergic fibers release epinephrine and norepinephrine as neurotransmitter substances.

The close functional relationship between the nervous and the endocrine systems is perhaps most noticeable in the body's response to stress. In stress conditions, the hypothalamus acts on the anterior pituitary gland to cause the release of ACTH, which stimulates the adrenal cortex to secrete glucocorticoids. At the same time, the sympathetic subdivision of the autonomic nervous system is stimulated with the adrenal medulla, so the release of epinephrine and norepinephrine occurs to assist the body in responding to the stressful stimulus.

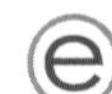
To learn more about the adrenal gland, go to AnimationDirect at *evolve.elsevier.com.*

QUICK CHECK

1. Why is the adrenal gland often thought of as two separate glands?
2. Name the hormones produced by the adrenal gland.
3. How does the pituitary gland influence adrenal function?

Pancreatic Islets

All the endocrine glands discussed so far are big enough to be seen without a magnifying glass. The **pancreatic islets,** or **islets of Langerhans,** in contrast, are too tiny to be seen without a microscope. These glands are merely little clumps of cells scattered like islands in a sea among the exocrine cells of the pancreas that secrete the pancreatic digestive juice (**Figure 11-11**).

Two of the most important kinds of cells in the pancreatic islets are the *alpha cells* (or *A cells*) and *beta cells* (or *B cells*). Alpha cells secrete a hormone called **glucagon,** whereas beta cells secrete one of the best known of all hormones, **insulin.**

Glucagon accelerates a process called **glycogenolysis** in the liver. Glycogenolysis is a chemical process by which the glucose stored in the liver cells in the form of glycogen is converted to glucose. This glucose then leaves the liver cells and enters the blood. Glucagon therefore increases blood glucose concentration.

Insulin and glucagon are antagonists. In other words, insulin decreases blood glucose concentration and glucagon

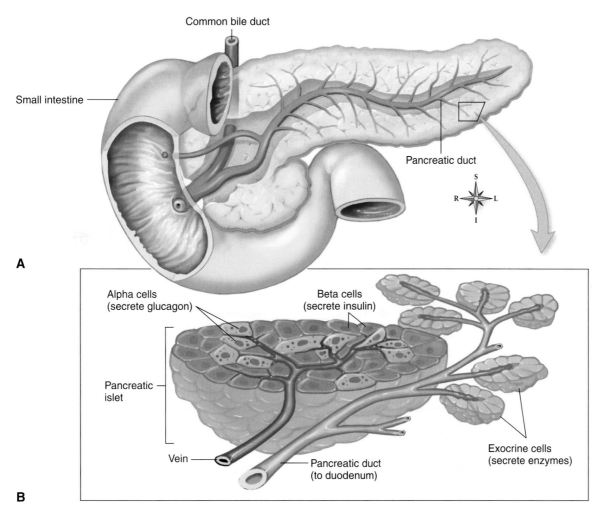

FIGURE 11-11 Pancreas. A, Location and structure of the pancreas (shown partially cut open). **B,** A pancreatic islet (of Langerhans) in enlarged cross section, showing the glucagon-producing alpha cells and insulin-producing beta cells. Notice the many exocrine cells surrounding the endocrine pancreatic islet.

increases it. Insulin is the only hormone that can decrease blood glucose concentration. Several hormones, however, increase glucose concentration, including glucocorticoids, growth hormone, and glucagon. Insulin decreases blood glucose by accelerating its movement out of the blood, through cell membranes, and into cells. As glucose enters the cells at a faster rate, the cells increase their metabolism of glucose.

Briefly then, insulin decreases blood glucose and increases glucose metabolism.

If the pancreatic islets secrete a normal amount of insulin, glucose enters the cells easily, and a normal amount of glucose stays behind in the blood. ("Normal" fasting blood glucose is about 70 to 100 mg of glucose in every 100 mL of blood.)

If the pancreatic islets secrete too much insulin, as they rarely do when a person has a tumor of the pancreas, more glucose than usual leaves the blood to enter the cells, and blood glucose decreases.

If the pancreatic islets secrete too little insulin, as they do in **type 1 diabetes mellitus,** less glucose leaves the blood to enter the cells, so the blood glucose increases, sometimes to even three or more times the normal amount.

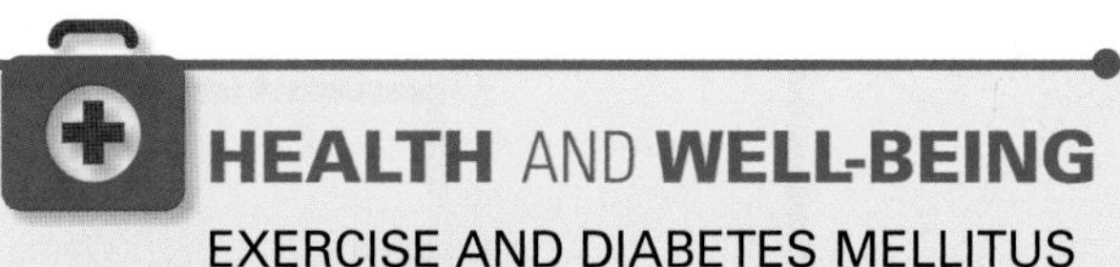

HEALTH AND WELL-BEING

EXERCISE AND DIABETES MELLITUS

Type 1 diabetes mellitus is characterized by high blood glucose concentration because the lack of sufficient insulin prevents glucose from entering cells. However, exercise physiologists have found that aerobic training increases the number of insulin receptors in target cells and the insulin affinity (attraction) of the receptors. This condition allows a small amount of insulin to have a greater effect than it would have otherwise had. Thus exercise reduces the severity of the diabetic condition.

All forms of diabetes benefit from properly planned exercise therapy. Not only is this form of treatment natural and cost effective, but it also helps reduce or prevent other problems such as obesity and heart disease.

Most cases of **type 2 diabetes mellitus** result from some decrease of insulin and an abnormality of the insulin receptors, preventing the normal effects of insulin on its target cells and thus also raising blood glucose levels.

Screening tests for all types of **diabetes mellitus (DM)** rely on the fact that the blood glucose level is elevated in this condition. Today, most screening is done with a simple test with a drop of blood. Subjects with a high blood glucose level are suspected of having diabetes mellitus. Testing for sugar in the urine is another common screening procedure. In diabetes mellitus, excess glucose is filtered out of the blood by the kidneys and lost in the urine, producing the condition **glycosuria**.

Figure 11-12 summarizes some of the many problems that can be caused by diabetes mellitus. A quick look at these problems underscores the importance of insulin and insulin receptors in healthy bodies.

QUICK CHECK

1. Name the two primary hormones of the pancreatic islets.
2. What effect does insulin have on the blood's glucose concentration?
3. How does diabetes produce glucose in the urine?

Female Sex Glands

A woman's primary sex glands are her two ovaries. Each ovary contains two different kinds of glandular structures: the ovarian follicles and the corpus luteum.

Ovarian follicles are little pockets in which egg cells, or **ova,** develop. Ovarian follicles also secrete **estrogen,** the "feminizing hormone." Estrogen is involved in the development and maturation of the breasts and external genitals. This

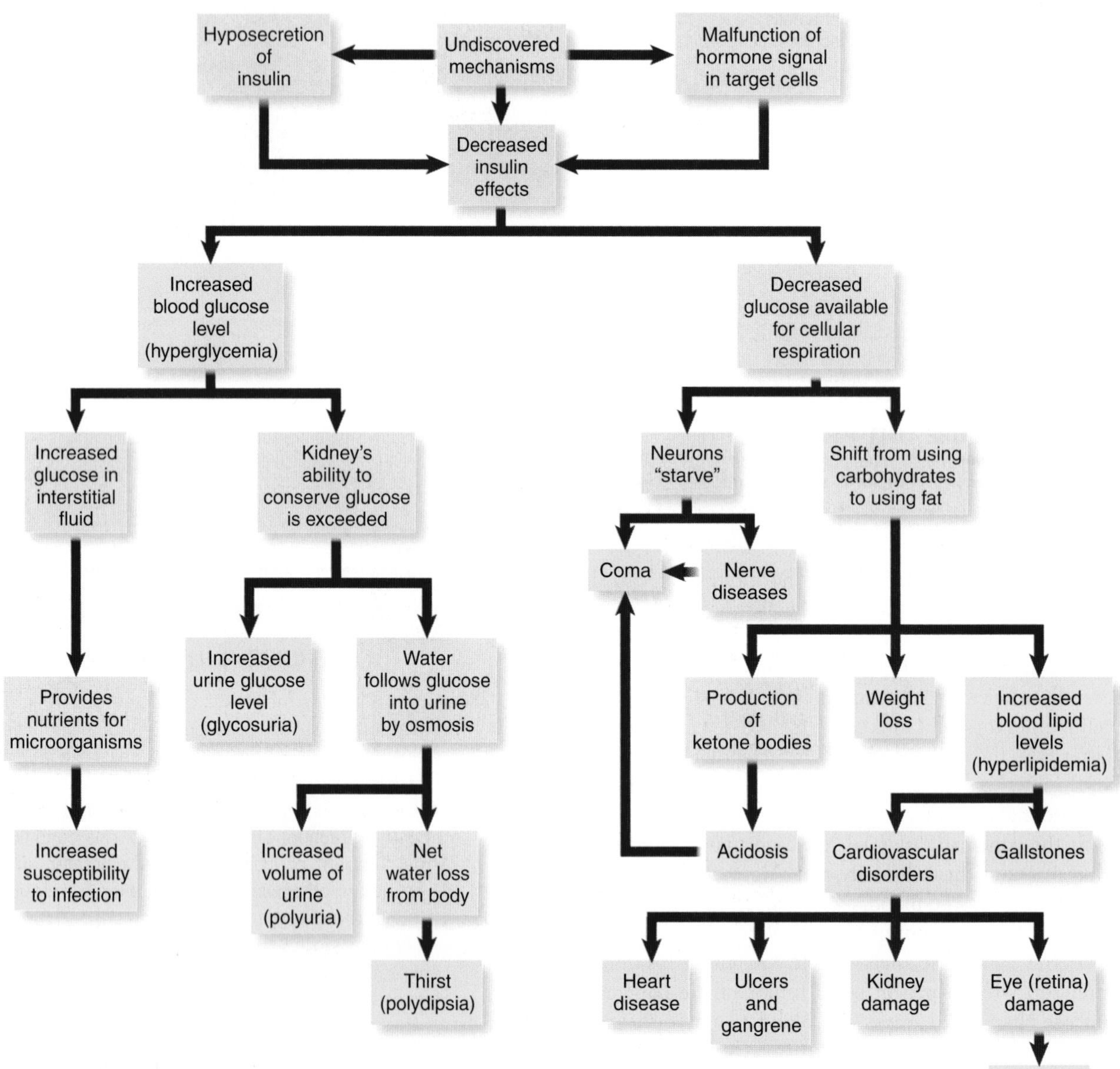

FIGURE 11-12 Diabetes mellitus. The signs and symptoms of this disorder *(highlighted in yellow)* all result from decreased insulin effects. Although this diagram may seem overwhelming at first glance, it is easy to follow if you trace each of the pathways step-by-step through to the end. By doing so, you will begin to appreciate how one event triggers another in human physiology.

hormone is also responsible for development of adult female body contours and initiation of the menstrual cycle.

The **corpus luteum** chiefly secretes **progesterone** but also some estrogen.

We shall save our discussion of the structure of these endocrine glands and the functions of their hormones for Chapter 21.

Male Sex Glands

Some of the cells of the testes produce the male sex cells called **sperm.** Other cells in the testes, male reproductive ducts, and glands produce the liquid portion of the male reproductive fluid called **semen.** The interstitial cells in the testes secrete the male sex hormone called **testosterone** directly into the blood. These cells of the testes are therefore the male endocrine glands.

Testosterone is the "masculinizing hormone." It is responsible for the maturation of the external genitals, beard growth, changes in voice at puberty, and for the muscular development and body contours typical of the male.

Chapter 21 contains more information about the structure of the testes and the functions of testosterone.

Thymus

The thymus is located in the mediastinum (see **Figure 11-1**), and in infants it may extend up into the neck as far as the lower edge of the thyroid gland. Like the adrenal gland, the thymus has a cortex and medulla. Both portions are composed largely of lymphocytes (white blood cells).

The thymus is the location where many of the body's cells of immunity develop. The hormone **thymosin** is actually a group of several hormones that together play an important role in regulating the development and function of *T cells*—an important category of immunity agents in the body. The function of T cells is discussed in detail in Chapter 14.

This small structure (it weighs about 20 grams) plays a critical part in the body's defenses against infections and cancer—it's a vital immunity mechanism.

Placenta

The placenta functions as a temporary endocrine gland.

During pregnancy, it produces **chorionic gonadotropins**, so called because they are tropic hormones secreted by cells of the **chorion,** the outermost membrane that surrounds the baby during development in the uterus. In addition to producing chorionic gonadotropins, the placenta also produces estrogen and progesterone.

During the earliest weeks of pregnancy, the kidneys excrete large amounts of chorionic gonadotropins in the urine. This fact, discovered more than a half century ago, led to the development of early pregnancy tests that are still in common use today.

Pineal Gland

The pineal gland is a small gland near the roof of the third ventricle of the brain (see **Figure 9-9**). It is named "pineal" because it resembles the pine nut (which looks like a kernel of corn). The pineal gland is easily located in a child but becomes fibrous and encrusted with calcium deposits as a person ages.

The pineal gland produces a number of hormones in very small quantities, with **melatonin** being the most significant. Melatonin inhibits the tropic hormones that affect the ovaries, and it is thought to be involved in regulating the onset of puberty and the menstrual cycle in women.

Because the pineal gland receives and responds to sensory information from the light-sensitive ganglion cells of the eye's retina, it is sometimes called the *third eye*. The pineal gland uses information regarding changing light levels to adjust its output of melatonin. Melatonin levels increase during the night and decrease during the day. This cyclic variation is an important timekeeping mechanism for the body's internal clock and sleep cycle.

Melatonin supplements are now widely used as an aid to induce sleep or to "reprogram" the sleep cycle as a treatment for jet lag.

Endocrine Functions Throughout the Body

Other Endocrine Tissues

Continuing research into the endocrine system has shown that nearly every organ and system has an endocrine function.

Tissues in the kidneys, stomach, intestines, and other organs secrete hormones that regulate a variety of essential human functions. For example, **ghrelin** is secreted by epithelial cells lining the stomach and boosts appetite, slows metabolism, and reduces fat burning. Ghrelin may, therefore, be involved in the development of obesity.

Another example, **atrial natriuretic hormone (ANH),** is secreted by cells in the wall of the heart's atria (upper chambers). ANH is an important regulator of fluid and electrolyte homeostasis and is an antagonist to aldosterone. Aldosterone stimulates the kidney to retain sodium ions and water, whereas ANH stimulates loss of sodium ions and water.

A more recently discovered hormone is **leptin,** which is secreted by fat-storing cells throughout the body. Leptin seems to regulate how hungry or full we feel and how fat is metabolized by the body. Researchers are now looking at how leptin works with other hormones in the hopes of finding ways to treat patients with obesity, diabetes mellitus, and other disorders involving fat storage.

Hormone Actions in Every Organ

This chapter has included a list of endocrine glands and hormones that may have seemed endless. Yet it is only a small fraction of the known hormones and hormone-producing cells.

We have mentioned the actions of hormones in previous chapters, and we will continue to discuss nearly all the hormones identified in this chapter as we proceed through the rest of this book. Why? Hormone actions are important regulators of homeostasis throughout the body. They play critical roles in the function of *every* organ of the body.

As you move forward in your course, always be on the lookout for the regulatory and coordinating roles of hormones. By doing so, you will have a more complete picture of whole-body function—a view that will serve you well in the future.

QUICK CHECK

1. Which hormones are produced by the male and female sex glands?
2. What is the role of thymosin?
3. Why is the placenta considered to be a gland?
4. Why is the pineal gland sometimes called the *timekeeper of the body?*
5. How many organs of the body are affected by hormone actions?

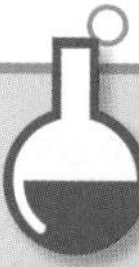

SCIENCE APPLICATIONS

ENDOCRINOLOGY

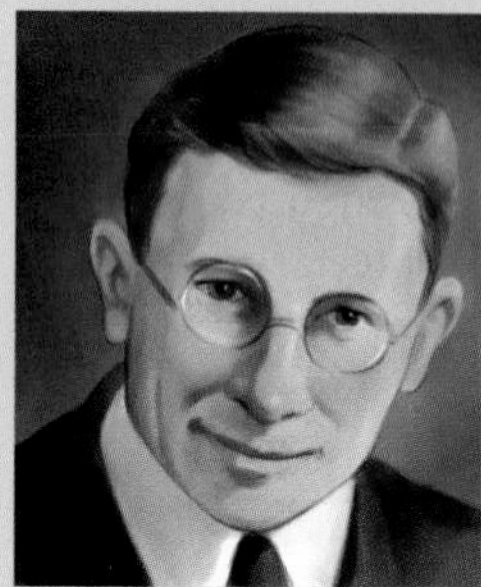

Frederick Banting (1891-1941)

Two of the undisputed heroes of **endocrinology** are Canadian surgeon Frederick Banting and his assistant Charles Best. Until the early twentieth century, children with type 1 diabetes mellitus died a slow, horrible death from their cells literally starving to death from lack of glucose. Acting on Banting's idea for removing insulin from the pancreatic islets of dogs, the two were the first to successfully isolate this important hormone. Chemist James Collip was able to purify the insulin sufficiently so that in 1921 their colleague, Scots physiologist John Macleod, could administer the insulin to a 14-year-old boy with diabetes. It worked! The treatment not only relieved the boy's suffering, but gave him a healthy, long life.

This breakthrough, for which Banting and Macleod received the 1923 Nobel Prize, was the start of a century of rapid progress in understanding and treating endocrine disorders.

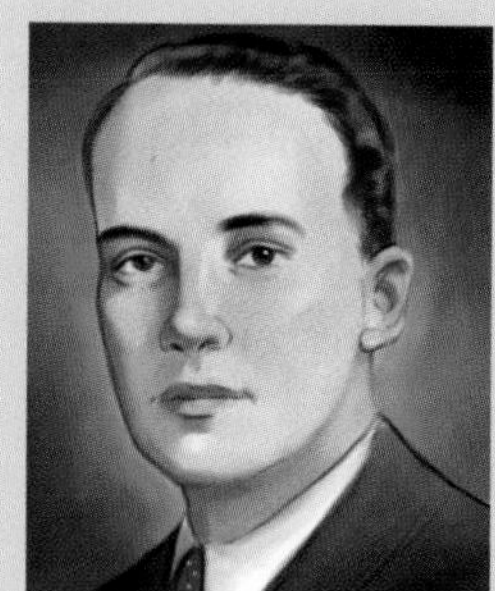

Charles Best (1899-1978)

Because hormones affect so many different body functions, nearly every kind of health professional, from *medical doctors* to *nurses* to *dietitians,* needs to be aware of their functions. Hormones and chemicals that influence hormone actions are often used in treatments, so *pharmacologists* and *pharmacists* must also have an excellent knowledge of endocrinology.

Some scientists have applied principles of endocrinology in a variety of unexpected ways, including the development of early pregnancy test kits, ovulation test kits, and the use of synthetic hormones in healthy people to control their fertility.

LANGUAGE OF SCIENCE AND MEDICINE *(continued from p. 237)*

antidiuretic hormone (ADH)
(an-tee-dye-yoo-RET-ik HOR-mohn)
[*anti-* **against,** *-dia-* **through,** *-uret-* **urination,** *-ic* **relating to,** *hormon-* **excite**]

atrial natriuretic hormone (ANH)
(AY-tree-al nay-tree-yoo-RET-ik HOR-mohn)
[*atria-* **entrance courtyard (atrium of heart),** *-al* **relating to,** *natri-* **natrium (sodium),** *-uret-* **urination,** *-ic* **relating to,** *hormon-* **excite**]

calcitonin (CT)
(kal-sih-TOH-nin)
[*calci-* **lime (calcium),** *-ton-* **tone,** *-in* **substance**]

chorion
(KOH-ree-on)
[*chorion* **skin**]

chorionic gonadotropin
(koh-ree-ON-ik goh-nah-doh-TROH-pin)
[*chorion-* **skin,** *-ic* **relating to,** *gon-* **offspring,** *-ad-* **relating to,** *-trop-* **nourish,** *-in* **substance**]

corpus luteum
(KOHR-pus LOO-tee-um)
pl., corpora lutea
(KOHR-por-ah LOO-tee-ah)
[*corpus* **body,** *lute-* **yellow,** *-um* **thing**]

corticoid
(KOHR-tih-koyd)
[*cortic-* **cortex (bark),** *-oid* **like**]

cortisol
(KOHR-tih-sol)
[*cortis-* **cortex (bark),** *-ol* **alcohol**]

cretinism
(KREE-tin-iz-em)
[*cretin-* **idiot,** *-ism* **condition**]

Cushing syndrome
(KOOSH-ing SIN-drohm)
[*Harvey W. Cushing* **American neurosurgeon,** *syn-* **together,** *-drome* **running or (race) course**]

cyclic AMP (cAMP)
(SIK-lik ay-em-pee)
[*cycl-* **circle,** *-ic* **relating to**]

diabetes insipidus
(dye-ah-BEE-teez in-SIP-ih-dus)
[*diabetes* **siphon,** *insipidus* **without zest**]

diabetes mellitus (DM)
(dye-ah-BEE-teez MELL-ih-tus)
[*diabetes* **pass-through or siphon,** *mellitus* **honey-sweet**]

dwarfism
(dwor-FIZ-em)
[*dwarf-* **something tiny,** *-ism* **condition**]

endocrine gland
(EN-doh-krin gland)
[*endo-* **inward or within,** *-crin-* **secrete,** *gland* **acorn**]

endocrine system
(EN-doh-krin SIS-tem)
[*endo-* **within,** *-crin-* **secrete**]

endocrinology
(en-doh-krin-OL-oh-jee)
[*endo-* **within,** *-crin-* **secrete,** *-log-* **words (study of),** *-y* **activity**]

epinephrine (Epi)
(ep-ih-NEF-rin)
[*epi-* **upon,** *-nephr-* **kidney,** *-ine* **substance**]

estrogen
(ES-troh-jen)
[*estro-* **frenzy,** *-gen* **produce**]

exocrine gland
(EK-soh-krin gland)
[*exo-* **outside or outward,** *-crin-* **secrete,** *gland* **acorn**]

follicle-stimulating hormone (FSH)
(FOL-lih-kul-STIM-yoo-lay-ting HOR-mohn)
[*foll-* **bag,** *-icle* **little,** *stimulate-* **urge,** *-ing* **action,** *hormon-* **excite**]

ghrelin
(GRAY-lin)
[*ghrel-* **grow (also acronym for "growth hormone releasing"),** *-in* **substance**]

gigantism
(jye-GAN-tiz-em)
[*gigant-* **great,** *-ism* **condition**]

glucagon
(GLOO-kah-gon)
[*gluca-* **sweet (glucose),** *-agon* **lead or bring**]

glucocorticoid (GC)
(gloo-koh-KOR-tih-koyd)
[*gluco-* **sweet (glucose),** *-cortic-* **cortex (bark),** *-oid* **like**]

gluconeogenesis
(gloo-koh-nee-oh-JEN-eh-sis)
[*gluco-* **sweet (glucose),** *-neo-* **new,** *-gen-* **produce,** *-esis* **process**]

glycogenolysis
(glye-koh-jeh-NOL-ih-sis)
[*glyco-* **sweet (glucose),** *-gen-* **produce,** *-o-* **combining form,** *-lysis* **loosening**]

glycosuria
(glye-koh-SOO-ree-ah)
[*glyco-* **sweet (glucose),** *-ur-* **urine,** *-ia* **condition**]

growth hormone (GH)
(grohth HOR-mohn)
[*hormon-* **excite**]

hormone
(HOR-mohn)
[*hormon-* **excite**]

hydrocortisone
(hye-droh-KOHR-tih-zohn)
[*hydro-* **water,** *-cortisone* **cortex of adrenal gland**]

hypercalcemia
(hye-per-kal-SEE-mee-ah)
[*hyper-* **excessive,** *calc-* **lime (calcium),** *-emia* **blood condition**]

hyperglycemia
(hye-per-glye-SEE-mee-ah)
[*hyper-* **excessive,** *-glyc-* **sweet (glucose),** *-emia* **blood condition**]

hypersecretion
(hye-per-seh-KREE-shun)
[*hyper-* **excessive,** *-secret-* **separate,** *-tion* **process**]

hyperthyroidism
(hye-per-THYE-royd-iz-em)
[*hyper-* **excessive,** *-thyr-* **shield (thyroid gland),** *-oid* **like,** *-ism* **condition**]

hypoglycemia
(hye-poh-glye-SEE-mee-ah)
[*hypo-* **under or below,** *-glyc-* **sweet (glucose),** *-emia* **blood condition**]

hyposecretion
(hye-poh-seh-KREE-shun)
[*hypo-* **under or below,** *-secret-* **separate,** *-tion* **process**]

hypothyroidism
(hye-poh-THYE-royd-iz-em)
[*hypo-* **under or below,** *-thyr-* **shield (thyroid gland),** *-oid* **like,** *-ism* **condition**]

inhibiting hormone (IH)
(in-HIB-ih-ting HOR-mohn)
[*inhib-* **restrain,** *-ing* **action,** *hormon-* **excite**]

insulin
(IN-suh-lin)
[*insul-* **island,** *-in* **substance**]

leptin
(LEP-tin)
[*lept-* **thin,** *-in* **substance**]

luteinization
(loo-tee-in-ih-ZAY-shun)
[*lute-* **yellow,** *-ization* **process**]

luteinizing hormone (LH)
(loo-tee-in-EYE-zing HOR-mohn)
[*lute-* **yellow,** *-izing* **process,** *hormon-* **excite**]

melatonin
(mel-ah-TOH-nin)
[*mela-* **black,** *-ton-* **tone,** *-in* **substance**]

mineralocorticoid (MC)
(MIN-er-al-oh-KOR-tih-koyd)
[*mineral-* **mine,** *-cortic-* **cortex (bark),** *-oid* **like**]

myxedema
(mik-seh-DEE-mah)
[*myx-* **mucus,** *-edema* **swelling**]

negative feedback
(NEG-ah-tiv FEED-bak)
[*negat-* **deny,** *-ive* **relating to,** *feedback* **information about the results of a process**]

neurohypophysis
(noo-roh-hye-POF-ih-sis)
[*neuro-* **nerve,** *-hypo-* **under or below,** *-physis* **growth**]

nonsteroid hormone
(non-STAYR-oyd HOR-mohn)
[*non-* **not,** *-stero-* **solid,** *-oid* **like,** *hormon-* **excite**]

norepinephrine (NR)
(nor-ep-ih-NEF-rin)
[*nor-* **chemical prefix (unbranched C chain),** *-epi-* **upon,** *-nephr-* **kidney,** *-ine* **substance**]

ova
(OH-vah)
sing., ovum
(OH-vum)
[*ovum* **egg**]

ovarian follicle
(oh-VAYR-ee-an FOL-ih-kul)
[*ov-* **egg,** *-arian* **relating to,** *foll-* **bag,** *-icle* **little**]

oxytocin (OT)
(ahk-see-TOH-sin)
[*oxy-* **sharp or quick,** *-toc-* **birth,** *-in* **substance**]

pancreatic islet (islet of Langerhans)
(pan-kree-AT-ik eye-let)
(EYE-let of lahn-GER-hans)
[*pan-* **all,** *-creat-* **flesh,** *-ic* **relating to,** *isl-* **island,** *-et* **little**] [*Paul Langerhans* **German pathologist**]

paracrine
(PAIR-ah-krin)
[*para-* **beside,** *-crin-* **secrete**]

parathyroid gland
(payr-ah-THYE-royd gland)
[*para-* **beside,** *-thyr-* **shield,** *-oid* **like,** *gland* **acorn**]

parathyroid hormone (PTH)
(payr-ah-THYE-royd HOR-mohn)
[*para-* **beside,** *-thyr-* **shield,** *-oid* **like,** *hormon-* **excite**]

pituitary gland
(pih-TOO-ih-tayr-ee gland)
[*pituit-* **phlegm,** *-ary* **relating to,** *gland* **acorn**]

positive feedback
(POZ-it-iv FEED-bak)
[*posit-* **put or place,** *-ive* **relating to,** *feedback* **information about the results of a process**]

progesterone
(proh-JES-ter-ohn)
[*pro-* **before,** *-gester-* **bearing (pregnancy),** *-stero-* **solid or steroid derivative,** *-one* **chemical**]

prolactin
(proh-LAK-tin)
[*pro-* **before,** *-lact-* **milk,** *-in* **substance**]

prostaglandin (PG)
(pross-tah-GLAN-din)
[*pro-* **before,** *-stat-* **set or place (prostate),** *-gland-* **acorn (gland),** *-in* **substance**]

releasing hormone (RH)
(ree-LEE-sing HOR-mohn)
[*hormon-* **excite**]

second messenger
(SEK-und MESS-en-jer)

sella turcica
(SEL-lah TER-sih-kah)
[*sella* **saddle,** *turcica* **Turkish**]

semen
(SEE-men)
[*semen* **seed**]

sex hormone
(seks HOR-mohn)
[*hormon-* **excite**]

signal transduction
(SIG-nul tranz-DUK-shen)
[*trans-* **across,** *-duc-* **transfer,** *-tion* **process**]

simple goiter
(SIM-pel GOY-ter)
[*goiter* **throat**]

sperm
(sperm)
pl., sperms or sperm
[*sperm* **seed**]

steroid hormone
(STAYR-oyd HOR-mohn)
[*ster-* **sterol,** *-oid* **like,** *hormon-* **excite**]

stress
(stress)
[*stress* **tighten**]

target cell
(TAR-get sel)
[*cell* **storeroom**]

testosterone
(tes-TOS-teh-rohn)
[*testo-* **witness (testis),** *-stero-* **solid or steroid derivative,** *-one* **chemical**]

thymosin
(THY-moh-sin)
[*thymos-* **thyme flower (thymus gland),** *-in* **substance**]

thyroid follicle
(THY-royd FOL-lih-kul)
[*thyro-* **shield (thyroid gland),** *-oid* **like,** *foll-* **bag,** *-icle* **little**]

thyroid-stimulating hormone (TSH)
(THY-royd STIM-yoo-lay-ting HOR-mohn)
[*thyro-* **shield,** *-oid* **like,** *stimulate-* **urge,** *-ing* **action,** *hormon-* **excite**]

thyroxine (T_4)
(thy-ROK-sin)
[*thyro-* **shield (thyroid gland),** *-ox-* **oxygen,** *-ine* **chemical**]

triiodothyronine (T_3)
(try-eye-oh-doh-THY-roh-neen)
[*tri-* **three,** *-iodo-* **violet (iodine),** *-thyro-* **shield (thyroid gland),** *-nine* **chemical**]

tropic hormone
(TROH-pik HOR-mohn)
[*trop-* **turn or change,** *-ic* **relating to,** *hormon-* **excite**]

type 1 diabetes mellitus
(type 1 dye-ah-BEE-teez MEL-ih-tus)
[*diabetes* **siphon,** *mellitus* **honey sweet**]

type 2 diabetes mellitus
(type 2-dye-ah-BEE-teez MEL-ih-tus)
[*diabetes* **siphon,** *mellitus* **honey sweet**]

❑ OUTLINE SUMMARY

To download a digital audio version of the chapter summary for use with your device, access the ***Audio Chapter Summaries*** *online at evolve.elsevier.com.*

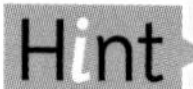

Scan this summary after reading the chapter to help you reinforce the key concepts. Later, use the summary as a quick review before your class or before a test.

Endocrine Glands

A. Exocrine glands are ducted glands and are not included in the endocrine system
B. Endocrine glands are ductless glands that secrete chemicals (hormones) into the blood (see **Figure 11-1**)
   1. Target cell — cell that has specific receptors for a particular hormone
   2. Endocrine glands are numerous and widespread in the body (see **Figure 11-1**)
   3. Diseases result from abnormal secretion of hormones
      a. Hypersecretion — oversecretion of a hormone
      b. Hyposecretion — undersecretion of a hormone

Mechanisms of Hormone Action

A. Hormones perform general functions of communication and control but a slower, longer-lasting type of control than that provided by nerve impulses
B. Cells that respond to hormones are called *target cells;* organs containing target cells are thus *target organs*
C. Nonsteroid hormones (first messengers) bind to receptors on the target cell membrane, triggering intracellular second messengers such as cyclic AMP to affect the cell's activities (see **Figure 11-2**)
D. Steroid hormones
   1. Primary effects produced by binding to receptors within the target cell nucleus and influence cell activity by acting on DNA — a slower process than nonsteroid action (see **Figure 11-3**)

2. Secondary effects may occur when steroid hormones bind to membrane receptors to rapidly trigger functional changes in the target cell

Regulation of Hormone Secretion

A. Hormone secretion is controlled by homeostatic feedback
B. Negative feedback — mechanisms that reverse the direction of a change in a physiological system (see **Figure 11-4**)
C. Positive feedback — (uncommon) mechanisms that amplify physiological changes
D. Levels of regulation — endocrine regulation of body function usually operates at multiple levels of control at the same time for better efficiency and precision

Prostaglandins

A. Prostaglandins (PGs) are powerful lipid substances found in a wide variety of body tissues; PGs are modified fatty acids
B. PGs are typically produced in a tissue and diffuse only a short distance to act on cells in that tissue; often called *tissue hormones* or *paracrine* agents
C. Several classes of PGs include prostaglandin A (PGA), prostaglandin E (PGE), and prostaglandin F (PGF)
D. PGs influence many body functions, including respiration, blood pressure, gastrointestinal secretions, and reproduction

Pituitary Gland

A. Structure of the pituitary gland (see **Figure 11-5**)
   1. Anterior pituitary — also called *adenohypophysis;* made up of glandular epithelium
   2. Posterior pituitary — also called *neurohypophysis;* made up of nervous tissue
   3. Location — in bony depression (sella turcica) of sphenoid bone in skull; connected to the hypothalamus by a pituitary stalk
B. Anterior pituitary gland (adenohypophysis)
   1. Names of major hormones
      a. Thyroid-stimulating hormone (TSH)
      b. Adrenocorticotropic hormone (ACTH)
      c. Follicle-stimulating hormone (FSH)
      d. Luteinizing hormone (LH)
      e. Growth hormone (GH)
      f. Prolactin (PRL) (lactogenic hormone)
   2. Functions of major hormones
      a. TSH — stimulates growth of the thyroid gland; also stimulates it to secrete thyroid hormone
      b. ACTH — stimulates growth of the adrenal cortex and stimulates it to secrete glucocorticoids (mainly cortisol)
      c. FSH — initiates growth of ovarian follicles each month in the ovary and stimulates one or more follicles to develop to the stage of maturity and ovulation; FSH also stimulates estrogen secretion by developing follicles; stimulates sperm production in the male
      d. LH — acts with FSH to stimulate estrogen secretion and follicle growth to maturity; causes ovulation; causes luteinization of the ruptured follicle and stimulates progesterone secretion by corpus luteum; causes interstitial cells in the testes to secrete testosterone in the male
      e. GH — stimulates growth by accelerating protein anabolism; also accelerates fat catabolism and slows glucose catabolism; by slowing glucose catabolism, tends to increase blood glucose to higher than normal level (hyperglycemia)
      f. PRL, or lactogenic hormone — stimulates breast development during pregnancy and secretion of milk after the delivery of the baby
C. Posterior pituitary gland (neurohypophysis)
   1. Names of hormones
      a. Antidiuretic hormone (ADH)
      b. Oxytocin (OT)
   2. Functions of hormones
      a. ADH — accelerates water reabsorption from urine in the kidney tubules into the blood, thereby decreasing urine secretion
      b. OT — stimulates the pregnant uterus to contract; may initiate labor; causes glandular cells of the breast to release milk into ducts; enhances social bonding

Hypothalamus

A. Produces posterior pituitary hormones
   1. Actual production of ADH and oxytocin occurs in the hypothalamus
   2. After production in the hypothalamus, hormones pass along axons into the pituitary gland
   3. The secretion and release of posterior pituitary hormones is controlled by nervous stimulation
B. Regulates anterior pituitary secretion
   1. Releasing hormones (RHs) and inhibiting hormones (IHs) control secretion by anterior pituitary
   2. RHs and IHs reach anterior pituitary through a direct capillary connection
C. The hypothalamus controls many body functions related to homeostasis (temperature, appetite, and thirst)

Thyroid Gland

A. Located in neck, just inferior to larynx (see **Figure 11-6**)
B. Tissue made up of thyroid follicles filled with colloid (see **Figure 11-7**)
C. Names of hormones
   1. Thyroid hormones — thyroxine (T_4) and triiodothyronine (T_3); produced by follicle cells and stored in colloid of follicles
   2. Calcitonin (CT) — made by CT cells outside the follicle walls
D. Functions of hormones
   1. Thyroid hormones — accelerate catabolism and energy production (increasing the body's metabolic rate)
   2. CT — decreases the blood calcium concentration by inhibiting breakdown of bone, which would release calcium into the blood

Parathyroid Glands (See **Figure 11-6**)

A. Small lumps of glandular tissue located on posterior surface of thyroid (see **Figure 11-6**)
B. Name of hormone — parathyroid hormone (PTH)
C. Function of hormone
   1. Increases blood calcium concentration by increasing the breakdown of bone with the release of calcium into the blood
   2. PTH and CT have antagonistic effects that help maintain stable blood calcium concentrations needed for good health (see **Figure 11-8**)

Adrenal Glands

A. Located on superior surface of each kidney; outer region is glandular and inner region is secretory nervous tissues (see **Figure 11-9**)
B. Adrenal cortex
   1. Names of hormones (corticoids)
      a. Mineralocorticoids (MCs) — chiefly aldosterone
      b. Glucocorticoids (GCs) — chiefly cortisol (hydrocortisone)
      c. Sex hormones — small amounts of male hormones (androgens) secreted by adrenal cortex of both sexes
   2. Three cell layers (zones)
      a. Outer layer, secretes mineralocorticoids
      b. Middle layer, secretes glucocorticoids
      c. Inner layer, secretes sex hormones
   3. Mineralocorticoids — increase blood sodium and decrease body potassium concentrations by accelerating kidney tubule reabsorption of sodium and excretion of potassium
   4. Functions of glucocorticoids
      a. Help maintain normal blood glucose concentration by increasing gluconeogenesis — the formation of "new" glucose from amino acids produced by the breakdown of proteins, mainly those in muscle tissue cells; also the conversion to glucose of fatty acids produced by the breakdown of fats stored in adipose tissue cells
      b. Play an essential part in maintaining normal blood pressure — make it possible for epinephrine and norepinephrine to maintain a normal degree of vasoconstriction, a condition necessary for maintaining normal blood pressure
      c. Act with epinephrine and norepinephrine to produce an anti-inflammatory effect, to bring about normal recovery from inflammations of various kinds
      d. Produce anti-immunity, antiallergy effect; bring about a decrease in the number of lymphocytes and plasma cells and therefore a decrease in the number of antibodies formed
      e. Secretion of glucocorticoid quickly increases when the body is thrown into a condition of stress; high blood concentration of glucocorticoids, in turn, brings about many other stress responses (see **Figure 11-10**)
      f. Chronic stress can disturb the body's balance of metabolic and immune functions
   5. Sex hormones — male androgens similar to testosterone are produced in both sexes; have a role in reproductive development
C. Adrenal medulla
   1. Names of hormones — epinephrine (Epi), or adrenaline, and norepinephrine (NR)
   2. Functions of hormones — help the body resist stress by intensifying and prolonging the effects of sympathetic stimulation; increased epinephrine secretion is the first endocrine response to stress

Pancreatic Islets

A. Islands of endocrine tissue scattered within the exocrine tissue of the pancreas, a digestive gland near the junction of the stomach and small intestine (see **Figure 11-11**)
B. Names of hormones
   1. Glucagon — secreted by alpha cells
   2. Insulin — secreted by beta cells
C. Functions of hormones
   1. Glucagon increases the blood glucose level by accelerating liver glycogenolysis (conversion of glycogen to glucose)
   2. Insulin decreases the blood glucose by accelerating the movement of glucose out of the blood into cells, which increases glucose metabolism by cells

Female Sex Glands

A. The ovaries contain two structures that secrete hormones — the ovarian follicles and the corpus luteum; see Chapter 21

B. Effects of estrogen (feminizing hormone)
   1. Development and maturation of breasts and external genitals
   2. Development of adult female body contours
   3. Initiation of menstrual cycle

Male Sex Glands

A. The interstitial cells of testes secrete the male hormone testosterone; see Chapter 21
B. Effects of testosterone (masculinizing hormone)
   1. Maturation of external genitals
   2. Beard growth
   3. Voice changes at puberty
   4. Development of musculature and body contours typical of the male

Thymus

A. Name of hormone — thymosin (group of related hormones)
B. Function of hormone — plays an important role in the development and function of T cells (agents of the body's immune system)

Placenta

A. Names of hormones — chorionic gonadotropins, estrogens, and progesterone
B. Function of hormones — maintain the corpus luteum during pregnancy

Pineal Gland

A. A small gland near the roof of the third ventricle of the brain
   1. Glandular tissue predominates in children and young adults
   2. Becomes fibrous and calcified with age
B. Called third eye because its influence on secretory activity is related to the amount of light entering the eyes
C. Secretes melatonin, which:
   1. Inhibits ovarian activity
   2. Regulates the body's internal clock

Endocrine Functions Throughout the Body

A. Many organs (for example, the stomach, intestines, and kidney) produce endocrine hormones
   1. Stomach lining produces ghrelin, which affects appetite and metabolism
   2. The atrial wall of the heart secretes atrial natriuretic hormone (ANH), which stimulates sodium loss from the kidneys
   3. Fat-storing cells secrete leptin, which controls how full or hungry we feel
B. Hormone actions occur in every organ of the body and will be addressed throughout the rest of this book

❑ ACTIVE LEARNING

STUDY TIPS

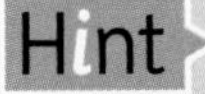

Use these tips to achieve success in meeting your learning goals.

To make the study of the endocrine system more efficient, we suggest these tips:

1. Before studying Chapter 11, review the synopsis of the endocrine system in Chapter 5.
2. The function of the endocrine system is similar to that of the nervous system. The differences are in the methods used to produce an effect and the extent of the effect. The endocrine system uses chemicals in the blood (hormones) rather than nerve impulses. Hormones can have a direct effect on almost every cell in the body, an impossible task for the nervous system. Steroid hormones can act directly because they can enter the cell; protein hormones cannot enter the cell so they need a second messenger system.
3. Material from earlier chapters regarding topics such as receptor proteins in the cell membrane, adenosine triphosphate (ATP), homeostasis, and negative feedback loops will help you understand the material in this chapter.
4. Use flash cards to learn the names of the hormones, what they do, and the names and locations of the glands that produce them. Remember that hormones released by the posterior pituitary gland are made in the hypothalamus.
5. In your study group, discuss the hormone mechanisms and the negative feedback loops involved in hormone regulation.
6. Review the hormone flash cards in your study group. A copy of **Figure 11-1** (showing the endocrine glands) may be helpful for reviewing the location of glands. Quiz each other on which gland produces what hormone.
7. Go over the questions at the end of the chapter and discuss possible test questions.

Review Questions

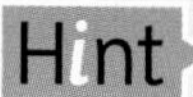

Write out the answers to these questions after reading the chapter and reviewing the Chapter Summary. If you simply think through the answer without writing it down, you won't retain much of your new learning.

1. Differentiate between endocrine and exocrine glands.
2. List the primary endocrine glands and identify the major hormones produced by each gland.
3. Define or explain *hormone, target cell, hypersecretion,* and *hyposecretion.*
4. Explain the mechanism of action of nonsteroid hormones.
5. Explain the mechanism of action of steroid hormones.
6. Explain and give an example of a negative feedback loop for the regulation of hormone secretion.
7. Explain and give an example of a positive feedback loop for the regulation of hormone secretion.
8. Explain the difference between prostaglandins and hormones. List some of the body functions that can be influenced by prostaglandins.
9. Describe the structure of the pituitary gland and where it is located.
10. Name the four tropic hormones released by the anterior pituitary gland and briefly explain their function.
11. Explain the function of growth hormone.
12. Explain the function of ADH.
13. Explain the function of prolactin and oxytocin.
14. Explain the function of the hypothalamus in the endocrine system.
15. Explain the difference between T_3 and T_4. What is unique about the thyroid gland?
16. Name the hormones produced by the zones or areas of the adrenal cortex.
17. Explain the function of aldosterone.
18. Explain the function of glucocorticoids.
19. List conditions that may occur from hyposecretion and hypersecretion of the: growth hormone (GH), thyroid gland, adrenal cortex, and pancreas.

Critical Thinking

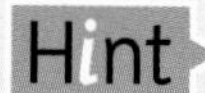

After finishing the Review Questions, write out the answers to these more in-depth questions to help you apply your new knowledge. Go back to sections of the chapter that relate to concepts that you find difficult.

20. Explain why a second messenger system is necessary for nonsteroid hormones but not for steroid hormones.
21. Pick a body function (regulation of glucose or calcium levels in the blood) and explain how the interaction of hormones is used to help maintain homeostasis.
22. What would be the effect on the body if the thyroid gland were removed?
23. If a doctor discovered a patient had very low levels of thyroxine but high levels of TSH, would the patient's problem be in the thyroid gland or the pituitary gland? Explain your answer.

Chapter Test

Hint *After studying the chapter, test your mastery by responding to these items. Try to answer them without looking up the answers. Then, verify the answers using the key in Appendix C at the back of this book.*

1. ______ glands secrete their products into ducts that empty onto a surface or into a cavity.
2. ______ glands are ductless and secrete their products, called ______, into intercellular spaces where they diffuse into the blood.
3. The two major classes of hormones are ______ hormones and ______ hormones.
4. A cell or body organ that has receptors for a hormone that triggers a reaction is called a ______.
5. One example of a second messenger system involves the conversion of ATP into ______.
6. The hormone receptors for nonsteroid hormones are located ______, whereas the receptors for steroid hormones are located ______.
7. "Tissue hormones" is another name for ______.
8. This part of the pituitary gland is made of nervous tissue: ______
9. This part of the pituitary gland is made of glandular tissue: ______
10. The hormone oxytocin is released by the ______ but is made in the ______
11. A tropic hormone secreted by the anterior pituitary gland is:
    a. thyroid-stimulating hormone
    b. adrenocorticotropic hormone
    c. luteinizing hormone
    d. all of the above
12. Antidiuretic hormone (ADH):
    a. is made in the posterior pituitary gland
    b. accelerates water reabsorption in the kidney
    c. in high concentrations causes diabetes insipidus
    d. all of the above
13. This hormone is released by the anterior pituitary and stimulates breast development during pregnancy and is necessary for eventual milk production:
    a. estrogen
    b. oxytocin
    c. prolactin
    d. progesterone
14. This hormone is released by the posterior pituitary and stimulates the contraction of the pregnant uterus:
    a. estrogen
    b. oxytocin
    c. prolactin
    d. progesterone
15. Thyroxine:
    a. is symbolized by T_3
    b. is made in the thyroid gland
    c. contains less iodine than triiodothyronine
    d. all of the above
16. Calcitonin:
    a. decreases the level of calcium in the blood
    b. increases the level of calcium in the blood
    c. stimulates the release of calcium from bone tissue
    d. both b and c

Match each function or source in Column B with the corresponding hormone in Column A.

Column A

17. ______ parathyroid hormone
18. ______ mineralocorticoids
19. ______ glucocorticoids
20. ______ epinephrine
21. ______ glucagon
22. ______ insulin
23. ______ chorionic gonadotropins
24. ______ melatonin
25. ______ atrial natriuretic hormone

Column B

a. released by the adrenal medulla; prolongs the effect of the sympathetic nervous system
b. made in the heart; helps regulate blood sodium
c. made in the pancreatic islets; decreases blood glucose levels
d. has the opposite effect of calcitonin
e. made by alpha cells in the pancreatic islets
f. made in the outermost layer of the adrenal cortex
g. the most significant hormone released by the pineal gland
h. the hormone made by the placenta and detected by home pregnancy tests
i. made by the middle layer of the adrenal cortex

Blood

OUTLINE

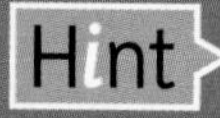

Scan this outline before you begin to read the chapter, as a preview of how the concepts are organized.

OBJECTIVES

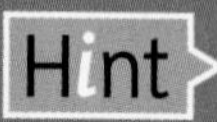

Before reading the chapter, review these goals for your learning.

After you have completed this chapter, you should be able to:

1. Describe the primary functions of blood.
2. Describe the characteristics of blood plasma.
3. List the formed elements of blood and identify the most important function of each.
4. Discuss the structure and function of red blood cells and how red blood cell numbers and hemoglobin content may change to produce anemia.
5. Describe ABO and Rh blood typing.
6. Discuss the structure and function of white blood cells.
7. Explain the steps involved in blood clotting.
8. Define the following medical terms associated with blood: *acidosis, serum, hematocrit, anemia, sickle cell, polycythemia, erythroblastosis fetalis, Rh factor, leukocytosis, leukopenia, phagocytosis, fibrinogen, thrombosis.*

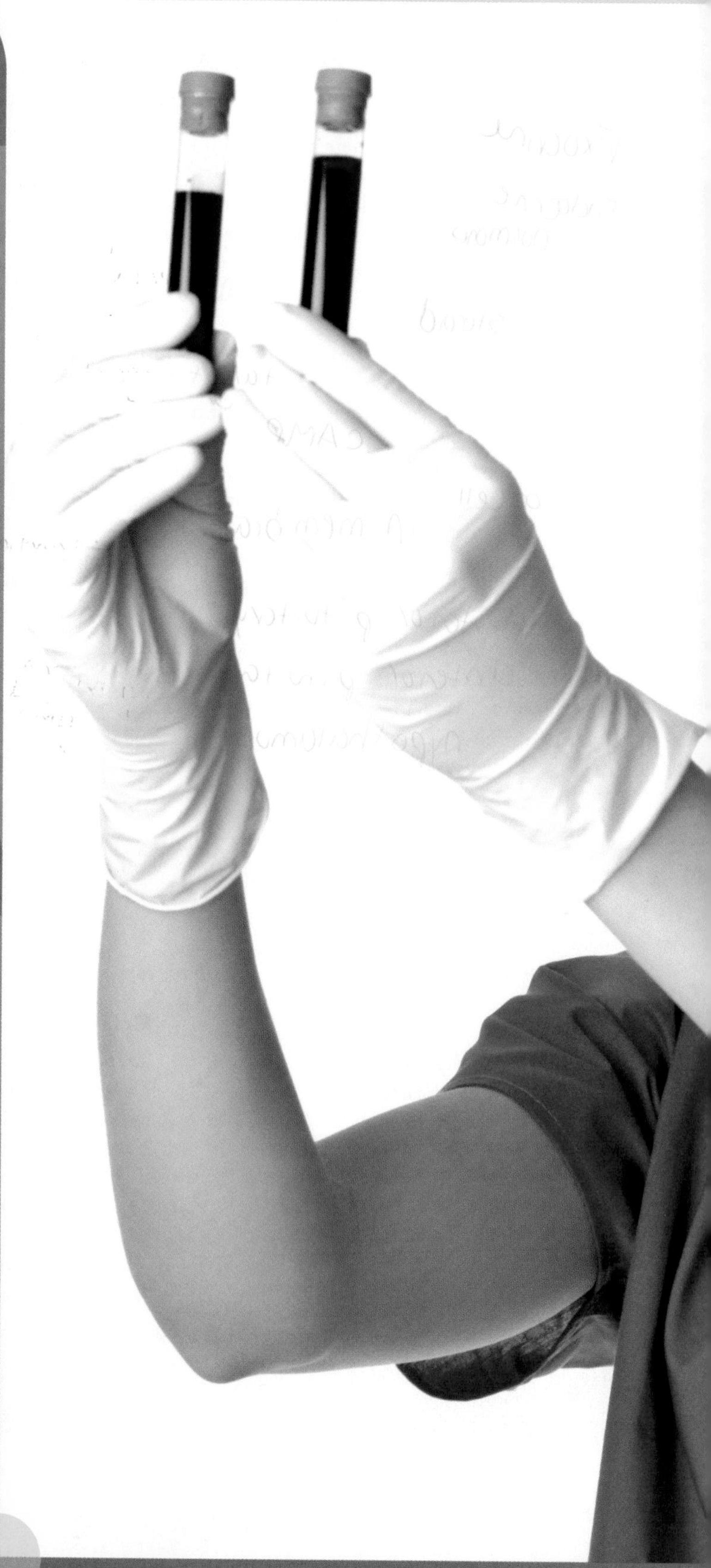

CHAPTER 12

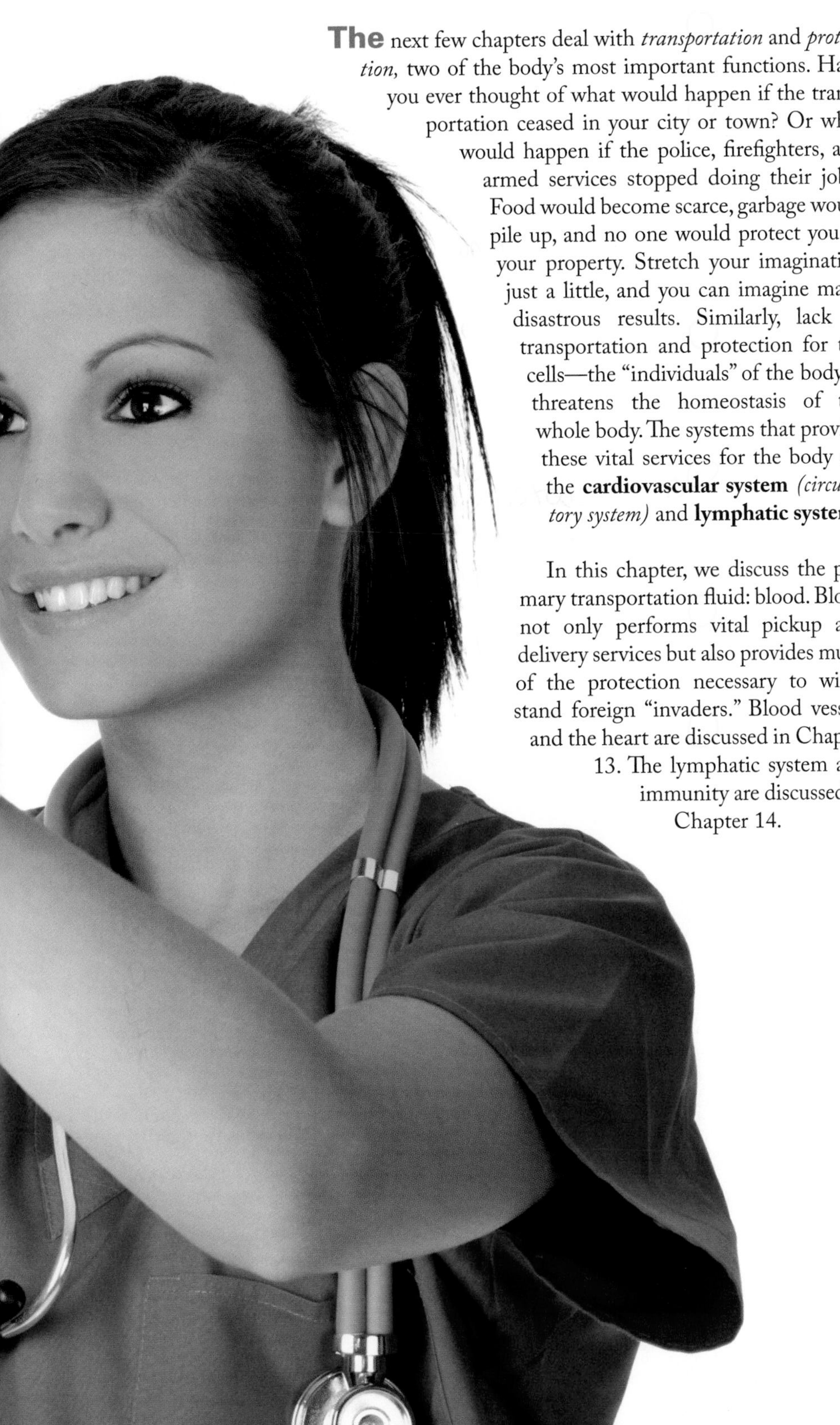

The next few chapters deal with *transportation* and *protection,* two of the body's most important functions. Have you ever thought of what would happen if the transportation ceased in your city or town? Or what would happen if the police, firefighters, and armed services stopped doing their jobs? Food would become scarce, garbage would pile up, and no one would protect you or your property. Stretch your imagination just a little, and you can imagine many disastrous results. Similarly, lack of transportation and protection for the cells—the "individuals" of the body—threatens the homeostasis of the whole body. The systems that provide these vital services for the body are the **cardiovascular system** *(circulatory system)* and **lymphatic system.**

In this chapter, we discuss the primary transportation fluid: blood. Blood not only performs vital pickup and delivery services but also provides much of the protection necessary to withstand foreign "invaders." Blood vessels and the heart are discussed in Chapter 13. The lymphatic system and immunity are discussed in Chapter 14.

LANGUAGE OF **SCIENCE** AND **MEDICINE**

Hint Before reading the chapter, say each of these terms out loud. This will help you to avoid stumbling over them as you read.

ABO system
(ay bee oh SIS-tem)

acidosis
(ass-ih-DOH-sis)
[*acid-* **sour,** *-osis* **condition**]

agglutinate
(ah-GLOO-tin-ayt)
[*agglutin-* **glue,** *-ate* **process**]

agranular leukocyte
(ay-GRAN-yoo-lar LOO-koh-syte)
[*a-* **without,** *-gran-* **grain,** *-ul-* **little,** *-ar* **relating to,** *leuko-* **white,** *-cyte* **cell**]

albumin
(al-BYOO-min)
[*alb-* **white,** *-in* **substance**]

anemia
(ah-NEE-me-ah)
[*an-* **without,** *-emia* **blood condition**]

antibody
(AN-tih-bod-ee)
[*anti-* **against,** *-body* **main part**]

anticoagulant
(an-tee-koh-AG-yoo-lant)
[*anti-* **against,** *-coagul-* **curdle,** *-ant* **agent**]

antigen
(AN-tih-jen)
[*anti-* **against,** *-gen* **produce**]

aplastic anemia
(ay-PLAS-tik ah-NEE-mee-ah)
[*a-* **without,** *-plast-* **form,** *-ic* **relating to,** *an-* **without,** *-emia* **blood condition**]

basophil
(BAY-so-fil)
[*bas-* **base (high pH),** *-phil* **love**]

blood doping
(blud DOH-ping)
[*dop-* **thick liquid (opium)**]

Continued on p. 276

Blood Composition

Blood Tissue

Blood is a fluid tissue that has many kinds of chemicals dissolved in it and millions upon millions of cells floating in it (**Figure 12-1**). The liquid (extracellular) part is called **plasma.** Suspended in the plasma are many different types of cells and cell fragments, which make up the **formed elements** of blood.

Many people seem curious about how much blood they have. The amount varies with how big they are and whether they are male or female. A big person has more blood than a small person, and a man has more blood than a woman. But as a general rule, most adults probably have between 4 and 6 liters of blood. It normally accounts for about 7% to 9% of the total body weight.

The volume of the plasma part of blood is usually a little more than half the entire volume of whole blood. An example of normal blood volumes for a person follows:

2.6 L Plasma
+2.4 L Formed elements
5.0 L Whole blood

Blood is slightly alkaline, with a pH between 7.35 and 7.45—always staying just above the chemically neutral point of 7.00 (see Chapter 2). If the alkalinity of your blood decreases toward neutral, you are a very sick person; in fact, you have **acidosis.** But even in this condition, blood almost never becomes the least bit acidic (below pH 7)—it just becomes less alkaline than normal.

Blood Plasma

Blood plasma is the liquid part of the blood, or blood minus its formed elements. It consists of water with many substances dissolved in it. All of the chemicals needed by cells to stay alive—nutrients, oxygen, and salts, for example—have to be brought to them by the blood.

Nutrients and salts are dissolved in plasma. A small amount of oxygen (O_2) is also transported in plasma. Wastes that cells must get rid of are dissolved in plasma and transported to the excretory organs. The hormones and other regulatory chemicals that help control cells' activities are also dissolved in plasma.

As **Figure 12-1** shows, the most abundant type of solute in the plasma is a group of **plasma proteins,** that together make up about 7% of the plasma by weight. These proteins include **albumins,** which help retain water in the blood by osmosis. **Globulins,** which include the antibodies that help protect us from infections, circulate in the plasma. The plasma also carries *fibrinogen* and *prothrombin,* which are necessary for blood clotting.

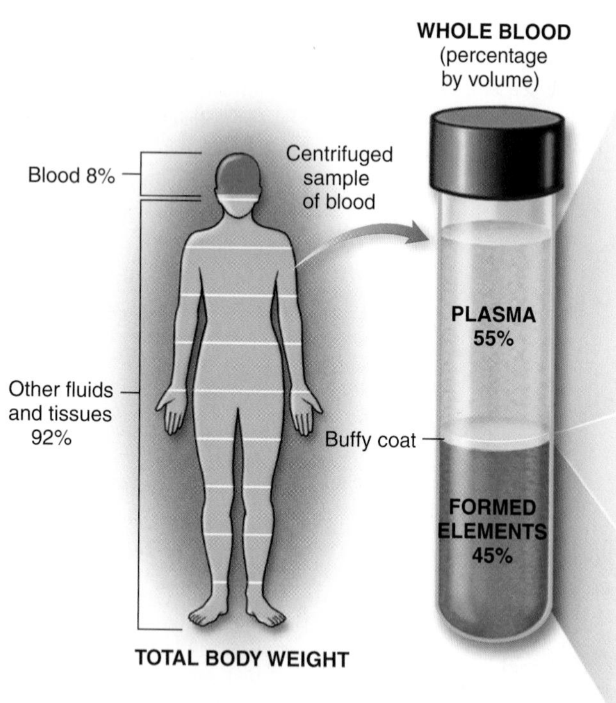

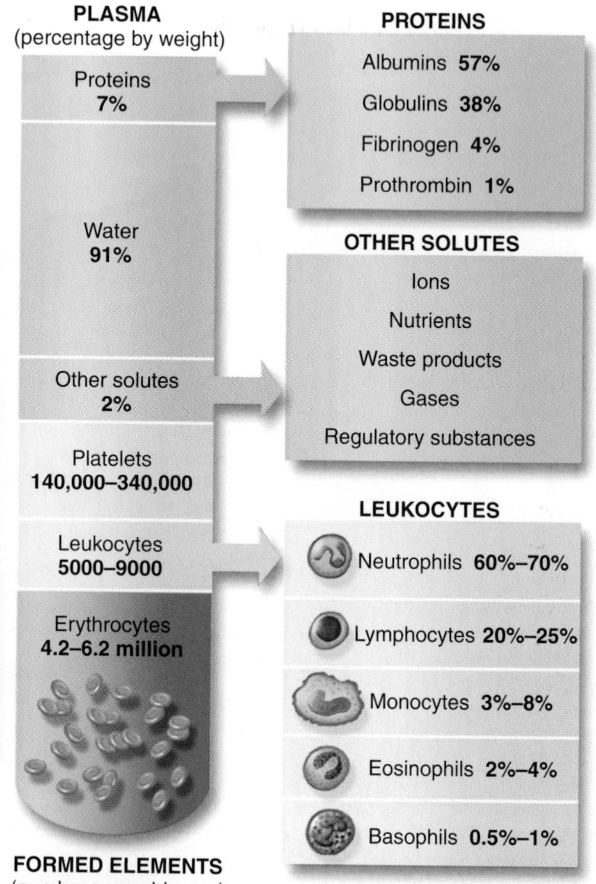

FIGURE 12-1 Components of blood. Approximate values for the components of blood in a normal adult. Values will vary with age, sex, and nutritional status.

Intravenous administration of albumin is sometimes used as a plasma volume expander in people with abnormally low blood volume. The injected albumin will draw about three to four times its volume of fluid into the blood through the process of osmosis. The result is an expansion of blood volume that can be lifesaving in cases of hemorrhage, severe burns, or kidney disease.

Blood **serum** is plasma minus its clotting factors, such as fibrinogen. Serum is obtained from whole blood by allowing it to clot in the bottom of a tube and then pouring off the liquid serum. Serum still contains antibodies, so it can be used to treat patients that have a need for specific antibodies.

Formed Elements

There are three main types and several subtypes of **formed elements:**

A. Red blood cells (RBCs), or erythrocytes
B. White blood cells (WBCs), or leukocytes
   1. Granular leukocytes (have granules in their cytoplasm)
      a. Neutrophils
      b. Eosinophils
      c. Basophils
   2. Agranular leukocytes (do not have granules in their cytoplasm)
      a. Lymphocytes
      b. Monocytes
C. Platelets, or thrombocytes

Figure 12-1 shows the breakdown of numbers and percentages of the formed elements. **Table 12-1** lists the functions of the formed elements of blood and shows what each looks like under the microscope.

It is difficult to believe how many blood cells and cell fragments there are in the body. For instance, 5,000,000 RBCs, 7500 WBCs, and 300,000 platelets in 1 cubic millimeter (mm^3) of blood (a tiny fraction of a drop) would be considered normal counts. Because RBCs, WBCs, and platelets are continually being destroyed, the body must continually make new ones to take their place at a really staggering rate: a few million RBCs are manufactured *each second!*

TABLE 12-1 Formed Elements of the Blood

BLOOD CELL	FUNCTION
Erythrocyte	Oxygen and carbon dioxide transport
Neutrophil	Immune defense (phagocytosis)
Eosinophil	Defense against parasites
Basophil	Inflammatory response
B lymphocyte	Antibody production
T lymphocyte	Cellular immune response; destroys virally infected cells and cancer cells
Monocyte	Immune defenses (phagocytosis)
Platelet	Blood clotting

Hematopoiesis

Recall from our previous discussion of bones in Chapter 7 that formation of new blood cells is called **hematopoiesis.** Two kinds of connective tissue—**myeloid tissue** and **lymphoid tissue**—make blood cells for the body.

Myeloid tissue is better known as *red bone marrow.* In the adult, it is found chiefly in the sternum, ribs, and coxal (hip) bones. A few other bones such as the vertebrae, clavicles, and cranial bones also contain small amounts of this important tissue.

Red bone marrow forms all types of blood cells except lymphocytes. These are formed by lymphoid tissue, which is found as white masses located chiefly in the lymph nodes, thymus, and spleen.

As blood cells mature, they move into the circulatory vessels. Erythrocytes circulate for up to 4 months before they break apart and their components are removed from the bloodstream by the spleen and liver. Granular leukocytes often have a life span of only a few days, but agranular leukocytes may live for more than 6 months.

QUICK CHECK

1. What are "formed elements" of blood?
2. What is the difference between blood *plasma* and blood *serum?*
3. What two kinds of connective tissue are responsible for hematopoiesis in the body?

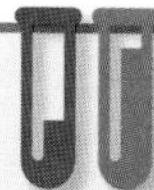

CLINICAL APPLICATION

BONE MARROW TRANSPLANTS

Bone marrow may be damaged by toxic chemicals or by high-dose x-ray and chemotherapy treatments. It can also be destroyed by diseases such as leukemia. Regardless of cause, if the bone marrow is severely damaged, a *bone marrow transplant* can be lifesaving. In this procedure, a needle is used to extract red marrow from the coxal or hipbone of a compatible donor who is under sedation, or anesthesia. The donated bone marrow is then processed and introduced into the recipient intravenously. Transplantation also may involve infusion of blood-forming *stem cells* (see Clinical Application: Stem Cells box, p. 58) harvested from the individual being treated, from a compatible donor, or from umbilical cord blood (see Research, Issues, and Trends: Freezing Umbilical Cord Blood Box, p. 493). If the recipient's immune system does not reject the new tissue or stem cells (always a danger in transplant procedures), a new colony of healthy tissue may become established in the bone marrow. As a result, destroyed or damaged myeloid tissue will be replaced and begin again to produce normal, functioning blood cells.

Red Blood Cells

RBC Structure and Function

The **red blood cell (RBC)** is an elegant example of how structural adaptation can impact biological function. Note in Figure 12-2 that the RBC, which is surrounded by a tough and flexible plasma membrane, is "caved in" on both sides so that each one has a thin center and thicker edges. This *biconcave* disk shape provides a large surface area for moving dissolved blood gases (O_2 and CO_2) and other solutes quickly in or out of the blood cell. It also helps keep the RBCs from spinning as they flow through the bloodstream.

Mature RBCs have no nucleus or cytoplasmic organelles. Because of this they are unable to reproduce themselves or replace lost or damaged cellular components. The result is a relatively short life span of about 80 to 120 days.

However, the additional intracellular space that becomes available in each cell when the nucleus and cytoplasmic organelles are lost is filled to capacity with an important red pigment called **hemoglobin (Hb).** The unique chemical properties of hemoglobin permit the RBC to perform several critically important functions required for maintenance of homeostasis, such as carrying oxygen and buffering blood. Because RBCs are completely filled with hemoglobin, they are often called **erythrocytes** (literally, "red cells").

During its short life span, each RBC travels around the entire cardiovascular system more than 100,000 times! It is the flexible plasma membrane that permits each cell to "deform" and undergo drastic changes in shape as it repeatedly passes through capillaries whose lumen is smaller than the red blood cell's diameter. Because of the large numbers of RBCs and their unique biconcave shape, the total surface area available for them to perform their biological functions is enormous.

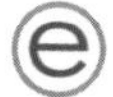

To learn more about how RBCs are formed, go to AnimationDirect at *evolve.elsevier.com.*

RBC Count

The **CBC,** or **complete blood cell count,** is a battery of tests used to measure the amounts or levels of many blood constituents and is often ordered as a routine part of the physical examination.

Measuring the *numbers* of circulating RBCs per unit of blood volume is a valuable part of the CBC. Values listed in CBC results as "normal" will vary slightly among laboratories and reference texts. For RBCs, a range of 4.2 to 6.2 million per cubic millimeter of blood (mm^3), with males generally having a higher number than females, is common. Normal deviations from average ranges often occur with age differences, level of hydration, altitude of residence, and other variables.

Originally RBC counts were done with a *hemocytometer,* a microscope slide with a counting grid etched on it. The current practice is to use a faster, more accurate automated blood cell counter.

The **hematocrit (Hct)** component of the CBC provides information about the *volume* of RBCs in a blood sample. If

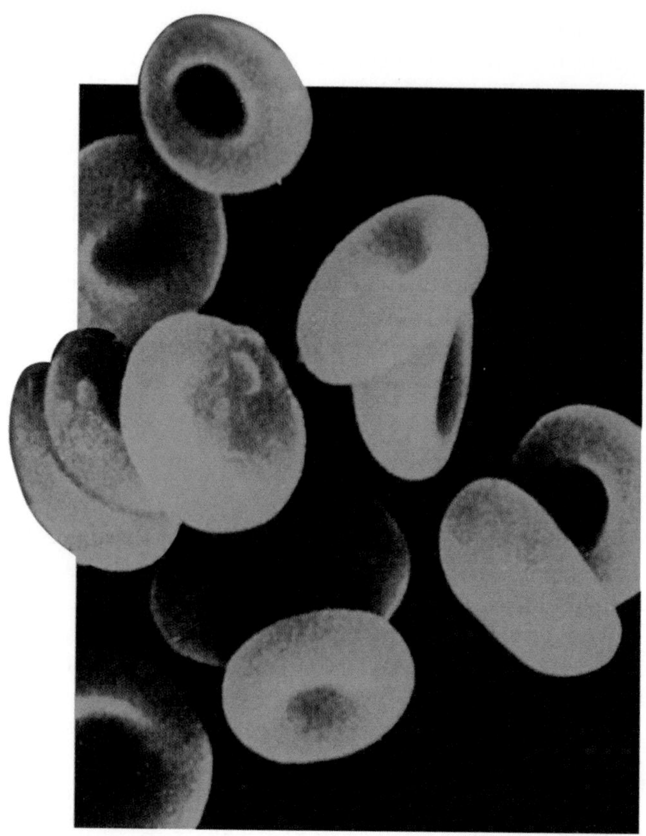

FIGURE 12-2 Red blood cells (RBCs). Color-enhanced scanning electron micrograph shows the detailed structure of normal RBCs. Note the biconcave shape of each RBC.

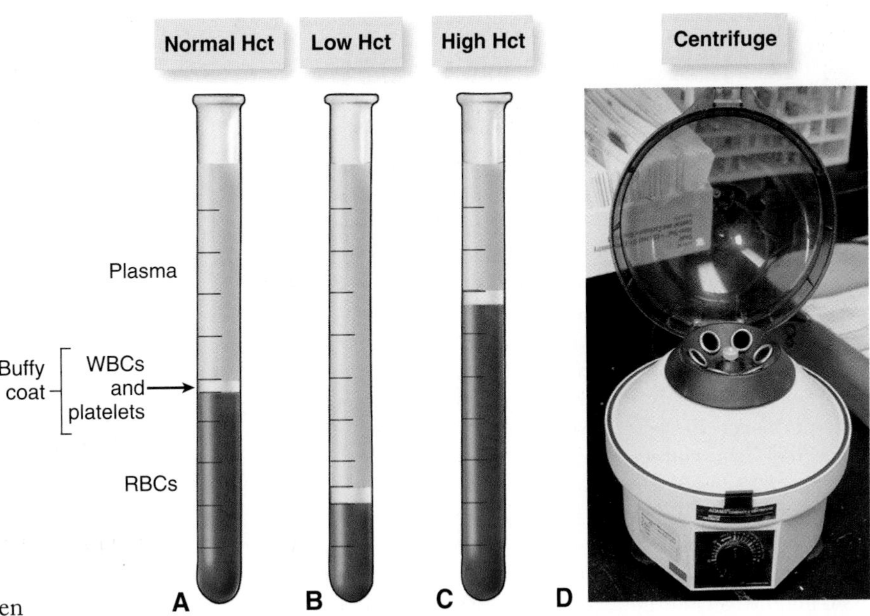

FIGURE 12-3 Hematocrit (Hct) test. Note the buffy coat located between the packed RBCs and the plasma. **A,** A normal percentage of RBCs. **B,** Anemia (a low percentage of RBCs). **C,** Polycythemia (a high percentage of RBCs). **D,** Photograph shows a laboratory centrifuge used to "spin down" tubes of whole blood to separate the formed elements from the plasma.

whole blood is placed in a special centrifuge tube and then "spun down," the heavier formed elements will quickly settle to the bottom of the tube.

During the procedure, RBCs are forced to the bottom of the tube first. The WBCs and platelets then settle out in a light-colored layer called the **buffy coat.** In Figure 12-3 the buffy coat can be seen between the packed RBCs on the bottom of the hematocrit tube and the liquid layer of plasma above.

The hematocrit test—also called *packed-cell volume (PCV)* test—gives an estimate of the proportion of RBCs to whole blood. Such information could help screen for dehydration, hemorrhaging, or other circumstances that affect the RBC ratio. Normally about 45% of the blood volume consists of RBCs (see Figure 12-1).

Hemoglobin

The hemoglobin molecules that fill the millions of RBCs are critical in the transport and exchange of oxygen and carbon dioxide between the blood and the body's cells. They also play a key role in maintenance of acid-base balance in the body.

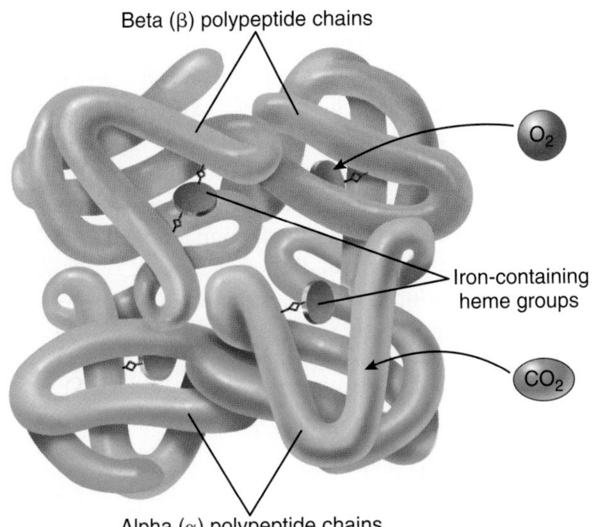

FIGURE 12-4 The hemoglobin (Hb) molecule. This large molecule is composed of four polypeptide subunits—the alpha (α) and beta (β) chains. Carbon dioxide may be carried on the amino acids of these chains. Each folded chain holds an iron-containing heme group *(red)* at its core. The iron (Fe) gives hemoglobin its oxygen-carrying capacity.

Hemoglobin is a quaternary protein made up of four folded polypeptide chains, two *alpha (α) chains* and two *beta (β) chains.* As you can see in Figure 12-4, there is a chemical structure called a *heme* group embedded within each folded chain. An iron (Fe) atom within each heme group attracts oxygen molecules to unite with hemoglobin and thus form an oxygen-hemoglobin complex called **oxyhemoglobin (HbO_2).**

Oxyhemoglobin makes possible the efficient transport of 98.5% of all of the oxygen required for the body cells (1.5% is dissolved in plasma).

Iron (Fe) is an essential nutrient needed to give hemoglobin its oxygen-carrying ability. Vitamin B_{12} and folate (also a B vitamin) are also among the critical nutrients needed by the red bone marrow to manufacture enough hemoglobin to maintain survival.

Carbon dioxide (CO_2) may attach to the amino acids within hemoglobin's alpha and beta chains to form **carbaminohemoglobin ($HbCO_2$).** This molecule transports about 20% of the carbon dioxide produced as a waste product of cellular metabolism to the lungs for disposal into the external environment. Recall that about 10% of CO_2 is transported in the blood dissolved in plasma. The majority of CO_2 (70%) carried in the blood is converted in RBCs to bicarbonate for its journey to the lungs for excretion (see Chapter 15).

Anemia

The term **anemia** is used to describe a number of different disease conditions caused by an inability of the blood to carry sufficient oxygen to the body cells. Anemias can result from inadequate numbers of RBCs or a deficiency of normal hemoglobin. Thus anemia can occur if the hemoglobin in RBCs is inadequate, even if adequate numbers of RBCs are present.

Hemorrhagic anemia results from a decrease in the number of RBCs caused by hemorrhage resulting from, for example, accidents or bleeding ulcers.

HEALTH AND WELL-BEING

BLOOD DOPING

A number of athletes have reportedly improved their performance by a practice called *blood boosting* or **blood doping.** A few weeks before an important event, an athlete has some blood drawn. The RBCs in this sample are separated and frozen. Just before competition, the RBCs are thawed and injected back into the athlete.

The increased hematocrit that results slightly improves the oxygen-carrying capacity of the blood, which theoretically improves performance. However, while the impact on performance is slight, the dangers to health and survival are real. This method is judged to be an unfair and unwise practice in athletics.

In addition to blood transfusions, injection of substances such as hormones that stimulate hematopoiesis (blood cell production) to increase RBC levels in an attempt to improve athletic performance has also been condemned by leading authorities in the area of sports medicine and by athletic organizations around the world. "Doping" with either the naturally occurring hormone erythropoietin (EPO) or with synthetic drugs that have similar biological effects—such as Epogen and Procrit—can result in devastating medical outcomes.

Aplastic anemia is characterized by a reduction in RBC numbers following destruction of the blood-forming elements in bone marrow. The cause is often related to exposure to certain toxic chemicals, high-dose irradiation (x-rays), certain drugs, and chemotherapy agents.

The term **pernicious anemia** is used to describe a deficiency of RBCs that results from a failure of the stomach lining to produce **intrinsic factor**—the substance that allows vitamin B_{12} to be absorbed from the foods we eat. Because RBC production requires adequate blood levels of this vitamin, red cell numbers will decrease in the absence of intrinsic factor even if the vitamin is present in the diet. Therefore successful long-term treatment requires repeated injections of vitamin B_{12} to maintain normal RBC production.

Iron is a critical component of the hemoglobin molecule. Without adequate iron in the diet, the body cannot manufacture enough hemoglobin. The result is **iron deficiency anemia,** a worldwide medical problem.

Sickle cell anemia is a genetic disease that results in the formation of limited amounts of an abnormal type of hemoglobin called *sickle hemoglobin,* or *hemoglobin S (HbS).* The genetic defect produces an amino acid substitution in one of the beta (β) polypeptide chains (see **Figure 12-4**), causing the resulting HbS to be less stable and less soluble than normal hemoglobin. The defective hemoglobin forms crystals and causes the red cell to become fragile and assume a sickle (crescent) shape when the blood oxygen level is low (**Figure 12-5**).

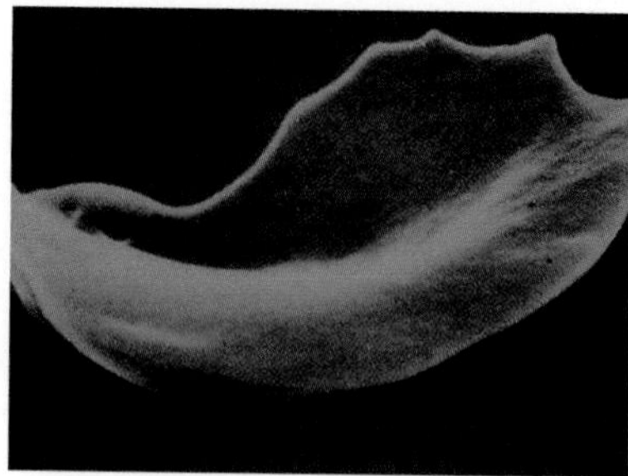

FIGURE 12-5 Sickle cell. A sickle-shaped red blood cell typical of sickle cell anemia.

A person who inherits only one defective gene develops only a small amount of HbS and has a form of the disease called **sickle cell trait.** Those with sickle cell trait most often have no symptoms at all. However, in some stressful or high-exertion situations, a person with sickle cell trait could become ill.

If two defective genes are inherited (one from each parent), then more HbS is produced and a much more severe condition called sickle cell disease develops. In addition to RBC sickling and rupture, high levels of HbS may cause reduction in blood flow; abnormal blood clotting; and in episodes of "crisis," severe pooling of red cells, particularly in the spleen, causing sudden death.

Treatment is primarily supportive because no effective anti-sickling drugs are currently available. However, patient education, early diagnosis, preventive measures to reduce dehydration and infection, and limited use of blood transfusions to treat episodes of crisis are improving survival rates.

Sickle cell anemia is found almost entirely in those of black African descent, and in the United States nearly 1 in every 600 African-American newborns is affected with sickle cell trait or disease.

If hemoglobin and RBC numbers fall below the normal levels, as they do in any type of anemia, it starts an unhealthy chain reaction: less hemoglobin, less oxygen transported to cells, slower use of nutrients by cells, less energy produced by cells, decreased cellular functions. If you understand this relationship between hemoglobin and energy, you can correctly guess that an anemic person's chief complaint will probably be that he or she feels "so tired all the time."

If bone marrow produces an excess of RBCs, the result is a condition called **polycythemia** (see **Figure 12-3,** *C*). The blood in individuals suffering from this condition may contain so many RBCs that it may become too thick to flow properly, resulting in a stroke or heart attack.

QUICK CHECK

1. How are RBCs different from most other cells of the body?
2. What protein in blood cells carries oxygen?
3. Can you give a broad definition of anemia?
4. Name two types of anemia and describe the primary characteristic of each type.

Blood Types

Blood is often identified as a specific "type" by using the **ABO system** and **Rh system** of classification.

Blood types are identified by certain antigen molecules on the plasma membrane surfaces of RBCs (**Figure 12-6**). An **antigen** is a substance that can stimulate the body to make antibodies. Almost all substances that act as antigens are foreign molecules—often on the surfaces of bacterial cells and viruses. That is, they are not the body's own natural molecules but instead are molecules that have entered the body from the outside by means of infection, transfusion, or some other method.

The word *antibody* can be defined in terms of what causes its formation or in terms of how it functions. Defined the first way, an **antibody** is a substance made by the body in response to stimulation by an antigen. Defined according to its functions, an antibody is a substance that reacts with the antigen that stimulated its formation. Many antibodies react with their antigens to cause clumping; that is, they **agglutinate** the antigens. In other words, the antibodies cause their targeted antigens to stick together in little clusters—a mechanism often used by the immune system to fight infections.

ABO System

Every person's blood is one of the following blood types in the ABO system of typing:

1. Type A
2. Type B
3. Type AB
4. Type O

Suppose that you have type A blood (as do about 41% of Americans). The letter *A* stands for a certain type of antigen in the plasma membrane of your RBCs that has been present since birth. Because you were born with type A antigen, your body does not form antibodies to react with it. In other words, your blood plasma contains no anti-A antibodies. It does, however, contain anti-B antibodies. For some unknown reason, these antibodies are present naturally in type A blood plasma. The body did not form them in response to the presence of the B antigen; they are simply part of the body's genetic makeup.

In summary, in type A blood the RBCs contain type A antigen and the plasma contains anti-B antibodies.

Recipient's blood		Reactions with donor's blood			
RBC antigens	Plasma antibodies	Donor type O	Donor type A	Donor type B	Donor type AB
None (Type O)	Anti-A Anti-B	No agglutination	Agglutination	Agglutination	Agglutination
A (Type A)	Anti-B	No agglutination	No agglutination	Agglutination	Agglutination
B (Type B)	Anti-A	No agglutination	Agglutination	No agglutination	Agglutination
A and B (Type AB)	(None)	No agglutination	No agglutination	No agglutination	No agglutination

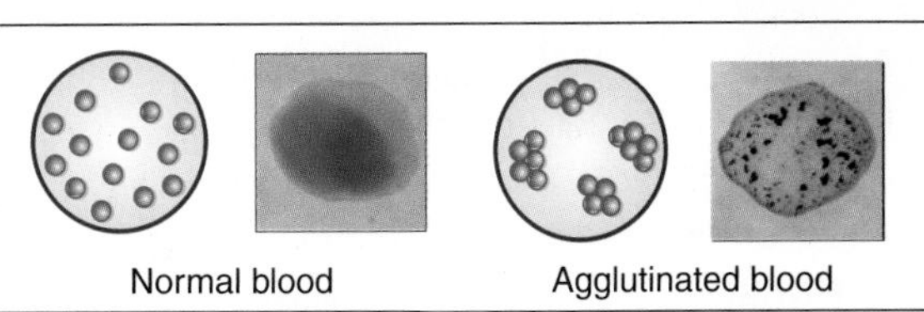

FIGURE 12-6 ABO blood typing. The left columns show the recipient's blood characteristics, and the top row shows the donor's blood type.

Similarly, in type B blood, the RBCs contain type B antigen, and the plasma contains anti-A antibodies. In type AB blood, as its name indicates, the RBCs contain both type A and type B antigens, and the plasma contains neither anti-A nor anti-B antibodies.

The opposite is true of type O blood; its RBCs contain neither type A nor type B antigens, and its plasma contains both anti-A and anti-B antibodies.

Figure 12-6 shows the results of different combinations of donor and recipient blood in the ABO system.

Rh System

You may be familiar with the term **Rh-positive** blood. It means that the RBCs of this blood type contain an antigen called the *Rh factor*. If, for example, a person has type AB, Rh-positive blood, his red blood cells contain type A antigen, type B antigen, and the Rh factor antigen. The term *Rh* is used because this important blood cell antigen was first discovered in the blood of Rhesus monkeys.

In **Rh-negative** blood, the RBCs do not have the Rh antigens on their surfaces. Plasma never naturally contains

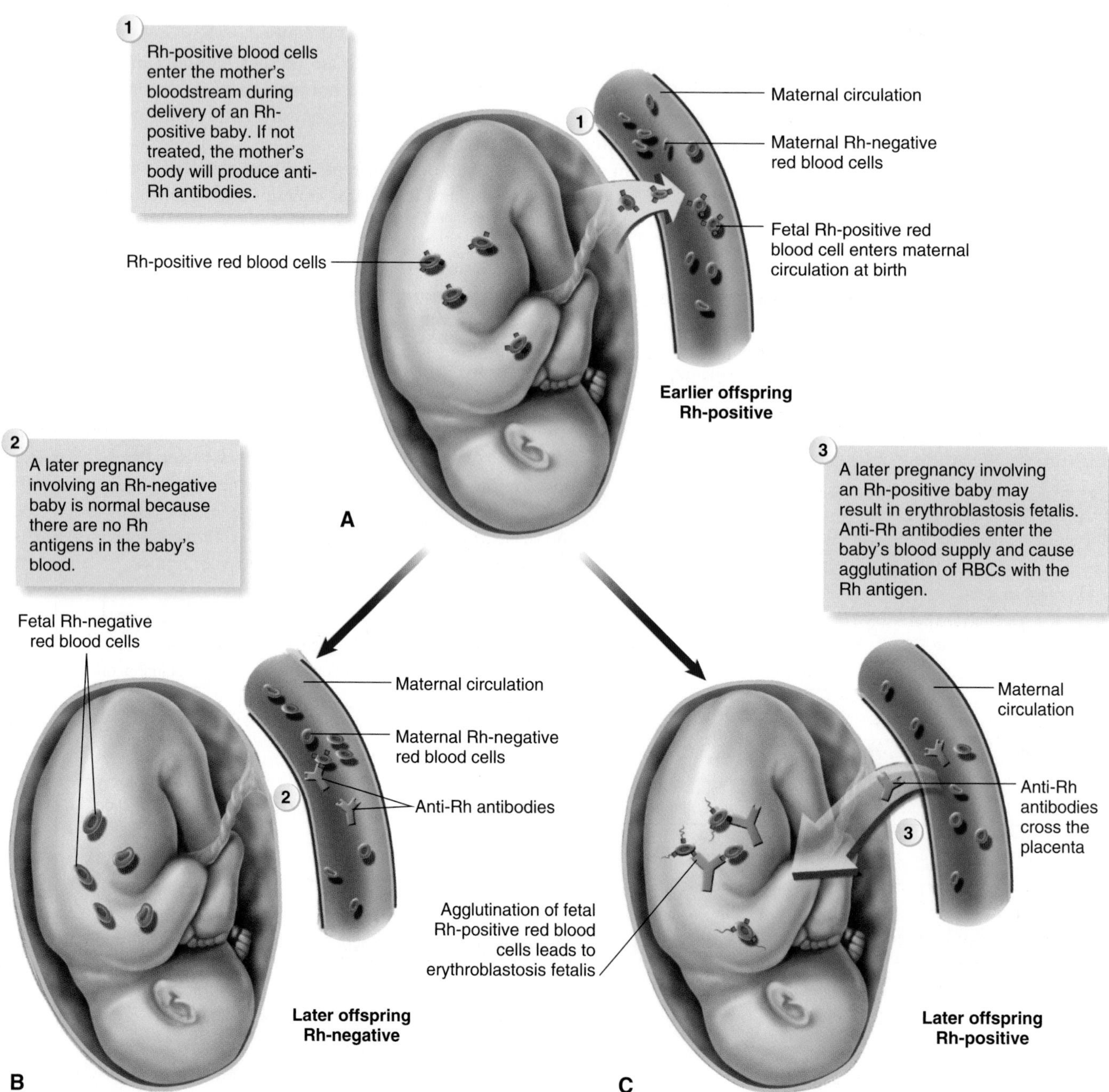
1
Rh-positive blood cells enter the mother's bloodstream during delivery of an Rh-positive baby. If not treated, the mother's body will produce anti-Rh antibodies.
Maternal circulation
Maternal Rh-negative red blood cells
Fetal Rh-positive red blood cell enters maternal circulation at birth
Rh-positive red blood cells
1
Earlier offspring Rh-positive
A
2
A later pregnancy involving an Rh-negative baby is normal because there are no Rh antigens in the baby's blood.
3
A later pregnancy involving an Rh-positive baby may result in erythroblastosis fetalis. Anti-Rh antibodies enter the baby's blood supply and cause agglutination of RBCs with the Rh antigen.
Fetal Rh-negative red blood cells
Maternal circulation
Maternal Rh-negative red blood cells
2
Anti-Rh antibodies
Agglutination of fetal Rh-positive red blood cells leads to erythroblastosis fetalis
Later offspring Rh-negative
B
Maternal circulation
Anti-Rh antibodies cross the placenta
3
Later offspring Rh-positive
C

FIGURE 12-7 Erythroblastosis fetalis. Under certain conditions, anti-Rh antibodies may enter the baby's blood supply and cause agglutination of RBCs with the Rh antigen.

anti-Rh antibodies. But if Rh-positive blood cells are introduced into an Rh-negative person's body, anti-Rh antibodies soon appear in the recipient's blood plasma.

Without appropriate precautions, there could be some danger for a baby born to an Rh-negative mother and an Rh-positive father. If the baby inherits the Rh-positive trait from his father, the Rh factor on his RBCs may stimulate the mother's body to form anti-Rh antibodies. Then, if she later carries another Rh-positive fetus, he may develop a type of **hemolytic anemia** called **erythroblastosis fetalis,** caused by the mother's Rh antibodies reacting with the baby's Rh-positive cells (**Figure 12-7**).

All Rh-negative mothers who carry an Rh-positive baby should be treated with an immunoglobulin (antibody) serum, widely marketed under the brand name **RhoGAM.** RhoGAM stops the mother's body from forming anti-Rh antibodies and thus prevents the possibility of harm to the next Rh-positive baby.

Likewise, a person with Rh-negative blood who receives a transfusion of Rh-positive blood will also develop anti-Rh antibodies and be at risk of an immune reaction if exposed to Rh-positive blood again later.

Combined ABO-Rh System

Both the ABO and Rh systems are often used in combination to identify a person's blood type, as you can see in **Table 12-2**. For example, the blood type AB+ refers to the ABO type "AB" and the Rh-positive type. Likewise, O− identifies the blood type of a person with the "O" version of ABO type and the Rh-negative version of Rh type.

Knowing one's blood type can be lifesaving in a medical emergency or during surgery, when a blood transfusion may be needed to maintain the total blood volume. Harmful effects or even death can result from a blood transfusion reaction if the donor's RBCs become agglutinated by antibodies in the recipient's plasma.

If a donor's RBCs do not contain any A, B, or Rh antigen, they cannot be clumped by anti-A, anti-B, or anti-Rh antibodies. For this reason, the type of blood that contains no A, B, or Rh antigens—type O−—can be used in an emergency as donor blood. With type O−, there is no danger of anti-A, anti-B, or anti-Rh antibodies clumping its RBCs. Type O− blood has therefore been called **universal donor blood.**

Similarly, blood type AB+ has been called **universal recipient blood** because it contains no anti-A, anti-B, or anti-Rh antibodies in its plasma. Therefore, type AB+ blood does not clump any donor's RBCs containing A, B, or Rh antigens.

In a normal clinical setting, however, all blood intended for transfusion is not only matched carefully to the blood of the recipient for ABO and Rh compatibility but also tested further in a process called *crossmatching* for a variety of so-called "minor antigens" that may also cause certain types of transfusion reactions.

Review **Figure 12-6**, which shows the results of different combinations of donor and recipient blood in the ABO system.

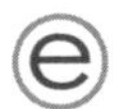
To learn more about erythroblastosis fetalis, go to AnimationDirect at *evolve.elsevier.com*.

QUICK CHECK

1. What is an *antigen* in blood typing?
2. What is meant when a person's blood is described as "Rh negative"?
3. What is the "universal recipient" blood and what is the reason for this name?

White Blood Cells

Introduction to White Blood Cells

Recall from the listing of formed elements found in the blood (see p. 265) that the **white blood cells (WBCs)** are also called **leukocytes.**

The WBC, when stained on a microscope slide, shows a prominent and sometimes oddly shaped nucleus—far different in appearance from the RBC, which has no nucleus. WBCs have no hemoglobin and thus are almost transparent when unstained. A mass of WBCs looks whitish in appearance because of the diffusion of light, much as clear snowflakes appear white when found in a mass.

Different types of WBCs are categorized by the presence or absence of stained granules in their cytoplasm. **Granular leukocytes** *(granulocytes)* have stained granules and **agranular leukocytes** *(agranulocytes)* do not. The granulocytes include the **neutrophils, eosinophils,** and **basophils** (**Figure 12-8**, *A, B,* and *C*). The **lymphocytes** and **monocytes** (**Figure 12-8**, *D* and *E*) are agranulocytes.

All of the WBCs are involved in immunity. However, each type and subtype of WBC has its own unique roles to play

TABLE 12-2 Blood Typing

BLOOD TYPE (ABO and Rh)	ANTIGENS PRESENT*	ANTIBODIES PRESENT*	PERCENT OF GENERAL POPULATION
O+	Rh	A, B	35%
O− (universal donor)	None	A, B, Rh?	7%
A+	A, Rh	B	35%
A−	A	B, Rh?	7%
B+	B, Rh	A	8%
B−	B	A, Rh?	2%
AB+ (universal recipient)	A, B, Rh	None	4%
AB−	A, B	Rh?	2%

Adapted from Pagana KD, Pagana TJ: *Mosby's manual of diagnostic and laboratory tests,* ed 5, St Louis, 2014, Mosby.
*Anti-Rh antibodies *may* be present, depending on exposure to Rh antigens.

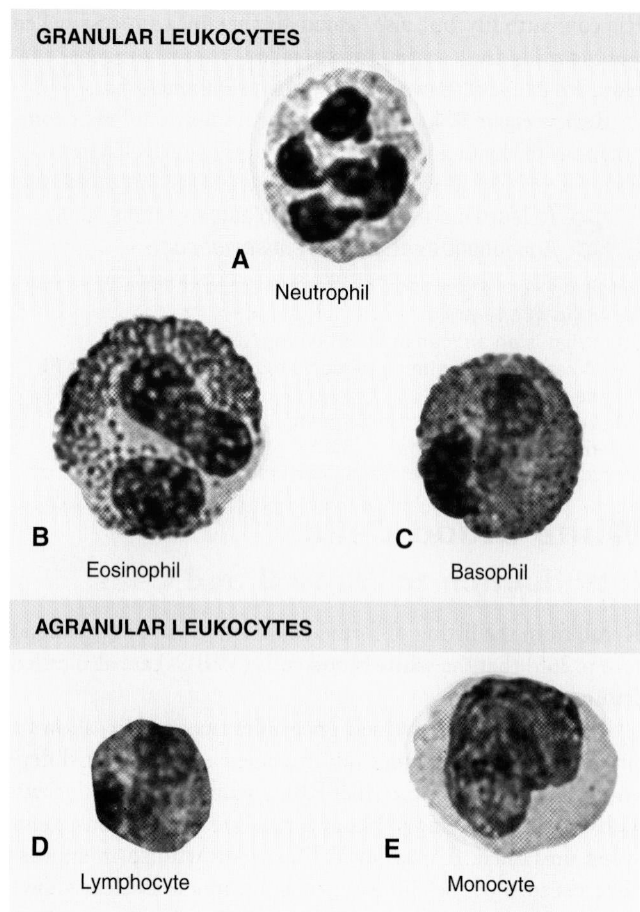

FIGURE 12-8 Leukocytes. A-E, Each light micrograph shows a different type of stained WBC.

in immunity, such as phagocytosis of foreign particles or virus-infected cells. Details of the roles of some WBCs are found in Chapter 14.

To learn more about WBCs, go to AnimationDirect at *evolve.elsevier.com.*

WBC Count

Normally, the total number of WBCs per cubic millimeter of whole blood (mm^3) ranges between 5000 and 10,000.

The term **leukopenia** is used to describe an abnormally *low* WBC count (less than 5000 WBCs/mm^3 of blood). Leukopenia does not occur often. However, malfunction of blood-forming tissues and cells and some diseases affecting the immune system, such as AIDS (discussed in Chapter 14), may lower WBC numbers.

Leukocytosis refers to an abnormally *high* WBC count (that is, more than 10,000 WBCs/mm^3 of blood). It is a much more common problem than leukopenia and almost always accompanies bacterial infections. In addition, leukocytosis is also seen in many forms of blood cancer (described later), which are often diagnosed when tremendous increases in WBC numbers are detected in blood tests.

A special type of white blood cell count called a **differential WBC count** reveals more information than simply counting the total number of all of the different types of WBCs in a blood sample. In a differential WBC count, a component test in the CBC test mentioned previously (see p. 266), the *proportions* of each type of white blood cell are reported as percentages of the total WBC count. Normal percentages are shown in **Figure 12-1**.

Because specific diseases affect each WBC type differently, the differential WBC count is a valuable diagnostic tool. For example, although some parasite infestations do not cause an increase in the total WBC count, they often do cause an increase in the proportion of eosinophils that are present. The reason? This type of WBC specializes in defending against parasites (see **Table 12-1**).

WBC Types

Granular Leukocytes

Neutrophils are the most numerous of the active WBCs called **phagocytes**, which protect the body from invading microorganisms by taking them into their own cell bodies and digesting them by the process of phagocytosis (**Figure 12-9**).

Eosinophils also serve as weak phagocytes. Perhaps their most important function involves protection against infections

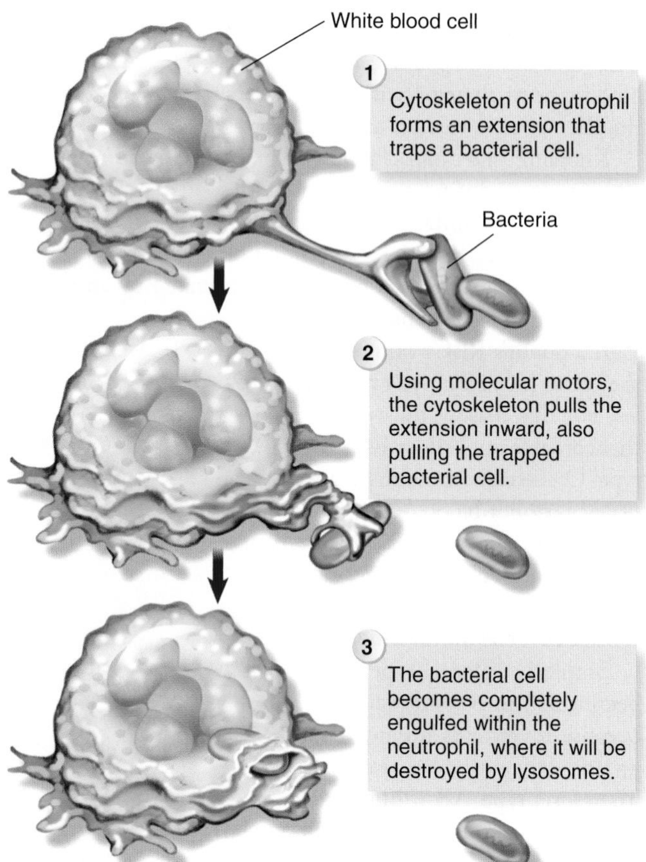

White blood cell
1
Cytoskeleton of neutrophil forms an extension that traps a bacterial cell.
Bacteria
2
Using molecular motors, the cytoskeleton pulls the extension inward, also pulling the trapped bacterial cell.
3
The bacterial cell becomes completely engulfed within the neutrophil, where it will be destroyed by lysosomes.

FIGURE 12-9 Phagocytosis. Diagrammatic representation of phagocytosis by a neutrophil (note the multilobed nucleus). Extension of cytoplasm envelopes the bacteria, which are drawn through the cell membrane and into the cytoplasm.

caused by certain parasites and parasitic worms. They also are involved in regulating allergic reactions, including asthma.

Basophils, in peripheral blood, and related **mast cells** found in the tissues, both secrete the chemical **histamine,** which is released during inflammatory reactions. Basophils also produce a potent **anticoagulant** called **heparin,** which helps prevent blood from clotting as it flows through the blood vessels of the body.

Agranular Leukocytes

Monocytes are the largest leukocytes. Like neutrophils, they are aggressive phagocytes. Because of their size, they are capable of engulfing larger bacterial organisms and cancerous cells. **Macrophages** (meaning "large eater") are monocytes that have grown to several times their original size after migrating out of the bloodstream. They are discussed further in Chapter 14.

Lymphocytes help protect us against infections, but they do it by a process different from phagocytosis. Lymphocytes function in the immune mechanism, the complex process that makes us immune to infectious diseases.

Lymphocytes called *B lymphocytes* develop within several lymphoid organs of the body. B lymphocytes (B cells) secrete plasma proteins called *antibodies* that attach to specific antigen molecules related to bacteria, viruses, chemical toxins, or other foreign substances. Active B lymphocytes, called **plasma cells,** are formed in unusually large numbers in a type of bone marrow cancer called *multiple myeloma,* which is described later.

Other lymphocytes, called *T lymphocytes,* mature in the thymus. T lymphocytes (T cells) do not secrete antibodies but instead protect us by directly attacking bacteria, virus-infected cells, or cancer cells.

Details of the role of lymphocytes in the immune system are discussed in Chapter 14.

WBC Disorders

Leukemia is the term used to describe a number of blood cancers affecting the WBCs. In almost every form of leukemia, marked leukocytosis (elevated WBC count) occurs. Leukocyte counts in excess of 100,000/mm^3 in circulating blood are common. Many of the additional WBCs do not function properly.

The different types of leukemia are identified as either *acute* or *chronic,* based on how quickly symptoms appear after the disease begins. Leukemias are referred to as *lymphocytic* or *myeloid* depending on where the disease develops in the body.

Platelets and Blood Clotting

Platelets

The **platelet,** the third main type of formed element, plays an essential part in blood clotting or *coagulation.* Your life might someday be saved just because your blood can clot. A clot plugs up torn or cut vessels and stops bleeding that otherwise might prove fatal. Platelets also are called **thrombocytes** from *thrombus* meaning "clot."

Much smaller than RBCs, platelets are tiny cell fragments that have broken away from a much larger precursor cell. Each tiny platelet is filled with chemicals necessary for triggering the formation of a blood clot.

Blood Clotting

The story of how we stop bleeding when an injury occurs—a process called **hemostasis**—is the story of a chain of rapid-fire reactions. All these reactions culminate in the formation of a blood clot.

When an injury occurs, smooth muscles around the wall of the vessel may reflexively contract and thereby constrict the diameter of the vessel—a process called **vasoconstriction.** The resulting pressure helps temporarily close any gaps in the vessel wall and reduces local blood flow until other measures come into play. Pressure applied from outside the wound by a first responder often enhances this effect.

As vessels constrict, damaged tissue cells release various clotting factors into the plasma. These factors rapidly react with other factors already present in the plasma to form **prothrombin activator.**

Normally the lining of blood vessels is extremely smooth, but an injury makes a rough spot with exposed collagen fibers. This attracts platelets to the site, which become "sticky" at the point of injury and rapidly accumulate near the break in the blood vessel, forming a soft, temporary **platelet plug.** As the platelets accumulate, they release additional clotting factors, forming even more prothrombin activator—a kind of self-amplifying, *positive-feedback* response.

If the normal amount of blood calcium is present, prothrombin activator triggers the next step of clotting by converting **prothrombin** (a protein in normal blood) to **thrombin.** In the last step, thrombin reacts with **fibrinogen** (a normal plasma protein) to change it to a fibrous gel called **fibrin.** Under the microscope, fibrin looks like a tangle of fine threads with RBCs caught in the tangle. **Figure 12-10** illustrates the steps in the blood-clotting mechanism.

The clotting mechanism contains clues for ways to stop bleeding by speeding up blood clotting. For example, you might simply apply gauze to a bleeding surface. Its slight roughness would cause more platelets to stick together and release more clotting factors. These additional factors would then make the blood clot more quickly.

Physicians sometimes prescribe vitamin K before surgery to make sure that the patient's blood will clot fast enough to prevent hemorrhage. Vitamin K stimulates liver cells to increase the synthesis of prothrombin. More prothrombin in blood allows faster production of thrombin during clotting and thus faster clot formation.

Abnormal Blood Clots

Unfortunately, clots sometimes form in unbroken blood vessels of the heart, brain, lungs, or some other organ—a dreaded thing because they may produce sudden death by shutting off the blood supply to a vital organ. When a clot stays in the

FIGURE 12-10 Blood clotting. A, The extremely complex clotting mechanism can be distilled into three basic steps outlined in the boxes. **B,** Color-enhanced scanning electron micrograph shows RBCs and WBCs entrapped in a fibrin *(yellow)* mesh during clot formation (platelets are *blue*).

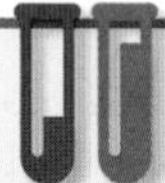

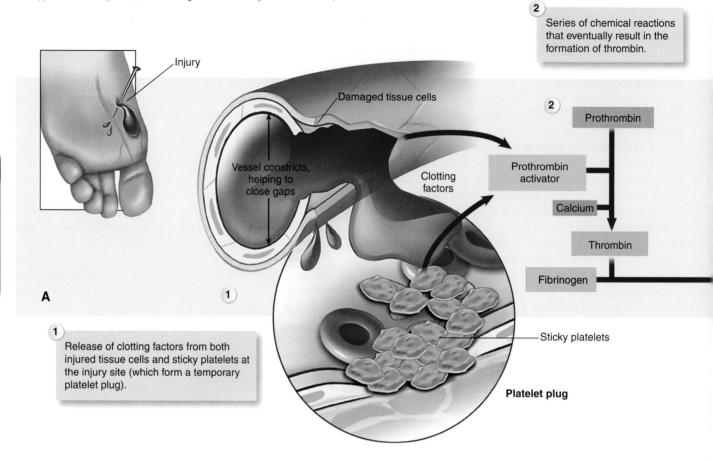

CLINICAL APPLICATION

ANTICOAGULANT THERAPY

The anticoagulant Coumadin (warfarin sodium) acts by inhibiting the synthesis of prothrombin and other vitamin K–dependent clotting factors. By doing so, Coumadin decreases the ability of blood to clot and is effective in preventing repeat thromboses after a heart attack or the formation of clots after surgical replacement of heart valves.

Heparin can also be used to prevent excessive blood clotting. Heparin inhibits the conversion of prothrombin to thrombin, thus preventing formation of a thrombus. The most widely used anticoagulant is low-dose (81-mg) aspirin. This readily available drug inhibits the formation of tiny platelet plugs and the subsequent formation of emboli, which may cause blockage of small blood vessels in the brain and lead to a stroke.

A laboratory test called the **prothrombin time (PT)** is often used to regulate dosage of anticoagulant drugs. In this test, thromboplastin (a blood clotting factor) and calcium are added simultaneously to a tube of the patient's plasma and a tube containing a normal control solution, and the time required for clot formation in both tubes is determined. A patient prothrombin time in excess of the standard control value (11 to 12.5 seconds) indicates the level of anticoagulant effect caused by the administered drug.

Unfortunately, PT test results may vary between different clinical laboratories. Variability is often caused by differing techniques or differences in the sensitivity of reagents used.

To minimize the effects of these and other variables and standardize the results of anticoagulation testing, a system called the **INR** (abbreviation for **I**nternational **N**ormalized **R**atio) has been developed. PT is reported in seconds. The INR is a mathematical calculation and is reported as a number. An INR of 0.8 to 1.2 is considered normal. In regulating anticoagulant therapy, keeping the INR between 1.5 and 3 will help ensure the prevention of unwanted blood coagulation in "at risk" individuals. By monitoring changes in the INR, a physician can adjust the dose of anticoagulant drug needed to maintain an appropriate level of anticoagulant effect.

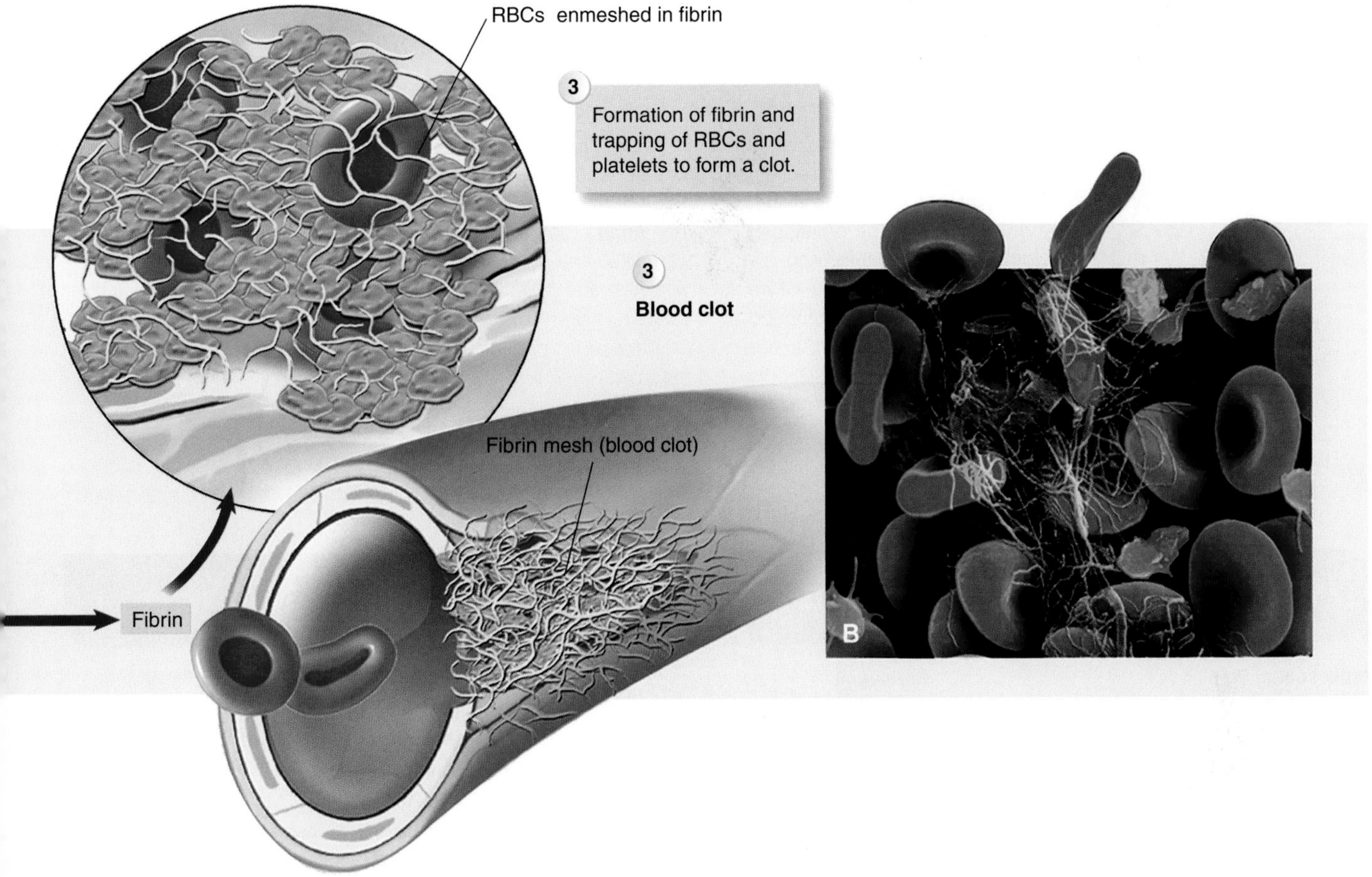

RBCs enmeshed in fibrin

3 Formation of fibrin and trapping of RBCs and platelets to form a clot.

3 Blood clot

Fibrin mesh (blood clot)

Fibrin

B

place where it formed, it is called a **thrombus**, and the condition is spoken of as **thrombosis**.

If part of the clot dislodges and circulates through the bloodstream, the dislodged part is then called an **embolus**, and the condition is called an **embolism**. For example, a clot fragment that lodges in the lung is called a *pulmonary embolism*—a situation that may prove fatal.

A number of drugs are now available to help dissolve abnormal clots. *Streptokinase* and *recombinant tissue plasminogen activator (t-PA or tPA)* are drugs frequently used in a variety of conditions, including treatment of clot-induced strokes, heart attacks, and other thrombus-induced and embolus-induced medical emergencies.

Suppose that your doctor told you that you had a clot in one of your coronary arteries. Which diagnosis would he or she make—coronary thrombosis or coronary embolism—if the physician thought that the clot had formed originally in the coronary artery as a result of the accumulation of fatty material in the vessel wall? Physicians now have effective drugs that they can use to help prevent thrombosis and embolism (see *Anticoagulant Therapy* in the box on the preceding page).

QUICK CHECK

1. Name the formed elements of blood.
2. In general, what is the function of WBCs?
3. What is the role of fibrin in blood clotting?
4. What is the structure and function of thrombocytes?
5. What is the difference between a thrombus and an embolus?

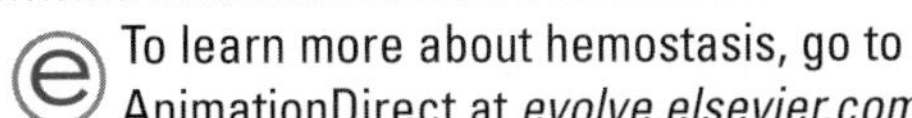

To learn more about hemostasis, go to AnimationDirect at *evolve.elsevier.com*.

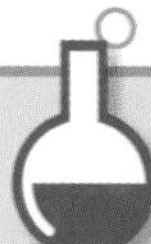

SCIENCE APPLICATIONS

HEMATOLOGY

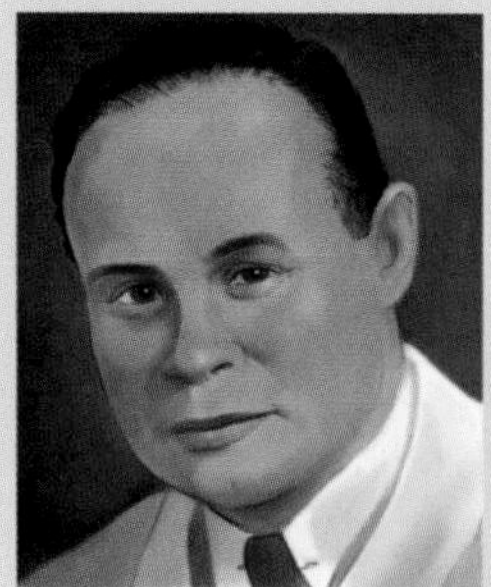

Charles Richard Drew (1904-1950)

African-American physician Charles Richard Drew was a pioneer in **hematology,** the study of blood. During World War II, he developed the idea of blood banks and researched the best way to store blood for transfusions to wounded soldiers. In New York, he set up the first blood bank ever, in 1941. This blood bank served as the model for a network of blood banks opened by the American Red Cross.

Many *hematologists* continue in Drew's footsteps, refining and perfecting the practice of blood science. Many professions benefit from this research. **Phlebotomists** collect blood for testing or storage, *clinical laboratory technicians* analyze blood samples, and many different health professionals use blood analysis and blood transfusions to help their patients. Of course, military **medics** still rely on blood banking technology to provide immediate aid to wounded combat and terrorism victims.

LANGUAGE OF SCIENCE AND MEDICINE (continued from p. 263)

buffy coat
(BUFF-ee koht)
[*buff-* **leather,** *-y* **characterized by**]

carbaminohemoglobin ($HbCO_2$)
(KAR-bam-ih-no-hee-moh-GLOH-bin)
[*carb-* **coal (carbon),** *-amino-* **ammonia compound (amino acid),** *-hemo-* **blood,** *-glob-* **ball,** *-in* **substance**]

cardiovascular system
(kar-dee-oh-VAS-kyoo-lar SIS-tem)
[*cardi-* **heart,** *-vas-* **vessel,** *-ular* **relating to**]

complete blood cell count (CBC)
(kom-PLEET blud sel kount)
[*cell-* **storeroom**]

differential WBC count
(dif-er-EN-shal DUB-el-yoo bee see kownt)
[*different-* **difference,** *-al* **relating to,** *WBC* **white blood cell**]

embolism
(EM-boh-liz-em)
[*embol-* **plug,** *-ism* **condition**]

embolus
(EM-boh-lus)
[embolus **plug**]

eosinophil
(ee-oh-SIN-oh-fil)
[*eos-* **dawn (red),** *-in-***substance,** *-phil* **love**]

erythroblastosis fetalis
(eh-rith-roh-blas-TOH-sis feh-TAL-is)
[*erythro-* **red,** *-blast-* **bud or sprout,** *-osis* **condition**]

erythrocyte
(eh-RITH-roh-syte)
[*erythro-* **red,** *-cyte* **cell**]

fibrin
(FYE-brin)
[*fibr-* **fiber,** *-in* **substance**]

fibrinogen
(fye-BRIN-oh-jen)
[*fibr-* **fiber,** *-in* **substance,** *-gen* **produce**]

formed element
(formd EL-eh-ment)

globulin
(GLOB-yoo-lin)
[*glob-* **ball,** *-ul-* **little,** *-in* **substance**]

granular leukocyte
(GRAN-yoo-lar LOO-koh-syte)
[*gran-* **grain,** *-ul-* **little,** *-ar* **relating to,** *leuko-* **white,** *-cyte* **cell**]

hematocrit (Hct)
(hee-MAT-oh-krit)
[*hemato-* **blood,** *-crit* **separate**]

hematology
(hee-mah-TOL-o-jee)
[*hemato-* **blood,** *-log-* **words (study of),** *-y* **activity**]

hematopoiesis
(hee-mat-oh-poy-EE-sis)
[*hemo-* **blood,** *-poiesis* **making**]

hemoglobin (Hb)
(hee-moh-GLOH-bin)
[*hemo-* **blood,** *-glob-* **ball,** *-in* **substance**]

hemolytic anemia
(hee-moh-LIT-ik)
[*hemo-* **blood,** *-lyt-* **loosen,** *-ic* **relating to,** *an-* **without,** *-emia* **blood condition**]

hemorrhagic anemia
(HEM-oh-raj-ick ah-NEEM-ee-ah)
[*hemo-* **blood,** *-rrh(e)a-* **flow,** *-ag(e)-* **process or state,** *-ic* **relating to,** *an-* **without,** *-emia* **blood condition**]

hemostasis
(hee-moh-STAY-sis)
[*hemo-* **blood,** *-stasis* **standing**]

heparin
(HEP-ah-rin)
[*hepar-* **liver,** *-in* **substance**]

histamine
(HIS-tah-meen)
[*hist-* **tissue,** *-amine* **ammonia compound**]

INR (International Normalized Ratio)
(in-ter-NASH-en-ul NOR-mah-lyzed RAY-shee-oh)

intrinsic factor
(in-TRIN-sik)
[*intr-* **inside or within,** *-insic* **beside**]

iron deficiency anemia
(EYE-ron deh-FISH-en-see ah-NEE-mee-ah)
[*iron* **element 26,** *de-* **down,** *-fic-* **perform,** *-ency* **state,** *an-* **without,** *-emia* **blood condition**]

leukemia
(loo-KEE-mee-ah)
[*leuk-* **white,** *-emia* **blood condition**]

leukocyte
(LOO-koh-syte)
[*leuko-* **white,** *-cyte* **cell**]

leukocytosis
(loo-koh-SYE-toh-sis)
[*leuko-* **white,** *-cyt-* **cell,** *-osis* **condition**]

leukopenia
(loo-koh-PEE-nee-ah)
[*leuko-* **white,** *-penia* **lack**]

lymphatic system
(lim-FAT-ik SIS-tem)
[*lymph-* **water,** *-atic* **relating to**]

lymphocyte
(LIM-foh-syte)
[*lymph-* **water (lymphatic system),** *-cyte* **cell**]

lymphoid tissue
(LIM-foyd TISH-yoo)
[*lymph-* **water (lymphatic system),** *-oid* **like,** *tissu* **fabric]**

macrophage
(MAK-roh-fayj)
[*macro-* **large,** *-phag-* **eat]**

mast cell
(mast sel)
[*mast* **fattening,** *cell* **storeroom]**

medic
(MED-ik)
[*med-* **heal,** *-ic-* **relating to]**

monocyte
(MON-oh-syte)
[*mono-* **single,** *-cyte* **cell]**

myeloid tissue
(MY-eh-loyd TISH-yoo)
[*myel-* **marrow,** *-oid* **of or like,** *tissu* **fabric]**

neutrophil
(NOO-troh-fil)
[*neutr-* **neither,** *-phil* **love]**

oxyhemoglobin (HbO_2)
(ahk-see-hee-moh-GLOH-bin)
[*oxy-* **sharp (oxygen),** *-hemo-* **blood,** *-glob-* **ball,** *-in* **substance]**

pernicious anemia
(per-NISH-us ah-NEE-mee-ah)
[*pernici-* **destruction,** *-ous* **relating to,** *an-* **without,** *-emia* **blood condition]**

phagocyte
(FAG-oh-syte)
[*phago-* **eat,** *-cyte* **cell]**

phlebotomist
(fleh-BOT-uh-mist)
[*phleb-* **vein,** *-tom-* **cut,** *-ist* **agent]**

plasma
(PLAZ-mah)
[*plasma* **something molded or created]**

plasma cell
(PLAZ-mah sel)
[*plasma* **something molded or created (blood plasma),** *cell* **storeroom]**

plasma protein
(PLAZ-mah PRO-teen)
[*plasma* **something molded or created (blood plasma),** *prote-* **primary,** *-in* **substance]**

platelet
(PLAYT-let)
[*plate-* **flat,** *-let* **small]**

platelet plug
(PLAYT-let plug)
[*plate-* **flat,** *-let* **small]**

polycythemia
(pahl-ee-sye-THEE-mee-ah)
[*poly-* **many,** *-cyt-* **cell,** *-emia* **blood condition]**

prothrombin
(proh-THROM-bin)
[*pro-* **before,** *-thromb-* **clot,** *-in* **substance]**

prothrombin activator
(proh-THROM-bin AK-tih-vay-tor)
[*pro-* **before,** *-thromb-* **clot,** *-in* **substance,** *act-* **perform,** *-iv-* **relating to,** *-at-* **process,** *-or* **condition]**

prothrombin time (PT)
(proh-THROM-bin tyme)
[*pro-* **before,** *-thromb-* **clot,** *-in* **substance]**

red blood cell (RBC)
(red blud sel)
[*cell-* **storeroom]**

Rh system
(ar aych SIS-tem)
[*Rh* **short for "rhesus monkey"]**

Rh-negative
(ar aych NEG-ah-tiv)
[*Rh* **short for "rhesus monkey,"** *negat-* **deny,** *-ive* **relating to]**

RhoGAM
(ROH-gam)
[brand name derived from *Rho,* 17th letter of Greek alphabet (refers to Rh antigen), *GAM* from gamma-globulin (Rh antibody)]

Rh-positive
(ar aych POZ-ih-tiv)
[*Rh* **short for "rhesus monkey,"** *posit-* **put or place,** *-ive* **relating to]**

serum
(SEER-um)
[*serum* **watery body fluid]**

sickle cell anemia
(SIK-ul sel ah-NEE-mee-ah)
[*sickle* **crescent-shaped tool,** *cell* **storeroom,** *an-* **without,** *-emia* **blood condition]**

sickle cell trait
(SIK-ul sel trayt)
[*sickle* **crescent,** *cell* **storeroom]**

thrombin
(THROM-bin)
[*thromb-* **clot,** *-in* **substance]**

thrombocyte
(THROM-boh-syte)
[*thromb-* **clot,** *-cyte* **cell]**

thrombosis
(throm-BOH-sis)
[*thrombo-* **clot,** *-osis* **condition]**

thrombus
(THROM-bus)
[*thrombus* **clot]**

universal donor blood
(yoo-neh-ver-sal DOH-nor blud)
[*uni-* **one,** *-vers-* **turn (into),** *-al* **relating to,** *don-* **give,** *-or* **agent]**

universal recipient blood
(yoo-neh-ver-sal REE-sip-ee-ahnt blud)
[*uni-* **one,** *-vers-* **turn (into),** *-al* **relating to,** *recip-* **take,** *-ent* **agent]**

vasoconstriction
(vay-soh-kon-STRIK-shun)
[*vas-* **vessel,** *-constrict-* **draw tight,** *-tion* **state]**

white blood cell (WBC)
(whyte blud sell)
[*cell* **storeroom]**

❑ OUTLINE SUMMARY

To download a digital audio version of the chapter summary for use with your device, access the ***Audio Chapter Summaries*** *online at evolve.elsevier.com.*

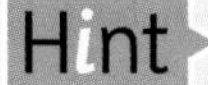

Scan this summary after reading the chapter to help you reinforce the key concepts. Later, use the summary as a quick review before your class or before a test.

Blood Composition

A. Blood tissue (see **Table 12-1**)
  1. Blood tissue composition
    a. Liquid fraction of whole blood (extracellular part) called *plasma*
    b. Cellular components suspended in the plasma make up the formed elements
  2. Normal volumes of blood
    a. Plasma — 2.6 L
    b. Formed elements — 2.4 L

c. Whole blood — 4 to 6 L average or 7% to 9% of total body weight
3. Blood pH
a. Blood is alkaline — pH 7.35 to pH 7.45
b. Blood pH decreased toward neutral creates a condition called *acidosis*

B. Blood plasma
1. Liquid fraction of whole blood minus formed elements (see **Figure 12-1**)
2. Composition — water containing many dissolved substances including:
a. Nutrients, salts
b. About 1.5% of total O_2 transported in blood
c. About 5% of total CO_2 transported in blood
d. Most abundant solutes dissolved in plasma are plasma proteins
(1) Albumins
(2) Globulins
(3) Fibrinogen
(4) Prothrombin
3. Plasma minus clotting factors is called *serum*
a. Serum is liquid remaining after whole blood clots
b. Serum contains antibodies

C. Formed elements
1. Types
a. Red blood cell also called RBC or erythrocyte
b. White blood cell also called WBC or leukocyte
(1) Granular leukocytes — neutrophils, eosinophils, and basophils
(2) Agranular leukocytes — lymphocytes and monocytes
c. Platelets or thrombocytes
2. Blood cells counts
a. RBCs — 4.5 to 5 million per mm^3 of blood
b. WBCs — 5000 to 10,000 per mm^3 of blood
c. Platelets — 300,000 per mm^3 of blood

D. Hematopoiesis — formation of new blood cells
1. Myeloid tissue (red bone marrow) — forms all blood cells except some lymphocytes; found within bones
2. Lymphoid tissue — forms additional white blood cells in the lymph nodes, thymus, and spleen
3. RBCs live about 4 months; WBCs live for a few days (granular) to over 6 months (agranular)

Red Blood Cells (Erythrocytes)

A. RBC structure and function
1. RBC offers excellent example of how structural adaptation affects biological function
2. Tough yet flexible plasma membrane deforms easily allowing RBCs to pass through small-diameter capillaries
3. Biconcave disk shape (thin center and thicker edges) results in large membrane surface area and reduced spinning as blood flows (see **Figure 12-2**)
4. Absence of nucleus and cytoplasmic organelles
a. Limits RBC life span to about 120 days
b. Provides more cellular space for hemoglobin (Hb)
5. Transport of respiratory gases (O_2 and CO_2)

B. RBC count
1. Complete blood cell count (CBC) — battery of laboratory tests used to measure the amounts or levels of many blood constituents
2. Hematocrit (Hct)
a. Also called packed cell volume (PCV)
b. Hct expressed as the percentage of whole blood that is RBCs (see **Figure 12-3**)

C. Hemoglobin (Hb)
1. Quaternary protein made up of four polypeptide chains, each with an oxygen-attracting heme group at center (see **Figure 12-4**)
2. Iron (Fe), folate (a B vitamin), and vitamin B_{12} are among the critical nutrients needed to manufacture Hb
3. Transport of respiratory gases (O_2 and CO_2)
a. Combined with hemoglobin
(1) Oxyhemoglobin (Hb + O_2)
(2) Carbaminohemoglobin (Hb + CO_2)
b. CO_2 converted to bicarbonate by the RBCs
4. Important role in homeostasis of acid-base balance

D. Anemia — inability of blood to carry adequate oxygen to tissues due to (1) inadequate RBC numbers or (2) a deficiency of normal hemoglobin
1. Types
a. Hemorrhagic — decreased RBC numbers caused by blood loss (hemorrhage)
b. Aplastic — decreased RBC numbers caused by destruction of blood-forming elements in bone marrow
c. Pernicious — lack of intrinsic factor in stomach reduces availability of vitamin B_{12} needed for RBC production
d. Sickle cell — inherited defective gene or genes produce an abnormal type of hemoglobin (HbS) that is less able to carry oxygen and which often forms clumps of RBCs that block blood vessels (see **Figure 12-5**)
e. Polycythemia — abnormally high RBC count; opposite of anemia

E. Blood types
1. ABO system (see **Figure 12-6**)
a. Antigen — substance that can activate immune system
b. Antibody — substance made by body in response to stimulation by an antigen
c. ABO blood types
(1) Type A blood — type A self-antigens in RBCs; anti–B type antibodies in plasma
(2) Type B blood — type B self-antigens in RBCs; anti–A type antibodies in plasma

(3) Type AB blood — type A and type B self-antigens in RBCs; no anti-A or anti-B antibodies in plasma

(4) Type O blood — no type A or type B self-antigens in RBCs; both anti-A and anti-B antibodies in plasma

2. Rh system
   a. Rh-positive blood — Rh factor antigen present in RBCs
   b. Rh-negative blood — no Rh factor present in RBCs; no anti-Rh antibodies present naturally in plasma; anti-Rh antibodies, however, appear in the plasma of Rh-negative persons if Rh-positive RBCs have been introduced into their bodies; a RH-negative person can generate anti-Rh antibodies following exposure to the Rh antigen
   c. Erythroblastosis fetalis — may occur when Rh-negative mother carries a second Rh-positive fetus; caused by mother's Rh antibodies reacting with the fetus's Rh-positive cells (see **Figure 12-7**)
3. Universal donor and universal recipient blood
   a. Type O− — universal donor blood
   b. Type AB+ — universal recipient blood

White Blood Cells (Leukocytes)

A. WBC structure and function
   1. Categorized by presence of stained nuclei and granules in translucent cytoplasm
      a. Granular leukocytes (granulocytes) — possess granules that stain
      b. Agranular leukocytes (agranulocytes) — absence of stained granules
   2. WBCs are all involved in immunity

B. WBC count
   1. Complete WBC count — normal range is 5000 to 10,000/mm³ of blood
   2. Leukopenia — abnormally low WBC count (below 5000/mm³ of blood)
      a. Occurs infrequently
      b. May occur with malfunction of blood-forming tissues or diseases affecting immune system, such as AIDS
   3. Leukocytosis — abnormally high WBC count (over 10,000/mm³ of blood)
      a. Frequent finding in bacterial infections
      b. Classic sign in blood cancers (leukemia)
   4. Differential WBC count — component test in CBC; measures proportions of each type of WBC in blood sample (see **Figure 12-1** and **Figure 12-8**)

C. WBC types
   1. Granular leukocytes (granulocytes)
      a. Neutrophils
         (1) Most numerous type of phagocyte
         (2) Numbers increase during bacterial infections
      b. Eosinophils
         (1) Weak phagocyte
         (2) Active against parasites and parasitic worms
         (3) Involved in allergic reactions
      c. Basophils
         (1) Related to mast cells in tissue spaces
         (2) Both mast cells and basophils secrete histamine (promotes inflammation)
         (3) Basophils also secrete heparin (an anticoagulant)
   2. Agranular leukocytes (agranulocytes)
      a. Monocytes
         (1) Largest leukocyte
         (2) Aggressive phagocyte — capable of engulfing larger bacteria and cancer cells (see **Figure 12-9**)
         (3) Develop into much larger cells called *macrophages* after leaving blood to enter tissue spaces
      b. Lymphocytes
         (1) B lymphocytes (B cells) involved in immunity against disease by secretion of antibodies
         (2) Mature B lymphocytes called *plasma cells*
         (3) T lymphocytes (T cells) involved in direct attack on bacteria or cancer cells (not antibody production)

D. WBC disorders
   1. Leukemia — cancer
      a. Elevated WBC count
      b. Cells do not function properly

Platelets and Blood Clotting

A. Platelets — also called thrombocytes
   1. Tiny cell fragments filled with clot-triggering chemicals
   2. Play essential role in blood clotting

B. Clotting mechanism (see **Figure 12-10**)
   1. Vasoconstriction of blood vessels helps close gaps in blood vessel wall and reduces local blood flow
   2. Blood vessel damage releases clotting factors that react with plasma factors to form prothrombin activator
   3. At the same time, platelets adhere to the break and form a "platelet plug" and release additional clotting factors promoting formation of prothrombin activator
   4. Prothrombin activator and calcium convert prothrombin to thrombin
   5. Thrombin reacts with fibrinogen to form fibrin
   6. Fibrin threads form a tangle to trap RBCs (and other formed elements) to produce a blood clot

C. Abnormal blood clots
   1. Thrombus — stationary blood clot
   2. Embolus — circulating blood clot (drug called *tissue plasminogen activator [TPA or tPA]* used to dissolve clots that have already formed)

ACTIVE LEARNING

STUDY TIPS

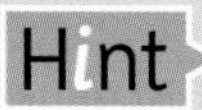

Use these tips to achieve success in meeting your learning goals.

To make the study of blood more efficient, we suggest these tips:

1. First, review terminology in the Language of Science and Medicine list.
2. Blood consists of a liquid portion, the plasma, and formed elements: the red blood cells, white blood cells, and platelets. The function of the blood is to carry substances from one part of the body to another.
3. Many transported materials are dissolved in the plasma, so the composition of the plasma varies based on what is going on in the body.
4. Because of its function, the blood plays an important role in a number of other systems such as the respiratory, digestive, urinary, and immune systems.
5. The process of blood clot formation is important, and it is necessary that you get the sequence of events correct. Develop a concept map that illustrates the sequence of events that lead to formation of a blood clot. For help with concept mapping go to *my-ap.us/conmapping*.
6. In studying the ABO blood typing system, the things you will need to remember are what antigens are on the red blood cell and what antibodies are in the plasma.
7. The antigens give the blood type its name: type A blood has A antigens and type B blood has B antigens. The antibodies are the opposite of the blood type. Type A blood has anti-B antibodies and type B blood has anti-A antibodies. Type O has no self-antigens and both antibodies, and type AB has both self-antigens and no antibodies.
8. In your study group, go over the flash cards with the functions of the various blood cells. Discuss the process of blood clot formation. Review the antigens and antibodies for the various blood types.
9. Review the Quick Check questions, go over the questions and the Outline Summary at the end of the chapter, and discuss possible test questions.

Review Questions

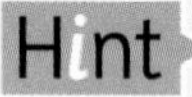

Write out the answers to these questions after reading the chapter and reviewing the Chapter Summary. If you simply think through the answer without writing it down, you won't retain much of your new learning.

1. Name the primary function of blood.
2. Name several substances found in blood plasma
3. Explain the function of albumins, globulins, and fibrinogen.
4. What is the difference between serum and plasma?
5. What two types of connective tissue form blood cells? Where are they found and what do each of them form?
6. Describe the structure of an RBC. What advantage does the unique shape of the RBC have?
7. What is anemia? Give two possible causes of anemia and identify two specific types.
8. What is the buffy coat?
9. Explain the function of neutrophils and monocytes.
10. Explain the function of lymphocytes.
11. What is leukemia? How is it classified?
12. Explain the function of eosinophils and basophils.
13. Explain fully the process of blood clot formation.
14. Differentiate between a thrombus and an embolus.
15. Explain how type A blood differs from type B blood.
16. Explain the cause of erythroblastosis fetalis.
17. Differentiate between Rh+ and Rh−.
18. Define leukopenia, phagocytosis, and thrombosis.

Critical Thinking

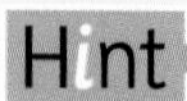

After finishing the Review Questions, write out the answers to these more in-depth questions to help you apply your new knowledge. Go back to sections of the chapter that relate to concepts that you find difficult.

19. Explain how heparin inhibits blood clot formation.
20. Differentiate between the process of blood clot formation and the process of blood agglutination.
21. Why is the first Rh-positive baby born to an Rh-negative mother usually unaffected?
22. Cyclists competing in past marathon events have sometimes been accused of using controversial and often illegal blood enhancing methods to gain a competitive edge. Explain this method and provide two variations of the practice. Do you believe that this practice might prove beneficial? Why or why not? Support your answer with examples or facts.
23. Arrange the following in chronological order to form a clot: platelet plug, fibrin, vasoconstriction, prothrombin activator, thrombin, prothrombin, fibrinogen, clot formation.

Chapter Test

Hint *After studying the chapter, test your mastery by responding to these items. Try to answer them without looking up the answers. Then, verify the answers using the key in Appendix C at the back of this book.*

1. The liquid part of the blood is called ________.
2. Three important plasma proteins are ________, ________, and ________.
3. Blood plasma without the clotting factors is called ________.
4. The three types of formed elements in the blood are ________, ________, and ________.
5. The two types of connective tissue that make blood cells are ________ and ________.
6. The red pigment in RBCs that carries oxygen is called ________.
7. The term ________ is used to describe a number of disease conditions caused by the inability of RBCs to carry a sufficient amount of oxygen.
8. If the body produces an excess of RBCs, the condition is called ________.
9. These WBCs are the most numerous of the phagocytes: ________.
10. These WBCs produce antibodies to fight microbes: ________.
11. Prothrombin activator and the mineral ________ in the blood convert prothrombin to thrombin in blood clot formation.
12. Thrombin converts the inactive plasma protein ________ into a fibrous gel called ________.
13. Vitamin ________ stimulates the liver to increase the synthesis of prothrombin.
14. A ________ is an unneeded blood clot that stays in the place where it was formed.
15. If part of a blood clot is dislodged and circulates through the bloodstream, it is called an ________.
16. ________ is a foreign substance that can cause the body to produce an antibody.
17. A person with type AB blood has ________ antigens on the blood cells and ________ antibodies in the plasma.
18. A person with type B blood has ________ antigens on the blood cells and ________ antibodies in the plasma.
19. Type ________ blood is considered the universal donor.
20. Type ________ blood is considered the universal recipient.
21. A condition called ________ can develop if an Rh-negative mother produces antibodies against an Rh-positive fetus.
22. The ________ test gives an estimate of the proportion of RBC's to whole blood.
23. ________ ________ ________ is a genetic disease that results in the formation of limited amounts of an abnormal hemoglobin known as hemoglobin S (HbS).
24. ________ occurs when blood pH decreases below 7.35 and 7.45 towards neutral (7.00).
25. ________ refers to an abnormally high WBC count.

Cardiovascular System

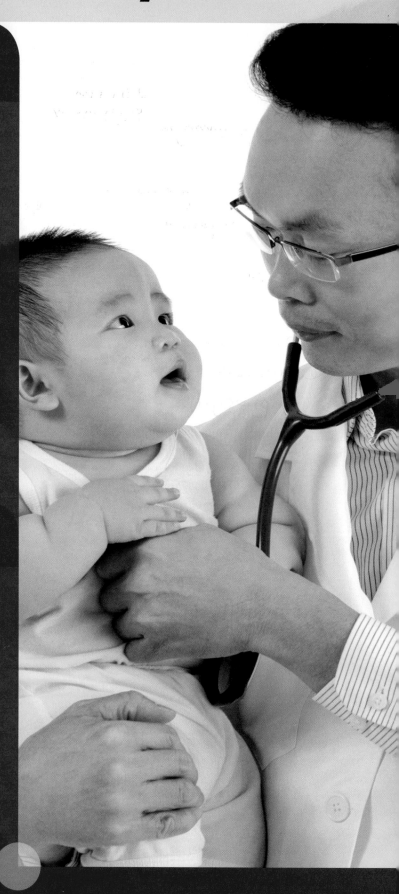

OUTLINE

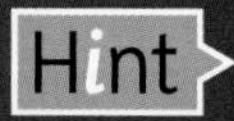

Scan this outline before you begin to read the chapter, as a preview of how the concepts are organized.

OBJECTIVES

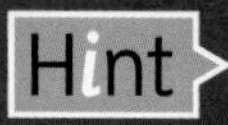

Before reading the chapter, review these goals for your learning.

After you have completed this chapter, you should be able to:

1. Discuss the location, size, and position of the heart in the thoracic cavity and identify the heart chambers, valves, and sounds.
2. Trace blood through the heart and compare the functions of the heart chambers on the right and left sides.
3. List the anatomical components of the heart conduction system and discuss the features of a normal electrocardiogram.
4. Explain the relationship between blood vessel structure and function.
5. Trace the path of blood through the systemic, pulmonary, hepatic portal, and fetal circulations.
6. Identify and discuss the primary factors involved in the generation and regulation of blood pressure and explain the relationships between these factors.

CHAPTER 13

The system that supplies our body's transportation needs is the **cardiovascular system.** We need such a system to make sure that each cell is surrounded by fluid that is constantly replenished with oxygen, water, and nutrients as they are used up by a cell. And we need to continually remove waste products from extracellular fluid as they are released from cells.

A circulating stream of blood can pick substances from various parts of the body and deliver them to others, thus allowing your body to move substances around in a way that helps you maintain a relative constancy of our internal environment. Clearly, circulation of the blood is critical to maintaining the homeostatic balance of your body.

We begin the study of the cardiovascular system with the heart—the pump that keeps blood moving through a closed circuit of blood vessels. Details related to heart structure are followed by a discussion of how the heart functions.

This chapter concludes with a study of the vessels through which blood flows as a result of the pumping action of the heart. As a group, these vessels are multipurpose structures. Some allow for rapid movement of blood from one body area to another. Others, such as the microscopic capillaries, permit the movement or exchange of many substances between the blood and fluid surrounding body cells.

Chapter 14 covers the lymphatic system and immunity topics that relate in many ways to the structure and functions of the cardiovascular system. Together the network of cardiovascular and lymphatic vessels make up what is often called the *circulatory system.*

To learn more about the cardiovascular system, go to AnimationDirect at *evolve.elsevier.com.*

LANGUAGE OF **SCIENCE** AND **MEDICINE**

Hint Before reading the chapter, say each of these terms out loud. This will help you to avoid stumbling over them as you read.

angina pectoris
(an-JYE-nah PEK-tor-is)
[*angina* **strangling,** *pect-* **breast,** *-oris* **relating to**]

aorta
(ay-OR-tah)
[*aort-* **lifted,** *-a* **thing**]

aortic semilunar valve
(ay-OR-tic sem-ee-LOO-nar valv)
[*aort-* **lifted,** *-ic* **relating to,** *semi-* **half,** *-luna* **moon,** *-ar* **relating to**]

apex
(AY-peks)
[*apex* **tip**]

arteriole
(ar-TEER-ee-ohl)
[*arteri-* **vessel,** *-ole* **little**]

artery
(AR-ter-ee)
[*arter-* **vessel,** *-y* **thing**]

atrioventricular (AV) bundle (bundle of His)
(ay-tree-oh-ven-TRIK-yoo-lar BUN-del)
[*atrio-* **entrance courtyard,** *-ventr-* **belly,** *-icul-* **little,** *-ar* **relating to** (*Wilhelm His, Jr.* **Swiss cardiologist**)]

atrioventricular (AV) node
(ay-tree-oh-ven-TRIK-yoo-lar nohd)
[*atrio-* **entrance courtyard,** *-ventr-* **belly,** *-icul-* **little,** *-ar* **relating to,** *nod-* **knot**]

atrioventricular (AV) valve
(ay-tree-oh-ven-TRIK-yoo-lar valv)
[*atrio-* **entrance courtyard,** *-ventr-* **belly,** *-icul-* **little,** *-ar* **relating to**]

Continued on p. 307

Heart

Location, Size, and Position

No one needs to be told where the heart is or what it does. Everyone knows that the heart is in the chest, that it beats night and day to keep the blood flowing, and that if it stops, life stops.

Most of us probably think of the heart as being located on the left side of the body. As you can see in **Figure 13-1**, the heart is located between the lungs in the lower portion of the mediastinum. Draw an imaginary line through the middle of the trachea in **Figure 13-1** and continue the line down through the thoracic cavity to divide it into right and left halves. Note that about two thirds of the mass of the heart is to the left of this line and one third is to the right.

The heart is often described as a triangular organ, shaped and sized roughly like a closed fist. In **Figure 13-1** you can see that the **apex,** or blunt point, of the lower edge of the heart lies on the diaphragm, pointing toward the left. Physicians and nurses often listen to the heart sounds by placing a stethoscope on the chest wall directly over the apex of the heart. Sounds of the so-called *apical beat* are easily heard in this area (that is, in the space between the fifth and sixth ribs on a line even with the midpoint of the left clavicle).

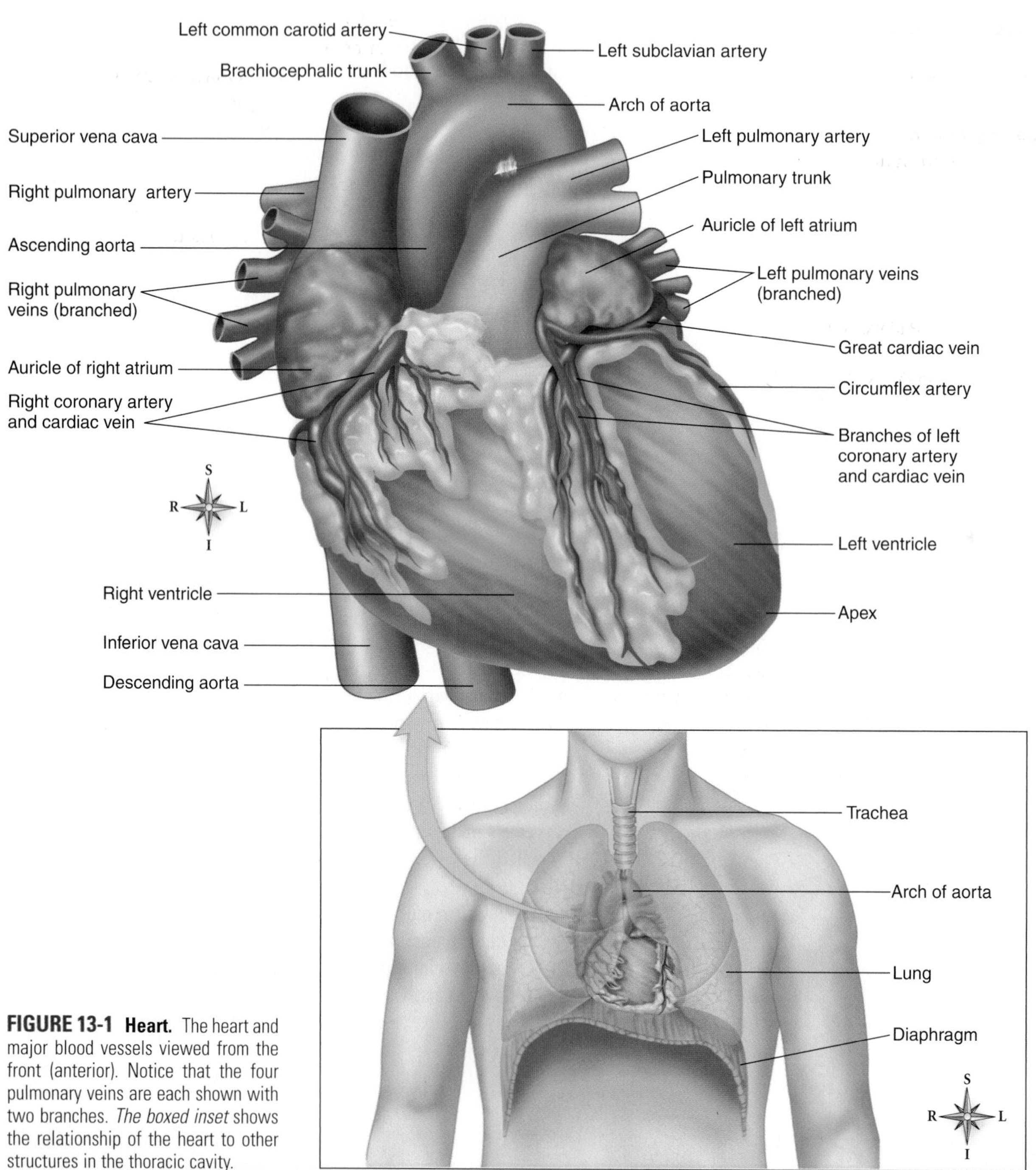

FIGURE 13-1 Heart. The heart and major blood vessels viewed from the front (anterior). Notice that the four pulmonary veins are each shown with two branches. *The boxed inset* shows the relationship of the heart to other structures in the thoracic cavity.

The heart is positioned in the thoracic cavity between the sternum in front and the bodies of the thoracic vertebrae behind. Because of this placement, it can be compressed or squeezed by application of pressure to the lower portion of the body of the sternum using the heel of the hand. Rhythmic compression of the heart in this way can maintain blood flow in cases of cardiac arrest, and if combined with effective artificial respiration, the resulting procedure, called **cardiopulmonary resuscitation (CPR),** can be lifesaving. The exact procedures for CPR change frequently as new research data become available, so it is important that individuals certified in CPR become recertified on a regular basis.

Functional Anatomy

Heart Chambers

If you cut open a heart, you can see many of its main structural features (**Figure 13-2**). This organ is hollow, not solid. A partition divides it into right and left sides. The heart contains four cavities, or hollow chambers. The two upper chambers are called **atria** (*singular,* **atrium**), and the two lower chambers are called **ventricles.**

The atria are smaller than the ventricles, and their walls are thinner and less muscular. Both atria have an earlike extension called an **auricle,** as you can see in **Figure 13-1**.

Atria are often called *receiving chambers* because blood enters the heart through veins that open into these upper cavities. Eventually, blood is pumped from the heart into arteries that exit from the ventricles. The ventricles are therefore sometimes referred to as the *discharging chambers* of the heart.

Each heart chamber is named according to its location. There are right and left atrial chambers above and right and left ventricular chambers below.

The wall of each heart chamber is composed of cardiac muscle tissue, usually referred to as the **myocardium**. The septum between the atrial chambers is called the *interatrial septum*. The *interventricular septum* separates the ventricles.

Each chamber of the heart is lined by a thin layer of very smooth tissue called the **endocardium** (see **Figure 13-2**). Inflammation of this lining is referred to as **endocarditis**. If inflamed, the endocardial lining can become rough and abrasive to red blood cells passing over its surface. Blood flowing over a rough surface is subject to clotting, and a **thrombus**, or clot, may form (see Chapter 12). Unfortunately, rough spots caused by endocarditis or injuries to blood vessel walls often

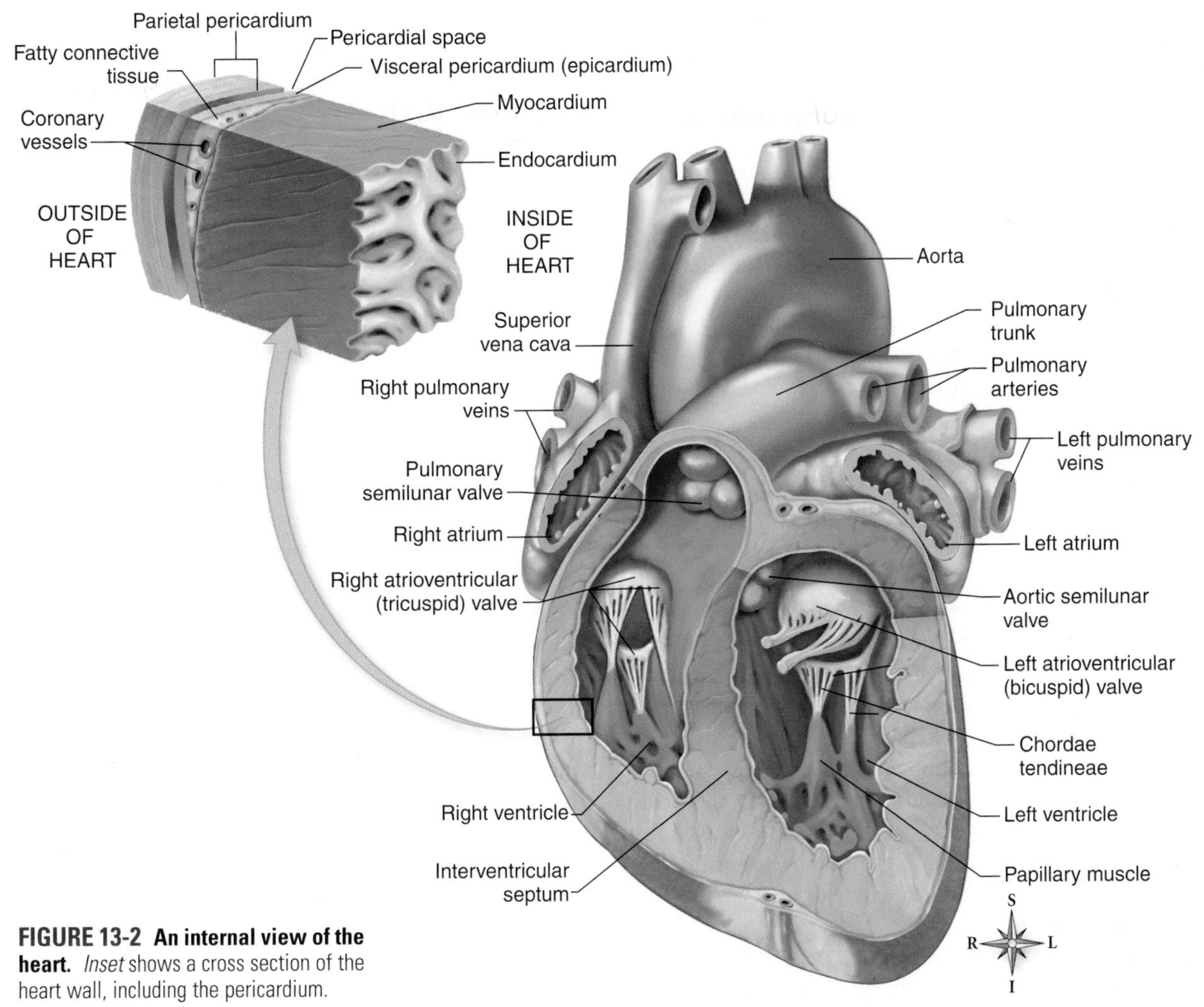

FIGURE 13-2 An internal view of the heart. *Inset* shows a cross section of the heart wall, including the pericardium.

cause the release of platelet factors. The result is often the formation of a fatal blood clot.

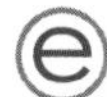
To learn more about the chambers of the heart, go to AnimationDirect at *evolve.elsevier.com*.

Pericardium

The heart has a covering and a lining. Its covering, called the **pericardium**, consists of two layers of fibrous tissue with a small space in between them. The inner layer of the pericardium is called the **visceral pericardium** or **epicardium**. It covers the heart the way an apple skin covers an apple. The outer layer of pericardium is called the **parietal pericardium.** It fits around the heart like a loose-fitting sack, allowing enough room for the heart to beat.

It is easy to remember the difference between the *endocardium*, which lines the heart chambers, and the *epicardium*, which covers the surface of the heart (see Figure 13-2), if you understand the meaning of the prefixes *endo-* and *epi-*. *Endo-* comes from the Greek word meaning "inside" or "within," and *epi-* comes from the Greek word meaning "upon" or "on."

The two pericardial layers slide over each other without friction when the heart beats because these are serous membranes with moist, not dry, surfaces. A thin film of pericardial fluid provides lubrication between the heart and its enveloping pericardial sac.

If the pericardium becomes inflamed, a condition called **pericarditis** results.

Heart Action

The heart serves as a muscular pumping device for distributing blood to all parts of the body. Contraction of the heart is called **systole**, and relaxation is called **diastole**. When the heart beats (that is, when it contracts), the atria contract first (atrial systole), forcing blood into the ventricles. Once filled, the two ventricles contract (ventricular systole) and force blood out of the heart (Figure 13-3).

For the heart to be efficient in its pumping action, more than just the rhythmic contraction of its muscular fibers is required. The direction of blood flow must be directed and controlled. This is accomplished by four sets of valves located at the entrance and near the exit of the ventricles.

Heart Valves

The two valves that separate the atrial chambers above from the ventricles below are called **atrioventricular (AV) valves.** The left AV valve is also known as the **bicuspid valve,** or **mitral valve,** and is located between the left atrium and ventricle. The right AV valve is also called the **tricuspid valve** and is located between the right atrium and ventricle.

The AV valves prevent backflow of blood into the atria when the ventricles contract. Locate the AV valves in Figure 13-2 and Figure 13-3. Note that a number of stringlike structures called **chordae tendineae** attach the AV valves to the wall of the ventricles.

The **semilunar (SL) valves** are located between each ventricular chamber and its large artery that carries blood away from the heart when contraction occurs (see Figure 13-3). The ventricles, like the atria, contract together; therefore, the two SL valves open and close at the same time.

The **pulmonary SL valve** is located at the beginning of the pulmonary artery and allows blood going to the lungs to flow out of the right ventricle during systole but prevents it from flowing back into the ventricle during diastole. The **aortic SL valve** is located at the beginning of the aorta and allows blood to flow out of the left ventricle up into the aorta but prevents backflow into this ventricle.

Heart Sounds

If a stethoscope is placed on the anterior chest wall, two distinct sounds can be heard. They are rhythmical and repetitive sounds that are often described as *lub dup*.

The first, or *lub*, sound is caused by the vibration and abrupt closure of the AV valves as the ventricles contract. Closure of the AV valves prevents blood from rushing back up into the atria during contraction of the ventricles. This first sound is of longer duration and lower pitch than the second. The pause between this first sound and the *dup*, or second, sound is shorter than that after the second sound and the *lub dup* of the next systole.

The second heart sound is caused by the closing of both SL valves when the ventricles undergo diastole (relax).

Physicians can use a stethoscope to detect many types of heart valve abnormalities as alterations of the normal lub dup pattern.

Later in the chapter, when you get to Figure 13-8 (p. 290), you will get the chance to compare the timing of the heart sounds to other events of the cardiac pumping cycle. This will further clarify the clinical importance of heart sounds as indicators of heart function.

Blood Flow Through the Heart

When the heart "beats," first the atria contract simultaneously. This is *atrial systole*. After the ventricles fill with blood, they, too, contract together during *ventricular systole*. Although the atria contract as a unit, followed by the ventricles below, the right and left sides of the heart act as separate pumps. As we study the blood flow through the heart, the separate functions of the two pumps will become clearer.

Note in Figure 13-3 that blood enters the right atrium through two large veins called the **superior vena cava** and **inferior vena cava.** The right heart pump receives oxygen-poor blood from the veins. After entering the right atrium, it is pumped through the right AV, or tricuspid valve, and enters the right ventricle. When the ventricles contract, blood in the right ventricle is pumped through the pulmonary SL valve into the **pulmonary artery** and eventually to the lungs, where oxygen is added and carbon dioxide is lost.

As you can see in Figure 13-3, blood rich in oxygen returns to the left atrium of the heart through four **pulmonary veins.** It then passes through the left AV, or bicuspid valve, into the left ventricle. When the left ventricle contracts, blood is

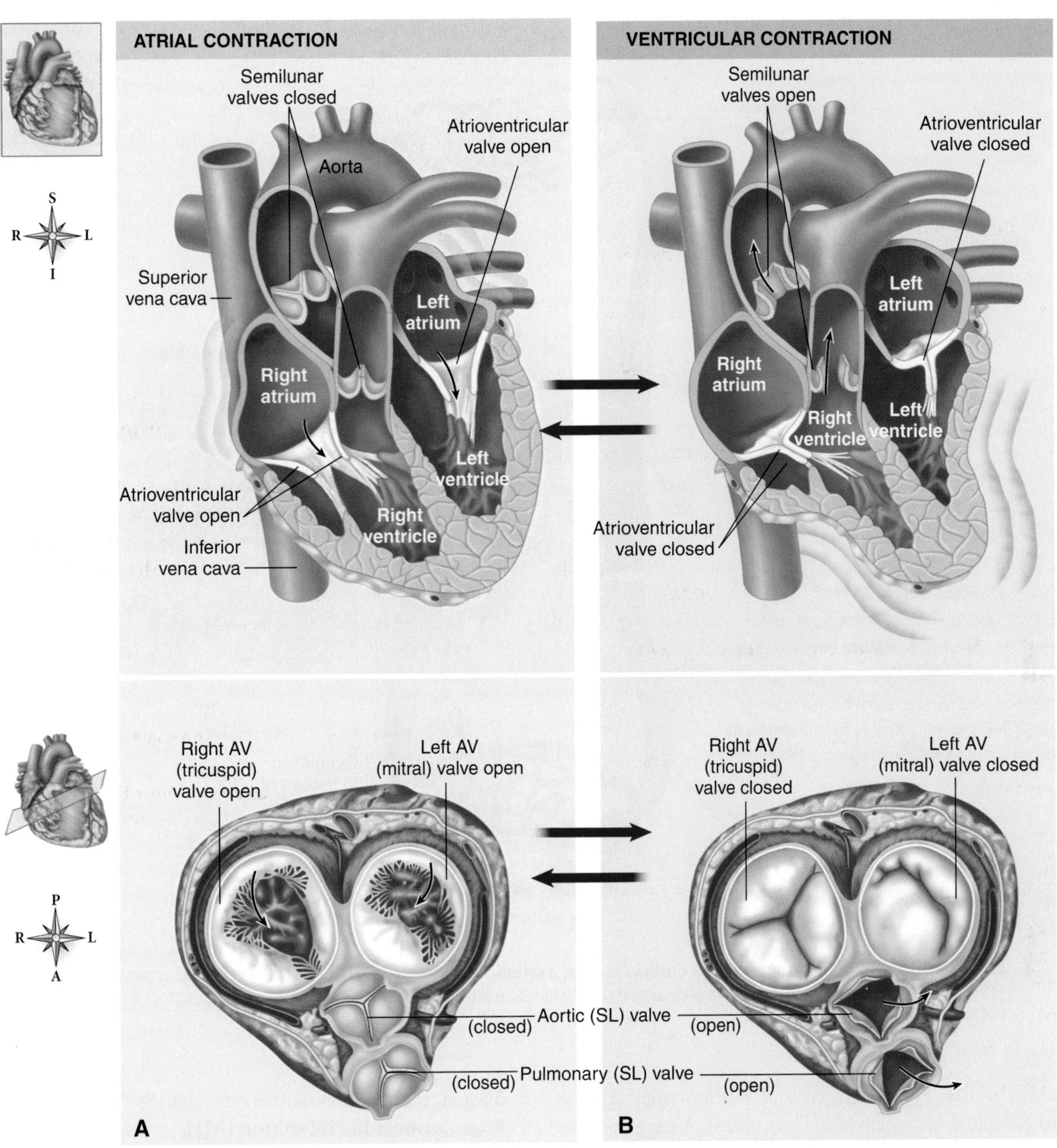

FIGURE 13-3 Heart action. A, During atrial systole (contraction), cardiac muscle in the atrial wall contracts, forcing blood through the atrioventricular (AV) valves and into the ventricles. Bottom illustration shows superior view of all four valves, with semilunar (SL) valves closed and AV valves open. **B,** During ventricular systole that follows, the AV valves close, and blood is forced out of the ventricles through the semilunar valves and into the arteries. Bottom illustration shows superior view of SL valves open and AV valves closed.

forced through the aortic SL valve into the **aorta** and is distributed to the body as a whole.

As you can tell from Figure 13-4, the two sides of the heart actually pump blood through two separate "circulations" and function as two separate pumps. The *pulmonary circulation* involves movement of blood from the right ventricle to the lungs and is shaded with blue in Figure 13-4. The *systemic circulation* involves movement of blood from the left ventricle throughout the body as a whole and is shaded with yellow in Figure 13-4. The vessels of the pulmonary and systemic circulations are discussed later in this chapter.

Blood Supply to the Heart Muscle

To sustain life, the heart must pump blood throughout the body on a regular and ongoing basis. As a result, the heart muscle, or myocardium, requires a constant supply of blood containing nutrients and oxygen to function effectively. The

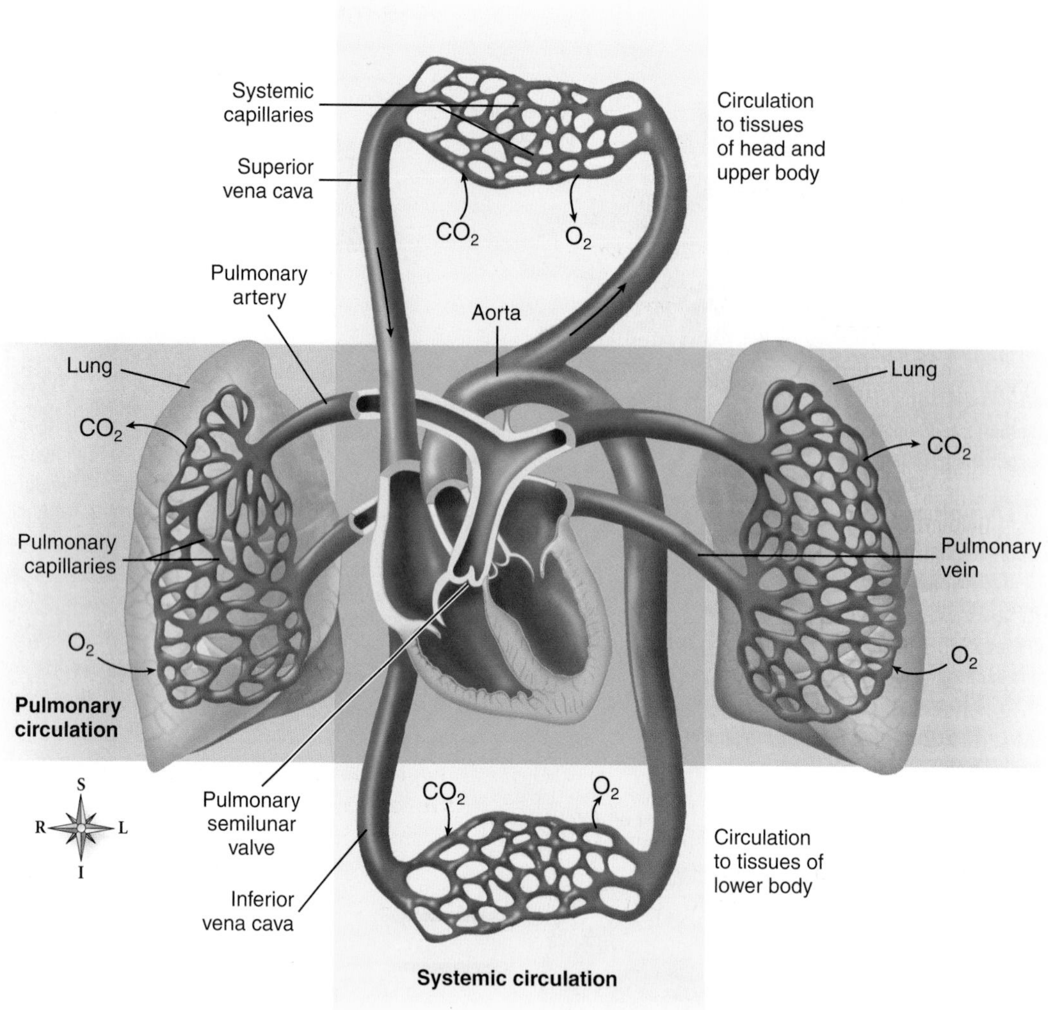

FIGURE 13-4 Blood flow through the cardiovascular system. In the pulmonary circulatory route, blood is pumped from the right side of the heart to the gas-exchange tissues of the lungs. In the systemic circulation, blood is pumped from the left side of the heart to all other tissues of the body.

process of the delivery of oxygen and nutrient-rich arterial blood to cardiac muscle tissue and the return of oxygen-poor blood from this active tissue to the venous system is called **coronary circulation.**

Blood flows into the heart muscle by way of two small vessels—the right and left **coronary arteries.** The coronary arteries are the aorta's first branches (**Figure 13-5,** *A*).

Figure 13-5, *B*, shows that the openings into these small vessels lie behind the flaps of the aortic SL valve. During ventricular systole, the myocardium is contracting and putting pressure on the coronary arteries, so little blood can enter them. However, during ventricular diastole, blood that backs up behind the aortic SL valve can flow easily into the coronary arteries.

In both coronary thrombosis and coronary **embolism,** a blood clot occludes or plugs up some part of a coronary artery. Blood cannot pass through the occluded vessel and so cannot reach the heart muscle cells it normally supplies. Deprived of oxygen, these cells soon become damaged or die. In medical terms, **myocardial infarction (MI),** or tissue death, occurs.

An MI, also referred to as a "heart attack," is a common cause of death during middle and late adulthood. Recovery from a myocardial infarction is possible if the amount of heart tissue damaged was small enough so that the remaining undamaged heart muscle can pump blood effectively enough to supply the needs of the rest of the heart and the body.

The term **angina pectoris** is used to describe the severe chest pain that occurs when the myocardium is deprived of adequate oxygen. It is often a warning that the coronary arteries are no longer able to supply enough blood and oxygen to the heart muscle.

Coronary bypass surgery is a common treatment for those who suffer from severely restricted coronary artery blood flow. In this procedure, veins or arteries are "harvested" or removed from other areas of the body and used to bypass partial blockages in coronary arteries (**Figure 13-6**). Another treatment used

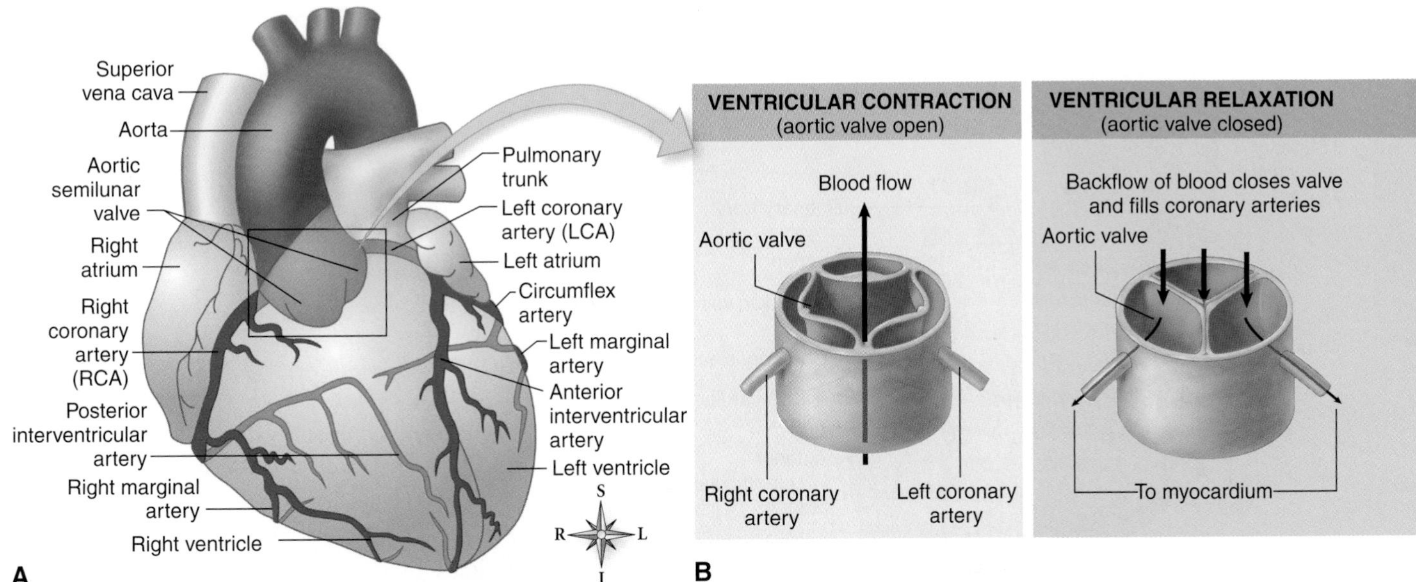

FIGURE 13-5 Coronary arteries. A, Diagram showing the major coronary arteries (anterior view). Clinicians often refer to the interventricular arteries as *descending* arteries. Thus a cardiologist would refer to the *left anterior descending (LAD) artery* and an anatomist would refer to the same vessel as the *anterior interventricular branch* or *artery.* **B,** The unusual placement of the coronary artery opening behind the leaflets of the aortic valve allows the coronary arteries to fill during ventricular relaxation.

to improve coronary blood flow is *angioplasty*, a procedure in which a device is inserted into a blood vessel to force open a channel for blood flow through a blocked artery.

After blood has passed through the capillary beds in the myocardium, it flows into **cardiac veins,** which empty into the **coronary sinus** and finally into the right atrium. Figure 13-7 shows how venous blood from the coronary circulation enters the right atrium through this "secret passage" rather than through the usual pathway through the superior or inferior vena cava.

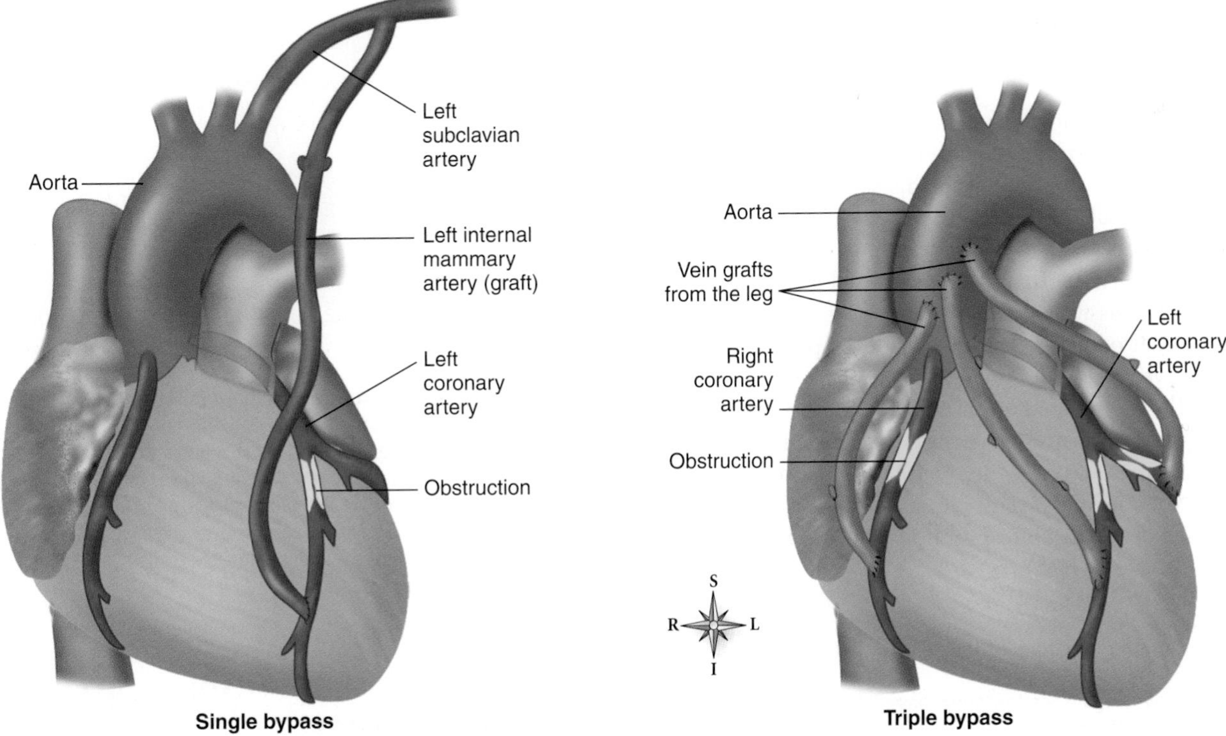

FIGURE 13-6 Coronary bypass. In coronary bypass surgery, blood vessels are "harvested" from other parts of the body and used to construct detours around blocked coronary arteries. Artificial vessels can also be used.

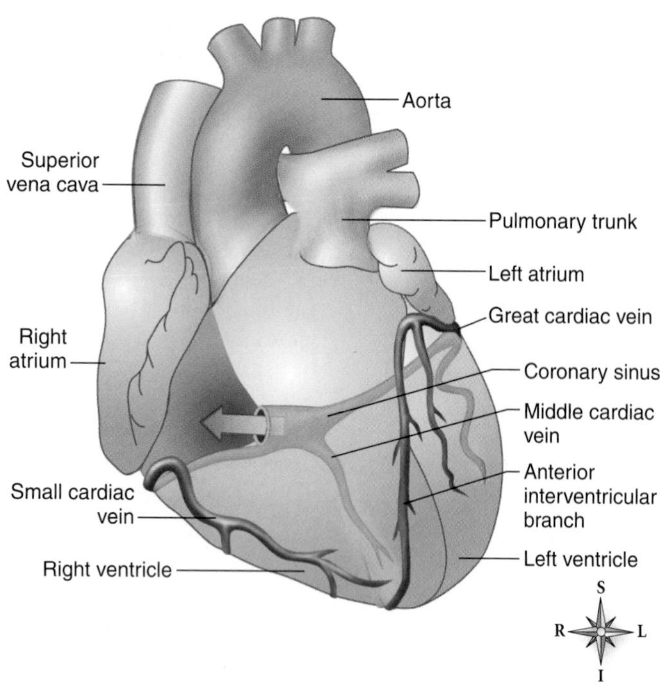

FIGURE 13-7 Coronary veins. Diagram showing the major veins of the coronary circulation (anterior view). Vessels near the anterior surface are more darkly colored than vessels of the posterior surface seen through the heart.

Cardiac Cycle

The beating of the heart is a regular and rhythmic process. Each complete heartbeat is called a **cardiac cycle** and includes the contraction (systole) and relaxation (diastole) of atria and ventricles. Each cycle takes about 0.8 second to complete if the heart is beating at an average rate of about 72 beats per minute.

Figure 13-8 summarizes some of the important events of the cardiac pumping cycle. Although it looks overly complicated at first, a few minutes exploring this set of graphs can help make sense of all the processes you are learning about the rhythm of the heart's pumping cycle.

For example, note that most of the atrial blood moves into the ventricles passively before the atria have a chance to contract. Another oddity is that there is a brief period at the beginning of ventricular contraction where there is no change in volume. This occurs because it takes a moment for the ventricular pressure to overcome the force needed to open the semilunar valves. You also can see there is another period of constant volume as the ventricles begin to relax—before the mitral valves open and blood gushes rapidly in from the atria.

QUICK CHECK

1. What are the functions of the atria and ventricles of the heart?
2. What coverings does the heart have? What is the heart's lining called?
3. What are systole and diastole of the heart?
4. What are the two major "circulations" of the body?
5. What are the auricles of the heart?

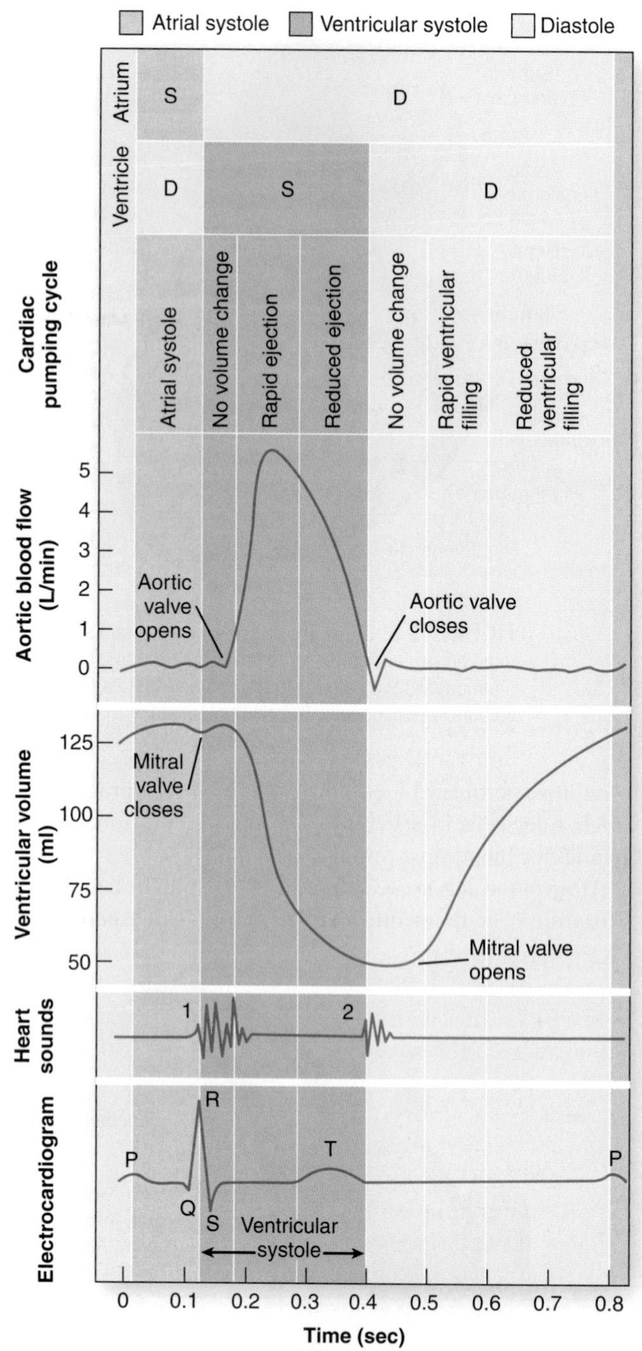

FIGURE 13-8 Composite chart of heart function. This chart is a composite of several diagrams of heart function during rest (72 beats/min). Along the top, *S* represents systole and *D* represents diastole of each heart chamber. Below that, details of the cardiac pumping cycle, aortic blood flow, ventricular volume, valve actions, heart sounds, and ECG are all adjusted to the same time scale. Although it appears overwhelming at first glance, this "stack of graphs" will be a valuable reference tool as you proceed through the rest of this chapter and try to "put it all together."

Electrical Activity of the Heart

Conduction System

Cardiac muscle fibers can contract rhythmically on their own. However, they must be coordinated by electrical signals (impulses) if the heart is to pump effectively.

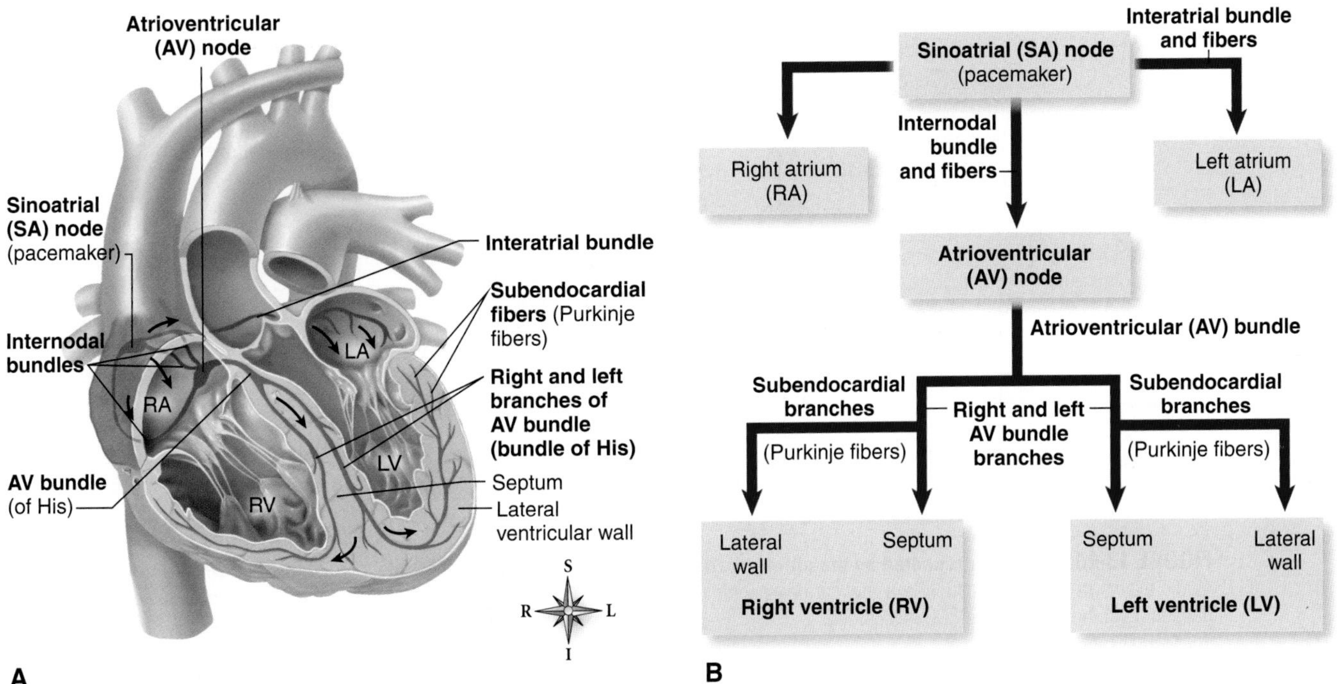

FIGURE 13-9 Conduction system of the heart. A, Specialized cardiac muscle cells in the wall of the heart rapidly conduct an electrical impulse throughout the myocardium. **B,** The signal is initiated by the SA node (pacemaker) and spreads to the rest of the atrial myocardium and to the atrioventricular (AV) node. The AV node then initiates a signal that is conducted through the ventricular myocardium by way of the AV bundle (of His) and subendocardial fibers (Purkinje fibers).

Although the rate of the cardiac muscle's rhythm is controlled by autonomic nerve signals, the heart has its own built-in conduction system for coordinating contractions during the cardiac cycle.

The most important thing to realize about this conduction system is that all of the cardiac muscle fibers in each region of the heart are electrically linked together. The *intercalated disks* that were first introduced in Chapter 4 (see **Figure 4-17**, p. 78) are actually connections that electrically join muscle fibers into a single unit that can conduct an impulse through the entire wall of a heart chamber without stopping. Thus both atrial walls will contract at about the same time because all of their fibers are electrically linked. Likewise, both ventricular walls will contract at about the same time.

Four structures embedded in the wall of the heart specialize in generating strong impulses and conduct them rapidly to certain regions of the heart wall. Thus they make sure that the atria contract and then the ventricles contract in an efficient manner. The main structures that make up this conduction system of the heart are as follows:

1. **Sinoatrial node,** which is sometimes called the SA node or the **pacemaker**
2. **Atrioventricular node,** or **AV node**
3. **AV bundle,** or **bundle of His**
4. **Subendocardial branches,** also called **Purkinje fibers**

Impulse conduction normally starts in the heart's pacemaker, namely, the SA node. From there, it spreads, as you can see in **Figure 13-9**, in all directions through the atria. This causes the atrial fibers to contract.

When impulses reach the AV node, it is triggered to relay its own impulse by way of the AV bundle and subendocardial branches to the ventricular myocardium, causing the ventricles to contract. Normally, therefore, a ventricular beat follows each atrial beat.

Various conditions such as endocarditis or myocardial infarction, however, can damage the heart's conduction system and thereby disturb its rhythmic beating. One such disturbance is the condition commonly called *heart block.* Impulses are blocked from getting through to the ventricles, resulting in the ventricles beating at a much slower rate than normal.

A physician may treat heart block by implanting in the heart an artificial pacemaker, an electrical device that causes ventricular contractions at a rate fast enough to maintain an adequate circulation of blood.

The heart's conduction system generates tiny electrical currents that spread through surrounding tissues and eventually to the surface of the body. This fact is of great clinical significance because these electrical signals can be picked up from the body surface and transformed into visible tracings by an instrument called an **electrocardiograph**.

Electrocardiogram

The **electrocardiogram** is a graphic record of the heart's electrical activity. This chart is also called an **ECG**—or **EKG** when spoken aloud. Skilled interpretation of these ECG records may sometimes make the difference between life and death. A normal ECG tracing is shown in **Figure 13-10**.

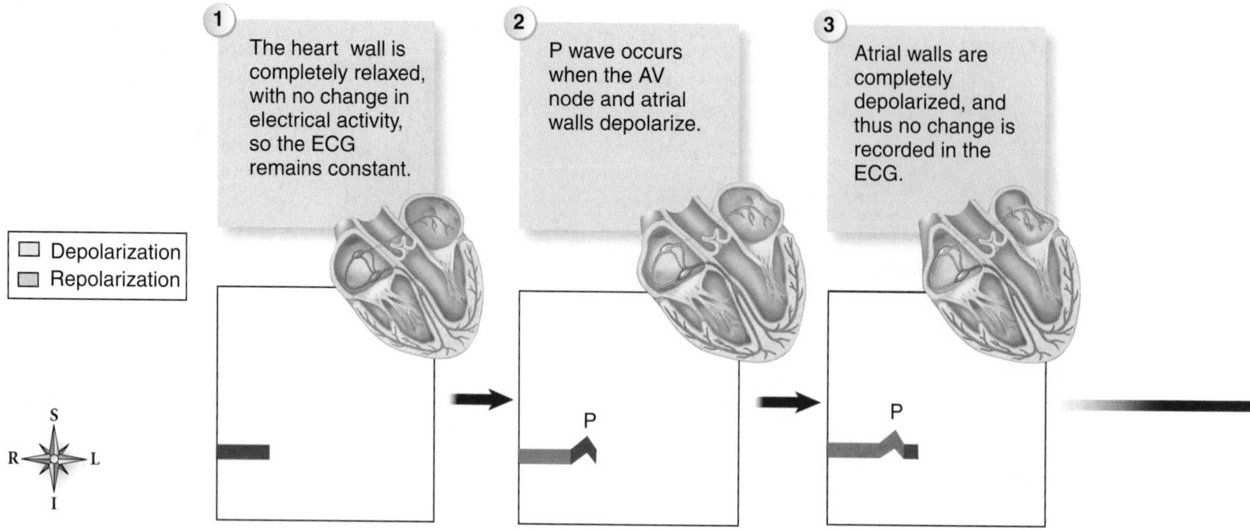

FIGURE 13-10 Events represented by the electrocardiogram (ECG). It is nearly impossible to illustrate the invisible, dynamic events of heart conduction in a few cartoon panels or "snapshots," but the sketches here give you an idea of what is happening in the heart as the ECG is recorded.

A normal ECG tracing has three very characteristic deflections, or waves, called the **P wave,** the **QRS complex,** and the **T wave.** These deflections represent the electrical activity that regulates the contraction or relaxation of the atria or ventricles. The term **depolarization** describes the electrical activity that triggers contraction of the heart muscle. **Repolarization** begins just before the relaxation phase of cardiac muscle activity.

In the normal ECG shown in **Figure 13-10**, the small P wave occurs with depolarization of the atria. The QRS complex occurs as a result of depolarization of the ventricles, and the T wave results from electrical activity generated by repolarization of the ventricles. You may wonder why no visible record of atrial repolarization is noted in a normal ECG. The reason is simply that the deflection is very small and is hidden by the large QRS complex that occurs at the same time.

Now is a good time to go back and review **Figure 13-8** and explore the relationship between the ECG and other events of the cardiac cycle. By looking at changes in blood flow and volume, for example, you will discover that ECG deflections occur *before* myocardial contractions—not *during* these contractions. This occurs because depolarizations trigger contractions and a trigger always comes before the event that is triggered.

Damage to cardiac muscle tissue that is caused by a myocardial infarction or disease affecting the heart's conduction system results in distinctive changes in the ECG. Therefore, ECG tracings are extremely valuable in the diagnosis and treatment of heart disease.

QUICK CHECK

1. What structure is the natural "pacemaker" of the heart?
2. What information is in an electrocardiogram?
3. What is heart block?

Cardiac Output

Definition of Cardiac Output

Cardiac output (CO) is the volume of blood pumped by one ventricle per minute. It averages about 5 L in a normal, resting adult. **Figure 13-11** shows the distribution of the heart's output to some of the major organs of the body.

The cardiac output is determined by the **heart rate (HR)** and **stroke volume (SV).** *Heart rate* refers to the number of heart beats (cardiac cycles) per minute. The term *stroke volume* refers to the volume of blood ejected from the ventricles during each beat. The heart rate is determined mostly by the natural rhythm of the heart created by the heart's own conduction system (see **Figure 13-9** on p. 291).

The relationship of CO to HR and SV is illustrated by this simple equation:

$$\text{HR}\left(\frac{\text{beats}}{\text{minute}}\right) \times \text{SV}\left(\frac{\text{volume}}{\text{beat}}\right) = \text{CO}\left(\frac{\text{volume}}{\text{minute}}\right)$$

Abnormally decreased CO can result in fatigue or, with a significant drop in CO, even death.

Heart Rate

As you learned in Chapter 9, however, the *autonomic nervous system (ANS)* may alter the heart's rhythm to increase or decrease HR. **Figure 9-19** on p. 200 shows that the *sympathetic* division of the ANS increases HR. Neurons of the sympathetic *cardiac nerve* release the neurotransmitter *norepinephrine (NE),* which causes the SA node to increase its usual pace and thereby increase HR.

The same figure also shows that the parasympathetic division of the ANS slows down HR. This happens when neurons of the *vagus nerve (cranial nerve X)* release *acetylcholine (ACh)* to decrease the pace of the SA node.

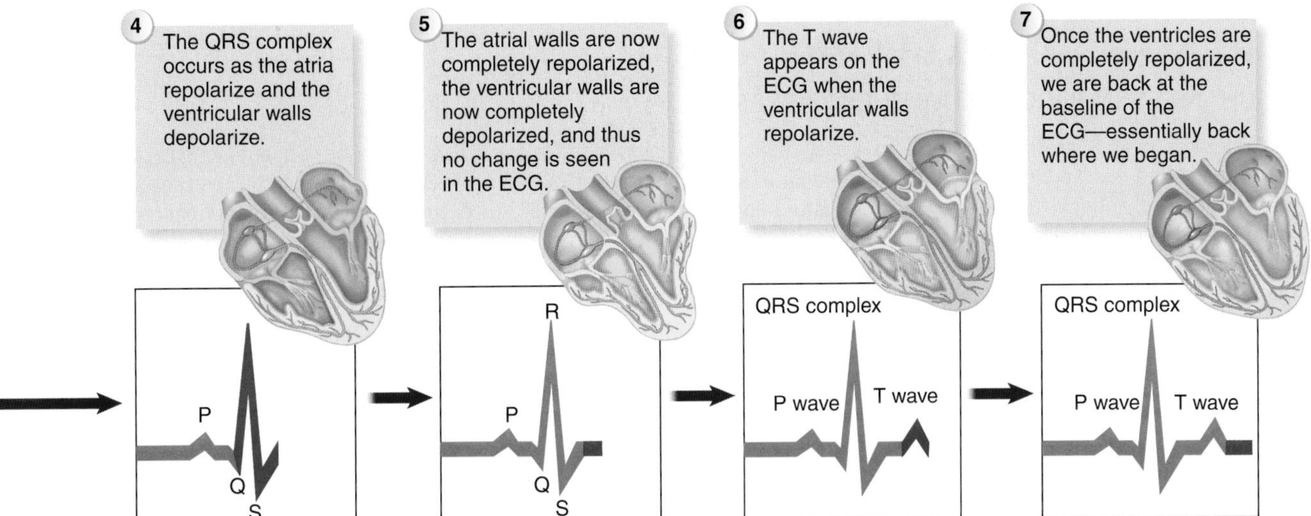

The balance between the antagonistic influence of sympathetic and parasympathetic signals to the heart can be shifted by a variety of factors. When blood CO_2 levels rise during exercise, for example, there is a reflexive rise in HR. This is an attempt by the body to restore homeostasis of blood gases.

A sudden drop in blood pressure triggers a reflexive increase in HR as the body attempts to restore normal blood flow out of the heart. Stress—the recognition of a threat to homeostatic balance—also can cause a sudden increase in HR so that skeletal muscles will be ready to resist or avoid the stressor.

Various dysrhythmias may affect HR by disrupting the normal rhythm of the heart.

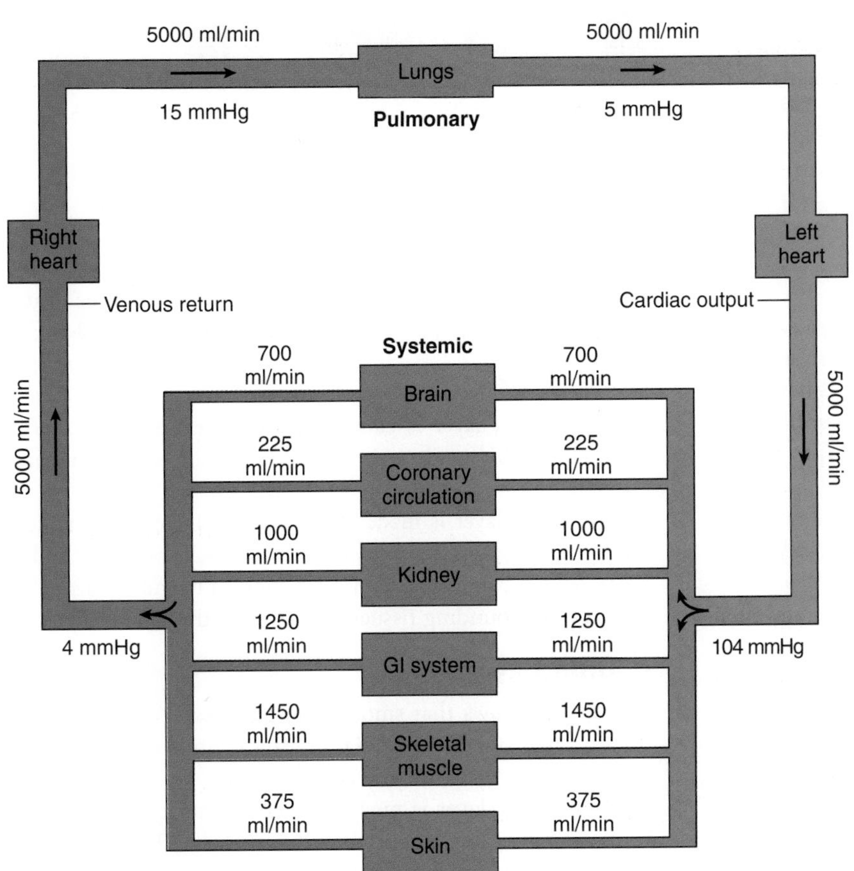

FIGURE 13-11 Cardiac output. This diagram shows that a typical resting cardiac output (CO) of 5000 mL/min (or 5 L/min) is distributed among the various systems and organs of the body. *GI,* Gastrointestinal.

Stroke Volume

The volume of blood ejected by the ventricles is determined by the volume of blood returned to the heart by the veins, or *venous return* (see **Figure 13-11**). Generally, the higher the venous return, the higher the SV.

Venous return can change when the volume of the blood changes, as in dehydration or blood loss due to hemorrhage. Various hormones, many of which are discussed in later chapters, can influence total blood volume and thus also affect SV.

The strength of myocardial contraction also helps determine SV. Ion imbalances can affect muscle fiber function and thus impair contraction—thus also decreasing SV. Valve disorders, coronary artery blockage, or myocardial infarction can all decrease stroke volume and thus may decrease cardiac output.

QUICK CHECK

1. What are the two main factors that affect cardiac output?
2. If a person's heart rate increases, what may happen to the cardiac output?
3. If a person bleeds excessively, what effect would that have on cardiac output?

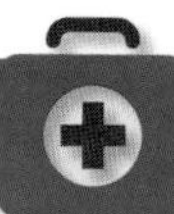

HEALTH AND WELL-BEING

CHANGES IN BLOOD FLOW DURING EXERCISE

Not only does the overall rate of blood flow increase during exercise, but also the relative blood flow through the different organs of the body changes. During exercise, blood is routed away from the kidneys and digestive organs and toward the skeletal muscles, cardiac muscle, and skin. Rerouting of blood is accomplished by contracting muscles in the arterioles of some tissues (thus reducing blood flow) while relaxing arterioles in other tissues (thus increasing blood flow).

How can homeostasis be better maintained by these changes? One reason is that glucose and oxygen levels drop rapidly in muscles as they use up these substances to produce energy for exercising. Increased blood flow restores normal levels of glucose and oxygen more rapidly. Blood that has been warmed up in active muscles flows to the skin for cooling. This helps keep the body temperature from getting too high. Can you think of other ways this change in blood flow helps maintain homeostasis? Typical changes in organ blood flow with exercise are shown in the illustration. The *red bar* in each pair shows the resting blood flow; the *blue bar* shows the flow during exercise.

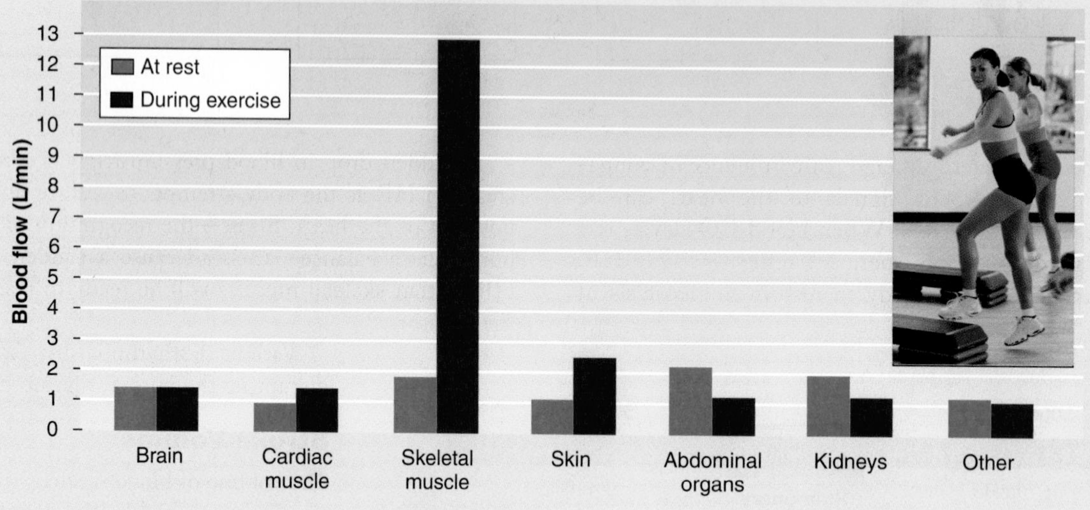

Blood Vessels

Types

Arterial blood is pumped from the heart through a series of large distribution vessels—the **arteries.** The largest artery in the body is the aorta. Arteries subdivide and blood flows into vessels that become progressively smaller arteries until finally it enters tiny **arterioles** that control blood flow into microscopic exchange vessels called **capillaries.**

In the so-called *capillary beds*, the exchange of nutrients and respiratory gases occurs between the blood and tissue fluid around the cells.

Blood exits or is drained from the capillary beds and then enters the small **venules**, which join with other venules and increase in size, becoming **veins.** The largest veins, often called *sinuses,* are the superior vena cava and the inferior vena cava.

As noted previously (see **Figure 13-4**), arteries carry blood away from the heart and toward capillaries. Veins carry blood toward the heart and away from capillaries, and capillaries carry blood from the tiny arterioles into tiny venules. The aorta carries blood out of the left ventricle of the heart, and the venae cavae return blood to the right atrium after the blood has circulated through the body.

Structure

Arteries, veins, and capillaries differ in structure. Three coats, or layers, are found in both arteries and veins (**Figure 13-12**).

Outer Layer

The outermost layer is called the **tunica externa** (or *tunica adventitia*). The word *tunica* means "coat" and *externa* means "outside."

This outer layer is made of connective tissue fibers, which reinforce the wall of the vessel so that it will not burst under pressure. The connective fibers also connect to the extracellular matrix of surrounding tissues to help hold the vessel in place.

Middle Layer

Figure 13-12 shows that smooth muscle tissue is found in the middle layer, or **tunica media,** of arteries and veins. The term *tunica media* means "middle coat."

This muscle layer is much thicker in arteries than it is in veins. Why is this important? Because the thicker muscle layer in the artery wall is able to resist great pressures generated by ventricular systole. In arteries, the tunica media plays a critical role in maintaining blood pressure and controlling blood distribution. This is a smooth muscle, so it is controlled

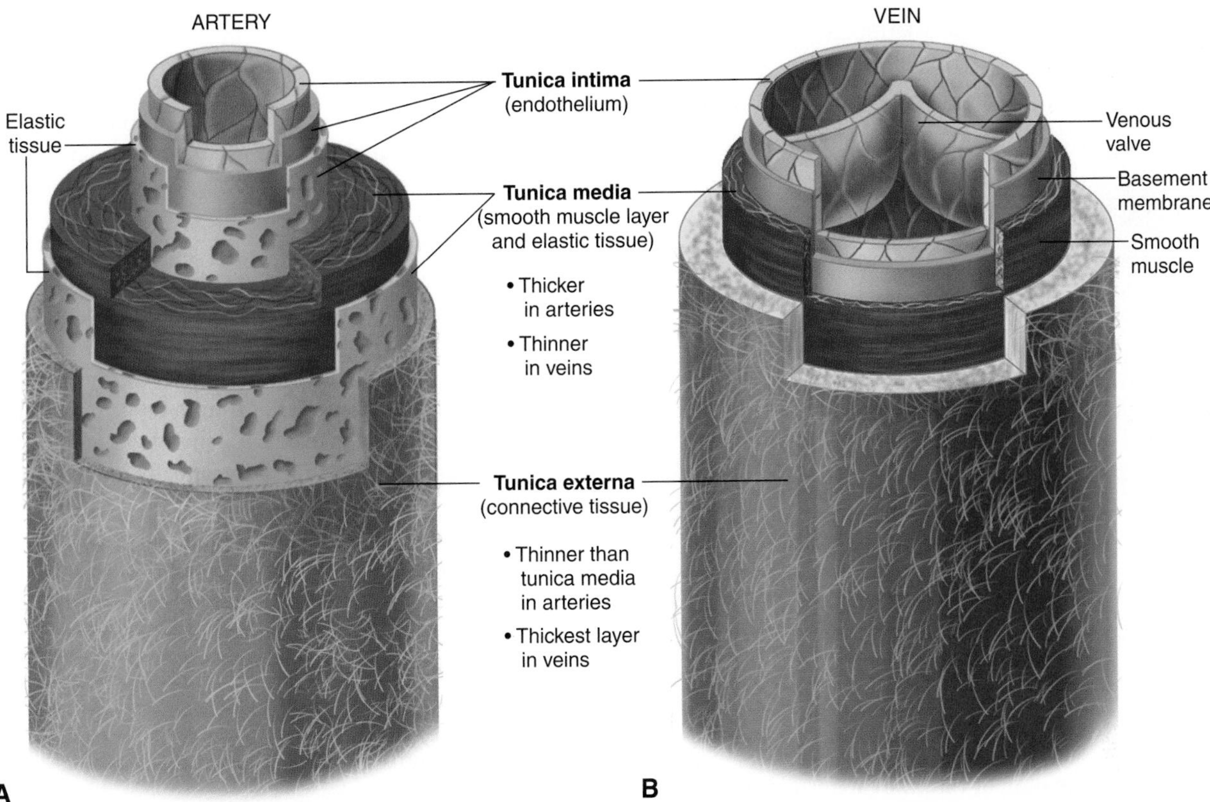

FIGURE 13-12 Artery and vein. Schematic drawings of an artery **(A)** and a vein **(B)** show comparative thicknesses of the three layers: the outer layer or *tunica externa*, the muscle layer or *tunica media*, and the *tunica intima* made of endothelium. Note that the muscle layer is much thinner in veins than in arteries and that veins have valves.

by the autonomic nervous system. The tunica media also sometimes includes a thin layer of elastic fibrous tissue.

Smooth muscle cells along the wall of arterioles are sometimes called **precapillary sphincters.** They encircle the arteriole walls and by contracting or relaxing, they regulate how much blood will flow into a capillary bed, as you can see in Figure 13-13.

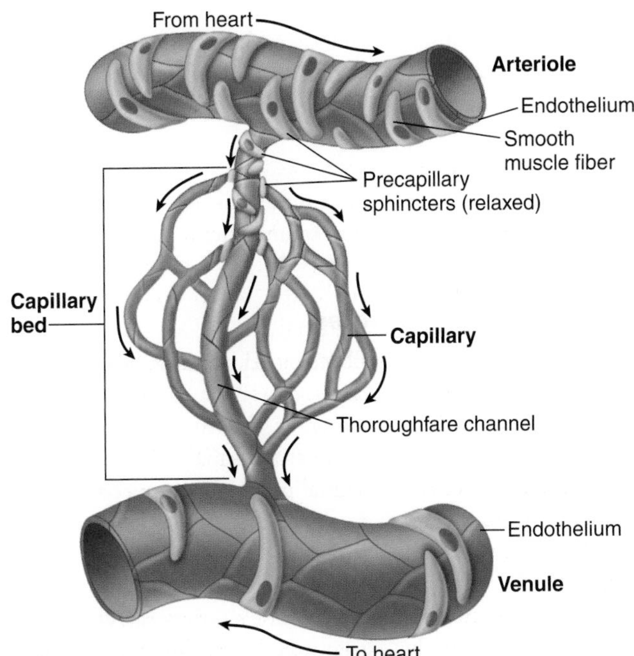

FIGURE 13-13 Capillaries. Capillaries are microscopic, thin-walled vessels that form networks joining arterioles to venules. Smooth muscle fibers (precapillary sphincters) around the arterioles can regulate how much blood flows into a capillary bed. Occasionally, these fibers wrap around the entrances to capillaries to more precisely control local blood flow.

Inner Layer

An inner layer of endothelial cells called the **tunica intima** ("innermost coat") lines arteries and veins.

The tunica intima is actually a single layer of squamous epithelial cells called **endothelium** that lines the inner surface of the entire cardiovascular system. The tunica intima also sometimes includes a thin layer of elastic fibrous tissue.

As you can see in Figure 13-12, veins have a unique structural feature not present in arteries. A vein's tunica intima is equipped with pockets that act as one-way valves. These valves prevent the backflow of blood—thus keeping blood flowing in one direction, back toward the heart.

These valves also allow veins to act as supplemental pumps that help maintain *venous return* of blood to the heart. Figure 13-14 shows how occasional activity of skeletal muscles surrounding the veins of the body create pressure on blood that drives these venous pumps. This explains why stretching, walking, and other activities helps improve blood circulation

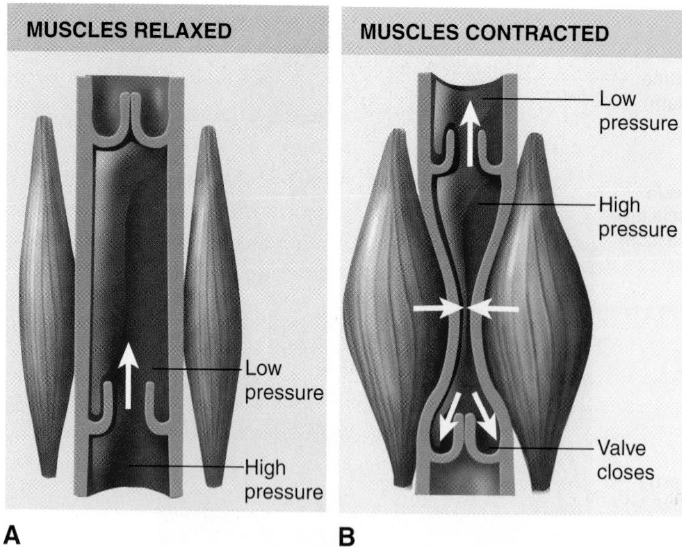

FIGURE 13-14 Venous valve function. Normal skeletal muscle contractions push on the walls of veins, which have one-way valves that allow the veins to act as pumps that push blood back toward the heart. This is similar to the action of the myocardium and heart valves acting together as a pump—except that this venous pump mechanism is not continuous and rhythmic.

and prevent the formation of thrombi (abnormal clots) in the veins.

When a surgeon cuts into the body, only arteries, arterioles, veins, and venules can be seen. Capillaries cannot be seen because they are microscopic. The most important structural feature of capillaries is their extreme thinness—only one layer of flat, endothelial cells composes the capillary membrane. Instead of three layers or coats, the capillary wall is composed of only one—the tunica intima. Substances such as glucose, oxygen, and wastes can quickly pass through it on their way to or from cells.

Functions

Together, arteries, capillaries, and veins all conduct blood around the body's circulatory routes. However, each has its own unique roles to play.

Arteries and Arterioles

Arteries and arterioles distribute blood from the heart to capillaries in all parts of the body.

In addition, by constricting or dilating, arterioles help maintain arterial blood pressure at a normal level. As we discuss later in this chapter, arterial pressure is a major force in keeping blood flowing.

Capillary Exchange

Capillaries function as exchange vessels—thus carrying out a central function of the cardiovascular system. For example, glucose and oxygen move out of the blood in capillaries into interstitial fluid and then on into cells. Carbon dioxide and other substances move in the opposite direction (that is, into the capillary blood from the cells). Fluid is also exchanged between capillary blood and interstitial fluid (see Chapter 19).

Figure 13-15 illustrates the concept that two opposing forces influence capillary exchange. These forces include osmosis and filtration. Recall from Chapter 3 that *osmosis* is passive movement of water when some solutes cannot cross the membrane and *filtration* is passive movement of fluid resulting from a hydrostatic pressure gradient (see p. 51).

Figure 13-15 shows that the capillary exchange forces vary, depending on location. At the arterial end of a capillary, the outwardly directed forces are dominant and tend to move fluids from blood to tissue. At the venous end of a capillary, the inwardly directed forces are greater and thus tend to move fluids from tissue to blood. Excess tissue fluids not moved into the blood are collected by the lymphatic system to be eventually returned to venous blood (see Chapter 14).

Factors that affect osmotic pressure (such as plasma albumin levels) or the hydrostatic pressure (such as blood pressure) that drives filtration can disrupt capillary exchange—perhaps resulting in dehydration or overhydration of tissue (see Chapter 19).

Veins and Venules

Venules and veins collect blood from capillaries and return it to the heart.

The larger veins also serve as blood reservoirs because they carry blood under lower pressure (than arteries) and can expand to hold a larger volume of blood or constrict to hold a much smaller amount. As noted previously, external pressure can turn veins, which have one-way valves, into pumps that help return blood to the heart.

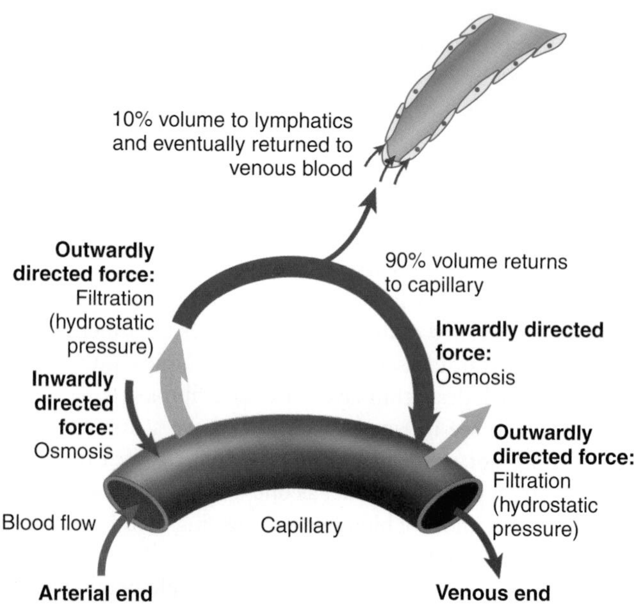

FIGURE 13-15 Capillary exchange. Osmosis (osmotic pressure) and filtration (hydrostatic pressure) are major forces that drive capillary exchange, tending to move fluids out of the capillary at the arterial end and into the capillary at the venous end. Excess tissue fluid can be collected by lymphatic vessels to be returned to the venous blood.

Study **Figure 13-16** and **Table 13-1** to learn the names of the main arteries of the body and **Figure 13-17** and **Table 13-2** for the names of the main veins.

To learn more about blood vessels, go to AnimationDirect at *evolve.elsevier.com*.

QUICK CHECK

1. What are the two main types of blood vessels in the body? How are they different?
2. Can you describe the three major layers of a large blood vessel?
3. What are capillaries? What is their role in the body?

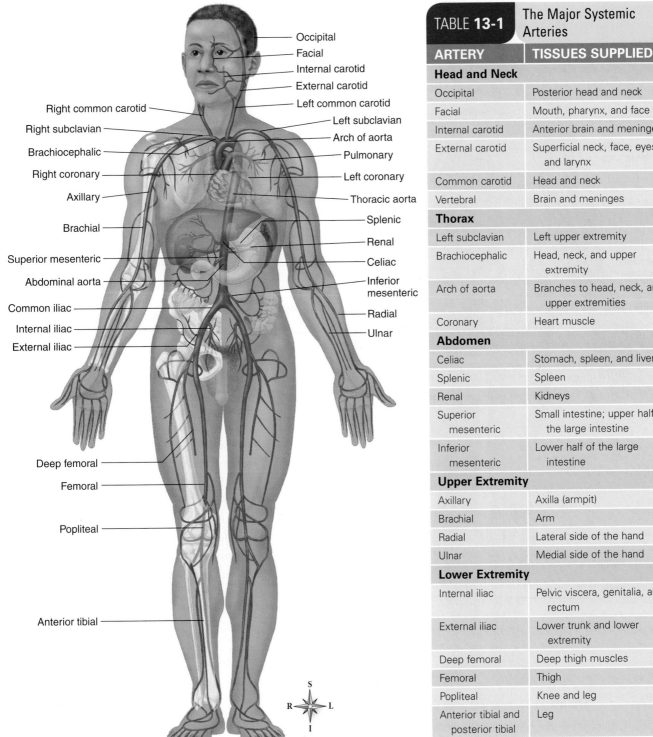

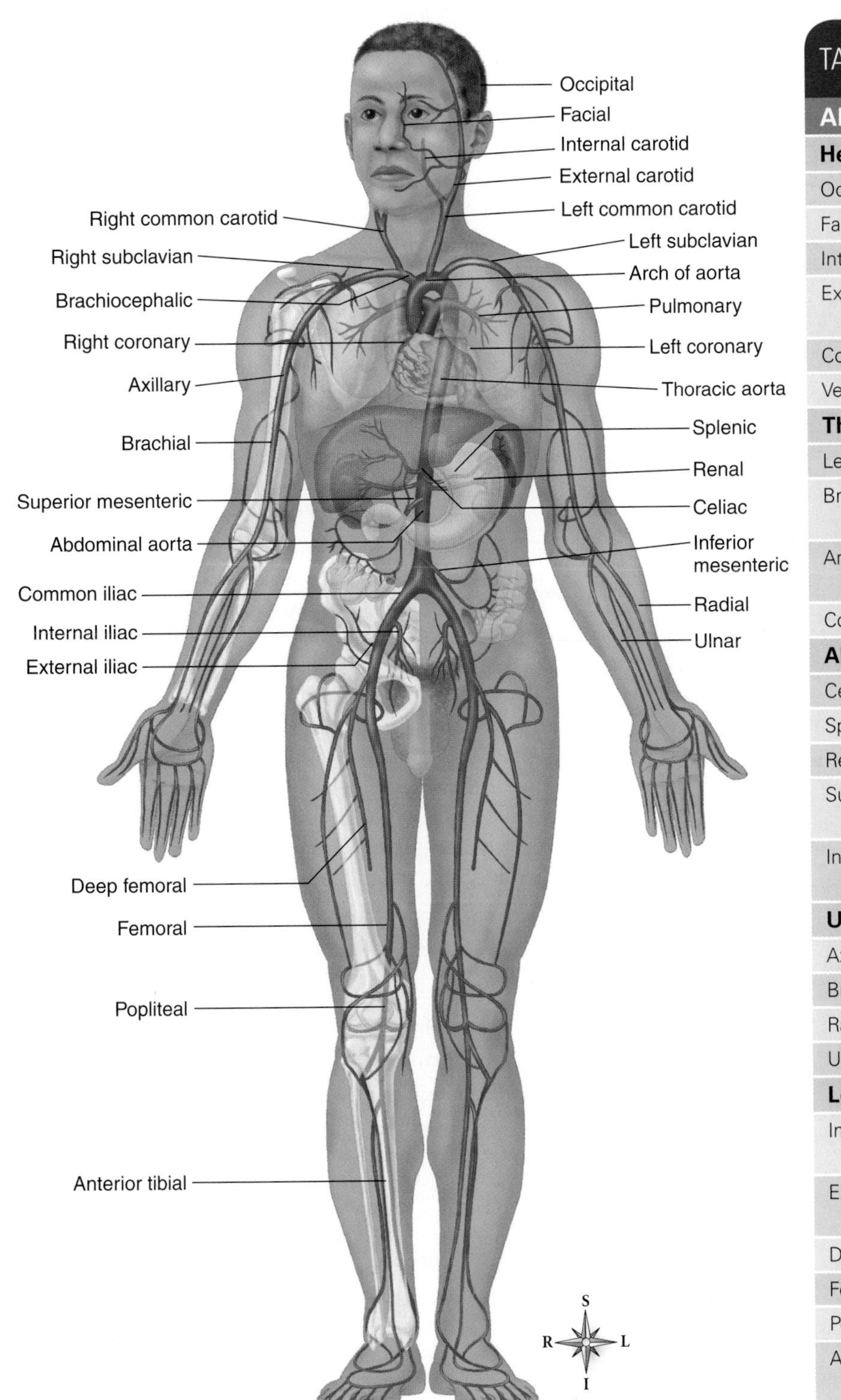

FIGURE 13-16 **Principal arteries of the body.**

TABLE 13-1 The Major Systemic Arteries

ARTERY	TISSUES SUPPLIED
Head and Neck	
Occipital	Posterior head and neck
Facial	Mouth, pharynx, and face
Internal carotid	Anterior brain and meninges
External carotid	Superficial neck, face, eyes, and larynx
Common carotid	Head and neck
Vertebral	Brain and meninges
Thorax	
Left subclavian	Left upper extremity
Brachiocephalic	Head, neck, and upper extremity
Arch of aorta	Branches to head, neck, and upper extremities
Coronary	Heart muscle
Abdomen	
Celiac	Stomach, spleen, and liver
Splenic	Spleen
Renal	Kidneys
Superior mesenteric	Small intestine; upper half of the large intestine
Inferior mesenteric	Lower half of the large intestine
Upper Extremity	
Axillary	Axilla (armpit)
Brachial	Arm
Radial	Lateral side of the hand
Ulnar	Medial side of the hand
Lower Extremity	
Internal iliac	Pelvic viscera, genitalia, and rectum
External iliac	Lower trunk and lower extremity
Deep femoral	Deep thigh muscles
Femoral	Thigh
Popliteal	Knee and leg
Anterior tibial and posterior tibial	Leg

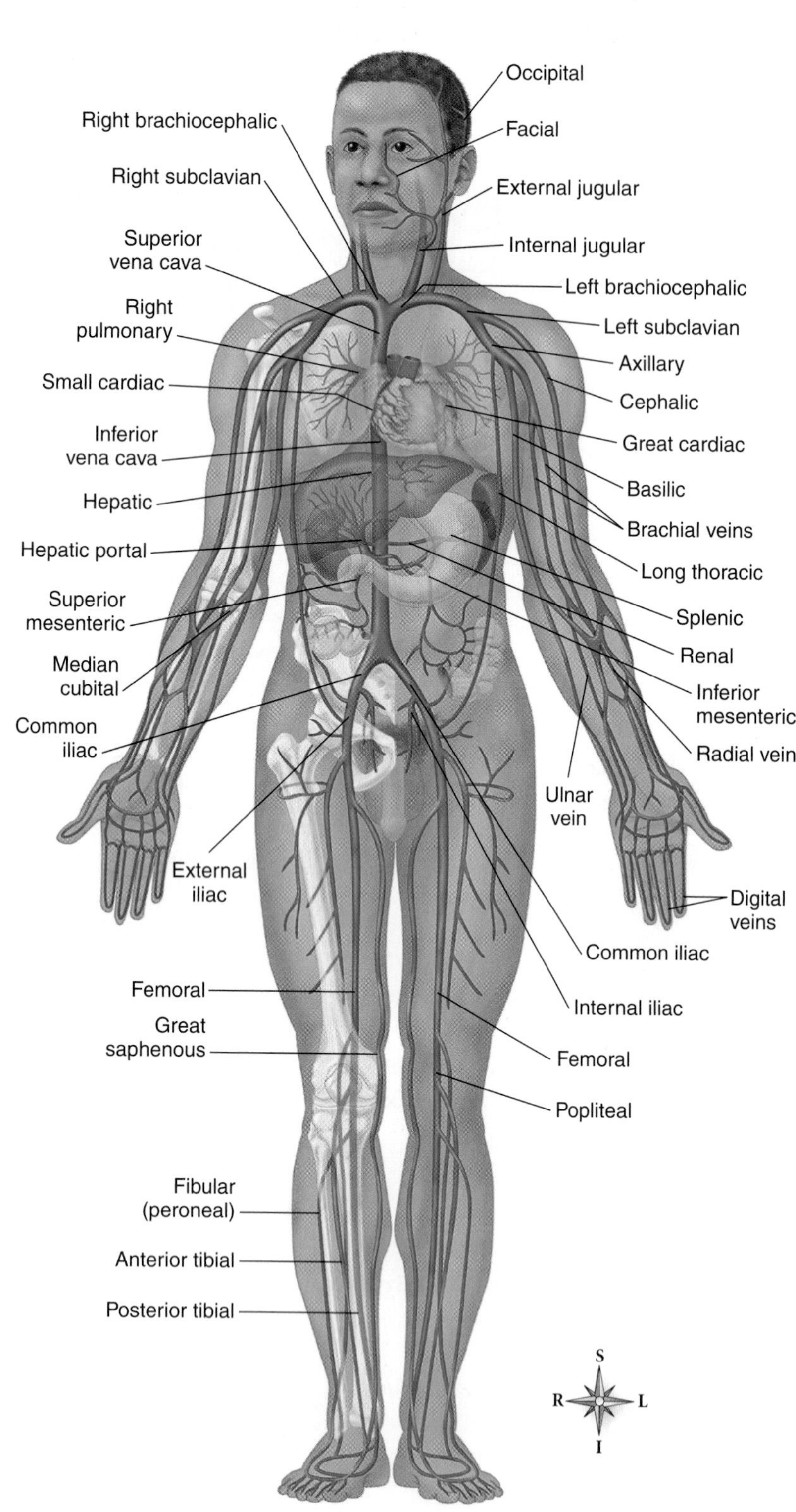

FIGURE 13-17 Principal veins of the body.

TABLE 13-2 The Major Systemic Veins

VEIN	TISSUES DRAINED
Head and Neck	
Facial and anterior facial	Anterior and superficial face
External jugular	Superficial tissues of the head and neck
Internal jugular	Sinuses of the brain
Thorax	
Brachiocephalic	Head, neck, upper extremity
Subclavian	Upper extremity
Superior vena cava	Head, neck, and upper extremities
Pulmonary	Lungs
Cardiac	Heart
Inferior vena cava	Lower body
Abdomen	
Hepatic	Liver
Long thoracic	Abdominal and thoracic muscles
Hepatic portal	Intestines and nearby internal organs
Splenic	Spleen
Superior mesenteric	Small intestine and most of the colon
Inferior mesenteric	Descending colon and rectum
Upper Extremity	
Cephalic	Lateral arm
Axillary	Axilla and arm
Basilic	Medial arm
Median cubital	Cephalic vein (to basilic vein)
Radial	Lateral forearm
Ulnar	Medial forearm
Lower Extremity	
External iliac	Lower limb
Internal iliac	Pelvic viscera
Femoral	Thigh
Great saphenous	Leg
Small saphenous	Foot
Popliteal	Leg
Peroneal (fibular)	Foot
Anterior tibial	Deep anterior leg and dorsal foot
Posterior tibial	Deep posterior leg and plantar aspect of foot

Routes of Circulation

Systemic and Pulmonary Routes of Circulation

The term *blood circulation* is self-explanatory, meaning that blood flows through vessels that are arranged in a complete circuit or circular pattern. Various sets of artery-capillary-vein pathways are called *routes of circulation.*

Blood flow from the left ventricle of the heart through blood vessels to all parts of the body and back to the right atrium of the heart has already been referred to as the **systemic circulation.**

Starting our story at the left ventricle, blood is pumped into the aorta. From there, it flows into arteries that carry it into the tissues and organs of the body. As indicated in **Figure 13-18**, within each structure, blood moves from arteries to arterioles to capillaries. There, the vital two-way exchange of substances occurs between blood and cells.

Next, blood flows out of each organ's capillary beds by way of its venules and then its veins to drain eventually into the inferior or superior venae cavae. These two great veins return venous blood to the right atrium of the heart.

At that point, the blood is short of coming full circle back to its starting point in the left ventricle. To reach the left ventricle and start on its way again, it must first flow through another circuit, referred to earlier as the **pulmonary circulation.**

Observe in **Figure 13-18** that venous blood moves from the right atrium to the right ventricle and then to the pulmonary artery to lung arterioles and capillaries. There, the exchange of gases between the blood and air takes place, converting the deep crimson color typical of venous blood to the scarlet color of arterial blood. This oxygenated blood then flows through lung venules into four pulmonary veins and returns to the left atrium of the heart. From the left atrium, it enters the left ventricle, from which it will once again be pumped throughout the body in the systemic circulation.

To learn more about pulmonary circulation and systemic circulation, go to AnimationDirect at *evolve.elsevier.com.*

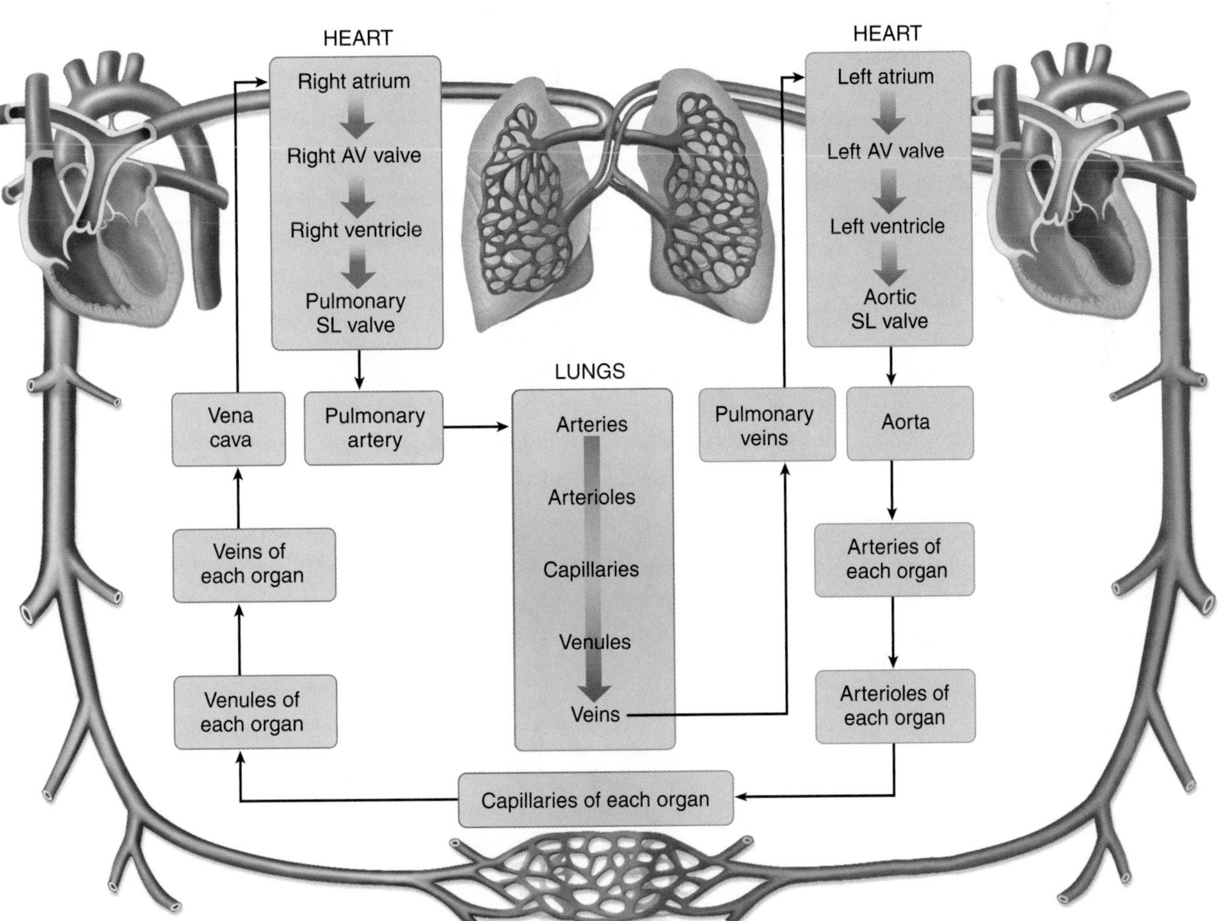

FIGURE 13-18 Diagram of blood flow in the cardiovascular system. Blood leaves the heart through arteries and then travels through arterioles, capillaries, venules, and veins before returning to the opposite side of the heart. Compare this figure with **Figure 13-4**.

Hepatic Portal Circulation

The term **hepatic portal circulation** refers to the route of blood flow to and through the liver. The term *portal* means "doorway" and refers to a systemic circulatory route that is a doorway to a second set of systemic tissues.

Veins from the spleen, stomach, pancreas, gallbladder, and intestines do not pour their blood directly into the inferior vena cava as do the veins from other abdominal organs. Instead, blood flow from these organs is detoured to the liver by means of the hepatic portal vein (**Figure 13-19**). The blood then passes through the capillary beds of the liver before it reenters the regular venous return pathway to the heart. Blood leaves the liver by way of the hepatic veins, which drain into the inferior vena cava.

As noted in **Figure 13-18**, most of the blood flows from arteries to arterioles to capillaries to venules to veins and back to the heart. Blood flow that is diverted to the hepatic portal circulation, however, does not follow this direct route. The diverted venous blood, instead of returning directly to the heart, is sent instead through a second capillary bed in the liver. The hepatic portal vein shown in **Figure 13-19** is located between two capillary beds—one located in the digestive organs and the other in the liver.

Once blood exits from the liver capillary beds, it returns to the systemic blood pathway returning to the right atrium of the heart.

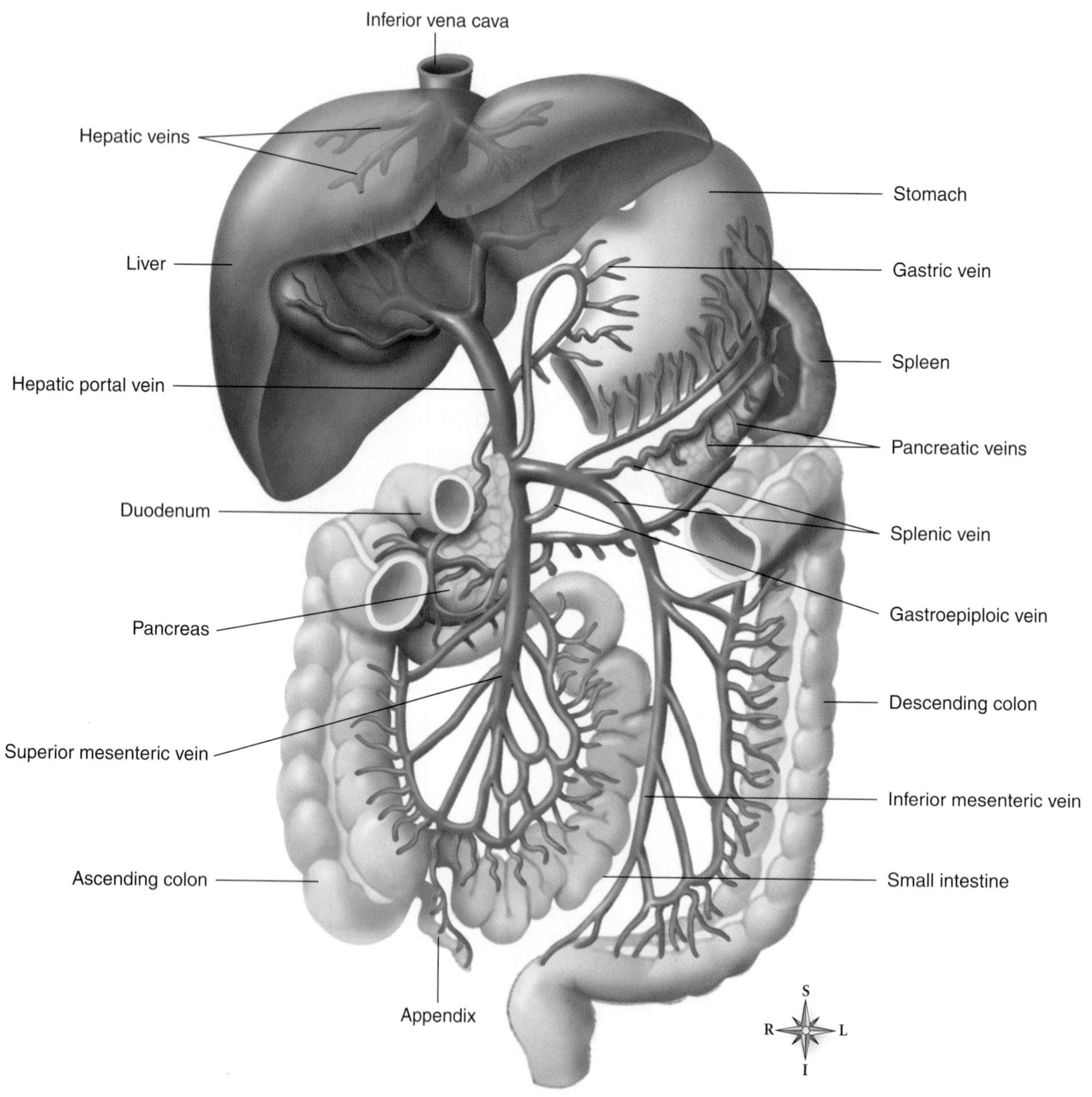

FIGURE 13-19 Hepatic portal circulation. In this very unusual circulation, a vein is located between two capillary beds. The hepatic portal circulation collects blood from capillaries in visceral structures located in the abdomen and delivers it to the liver through the hepatic portal vein. The blood leaves the liver through hepatic veins, which deliver it to the inferior vena cava. (Organs are not drawn to scale here.)

The detour of venous blood through a second capillary bed in the liver before its return to the heart serves some valuable purposes. For example, when nutrients from a meal are being absorbed, the blood in the portal vein contains a higher-than-normal concentration of glucose. Recall from Chapter 11 (see **Figure 11-4**, p. 242) that such high glucose levels trigger the secretion of insulin from pancreatic islets. Influenced by insulin, liver cells remove the excess glucose and store it as glycogen. Therefore blood leaving the liver usually has a lower blood glucose concentration than blood entering the liver.

Liver cells also remove and detoxify various poisonous substances that may be present in the blood. The hepatic portal circulation brings any new toxins absorbed from food directly to the liver where they can be detoxified.

The hepatic portal system is an excellent example of how "structure fits function" in helping the body maintain homeostasis.

Fetal Circulation

Circulation in the body before birth differs from circulation after birth because the fetus must secure oxygen and nutrients from maternal blood instead of from its own lungs and digestive organs.

For the exchange of nutrients and oxygen to occur between fetal and maternal blood, blood vessels must carry the fetal blood to the **placenta**, where the exchange occurs, and then return it to the fetal body. Three vessels (shown in **Figure 13-20** as part of the **umbilical cord**) accomplish this purpose. They are the two small **umbilical arteries** and a single, much larger **umbilical vein.**

The movement of blood in the umbilical vessels may seem unusual at first in that the umbilical vein carries oxygenated blood, and the umbilical artery carries oxygen-poor blood. Remember that arteries are vessels that carry blood away from

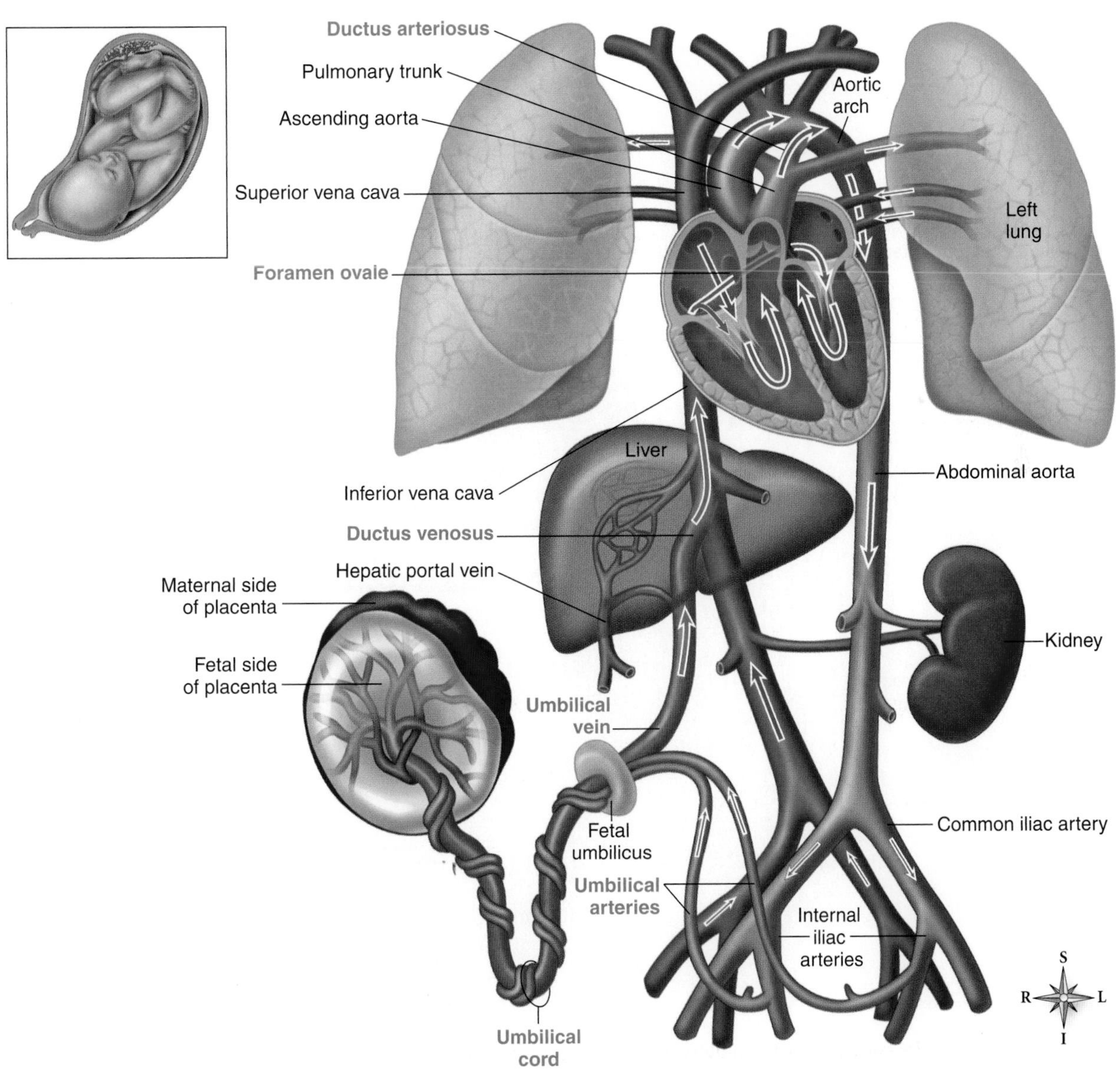

FIGURE 13-20 Fetal circulation. Before birth, the source of oxygen and nutrients is the placenta, giving umbilical arteries a vital role in survival of the fetus.

the heart, whereas veins carry blood toward the heart, regardless of the oxygen content these vessels may have.

Another structure unique to fetal circulation is called the **ductus venosus**. As you can see in Figure 13-20, it is actually a continuation of the umbilical vein. It serves as a shunt, allowing most of the blood returning from the placenta to bypass the immature liver of the developing fetus and empty directly into the inferior vena cava.

Two other structures in the developing fetus allow most of the blood to bypass the developing lungs, which remain collapsed until birth. The **foramen ovale** shunts blood from the right atrium directly into the left atrium, and the **ductus arteriosus** connects the aorta and the pulmonary artery.

At birth, the baby's umbilical blood vessels and shunts must be rendered nonfunctional. When the newborn infant takes its first deep breaths, the cardiovascular system is subjected to increased pressure. The result is closure of the foramen ovale and rapid collapse of the umbilical blood vessels, the ductus venosus, and ductus arteriosus.

To learn more about fetal circulation, go to AnimationDirect at *evolve.elsevier.com*.

QUICK CHECK

1. How do systemic and pulmonary circulations differ?
2. What is the hepatic portal circulation?
3. How is fetal circulation different from circulation after birth?

Hemodynamics

The term **hemodynamics** refers to the set of processes that influence the flow of blood. As we shall see, the main force that drives the continuous flow of blood through its circulatory routes is *blood pressure.*

Defining Blood Pressure

A good way to explain blood pressure might be to first answer a few questions about it. What is blood pressure? Just what the words indicate—blood pressure is the pressure or "push" of blood as it flows through the cardiovascular system.

Where does blood pressure exist? It exists in all blood vessels, but it is highest in the arteries and lowest in the veins. In fact, if we list blood vessels in order according to the amount of blood pressure in them and draw a graph, as in Figure 13-21, the graph looks like a hill, with aortic blood pressure at the top and vena caval pressure at the bottom. This blood pressure "hill" is spoken of as the **blood pressure gradient.**

More precisely, the blood pressure gradient is the difference between two blood pressures. The blood pressure gradient for the entire systemic circulation is the difference between the average or mean blood pressure in the aorta and the blood pressure at the termination of the venae cavae where they join the right atrium of the heart. The mean blood pressure in the aorta, given in Figure 13-21, is 100 millimeters of mercury (mm Hg), and the pressure at the termination of

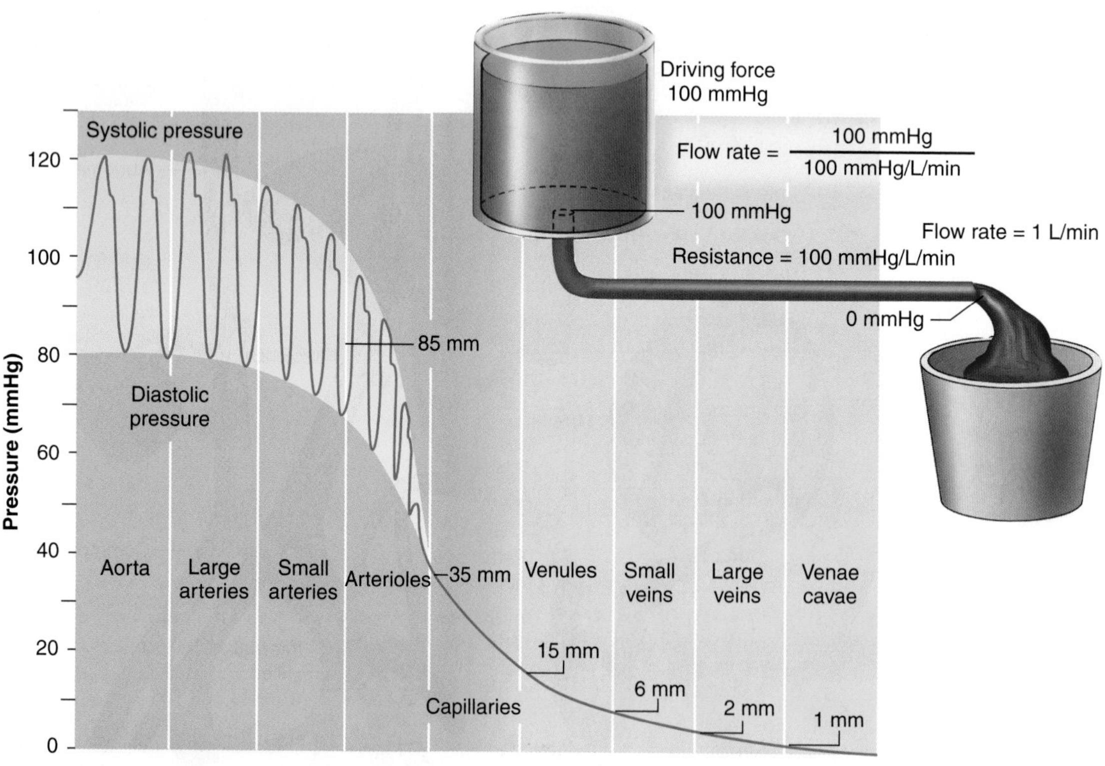

FIGURE 13-21 Pressure gradients in blood flow. Blood flows down a "blood pressure hill" from arteries, where blood pressure is highest, into arterioles, where it is somewhat lower, into capillaries, where it is still lower, and so on. All numbers on the graph indicate blood pressure measured in millimeters of mercury (mm Hg). The broken line, starting at 100 mm Hg, represents the average pressure in each part of the cardiovascular system.

the venae cavae is 0. Therefore, with these typical normal figures, the systemic blood pressure gradient is 100 mm Hg (100 minus 0).

Why is it important to understand how blood pressure functions? The blood pressure gradient is vitally involved in keeping the blood flowing. When a blood pressure gradient is present, blood circulates; conversely, when a blood pressure gradient is not present, blood does not circulate.

For example, suppose that the blood pressure in the arteries were to decrease to a point at which it became equal to the average pressure in arterioles. The result would be that there would be no blood pressure gradient between arteries and arterioles, and therefore no force would be available to move blood out of arteries into arterioles. Circulation would stop, in other words, and very soon life itself would cease. That is why when arterial blood pressure is observed to be falling rapidly, whether during surgery or in some other circumstance, emergency measures must be started quickly to try to reverse this fatal trend.

What we have just said may start you wondering about why high blood pressure (meaning, of course, high arterial blood pressure) and low blood pressure are bad for circulation. High blood pressure, or **hypertension (HTN),** is bad for several reasons. For one thing, if blood pressure becomes too high, it may cause the rupture of one or more blood vessels (for example, in the brain, as happens in a stroke). Chronic HTN can also increase the load on the heart, causing abnormal thickening of the myocardium—and perhaps eventually lead to heart failure.

But low blood pressure can be dangerous too. If arterial pressure falls low enough, then blood will not flow through, or *perfuse*, the vital organs of the body. Circulation of blood and thus life will cease. Massive hemorrhage, which dramatically reduces blood pressure, kills in this way.

Factors That Influence Blood Pressure

What causes blood pressure? What makes blood pressure change from time to time? Factors such as blood volume, the strength of each heart contraction, heart rate, and the thickness of blood are all part of the answers to these questions. We explain further in the paragraphs that follow.

Blood Volume

The direct cause of blood pressure is the volume of blood in the vessels. The larger the volume of blood is in the arteries, for example, the more pressure the blood exerts on the walls of the arteries, or the higher the arterial blood pressure will be.

Conversely, the less blood there is in the arteries, the lower the blood pressure tends to be.

Hemorrhage demonstrates this relationship between blood volume and blood pressure. Hemorrhage is a pronounced loss of blood, and this decrease in the volume of blood causes blood pressure to drop. In fact, the major sign of hemorrhage is a rapidly falling blood pressure.

Another example is the fact that **diuretics**—drugs that promote water loss by increasing urine output—are often used to treat hypertension (high blood pressure). As water is lost from the body, blood volume decreases, and thus blood pressure decreases to a lower level.

The volume of blood in the arteries is determined by how much blood the heart pumps into the arteries and how much blood the arterioles drain out of them. The diameter of the arterioles plays an important role in determining how much blood drains out of arteries into arterioles.

Figure 13-22 summarizes some of the major factors that affect arterial blood volume, which influences arterial blood pressure, which is in turn the main factor driving continued blood flow in the body.

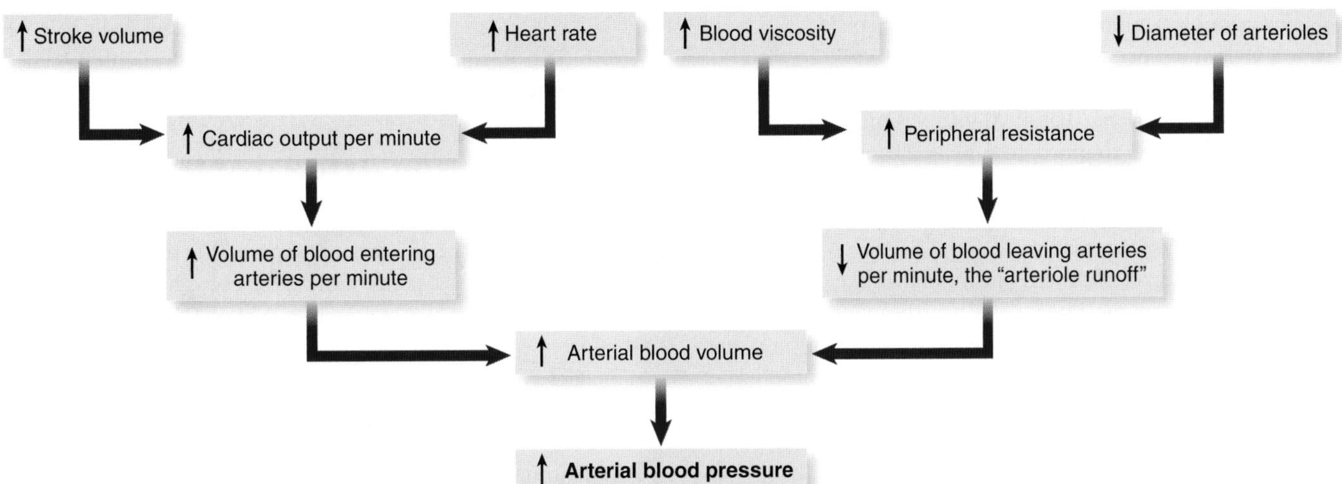

FIGURE 13-22 Relationship between arterial blood volume and blood pressure. Arterial blood pressure is directly proportional to arterial blood volume. Cardiac output (CO) and peripheral resistance (PR) are directly proportional to arterial blood volume, but for opposite reasons: CO affects blood *entering* the arteries, and PR affects blood *leaving* the arteries. If cardiac output increases, the amount of blood entering the arteries increases and tends to increase the volume of blood in the arteries. If peripheral resistance increases, it decreases the amount of blood leaving the arteries, which tends to increase the amount of blood left in them. Thus an increase in either CO or PR results in an increase in arterial blood volume, which increases arterial blood pressure.

Strength of Heart Contractions

The strength and the rate of the heartbeat affect cardiac output and therefore blood pressure. Each time the left ventricle contracts, it squeezes a certain volume of blood (the stroke volume) into the aorta and into other arteries. The stronger each contraction is, the more blood it pumps into the aorta and arteries. Conversely, the weaker that each contraction is, the less blood it pumps.

Suppose that one contraction of the left ventricle pumps 70 mL of blood into the aorta, and suppose that the heart beats 70 times a minute; 70 mL × 70 equals 4900 mL. Almost 5 liters of blood would enter the aorta and arteries every minute (the cardiac output). Now suppose that the heartbeat were to become weaker and that each contraction of the left ventricle pumps only 50 mL instead of 70 mL of blood into the aorta. If the heart still contracts just 70 times a minute, it will obviously pump much less blood into the aorta—only 3500 mL instead of the more normal 4900 mL per minute. This decrease in the heart's output decreases the volume of blood in the arteries, and the decreased arterial blood volume decreases arterial blood pressure.

In summary, the strength of the heartbeat affects blood pressure in this way: a stronger heartbeat increases blood pressure, and a weaker beat decreases it.

Heart Rate

The rate of the heartbeat also may affect arterial blood pressure. You might reason that when the heart beats faster, more blood enters the aorta, and therefore the arterial blood volume and blood pressure would increase.

This is true only if the stroke volume does not decrease sharply when the heart rate increases. Often, however, when the heart beats very fast, each contraction of the left ventricle takes place so rapidly that it has little time to fill with blood and therefore squeezes out much less blood than usual into the aorta.

For example, suppose that the heart rate speeded up from 70 to 100 times per minute and that, at the same time, its stroke volume decreased from 70 mL to 40 mL. Instead of a cardiac output of 70 × 70 or 4900 mL per minute, the cardiac output would have changed to 100 × 40 or 4000 mL per minute. Arterial blood volume decreases under these conditions, and therefore blood pressure also decreases, even though the heart rate has increased.

What generalization, then, can we make? We can say only that an increase in the rate of the heartbeat increases blood pressure, and a decrease in the rate decreases blood pressure. But whether a change in the heart rate actually produces a similar change in blood pressure depends on whether the stroke volume also changes and by how much.

Blood Viscosity

Another factor that needs to be mentioned in connection with blood pressure is the viscosity of blood, or in plainer language, its thickness. If blood becomes less viscous than normal, blood pressure decreases.

For example, if a person suffers a hemorrhage, fluid moves into the blood from the interstitial fluid. This dilutes the blood and decreases its viscosity, and blood pressure then falls because of the decreased viscosity. After hemorrhage, transfusion of whole blood or plasma is preferred to infusion of saline solution. The reason is that saline solution is not a viscous liquid and so cannot keep blood pressure at a normal level.

In a condition called *polycythemia*, the number of red blood cells increases beyond normal and thus increases blood viscosity (see **Figure 12-3** on p. 267). This in turn increases blood pressure. Polycythemia can occur when oxygen levels in the air decrease and the body attempts to increase its ability to attract oxygen to the blood, as happens in working at high altitudes.

Resistance to Blood Flow

A factor that has a huge impact on local blood pressure gradients, and thus on blood flow, is any factor that changes the resistance to blood flow. The term **peripheral resistance (PR)** describes any force that acts against the flow of blood in a blood vessel. Viscosity of blood, for example, affects PR by influencing the ease with which blood flows through blood vessels.

Another factor that affects PR is the tension in smooth muscles of the blood vessel wall (**Figure 13-23**). When these muscles are relaxed, resistance is low and therefore blood pressure is low—thus blood may flow easily down its pressure gradient and into the vessel. When vessel wall muscles are contracted, however, resistance increases and therefore so does the blood pressure—thus the pressure gradient is reduced and blood will not flow so easily into the vessel.

Notice also in **Figure 13-23** that relatively minor changes in vessel diameter cause dramatic changes in blood flow. This fact means that with very slight adjustments of muscle tension in blood vessels, a wide range of different rates of blood flow can be achieved.

Such adjustment of muscle tension in vessel walls to control blood pressure, and therefore blood flow, is often called the **vasomotor mechanism**.

Fluctuations in Arterial Blood Pressure

No one's blood pressure stays the same all the time. It fluctuates, even in a perfectly healthy individual. For example, it goes up when a person exercises strenuously. Not only is this normal, but the increased blood pressure serves a good purpose. It increases circulation to bring more blood to muscles each minute and thus supplies them with more oxygen and nutrients for more energy.

A normal, resting arterial blood pressure is below 120/80, or 120 mm Hg systolic pressure (as the ventricles contract) and 80 mm Hg diastolic pressure (as the ventricles relax). Remember, however, that what is "normal" varies somewhat among individuals and also varies with age.

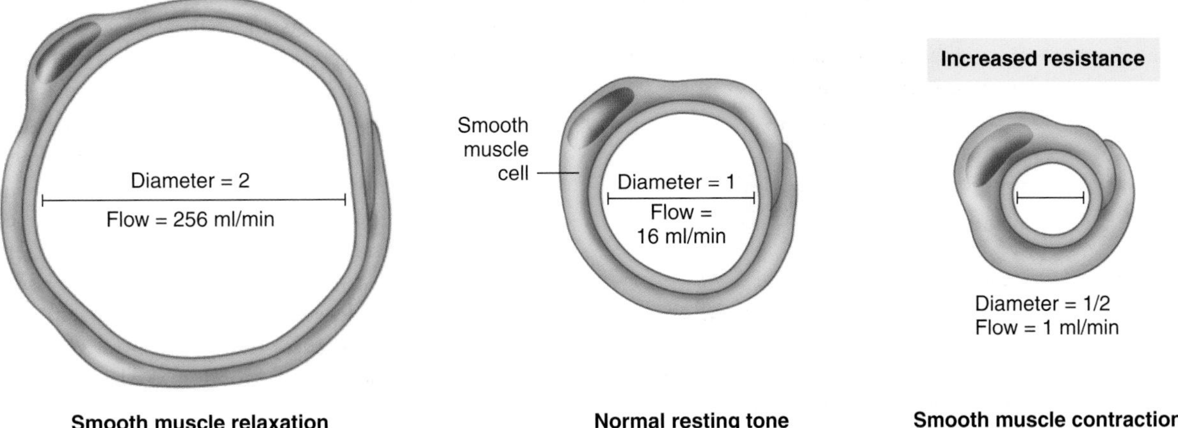

FIGURE 13-23 Vasomotor mechanism. Changes in smooth muscle tension in the wall of an arteriole influence the resistance of the vessel to blood flow. Relaxation of muscle results in decreased resistance; contraction of muscle results in increased resistance. Note also that resulting changes in blood flow are large compared to the amount of change in vessel diameter.

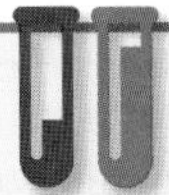

CLINICAL APPLICATION

BLOOD PRESSURE READINGS

A device called a **sphygmomanometer** is often used to measure blood pressures in both clinical and home health care situations. The traditional sphygmomanometer is an inverted tube of mercury (Hg) with a balloonlike air cuff attached via an air hose.

The air cuff is placed around a limb, usually the subject's arm as shown in the figure. A stethoscope sensor is placed over a major artery (the *brachial artery* in the figure) to listen for the arterial pulse. A hand-operated pump fills the air cuff, increasing the air pressure and pushing the column of mercury higher.

While listening through the stethoscope, the operator opens the air cuff's outlet valve and slowly reduces the air pressure around the limb. Loud, tapping *Korotkoff sounds* suddenly begin when the cuff pressure measured by the mercury column equals the **systolic pressure**—often below 120 mm Hg. As the air pressure surrounding the arm continues to decrease, the Korotkoff sounds continue with each pulse of blood pressure, then eventually disappear.

The pressure measurement at which the sounds disappear is equal to the **diastolic pressure**—often 70 to 80 mm Hg. The subject's blood pressure is then expressed as systolic pressure (the maximum arterial pressure during each cardiac cycle) over the diastolic pressure (the minimum arterial pressure), such as 120/80 (read "one-twenty over eighty").

The final reading is then compared with the expected range, which is based on the patient's age and various other individual factors. Mercury sphygmomanometers have been replaced in many clinical settings by nonmercury devices that similarly measure the maximum and minimum arterial blood pressures. In home health care settings, patients are often taught how to monitor their own blood pressure.

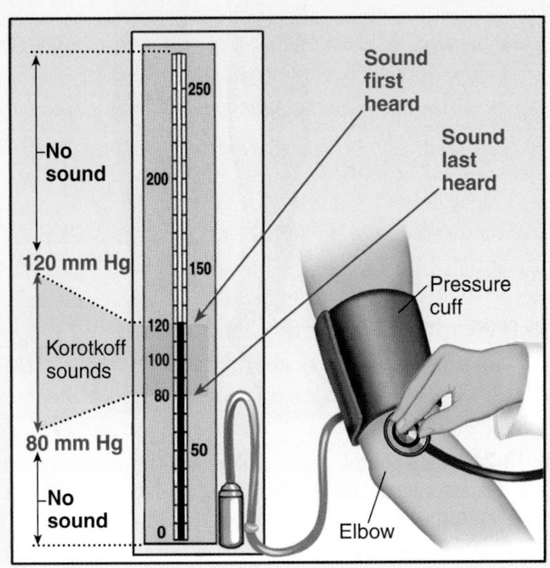

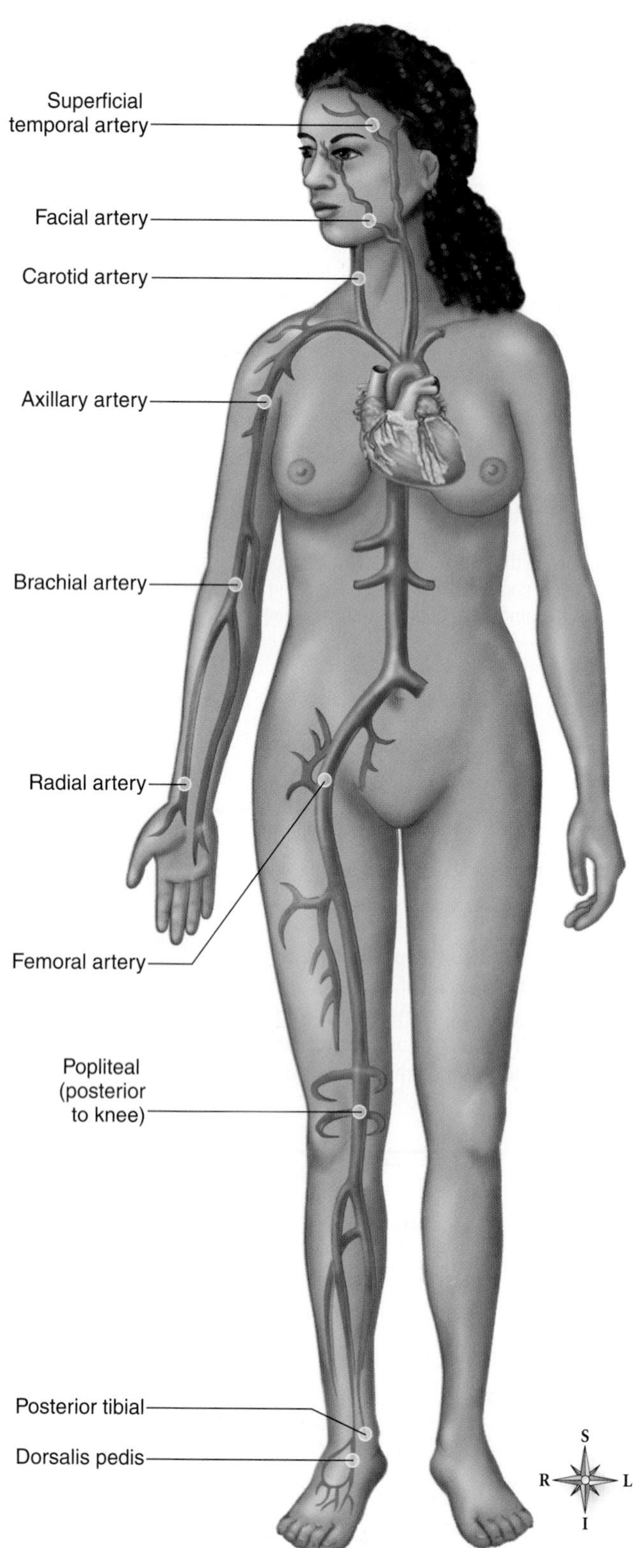

FIGURE 13-24 Pulse points. Each pulse point is named after the artery with which it is associated. External pressure applied to a pulse point can be used by first responders to slow bleeding from an injury distal to the pulse point or *pressure point.*

Central Venous Blood Pressure

The venous blood pressure, as you can see in Figure 13-21, is very low in the large veins and falls almost to 0 by the time blood leaves the venae cavae and enters the right atrium. The venous blood pressure within the right atrium is called the **central venous pressure.** The central venous pressure represents the "low end" of the pressure gradient needed to drive blood flow all the way back to the heart.

The central venous pressure level is important because it influences the pressure that exists in the large peripheral veins. If the heart beats strongly, the central venous pressure is low as blood enters and leaves the heart chambers efficiently.

If the heart is weakened, however, central venous pressure increases, and the flow of blood into the right atrium is slowed. As a result, a person suffering heart failure, who is sitting at rest in a chair, often has distended external jugular veins as blood "backs up" in the venous network.

At least five mechanisms help keep venous blood moving back through the cardiovascular circuit and back to the right atrium. They are the following:

1. Continued beating of the heart, which pumps blood through the entire cardiovascular system
2. Adequate blood pressure in the arteries, to push blood to and through the veins
3. Semilunar valves in the veins that ensure continued blood flow in one direction (toward the heart)
4. Contraction of skeletal muscles, which squeeze veins, producing a kind of pumping action
5. Changing pressures in the chest cavity during breathing that produce a kind of pumping action in the veins in the thorax

Pulse

What you feel when you take a **pulse** is an artery expanding and then recoiling alternately because of the changing arterial blood pressures that result from the left ventricle contracting and relaxing. To feel a pulse, you must place your fingertips over an artery that lies near the surface of the body and over a bone or other firm base.

The pulse is a valuable clinical sign. It can provide information, for example, about the rate, strength, and rhythmicity of the heartbeat. It also can provide information about blood pressure.

Pulse is easily determined with little or no danger or discomfort. The nine major "pulse points" are named after the arteries over which they are felt. Locate each pulse point on Figure 13-24 and on your own body.

Three pulse points are located on each side of the head and neck:

- Superficial temporal artery in front of the ear
- Common carotid artery in the neck along the front edge of the sternocleidomastoid muscle
- Facial artery at the lower margin of the mandible at a point below the corner of the mouth

A pulse is also detected at three points in the upper limb:

- Axillary artery in the armpit
- Brachial artery at the bend of the elbow along the inner or medial margin of the biceps brachii muscle
- Radial artery at the wrist

The so-called *radial pulse* is the most frequently monitored and easily accessible in the body.

The pulse also can be felt at three locations in the lower extremity:

- Femoral artery in the groin
- Popliteal artery behind and just proximal to the knee
- Posterior tibial artery just behind the medial malleolus (inner bump of the ankle)
- Dorsalis pedis artery on the front surface of the foot, just below the bend of the ankle joint.

QUICK CHECK

1. How does the blood pressure gradient explain blood flow?
2. Name four factors that influence blood pressure.
3. Does a person's blood pressure stay the same all the time?
4. Where are the places on your body that you can likely feel your pulse?

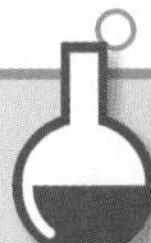

SCIENCE APPLICATIONS

CARDIOLOGY

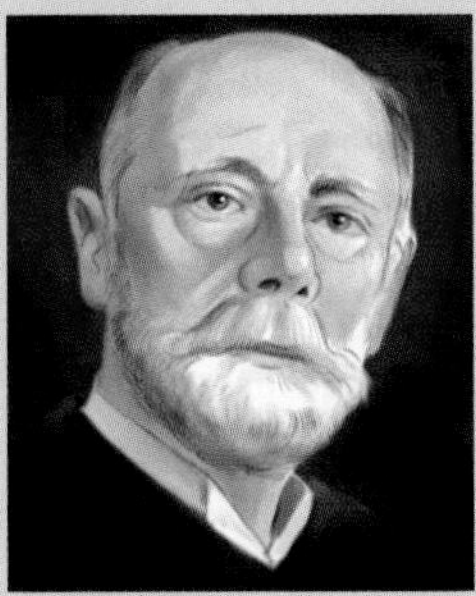

Willem Einthoven (1860-1927)

Cardiology, the study and treatment of the heart, owes much to Dutch physiologist Willem Einthoven and his invention of the modern electrocardiograph in 1903. Einthoven's first major contribution was the invention of a machine that could record electrocardiograms (ECGs) with far greater sensitivity than the crude machines of the nineteenth century.

Then, with the help of British physician Thomas Lewis, Einthoven demonstrated and named the P, Q, R, S, and T waves and proved that these waves precisely record the electrical activity of the heart (see **Figure 13-10**). In 1905, he even invented a way that ECG data could be sent from a patient over the telephone to his laboratory where they could be recorded and analyzed—a technique now called *telemetry.*

Einthoven's detailed studies of ECG recordings changed the practice of heart medicine forever. In fact, his invention was later applied to the study of nerve impulses and led to breakthrough discoveries in the neurosciences.

Cardiologists today still use modern versions of Einthoven's machine to diagnose heart disorders. Of course, *biomedical engineers* continue to develop refinements to electrocardiograph equipment and to invent new machines to monitor heart function. In fact, engineers and *designers* have worked with cardiologists to develop artificial heart valves, artificial pacemakers, and even artificial hearts. With all of this medical equipment being used in cardiology, and medicine in general, there is a need for many *technicians* working to keep it all in good repair.

LANGUAGE OF SCIENCE AND MEDICINE *(continued from p. 283)*

atrium
(AY-tree-um)
pl., atria
(AY-tree-ah)
[*atrium* **entrance courtyard**]

auricle
(AW-rih-kul)
[*auri-* **ear,** *-icle* **little**]

bicuspid (mitral) valve
(bye-KUS-pid [MY-tral] valv)
[*bi-* **double,** *-cusp-* **point,** *-id* **characterized by,** (*mitr-* **bishop's hat,** *-al* **relating to**)]

blood pressure gradient
(blud PRESH-ur GRAY-dee-ent)
[*gradi-* **step,** *-ent* **state**]

capillary
(KAP-ih-layr-ee)
[*capill-* **hair of head,** *-ary* **relating to**]

cardiac cycle
(KAR-dee-ak SYE-kul)
[*cardi-* **heart,** *-ac* **relating to,** *cycle* **circle**]

cardiac output (CO)
(KAR-dee-ak OUT-put)
[*cardi-* **heart,** *-ac* **relating to**]

cardiac vein
(KAR-dee-ak vayn)
[*cardi-* **heart,** *-ac* **relating to,** *cycle* **circle,** *vena* **blood vessel**]

cardiologist
(kar-dee-AHL-uh-jist)
[*cardi-* **heart,** *-o-* **combining form,** *-log-* **words (study of),** *-ist* **agent**]

cardiology
(kar-dee-AHL-uh-jee)
[*cardio-* **heart,** *-log-* **words (study of),** *-y* **activity**]

cardiopulmonary resuscitation (CPR)
(kar-dee-oh-PUL-moh-nayr-ree ree-sus-ih-TAY-shun)
[*cardio-* **heart,** *-pulmon-* **lung,** *-ary* **relating to,** *resuscitat-* **revive,** *-tion* **process**]

cardiovascular system
(kar-dee-oh-VAS-kyoo-lar SIS-tem)
[*cardi-* **heart,** *-vas-* **vessel,** *-ular* **relating to**]

central venous pressure
(SEN-tral VEE-nus PRESH-ur)
[*centr-* **center,** *-al* **relating to,** *ven-* **vein,** *-ous* **relating to**]

chordae tendineae
(KOR-dee ten-DIN-ee)
[*chorda* **string or cord,** *tendinea* **pulled tight**]

coronary artery
(KOHR-oh-nayr-ee AR-ter-ee)
[*corona-* **crown,** *-ary* **relating to,** *arteri-* **vessel**]

coronary bypass surgery
(KOHR-oh-nayr-ee BYE-pass SER-jer-ee)
[*corona-* **crown,** *-ary* **relating to**]

coronary circulation
(KOHR-oh-nayr-ee ser-kyoo-LAY-shun)
[*corona-* **crown,** *-ary* **relating to,** *circulat-* **go around,** *-tion* **process**]

coronary sinus
(KOHR-oh-nayr-ee SYE-nus)
[*corona-* **crown,** *-ary* **relating to,** *sinus* **hollow**]

depolarization
(dee-poh-lar-ih-ZAY-shun)
[*de-* **opposite,** *-pol-* **pole,** *-ar-* **relating to,** *-ization* **process**]

diastole
(dye-AS-toh-lee)
[*dia-* **through,** *-stole* **contraction**]

diastolic blood pressure
(dye-ah-STOL-ik blud PRESH-ur)
[*dia-* **apart,** *-stol-* **position,** *-ic* **relating to**]

diuretic
(dye-yoo-RET-ik)
[*dia-* **through,** *-ure-* **urine,** *-ic* **relating to**]

ductus arteriosus
(DUK-tus ar-teer-ee-OH-sus)
[*ductus* **duct,** *arteri-* **vessel,** *-osus* **relating to**]

ductus venosus
(DUK-tus veh-NO-sus)
[*ductus* **duct,** *ven-* **vessel (vein),** *-osus* **relating to**]

electrocardiogram (ECG or EKG)
(eh-lek-troh-KAR-dee-oh-gram)
[*electro-* **electricity,** *-cardio-* **heart,** *-gram* **drawing**]

electrocardiograph
(eh-lek-troh-KAR-dee-oh-graf)
[*electro-* **electricity,** *-cardio-* **heart,** *-graph* **draw**]

embolism
(EM-boh-liz-em)
[*embol-* **plug,** *-ism* **condition**]

endocarditis
(en-doh-kar-DYE-tis)
[*endo-* **within,** *-cardi-* **heart,** *-itis* **inflammation**]

endocardium
(en-doh-KAR-dee-um)
[*endo-* **within,** *-cardi-* **heart,** *-um* **thing**]

endothelium
(en-doh-THEE-lee-um)
[*endo-* **within,** *-theli-* **nipple,** *-um* **thing**]

epicardium (visceral pericardium)
(ep-ih-KAR-dee-um)
(VISS-er-al pair-ih-KAR-dee-um)
[*epi-* **on or upon,** *-cardi-* **heart,** *-um* **thing,** (*viscer-* **internal organ,** *-al* **relating to,** *peri-* **around,** *-cardi-* **heart,** *-um* **thing**)]

foramen ovale
(foh-RAY-men oh-VAL-ee)
[*foramen* **opening,** *ovale* **egg shaped**]

heart rate (HR)
(hart rayt)

hemodynamics
(hee-moh-dye-NAM-iks)
[*hemo-* **blood,** *-dynam-* **moving force,** *-ic* **relating to**]

hepatic portal circulation
(heh-PAT-ik POR-tall ser-kyoo-LAY-shun)
[*hepa-* **liver,** *-ic* **relating to,** *port-* **doorway,** *-al* **relating to,** *circulat-* **go around,** *-tion* **process**]

hypertension (HTN)
(hye-per-TEN-shun)
[*hyper-* **excessive,** *-tens-* **stretch or pull tight,** *-sion* **state**]

inferior vena cava
(in-FEER-ee-or VEE-nah KAY-vah)
pl., venae cavae
(VEE-nee KAY-vee)
[*infer-* **lower,** *-or* **quality,** *vena* **vein,** *cava* **hollow**]

mitral valve
(MY-tral valv)
[*mitr-* **bishop's hat,** *-al* **relating to**]

myocardial infarction (MI)
(my-oh-KAR-dee-al in-FARK-shun)
[*myo-* **muscle,** *-cardi-* **heart,** *-al* **relating to,** *in-* **in,** *-farc-* **stuff,** *-tion* **process**]

myocardium
(my-oh-KAR-dee-um)
[*myo-* **muscle,** *-cardi-* **heart,** *-um* **thing**]

P wave
(pee wave)
[**named for letter of Roman alphabet**]

pacemaker
(PAYS-may-ker)

parietal pericardium
(pah-RYE-ih-tal payr-ih-KAR-dee-um)
[*pariet-* **wall,** *-al* **relating to,** *peri-* **around,** *-cardi-* **heart,** *-um* **thing**]

pericarditis
(payr-ih-kar-DYE-tis)
[*peri-* **around,** *-cardi-* **heart,** *-itis* **inflammation**]

pericardium
(payr-ih-KAR-dee-um)
[*peri-* **around,** *-cardi-* **heart,** *-um* **thing**]

peripheral resistance (PR)
(peh-RIF-er-all rih-ZIS-tens)
[*peri-* **around,** *-pher-* **boundary,** *-al* **relating to,** *re-* **against,** *-sist-* **take a stand,** *-ance* **state**]

placenta
(plah-SEN-tah)
[*placenta* **flat cake**]

precapillary sphincter
(pree-CAP-pih-layr-ee SFINGK-ter)
[*pre-* **before,** *-capill-* **hair of head,** *-ary* **relating to,** *sphincter* **tight band**]

pulmonary artery
(PUL-moh-nayr-ee AR-ter-ee)
[*pulmon-* **lung,** *-ary* **relating to,** *arteri-* **vessel**]

pulmonary circulation
(PUL-moh-nayr-ee ser-kyoo-LAY-shun)
[*pulmon-* **lung,** *-ary* **relating to,** *circulat-* **go around,** *-tion* **process**]

pulmonary semilunar valve
(PUL-moh-nair-ee sem-ee-LOO-nar valv)
[*pulmon-* **lung,** *-ary* **relating to,** *semi-* **half,** *-luna* **moon,** *-ar* **relating to**]

pulmonary vein
(PUL-moh-nayr-ee vayn)
[*pulmon-* **lung,** *-ary* **relating to,** *vena* **blood vessel**]

pulse
(puls)

Purkinje fiber
(pur-KIN-jee FYE-ber)
[*Johannes E. Purkinje* **Czech physiologist,** *fiber* **thread**]

QRS complex
(kyoo ar es KOM-pleks)
[**named for letters of Roman alphabet**]

repolarization
(ree-poh-lah-rih-ZAY-shun)
[*re-* **back or again,** *-pol-* **pole,** *-ar-* **relating to,** *-ization* **process**]

semilunar (SL) valve
(sem-ee-LOO-nar valv)
[*semi-* **half,** *-luna-* **moon,** *-ar* **relating to**]

sinoatrial (SA) node
(sye-no-AY-tree-al nohd)
[*sin-* **hollow (sinus),** *atri-* **entrance courtyard,** *-al* **relating to,** *nod-* **knot**]

sphygmomanometer
(sfig-moh-mah-NOM-eh-ter)
[*sphygmo-* **pulse,** *-mano-* **thin,** *-meter* **measure**]

stroke volume (SV)
(strowk VOL-yoom)
[*stroke* **a striking**]

subendocardial branch
(sub-en-doh-KAR-dee-al)
[*sub-* **under,** *-endo-* **within,** *-cardi-* **heart,** *-al* **relating to**]

superior vena cava
(soo-PEER-ee-or VEE-nah KAY-vah)
pl., venae cavae
(VEE-nee KAY-vee)
[*super-* **over or above,** *-or* **quality,** *vena* **vein,** *cava* **hollow**]

systemic circulation
(sis-TEM-ik ser-kyoo-LAY-shun)
[*system-* **organized whole (body system),** *-ic* **relating to,** *circulat-* **go around,** *-tion* **process**]

systole
(SIS-toh-lee)
[*systole* **contraction**]

systolic blood pressure
(sis-TOL-ik blud PRESH-ur)
[*sy(n)-* **together,** *-stol-* **position,** *-ic* **relating to**]

T wave
(tee wave)
[**named for letter of Roman alphabet**]

thrombus
(THROM-bus)
pl., thrombi
(THROM-bye)
[thrombus **clot**]

tricuspid valve
(try-KUS-pid valv)
[*tri-* **three,** *-cusp-* **point,** *-id* **characterized by**]

tunica externa
(TOO-nih-kah ex-TER-nah)
[*tunica* **tunic or coat,** *extern-* **outside**]

tunica intima
(TOO-nih-kah IN-tih-mah)
[*tunica* **tunic or coat,** *intima* **innermost**]

tunica media
(TOO-nih-kah MEE-dee-ah)
[*tunica* **tunic or coat,** *media* **middle**]

umbilical artery
(um-BIL-ih-kul AR-ter-ee)
[*umbilic-* **navel,** *-al* **relating to,** *arteri-* **vessel,** *-y* **thing**]

umbilical cord
(um-BIL-ih-kul)
[*umbilic-* **navel,** *-al* **relating to**]

umbilical vein
(um-BIL-ih-kul)
[*umbilic-* **navel,** *-al* **relating to,** *vein* **blood vessel**]

vasomotor mechanism
(vay-so-MOH-tor MEK-ah-niz-em)
[*vas-* **vessel,** *-motor* **move**]

vein
(vayn)
[*vein* **blood vessel**]

ventricle
(ven-TRIK-ul)
[*ventr-* **belly,** *-icle* **little**]

venule
(VEN-yool)
[*ven-* **vessel (vein),** *-ule* **little**]

❑ OUTLINE SUMMARY

To download a digital audio version of the chapter summary for use with your device, access the ***Audio Chapter Summaries*** *online at evolve.elsevier.com.*

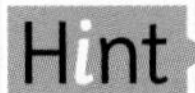

Scan this summary after reading the chapter to help you reinforce the key concepts. Later, use the summary as a quick review before your class or before a test.

Heart

A. Location, size, and position
  1. Triangular organ located in mediastinum with two thirds of the mass to the left of the body midline and one third to the right; the apex on the diaphragm; shape and size of a closed fist (see **Figure 13-1**)
  2. Cardiopulmonary resuscitation (CPR) — the heart lies between the sternum in front and the bodies of the thoracic vertebrae behind; rhythmic compression of the heart between the sternum and vertebrae can maintain some blood flow during cardiac arrest; when combined with an artificial respiration procedure, CPR can be lifesaving

B. Anatomy
  1. Heart chambers (see **Figure 13-2**)
    a. Two upper chambers called *atria* (receiving chambers) — right and left atria
    b. Two lower chambers called *ventricles* (discharging chambers) — right and left ventricles
    c. Wall of each heart chamber is composed of cardiac muscle tissue called *myocardium*
    d. Endocardium — smooth lining of heart chambers
      (1) Inflammation of endocardium called *endocarditis*
      (2) Inflamed endocardium can be become rough and thereby cause a *thrombus*
  2. Pericardium
    a. Pericardium is a two-layered fibrous sac with a lubricated space between the two layers
    b. Inner layer called *visceral pericardium* or *epicardium*
    c. Outer layer called *parietal pericardium*
    d. Inflammation of pericardium is called *pericarditis*
  3. Heart action
    a. Contraction of the heart is called *systole*
    b. Relaxation of the heart is called *diastole*
  4. Heart valves (see **Figure 13-3**)
    a. Valves keep blood flowing through the heart and prevent backflow

b. Consist of two atrioventricular (AV) and two semilunar (SL) valves
   (1) Tricuspid valve — at the opening of the right atrium into the ventricle
   (2) Bicuspid (mitral) valve — at the opening of the left atrium into the ventricle
   (3) Pulmonary semilunar valve — at the beginning of the pulmonary artery
   (4) Aortic semilunar valve — at the beginning of the aorta
c. Stringlike structures called *chordae tendineae* attach the AV valves to the wall of the ventricles

C. Heart sounds
   1. Two distinct heart sounds in every heartbeat or cycle — "lub dup"
   2. First sound (lub) is caused by the vibration and closure of AV valves during contraction of the ventricles
   3. Second sound (dup) is caused by the closure of the semilunar valves during relaxation of the ventricles

D. Blood flow through the heart (see **Figure 13-4**)
   1. The heart acts as two separate pumps — the right atrium and right ventricle performing different functions from the left atrium and left ventricle
   2. Sequence of blood flow
      a. Systemic venous blood enters the right atrium through the superior and inferior venae cavae — passes from the right atrium through the tricuspid valve to the right ventricle
      b. From the right ventricle it passes through the pulmonary semilunar valve to the pulmonary artery to the lungs
      c. Blood moves from the lungs through pulmonary veins to the left atrium, passing through the bicuspid (mitral) valve to the left ventricle
      d. Blood in the left ventricle is pumped through the aortic semilunar valve into the aorta and is distributed to the body as a whole by the systemic arteries

E. Blood supply to the heart muscle
   1. Blood, which supplies oxygen and nutrients to the myocardium of the heart, flows through the right and left coronary arteries (see **Figure 13-5**); called *coronary circulation*
   2. Blockage of blood flow through the coronary arteries is called *myocardial infarction (heart attack)*
   3. Angina pectoris — chest pain caused by inadequate oxygen to the heart
   4. Coronary bypass surgery — veins from other parts of the body are used to bypass blockages in coronary arteries (see **Figure 13-6**)
   5. Coronary veins collect blood from the myocardium and return it to the right atrium through the coronary sinus (see **Figure 13-7**)

F. Cardiac cycle
   1. Heartbeat is regular and rhythmic — each complete beat is called a *cardiac cycle* — average is about 72 beats per minute
   2. Each cycle, about 0.8 second long, is subdivided into systole (contraction phase) and diastole (relaxation phase)
   3. Events of the cardiac cycle are correlated with heart sounds, changes in blood flow and volume, and electrical activity of the heart (see **Figure 13-8**)

G. Electrical activity of the heart
   1. Conduction system of the heart (see **Figure 13-9**)
      a. Intercalated disks electrically connect all the cardiac muscle fibers in a region together so that they receive impulses, and thus contract, at about the same time
      b. Specialized conduction system structures generate and transmit the electrical impulses that result in contraction of the heart
         (1) SA (sinoatrial) node, the pacemaker — located in the wall of the right atrium near the opening of the superior vena cava
         (2) AV (atrioventricular) node — located in the right atrium along the lower part of the interatrial septum
         (3) AV bundle (bundle of His) — located in the septum of the ventricle
         (4) Subendocardial branches (Purkinje fibers) — located in the walls of the ventricles
   2. Electrocardiogram (see **Figure 13-10**)
      a. The tiny electrical impulses traveling through the heart's conduction system can be picked up on the surface of the body and transformed into visible tracings by a machine called an *electrocardiograph*
      b. The visible tracing of these electrical signals is called an *electrocardiogram,* or *ECG*
      c. The normal ECG has three deflections or waves
         (1) P wave — associated with depolarization of the atria
         (2) QRS complex — associated with depolarization of the ventricles
         (3) T wave — associated with repolarization of the ventricles
   3. Damaged heart muscle can result in disturbance to the conduction system
      a. Example — heart block, in which the ventricles beat slower than normal
      b. An artificial pacemaker may be implanted to restore normal function

H. Cardiac output
   1. Definition of cardiac output (CO)
      a. Amount of blood that one ventricle can pump each minute — average is about 5 L per minute at rest (see **Figure 13-11**)

b. Cardiac output is determined by heart rate (HR) and stroke volume (SV)
   (1) Relationship can be expressed mathematically as $CO = HR \times SV$
   (2) Heart rate is the number of beats (cardiac cycles) per minute
   (3) Stroke volume is the volume of blood ejected from one ventricle with each beat (cycle)
   (4) Any factor that affects HR or SV may thus also affect CO
2. Factors that affect heart rate
   a. HR determined mainly by heart's pacemaker
   b. Autonomic nervous system (ANS) can influence pacemaker
      (1) Sympathetic cardiac nerve releases norepinephrine (NE) to increase HR
      (2) Parasympathetic vagus nerve (cranial nerve X) releases acetylcholine (ACh) to decrease HR
      (3) Exercise, change in blood pressure, stress, and dysrhythmias can cause changes in HR
3. Factors that affect stroke volume
   a. Venous return — volume of blood returned to the heart by veins (see **Figure 13-11**)
      (1) A high venous return results in a high SV
      (2) Affected by total blood volume, which in turn can be affected by dehydration, hemorrhage, or various hormones
   b. Strength of myocardial contraction
      (1) Impaired contractions reduce SV
      (2) Can be influenced by ion imbalances, valve disorders, coronary artery blockage, or MI

Blood Vessels

A. Types
   1. Arteries — carry blood away from the heart and toward capillaries
   2. Capillaries — carry blood from the arterioles to the venules
   3. Veins — carry blood toward the heart and away from veins
B. Structure
   1. Arteries (see **Figure 13-12**)
      a. Tunica intima — inner layer of endothelial cells
      b. Tunica media — smooth muscle with some elastic tissue, thick in arteries; important in blood pressure regulation
      c. Tunica externa — thin layer of fibrous elastic connective tissue; may have some elastic tissue
   2. Capillaries — microscopic vessels with only one layer — tunica intima; blood flow in capillaries regulated by smooth muscle in arterioles (see **Figure 13-13**)
   3. Veins (see **Figure 13-12**)
      a. Tunica intima — inner layer; valves prevent retrograde movement of blood (see **Figure 13-14**)
      b. Tunica media — smooth muscle; thin in veins
      c. Tunica externa — heavy layer of fibrous connective tissue in many veins
C. Functions
   1. Arteries — distribution of nutrients, gases, etc., with movement of blood under high pressure; assist in maintaining the arterial blood pressure and thus maintain blood flow
   2. Capillaries — serve as exchange vessels for nutrients, wastes, and fluids (a central cardiovascular function)
      a. Osmosis and filtration are major forces that drive capillary exchange (see **Figure 13-15**)
      b. Outwardly directed forces are greater at arterial end of capillary, moving fluid from blood to tissue
      c. Inwardly directed forces are greater at venous end of capillary, moving fluid from tissue to blood
      d. Excess tissue fluid not returned to blood is collected by lymphatic system (see Chapter 14)
   3. Veins — collect blood for return to the heart; low pressure vessels (see **Figure 13-14**)
D. Names of main arteries — see **Figure 13-16** and **Table 13-1**
E. Names of main veins — see **Figure 13-17** and **Table 13-2**

Routes of Circulation

A. Systemic and pulmonary routes of circulation
   1. Blood circulation — refers to the flow of blood through all the vessels, which are arranged forming a complete circuit or circular pattern (see **Figure 13-18**)
   2. Systemic circulation
      a. Carries blood throughout the body
      b. Path goes from left ventricle through aorta, smaller arteries, arterioles, capillaries, venules, venae cavae, to right atrium
   3. Pulmonary circulation
      a. Carries blood to and from the lungs
      b. Arteries deliver deoxygenated blood to the lungs for gas exchange
      c. Path goes from right ventricle through pulmonary arteries, lungs, pulmonary veins, to left atrium
B. Special circulatory routes
   1. Hepatic portal circulation (see **Figure 13-19**)
      a. Unique blood route through the liver
      b. Vein (hepatic portal vein) exists between two capillary beds
      c. Assists with homeostasis of blood glucose levels
   2. Fetal circulation (see **Figure 13-20**)
      a. Refers to circulation before birth
      b. Modifications required for fetus to efficiently secure oxygen and nutrients from the maternal blood

c. Unique structures include the placenta, umbilical arteries and vein, ductus venosus, ductus arteriosus, and foramen ovale

Hemodynamics

A. Defining blood pressure — push, or force, of blood in the blood vessels
   1. Highest in arteries, lowest in veins (see **Figure 13-21**)
   2. Blood pressure gradient causes blood to circulate — liquids can flow only from the area where pressure is higher to where it is lower
   3. Abnormally low blood pressure results in reduced blood flow to tissues
   4. Hypertension (HTN) — high blood pressure
      a. Can cause vessels to rupture
      b. Can increase workload of heart, causing abnormally thickening of myocardium

B. Factors that influence blood pressure
   1. Blood volume
      a. The larger the volume, the more pressure is exerted on vessel walls (see **Figure 13-22**)
      b. Diuretics — drugs that promote water loss and thus loss of total blood volume
   2. Strength of heart contractions — affect cardiac output; stronger heartbeat increases pressure; weaker beat decreases it
   3. Heart rate — increased rate increases pressure; decreased rate decreases pressure
   4. Blood viscosity (thickness)
      a. Less-than-normal viscosity decreases pressure, more-than-normal viscosity increases pressure
      b. Polycythemia — abnormally high hematocrit, which increases blood viscosity and thus increases blood pressure
   5. Resistance to blood flow (peripheral resistance [PR]) — affected by many factors, including the vasomotor mechanism (vessel muscle contraction/relaxation) (see **Figure 13-23**)

C. Fluctuations in arterial blood pressure
   1. Blood pressure varies within normal range
   2. Normal systemic arterial blood pressure is below 120/80 at rest

D. Central venous pressure
   1. Venous blood pressure within right atrium, the "low end" of the pressure gradient that drives blood flow
   2. Venous return of blood to the heart depends on at least five mechanisms:
      a. A strongly beating heart
      b. An adequate arterial blood pressure
      c. Valves in the veins
      d. Pumping action of skeletal muscles as they contract
      e. Changing pressures in the chest cavity caused by breathing

Pulse

A. Definition — alternate expansion and recoil of the blood vessel wall

B. Nine major "pulse points" named after arteries over which they are felt (see **Figure 13-24**)

❑ ACTIVE LEARNING

STUDY TIPS

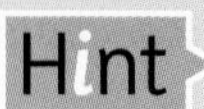

Use these tips to achieve success in meeting your learning goals.

To make the study of the cardiovascular system more efficient, we suggest these tips:

1. Before studying Chapter 13, review the synopsis of the cardiovascular system in Chapter 5. Chapter 13 deals with the heart, which is the pump that moves the blood, and the vessels, which are the tubing that carries the blood.
2. The prefix *cardio-* refers to the heart; in Chapter 8 you learned that *myo-* means muscle. *Myocardium* is the heart muscle.
3. The arteries and veins are composed of three layers of tissue. There is a difference in thickness in these vessels because the arteries carry blood under higher pressure. Arteries and veins carry blood in opposite directions—arteries away from the heart, veins toward the heart. Capillaries need to be thin-walled because this is where the exchange of material between the blood and the tissues takes place.
4. A liquid moves from high to low pressure, so it is logical that the blood pressure in the cardiovascular system is highest just after leaving the heart and is lowest just before returning to the heart.
5. The structures of the heart can be learned with flash cards. The location of the semilunar valves should be easy to remember because their names tell you where they are. It is harder to remember where the tricuspid and mitral valves are because the names do not help. An easier way to remember them is to use their other names: the right and left atrioventricular valves, respectively. This name tells you exactly where they are: between the atria and ventricles on the right or left side. Blood moves through the cardiovascular system in one direction, from the right heart, to the lungs, to the left heart, to the rest of the body, and back to the right heart.
6. Electrical conduction through the heart wall may make more sense if you remember that atria contract from the top down but ventricles must contract from the bottom up so the electrical impulse for contraction must be carried to the bottom of the ventricles before they start contracting. *my-ap.us/QmBof4* offers a tutorial on the electrical conduction pathways of the heart. The letters for the electrocardiogram (ECG) waves do not stand for anything; they are arbitrary, but they do indicate a sequence of events (that is, the P tracing comes before the QRS complex). Check out *my-ap.us/L2JjzP* for a tutorial on ECG. Find additional online tips at *my-ap.us/LDwVq7*.
7. If you are asked to learn the names and locations of specific blood vessels, use flash cards and the figures in this chapter. Note that most arteries and the veins near them have similar names; then pay special attention to places where that pattern varies.
8. Fetal circulation makes sense if you remember the environment in which the fetus is living. Fetal blood returning from the placenta is oxygenated and full of nutrients, so it does not have to go to the lungs or the liver.
9. In your study groups, bring copies of the figures of the heart and of the blood vessels if you need to learn them. Blacken out the labels and quiz each other on the names of each structure and their functions.
10. Discuss the sequence of heart circulation, the parts of an ECG, the heart conduction system, the structure and function of the blood vessels, and the structures in fetal circulation.
11. Refer to the Language of Science and Medicine terms and review the questions and the outline summary at the end of the chapter and discuss possible test questions.

Review Questions

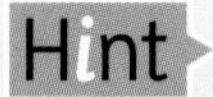

Write out the answers to these questions after reading the chapter and reviewing the Chapter Summary. If you simply think through the answer without writing it down, you won't retain much of your new learning.

1. Describe the heart and its position in the body.
2. Name the four chambers of the heart.
3. Describe the myocardium and the endocardium.
4. Describe the two layers of the pericardium. What is the function of pericardial fluid?
5. Define *systole* and *diastole.*
6. Name and give the location of the four heart valves.
7. Trace the flow of blood from the superior vena cava to the aorta.
8. Describe *angina pectoris.*
9. Differentiate between stroke volume and cardiac output.
10. Trace the path and name the structures involved in the conduction system of the heart.
11. Describe the features of a normal ECG or EKG.
12. Name and describe the main types of blood vessels in the body.
13. Name the three tissue layers that make up arteries and veins.
14. Describe systemic circulation and pulmonary circulation.
15. Name and briefly explain the four factors that influence blood pressure.
16. List the five mechanisms that keep the venous blood moving toward the right atrium.
17. Name four locations in the body where the pulse can be felt.

Critical Thinking

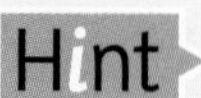

After finishing the Review Questions, write out the answers to these more in-depth questions to help you apply your new knowledge. Go back to sections of the chapter that relate to concepts that you find difficult.

18. Explain how the traces on an ECG relate to what is occurring in the heart.
19. Explain hepatic portal circulation. How is it different from typical systemic circulation, and what advantages are gained from this type of circulation?
20. Explain the differences between normal postnatal circulation and fetal circulation. Based on the environment of the fetus, explain how these differences make fetal circulation more efficient.
21. Explain why a pressure difference must exist between the aorta and the right atrium.

Chapter Test

Hint *After studying the chapter, test your mastery by responding to these items. Try to answer them without looking up the answers. Then, verify the answers using the key in Appendix C at the back of this book.*

1. ________ are the thicker chambers of the heart, which are sometimes called the *discharging chambers.*
2. The ________ are the thinner chambers of the heart, which are sometimes called the *receiving chambers* of the heart.
3. Cardiac muscle tissue is called ________.
4. The ventricles of the heart are separated into right and left sides by the ________.
5. The thin layer of tissue lining the interior of the heart chambers is called the ________.
6. Another term for the visceral pericardium is the ________.
7. Contraction of the heart is called ________.
8. Relaxation of the heart is called ________.
9. The heart valve located between the right atrium and right ventricle is called the ________ valve.
10. The term ________ refers to the volume of blood ejected from the ventricle during each beat.
11. The ________ is the pacemaker of the heart and causes the contraction of the atria.
12. The ________ are extensions of the atrioventricular fibers and cause the contraction of the ventricles.
13. The ECG tracing that occurs when the ventricles depolarize is called the ________.
14. The ECG tracing that occurs when the atria depolarize is called the ________.
15. The ________ are the blood vessels that carry blood back to the heart.
16. The ________ are the blood vessels that carry blood away from the heart.
17. The ________ are the microscopic blood vessels in which substances are exchanged between the blood and tissues.
18. The innermost layer of tissue in an artery is called the ________.
19. The outermost layer of tissue in an artery is called the ________.
20. Systemic circulation involves the moving of blood throughout the body; ________ involves moving blood from the heart to the lungs and back.
21. The two structures in the developing fetus that allow most of the blood to bypass the lungs are the ________ and the ________.
22. The strength of the heart contraction and blood volume are two factors that influence blood pressure. Two other factors that influence blood pressure are ________ and ________.
23. The venous blood pressure within the right atrium is called the ________.
24. A device used to measure blood pressure in clinical and home health care situations is called a ________.
25. Place the following structures in their proper order in blood flow through the heart by putting a 1 in front of the first structure the blood would pass through and ending with a 10 in front of the last structure the blood would pass through.
    a. ________ left atrium
    b. ________ tricuspid valve (right atrioventricular valve)
    c. ________ right ventricle
    d. ________ pulmonary vein
    e. ________ aortic semilunar valve
    f. ________ mitral valve (left atrioventricular valve)
    g. ________ left ventricle
    h. ________ pulmonary artery
    i. ________ right atrium
    j. ________ pulmonary semilunar valve

Lymphatic System and Immunity

OUTLINE

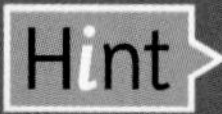

Scan this outline before you begin to read the chapter, as a preview of how the concepts are organized.

OBJECTIVES

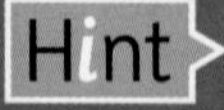

Before reading the chapter, review these goals for your learning.

After you have completed this chapter, you should be able to:

1. Describe the generalized functions of the lymphatic system and list the primary lymphatic structures.
2. Discuss the immune system, and compare nonspecific and specific immunity, natural and artificial immunity, and active and passive immunity.
3. Discuss the major types of immune system molecules and indicate how antibodies and complement proteins function.
4. Discuss the development and functions of B and T cells, and compare and contrast humoral and cell-mediated immunity.

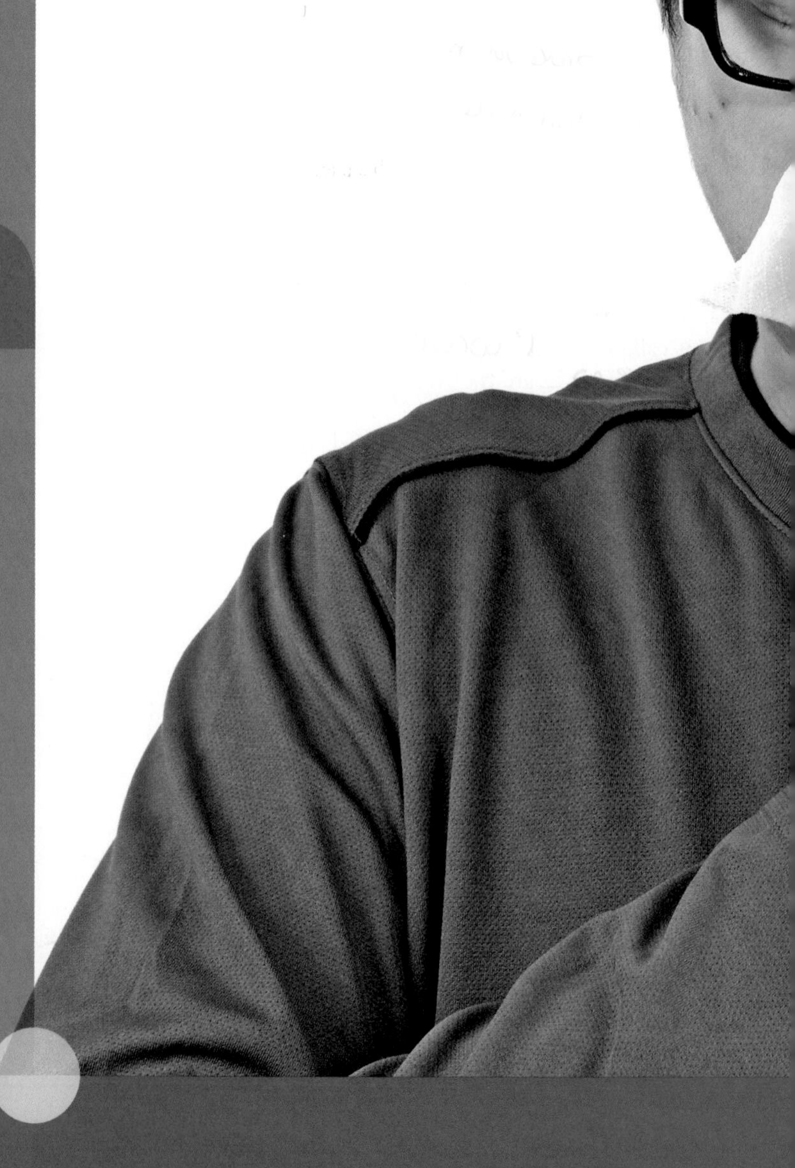

CHAPTER 14

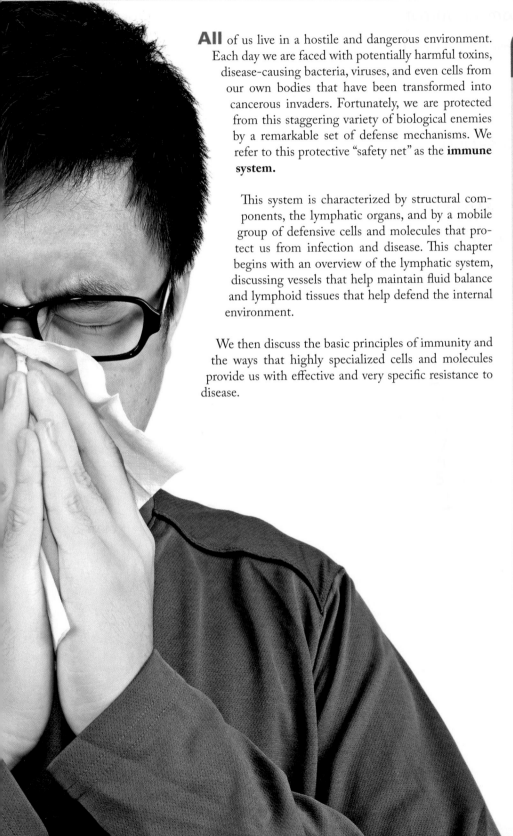

All of us live in a hostile and dangerous environment. Each day we are faced with potentially harmful toxins, disease-causing bacteria, viruses, and even cells from our own bodies that have been transformed into cancerous invaders. Fortunately, we are protected from this staggering variety of biological enemies by a remarkable set of defense mechanisms. We refer to this protective "safety net" as the **immune system.**

This system is characterized by structural components, the lymphatic organs, and by a mobile group of defensive cells and molecules that protect us from infection and disease. This chapter begins with an overview of the lymphatic system, discussing vessels that help maintain fluid balance and lymphoid tissues that help defend the internal environment.

We then discuss the basic principles of immunity and the ways that highly specialized cells and molecules provide us with effective and very specific resistance to disease.

LANGUAGE OF SCIENCE AND MEDICINE

Hint Before reading the chapter, say each of these terms out loud. This will help you to avoid stumbling over them as you read.

acquired immunodeficiency syndrome (AIDS)
(ah-KWYERD IM-yoo-noh-deh-FISH-en-see SIN-drohm)
[*immuno-* **free,** *-defici-* **fail,** *-y* **state,** *syn-* **together,** *-drome* **running or (race) course**]

adaptive immunity
(ah-DAP-tiv ih-MYOO-nih-tee)
[*adapt-* **fit to,** *-ive* **relating to,** *immun-* **free,** *-ity* **state**]

adenoid
(AD-eh-noyd)
[*adeno-* **gland,** *-oid* **like**]

afferent lymphatic vessel
(AF-fer-ent lim-FAT-ik VES-el)
[*a[d]-* **toward,** *-fer-* **carry,** *-ent* **relating to,** *lymph-* **water,** *-atic* **relating to**]

agglutinate
(ah-GLOO-tin-ayt)
[*agglutin-* **glue,** *-ate* **process**]

allergy
(AL-er-jee)
[*all-* **other,** *-erg-* **work,** *-y* **state**]

anaphylactic shock
(an-ah-fih-LAK-tik)
[*ana-* **without,** *-phylact-* **protection,** *-ic* **relating to**]

antibody
(AN-tih-bod-ee)
[*anti-* **against**]

antibody-mediated (humoral) immunity
(AN-tih-bod-ee-MEE-dee-ayt-ed [HYOO-mor-al] ih-MYOO-nih-tee)
[*anti-* **against,** *-medi-* **middle,** *-ate* **process,** (*humor-* **liquid,** *-al* **relating to**) *immun-* **free,** *-ity* **state**]

Continued on p. 333

Lymphatic System

Organization of the Lymphatic System

Maintaining the constancy of the fluid around each body cell is possible only if numerous homeostatic mechanisms function effectively together in a controlled and integrated response to changing conditions. We know from Chapter 13 that the cardiovascular system plays a key role in bringing needed substances to cells and then removing the waste products that accumulate as a result of metabolism. This exchange of substances between blood and tissue fluid occurs in capillary beds. Many additional substances that cannot enter or return through the capillary walls, including excess fluid and protein molecules, are returned to the blood as **lymph.**

Lymph is the excess fluid left behind by capillary exchange that drains from tissue spaces and is transported by way of **lymphatic vessels** to eventually reenter the bloodstream. Thus the lymphatic system is an important partner of the *cardiovascular system*—both vital components of the *circulatory system.*

In addition to lymph and the lymphatic vessels, the lymphatic system includes lymph nodes and lymphatic organs such as the thymus and spleen (Figure 14-1). Such lymphatic

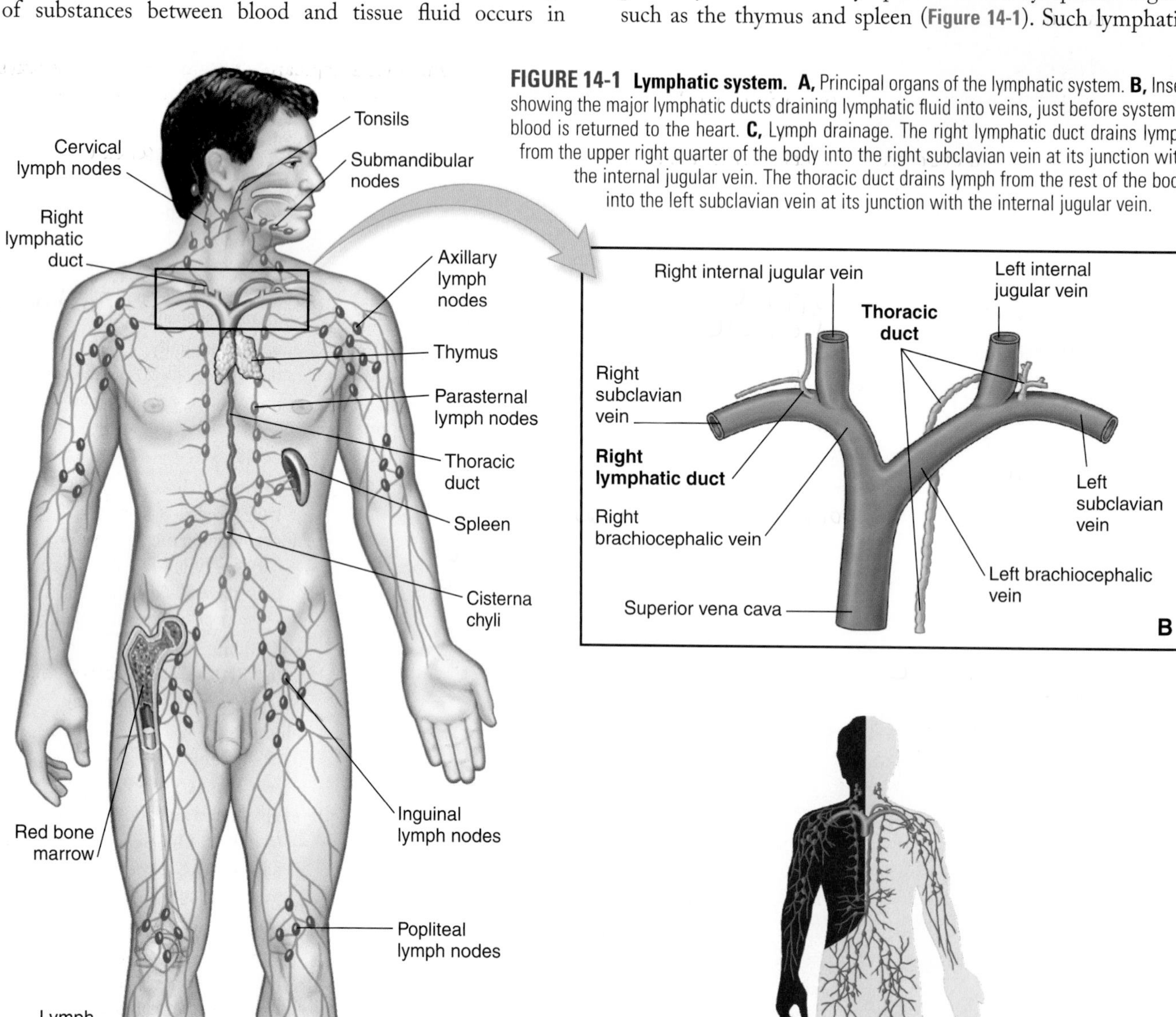

FIGURE 14-1 Lymphatic system. A, Principal organs of the lymphatic system. **B,** Inset showing the major lymphatic ducts draining lymphatic fluid into veins, just before systemic blood is returned to the heart. **C,** Lymph drainage. The right lymphatic duct drains lymph from the upper right quarter of the body into the right subclavian vein at its junction with the internal jugular vein. The thoracic duct drains lymph from the rest of the body into the left subclavian vein at its junction with the internal jugular vein.

organs help to filter the body's fluids, removing harmful particles before they can cause significant damage to other parts of the body.

To learn more about the lymphatic system, go to AnimationDirect at *evolve.elsevier.com.*

Lymph

Lymph forms in this way: blood plasma filters out of the capillaries into the microscopic spaces between tissue cells because of the hydrostatic pressure generated by the pumping action of the heart (see **Figure 13-15** on p. 296). There, the liquid is called **interstitial fluid (IF),** or tissue fluid. Much of the interstitial fluid goes back into the blood by the same route it came out (that is, through the capillary membrane). The remainder of the interstitial fluid enters the lymphatic system before it returns to the blood.

The fluid, called *lymph* at this point, enters a network of tiny blind-ended tubes distributed in the tissue spaces. These tiny vessels, called **lymphatic capillaries,** permit excess tissue fluid along with some other substances such as dissolved protein molecules to leave the tissue spaces. **Figure 14-2** shows how lymph forms as part of the process that maintains fluid homeostasis in the tissues of the body.

Lymphatic Vessels

Lymphatic and blood capillaries are similar in many ways. Both types of vessels are microscopic and both are formed from sheets that consist of a single cell layer of simple squamous epithelium called *endothelium.* The flattened endothelial

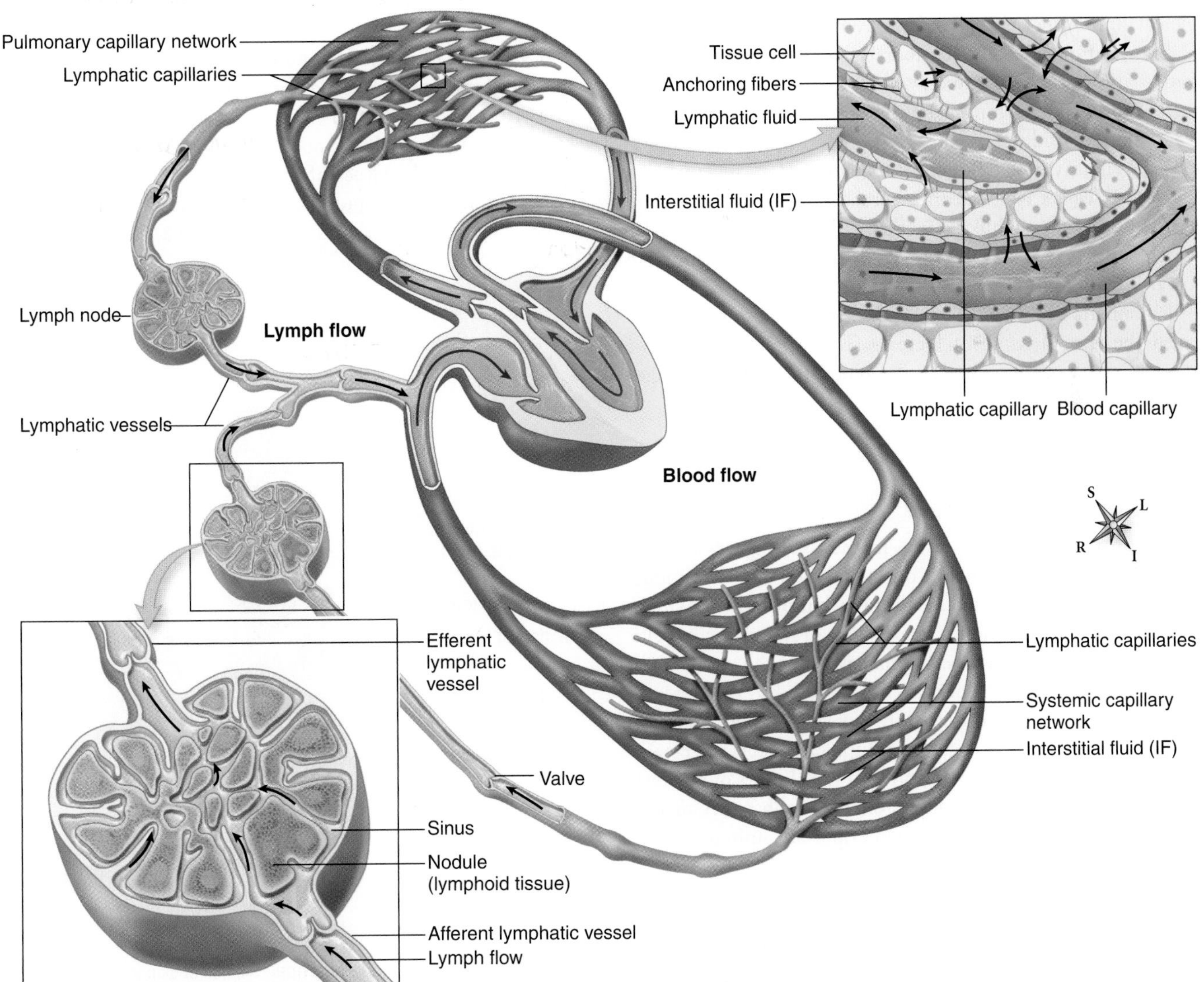

FIGURE 14-2 Role of lymphatic system in fluid homeostasis. Fluid filtered from blood plasma that is not reabsorbed by blood vessels drains into lymphatic vessels. Lymphatic drainage prevents accumulation of too much tissue fluid. Lymph nodes and other lymphoid structures filter the lymphatic fluid before it is returned to the bloodstream.

cells that form blood capillaries, however, fit tightly together so that large molecules cannot easily enter or exit from the vessel. The "fit" between endothelial cells forming the lymphatic capillaries is not as tight. As a result, the lymphatic capillaries are more porous and allow larger molecules, including proteins and other substances, as well as the fluid itself, to enter the vessel and eventually return to the general circulation.

The movement of lymph in the lymphatic vessels goes one way only. Unlike blood, lymph does not flow over and over again through vessels that form a circular route. The lymphatic vessels often have a "beaded" appearance, resulting from the presence of valves that assist in maintaining a one-way flow of lymph. These valves, similar to those in veins, sometimes cause lymph to back up behind them and cause swellings that look like beads.

Lymph flowing through the lymphatic capillaries next moves into successively larger and larger vessels sometimes called *lymphatic venules* and lymphatic *veins*. These lymphatic vessels eventually empty into one of two terminal vessels called the **right lymphatic duct** and the **thoracic duct,** which return their lymph into the blood in large veins in the neck region.

Lymph from about three fourths of the body eventually drains into the thoracic duct, which is the largest lymphatic vessel in the body. Lymph from the right upper extremity and from the right side of the head, neck, and upper torso flows into the right lymphatic duct (see **Figure 14-1**).

Note in **Figure 14-1** that the thoracic duct in the abdomen has an enlarged pouchlike structure called the **cisterna chyli,** which serves as a temporary holding area for lymph moving toward its point of entry into the veins.

Lymphatic capillaries in the wall of the small intestine are given the special name of **lacteals**. They transport fats obtained from food nutrients to the bloodstream and are discussed further in Chapter 16.

Lymph Nodes

Location and Structure

As lymph travels from its origin in the tissue spaces toward the thoracic or right lymphatic ducts and then into the venous blood, it is filtered by passing through **lymph nodes,** which are located in clusters along the pathway of lymphatic vessels. Some of these nodes may be as small as a pinhead, and others may be as large as a lima bean.

With the exception of relatively few single nodes, most of the larger lymph nodes occur in groups or clusters in certain areas. **Figure 14-1** shows the locations of the clusters of greatest clinical importance. The structure of the lymph nodes makes it possible for them to perform two important immune functions: defense and white blood cell formation.

Lymph nodes are *lymphoid organs* because they contain **lymphoid tissue,** which is a white mass of developing lymphocytes and related cells. Lymphoid organs such as lymph nodes, tonsils, thymus, and spleen are important structural components of the immune system because they provide immune defense and development of immune cells.

An inset in **Figure 14-2** shows the structure of a typical lymph node. This structural pattern of a hollow capsule with nodules of lymphoid tissue suspended by reticular fibers is repeated in all the lymphoid organs.

Biological Filtration

In **Figure 14-3**, a small node located next to an infected hair follicle is shown filtering bacteria from lymph. Lymph nodes perform biological filtration, a process in which cells (phagocytic cells in this case) alter the contents of the filtered fluid. Biological filtration of bacteria and other abnormal cells by phagocytosis prevents local infections from spreading.

Figure 14-2 shows that lymph enters the node through one or more **afferent lymphatic vessels.** *Afferent* is from the Latin term for "carry toward." These vessels deliver lymph to the node.

Once lymph enters the node, it "percolates" slowly through spaces called *sinuses* that surround *nodules* found in the outer (cortex) and inner (medullary) areas of the node (see **Figure 14-2**). At the core of each nodule is a *germinal center* where new cells are produced.

Lymph exits from the node through a single **efferent lymphatic vessel.** *Efferent* is from the Latin term for "carry away from."

In passing through the node, lymph is filtered so that bacteria, cancer cells, virus-infected cells, and damaged tissue cells are removed and prevented from entering the blood and circulating all over the body (**Figure 14-3**). Lymph nodes

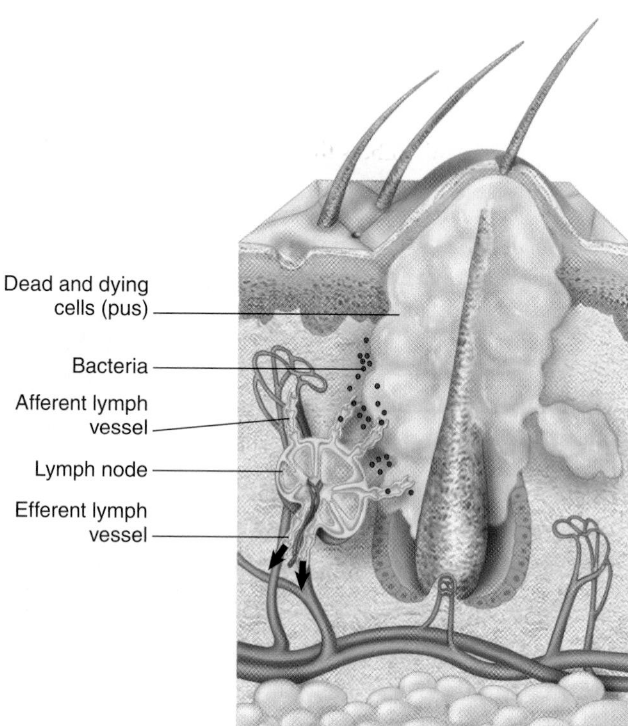

FIGURE 14-3 Lymph node function. Section of skin in which an infection surrounds a hair follicle. The yellow areas represent dead and dying cells (pus). The black dots around the yellow areas represent bacteria. Bacteria entering the node via the afferent lymphatics are filtered out.

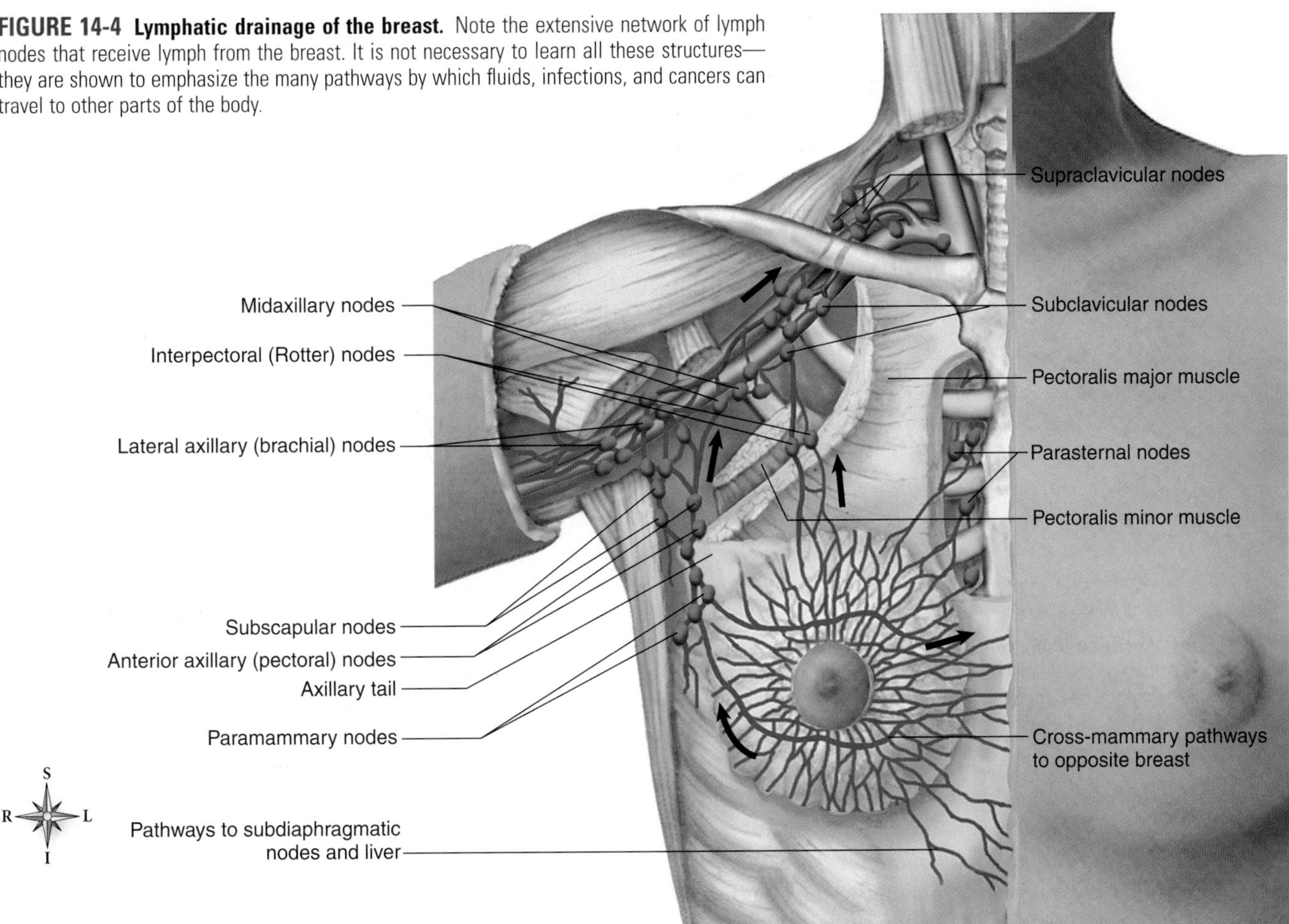

FIGURE 14-4 Lymphatic drainage of the breast. Note the extensive network of lymph nodes that receive lymph from the breast. It is not necessary to learn all these structures—they are shown to emphasize the many pathways by which fluids, infections, and cancers can travel to other parts of the body.

accomplish this by a two-step process. First, debris is trapped by the web of reticular fibers that suspend the lymph nodules. Next, immune cells destroy and break apart the debris by phagocytosis and other biological processes.

Knowledge of lymph node location and function is important in clinical medicine. For example, the breast has a uniquely extensive network of lymphatic drainage and filtration (**Figure 14-4**). This arrangement helps efficiently drain excess fluids that may accumulate when the breasts are producing milk, but it can also serve as a pathway for the spread of infections and cancer.

A surgeon uses knowledge of lymph node function when removing lymph nodes under the arms (axillary nodes) and in other nearby areas during an operation for breast cancer. These nodes may contain cancer cells filtered out of the lymph drained from the breast and are removed to prevent further spread of cancer to other parts of the body.

Clusters of lymph nodes in the neck may become infected and swell when there are infections in the ears or throat. This is why the neck may be palpated to check for swollen lymph nodes when a throat or ear infection is suspected.

To learn more about lymphatic vessels and lymph nodes, go to AnimationDirect at *evolve.elsevier.com*.

Thymus

As you can see in **Figure 14-1**, the **thymus** is a small lymphoid tissue organ located in the mediastinum, extending upward in the midline of the neck. It is composed of lymphocytes in a meshlike framework of reticular fibers. The thymus, also called the *thymus gland,* is largest at puberty and even then weighs only about 35 or 40 grams—a little more than an ounce.

Although small in size, the thymus plays a central and critical role in the body's vital immunity mechanism. First, it is a source of lymphocytes before birth and is then especially important in the "maturation," or development, of a type of lymphocyte that then leaves the thymus and circulates to the spleen, tonsils, lymph nodes, and other lymphoid tissues.

These **T lymphocytes,** or **T cells,** are critical to the functioning of the immune system and are discussed in more detail later. A group of hormones secreted by the thymus called **thymosins** influences the development of T cells.

The thymus appears to complete much of its work early in childhood, reaching its maximum size at puberty. The thymus tissue is then gradually replaced by fat and connective tissue, a process called *involution.* By age 60, the lymphoid tissue is about half its maximum and is virtually gone by age 80 or so.

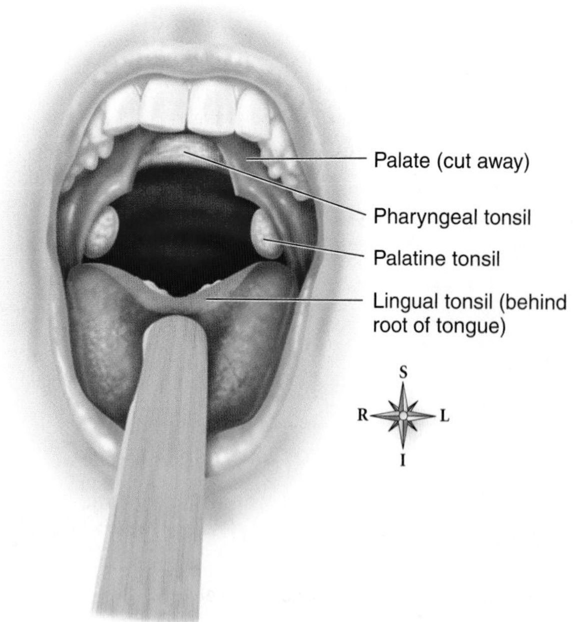

FIGURE 14-5 Location of the tonsils. Small segments of the roof and floor of the mouth have been removed to show the protective ring of tonsils (lymphoid tissue) around the internal opening of the nose and throat.

Tonsils

Masses of lymphoid tissue called *tonsils* are located in a protective ring under the mucous membranes in the mouth and back of the throat (**Figure 14-5**). They help protect against bacteria that may invade tissues in the area around the openings between the nasal and oral cavities.

The **palatine tonsils** are located on each side of the throat. The **pharyngeal tonsils,** known as **adenoids** when they become swollen, are near the posterior opening of the nasal cavity. A third type of tonsil, the **lingual tonsils,** is near the base of the tongue.

The tonsils serve as the first line of defense from the exterior and as such are subject to chronic infection. In rare cases, they may be removed surgically if antibiotic therapy is not successful at treating the chronic infection or if swelling impairs breathing.

Spleen

The **spleen** is the largest lymphoid organ in the body. It is located high in the upper left quadrant of the abdomen lateral to the stomach (see **Figure 14-1** and **Figure 1-6**). Although the spleen is protected by the lower ribs, it can be injured by abdominal trauma.

The spleen has a very large network of reservoir veins and may contain more than 500 mL (about 1 pint) of blood. The spleen serves as a reservoir for blood that can be returned to the cardiovascular system when needed. If the spleen is damaged and bleeding, a surgical removal called a **splenectomy** may be required to stop the loss of blood and ensure survival.

After entering the spleen, blood flows through white, pulp-like accumulations of lymphocytes. As blood flows through the *white pulp,* the spleen removes by mechanical and biological filtration many bacteria and other debris. The spleen also destroys worn out red blood cells (RBCs), which often fall apart when passing through the spleen's meshwork, and salvages the iron found in hemoglobin for future use.

The white pulp of the spleen also serves as a reservoir for monocytes, which can quickly leave the spleen to help repair damaged tissue anywhere in the body during an emergency.

Although the spleen provides useful functions in maintaining the healthy stability of the body, other organs can also perform these functions. Thus, we can survive without our spleen if surgical removal is required to preserve our overall health.

QUICK CHECK

1. How does the lymphatic system return fluid to the blood?
2. What is the role of lymph nodes in the body?
3. Why is the thymus important for immunity?

Immune System

Function of the Immune System

The body's defense mechanisms protect us from disease-causing microorganisms that invade our bodies, from foreign tissue cells that may have been transplanted into our bodies, and from our own cells when they have turned malignant or cancerous. The body's overall defense system is called the *immune system.* The immune system makes us immune—that is, able to resist these threats to our health and survival.

In the lymphatic system, we have seen many organs that help provide defense: lymph nodes, tonsils, thymus, and spleen. The immune system is not simply a small group of organs working together. Instead, it is an interactive network of many organs and billions of freely moving cells and trillions of free-floating molecules in many different areas of the body.

Nonspecific Immunity

Nonspecific immunity is maintained by mechanisms that attack any irritant or abnormal substance that threatens the internal environment. In other words, nonspecific immunity confers general protection rather than protection from a specific threatening cell or chemical. Because we are born with nonspecific defenses that do not require prior exposure to a harmful substance or threatening cell, nonspecific immunity is often called **innate immunity.**

As you can see in **Table 14-1**, the innate, nonspecific immune responses are more rapid than specific immune responses, so they are often the "first responders" when threats occur in the body. Many of the innate immune mechanisms also trigger the specific immune mechanisms, which are slower to respond but have additional, complex strategies to help eliminate the threat.

TABLE 14-1 Nonspecific and Specific Immunity

	NONSPECIFIC IMMUNITY	SPECIFIC IMMUNITY
Synonyms	Innate immunity, native immunity, genetic immunity	Adaptive immunity, acquired immunity
Specificity	Not specific—recognizes variety of nonself or abnormal cells and particles	Specific—recognizes only specific antigens on certain cells or particles
Speed of reaction	Rapid—immediate up to several hours	Slower—several hours to several days
Memory	None—same response to repeated exposures to same antigen	Yes—enhanced response to repeated exposures to same antigen
Chemicals	Complement proteins, interferons, others	Antibodies, various signaling chemicals
Cells	Phagocytes (neutrophils, macrophages, dendritic cells)	Lymphocytes (B cells and T cells)

There are many types of nonspecific immune defenses in the body, as you can see by scanning **Table 14-2**. The skin and mucous membranes, for example, are nonspecific mechanical barriers that prevent entry into the body by bacteria and many other substances such as toxins and harmful chemicals. Tears and mucus also contribute to nonspecific immunity. Tears wash harmful substances from the eyes, and mucus traps foreign material that may enter through the respiratory tract. Phagocytosis of bacteria by white blood cells (WBCs) is a nonspecific form of immunity.

HEALTH AND WELL-BEING

EFFECTS OF EXERCISE ON IMMUNITY

Exercise physiologists have found that moderate exercise increases the number of white blood cells (WBCs), specifically granular leukocytes and lymphocytes. Not only is the number of circulating immune cells higher after exercise, but the activity of sensitized T cells is also increased. But at the same time, research also shows that strenuous exercise may actually inhibit immune function. Nevertheless, moderate exercise such as walking, when engaged in immediately after a trauma such as surgery, is often encouraged because of its immunity-strengthening effects.

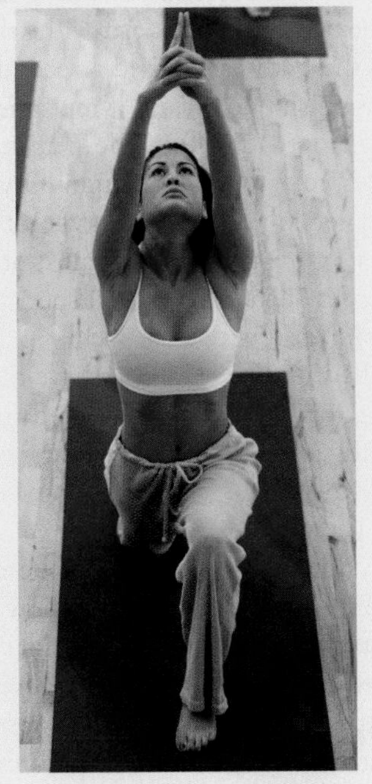

TABLE 14-2 Mechanisms of Nonspecific Defense

MECHANISM	DESCRIPTION
Mechanical and Chemical Barriers	Physical impediments to the entry of foreign cells or substances
Skin and mucous membranes	Forms a continuous wall that separates the internal environment from the external environment, preventing the entry of pathogens
Secretions	Secretions such as sebum, mucus, acids, and enzymes chemically inhibit the activity of pathogens
Inflammation	The inflammatory response isolates the pathogens and stimulates the speedy arrival of large numbers of immune cells
Fever	Fever may enhance immune reactions and inhibit pathogens
Phagocytosis	Ingestion and destruction of pathogens by phagocytic cells
Neutrophils	Granular leukocytes that are usually the first phagocytic cell to arrive at the scene of an inflammatory response
Macrophages	Monocytes that have enlarged to become giant phagocytic cells capable of consuming many pathogens; often called by other, more specific names when found in specific tissues of the body
Complement	Group of plasma proteins (inactive enzymes) that produce a cascade of chemical reactions that ultimately causes lysis (rupture) of a foreign cell; the complement cascade can be triggered by adaptive or innate immune mechanisms
Interferon (IF)	Protein produced by cells after they become infected by a virus; inhibits the spread or further development of a viral infection (see box on p. 326)

The **inflammatory response** is a set of nonspecific responses that often occurs in the body. In the example shown in **Figure 14-6**, bacteria cause tissue damage that, in turn, triggers the release of mediators from any of a variety of immune cells. Such signal molecules sent by cells are often called **cytokines.** Some of the cytokines attract WBCs to the area. Many of these factors produce the characteristic signs of inflammation: *heat, redness, pain,* and *swelling.*

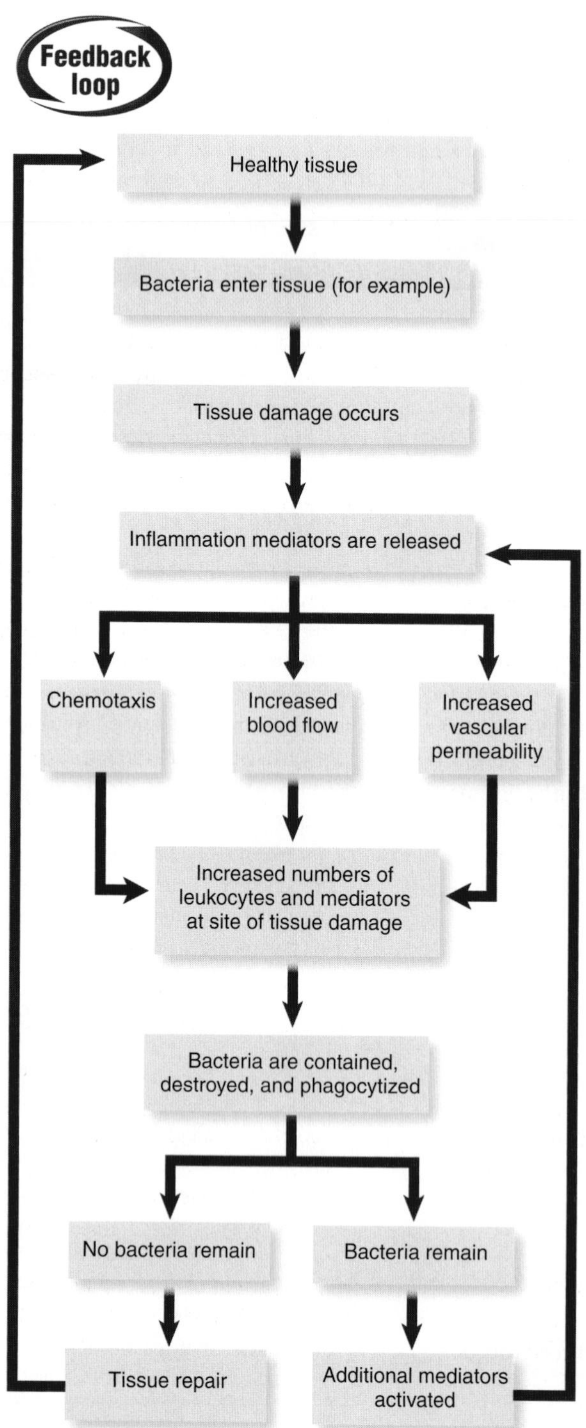

FIGURE 14-6 Inflammatory response. In this example, bacterial infection triggers a set of responses that tend to inhibit or destroy the bacteria.

These signs of inflammation are caused by increased blood flow (resulting in heat and redness) and vascular permeability (resulting in tissue swelling and the pain that it causes) in the affected region. Such changes help phagocytic WBCs and beneficial proteins reach the general area and enter the affected tissue.

Besides local inflammation, systemic inflammation may occur when the inflammation mediators—cytokines and other chemical signals—trigger responses that occur on a body-wide basis. A systemic (body-wide) inflammatory response may be manifested by a **fever**—a state of abnormally high body temperature. The elevated temperature of a low to moderate fever may facilitate some immune reactions and may also inhibit the reproduction of some bacteria. However, immunologists still debate the role of fever in protecting the body.

A class of enzymes in blood plasma called complement can trigger a cascade of chemical reactions that literally punch holes in abnormal cells and regulate other immune mechanisms. Complement can be triggered by both innate, nonspecific mechanisms and by specific immune mechanisms—as we discuss later in this chapter.

Specific Immunity

Specific immunity includes protective mechanisms that confer very specific protection against certain types of threatening microorganisms or other toxic materials. Specific immunity includes a long-term protective function called *immune memory,* which allows the immune system to effectively stop a second attack by the same specific pathogen. Because it is able to adapt to newly encountered "enemies," specific immunity is often called **adaptive immunity.**

In specific immunity, when the body is first attacked by particular bacteria or viruses, disease symptoms may occur as the body fights to destroy the threatening organism. However, if the body is exposed a second time to the same threatening organism, no serious symptoms occur because the organism is destroyed quickly—the person is said to be *immune* to that particular organism. Immunity is said to be specific because protection against one type of disease-causing microbe does not protect the body against others.

As **Table 14-1** shows, specific immune responses are slow compared with nonspecific immune responses. However, specific immune responses have memory—the ability to produce a stronger, faster response to repeated exposure to the same antigen. **Table 14-1** summarizes other important features of both types of immunity, some of which are discussed later in this chapter.

Specific immunity may be classified as either "natural" or "artificial" depending on how the body is exposed to the harmful agent (**Table 14-3**). Natural exposure is not deliberate and occurs in the course of everyday living. We are naturally exposed to many disease-causing agents on a regular basis. Artificial exposure is called **immunization** and is the deliberate exposure of the body to a potentially harmful agent.

TABLE 14-3 Types of Specific Immunity

TYPE	EXAMPLE
Natural immunity	Exposure to the causative agent is not deliberate, happens naturally in course of living.
Active immunity	A child develops measles and acquires immunity to a subsequent infection.
Passive immunity	A fetus receives protection from the mother through the placenta, or an infant receives protection via the mother's milk.
Artificial immunity	Exposure to the causative agent is deliberate.
Active immunity	Injection of the causative agent, such as a vaccination against polio, activates the immune system and thus confers immunity.
Passive immunity	Injection of protective material (antibodies) that was developed by another individual's immune system is given.

Natural and artificial immunity may be "active" or "passive."

- Active immunity occurs when an individual's own immune system responds to an agent that produces an immune response, regardless of whether that agent was naturally or artificially encountered.
- Passive immunity results when immunity to a disease that has developed in another individual or animal is transferred to an individual who was not previously immune. For example, antibodies in a mother's milk confer passive immunity to her nursing infant.
- Active immunity generally lasts longer than passive immunity. Passive immunity, although temporary, provides immediate protection.

Table 14-3 lists the various forms of specific immunity and gives examples of each.

QUICK CHECK

1. What is the difference between *specific immunity* and *nonspecific* immunity?
2. What are the changes that occur in the body's inflammatory response?

Immune System Molecules

The immune system functions because of adequate amounts of defensive protein molecules and protective cells. Molecules critical to immune system functioning include **cytokines, antibodies,** and **complement** proteins.

Cytokines

As mentioned earlier in this chapter, cytokines are chemicals released from cells to act as direct agents of innate, nonspecific immunity. They can also trigger or regulate many innate and adaptive immune responses. Often cytokines are critical to the cell-to-cell communication that is needed to coordinate the combined innate and adaptive actions that are unleashed during any immune response.

Many of the cytokines are proteins called **interleukins (ILs).** This name is apt for a substance used by WBCs to communicate between cells, because *inter-* means "between," *-leuk-* refers to leukocytes, and *-in* means "substance." ILs are often involved in signaling in both innate and adaptive immune mechanisms. For example, ILs are involved in producing a fever and in activating the cells of adaptive, specific immunity.

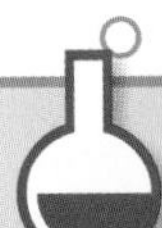

SCIENCE APPLICATIONS

VACCINES

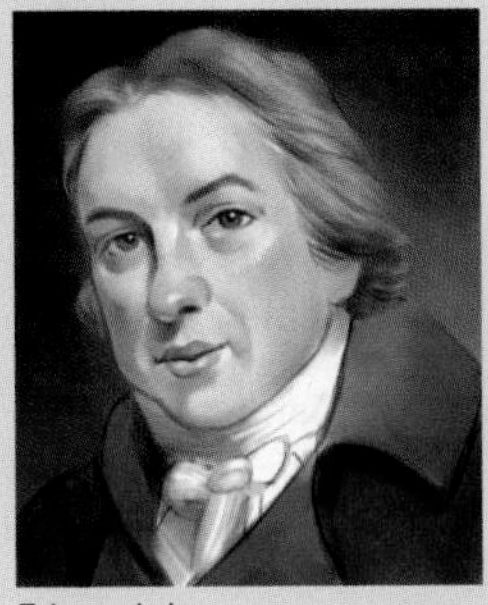

Edward Jenner (1749–1823)

English surgeon Edward Jenner changed the world forever in 1789 when he inoculated his young son and two others against the terrible viral disease smallpox. Using material from the blisters of a patient with the milder disease swinepox, he was able to trigger immunity to smallpox—the world's first vaccination. Later, in 1796, he found that vaccination with material from cowpox blisters worked even better in protecting people from smallpox. A disease that had formerly killed millions of people worldwide eventually disappeared from the human population in the twentieth century because of Jenner's pioneering efforts.

In this century, interest in smallpox vaccinations has resurfaced because of the threat of smallpox as a weapon. Immunologists are at work improving on this important vaccine to protect people against such weapons. They also continue to work on vaccines for other infectious diseases such as Ebola, malaria, acquired immunodeficiency syndrome (AIDS), and even disorders such as heart disease and cancer. Many health care professionals use vaccines in their practice to boost the immune systems of their clients.

Many *physicians* also treat disorders of the immune system itself. For example, immune deficiencies such as AIDS, allergies such as "hay fever," and autoimmune disorders such as lupus and rheumatoid arthritis are treated every day by physicians and other health professionals.

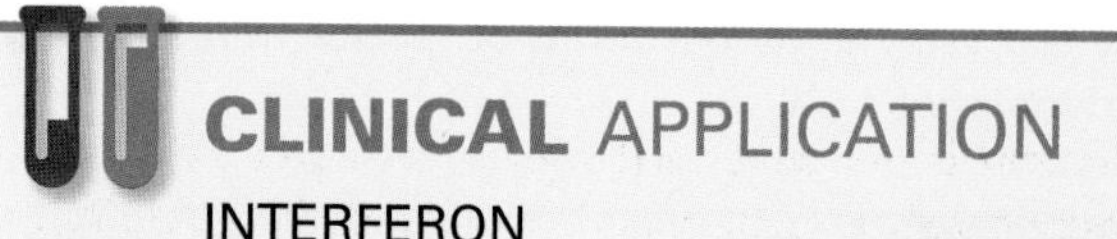

CLINICAL APPLICATION

INTERFERON

Interferon (IF) is a type of small protein compound that plays a very significant role in producing innate immunity against viral infections. It is a cytokine produced by body cells within hours after they have been infected by a virus. The IF released from the virus-infected cells protects other cells by interfering with the ability of the virus to reproduce as it moves from cell to cell.

In the past, thousands of pints of blood had to be processed to harvest tiny quantities of leukocyte interferon for study. Synthetic human IF is now being "manufactured" in bacteria as a result of gene-splicing techniques and is available in quantities sufficient for clinical use. Synthetic IF decreases the severity of many virus-related diseases, including chickenpox, measles, and hepatitis C. Interferon also shows promise as an anticancer agent. It has been shown to be effective in treating breast, skin, and other forms of cancer.

Antibodies

Definition

Antibodies are a class of proteins that are normally present in the body. A defining characteristic of an antibody molecule is the uniquely shaped concave regions, called **combining sites,** on its surface. Another defining characteristic is the ability of an antibody molecule to combine with a specific compound called an **antigen.**

All antigens are compounds whose molecules have small regions on their surfaces that are uniquely shaped to fit into the combining sites of a specific antibody molecule as precisely as a key fits into a specific lock. Antigens are often protein molecules embedded in the surface membranes of threatening or diseased cells, such as microorganisms or cancer cells.

Functions

In general, antibodies produce **humoral immunity,** or **antibody-mediated immunity,** by changing the antigens in a way that prevents them from harming the body (**Figure 14-7**). To do this, an antibody must first bind to its specific antigen. This forms an antigen-antibody complex. The antigen-antibody complex then acts in one or more ways to make the antigen, or the cell on which it is present, harmless.

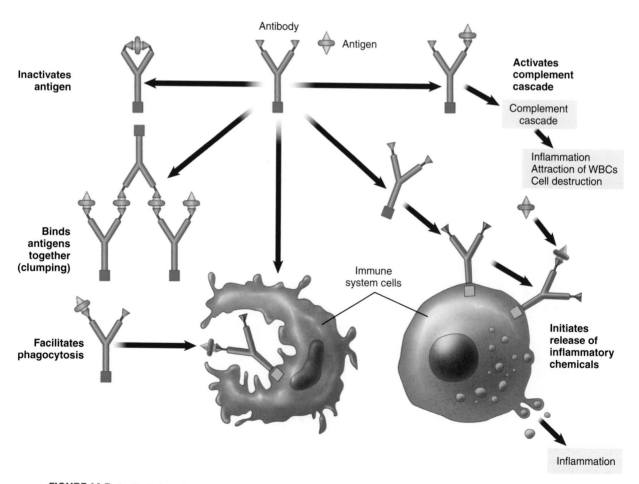

FIGURE 14-7 Antibody function. Antibodies produce humoral immunity by binding to specific antigens to form antigen-antibody complexes. These complexes produce a variety of changes that inactivate or kill threatening cells. *WBCs,* White blood cells.

For example, if the antigen is a toxin (that is, a substance poisonous to body cells), the toxin is neutralized or made nonpoisonous by becoming part of an antigen-antibody complex. Or if antigens are molecules in the surface membranes of threatening cells, when antibodies combine with them, the resulting antigen-antibody complexes may **agglutinate** the enemy cells (that is, make them stick together in clumps). Then macrophages or the other phagocytes can rapidly destroy them by ingesting and digesting large numbers of them at one time.

Another important function of antibodies is promotion and enhancement of phagocytosis. Certain antibody fractions help promote the attachment of phagocytic cells to the object they will engulf. As a result, the contact between the phagocytic cell and its victim is enhanced, and the object is more easily ingested. This process contributes to the efficiency of immune system phagocytic cells, which is described on p. 323.

Probably the most important way in which antibodies act is a process called the **complement cascade.** Often when antigens that are molecules on an antigenic or foreign cell's surface combine with antibody molecules, they change the shape of the antibody molecule slightly but just enough to expose two previously hidden regions. These are called **complement-binding sites.** The exposure of the complement-binding sites of an antibody that is attached to an antigen on the surface of a threatening cell then permits complement proteins to initiate a series of events that kill the cell. The next section describes these events.

To learn more about antibodies and antigens, go to AnimationDirect at *evolve.elsevier.com*.

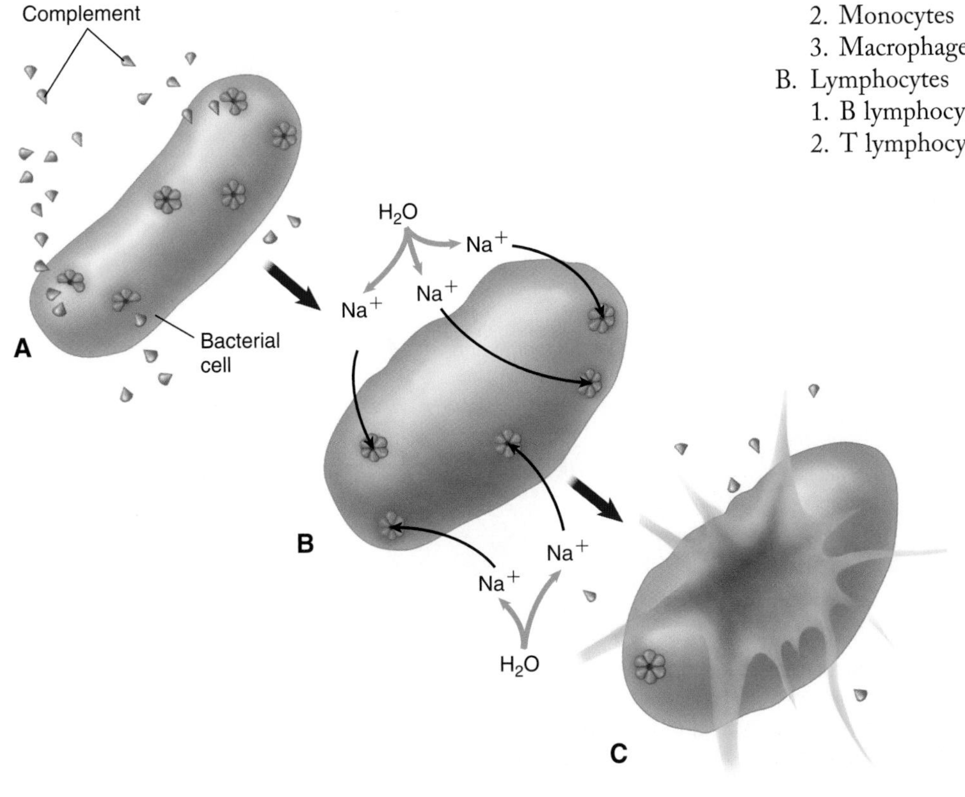

Complement Proteins

Complement is the name used to describe a group of protein enzymes normally present in an inactive state in blood. These proteins may be activated by several triggers, including exposure of complement-binding sites on antibodies when they attach to antigens. The result is formation of highly specialized protein molecules that target foreign cells for destruction. The process is a rapid-fire cascade or sequence of events collectively called the **complement cascade.** The end result of this process is that doughnut-shaped protein rings (complete with a hole in the middle) are formed and literally bore holes in the foreign cell!

The tiny holes allow sodium to rapidly diffuse into the cell. Water follows, through the process of osmosis. The cell literally bursts as the internal osmotic pressure increases (**Figure 14-8**).

Complement proteins also serve other roles in the immune system, such as attracting immune cells to a site of infection, activating immune cells, marking foreign cells for destruction, and increasing permeability of blood vessels. Complement proteins also play a vital role in producing the inflammatory response.

QUICK CHECK

1. What are antibodies? How do they function in the body?
2. What are complement proteins? How do they function in the body?

Immune System Cells

The primary cells of the immune system include the following:

A. Phagocytes
   1. Neutrophils
   2. Monocytes
   3. Macrophages
B. Lymphocytes
   1. B lymphocytes
   2. T lymphocytes

FIGURE 14-8 Complement cascade. **A,** Complement molecules activated by antibodies form doughnut-shaped complexes in a bacterium's plasma membrane. **B,** Holes in the complement complex allow sodium (Na^+) and then water (H_2O) to diffuse into the bacterium. **C,** After enough water has entered, the swollen bacterium bursts. This is just one of many functions of the complement proteins.

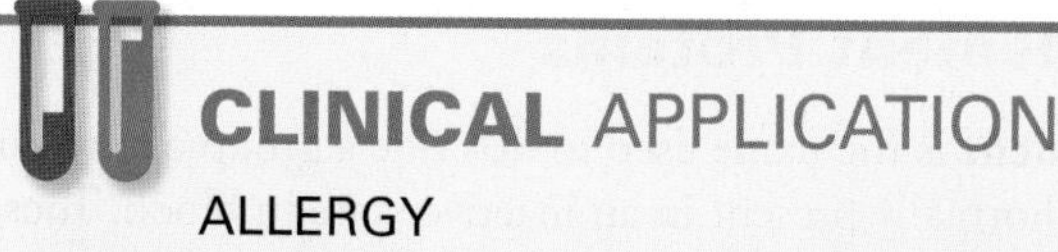

CLINICAL APPLICATION

ALLERGY

The term **allergy** is used to describe hypersensitivity of the immune system to relatively harmless environmental antigens. One in six Americans has a genetic predisposition to an allergy. Immediate allergic responses involve antigen-antibody reactions that trigger the release of histamine, kinins, and other inflammatory substances. These responses usually cause symptoms such as a runny nose, conjunctivitis, and hives. In some cases, these substances may cause constriction of airways, relaxation of blood vessels, and irregular heart rhythms that can lead to a life-threatening condition called **anaphylactic shock.** Delayed allergic responses, on the other hand, involve cell-mediated immunity. In contact dermatitis, for example, T lymphocytes trigger events that lead to local skin inflammation a few hours or even days after initial exposure.

Phagocytes

Phagocytic WBCs are an important part of the immune system. In Chapter 12, phagocytes were described as bone-marrow–derived cells that carry on phagocytosis, or ingestion and digestion of foreign cells or particles.

Antibody molecules that bind to and coat certain foreign particles help macrophages function effectively. They serve as "flags" that alert the macrophage to the presence of foreign material, infectious bacteria, or cellular debris. They also help bind the phagocyte to the foreign material so that it can be engulfed more effectively (**Figure 14-9**).

Two important phagocytes are neutrophils and monocytes (see **Figure 12-8**, p. 272). These blood phagocytes migrate out of the blood and into the tissues in response to an infection.

The neutrophils are functional but short lived in the tissues. The pus found at some infection sites is mostly dead neutrophils.

Once in the tissues, monocytes develop into phagocytic cells called **macrophages**. Most macrophages then "wander"

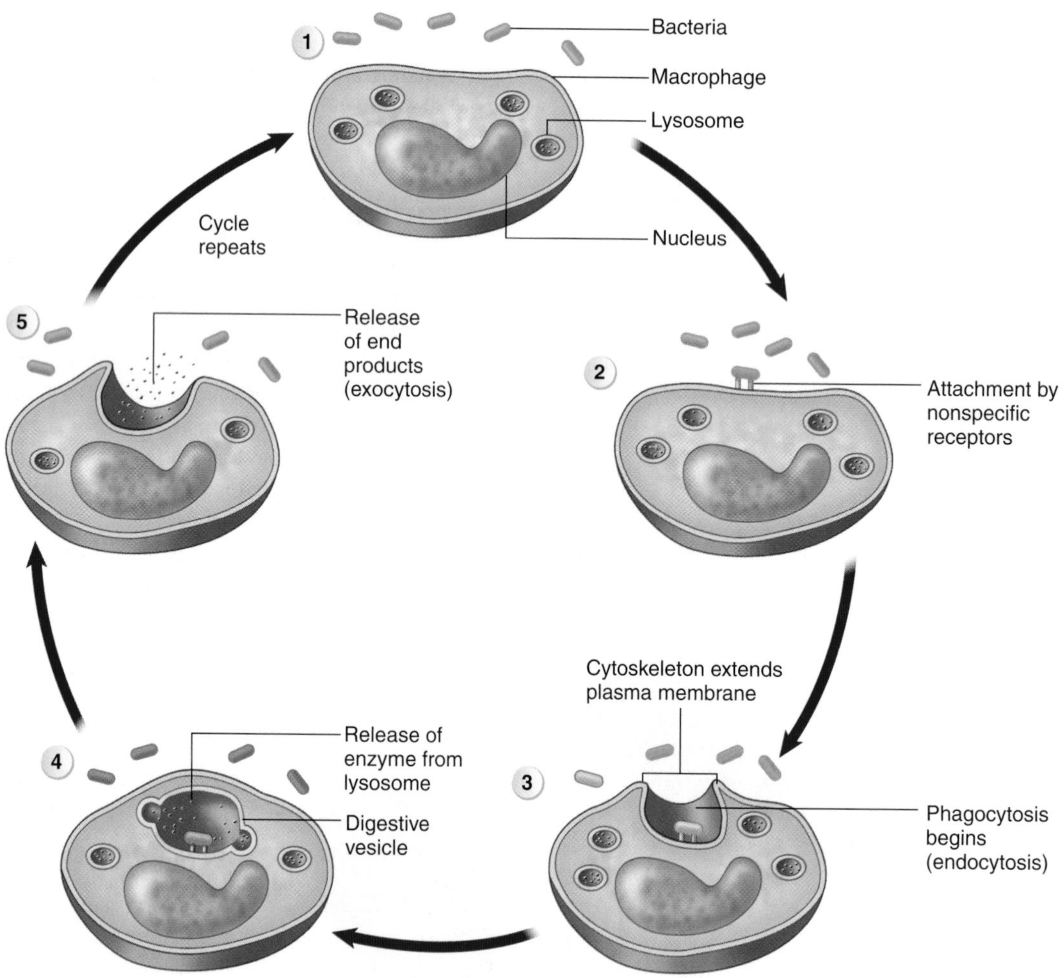

FIGURE 14-9 Phagocytosis of bacteria. Drawing shows sequence of steps in phagocytosis of bacteria. The plasma membrane extends toward the bacterial cells, then envelops them. Once trapped, they are engulfed by the cell and destroyed by lysosomal enzymes.

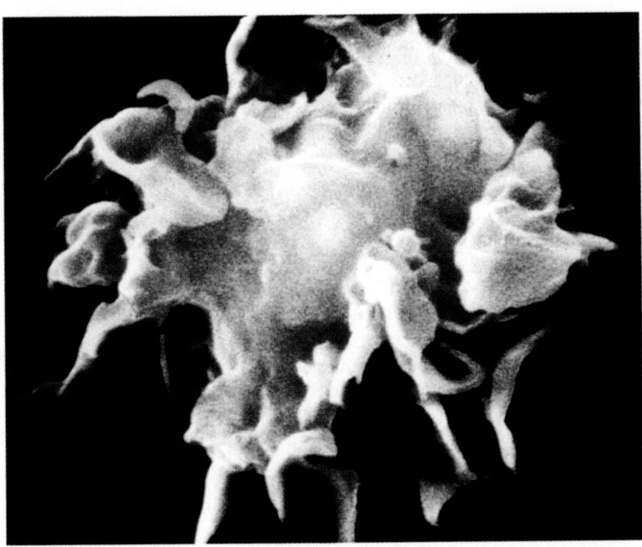

FIGURE 14-10 Dendritic cell (DC). Scanning electron micrograph showing the detail of projections of the plasma membrane. DCs are phagocytic antigen-presenting cells (APCs) that are found in many areas of the body.

through the tissues to engulf bacteria wherever they find them.

Another type of phagocytic cell is called the **dendritic cell (DC)**. These highly branched (*dendrite* "branch") cells are produced in bone marrow and are released into the bloodstream (**Figure 14-10**). Some remain in the blood, but many migrate to tissues in contact with the external environment—the skin, respiratory lining, digestive lining, and so on. Resident DCs in these barrier regions help protect us from threatening particles and cells.

Macrophages and DCs perform another important immune function besides destruction of threatening cells and particles. They also act as **antigen-presenting cells (APCs)**. Macrophages and DCs ingest a cell or particle, remove its antigens, and display some of them on their cell surfaces. The displayed antigens can then be presented to other immune cells to trigger additional, specific immune responses.

Lymphocytes

The most numerous cells of the immune system are the lymphocytes (**Figure 14-11**). Lymphocytes are responsible for antibody production and other adaptive immune mechanisms. Lymphocytes circulate in the body's fluids. Huge numbers of them wander vigilantly throughout most of its tissues. Several million strong, lymphocytes continually patrol the body, searching out any enemy cells that may have entered or threatening virus-infected cells and cancer cells.

Developing and reserve lymphocytes densely populate the body's widely scattered lymph nodes and its other lymphoid tissues, especially the thymus gland in the chest and the spleen and liver in the abdomen.

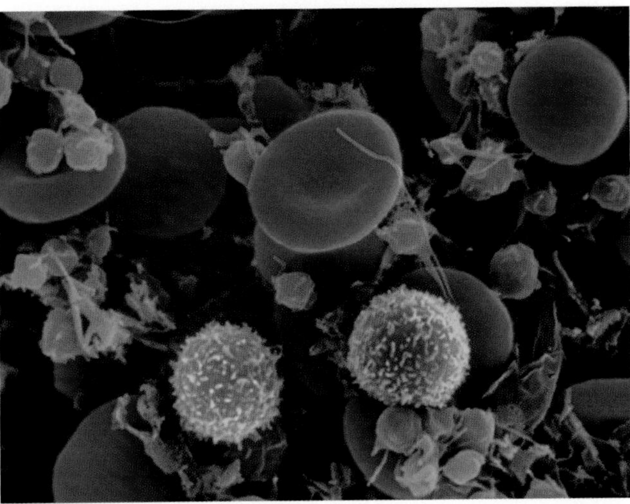

FIGURE 14-11 Lymphocytes. Color-enhanced scanning electron micrograph showing lymphocytes in yellow, red blood cells in red, and platelets in green.

There are two major types of lymphocytes sometimes designated as **B lymphocytes** and **T lymphocytes** but usually called **B cells** and **T cells.** Each type of lymphocyte has the same appearance, but has a different set of roles to play in immunity.

B Cells

Development of B Cells

All lymphocytes that circulate in the tissues arise from primitive cells in the bone marrow called *stem cells* and go through two stages of development. The first stage of B-cell development—transformation of stem cells into immature B cells—occurs in the liver and bone marrow before birth but only in the bone marrow in adults. Because this process was first discovered in a bird organ called the *bursa*, these cells were named *B cells*.

Immature B cells are small lymphocytes that have synthesized and inserted into their cytoplasmic membranes numerous molecules of one specific kind of antibody (**Figure 14-12**).

After they mature, B cells eventually leave the tissue where they were formed. Each mature, but inactive, B cell carries a different type of antibody. The various B cells then enter the blood and are transported to their new place of residence, chiefly the lymph nodes.

The second stage of B-cell development changes a mature, inactive B cell into an activated B cell. Not all B cells undergo this change. They do so only if an inactive B cell comes in contact with certain nonself or abnormal molecules—antigens—whose shape fits into the shape of the B cell's surface antibody molecules. If this happens, the antigens lock onto the antibodies and, by so doing, change the inactive B cell into an activated B cell. B-cell activation also requires a chemical signal (cytokine) from another immune cell—a type of T cell. Then the activated B cell, by dividing rapidly and repeatedly, develops into groups or clones of many identical

FIGURE 14-12 B-cell development. B-cell development takes place in two stages. *First stage:* Shortly before and after birth, stem cells develop into immature B cells, which then mature into inactive B cells that migrate to lymphoid organs. *Second stage* (occurs only when the inactive B cell contacts its specific antigen): Inactive B cell develops into activated B cell, which divides rapidly and repeatedly to form a clone of plasma cells and a clone of memory cells. Plasma cells then secrete antibodies capable of combining with the specific antigen that began the process. Stem cells maintain a constant population of newly differentiating inactive B cells.

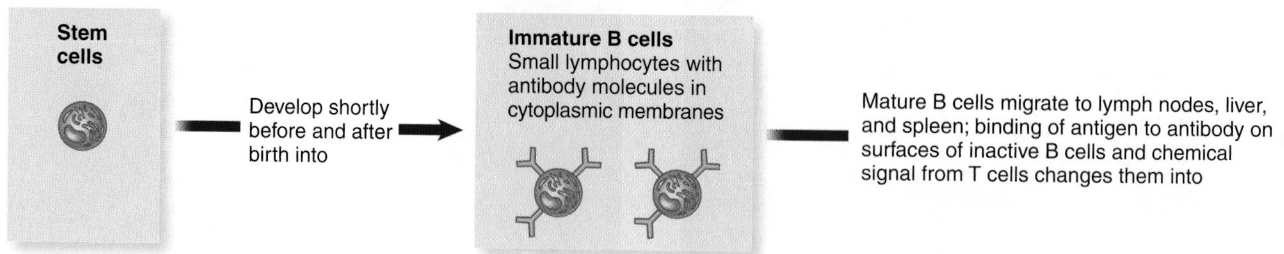

cells—all having the same type of antibody. A **clone** is a family of many identical cells, all descended from one cell.

Each clone of B cells is made up of two kinds of cells, **plasma cells** (also called **effector cells**) and **memory cells,** as you can see in **Figure 14-12**. Plasma cells secrete huge amounts of antibody into the blood—reportedly, 2000 antibody molecules per second by each plasma cell for every second of the few days that it lives. Antibodies circulating in the blood constitute an enormous, mobile, ever-on-duty army.

Memory cells can secrete antibodies but do not immediately do so. They remain in reserve in the lymph nodes until they are contacted by the same antigen that led to their formation. Then, very quickly, the memory cells develop into plasma cells and secrete large numbers of antibodies. Memory cells, in effect, seem to "remember" their ancestor-activated B cell's encounter with its appropriate antigen. They stand ready, at a moment's notice, to produce antibodies that will combine with this antigen.

Function of B Cells

B cells function indirectly to produce humoral immunity. Recall that humoral immunity is resistance to disease organisms produced by the actions of antibodies binding to specific antigens while circulating in body fluids. Activated B cells develop into plasma cells. **Plasma cells** secrete antibodies into the blood; they are the "antibody factories" of the body. These antibodies, like other proteins manufactured for extracellular use, are formed on the endoplasmic reticulum of the cell.

T Cells

Development of T Cells

T cells are lymphocytes that have undergone their first stage of development in the thymus gland. Stem cells from the bone marrow seed the thymus, and shortly before and after birth, they develop into T cells. The newly formed T cells stream out of the thymus into the blood and migrate chiefly to the lymph nodes, where they take up residence. Embedded in each T cell's cytoplasmic membrane are protein molecules shaped to fit only one specific kind of antigen molecule.

The second stage of T-cell development takes place when and if a T cell comes into contact with its specific antigen. If this happens, the antigen binds to the protein on the T cell's surface, thereby changing the T cell to an activated T cell (**Figure 14-13**).

As with B cells, T cells must also receive a chemical (cytokine) signal from another T cell to become activated. Likewise, T cells also produce a clone of identical cells, all able to react with the same antigen.

And as with B cells, T cells form a group of *effector cells* along with *memory cells*. The effector T cells actively engage in immune responses, whereas the memory T cells do not. Later,

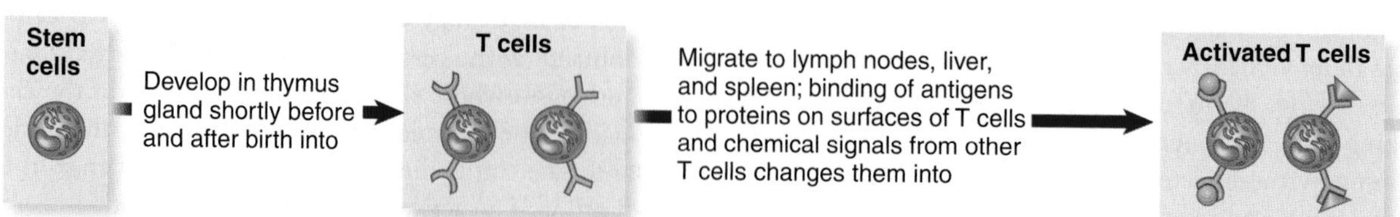

FIGURE 14-13 T-cell development. The first stage takes place in the thymus gland shortly before and after birth. Stem cells maintain a constant population of newly differentiating cells as they are needed. The second stage occurs only if a T cell contacts an antigen, which combines with certain proteins on the T cell's surface.

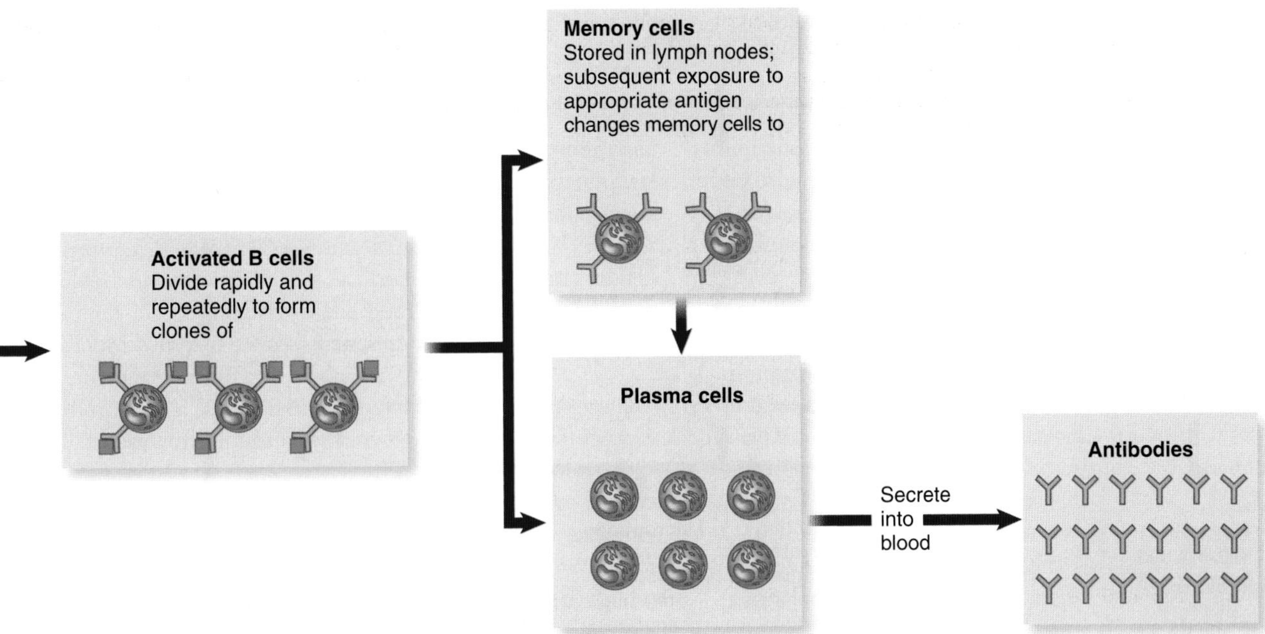
Memory cells
Stored in lymph nodes; subsequent exposure to appropriate antigen changes memory cells to
Activated B cells
Divide rapidly and repeatedly to form clones of
Plasma cells
Secrete into blood
Antibodies

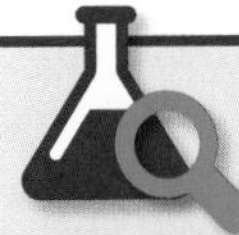

RESEARCH, ISSUES, AND TRENDS

MUCOSAL IMMUNITY

The *mucosal immune system* is a complex system of defense distinct from the systemic (internal) immune system, which has been discussed in most of this chapter. It includes both innate (nonspecific) and adaptive (specific) mechanisms that are found within the mucous barriers of the body: digestive tract, urinary/reproductive tracts, respiratory tract, exocrine ducts, conjunctiva (eye covering), middle ear, and so on. The immune cells that make up the mucosal immune system are located mainly in or near *mucosal-associated lymphoid tissue (MALT)*.

The main functions of the mucosal immune system involve preventing pathogens from colonizing the mucous surfaces of the body, preventing the accidental absorption of antigens from outside the body, and blocking inappropriate or intense responses of the systemic immune system to these external antigens.

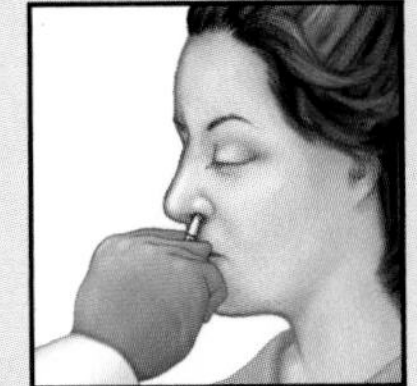

Understanding the mucosal immune system and its cooperation with the systemic (internal) immune system promises to reveal new strategies of immunization. For example, researchers have found that immunizing through the bloodstream activates only the internal (systemic) B cells and T cells. Thus a pathogen would have to actually enter our internal environment before this type of specific immunity could protect us. Immunization of the mucosal lymphocytes, however, can activate both mucosal and systemic lymphocytes, providing a more thorough type of protection. Another advantage of mucosal immunization is that it is easier to administer to patients than immunizations injected under the skin or into the bloodstream. For example, immunization can be delivered by nasal sprays or drops instead of "shots."

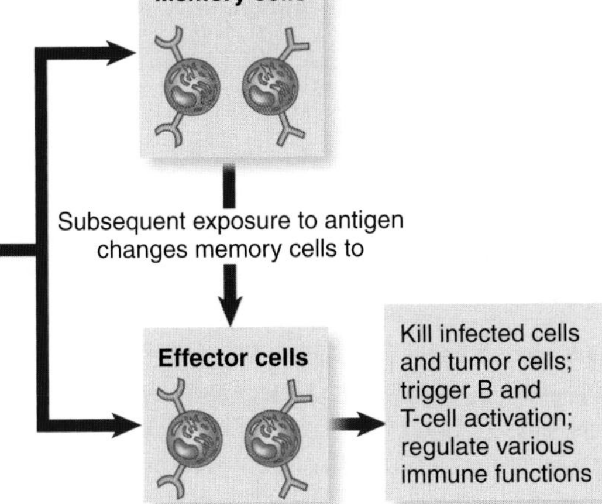
Memory cells
Subsequent exposure to antigen changes memory cells to
Effector cells
Kill infected cells and tumor cells; trigger B and T-cell activation; regulate various immune functions

if more effector T cells are needed, the memory T cells can produce additional clones that include more effector T cells.

Functions of T Cells

Activated T cells produce cell-mediated immunity. As the name suggests, **cell-mediated immunity** is resistance to disease organisms that results from the actions of cells—chiefly, sensitized T cells. One group of activated T cells kills infected cells and tumor cells directly. When bound to antigens, these *cytotoxic T cells* release a substance that acts as a specific and lethal poison against the abnormal cell.

Activated T cells called *helper T cells* produce their deadly effects indirectly by means of chemical signals that they release into the area around enemy cells. Among these is a

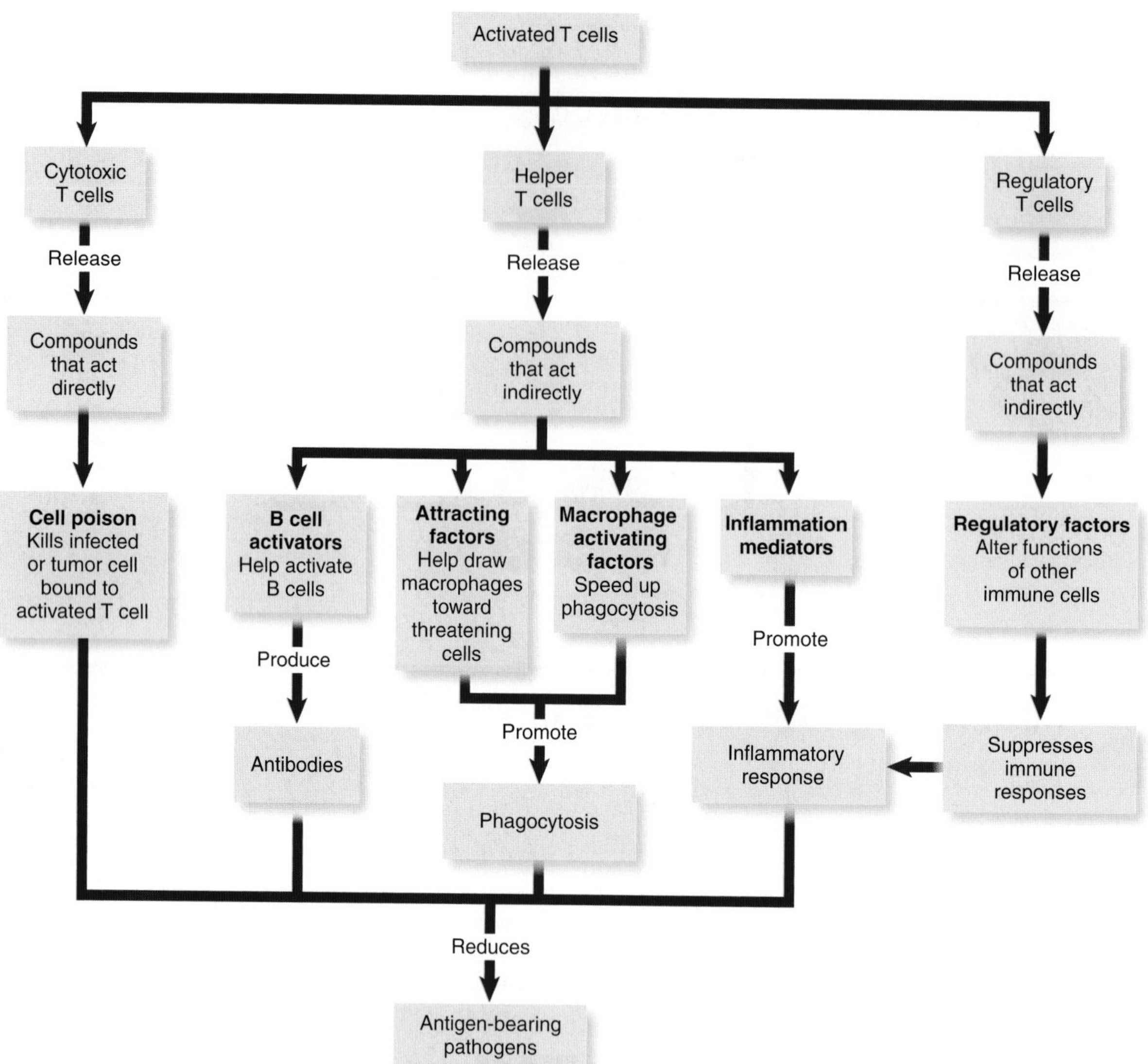

FIGURE 14-14 T-cell function. Activated T cells produce cell-mediated immunity by releasing various compounds near infected or tumor cells. Some compounds act directly, and some act indirectly on these cells.

substance that attracts macrophages into the vicinity of the enemy cells. The assembled macrophages then destroy the cells by phagocytosing (ingesting and digesting) them (**Figure 14-14**). Helper T cells also release the cytokines needed to help trigger the activation of B cells.

A third group of T cells called *regulatory T cells* helps shut down an immune reaction after the antigens have been destroyed and also helps prevent inappropriate immune reactions.

QUICK CHECK

1. What are phagocytes and how do they function in the body?
2. What is the role of B cells in immunity?
3. What is the role of T cells in immunity?
4. What are memory cells?

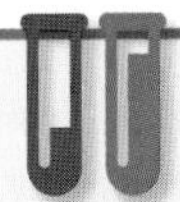

CLINICAL APPLICATION

HUMAN IMMUNODEFICIENCY VIRUS INFECTION

Infection by **HIV** (**human immunodeficiency virus**) is a worldwide health concern. HIV infection has reached epidemic proportions in many countries, thus qualifying as a *pandemic.*

HIV, a retrovirus, contains RNA that undergoes reverse transcription inside infected cells to form its own DNA. The viral DNA often becomes part of the cell's DNA. When the viral DNA is activated, it directs the synthesis of its own RNA and protein coat, thus "stealing" raw materials from the cell. When this occurs in certain T cells, the cell is destroyed, and immunity is impaired. As the T cell dies, it releases new retroviruses that can spread the HIV infection.

Although HIV can invade several types of cells, it has its most obvious effects in a certain type of T cell called a *CD4*$^{+}$ T cell. The CD4^{+} cells give rise to helper T cells, and when they are not able to complete their normal functions, infectious organisms and cancer cells can grow and spread much more easily than normal. Unusual conditions, such as *pneumocystosis* (a protozoan infection) and *Kaposi sarcoma* (a type of skin cancer), may also appear. Because their immune systems are deficient, AIDS patients may eventually die from one of these infections or cancers.

HIV infection sometimes progresses to a collection of symptoms called **AIDS,** or **acquired immunodeficiency syndrome.** After infection with HIV, an untreated person may not show signs of AIDS for months or years. This is because the immune system can hold the infection at bay for a long time before finally succumbing to it.

There are several strategies for preventing the development of AIDS. Many agencies are trying to reduce the incidence of AIDS by educating people about how to avoid contact with the HIV retrovirus. HIV is spread by means of direct contact of body fluids, so preventing such contact reduces HIV transmission. Sexual relations, contaminated blood transfusions, and intravenous use of contaminated needles are the usual modes of HIV transmission. HIV can also be a *perinatal infection,* that is, an infection passing from mother to infant during birth. Many researchers are working on HIV vaccines. Like many viruses, including those that cause the common cold, HIV changes rapidly enough to make development of a vaccine very challenging.

Another way to inhibit the progress of an HIV infection is by means of chemicals such as azidothymidine (AZT) and ritonavir (Norvir) that block HIV's ability to reproduce within infected cells. A "cocktail" of several antiviral drugs working together greatly reduces the number of virus particles in a patient's blood, thus reducing the effects of HIV infection. More than 100 such compounds in various combinations are being evaluated for use in halting the progress of HIV infections.

LANGUAGE OF SCIENCE AND MEDICINE *(continued from p. 317)*

antigen
(AN-tih-jen)
[*anti-* **against,** *-gen* **produce**]

antigen-presenting cell (APC)
(AN-tih-jen prih-ZENT-ing sel)
[*anti-* **against,** *-gen* **produce,** *present-* **place before,** *-ing* **result,** *cell-* **storeroom**]

B cell (B lymphocyte)
(bee sel [bee LIM-foh-syte])
[*B* **bursa-equivalent tissue,** *cell* **storeroom** (*lympho-* **water (lymphatic system),** *-cyte* **cell**)]

cell-mediated immunity
(sel-MEE-dee-ayt-ed ih-MYOO-nih-tee)
[*cell* **storeroom,** *-medi-* **middle,** *-ate* **process,** *immun-* **free,** *-ity* **state**]

cisterna chyli
(sis-TER-nah KYE-lye)
[*cisterna* **vessel,** *chyli* **of juice**]

clone
(klohn)
[*clon-* **plant cutting**]

combining site
(kom-BINE-ing syte)

complement
(KOM-pleh-ment)
[*comple-* **complete,** *-ment* **result of action**]

complement cascade
(KOM-pleh-ment kas-KAYD)
[*comple-* **complete,** *-ment* **result of action,** *cascade* **waterfall**]

complement-binding site
(KOM-pleh-ment BIND-ing syte)
[*comple-* **complete,** *-ment* **result of action**]

cytokine
(SYE-toh-kyne)
[*cyto-* **cell,** *-kine* **movement**]

dendritic cell (DC)
(DEN-drih-tik sell)
[*dendrit-* **tree branch,** *-ic* **relating to,** *cell* **storeroom**]

effector cell
(ef-FEK-tor sel)
[*effect-* **accomplish,** *-or* **agent,** *cell* **storeroom**]

efferent lymphatic vessel
(EF-fer-ent lim-FAT-ik VES-el)
[*e-* **away,** *-fer-* **carry,** *-ent* **relating to,** *lymph-* **water,** *-atic* **relating to**]

fever
(FEE-ver)

human immunodeficiency virus (HIV)
(imyoo-no-deh-FISH-en-see)
[*immuno-* **free (immunity),** *-de-* **down,** *-fic-* **perform,** *-ency* **state,** *virus* **poison**]

humoral immunity
(HYOO-mor-al ih-MYOO-nih-tee)
[*humor-* **liquid,** *-al* **relating to,** *immun-* **free,** *-ity* **state**]

immune system
(ih-MYOON)
[*immun-* **free (immunity)**]

immunization
(ih-myoo-nih-ZAY-shun)
[*immun-* **free (immunity),** *-tion* **process**]

inflammatory response
(in-FLAM-ah-toh-ree ree-SPONS)
[*inflam-* **set afire,** *-ory* **relating to**]

innate immunity
(IN-ayt ih-MYOO-nih-tee)
[*innat-* **inborn,** *immun-* **free,** *-ity* **state**]

interferon (IF)
(in-ter-FEER-on)
[*inter-* **between,** *-fer-* **strike,** *-on* **substance**]

interleukins
(in-ter-LOO-kin)
[*inter-* **between,** *-leuk-* **white (blood cell),** *-in* **substance**]

interstitial fluid (IF)
(in-ter-STISH-al)
[*inter-* **between,** *-stit-* **stand,** *-al* **relating to**]

lacteal
(LAK-tee-al)
[*lact-* **milk,** *-al* **relating to**]

lingual tonsil
(LING-gwal TAHN-sil)
[*lingua-* **tongue,** *-al* **relating to,** *tons-* **goiter,** *-il* **little**]

lymph
(limf)
[*lymph* **water**]

lymph node
(limf nohd)
[*lymph* **water,** *nod-* **knot**]

lymphatic capillary
(lim-FAT-ik KAP-ih-layr-ee)
[*lymph-* **water,** *-atic* **relating to,** *capill-* **hair,** *-ary* **relating to**]

lymphatic vessel
(lim-FAT-ik)
[*lymph-* **water,** *-atic* **relating to**]

lymphoid tissue
(LIM-foyd)
[*lymph-* **water (lymphatic system),** *-oid* **like,** *tissu* **fabric**]

macrophage
(MAK-roh-fayj)
[*macro-* **large,** *-phag-* **eat**]

memory cell
(MEM-oh-ree sel)
[*cell* **storeroom**]

nonspecific immunity
(non-speh-SIF-ik ih-MYOO-nih-tee)
[*non-* **not,** *-spec-* **form or kind,** *-ific* **relating to,** *immun-* **free,** *-ity* **state**]

palatine tonsil
(PAL-ah-tine TAHN-sil)
[*palat-* **palate,** *-ine* **relating to,** *tons-* **goiter,** *-il* **little**]

pharyngeal tonsil
(fah-RIN-jee-al TAHN-sil)
[*pharyng-* **throat,** *-al* **relating to,** *tons-* **goiter,** *-il* **little**]

plasma cell (effector B cell)
(PLAZ-mah sell [ef-FEK-tor bee sel])
[*plasma* **something molded (blood plasma),** *cell* **storeroom (***effect-* **accomplish,** *-or* **agent,** *B* **bursa-equivalent tissue**]

right lymphatic duct
(lim-FAT-ik)
[*lymph-* **water,** *-atic* **relating to**]

specific immunity
(speh-SIF-ik ih-MYOO-nih-tee)
[*spec-* **form or kind,** *-ific* **relating to,** *immun-* **free,** *-ity* **state**]

spleen

splenectomy
(spleh-NEK-toh-mee)
[*splen-* **spleen,** *-ec-* **out,** *-tom-* **cut,** *-y* **action**]

T cell (T lymphocyte)
(tee sel [tee LIM-foh-syte])
[*T* **thymus gland,** *cell* **storeroom (***T* **thymus gland,** *lymph-* **water [lymphatic system]),** *-cyte* **cell**]

thoracic duct
(thoh-RASS-ik)
[*thorac-* **chest (thorax),** *-ic* **relating to,** *duct* **lead**]

thymosin
(THY-moh-sin)
[*thymos-* **thyme flower (thymus gland),** *-in* **substance**]

thymus
(THY-mus)
pl., thymuses or thymi
(THY-muss-ez or THY-mye)
[*thymus* **thyme flower**]

❑ OUTLINE SUMMARY

To download a digital audio version of the chapter summary for use with your device, access the ***Audio Chapter Summaries*** *online at evolve.elsevier.com.*

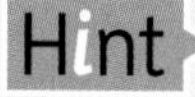

Scan this summary after reading the chapter to help you reinforce the key concepts. Later, use the summary as a quick review before your class or before a test.

The Lymphatic System

A. Organization of the lymphatic system — lymphatic fluid (lymph), lymphatic vessels, and many lymph organs make up this system (see **Figure 14-1**)
B. Lymph — excess fluid left behind by capillary exchange that drains from tissue spaces and is transported by *lymphatic vessels* back to the bloodstream
C. Lymphatic vessels — permit only one-way movement of lymph
   1. Lymphatic capillaries — tiny blind-ended tubes distributed in tissue spaces (see **Figure 14-2**)
      a. Microscopic in size
      b. Sheets consisting of one cell layer of simple squamous epithelium
      c. Poor "fit" between adjacent cells results in porous walls
      d. Called *lacteals* in the intestinal wall (fat transportation from digestive tract to bloodstream)
   2. Right lymphatic duct
      a. Drains lymph from the right upper extremity and right side of head, neck, and upper torso
   3. Thoracic duct
      a. Largest lymphatic vessel
      b. Has an enlarged pouch along its course, called *cisterna chyli*
      c. Drains lymph from about three fourths of the body

D. Lymph nodes
   1. Filter lymph (see **Figure 14-2** and **Figure 14-3**)
   2. Located in clusters along the pathway of lymphatic vessels (see **Figure 14-1** and **Figure 14-4**)
   3. Lymphoid tissue — mass of lymphocytes and related cells inside a lymphoid organ; provides immune function and development of immune cells
   4. Lymph nodes and other lymphoid organs have functions that include defense and WBC formation
   5. Flow of lymph: to node via several afferent lymphatic vessels and drained from node by a single efferent lymphatic vessel

E. Thymus (see **Figure 14-1**)
   1. Lymphoid tissue organ located in mediastinum
   2. Total weight of 35 to 40 grams — a little more than an ounce
   3. Plays a vital and central role in immunity
   4. Produces T lymphocytes, or T cells
   5. Secretes hormones called *thymosins*, which influence T-cell development
   6. Lymphoid tissue is eventually replaced by fat in the process called *involution*

F. Tonsils (see **Figure 14-5**)
   1. Composed of three masses of lymphoid tissue around the openings of the mouth and throat
      a. Palatine tonsils ("the tonsils")
      b. Pharyngeal tonsils (also known as *adenoids*)
      c. Lingual tonsils
   2. Subject to chronic infection
   3. Enlargement of pharyngeal tonsils may impair breathing

G. Spleen (see **Figure 14-1**)
   1. Largest lymphoid organ in body
   2. Located in upper left quadrant of abdomen
   3. Often injured by trauma to abdomen; surgical removal called *splenectomy*
   4. Functions include phagocytosis of bacteria and old RBCs; monocyte reservoir; acts as a blood reservoir
   5. Because spleen functions can be done by other organs, one can survive without it

The Immune System

A. Protects body from pathological bacteria, foreign tissue cells, and cancerous cells

B. Made up of defensive cells and molecules

C. Two main strategies — nonspecific defenses and specific defenses (see **Table 14-1**)

D. Nonspecific immunity (innate immunity)
   1. Nonspecific immunity is called *innate immunity* because it does not require prior exposure to an antigen
   2. Many types of innate immunity occur in the body (see **Table 14-2**)
      a. Nonspecific immunity is the rapid first response and often triggers slower specific responses
      b. May involve signaling chemicals called cytokines
   3. Skin — mechanical barrier to bacteria and other harmful agents
   4. Tears and mucus — wash eyes and trap and kill bacteria
   5. Inflammation
      a. Inflammatory response — attracts immune cells to site of injury, increases local blood flow, increases vascular permeability; promotes movement of WBCs to site of injury or infection (see **Figure 14-6**)
      b. Fever — systemic effect of increased body temperature; may increase immune efficiency or inhibit infectious agents
   6. Complement — class of enzymes in blood plasma that can trigger a variety of immune responses; also involved in specific (adaptive) mechanisms

E. Specific immunity (adaptive immunity)
   1. Specific immunity is also called *adaptive immunity* because of its ability to recognize, respond to, and remember harmful substances or bacteria
   2. Types of specific immunity (see **Table 14-3**)
      a. Natural immunity — exposure to causative agent is not deliberate
         (1) Active — active disease produces immunity
         (2) Passive — immunity passes from mother to fetus through placenta or from mother to child through mother's milk
      b. Artificial immunity — exposure to causative agent is deliberate
         (1) Active — vaccination results in activation of immune system and long-term protection
         (2) Passive — protective material developed in another individual's immune system and given to previously nonimmune individual, giving short-term protection

Immune System Molecules

A. Cytokines
   1. Cytokines are molecules that communicate among cells, coordinating immune responses
   2. Interleukins (ILs) are an example of cytokines

B. Antibodies
   1. Protein molecules with specific combining sites
   2. Combining sites attach antibodies to specific antigens (foreign proteins), forming an antigen-antibody complex — this provides *humoral,* or *antibody-mediated, immunity* (see **Figure 14-7**)

3. Antigen-antibody complexes may do the following:
   a. Neutralize toxins
   b. Clump or agglutinate enemy cells
   c. Promote phagocytosis

C. Complement proteins
1. Group of proteins normally present in blood in inactive state
2. Complement cascade
   a. Important mechanism of action for antibodies
   b. Causes cell lysis by permitting entry of water through a defect created in the plasma membrane (see **Figure 14-8**)
3. Also helps perform other functions (*examples:* attracting immune cells to a site of infection, activating immune cells, marking foreign cells for destruction, increasing permeability of blood vessels), the inflammatory response

Immune System Cells

A. Phagocytes
1. Ingest and destroy foreign cells or other harmful substances via phagocytosis (see **Figure 14-9**)
2. Types
   a. Neutrophils — short-lived phagocytic cells
   b. Monocytes — develop into phagocytic macrophages and migrate to tissues (see **Figure 14-14**)
   c. Dendritic cells (DCs) — often found at or near external surfaces (see **Figure 14-10**)
3. Macrophages and DCs act as antigen-presenting cells (APCs) by displaying ingested antigens on their outer surface to trigger specific immune cells

B. Lymphocytes (see **Figure 14-11**)
1. Most numerous of immune system cells
2. B cells
   a. Development of B cells — primitive stem cells migrate from bone marrow and go through two stages of development (see **Figure 14-12**)
      (1) First stage — stem cells develop into immature B cells
         (a) Takes place in the liver and bone marrow before birth and in the bone marrow only in adults
         (b) B cells are small lymphocytes with antibody molecules (which they have synthesized) in their plasma membranes
         (c) After they mature, inactive B cells migrate chiefly to lymph nodes
      (2) Second stage — inactive B cell develops into activated B cell
         (a) Initiated by inactive B cell's contact with antigens, which bind to its surface antibodies, plus cytokines (signal chemicals) from T cells
         (b) Activated B cell, by dividing repeatedly, forms two clones of cells — plasma (effector) cells and memory cells
         (c) Plasma cells secrete antibodies into blood; memory cells are stored in lymph nodes
         (d) If subsequent exposure to antigen that activated B cell occurs, memory cells become plasma cells and secrete antibodies
   b. Function of B cells — indirectly, B cells produce humoral immunity
      (1) Activated B cells develop into plasma cells
      (2) Plasma cells secrete antibodies into the blood
      (3) Circulating antibodies produce humoral immunity (see **Figure 14-12**)
3. T cells
   a. Development of T cells — stem cells from bone marrow migrate to thymus gland (see **Figure 14-13**)
      (1) First stage — stem cells develop into T cells
      (2) T cells mature in the thymus during few months before and after birth
      (3) Mature T cells migrate chiefly to lymph nodes
      (4) Second stage — T cells develop into activated T cells
         (a) Occurs when, and if, antigen binds to T cell's surface proteins and a cytokine (chemical signal) is received from another T cell
         (b) As with B cells, clones made up of effector cells and memory cells are formed
   b. Functions of T cells — produce cell-mediated immunity (see **Figure 14-13** and **Figure 14-14**)
      (1) Cytotoxic T cells — kill infected or tumor cells by releasing a substance that poisons infected or tumor cells
      (2) Helper T cells — release cytokines that attract and activate macrophages to kill cells by phagocytosis; produce cytokines that help activate B cells
      (3) Regulatory T cells — release cytokines to suppress immune responses

❑ ACTIVE LEARNING

STUDY TIPS

Hint *Use these tips to achieve success in meeting your learning goals.*

To make the study of the lymphatic system and immunity more efficient, we suggest these tips:

1. Before studying Chapter 14, review the synopsis of the lymphatic system in Chapter 5.
2. The lymphatic system is the "drainage" system of the body. Fluid is pushed out of the capillaries and washes over the tissue cells. The fluid carries bacteria and cellular debris into the open-ended capillaries in the lymphatic system. Much of the fluid is reabsorbed by the capillaries but some is not. The remaining fluid is then called *lymph*. It is carried to the lymph node, where it is filtered, cleaned, and carried in the ducts back to the blood. Keep this process in mind when you study the structures of the lymphatic system.
3. Several specific organs make up the lymphatic system. Flash cards with their names, locations, and functions will help you learn them.
4. Immune system actions can be divided into nonspecific immunity and specific immunity, according to differences in function. If you keep this division of immunity "styles" in mind, immune function is easier to understand.
5. Specific immunity can be classified as natural or artificial depending on how the body was exposed to the antigen, and active or passive depending on how much work the body had to do to develop the response. The natural, active immune response is divided into two parts also: humoral immunity and cell-mediated immunity. Humoral immunity is mediated by B lymphocytes, or B cells. They stay in the lymph node and secrete antibodies into the blood, a body humor. They also form memory cells for lifelong immunity. T lymphocytes, or T cells, provide the cell-mediated immunity. They leave the lymph node and actively engage antigens.
6. In your study groups, use flash cards or online resources to quiz each other on the terms and structures of the lymphatic and immune systems. Discuss the process of how lymph is formed, filtered, and returned to the blood. Discuss nonspecific immunity, especially the inflammatory response. Discuss the steps in humoral and cell-mediated immunity.
7. In your study group, go over the Language of Science and Medicine terms, review the questions in the back of the chapter, and discuss possible test questions.

Review Questions

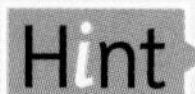

Write out the answers to these questions after reading the chapter and reviewing the Chapter Summary. If you simply think through the answer without writing it down, you won't retain much of your new learning.

1. Define *lymph* and explain its function.
2. Name the two lymphatic ducts and the areas of the body each of them drain.
3. Describe the structure of the lymph node.
4. Explain the defense function of the lymph node.
5. Locate the thymus gland in the body and list its functions.
6. Name and locate the three pairs of tonsils.
7. Give the location and function of the spleen.
8. Explain the types of nonspecific immunity.
9. Name and differentiate between the four types of specific immunity.
10. Explain how antibodies and antigens differ.
11. Explain the role of complement in the immune system.
12. Explain the role of macrophages in the immune system.
13. Explain the development and functioning of B cells.
14. Explain the development and functioning of T cells.
15. Differentiate between humoral (antibody-mediated) and cell-mediated immunity.

Critical Thinking

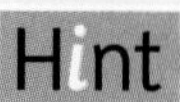

After finishing the Review Questions, write out the answers to these more in-depth questions to help you apply your new knowledge. Go back to sections of the chapter that relate to concepts that you find difficult.

16. Differentiate between lymphatic capillaries and blood capillaries. Explain how the differences in structure relate to their function.
17. Explain the role of lymph nodes in the possible spread of cancer.
18. Explain some possible reasons to avoid surgical removal of the tonsils.

Chapter Test

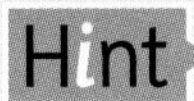

After studying the chapter, test your mastery by responding to these items. Try to answer them without looking up the answers. Then, verify the answers using the key in Appendix C at the back of this book.

1. ________ is the fluid that leaves the blood capillaries and may eventually be returned to the blood through lymphatic vessels.
2. Lymph from about three fourths of the body drains into the ________.
3. Lymph from the right upper extremity and the right side of the head drains into the ________.
4. The enlarged, pouchlike structure in the abdomen that serves as a storage area for lymph is called the ________.
5. The function of the ________ is to filter and clean the lymph.
6. The many lymphatic vessels that enter the lymph node are called the ________ vessels. The single vessel leaving the lymph node is called the ________ vessel.
7. The thymus gland is the site of maturation for these WBCs: ________. It also produces the hormone ________.
8. The three pairs of tonsils are the ________ tonsils, the ________ tonsils, and the ________ tonsils.
9. The largest lymphoid organ is the ________.
10. The signs of ________ are heat, redness, pain, and swelling.
11. ________ kills threatening cells by drilling holes in their plasma membrane, which disrupts the sodium and water balance.
12. Macrophages were originally ________ that migrated into the tissues.
13. The immunity that develops against polio after receiving a polio vaccination is an example of:
    a. active natural immunity
    b. passive natural immunity
    c. active artificial immunity
    d. passive artificial immunity
14. The immunity that is given to the fetus or newborn by the immune system of the mother is an example of:
    a. active natural immunity
    b. passive natural immunity
    c. active artificial immunity
    d. passive artificial immunity
15. The immunity that comes from the injection of antibodies made by another individual's immune system is an example of:
    a. active natural immunity
    b. passive natural immunity
    c. active artificial immunity
    d. passive artificial immunity
16. The immunity that develops after a person has had a disease is an example of:
    a. active natural immunity
    b. passive natural immunity
    c. active artificial immunity
    d. passive artificial immunity

If the following statement describes the development or functioning of a B cell, write a B in front of it. If it describes the development or functioning of a T cell, write a T in front of it.

17. ________ produces antibodies
18. ________ some develop into plasma cells
19. ________ the main cell involved in cell-mediated immunity
20. ________ the main cell involved in humoral immunity
21. ________ develops in the thymus gland
22. ________ moves to the site of the antigen and releases cell poison
23. ________ divides rapidly into clones once it is activated
24. ________ releases a substance that attracts macrophages
25. ________ some of these cells develop into memory cells

Respiratory System

OUTLINE

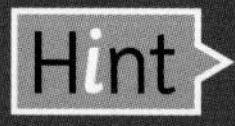

Scan this outline before you begin to read the chapter, as a preview of how the concepts are organized.

OBJECTIVES

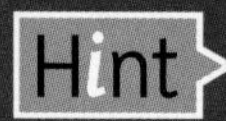

Before reading the chapter, review these goals for your learning.

After you have completed this chapter, you should be able to:

1. Discuss the major functions of the respiratory system.
2. List the major organs of the respiratory system and describe the functions of each.
3. Compare, contrast, and explain the mechanism responsible for the exchange of gases that occurs during external and internal respiration.
4. List and discuss the volumes of air exchanged during pulmonary ventilation.
5. Identify and discuss the mechanisms that regulate respiration.

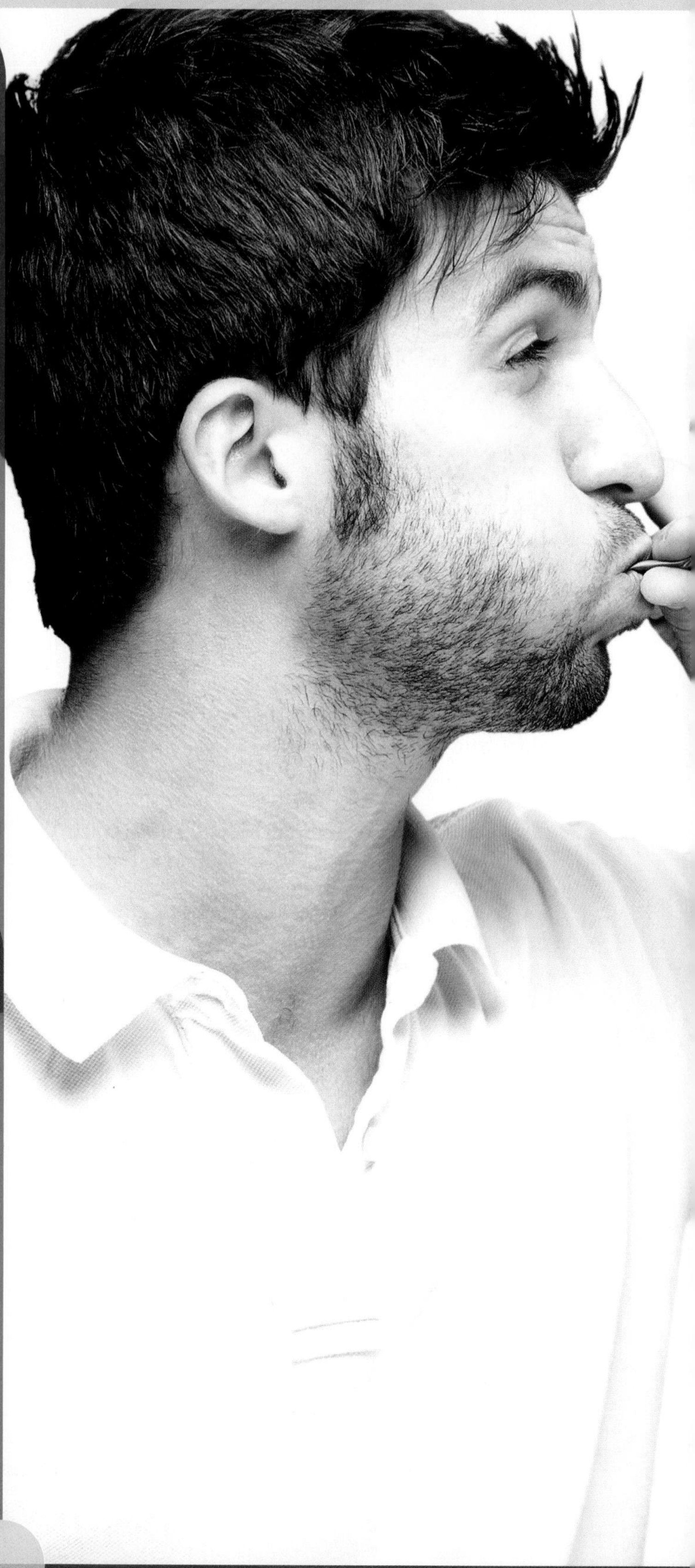

CHAPTER 15

No one needs to be told how important the **respiratory system** is. The respiratory system serves the body much as a lifeline to an air pump serves a deep-sea diver. Think how panicked you would feel if suddenly your lifeline became blocked—if you could not breathe for a few seconds!

Of all the substances that cells and therefore the body as a whole must have to survive, oxygen is by far the most crucial. A person can live a few weeks without food, a few days without water, but only a few minutes without oxygen. Constant removal of carbon dioxide from the body is just as important for survival as a constant supply of oxygen.

The respiratory system ensures that oxygen is supplied to, and carbon dioxide (a waste product) is removed from, the body's cells. The process of respiration therefore is a vital homeostatic mechanism. By constantly supplying adequate oxygen and by removing carbon dioxide as it forms, the respiratory system helps maintain a constant environment that enables your body cells to function effectively.

To accomplish its functions, the respiratory system effectively *filters, warms,* and *humidifies* the air we breathe. Respiratory organs such as vocal cords, sinuses, and specialized epithelium, also help produce speech and make possible the sense of smell, or *olfaction.* Even the primary function of gas exchange has a secondary effect—the removal of excess acid from the body. This pH-balancing function of the respiratory system will be discussed further in Chapter 20.

In this chapter, the overall structural plan of the respiratory system is considered first, then the organs of the upper and lower respiratory tract. The last half of this chapter focuses on moving air through the tract—a process called *ventilation*—and mechanisms of gas exchange and transport.

LANGUAGE OF **SCIENCE** AND **MEDICINE**

Hint Before reading the chapter, say each of these terms out loud. This will help you to avoid stumbling over them as you read.

adenoid
(AD-eh-noyd)
[*adeno-* **gland,** *-oid* **like**]

alveolar duct
(al-VEE-oh-lar dukt)
[*alve-* **hollow,** *-ol-* **little,** *-ar* **relating to**]

alveolar sac
(al-VEE-oh-lar sak)
[*alve-* **hollow,** *-ol-* **little,** *-ar* **relating to**]

alveoli
(al-VEE-oh-lye)
sing., alveolus
(al-VEE-oh-lus)
[*alve-* **hollow,** *-olus* **little**]

aortic body
(ay-OR-tik BOD-ee)
[*aort-* **lifted,** *-ic* **relating to**]

apnea
(AP-nee-ah)
[*a-* **not,** *-pne-* **breathe,** *-a* **condition**]

auditory tube (eustachian tube)
(AW-dih-tohr-ee [yoo-STAY-shun] toob)
[*audit-* **listen,** *-or-* **agent,** *-y* **relating to,** *Bartolomeo Eustachio* **Italian anatomist,** *-an* **relating to**]

bicarbonate ion
(bye-KAR-boh-net)
[*bi-* **two,** *-carbon-* **coal (carbon),** *-ate* **oxygen compound**]

bronchi
(BRONG-kye)
sing., bronchus
(BRONG-kus)
[*bronchus* **windpipe**]

bronchiole
(BRONG-kee-ohl)
[*bronch-* **windpipe,** *-ol-* **little**]

Continued on p. 360

Structural Plan

Overview

Respiratory organs include the **nose, pharynx** *(throat),* **larynx** *(voice box),* **trachea** *(windpipe),* **bronchi** *(branches),* and **lungs.** The basic structural scheme of this organ system is that of a tube with many branches ending in millions of extremely tiny, very thin-walled sacs called **alveoli.** Figure 15-1 shows the extensive branching of the "respiratory tree" in both lungs. Think of this air distribution system as an "upside-down tree."

The trachea, or windpipe, then becomes the trunk and the bronchial tubes the branches. This idea is developed further when the types of bronchi and the alveoli are studied in more detail later in the chapter.

A network of capillaries fits like a hairnet around each microscopic alveolus. Incidentally, this is a good place for us to think again about a principle already mentioned several times—namely, that structure and function are intimately related. The function of alveoli—in fact, the function of the entire respiratory system—is to distribute air close enough to blood for a gas exchange to take place between air and blood. The passive transport process of **diffusion,** which was described in Chapter 3, is the mode for the exchange of gases that occurs in the respiratory system. You may want to review the discussion of diffusion on pp. 48-50 before you study the mechanism of gas exchange that occurs in the lungs and body tissues.

To learn more about the respiratory tract, go to AnimationDirect at *evolve.elsevier.com.*

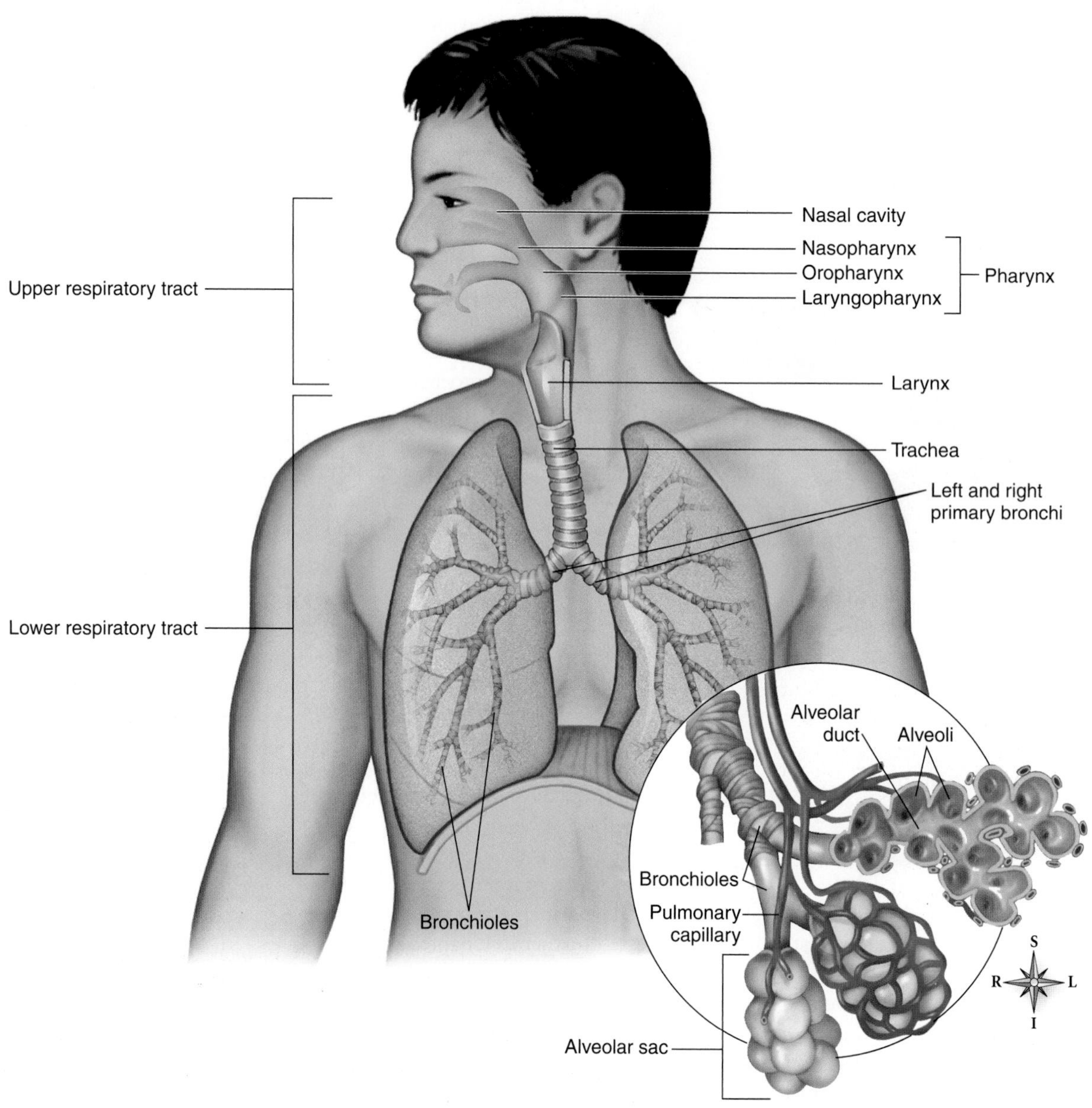

FIGURE 15-1 Structural plan of the respiratory system. *Inset* shows the alveolar sacs where the exchange of oxygen and carbon dioxide takes place through the walls of the grapelike alveoli. Capillaries surround the alveoli.

Respiratory Tract

The respiratory tract—the pathway of air flow—is often divided into upper and lower tracts or divisions to assist in the description of symptoms associated with common respiratory problems such as a cold. The organs of the upper respiratory tract are located outside of the thorax, or chest cavity, whereas those in the lower tract or division are located almost entirely within it.

The **upper respiratory tract** is composed of the nose, pharynx, and larynx. The **lower respiratory tract,** or division, consists of the trachea, all segments of the bronchial tree, and the lungs.

The designation *upper respiratory infection,* or URI, is often used to describe what many patients call a "head cold." Typically the symptoms of an upper respiratory infection involve the sinuses, nasal cavity, pharynx, and/or larynx, whereas the symptoms of what is often referred to as a "chest cold" are similar to pneumonia and involve the organs of the lower respiratory tract.

Respiratory Mucosa

Structure

Before beginning the study of individual organs in the respiratory system, it is important to review the histology or microscopic anatomy of the **respiratory mucosa**—the membrane that lines most of the air distribution tubes in the system.

Respiratory mucosa is typically *ciliated pseudostratified epithelium,* as you can see in Figure 15-2. As its name implies, this type of tissue is covered with *cilia.* Look back at Figure 3-4 on p. 46 and Figure 3-5 on p. 47 to see the structure of these tiny cell projections and how they can move fluids along the surfaces of a layer of cells. Figure 15-2 also shows the presence of *goblet cells,* which can produce and release huge amounts of **mucus.** Mucus varies in composition from very watery to very thick and sticky, depending on the specific location of the mucosa.

Although most of the respiratory passages are lined with ciliated pseudostratified epithelium, there are a few areas lined with other tissues. For example, protective *stratified squamous epithelium* is found just inside the nostrils, covering the vocal folds of the larynx, and lining the pharynx. Look back at Figure 4-4 on p. 70 to see the many layers of this thicker type of epithelium.

Simple squamous epithelium—an extremely thin tissue—lines the alveoli of the lungs where gas exchange occurs.

Function

Recall that in addition to serving as air distribution passageways or gas exchange surfaces, the structures of the respiratory tract and lungs cleanse, warm, and humidify inspired air. Air entering the nose is generally contaminated with one or more common irritants; examples include insects, dust, pollen, and bacterial organisms. A remarkably effective air purification mechanism removes almost every form of contaminant before inspired air reaches the alveoli, or terminal air sacs, in the lungs.

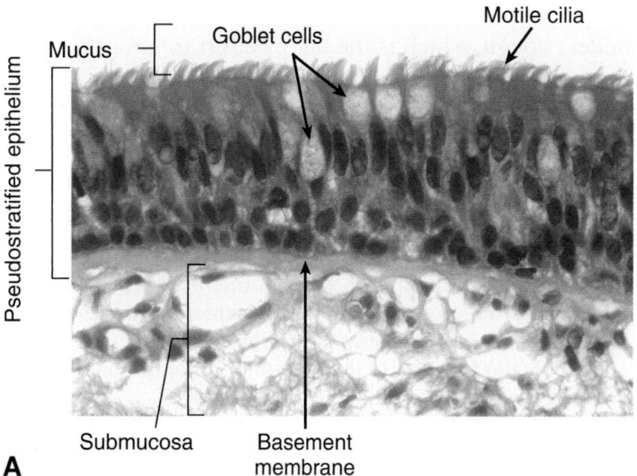

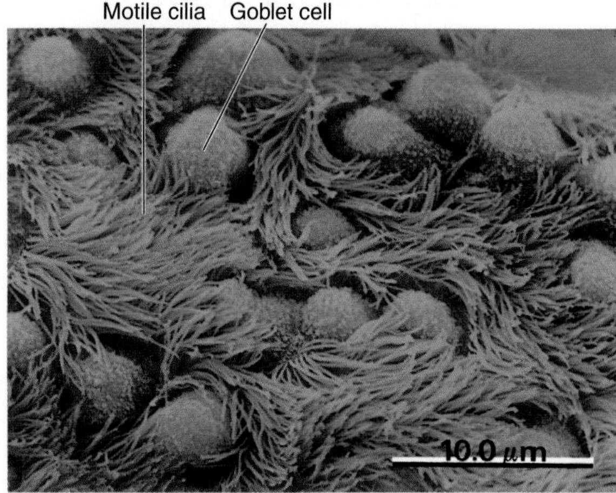

FIGURE 15-2 Respiratory mucosa. A, Light micrograph (×200) and **B,** scanning electron micrograph (×2000) of the ciliated pseudostratified epithelium typical of the respiratory lining. Note the numerous motile (moving) cilia and mucus-producing goblet cells.

A layer of protective mucus, called a *mucous blanket,* covers nearly the entire ciliated pseudostratified epithelial lining of the air distribution tubes in the respiratory tree. More than 125 mL of respiratory mucus is produced daily. It serves as the most important air purification mechanism. Air is purified when contaminants such as dust, pollen, and smoke particles stick to the mucus and become trapped.

Normally, the cleansing layer of mucus containing inhaled contaminants moves upward to the pharynx from the lower portions of the bronchial tree on the millions of hairlike cilia that beat or move only in one direction. This mechanism is often called the **ciliary escalator.**

Cigarette smoke and other irritants are detected by the cilia, which beat rapidly in response—an attempt to clear out the contaminants more efficiently. Prolonged exposure to cigarette smoke both increases production of mucus and eventually paralyzes cilia, thus causing accumulations of contaminated mucus to build up and remain in the respiratory passageways for longer periods of time. The result is a typical smoker's cough, which is the body's effort to clear these large quantities of contaminated mucus.

To learn more about respiratory mucosa, go to AnimationDirect at *evolve.elsevier.com.*

QUICK CHECK

1. What are the primary functions of the respiratory system?
2. What are the organs of the upper respiratory tract? What are the organs of the lower respiratory tract?
3. What is the function of the respiratory membrane?
4. What is the function of the ciliary escalator?

Upper Respiratory Tract

Nose

Air enters the respiratory tract through the **external nares,** or nostrils. It then flows into the right and left **nasal cavities,** which are lined by respiratory mucosa. A partition called the **nasal septum** separates these two cavities.

The surface of the nasal cavities is moist from mucus and warm from blood flowing just under it. Nerve endings responsible for the sense of smell (olfactory receptors) are also located in the nasal mucosa.

Four **paranasal sinuses**—frontal, maxillary, sphenoidal, and ethmoidal—drain into the nasal cavities (**Figure 15-3**). The paranasal sinuses are lined with a mucous membrane that assists in the production of mucus for the respiratory tract. In addition, these hollow spaces help lighten the skull bones and serve as resonant chambers that enhance the production of sound.

Because the mucosa that lines the sinuses is continuous with the mucosa that lines the nose, sinus infections, called **sinusitis,** often develop from colds in which the nasal mucosa is inflamed. Symptoms of sinusitis include pressure, pain, headache, and often external tenderness, swelling, and redness. In chronic cases, infection may spread to adjacent bone or into the cranial cavity inflaming meninges or brain tissue. Treatment includes decongestants; analgesics; antibiotics; and in some cases, surgery to improve drainage.

Two ducts from the **lacrimal sacs** also drain into the nasal cavity, as **Figure 15-3** shows. The lacrimal sacs collect tears from the corner of each eyelid and drain them into the nasal cavity.

Note in **Figure 15-4** that three shelflike structures called **conchae** protrude into the nasal cavity on each side. The nasal conchae are sometimes called nasal **turbinates.** The mucosa-covered conchae greatly increase the surface over which air must flow as it passes through the nasal cavity. As air moves over the conchae and through the nasal cavities, it is warmed and humidified. This helps explain why breathing through the nose is more effective in humidifying inspired air than is breathing through the mouth.

Pharynx

The **pharynx** is the structure that many of us call the throat. It is about 12.5 cm (5 inches) long and can be divided into three portions (see **Figure 15-4**). The uppermost part of the tube just behind the nasal cavities is called the **nasopharynx.** The portion behind the mouth is called the **oropharynx.** The last or lowest segment is called the **laryngopharynx.**

The pharynx as a whole serves the same purpose for the respiratory and digestive tracts as a hallway serves for a house. Air and food pass through the pharynx on their way to the lungs and the stomach, respectively. Air enters the pharynx from the two nasal cavities or the oral cavity and leaves it by way of the larynx. Food enters the pharynx from the mouth and leaves it by way of the esophagus.

The right and left **auditory tubes,** or **eustachian tubes,** open into the nasopharynx; they connect the middle ears with the nasopharynx (see **Figure 15-4**). This connection permits

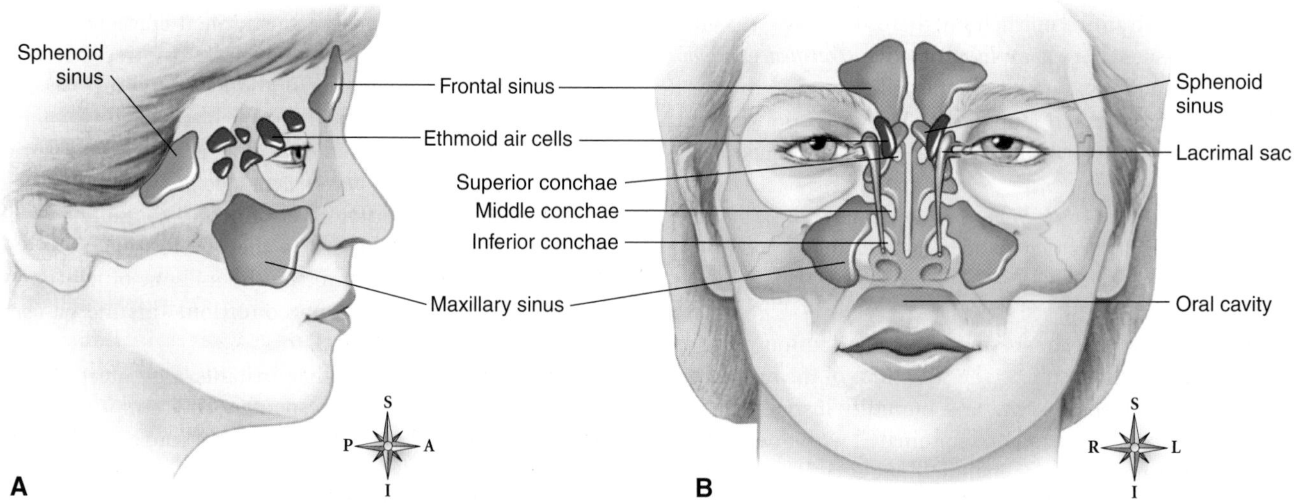

FIGURE 15-3 The paranasal sinuses. A, Lateral view of the position of the sinuses. **B,** The anterior view shows the anatomical relationship of the paranasal sinuses to each other and to the nasal cavity.

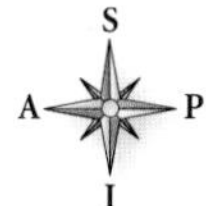

FIGURE 15-4 Sagittal section of the head and neck. The nasal septum has been removed, exposing the right lateral wall of the nasal cavity so that the nasal conchae can be seen. Note also the divisions of the pharynx and the position of the tonsils.

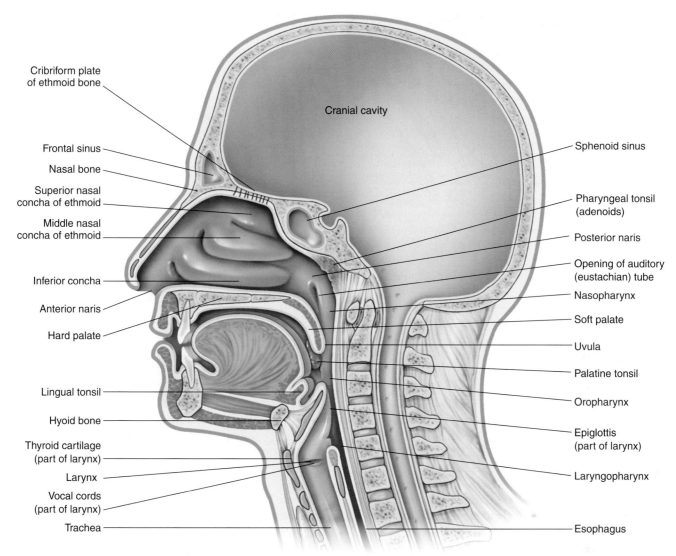

equalization of air pressure between the middle and the exterior ear. The lining of the auditory tubes is continuous with the lining of the nasopharynx and middle ear. Thus, just as sinus infections can develop from colds in which the nasal mucosa is inflamed, middle ear infections can develop from inflammation of the nasopharynx.

Masses of lymphoid tissue called **tonsils** are embedded in the mucous membrane of the pharynx (see **Figure 14-5**). Recall the location of the tonsils from the previous chapter (see p. 322). The **lingual tonsils** and **palatine tonsils** are located in the oropharynx and the **pharyngeal tonsils,** also called the **adenoids,** are located in the nasopharynx.

As you read in Chapter 14, these tonsils form a ring of lymphoid tissue in the throat that provides immune protection at a critical boundary with the external environment. Although the tonsils usually protect us, they can also become infected and inflamed themselves—a condition called **tonsillitis.** Swelling of the pharyngeal tonsils caused by infections may make it difficult or impossible for air to travel from the nose into the throat. In these cases the individual is forced to breathe through the mouth.

Larynx

The **larynx,** or voice box, is located just below the pharynx. It is composed of nine pieces of cartilage. You know the largest of these (the *thyroid cartilage*) as the "Adam's apple" (**Figure 15-5**).

Two short fibrous bands, the **vocal cords,** stretch across the interior of the larynx. Muscles that attach to the larynx cartilages can pull on these cords in such a way that they become tense or relaxed. When they are tense, the voice is high pitched; when they are relaxed, it is low pitched. The space between the vocal cords is the **glottis.**

Another cartilage called the **epiglottis** partially covers the opening of the larynx (see **Figure 15-5**). The epiglottis acts like

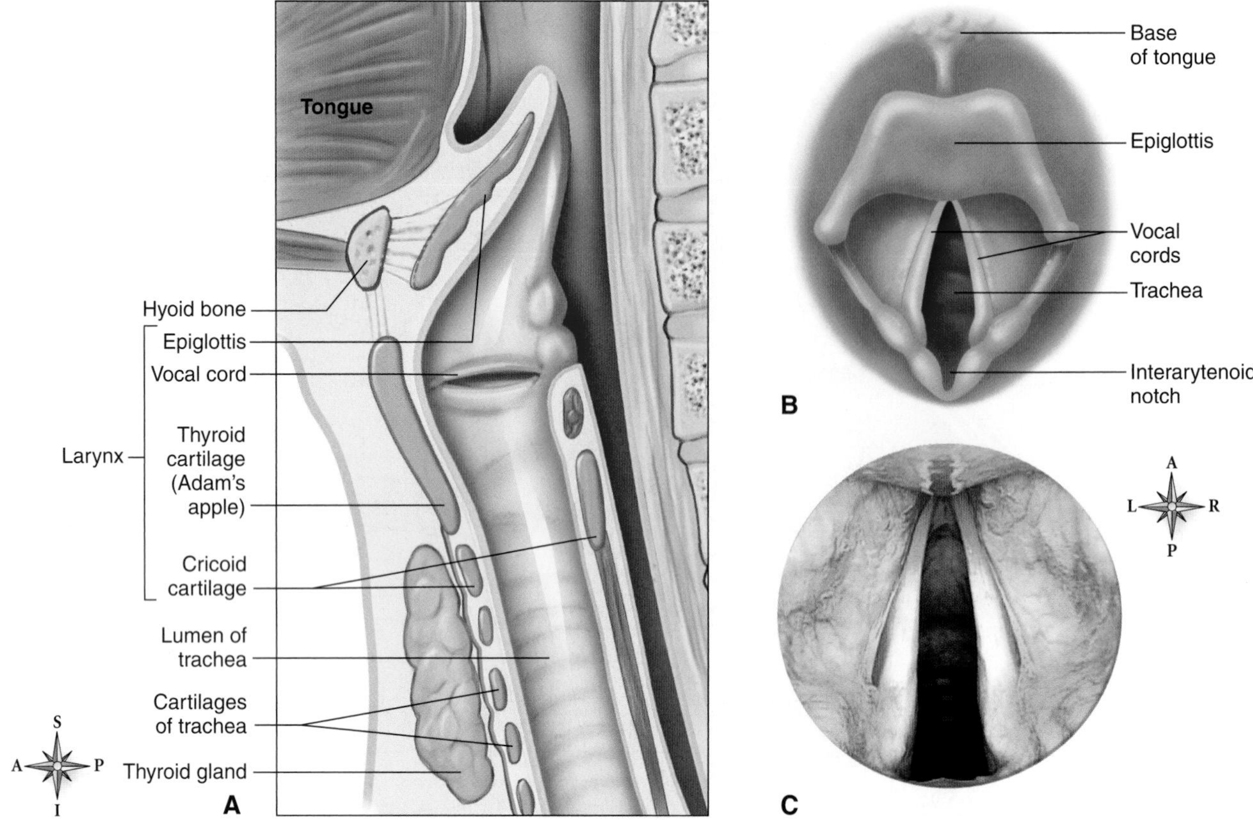

FIGURE 15-5 The larynx. A, Sagittal section of the larynx. **B,** Superior view of the larynx. **C,** Photograph of the larynx taken with an endoscope (optical device) inserted through the mouth and pharynx to the epiglottis.

a trapdoor, closing off the larynx during swallowing and preventing food and liquids from entering the trachea.

Lower Respiratory Tract

Trachea

The **trachea,** or windpipe, is a tube about 11 cm (4.5 in) long and 2.5 cm (1 in) wide. It extends from the larynx in the neck to the bronchi in the chest cavity (**Figure 15-1** and **Figure 15-6**).

The trachea performs a simple but vital function: it provides part of the open passageway through which air can reach the lungs from the outside.

Additional functional significance is related to the fact that the trachea is lined by the typical respiratory mucosa, which contains numerous mucus-producing glands and is covered by cilia. The glands help produce part of the blanket of mucus that is continually moved by the beating cilia in one direction—upward and toward the pharynx—as part of the *ciliary escalator* mechanism. Therefore, in addition to its role in air distribution, the trachea serves a protective function by production and movement of mucus important in trapping and eliminating airborne contaminants.

By pushing with your fingers against your throat about an inch above the sternum, you can feel the shape of the trachea or windpipe. Only if you use considerable force can you squeeze it closed. Nature has taken precautions to keep this lifeline open. Its framework is made of an almost noncollapsible material—15 or 20 C-shaped rings of cartilage placed one above the other with only a little soft tissue between them.

Figure 15-6, *B*, shows how the incomplete cartilage rings permit easy swallowing by allowing the esophagus (food tube) to stretch within the narrow space in the neck between the trachea and the vertebrae.

Despite the structural safeguard of cartilage rings, blockage of the trachea sometimes occurs. A tumor or an infection may enlarge the lymph nodes of the neck so much that they squeeze the trachea shut, or a person may aspirate (breathe in) a piece of food or something else that blocks the windpipe. Because air has no other way to get to the lungs, complete tracheal obstruction causes death in a matter of minutes.

Suffocation from all causes, including choking on food and other substances caught in the trachea, kills more than 4000 people each year and is the fifth major cause of accidental death in the United States.

QUICK CHECK

1. What are the paranasal sinuses? What is the function of these sinuses?
2. What are the three divisions of the pharynx?
3. What is the scientific term for the voice box?
4. What keeps the trachea from collapsing?

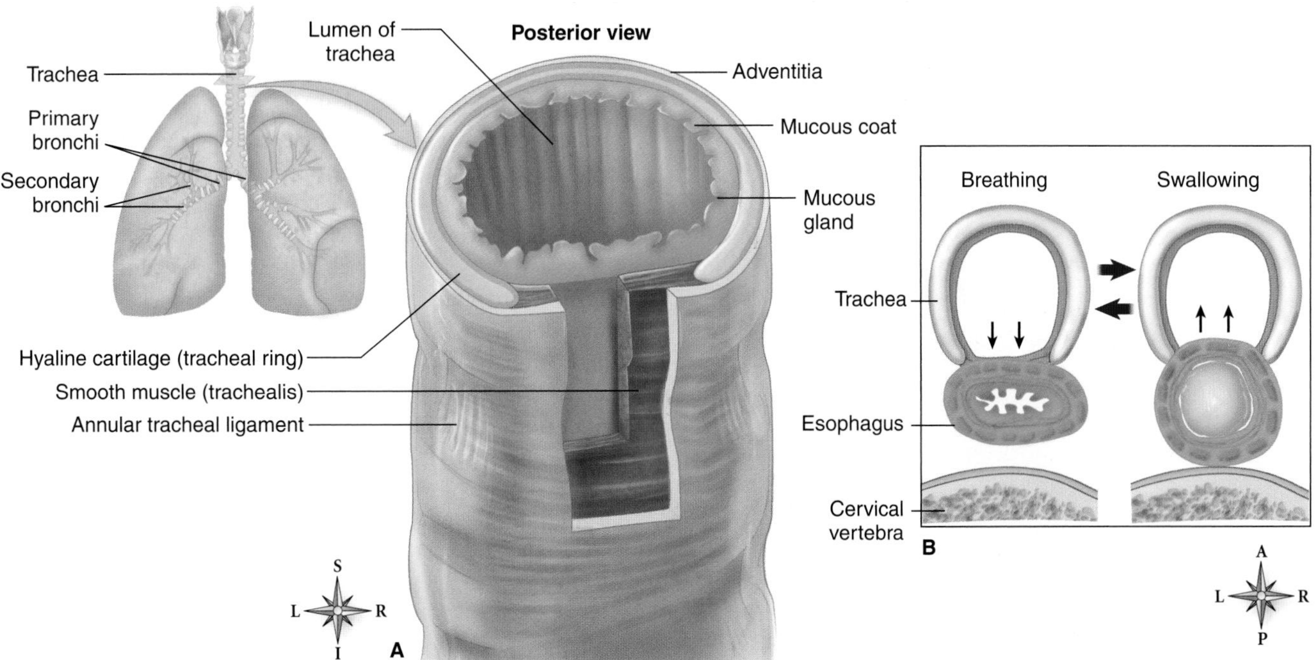

FIGURE 15-6 Cross section of the trachea. *Inset* at top shows from where the section was cut. **A,** Structure of trachea. **B,** Incomplete cartilage rings and elasticity of posterior tracheal wall allow the esophagus to expand during swallowing.

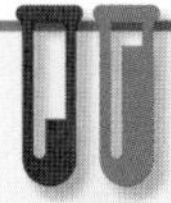

CLINICAL APPLICATION

KEEPING THE TRACHEA OPEN

Often a tube is placed through the mouth, pharynx, and larynx into the trachea of surgery patients, especially if they have been given a muscle relaxant. This procedure is called **endotracheal intubation.** The purpose of the tube is to ensure an open airway (see part *A* of the figure).

To ensure that the tube enters the trachea rather than the nearby esophagus (which leads to the stomach), anatomical landmarks such as the vocal folds are used. Likewise, the distinct feel of the V-shaped posterior groove called the **interarytenoid notch** (Figure 15-5, *B*) can help guide the proper insertion of the tube.

Another procedure done frequently in today's modern hospitals is a **tracheostomy.** This procedure involves the cutting of an opening into the trachea (part *B* of the figure). A surgeon may perform this procedure so that a suction device can be inserted to remove secretions from the bronchial tree or so that an *intermittent positive-pressure breathing (IPPB)* machine can be used to improve ventilation of the lungs.

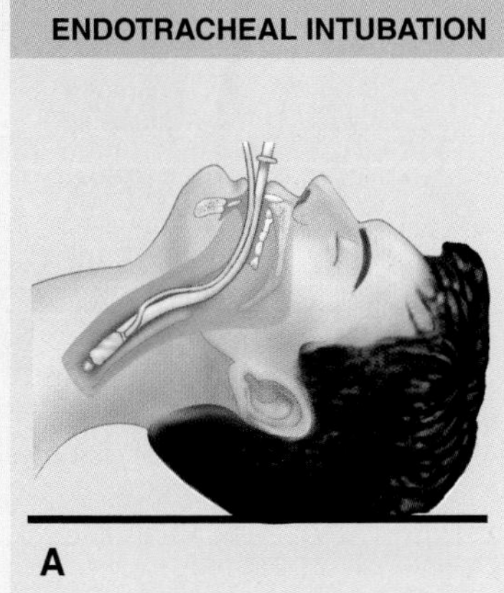

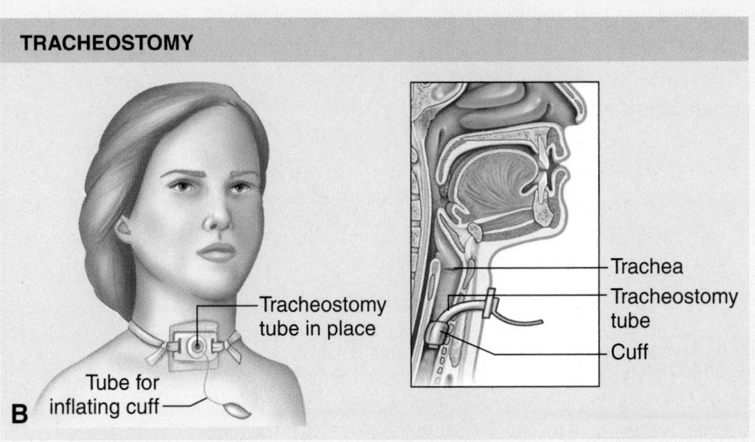

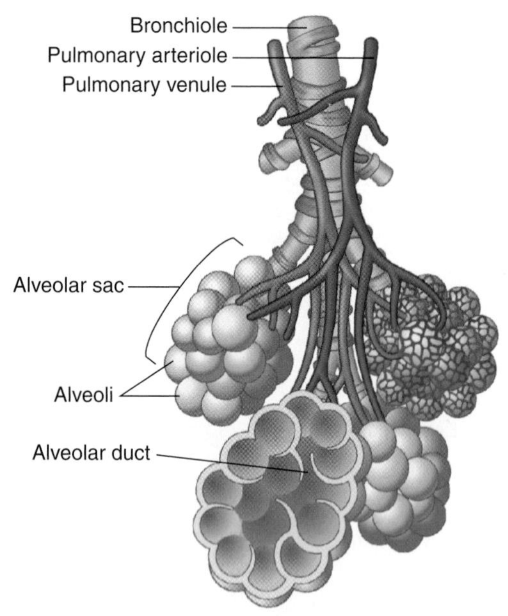

FIGURE 15-7 Bronchioles and alveoli. Bronchioles subdivide to form tiny tubes called *alveolar ducts,* which end in clusters of alveoli called *alveolar sacs.*

Bronchial Tree

Recall that one way to picture the thousands of air passages that make up the lungs is to think of an upside-down tree. The trachea is the main trunk of this tree; the right bronchus (the tube leading into the right lung) and the left bronchus (the tube leading into the left lung) are the trachea's first branches, or **primary bronchi.**

In each lung, they branch into smaller **secondary bronchi** (*singular,* bronchus) whose walls, as with those of the trachea and bronchi, are kept open by rings of cartilage for air passage. These bronchi divide into smaller and smaller tubes, ultimately branching into tiny tubes whose walls contain only smooth muscle. These very small passageways are called **bronchioles.**

The bronchioles subdivide into microscopic tubes called **alveolar ducts,** which resemble the main stem of a bunch of grapes (**Figure 15-7**). Each alveolar duct ends in several **alveolar sacs,** each of which resembles a cluster of grapes, and the wall of each alveolar sac is made up of numerous **alveoli,** each of which resembles a single, hollow grape.

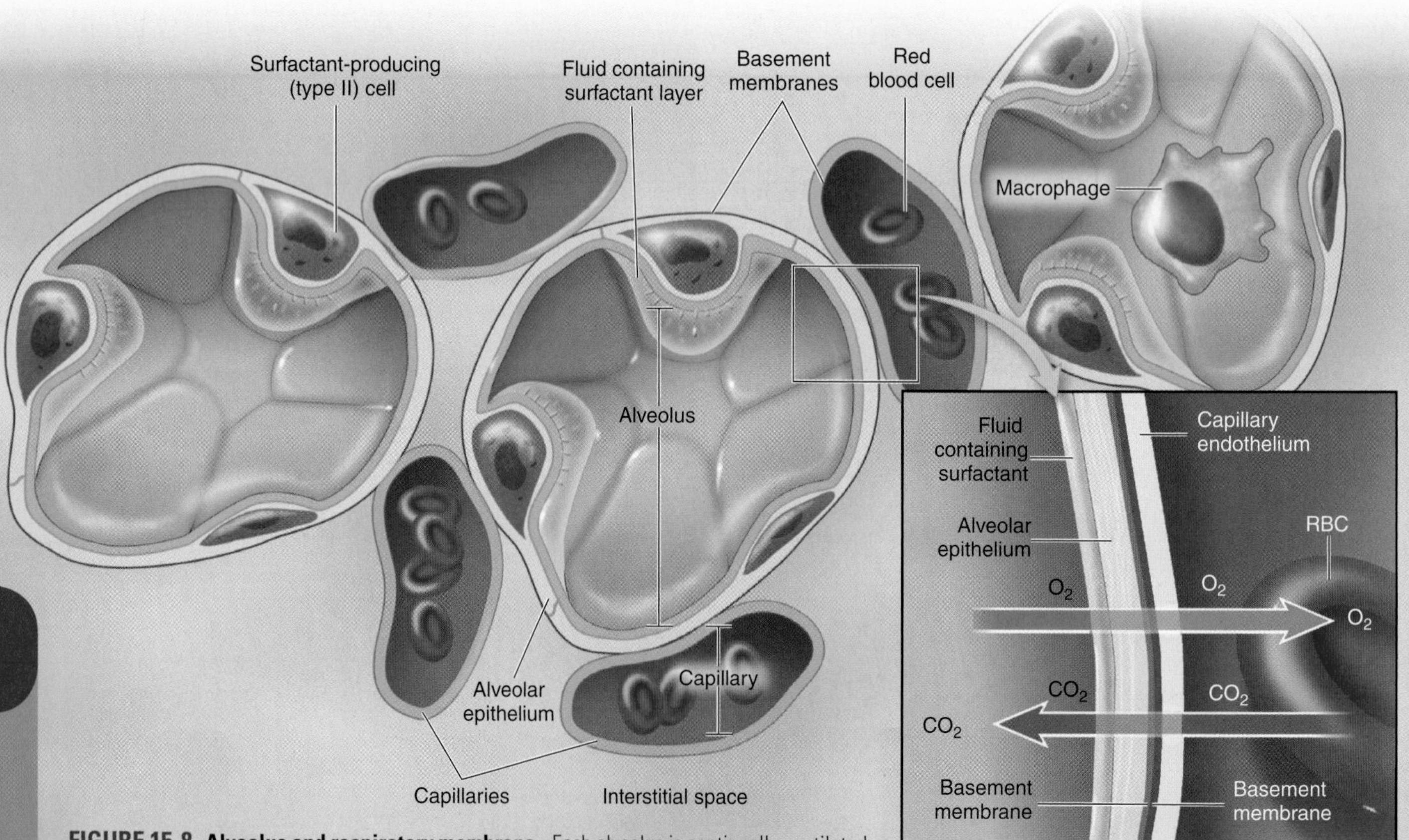

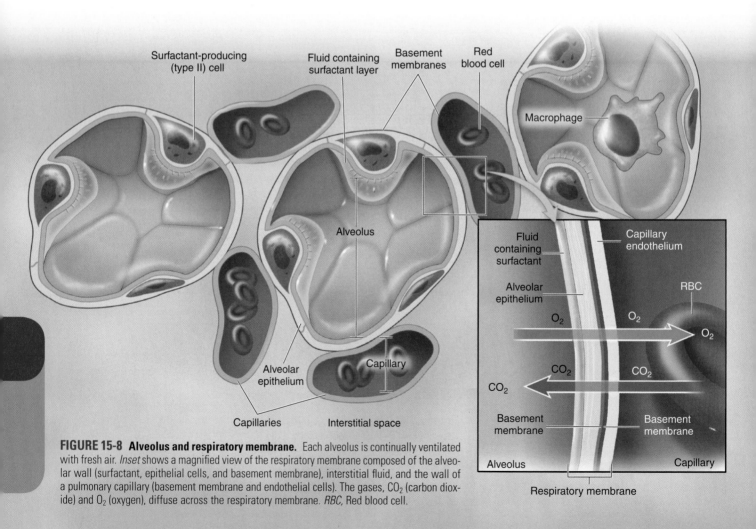

FIGURE 15-8 Alveolus and respiratory membrane. Each alveolus is continually ventilated with fresh air. *Inset* shows a magnified view of the respiratory membrane composed of the alveolar wall (surfactant, epithelial cells, and basement membrane), interstitial fluid, and the wall of a pulmonary capillary (basement membrane and endothelial cells). The gases, CO_2 (carbon dioxide) and O_2 (oxygen), diffuse across the respiratory membrane. *RBC,* Red blood cell.

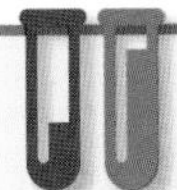

CLINICAL APPLICATION

INFANT RESPIRATORY DISTRESS SYNDROME

Infant respiratory distress syndrome, or **IRDS,** is a serious, life-threatening condition that often affects prematurely born infants or those who weigh less than 2.2 kg (5 lb) at birth. IRDS is the leading cause of death among premature infants in the United States, claiming more than 5000 premature babies each year. The disease, characterized by a lack of **surfactant** in the alveolar air sacs, affects 50,000 babies annually.

Surfactant is manufactured by specialized cells in the walls of the alveoli. Surfactant reduces the surface tension of the fluid on the free surface of the alveolar walls and permits easy movement of air into and out of the lungs. The ability of the body to manufacture this important substance is not fully developed until shortly before birth—normally about 38 weeks after conception.

In newborn infants who are unable to manufacture surfactant, many air sacs collapse during expiration because of the increased surface tension. The effort required to reinflate these collapsed alveoli is much greater than that needed to reinflate normal alveoli with adequate surfactant. The baby soon develops labored breathing, and symptoms of respiratory distress appear shortly after birth.

In the past, treatment of IRDS was limited to keeping the alveoli open so that delivery and exchange of oxygen and carbon dioxide could occur. To accomplish this, a tube was inserted into the respiratory tract, and oxygen-rich air was delivered under sufficient pressure to keep the alveoli from collapsing at the end of expiration. A newer treatment involves delivering air under pressure and applying prepared surfactant directly into the baby's airways by means of a tube.

Alveoli

Alveoli are very effective in promoting the rapid and effective exchange of oxygen and carbon dioxide between blood circulating through the lung capillaries and alveolar air.

Once again, structure and function are closely related. Two characteristics about the structure of alveoli assist in diffusion and make them able to perform this function admirably.

First, the wall of each alveolus is made up of a single layer of simple squamous epithelial cells—and so are the walls of the capillaries that surround and lie in contact with them. This means that, between the blood in the capillaries and the air in each alveolus, there is a barrier less than 1 micron thick. This extremely thin barrier is called the **respiratory membrane** (**Figure 15-8**).

Second, there are millions of alveoli. This means that together they make an enormous surface. The total surface area of all the alveoli together is approximately 84 square meters (915 square feet)—about the size of a small home's floor plan. This huge surface area allows large amounts of oxygen and carbon dioxide to be rapidly exchanged.

The surface of the respiratory membrane inside each alveolus is covered by a substance called **surfactant.** Surfactant helps reduce *surface tension* or "stickiness" of the watery mucus lining the alveoli—keeping the alveoli from collapsing as air moves in and out during respiration. Note the difference in appearance between the surfactant-producing cells and the flattened alveolar epithelial cells shown in **Figure 15-8**.

Do not confuse the *respiratory membrane* separating air in the alveoli from blood in the surrounding pulmonary capillaries with the *respiratory mucosa* (see **Figure 15-2**) that lines the tubes of the respiratory tree.

To learn more about the respiratory membrane, go to AnimationDirect at *evolve.elsevier.com*.

Lungs

The **lungs** are fairly large organs. Note in **Figure 15-9** that deep grooves called *fissures* subdivide each lung into lobes. The right lung has three lobes and the left lung has two.

Figure 15-9 shows the relationship of the lungs to the rib cage at the end of a normal expiration. The narrow, superior position of each lung, up under the collarbone, is the *apex*. The broad, inferior portion resting on the diaphragm is the *base*.

Each lung is made up of all the elements of the bronchial tree, alveoli, and pulmonary blood vessels—along with connective tissues, lymphatic vessels, and nerves. The lung, therefore, is a combination of several kinds of structures that form a unit for respiration.

A **pleura** is a serous membrane that covers the outer surface of each lung and lines the inner surface of the rib cage. The pleura resembles other serous membranes in structure and function. As with the peritoneum or pericardium, the pleura is an extensive, thin, moist, slippery membrane. It lines a large, closed cavity of the body and covers the organs located within it.

The *parietal pleura* lines the walls of the thoracic cavity. The *visceral pleura* covers the lungs, and the intrapleural space lies between the two pleural membranes (**Figure 15-10**).

Normally the intrapleural space contains just enough serous fluid to make both portions of the pleura moist and slippery and able to glide easily over each other as the lungs expand and deflate with each breath. **Pleurisy** is an inflammation of the pleura that causes pain when the parietal and visceral pleural membranes rub together.

Pneumothorax is the presence of air in the intrapleural space on one side of the chest. The additional air increases the pressure on the lung on that side and causes it to collapse. While collapsed, the lung does not function in breathing.

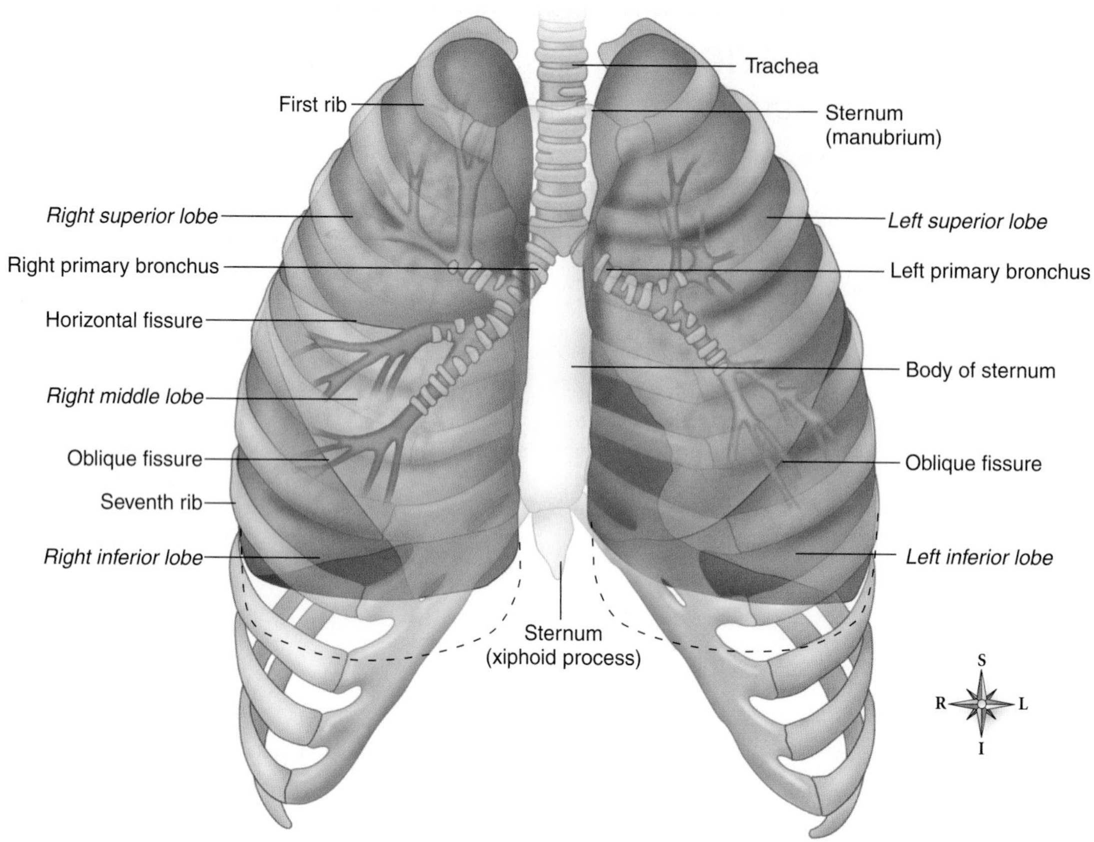

FIGURE 15-9 Lungs. The trachea is an airway that branches to form an inverted tree of bronchi and bronchioles. Note that the right lung has three lobes and the left lung has two lobes. The rib cage is semi-transparent so that lung structures are easily visible.

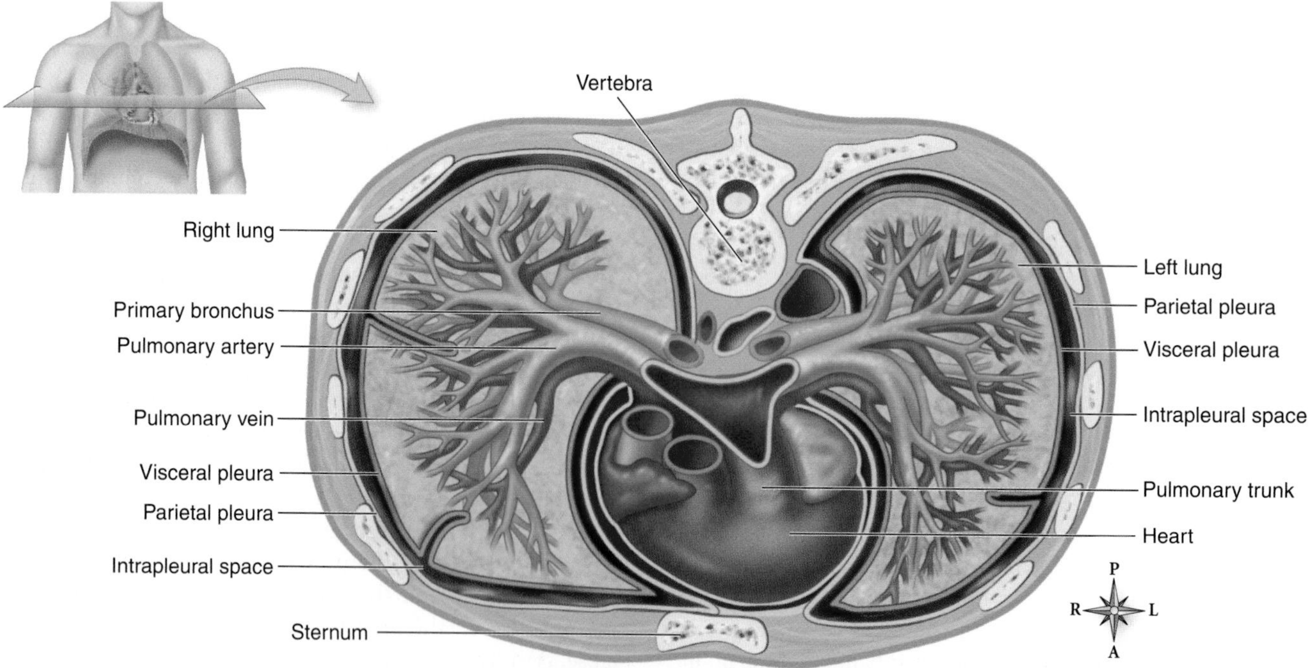

FIGURE 15-10 Lungs and pleura. *Inset* shows from where in the body this transverse section of the thorax was cut. A serous membrane lines the thoracic wall (parietal pleura) and then folds inward near the bronchi to cover the lung (visceral pleura). The intrapleural space contains a small amount of serous pleural fluid.

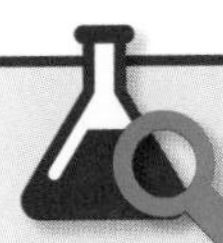

RESEARCH, ISSUES, AND TRENDS

LUNG VOLUME REDUCTION SURGERY

Lung volume reduction surgery (LVRS) is a "treatment of last resort" for severe cases of emphysema. It involves the removal of 20% to 30% of each lung. Diseased tissue is generally removed from the upper, or apical, areas of the superior lobes. Evidence from a number of large clinical trials has now shown that the LVRS procedure may benefit or at least help stabilize selected emphysema patients whose lung function continues to decline despite aggressive pulmonary rehabilitation efforts and other, more conservative forms of treatment.

More than 2 million Americans, who are older than age 50 and current or former smokers, have **emphysema**—a major cause of disability and death in the United States. Emphysema is one of a number of conditions classified as a **chronic obstructive pulmonary disease** (**COPD**). Emphysema is characterized by the trapping of air in alveoli of the lung, which causes them to rupture and fuse to other alveoli.

Although lung damage caused by emphysema is irreversible, in some cases the disease may be halted or its progression slowed by LVRS. In the end stages of this chronic disease, breathing becomes labored as the lungs fill with large, irregular spaces resulting from the enlargement and rupture of many alveoli (see illustration). The LVRS procedure removes part of the diseased lung tissue and increases available space in the pleural cavities. As a result, the diaphragm and other respiratory muscles can more effectively move air into and out of the remaining lung tissue, thereby improving pulmonary function and making breathing easier.

LVRS may reduce the need for lung transplantation procedures and augment the effectiveness of such supporting medical treatments as nutritional supplementation and exercise training in the treatment of selected late-stage emphysema patients. Newer and less invasive techniques involving smaller incisions and specialized video equipment inserted into the thoracic cavity (video-assisted thoracic surgery) are now being used for many LVRS procedures. As a result, the relatively long hospital stays and home recovery periods previously required after more traditional open-chest surgery have been shortened.

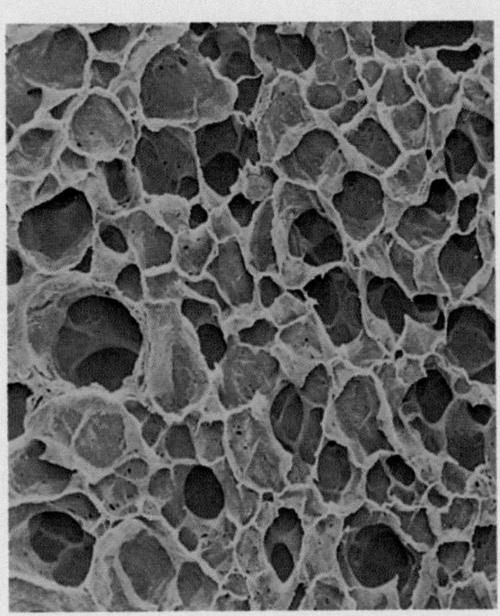

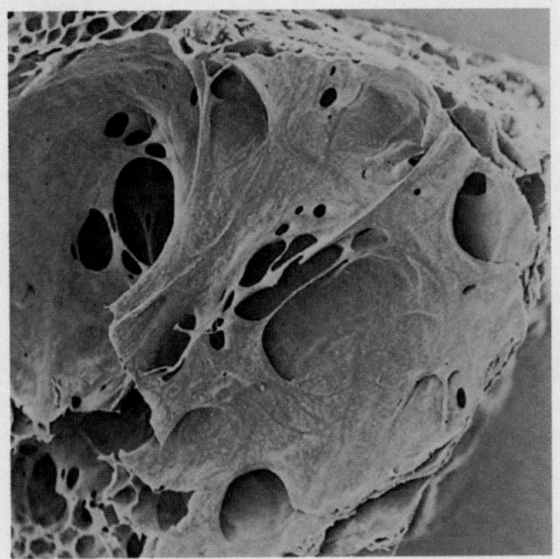

Emphysema. The effects of emphysema can be seen in these scanning electron micrographs of lung tissue. **A,** Normal lung with many small alveoli. **B,** Lung tissue affected by emphysema. Notice that the alveoli have merged into larger air spaces, thereby greatly reducing the surface area available for gas exchange.

QUICK CHECK

1. What are bronchi? What is their function?
2. What is the function of the alveoli?
3. Can you describe the structure and function of the pleura?
4. What is the difference between the respiratory membrane and respiratory mucosa?

Respiration

Respiration means exchange of gases (oxygen and carbon dioxide) between a living organism and its environment. If the organism consists of only one cell, gases can move directly between it and the environment. If, however, the organism consists of billions of cells, as do our bodies, most of its cells are too far from the air for a direct exchange of gases. To overcome this difficulty, a pair of organs—the lungs—provides a place where air and a circulating fluid (blood) can come close enough to each other for oxygen to move out of the air into the blood while at the same time carbon dioxide moves out of the blood into air.

Breathing, or **pulmonary ventilation,** is the process that moves air into and out of the lungs. It makes possible the exchange of gases between air in the lungs and in the blood. Together, these processes are often called **external respiration.**

In addition, exchange of gases occurs between the blood and the cells of the systemic tissues of the body, which then use the oxygen in the biochemical pathways that transfer energy from nutrient molecules to ATP. Together, these processes are called **internal respiration.** The term **cellular respiration** refers to the use of oxygen by cells in the process of metabolism, which is discussed further in Chapter 17.

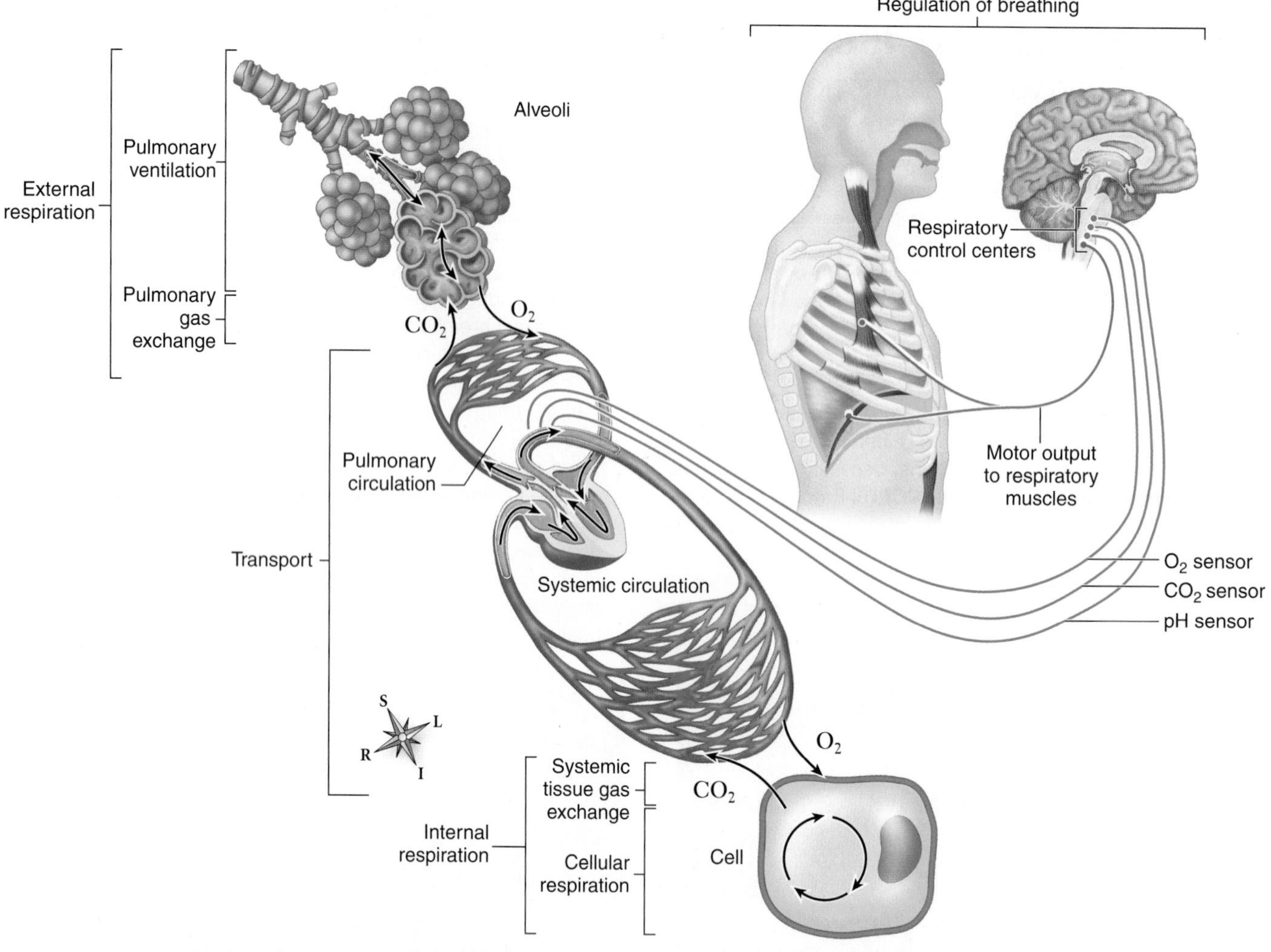

FIGURE 15-11 Overview of respiratory physiology. This chapter is organized around the principle that respiratory function includes external respiration (ventilation and pulmonary gas exchange), transport of gases by blood, and internal respiration (systemic tissue gas exchange and cellular respiration). Cellular respiration is discussed separately (see Chapter 17). Regulatory mechanisms centered in the brainstem use feedback from blood gas sensors to regulate ventilation.

All of these respiratory processes require transport of gases (oxygen and carbon dioxide) by the blood. And because a relatively constant set point concentration of these blood gases is required for survival, there are complex regulatory mechanisms that control them.

Figure 15-11 summarizes the major concepts of respiratory physiology, and we use it as the basis of discussion in the remaining sections of this chapter. Refer to this figure after reading each section to help you put your new learning into a useful "big picture" and deepen your understanding.

Pulmonary Ventilation

Mechanics of Breathing

Pulmonary ventilation, or breathing, has two phases. **Inspiration,** or **inhalation,** moves air into the lungs, and **expiration,** or **exhalation,** moves air out of the lungs.

The lungs are enclosed within the thoracic cavity. Thus changes in the shape and size of the thoracic cavity result in changes in the air pressure within that cavity and in the lungs. This difference in air pressure is the driving force of movement of air into and out of the lungs. Air moves from an area where pressure is high to an area where pressure is lower. Anything that flows—whether it is blood, lymph, or air—follows this primary principle: a fluid always flows down a pressure gradient.

Respiratory muscles are responsible for the changes in the shape of the thoracic cavity that change the internal air pressures involved in breathing.

Inspiration

Inspiration occurs when the chest cavity enlarges. As the thorax enlarges, the lungs expand along with it, and air rushes into them and down into the alveoli. This happens because of a very important law of physics: the volume and pressure of a gas are inversely proportional. That means that when the volume of a gas goes up, as lung volume goes up when we expand

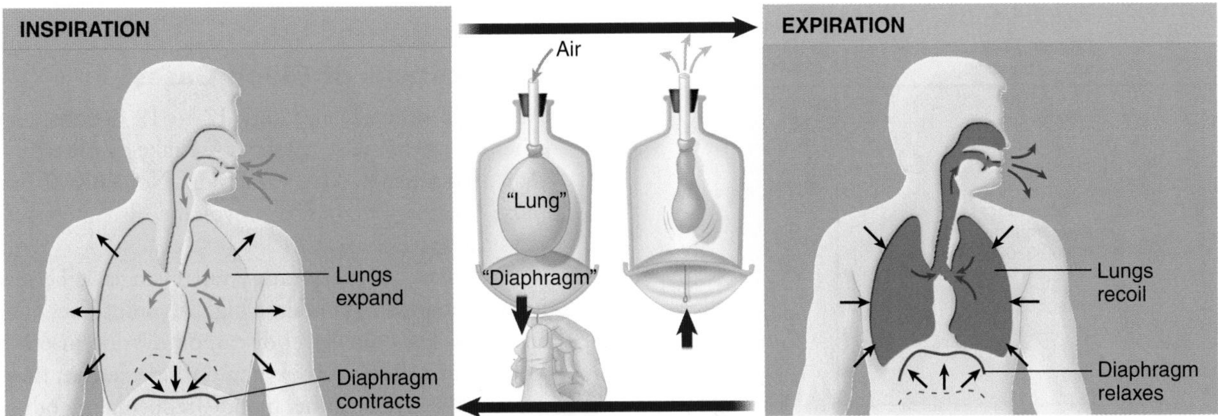

FIGURE 15-12 Mechanics of breathing. During *inspiration,* the diaphragm contracts, increasing the volume of the thoracic cavity. This increase in volume results in a decrease in pressure, which causes air to rush into the lungs. During *expiration,* the diaphragm returns to an upward position, reducing the volume in the thoracic cavity. Air pressure increases then, forcing air out of the lungs. *Insets* show the classic model in which a jar represents the rib cage, a rubber sheet represents the diaphragm, and a balloon represents the lungs.

the thorax, then the pressure goes down. Thus air pressure in the lungs decreases during inspiration. When air pressure in the lungs is less than atmospheric air pressure, air rushes down its pressure gradient into the lungs.

Muscles that increase the volume of the thorax are classified as **inspiratory muscles** and include the **diaphragm** and the *external intercostal muscles.*

The diaphragm is the dome-shaped muscle separating the abdominal cavity from the thoracic cavity. The diaphragm flattens out when it contracts during inspiration. Instead of protruding up into the chest cavity, as it does at rest, it moves down toward the abdominal cavity as it contracts. Thus the contraction or flattening of the diaphragm makes the chest cavity longer from top to bottom. The diaphragm is the most important muscle of inspiration. Nerve impulses passing through the **phrenic nerve** stimulate the diaphragm to contract.

The external intercostal muscles are located between the ribs. When they contract, they enlarge the thorax by increasing the size of the cavity from front to back and from side to side. Contraction of the inspiratory muscles increases the volume of the thoracic cavity and reduces lung air pressure below atmospheric pressure, drawing air into the lungs (**Figure 15-12**).

Expiration

Quiet, resting expiration is ordinarily a passive process that begins when the inspiratory muscles relax and return to their resting length. The thoracic cavity returns to its smaller volume. The elastic nature of thoracic and lung tissue also causes these organs to "recoil" and decrease in size. Because volume and pressure are inversely proportional (one goes up as the other goes down), the decrease in lung volume causes an increase in lung air pressure. As the lung air pressure rises above atmospheric air pressure, air flows down its pressure gradient and outward through the respiratory passageways.

When we speak, sing, or do heavy work, we may need more forceful expiration to increase the rate and depth of ventilation. During more forceful expiration, the **expiratory muscles** (*internal intercostal muscles* and *abdominal muscles*) contract.

When contracted, the internal intercostal muscles pull the rib cage inward and decrease the front-to-back size of the thorax. Contraction of the abdominal muscles pushes the abdominal organs against the underside of the diaphragm, pushing it farther upward into the thoracic cavity. As the thoracic cavity decreases in size, the air pressure within it increases above atmospheric air pressure and air flows out of the lungs (see **Figure 15-12**).

Pulmonary Volumes

A special device called a **spirometer** is used to measure the amount of air exchanged in breathing. **Figure 15-13** illustrates the various pulmonary volumes, which can be measured as a subject breathes into a spirometer.

We take 500 mL (about a pint) of air into our lungs with each normal inspiration and expel it with each normal expiration. Because this amount comes and goes regularly like the tides of the sea, it is referred to as the **tidal volume (TV)**. The largest amount of air that we can breathe out in one expiration—by inhaling as deeply as possible, then exhaling fully—is known as the **vital capacity** (**VC**). In young men, this is normally about 4800 mL.

Tidal volume and vital capacity are frequently measured in patients with lung disease such as emphysema or heart problems, conditions that often lead to abnormally low volumes of air being moved in and out of the lungs.

Observe the area in **Figure 15-13** that represents the **expiratory reserve volume** (**ERV**). This is the amount of air that can be forcibly exhaled after expiring the tidal volume. Compare this with the area in **Figure 15-13** that represents the **inspiratory reserve volume** (**IRV**). The IRV is the amount of air that can be forcibly inspired over and above a normal inspiration. As the tidal volume increases, the ERV and IRV decrease.

Note in **Figure 15-13** that VC is the total of tidal volume, inspiratory reserve volume, and expiratory reserve volume—or expressed in another way: VC = TV + IRV + ERV.

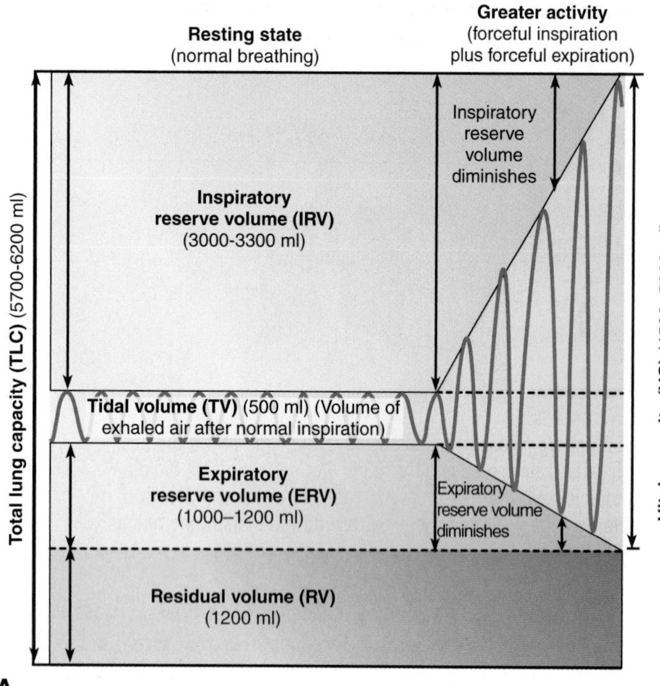

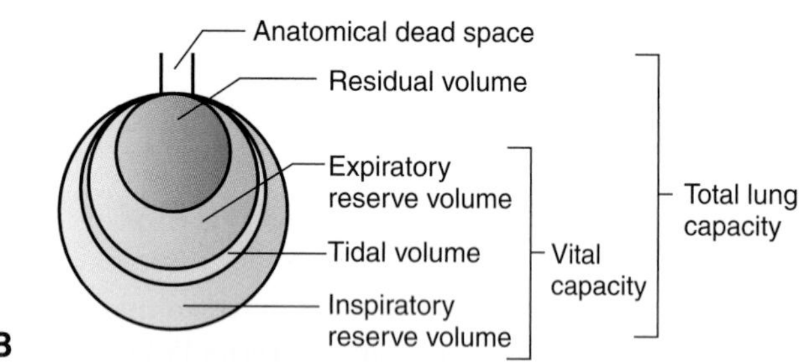

FIGURE 15-13 Pulmonary ventilation volumes. The chart in **A** shows a tracing like that produced with a spirometer. The diagram in **B** shows the pulmonary volumes as relative proportions of an inflated balloon (see **Figure 15-12**). During normal, quiet breathing, about 500 mL of air is moved into and out of the respiratory tract, an amount called the *tidal volume*. During forceful breathing (like that during and after heavy exercise), an extra 3300 mL can be inspired (the inspiratory reserve volume), and an extra 1000 mL or so can be expired (the expiratory reserve volume). The largest volume of air that can be moved in and out during ventilation is called the *vital capacity*. Air that remains in the respiratory tract after a forceful expiration is called the *residual volume*.

Residual volume (**RV**) is simply the air that remains in the lungs after the most forceful expiration.

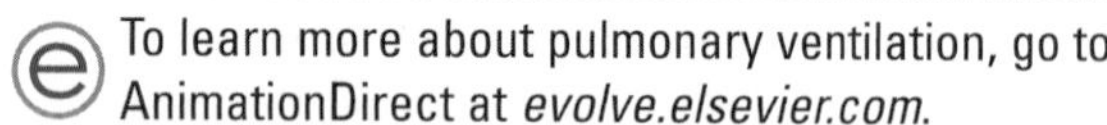
To learn more about pulmonary ventilation, go to AnimationDirect at *evolve.elsevier.com*.

QUICK CHECK

1. How does the diaphragm operate during inspiration? During expiration?
2. In what form does oxygen travel in the blood? What form of carbon dioxide?
3. What is the vital capacity? How is it measured?
4. What is external respiration?

Regulation of Ventilation

Homeostasis of Blood Gases

Although we may take only 12 to 18 breaths a minute when we are not moving about, we take considerably more than that when we are exercising. Not only do we take more breaths, but our tidal volume also increases with physical activity.

The reason our respiratory rate changes is because our body attempts to maintain a high set point level of oxygen and a low set point level of carbon dioxide in our blood. When our cells use up oxygen during exercise, they draw more oxygen from the blood—reducing blood oxygen concentration below its set point. Likewise, cells release more carbon dioxide into the blood during exercise—thus raising the blood carbon dioxide concentration above its set point. Various regulatory mechanisms respond to these changes in negative feedback loops that reverse blood gas concentrations back toward their set point values—by changing our respiratory rate and depth of breathing.

Brainstem Control of Respiration

Changes in respiration depend on proper functioning of the muscles of respiration. These muscles are stimulated by nervous impulses that originate in **respiratory control centers** located in the brainstem.

The brainstem centers are influenced by input from a number of sensory receptors located in different areas of the body. These receptors can sense the need for changing the rate or depth of respirations to maintain homeostasis. Certain receptors sense carbon dioxide or oxygen levels, whereas others sense blood acid levels or the amount of stretch in lung tissues.

CLINICAL APPLICATION

OXYGEN THERAPY

Oxygen therapy is the administration of oxygen to individuals suffering from **hypoxia**—an insufficient oxygen supply to the tissues. Individuals with certain respiratory problems, such as emphysema, may require supplemental oxygen in order to maintain a normal lifestyle.

Oxygen (O_2) in the form of compressed gas is commonly stored in and dispensed from small, green, metal cylinders or tanks. Because the oxygen dispensed from such tanks is often cold and dry, it is often warmed and moistened, generally by bubbling the released gas through water, to prevent damage to the respiratory tract. Supplemental oxygen is delivered through a mask or tubes that lead into the nasal passage (nasal prongs).

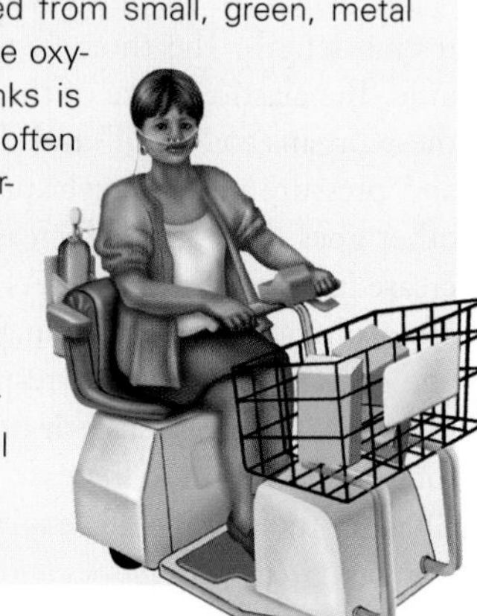

A group of control centers in the medulla—the *medullary rhythmicity area*—seem to produce the basic rhythm of breathing. A normal resting breathing rate is about 12 to 18 breaths a minute. The two most important control centers in the medulla for regulating breathing rhythm are called the *ventral respiratory group (VRG)* and the *dorsal respiratory group (DRG)*. The VRG provides the basic rhythm generator for breathing. The DRG adjusts the breathing rhythm when blood pH or carbon dioxide levels change—as they would during exercise.

Several control centers in the pons—the *pontine respiratory group (PRG)*—seem to provide input to the DRG and thus help modulate the basic rhythm as needed under a variety of changing conditions in the body.

The depth and rate of respiration can be influenced by many "inputs" to the brainstem's respiratory control centers from other areas of the brain or from sensory receptors located outside of the central nervous system (**Figure 15-14**).

Cerebral Cortex Control of Respiration

The cerebral cortex can influence respiration by sending nerve signals that affect the function of the respiratory centers of the brainstem. In other words, an individual may voluntarily override the "automatic" brainstem rhythm of breathing and speed up or slow down the breathing rate—or greatly change the pattern of respiration during activities. This ability permits us to change respiratory patterns and even to hold our breath for short periods to accommodate activities such as speaking, eating, or swimming under water.

This voluntary control of respiration, however, has limits. As discussed in a later section, other factors such as blood carbon dioxide levels are much more powerful in controlling respiration than is conscious control. Regardless of cerebral intent to the contrary, we resume breathing when our bodies sense the need for more oxygen or if carbon dioxide levels increase to certain levels.

Respiratory Reflexes

Chemoreflexes

Chemoreceptors located in the **carotid** and **aortic bodies** are specialized sensory receptors that are sensitive to increases in blood carbon dioxide level and decreases in blood oxygen level. Such **chemoreflexes** can also sense and respond to increasing blood acid levels.

The carotid body chemoreceptors are found at the point where the common carotid arteries divide. The aortic bodies are small clusters of chemosensitive cells that lie adjacent to the aortic arch near the heart (see **Figure 15-14**). When stimulated by increasing levels of blood carbon dioxide, decreasing

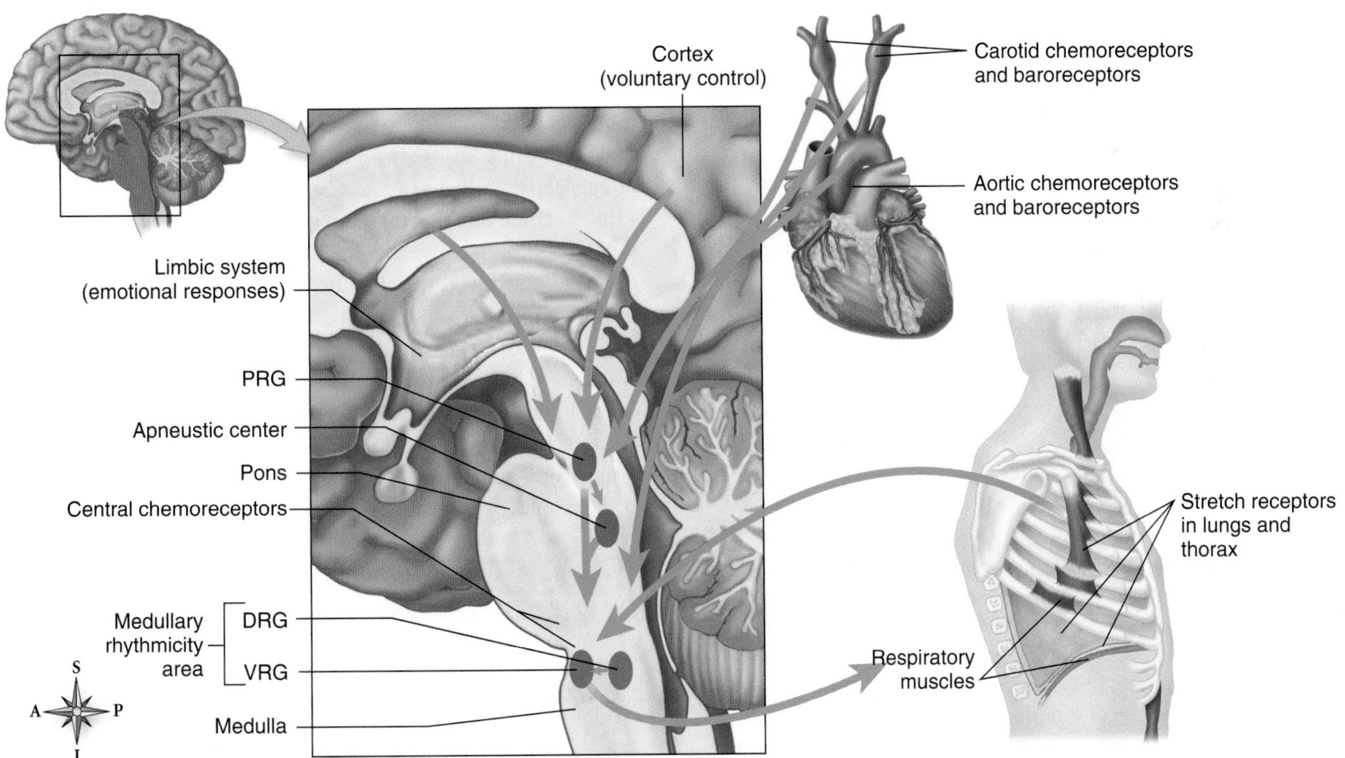

FIGURE 15-14 Regulation of respiration. Respiratory control centers in the brainstem control the basic rate and depth of breathing. The brainstem also receives input from other parts of the body: information from chemoreceptors and stretch receptors can alter the basic breathing pattern, as can emotional and sensory input. Despite these controls, the cerebral cortex can override the "automatic" control of breathing to some extent to accomplish activities such as singing or blowing up a balloon. *Green arrows* show how regulatory information flows into the respiratory control centers. The *purple arrow* shows the flow of regulatory information from the control centers to the respiratory muscles that drive breathing. *DRG,* Dorsal respiratory group; *PRG,* pontine respiratory group; *VRG,* ventral respiratory group.

oxygen levels, or increasing blood acidity, these receptors send nerve impulses to the respiratory regulatory centers that in turn modify respiratory rates.

The blood P_{CO_2} level is the most powerful stimulus driving respiration.

Pulmonary Stretch Reflexes

Stretch receptors in the lungs are located throughout the pulmonary airways and in the alveoli (see **Figure 15-14**). Nervous impulses generated by these receptors influence the normal pattern of breathing and protect the respiratory system from excess stretching caused by harmful overinflation.

When the tidal volume of air has been inspired, the lungs are expanded enough to stimulate stretch receptors that then send inhibitory impulses to the inspiratory center. Relaxation of inspiratory muscles occurs, and expiration follows. After expiration, the lungs are sufficiently deflated to inhibit the stretch receptors, and inspiration is then allowed to start again.

Breathing Patterns

Several terms are used to describe different breathing patterns. These are clinically useful, because they exactly describe respiratory patterns that help assess a person's health state.

Eupnea, for example, refers to a normal respiratory rate. During eupnea, the need for oxygen and carbon dioxide exchange is being met, and the individual is usually not aware of the breathing pattern.

The terms **hyperventilation** and **hypoventilation** describe very rapid and deep or slow and shallow respirations, respectively. Hyperventilation sometimes results from a conscious voluntary effort preceding exertion or from psychological factors—"hysterical hyperventilation."

Dyspnea refers to labored or difficult breathing and is often associated with hypoventilation.

If breathing stops completely for a brief period, regardless of cause, it is called **apnea.** *Sleep apnea* is a condition that results in brief but often frequent pauses in breathing during sleep. It is often caused by enlarged tonsil tissue and may necessitate tonsillectomy. Failure to resume breathing after a prolonged period of apnea is called **respiratory arrest.**

A series of cycles of alternating apnea and hyperventilation is called **Cheyne-Stokes respiration** (**CSR**). CSR may also occur in critical diseases such as congestive heart failure, brain injuries, or brain tumors. CSR also may occur in the case of a drug overdose.

Examples of breathing patterns are summarized in **Table 15-1**.

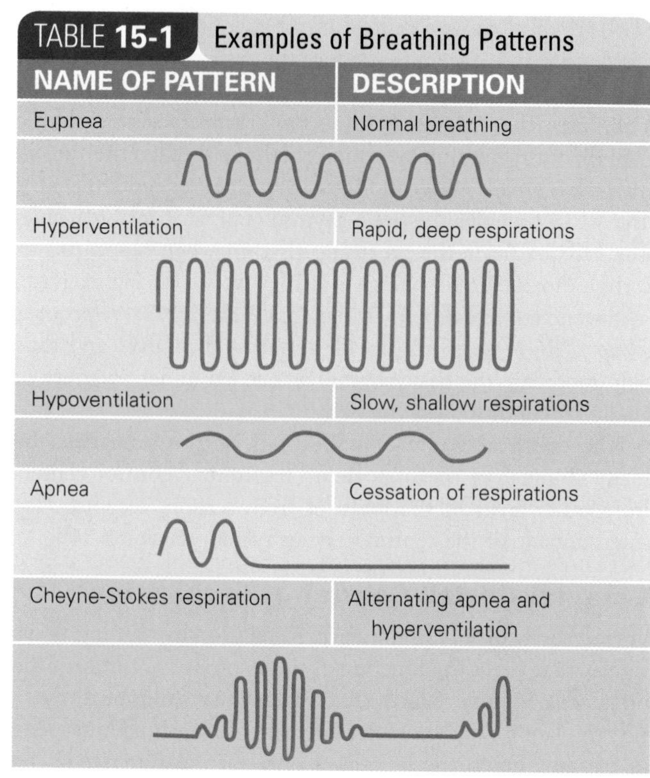

TABLE 15-1 Examples of Breathing Patterns

NAME OF PATTERN	DESCRIPTION
Eupnea	Normal breathing
Hyperventilation	Rapid, deep respirations
Hypoventilation	Slow, shallow respirations
Apnea	Cessation of respirations
Cheyne-Stokes respiration	Alternating apnea and hyperventilation

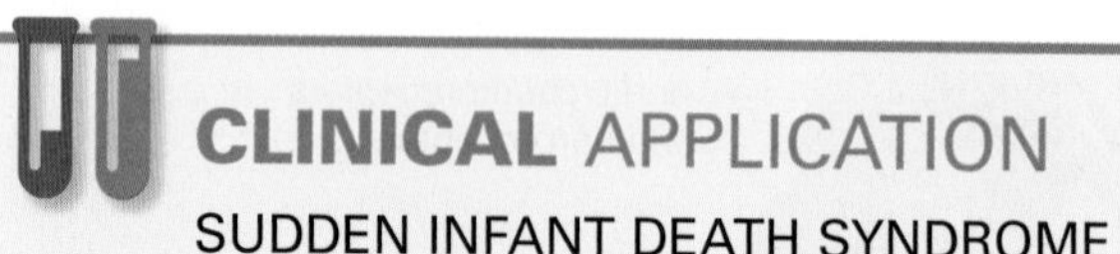

CLINICAL APPLICATION

SUDDEN INFANT DEATH SYNDROME

Sudden infant death syndrome (**SIDS**) is the third-ranking cause of infant death and accounts for about 1 in 9 of the nearly 30,000 infant deaths reported each year in the United States. Sometimes called "crib-death," SIDS occurs most frequently in babies with no obvious medical problems who are younger than 3 months of age. The exact cause of death can seldom be determined, even after extensive testing and autopsy.

SIDS occurs at a higher rate in African American and Native American babies than in white, Hispanic, or Asian infants, although the reasons remain a mystery. Regardless of infant ethnicity, recent data suggest that certain precautions, such as having babies sleep only on their backs and keeping cribs free of pillows or plush toys that might partially cover the nose or mouth, may reduce the incidence of SIDS. Also important is the elimination of smoking during pregnancy and protecting infants from exposure to "secondhand" cigarette smoke after birth. Although the exact cause of SIDS remains unknown, genetic defects involving the structure and function of the respiratory system or unusual physiological responses to common flu or cold viruses may also play a role in this tragic problem.

QUICK CHECK

1. Where are the respiratory control centers located?
2. What is a chemoreceptor? How does it influence breathing?
3. What is hyperventilation? Hypoventilation?

Gas Exchange and Transport

Pulmonary Gas Exchange

Blood pumped from the right ventricle of the heart enters the pulmonary artery and eventually enters the lungs. It then flows through the thousands of tiny pulmonary capillaries that are in close proximity to the air-filled alveoli (see **Figure 15-8**).

External respiration, or the exchange of gases between the blood and alveolar air, occurs by diffusion. Diffusion is a passive process resulting in movement down a concentration gradient (see **Table 3-2** on p. 49). That is, substances move from an area of high concentration to an area of lower concentration of the diffusing substance.

The amounts or concentrations of some blood substances are measured in terms of weight. Reporting how many milligrams of a particular substance are present in 100 mL of blood (mg/dL) is one example. However, the concentration of a particular gas in air or within the blood is expressed as the *pressure* exerted by that gas and is reported in millimeters of mercury (mm Hg). Recall from Chapter 13 that blood pressure levels are also reported in mm Hg.

Several different gases are present in both air and blood. The total pressure of all gases present in an air or blood sample is, of course, the sum of the pressures exerted by each of the gases present. Because the pressure of the so-called *respiratory gases*—oxygen (O_2) and carbon dioxide (CO_2)—in air or blood constitutes only a part of the total pressure present, their concentration is reported as a **partial pressure (P)**. The symbol used to designate partial pressure is the capital letter P preceding the chemical symbol for the gas. For respiratory gases the symbols Po_2 and Pco_2 are used.

Instead of referring directly to "concentration," respiratory physiologists state that blood gas particles diffuse from an area of high *partial pressure* to an area of lower *partial pressure.* Understanding the role of partial pressures of blood gases in normal gas exchange is necessary before considering the diagnosis and treatment of many respiratory disease conditions.

O_2 is continually removed from the blood and used by the body cells. By the time blood flows into the pulmonary capillaries, it has a Po_2 of about 40 mm Hg. Because alveolar air is rich in oxygen (Po_2 100 mm Hg), diffusion causes movement of oxygen from the area of high partial pressure (alveolar air) to the area of lower partial pressure (capillary blood). Put another way, oxygen diffuses "down" its partial pressure gradient.

Diffusion of carbon dioxide also occurs between blood in pulmonary capillaries and alveolar air. Blood flowing through the pulmonary capillaries is high in CO_2, having a Pco_2 of 46 mm Hg. The Pco_2 of alveolar air is about 40 mm Hg. Therefore, diffusion of carbon dioxide results in its movement from an area of high partial pressure in the pulmonary capillaries to an area of lower partial pressure in alveolar air. Once in the alveoli, carbon dioxide leaves the body in expired air (**Figure 15-15**, *top panel*).

Systemic Gas Exchange

The exchange of gases that occurs between blood in systemic capillaries and the body cells is called internal respiration. As you would expect, the direction of movement of oxygen and carbon dioxide during internal respiration is just the opposite of that noted in the exchange that occurs during external respiration, when gases are exchanged between the blood in the pulmonary capillaries and the air in alveoli.

During the process of internal respiration oxygen molecules move rapidly out of the blood through the systemic capillary membrane into the interstitial fluid and on into the cells that make up the tissues. At the same time, carbon dioxide molecules leave the cells, diffuse through the interstitial fluid and then enter the systemic capillaries, eventually being transported to the lungs for elimination from the body. The oxygen is used by the cells in their metabolic activities. Trace these movements of blood gases for yourself using **Figure 15-15**, *bottom panel.*

Diffusion results in the movement of oxygen from an area of high partial pressure in the systemic capillaries (Po_2 100 mm Hg) to an area of lower partial pressure (Po_2 40 mm Hg) in the cells where it is needed. Diffusion is also responsible for the movement of CO_2 from an area of high partial pressure in the cells (Pco_2 46 mm Hg) to an area of lower partial pressure (Pco_2 43 mm Hg) in the systemic capillaries.

Simply stated, during internal respiration oxygenated blood enters systemic capillaries and is changed into deoxygenated blood as it flows through them. During the process of delivering oxygen, the waste product carbon dioxide is also picked up and transported to the lungs for removal from the body.

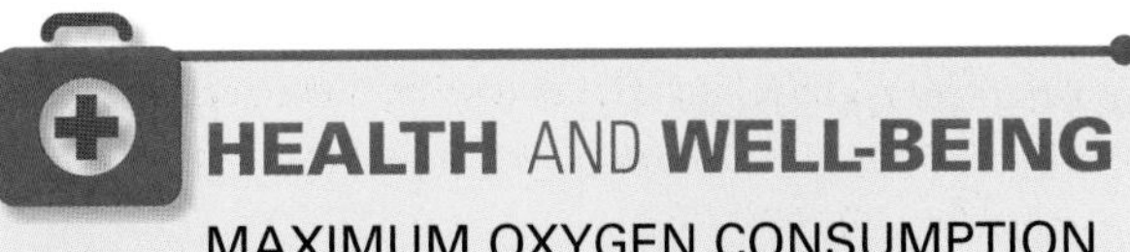

HEALTH AND WELL-BEING

MAXIMUM OXYGEN CONSUMPTION

Exercise physiologists use **maximum oxygen consumption** ($Vo_{2\ max}$) as a predictor of a person's capacity to do aerobic exercise. An individual's $Vo_{2\ max}$ represents the amount of oxygen taken up by the lungs, transported to the tissues, and used to do work. $Vo_{2\ max}$ is determined largely by hereditary factors, but aerobic (endurance) training can increase it by as much as 35%. Many endurance athletes are now using $Vo_{2\ max}$ measurements to help them determine and then maintain their peak condition.

Blood Transportation of Gases

Blood transports the respiratory gases, oxygen and carbon dioxide, either in a dissolved state or combined with other chemicals. Immediately on entering the blood, both oxygen and carbon dioxide dissolve in the plasma, but because fluids can hold only small amounts of gas in solution, most of the oxygen and carbon dioxide rapidly form a chemical union with hemoglobin or water. Once gas molecules are bound to another molecule, their plasma concentration (partial pressure) decreases and more gas can diffuse into the plasma. In this way, comparatively large volumes of the gases can be transported.

Transport of Oxygen

Only very limited amounts of oxygen can be dissolved in the blood. Of the total amount of oxygen that blood can

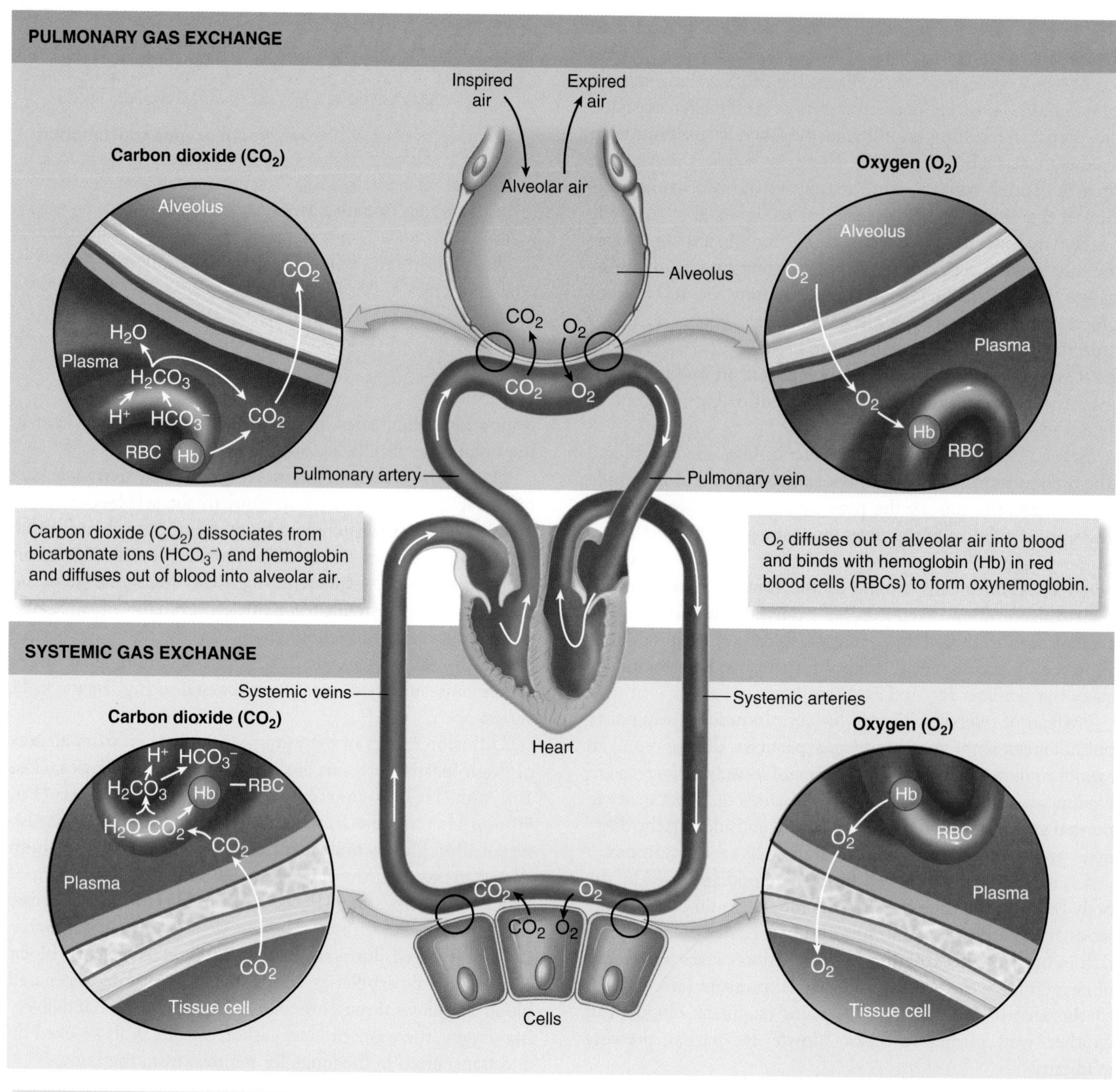

FIGURE 15-15 Exchange and transport of gases. The *top panel* of the diagram shows pulmonary gas exchange and the *bottom panel* shows systemic gas exchange. In each, the *left inset* shows the transport and movement of carbon dioxide (CO_2) and the *right inset* shows the transport and movement of oxygen (O_2).

transport, about 20.4 mL in 100 mL of blood, only about 1.5% or 0.3 mL is actually dissolved. Many times that amount, about 21.1 mL, combines with the hemoglobin (Hb) in 100 mL of blood to form **oxyhemoglobin (HbO_2)** so that it can be carried to the tissues and used by the body cells.

To combine with hemoglobin, oxygen must first diffuse into the RBCs to form oxyhemoglobin. Hemoglobin molecules are large proteins that contain four iron-containing **heme** components, each of which is capable of combining with an oxygen molecule (see **Figure 12-4** on p. 267).

In many ways each hemoglobin molecule acts as a kind of "oxygen sponge." Oxygen associates with hemoglobin rapidly—so rapidly, in fact, that about 97% of the blood's hemoglobin has united with oxygen and become "oxygenated blood" by the time it leaves the pulmonary capillaries to return to the heart.

Oxygenated blood is found in the systemic arteries and pulmonary veins. Normally, oxygenated blood is 97% "saturated." So-called deoxygenated blood, found in the systemic veins and pulmonary arteries, is still about 75% saturated with oxygen. The difference in oxygen saturation results from the release of oxygen from oxyhemoglobin to supply the body cells. Therefore the binding of oxygen to hemoglobin is said to be reversible, with oxyhemoglobin formation or oxygen release dependent on the partial pressure of oxygen driving the reaction.

Summing up, we can say that oxygen travels in two forms: (1) as dissolved O_2 in the plasma and (2) as a combination of O_2 and hemoglobin (oxyhemoglobin). Of these two forms of transport, oxyhemoglobin carries the vast majority of the total oxygen transported by the blood.

Transport of Carbon Dioxide

Carbon dioxide is a by-product of cellular metabolism and plays an important and necessary role in regulating the pH of body fluids. However, if it accumulates in the body beyond normal limits (40 to 50 mm Hg in venous blood), it can quickly become toxic. Elimination of excess CO_2 from the body occurs when it enters the alveoli and is expelled during expiration. For this to occur, CO_2 must be transported in the blood to the lungs in one of three forms, as described in the following sections.

Carbon Dioxide

About 10% of the total amount of carbon dioxide in blood is carried in the *dissolved form*. It is this dissolved CO_2 that produces the P_{CO_2} of blood plasma. However, all CO_2 in the blood must pass through the dissolved state before moving into or out of any of the states described in the following sections.

Carbaminohemoglobin

About 20% of the total CO_2 transported in the blood is in the form of **carbaminohemoglobin ($HbCO_2$)**. **$HbCO_2$** is formed by the union of carbon dioxide and hemoglobin.

The formation of this compound is accelerated by an increase in P_{CO_2}—as the extra dissolved CO_2 binds to hemoglobin. Likewise, formation of $HbCO_2$ is slowed—or even reversed—by a decrease in P_{CO_2}.

Bicarbonate

About 70% of the total CO_2 transported in the blood is carried in the form of **bicarbonate ions (HCO_3^-)**.

When CO_2 dissolves in water (as in blood plasma), some of the CO_2 molecules associate with water (H_2O) to form *carbonic acid (H_2CO_3)*. Once formed, some of the H_2CO_3 molecules dissociate to form hydrogen (H^+) and bicarbonate (HCO_3^-) ions. The speed of this process is quite slow when it occurs in the plasma, but the rate of reaction increases dramatically within RBCs because of the presence of an enzyme called **carbonic anhydrase (CA)**. The reaction is summarized by the following chemical equation:

$$\underset{\text{Carbon dioxide}}{CO_2} + \underset{\text{Water}}{H_2O} \rightleftharpoons \underset{\text{Carbonic acid}}{H_2CO_3} \rightleftharpoons \underset{\text{Hydrogen ion}}{H^+} + \underset{\text{Bicarbonate ion}}{HCO_3^-}$$

Note that the arrows go in both directions. This indicates that the reaction is *reversible*—it can go in either direction. If bicarbonate is being formed, CO_2 molecules entering into plasma can continually be removed from the blood and transported to the lungs. And, when the process is reversed in the

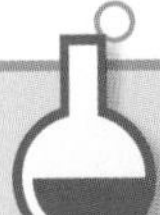

SCIENCE APPLICATIONS

RESPIRATORY MEDICINE

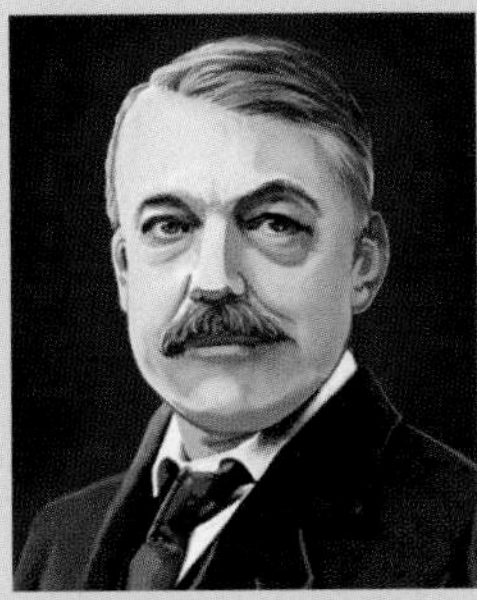

Christian Bohr (1855-1911)

The Danish physician Christian Bohr left a legacy of achievement in science in more ways than one. His son Niels Bohr (creator of the *Bohr model* of the atom seen in **Figure 2-4** on p. 26) and his grandson Aage Bohr both won Nobel Prizes in science, as did his student August Krogh. Christian Bohr's contributions to understanding respiration, however, have also left a lasting mark on respiratory physiology and medicine—resulting in three Nobel Prize nominations of his own.

Bohr's most famous discovery was the fact that a decrease in plasma pH or an increase in P_{CO_2} will decrease hemoglobin's binding affinity with oxygen. Called the *Bohr effect,* this phenomenon explains how Hb so easily gives up its oxygen in very active tissues like muscles during exercise—where an increase in CO_2 and the accompanying acidity reflects the amount of cellular work and thus an increased use of oxygen.

The contributions of Bohr and many others to today's understanding of the relationship of respiration, blood gases, and pH continue to play a central role in health care. Today, countless *physicians, nurses,* **respiratory therapists, emergency medical technicians,** and **paramedics**, continue to benefit from an understanding of these fundamental principles of physiology.

lungs, CO_2 can be released to enter the alveolar air and then be exhaled.

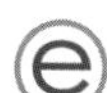
To learn more about gas exchange, go to AnimationDirect at *evolve.elsevier.com*.

QUICK CHECK

1. What is internal respiration?
2. In what form does most oxygen travel in the blood?
3. In what 3 forms does carbon dioxide travel in the blood?

LANGUAGE OF SCIENCE AND MEDICINE *(continued from p. 341)*

carbaminohemoglobin ($HbCO_2$)
(kahr-bam-ih-no-hee-moh-GLOH-bin)
[*carb-* **coal (carbon)**, *-amino-* **ammonia compound (amino acid)**, *-hemo-* **blood**, *-glob-* **ball**, *-in* **substance**]

carbonic anhydrase (CA)
(kar-BON-ik an-HYE-drayz)
[*carbo-* **coal**, *-ic* **relating to**, *a-* **without**, *-hydr-* **water**, *-ase* **enzyme**]

carotid body
(kah-ROT-id BOD-ee]
[*caro-* **heavy sleep**, *-id* **relating to**]

cellular respiration
(SEL-yoo-lar res-pih-RAY-shun)
[*cell* **storeroom**, *-ular* **relating to**, *re-* **again**, *-spir-* **breathe**, *-ation* **process**]

chemoreceptor
(kee-moh-ree-SEP-tor)
[*chemo-* **chemical**, *-recept-* **receive**, *-or* **agent**]

chemoreflex
(kee-moh-REE-fleks)
[*chemo-* **chemical**, *-re-* **back or again**, *-flex* **bend**]

Cheyne-Stokes respiration (CSR)
(chayn stohks res-pih-RAY-shun)
[*John Cheyne* **Scots physician**, *William Stokes* **Irish physician**, *re-* **again**, *-spir-* **breathe**, *-ation* **process of**]

chronic obstructive pulmonary disease (COPD)
(KRON-ik ob-STRUK-tiv PUL-moh-nayr-ee dih-ZEEZ)
[*chron-* **time**, *-ic* **relating to**, *obstruct-* **block**, *-ive* **relating to**, *pulmon-* **lung**, *-ary* **relating to**, *dis-* **opposite of**, *-ease* **comfort**]

ciliary escalator
(SIL-ee-ayr-ee ES-kuh-lay-ter)
[*cili-* **eyelash**, *-ary* **relating to**, *escalat-* **scale**, *-or* **agent**]

conchae
(KONG-kee or KONG-kay)
sing., concha
(KONG-kah)
[*concha* **sea shell**]

diaphragm
(DYE-ah-fram)
[*dia-* **across**, *-phrag-* **enclose**, *-(u)m* **thing**]

diffusion
(dih-FYOO-shun)
[*diffus-* **spread out**, *-sion* **process**]

dyspnea
(DISP-nee-ah)
[*dys-* **painful**, *-pne-* **breathe**, *-a* **condition**]

emergency medical technician
(eh-MER-jen-see MED-ih-kal tek-NISH-en)
[*medic-* **heal**, *-al* **relating to**, *techn-* **art or skill**, *-ic* **relating to**, *-ian* **practitioner**]

emphysema
(em-fih-ZEE-mah)
[*em-* **in**, *-physema* **blowing or puffing up**]

endotracheal intubation
(en-doh-TRAY-kee-al in-too-BAY-shun)
[*endo-* **within**, *-trache-* **rough duct**, *-al* **relating to**, *in-* **within**, *-tub-* **tube**, *-ation* **process**]

epiglottis
(ep-ih-GLOT-is)
[*epi-* **upon**, *-glottis* **mouth of windpipe**]

eupnea
(YOOP-nee-ah)
[*eu-* **easily**, *-pne-* **breathe**, *-a* **condition**]

eustachian tube
(yoo-STAY-shun toob)
[*Bartolomeo Eustachio* **Italian anatomist**, *-an* **relating to**]

expiration (exhalation)
(eks-pih-RAY-shun [eks-huh-LAY-shun])
[*ex-* **out**, *-pir-* **breathe**, *-ation* **process** (*ex-* **out**, *-hal-* **breathe**, *-ation* **process**)]

expiratory muscle
(eks-PYE-rah-tor-ee MUS-el)
[*ex-* **out of**, *-[s]pir-* **breathe**, *-tory* **relating to**, *musc-* **mouse**, *-cle* **little**]

expiratory reserve volume (ERV)
(eks-PYE-rah-tor-ee ree-ZERV VOL-yoom)
[*ex-* **out of**, *-[s]pir-* **breathe**, *-tory* **relating to**]

external nares
(eks-TER-nal NAY-reez)
sing., naris
(NAY-ris)
[*extern-* **outside**, *-al* **relating to**, *naris* **nostril**]

external respiration
(eks-TER-nal res-pih-RAY-shun)
[*extern-* **outside**, *-al* **relating to**, *re-* **again**, *-spir-* **breathe**, *-ation* **process of**]

glottis
(GLOT-iss)
[*glottis* **mouth of windpipe**]

heme
(heem)
[*hem-* **blood**]

hyperventilation
(hye-per-ven-tih-LAY-shun)
[*hyper-* **excessive**, *-vent-* **fan or create wind**, *-tion* **process**]

hypoventilation
(hye-poh-ven-tih-LAY-shun)
[*hypo-* **under or below**, *-vent-* **fan or create wind**, *-tion* **process**]

hypoxia
(hye-POK-see-ah)
[*hypo-* **under or below**, *-ox-* **oxygen**, *-ia* **condition**]

infant respiratory distress syndrome (IRDS)
(IN-fant RES-pih-rah-toh-ree dih-STRESS SIN-drohm)
[*re-* **again**, *-spir-* **breathe**, *-tory* **relating to**, *syn-* **together**, *-drome* **course**]

inspiration (inhalation)
(in-spih-RAY-shun)
[*in-* **in**, *-spir-* **breathe**, *-ation* **process**]

inspiratory muscle
(in-SPY-rah-tor-ee MUS-el)
[*in-* **in**, *-spir-* **breathe**, *-tory* **relating to**, *mus-* **mouse**, *-cle* **little**]

inspiratory reserve volume (IRV)
(in-SPY-rah-tor-ee ree-SERV VOL-yoom)
[*in-* **in**, *-spir-* **breathe**, *-tory* **relating to**]

interarytenoid notch
(IN-ter-ar-ih-tee-noyd notch)
[*inter-* **among**, *-aryten-* **ladle**, *-oid* **like**]

internal respiration
(in-TER-nal res-pih-RAY-shun)
[*intern-* **inside**, *-al* **relating to**, *re-* **again**, *-spir-* **breathe**, *-ation* **process**]

lacrimal sac
(LAK-rih-mal sak)
[*lacrima-* **tear**, *-al* **relating to**]

laryngopharynx
(lah-ring-go-FAYR-inks)
[*laryng-* **voice box (larynx)**, *-pharynx* **throat**]

larynx
(LAYR-inks)
[*larynx* **voice box**]

lingual tonsil
(LING-gwal TAHN-sil)
[*ling-* **tongue,** *-al* **relating to,** *tons-* **goiter,** *-il* **little**]

lower respiratory tract
(LOW-er RES-pih-rah-tor-ee trakt)
[*re-* **again,** *-spir-* **breathe,** *-tory* **relating to,** *tract* **trail**]

lung

maximum oxygen consumption
[*maximum* **greatest,** *oxy-* **sharp,** *-gen* **produce,** *con-* **with or in,** *-sum-* **take,** *-tion* **process**]

mucus
(MYOO-kus)
[*mucus* **slime**]

nasal cavity
(NAY-zal KAV-ih-tee)
[*nas-* **nose,** *-al* **relating to,** *cav-* **hollow,** *-ity* **state**]

nasal septum
(NAY-zal SEP-tum)
[*nas-* **nose,** *-al* **relating to,** *septum* **wall**]

nasopharynx
(nay-zoh-FAYR-inks)
[*naso-* **nose,** *-pharynx* **throat**]

nose

oropharynx
(or-oh-FAYR-inks)
[*oro-* **mouth,** *-pharynx* **throat**]

oxyhemoglobin (HbO_2)
(ahk-see-hee-moh-GLOH-bin)
[*oxy-* **sharp,** *-hemo-* **blood,** *-glob-* **ball,** *-in* **substance**]

palatine tonsil
(PAL-ah-tine TAHN-sil)
[*palat-* **palate,** *-ine* **relating to,** *tons-* **goiter,** *-il* **little**]

paramedic
(payr-ah-MED-ik)
[*para-* **beside,** *-med-* **heal,** *-ic-* **relating to**]

paranasal sinus
(payr-ah-NAY-zal SYE-nus)
[*para-* **beside,** *-nas-* **nose,** *-al* **relating to,** *sinus* **hollow**]

partial pressure (P)
(PAR-shal PRESH-ur)

pharyngeal tonsil
(fah-RIN-jee-al TAHN-sil)
[*pharyng-* **throat,** *-al* **relating to,** *tons-* **goiter,** *-il* **little**]

pharynx
(FAYR-inks)
[*pharynx* **throat**]

phrenic nerve
(FREN-ik)
[*phren-* **mind,** *-ic* **relating to**]

pleura
(PLOO-rah)
pl., plurae
(PLOO-ree)
[*pleura* **side of body (rib)**]

pleurisy
(PLOOR-ih-see)
[*pleur-* **side of body (rib),** *-itis* **inflammation**]

pneumothorax
(noo-moh-THOH-raks)
[*pneumo-* **air or wind,** *-thorax* **chest**]

primary bronchi
(PRYE-mayr-ee BRONG-kye)
sing., bronchus
(BRONG-kus)
[*prim-* **first,** *-ary* **relating to,** *bronchus* **windpipe**]

pulmonary ventilation
(PUL-moh-nayr-ee ven-tih-LAY-shun)
[*pulmon-* **lung,** *-ary* **relating to,** *vent-* **fan or create wind,** *-tion* **process**]

residual volume (RV)
(reh-ZID-yoo-al VOL-yoom)
[*residu-* **remainder,** *-al* **relating to**]

respiration
(res-pih-RAY-shun)
[*re-* **again,** *-spir-* **breathe,** *-ation* **process**]

respiratory arrest
(RES-pih-rah-tor-ee ah-REST)
[*re-* **again,** *-spir-* **breathe,** *-tory* **relating to**]

respiratory control center
(RES-pih-rah-tor-ee kon-TROL SEN-ter)
[*re-* **again,** *-spir-* **breathe,** *-tory* **relating to**]

respiratory membrane
(RES-pih-rah-tor-ee MEM-brayn)
[*re-* **again,** *-spir-* **breathe,** *-tory* **relating to,** *membran-* **thin skin**]

respiratory mucosa
(RES-pih-rah-tor-ee myoo-KOH-sah)
[*re-* **again,** *-spir-* **breathe,** *-tory* **relating to,** *mucus* **slime**]

respiratory system
(RES-pih-rah-tor-ee SIS-tem)
[*re-* **again,** *-spir-* **breathe,** *-tory* **relating to**]

respiratory therapist
(RES-pih-rah-tor-ee THAYR-ah-pist)
[*re-* **again,** *-spir-* **breathe,** *-tory* **relating to,** *therap-* **treatment,** *-ist* **agent**]

secondary bronchi
(SEK-on-dayr-ee BRONG-kye)
sing., bronchus
(BRONG-kus)
[*second-* **second,** *-ary* **relating to,** *bronchus* **windpipe**]

sinusitis
(sye-nyoo-SYE-tis)
[*sinus-* **hollow,** *-itis* **inflammation**]

spirometer
(spih-ROM-eh-ter)
[*spir-* **breathe,** *-meter* **measure**]

sudden infant death syndrome (SIDS)
(SUD-den IN-fant deth SIN-drohm)
[*syn-* **together,** *-drome* **running or (race) course**]

surfactant
(sur-FAK-tant)
[**combination of surf(ace) act(ive) a(ge)nt**]

tidal volume (TV)
(TYE-dal VOL-yoom)
[*tid-* **time,** *-al* **relating to**]

tonsillitis
(tahn-sih-LYE-tis)
[*tonsil-* **tonsil,** *-itis* **inflammation**]

tonsils
(TAHN-silz)
[*tons-* **goiter,** *-il* little]

trachea
(TRAY-kee-ah)
[*trachea* **rough duct**]

tracheostomy
(tray-kee-OS-toh-mee)
[*trache-* **rough duct (trachea),** *-os-* **mouth or opening,** *-tom-* **cut,** *-y* **action**]

turbinate
(TUR-bih-nayt)
[*turbin-* **top (spinning toy),** *-ate* **of or like**]

upper respiratory tract
(UP-er RES-pih-rah-tor-ee trakt)
[*re-* **again,** *-spir-* **breathe,** *-tory* **relating to,** *tract* **trail**]

vital capacity (VC)
(VYE-tal kah-PASS-ih-tee)
[*vita-* **life,** *-al* **relating to,** *capac-* **hold,** *-ity* **state**]

vocal cords
(VOH-kul kords)
[*voca-* **voice,** *-al* **relating to,** *cord-* **string**]

OUTLINE SUMMARY

To download a digital audio version of the chapter summary for use with your device, access the ***Audio Chapter Summaries*** *online at evolve.elsevier.com.*

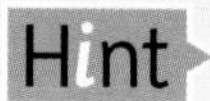

Scan this summary after reading the chapter to help you reinforce the key concepts. Later, use the summary as a quick review before your class or before a test.

Structural Plan

A. Overview
   1. Basic plan of respiratory system would be similar to an inverted tree if it were hollow; leaves of the tree would be comparable to alveoli, with the microscopic sacs enclosed by networks of capillaries (see **Figure 15-1**)
   2. Passive transport process of diffusion is responsible for the exchange of gases that occurs during respiration

B. Respiratory tract
   1. Upper respiratory tract — nose, pharynx, and larynx
   2. Lower respiratory tract — trachea, bronchial tree, and lungs

C. Respiratory mucosa
   1. Structure
      a. Specialized membrane that lines the air distribution tubes in the respiratory tree (see **Figure 15-2**)
      b. Ciliated pseudostratified epithelium — lines most of tract; produces mucus
      c. Stratified squamous epithelium — lines nostrils, vocal folds, pharynx; protective function
      d. Simple squamous epithelium — lines alveoli; facilitates gas exchange
   2. Function
      a. More than 125 mL of mucus produced each day forms a "mucous blanket" over much of the respiratory mucosa
      b. Mucus serves as an air purification mechanism by trapping inspired irritants such as dust and pollen
      c. Ciliary escalator — cilia on mucosal cells beat in only one direction, moving mucus upward to pharynx for removal

Upper Respiratory Tract

A. Nose
   1. Structure
      a. Nasal septum separates interior of nose into two cavities
      b. Mucous membrane lines nose
      c. Frontal, maxillary, sphenoidal, and ethmoidal sinuses drain into nose (see **Figure 15-3**)
   2. Functions
      a. Warms and moistens inhaled air
      b. Contains sense organs of smell

B. Pharynx
   1. Structure (see **Figure 15-4**)
      a. Pharynx (throat) about 12.5 cm (5 inches) long
      b. Divided into nasopharynx, oropharynx, and laryngopharynx
      c. Two nasal cavities, mouth, esophagus, larynx, and auditory tubes all have openings into pharynx
      d. Pharyngeal tonsils and openings of auditory tubes open into nasopharynx; tonsils found in oropharynx
      e. Mucous membrane lines pharynx
   2. Functions
      a. Passageway for food and liquids
      b. Air distribution; passageway for air

C. Larynx
   1. Structure (see **Figure 15-5**)
      a. Nine pieces of cartilage form framework
         (1) Thyroid cartilage (Adam's apple) is largest
         (2) Epiglottis partially covers opening into larynx
      b. Mucous lining
      c. Vocal cords stretch across interior of larynx
   2. Functions
      a. Air distribution; passageway for air to move to and from lungs
      b. Voice production

Lower Respiratory Tract

A. Trachea
   1. Structure (see **Figure 15-6**)
      a. Tube about 11 cm (4.5 in) long and 2.5 cm (1 in) wide
      b. Extends from larynx into the thoracic cavity
      c. Mucous lining
      d. C-shaped rings of cartilage hold trachea open (but allow for swallowing)
   2. Function — passageway for air to move to and from lungs
   3. Obstruction
      a. Blockage of trachea occludes the airway and, if complete, causes death in minutes
      b. Tracheal obstruction causes more than 4000 deaths annually in the United States

B. Bronchial tree
   1. Structure
      a. Trachea branches into right and left bronchi
      b. Each bronchus branches into smaller and smaller tubes eventually leading to bronchioles
      c. Bronchioles end in clusters of microscopic alveolar sacs, the walls of which are made up of alveoli (see **Figure 15-7**)
   2. Function — air distribution; passageway for air to move to and from alveoli

C. Alveoli
1. Respiratory membrane — thin wall that separates pulmonary blood from alveolar air, allowing diffusion of gases
2. Function — exchange of gases between air and blood (see **Figure 15-8**)
3. Surfactant — substance released into alveoli to reduce surface tension and thus prevent collapse of alveoli

D. Lungs
1. Structure (see **Figure 15-9**)
   a. Size — large enough to fill the chest cavity, except for middle space occupied by heart, large blood vessels, thymus, and esophagus
   b. Apex — narrow upper part of each lung, under collarbone
   c. Base — broad lower part of each lung; rests on diaphragm
   d. Pleura — moist, smooth, slippery membrane that lines chest cavity (parietal) and covers outer surface of lungs (visceral); reduces friction between the lungs and chest wall during breathing (see **Figure 15-10**)
2. Function — respiration

Respiration

A. Respiration involves several processes and mechanisms
1. External respiration — pulmonary ventilation (breathing) and pulmonary gas exchange
2. Transport of gases by blood and regulation of set point levels of blood gases
3. Internal respiration — systemic gas exchange and cellular respiration

B. **Figure 15-11** summarizes all these processes and thus serves as a "big picture" view of respiration

Pulmonary Ventilation

A. Mechanics of breathing (see **Figure 15-12**)
1. Basic principles
   a. Pulmonary ventilation includes two phases called *inspiration* (movement of air into lungs) and *expiration* (movement of air out of lungs)
   b. Changes in size and shape of thorax cause changes in air pressure within that cavity and in the lungs
   c. Pressure differences (gradients) cause air to move into and out of the lungs
2. Inspiration
   a. Active process — air moves into lungs
   b. Inspiratory muscles include diaphragm and external intercostals
      (1) Diaphragm flattens when stimulated by phrenic nerve during inspiration — increases top-to-bottom length of thorax
      (2) External intercostal muscles contract and elevate the ribs — increases the size of the thorax from the front to the back and from side to side
   c. Increase in the size of the chest cavity reduces pressure within it; air then enters the lungs by moving down its pressure gradient
3. Expiration
   a. Quiet expiration is ordinarily a passive process
   b. During expiration, thorax returns to its resting size and shape
   c. Elastic recoil of lung tissues aids in expiration
   d. Expiratory muscles used in forceful expiration are internal intercostals and abdominal muscles
      (1) Internal intercostals — contraction depresses the rib cage and decreases the size of the thorax from the front to back
      (2) Contraction of abdominal muscles elevates the diaphragm, thus decreasing size of the thoracic cavity from the top to bottom
   e. Reduction in the size of the thoracic cavity increases its pressure and air leaves the lungs

B. Pulmonary volumes (see **Figure 15-13**)
1. Volumes of air exchanged in breathing can be measured with a spirometer
2. Tidal volume (TV) — amount normally breathed in or out with each breath
3. Vital capacity (VC) — greatest amount of air that one can breathe out in one expiration
4. Expiratory reserve volume (ERV) — amount of air that can be forcibly exhaled after expiring the tidal volume
5. Inspiratory reserve volume (IRV) — amount of air that can be forcibly inhaled after a normal inspiration
6. Residual volume (RV) — air that remains in the lungs after the most forceful expiration

C. Regulation of ventilation
1. Regulation of respiration permits the body to adjust to varying demands for oxygen supply and carbon dioxide removal by maintaining set point concentrations of blood gases
2. Brainstem control of respiration (see **Figure 15-14**)
   a. Most important central regulatory centers in brainstem are called *respiratory control centers*
   b. Medullary centers — under resting conditions the medullary rhythmicity area produces a normal rate and depth of respirations (12 to 18 per minute)
   c. Pontine centers — as conditions in the body vary, these centers in the pons can alter the activity of the medullary rhythmicity area, thus adjusting breathing rhythm
   d. Brainstem centers are influenced by information from other parts of the brain and from sensory receptors located in other body regions
3. Cerebral cortex — voluntary (but limited) control of respiratory activity
4. Respiratory reflexes
   a. Chemoreflexes — chemoreceptors respond to changes in carbon dioxide, oxygen, and blood acid levels — receptors located in carotid and aortic bodies

b. Pulmonary stretch reflexes — respond to the stretch receptors in lungs, thus protecting respiratory organs from overinflation

D. Breathing patterns (see **Table 15-1**)
1. Eupnea — normal breathing
2. Hyperventilation — rapid and deep respirations
3. Hypoventilation — slow and shallow respirations
4. Dyspnea — labored or difficult respirations
5. Apnea — stopped respiration
6. Respiratory arrest — failure to resume breathing after a period of apnea
7. Cheyne-Stokes respiration (CSR) — cycles of alternating apnea and hyperventilation associated with critical conditions

Gas Exchange and Transport

A. Pulmonary gas exchange — exchange of gases in lungs (see **Figure 15-15**)
1. Carbaminohemoglobin breaks down into carbon dioxide and hemoglobin
2. Carbon dioxide moves out of lung capillary blood into alveolar air and out of body in expired air
3. Oxygen moves from alveoli into lung capillaries
4. Hemoglobin combines with oxygen, producing oxyhemoglobin

B. Systemic gas exchange — exchange of gases in tissues (see **Figure 15-15**)
1. Oxyhemoglobin breaks down into oxygen and hemoglobin
2. Oxygen moves out of tissue capillary blood into tissue cells
3. Carbon dioxide moves from tissue cells into tissue capillary blood
4. Hemoglobin combines with carbon dioxide, forming carbaminohemoglobin

C. Blood transportation of gases
1. Transport of oxygen
   a. Only small amounts of oxygen (O_2) can be dissolved in blood
   b. Most oxygen combines with hemoglobin to form oxyhemoglobin (HbO_2) to be carried in blood
2. Transport of carbon dioxide
   a. Dissolved carbon dioxide (CO_2) — 10%
   b. Carbaminohemoglobin ($HbCO_2$) — 20%
   c. Bicarbonate ions (HCO_3^-) — 70%

❑ ACTIVE LEARNING

STUDY TIPS

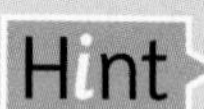

Use these tips to achieve success in meeting your learning goals.

To make the study of the respiratory system more efficient, we suggest these tips:

1. Before you begin or during your more in-depth study of the respiratory system, take time to briefly review helpful information presented in Chapter 2 (chemical reactions and pH), Chapter 3 (diffusion), Chapter 4 (epithelium), Chapter 5 (synopsis of respiratory system), Chapter 6 (mucous and serous membranes), Chapter 12 (red blood cell [RBC] and hemoglobin functions), and Chapter 13 (systemic vs. pulmonary circulation).
2. Think of the respiratory system as a series of tubes serving as an air distribution system. The distribution tubes resemble an "upside-down tree" with the trachea as the trunk and the bronchial tubes being the branches. Ultimately, the very smallest tubes end in millions of tiny, thin-walled sacs (alveoli) that serve as air exchangers for transfer of oxygen and carbon dioxide. Discuss the difference between the respiratory mucosa and the respiratory membrane.
3. Learn how to correlate the movement of air into and out of the lungs (breathing or pulmonary ventilation) with measurement of pressure changes in the chest cavity. To move air in or out of the lungs, the pressure of the chest cavity must be lowered or raised. Changes in pressure are caused by changes in the size (volume) of the thorax, which, in turn, are caused by alternate contraction and relaxation of the inspiratory (diaphragm/external intercostal) and expiratory (internal intercostal and abdominal) respiratory muscles. Expiration can also occur because the elastic nature of lung tissues causes them to "recoil" as air leaves the alveoli, thus assisting in expiration. Flash cards can help you learn the names and definitions of the various pulmonary volumes and types of breathing.
4. In your study group, define the term *partial pressure* of a gas and discuss how the partial pressure of oxygen and of carbon dioxide influence the exchange of these gases in the lungs and tissues. Remember, gases diffuse "down their partial pressure gradients." Flash cards can help you review the various ways that oxygen and carbon dioxide are transported in the blood and can also help you learn the names and locations of the control centers and specialized receptors that influence respiration.
5. As you read and study the chapter, carefully check your understanding of each section by answering the Quick Check questions. Go over the questions at the end of the chapter and discuss possible test questions in your study group. Review the Language of Science and and Medicine terms. Check out *my-ap.us/M0GBpB* for respiratory system tutorials.

Review Questions

Hint

Write out the answers to these questions after reading the chapter and reviewing the Chapter Summary. If you simply think through the answer without writing it down, you won't retain much of your new learning.

1. Differentiate between the respiratory membrane and the respiratory mucosa.
2. List the functions of the paranasal sinuses.
3. List the organs of the upper respiratory system and briefly describe the function of each organ.
4. List the organs of the lower respiratory system and briefly describe the function of each organ.
5. Describe the function of the auditory tube.
6. Describe the function of the epiglottis.
7. Describe, in decreasing order of size, the structures that make up the air tubes of the lung.
8. Describe the pleura and the function of pleural fluid.
9. Differentiate between external respiration, internal respiration, and cellular respiration.
10. Explain the mechanical process of inspiration.
11. Explain the mechanical process of expiration.
12. Define the term *partial pressure (P)* of a gas and explain how the partial pressure of oxygen (Po_2) and carbon dioxide (Pco_2) influence their diffusion.
13. Explain how gas is exchanged between the lung and the blood, and between the blood and the tissues.
14. Name the form that oxygen is carried in the blood. Name how carbon dioxide is carried in the blood.
15. Name and explain the volumes that make up vital capacity.
16. Explain the function of chemoreceptors in regulating respiration.
17. Explain the function of stretch receptors in the lung.

Critical Thinking

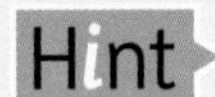

After finishing the Review Questions, write out the answers to these more in-depth questions to help you apply your new knowledge. Go back to sections of the chapter that relate to concepts that you find difficult.

18. Explain the effect smoking has on the body's ability to remove trapped material in the respiratory mucosa.
19. The developing fetus does not produce lung surfactant until late in its development. Explain what problem a premature infant would have if born before surfactant had been produced.
20. Explain the role of other systems in the regulation of respiration.
21. Explain what occurs at the cellular level during carbon monoxide poisoning and why it is so dangerous and can cause death.

Chapter Test

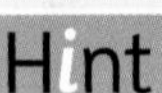

After studying the chapter, test your mastery by responding to these items. Try to answer them without looking up the answers. Then, verify the answers using the key in Appendix C at the back of this book.

1. The organs of the respiratory system are structured to perform two basic functions: ________ and ________.
2. The upper respiratory tract consists of the ________, the ________, and the ________.
3. The lower respiratory tract consists of the ________, the ________, and the ________.
4. The membrane that separates the air in the alveoli from the blood in the surrounding capillaries is called the ________.
5. The membrane that lines most of the air distribution tubes in the respiratory system is called the ________.
6. The frontal, maxillary, sphenoidal, and ethmoidal cavities make up the ________.
7. The ________ sacs drain tears into the nasal cavity.
8. The ________ protrude into the nasal cavities and function to warm and humidify the air.
9. The ________ is the structure that can also be called the *throat*.
10. The ________ is also called the *voice box*.
11. The ________ is the large air tube in the neck.
12. The four progressively smaller air tubes that connect the trachea and the alveolar sacs are the ________, ________, ________, and the ________.
13. ________ is a substance made by the lungs to help reduce the surface tension of water in the alveoli.
14. The right lung is made up of ________ lobes, whereas the left lung is made up of ________ lobes.
15. The exchange of gases between the blood and the tissues is called ________.
16. The exchange of gases between the blood and the air in the lungs is called ________.
17. The ________ is the most important muscle in respiration.
18. Oxygen is carried in the blood as ________.
19. Carbon dioxide can be carried in the blood as the ________ ion or combined with hemoglobin as ________.
20. The inspiratory and expiratory centers are located in the ________ of the brain.
21. ________ are the receptors that inhibit the inspiratory center that keeps the lungs from overexpanding.
22. ________ are the receptors that modify respiratory rates by responding to the amount of carbon dioxide, oxygen, or acid levels in the blood.
23. The amount of air that is moved in and out of the lung during normal breathing is called ________ volume.
24. The three volumes that make up vital capacity are ________, ________, and ________.
25. The volume included in total lung capacity but not vital capacity is ________ volume.

Digestive System

OUTLINE

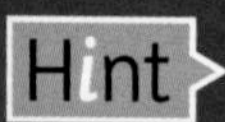

Scan this outline before you begin to read the chapter, as a preview of how the concepts are organized.

OBJECTIVES

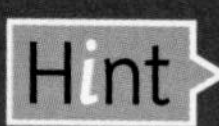

Before reading the chapter, review these goals for your learning.

After you have completed this chapter, you should be able to:

1. List and describe the four layers of the wall of the alimentary canal. Compare the lining layer in the esophagus, stomach, small intestine, and large intestine.
2. Define and contrast mechanical and chemical digestion.
3. Discuss the basics of carbohydrate, protein, and fat digestion and give the end products of each process.
4. List in sequence each of the component parts or segments of the alimentary canal from the mouth to the anus and identify the accessory organs of digestion.
5. Define *peristalsis, bolus, chyme, jaundice, ulcer,* and *diarrhea.*

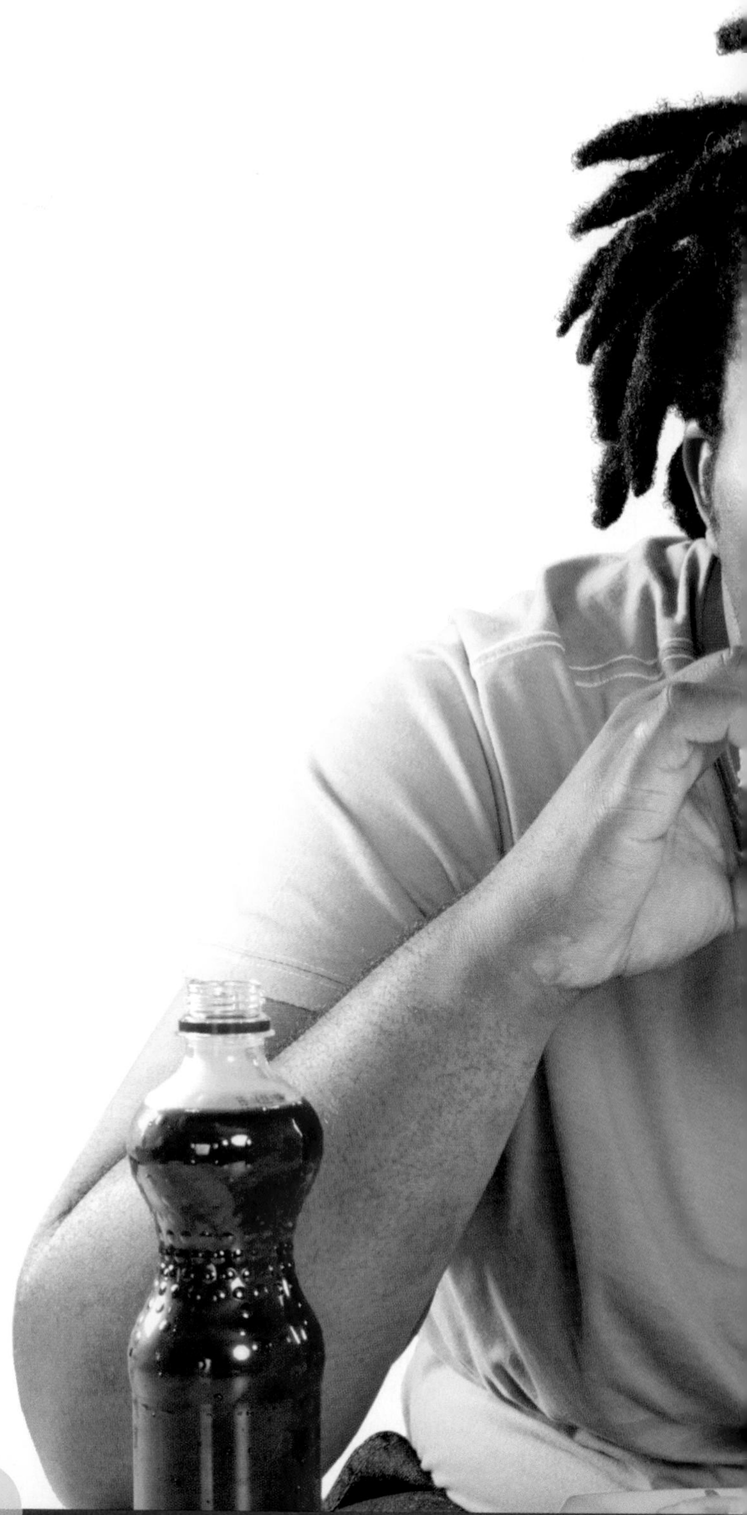

CHAPTER 16

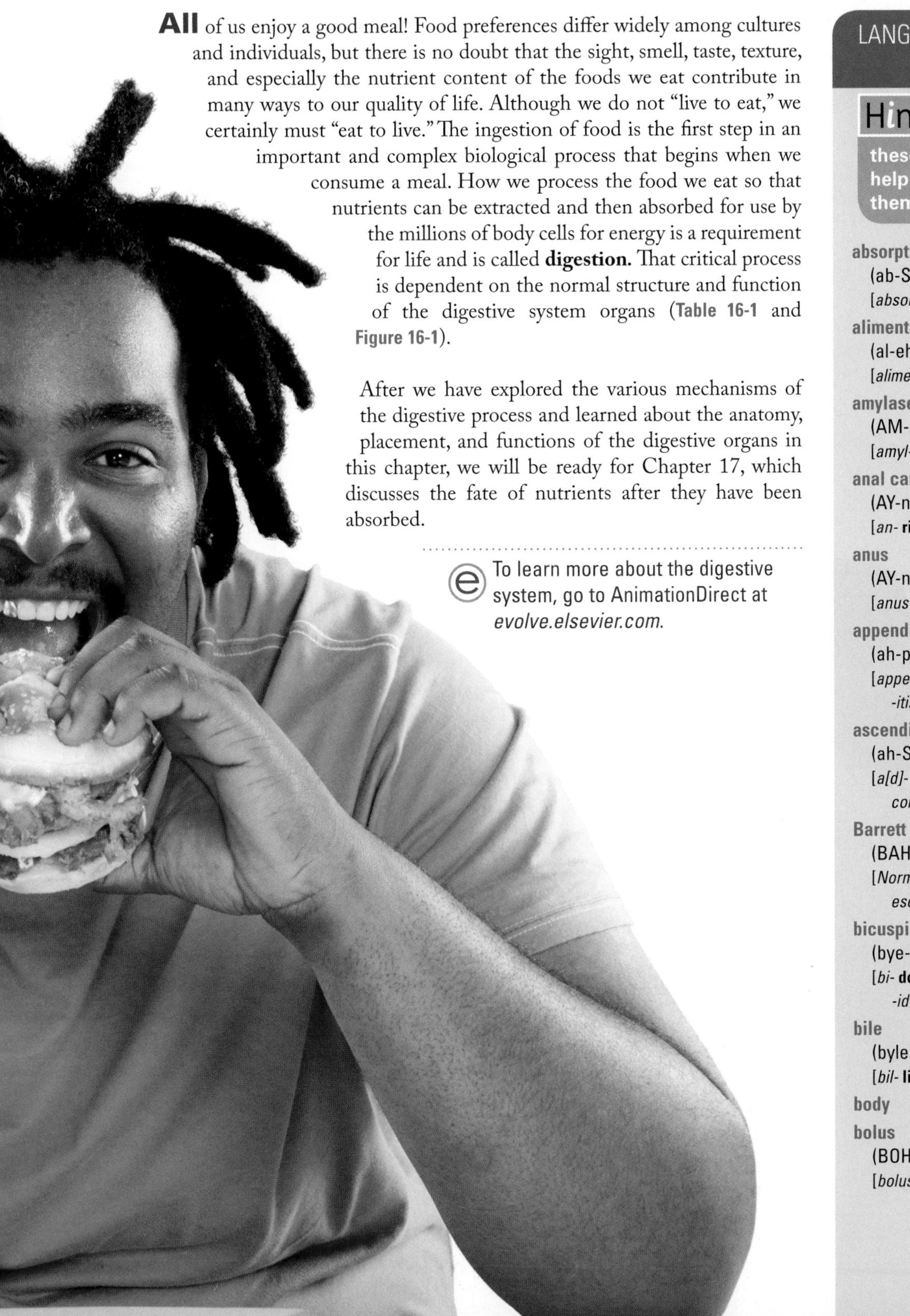

All of us enjoy a good meal! Food preferences differ widely among cultures and individuals, but there is no doubt that the sight, smell, taste, texture, and especially the nutrient content of the foods we eat contribute in many ways to our quality of life. Although we do not "live to eat," we certainly must "eat to live." The ingestion of food is the first step in an important and complex biological process that begins when we consume a meal. How we process the food we eat so that nutrients can be extracted and then absorbed for use by the millions of body cells for energy is a requirement for life and is called **digestion.** That critical process is dependent on the normal structure and function of the digestive system organs (**Table 16-1** and **Figure 16-1**).

After we have explored the various mechanisms of the digestive process and learned about the anatomy, placement, and functions of the digestive organs in this chapter, we will be ready for Chapter 17, which discusses the fate of nutrients after they have been absorbed.

To learn more about the digestive system, go to AnimationDirect at *evolve.elsevier.com.*

LANGUAGE OF **SCIENCE** AND **MEDICINE**

Hint Before reading the chapter, say each of these terms out loud. This will help you to avoid stumbling over them as you read.

absorption
(ab-SORP-shun)
[*absorp-* **swallow,** *-tion* **process**]

alimentary canal
(al-eh-MEN-tar-ee kah-NAL)
[*aliment-* **nourishment,** *-ary* **relating to**]

amylase
(AM-eh-lays)
[*amyl-* **starch,** *-ase* **enzyme**]

anal canal
(AY-nal kah-NAL)
[*an-* **ring (anus),** *-al* **relating to**]

anus
(AY-nus)
[*anus* **ring**]

appendicitis
(ah-pen-dih-SYE-tis)
[*appendic-* **hang upon,** *-itis* **inflammation**]

ascending colon
(ah-SEND-ing KOH-lon)
[*a[d]-* **toward,** *-scend-* **climb,** *colon* **large intestine**]

Barrett esophagus
(BAHR-et ee-SOF-ah-gus)
[*Norman R. Barrett* **English surgeon,** *eso-* **carry,** *-phag-* **food (eat)**]

bicuspid
(bye-KUS-pid)
[*bi-* **double,** *-cusp-* **point,** *-id* **characterized by**]

bile
(byle)
[*bil-* **liver secretion**]

body

bolus
(BOH-lus)
[*bolus* **lump**]

Continued on p. 386

TABLE 16-1 Organs of the Digestive System

MAIN ORGAN	ACCESSORY ORGAN
Mouth	Teeth and tongue Salivary glands Parotid Submandibular Sublingual
Pharynx (throat)	Tonsils
Esophagus	
Stomach	
Small intestine Duodenum Jejunum Ileum	Liver Gallbladder Pancreas
Large intestine Cecum Colon Ascending colon Transverse colon Descending colon Sigmoid colon Rectum Anal canal	Vermiform appendix

Overview of Digestion

The principal structure of the **digestive system** is an irregular tube, open at both ends, called the **alimentary canal.** The term **gastrointestinal (GI) tract** technically refers only to the portion that includes the stomach and intestines but is often used to designate the entire *digestive tract.*

In the adult, this hollow tube is about 9 meters (29 feet) long. Think of the tube as a passageway that extends through the body like a hallway through a building. Thus the food we eat and even the nutrient materials released by the digestive process are not truly "part of the body" until they have passed through the wall of the GI tract and entered the internal environment.

To accomplish the function of making nutrients available to each cell of the body, the digestive system uses various mechanisms (**Table 16-2**).

First, complex foods must be taken into the GI tract in a process called **ingestion.**

Then, the ingested food material must be broken down into simpler nutrients in the process that gives this system its name: **digestion.** The breakdown, or digestion, of food material is both *mechanical* and *chemical* in nature.

The teeth are used to physically break down large chunks of food before it is swallowed. The churning of food in the stomach then continues the mechanical digestive process. To physically break down large chunks of food into smaller bits and to move it along the tract, movement or **motility** of the GI wall is required.

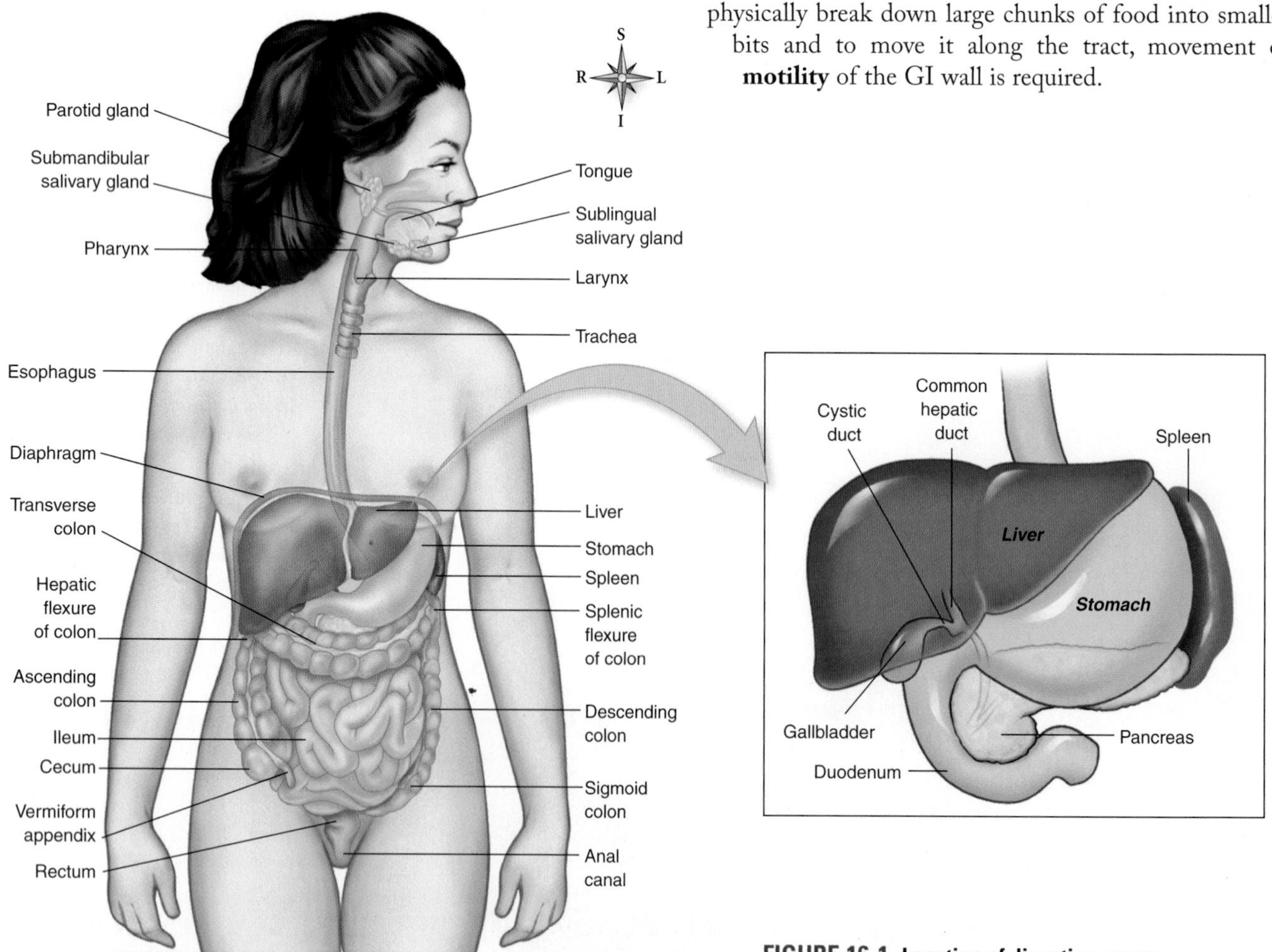

FIGURE 16-1 Location of digestive organs.

TABLE 16-2 Primary Mechanisms of the Digestive System

MECHANISM	DESCRIPTION
Ingestion	Process of taking food into the mouth, starting it on its journey through the digestive tract
Digestion	A group of processes that break complex nutrients into simpler ones, thus facilitating their absorption; *mechanical digestion* physically breaks large chunks into small bits; *chemical digestion* breaks molecules apart
Motility	Movement by the muscular components of the digestive tube, including processes of mechanical digestion; examples include *peristalsis* and *segmentation*
Secretion	Release of digestive juices (containing enzymes, acids, bases, mucus, bile, or other products that facilitate digestion); some digestive organs also secrete endocrine hormones that regulate digestion or metabolism of nutrients
Absorption	Movement of digested nutrients through the gastrointestinal (GI) mucosa and into the internal environment
Elimination	Excretion of the residues of the digestive process (feces) from the rectum, through the anus; defecation
Regulation	Coordination of digestive activity (motility, secretion, other digestive processes)

In chemical digestion, large nutrient molecules are reduced to smaller molecules. This process requires **secretion** of digestive enzymes and other products into the lumen of the GI tract. After the digestive processes have altered the physical and chemical composition of ingested food, the resulting nutrients are ready for the process of **absorption,** or movement through the GI mucosa into the internal environment.

Part of the digestive system, the large intestine, also serves as an organ of **elimination,** ridding the body of waste material, or **feces,** resulting from the digestive process.

Regulation of activities such as motility and secretion is required to coordinate the various mechanisms of digestion.

Wall of the Digestive Tract

The digestive tract has been described as a tube that extends from the mouth to the anus. The wall of this digestive tube is fashioned of four layers of tissue (**Figure 16-2**). The inside, or hollow space within the tube, is called the **lumen.** The four layers, named from the inside coat to the outside of the tube, are as follows:

1. Mucosa or mucous membrane
2. Submucosa
3. Muscularis
4. Serosa

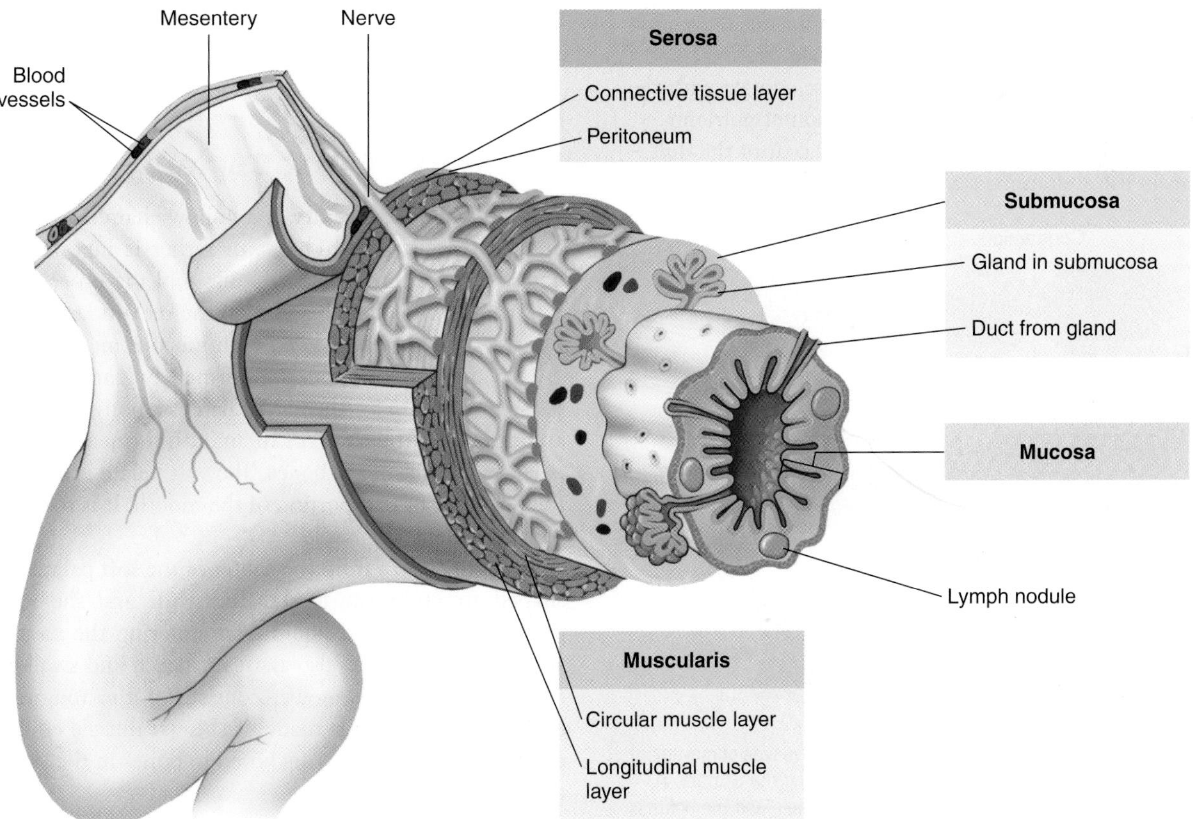

FIGURE 16-2 Section of the small intestine. The four layers typical of walls of the GI tract are shown. Circular folds of mucous membrane called *plicae* increase the surface area of the lining coat.

Although the same four tissue coats form every organ of the alimentary tract, their structure varies from organ to organ. The **mucosa** of the esophagus, for example, is composed of tough and abrasion-resistant stratified epithelium. The mucosa of the remainder of the tract is a delicate layer of simple columnar epithelium structured for absorption and secretion. The mucus produced by either type of epithelium coats the lining of the alimentary canal.

The **submucosa,** as the name implies, is a connective tissue layer that lies just below the mucosa. It contains many blood vessels and nerves.

The two or three layers of muscle tissue make up the **muscularis** (see Figure 16-2). These muscle layers have an important role to play in producing *motility* or movement of the GI tract during the digestive process. **Peristalsis** is a rhythmic, wavelike contraction of the gut wall caused by alternating a wavelike contraction along the circular muscle layer in the muscularis. This type of sequenced contraction squeezes and pushes ingested food material forward through the digestive tube's internal pathway—similar to how you might squeeze toothpaste out of its tube (Figure 16-3).

In addition to peristaltic contractions that cause material to move forward, alternating contraction of fibers of the muscularis within a single region, or segment, of the GI tract also produces a "back-and-forth" or "swishing" type of intestinal motility called **segmentation** (Figure 16-4). As peristaltic movement pushes food down the GI tract, segmentation contractions assist in mixing food with digestive juices and helps continue the mechanical breakdown of larger food particles.

Peristalsis and segmentation can occur in an alternating sequence. When this happens, food is churned and mixed as it slowly progresses along the GI tract in close contact with the intestinal mucosa, which facilitates absorption of nutrients.

The **serosa** is the outermost covering or coat of the digestive tube. In the abdominal cavity, this serosa covering is called the *visceral peritoneum*. The loops of the digestive tract are anchored to the posterior wall of the abdominal cavity by a large double fold of peritoneal tissue called the **mesentery.**

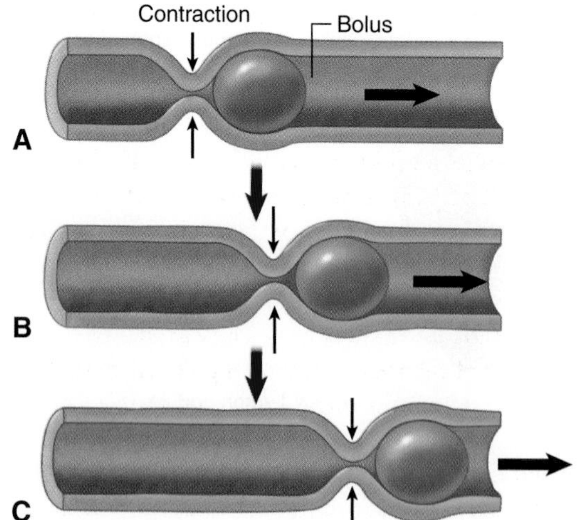

FIGURE 16-3 Peristalsis. Peristalsis is a progressive type of movement in which material is propelled from point to point along the GI tract. **A,** A ring of contraction occurs where the GI wall is stretched, and the bolus is pushed forward. **B,** The moving bolus triggers a ring of contraction in the next region that pushes the bolus even farther along. **C,** The ring of contraction moves like a wave along the GI tract to push the bolus forward.

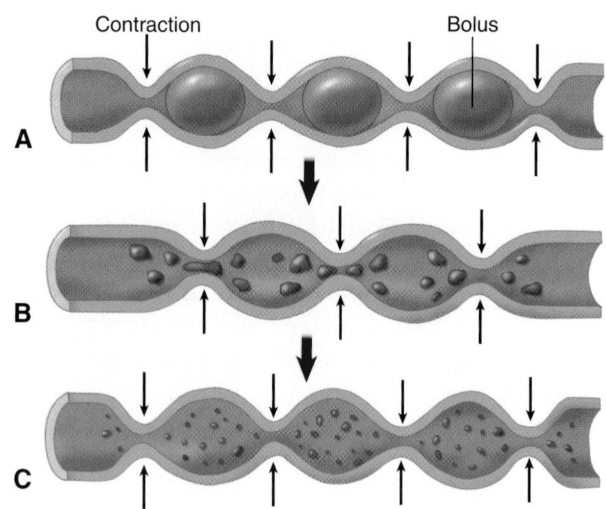

FIGURE 16-4 Segmentation. Segmentation is a back-and-forth action that breaks apart chunks of food and mixes in digestive juices. **A,** Ringlike regions of contraction occur at intervals along the GI tract. **B,** Previously contracted regions relax and adjacent regions now contract, effectively "chopping" the contents of each segment into smaller chunks. **C,** The location of the contracted regions continues to alternate back and forth, chopping and mixing the contents of the GI lumen.

To learn more about intestinal motility, go to AnimationDirect at *evolve.elsevier.com*.

Mouth

Structure of Oral Cavity

The **mouth,** or **oral cavity,** is a hollow chamber with a roof, a floor, and walls. Food enters, or rather is ingested into, the digestive tract through the mouth, and the process of digestion begins immediately. As with the remainder of the digestive tract, the mouth is lined with mucous membrane.

The roof of the mouth is formed by the **hard** and **soft palates** (Figure 16-5). The hard palate is a bony structure in the anterior or front portion of the mouth formed by parts of the palatine and maxillary bones. The soft palate is located above the posterior or rear portion of the mouth. It is soft because it consists chiefly of muscle.

Hanging down from the center of the soft palate is a cone-shaped structure, the **uvula.** The uvula and the soft palate prevent any food and liquid from entering the nasal cavities above the mouth and also assist in speech and swallowing.

The floor of the mouth consists of the tongue and its muscles. The tongue is made of skeletal muscle covered with mucous membrane. It is anchored to bones in the skull and to the hyoid bone in the neck.

A thin membrane called the **frenulum** attaches the tongue to the floor of the mouth. Occasionally a person is born with a frenulum that is too short to allow free movement of the

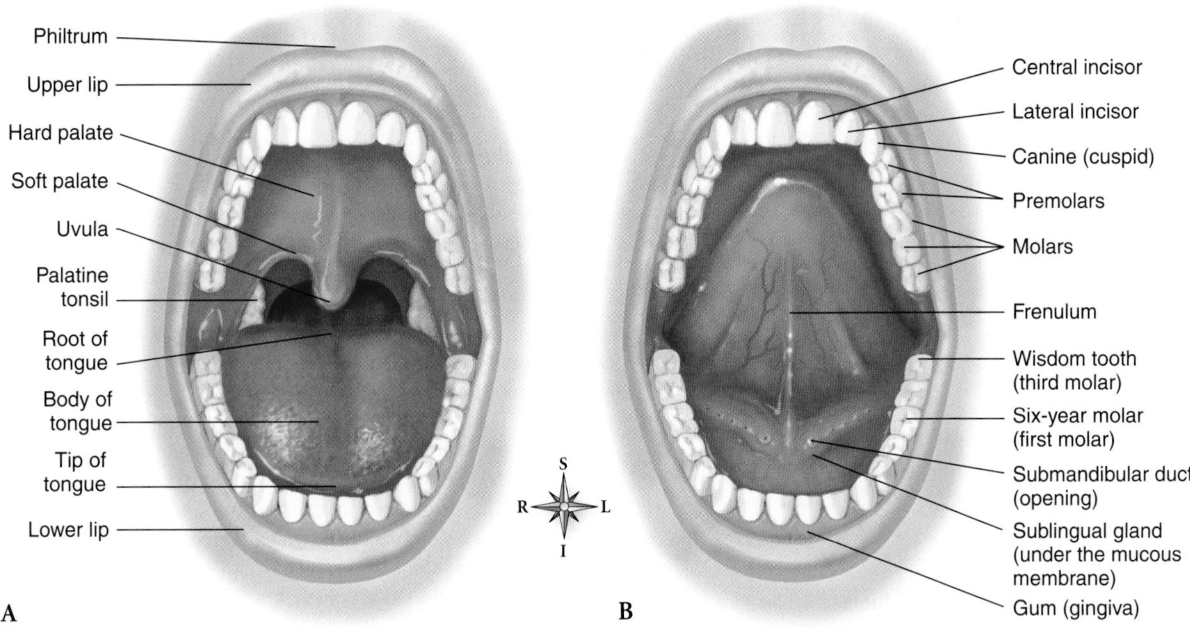

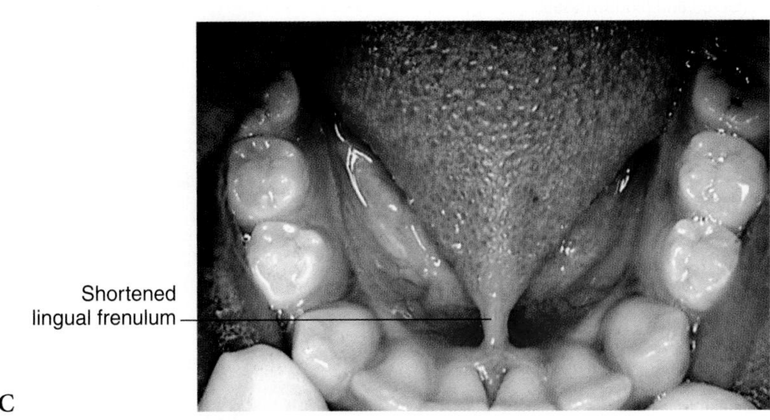

FIGURE 16-5 Mouth cavity and tongue. A, Mouth cavity showing hard and soft palates, tongue surface, and uvula. **B,** Types of adult teeth, undersurface of tongue showing frenulum, sublingual gland, and opening of sublingual duct. **C,** Photograph shows an abnormally short lingual frenulum, which may result in faulty speech.

tongue (**Figure 16-5**, *C*). Individuals with this condition cannot enunciate words normally.

Note in **Figure 16-5**, *A*, that the tongue can be divided into a blunt rear portion called the *root*, a pointed *tip*, and a central *body*.

QUICK CHECK

1. What is the alimentary canal?
2. What kinds of processing does food undergo in the body?
3. Describe the layers of the digestive tract's wall.
4. What is the uvula? What function does it perform?

Teeth

Typical Tooth

A typical tooth can be divided into three main parts: crown, neck, and root.

The **crown** is the portion that is exposed and visible in the mouth. It is largely made of a bone-like material called **dentin** that is covered by **enamel**—the hardest tissue in the body. Enamel is ideally suited to withstand the grinding that occurs during the chewing of hard and brittle foods. The root and neck of each tooth are covered by **cementum** (**Figure 16-6**).

The center of the tooth contains a pulp cavity that consists of connective tissue, blood and lymphatic vessels, and sensory nerves.

The **neck** of a tooth is the narrow portion that joins the crown of the tooth to the root. The neck is surrounded by the pink **gingiva** or *gum* tissue. A general term for mild, localized, and often transitory inflammation of the gums or gingiva is called **gingivitis.**

The **root** of the tooth fits into the bony socket that surrounds it in either the upper or lower jaw bone. A fibrous **periodontal membrane** lines each tooth socket and anchors

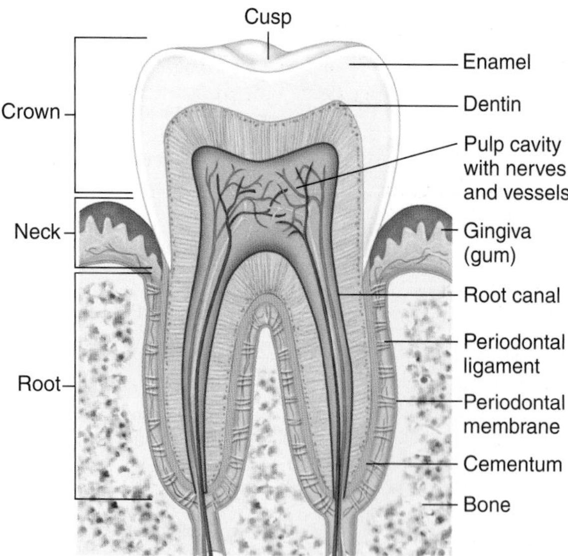

FIGURE 16-6 Longitudinal section of a tooth. A molar is sectioned to show its bony socket and details of its three main parts: crown, neck, and root. Enamel (over the crown) and cementum (over the neck and root) surround the dentin layer. The pulp contains nerves and blood vessels.

the tooth to the bone. **Periodontitis** is a generalized and serious type of inflammation and infection of this membrane and surrounding bone. It is often a complication of untreated gingivitis. As the infection worsens, it will cause loss of both periodontal membrane and bone, resulting in loosening and eventually complete loss of teeth. Periodontitis is the leading cause of tooth loss among adults.

Tooth decay, or **dental caries,** is a disease of the enamel, dentin, and cementum of teeth that results in the formation of a permanent defect called a *dental cavity.* The incidence of gingivitis, dental caries, and periodontitis can be reduced by good dental health practices, which include regular and thorough brushing and flossing of the teeth.

Types of Teeth

The shape and placement of the teeth (see **Figure 16-5**, *B*) assist in their functions. The four major types of teeth are as follows:

1. Incisors
2. Canines or cuspids
3. Premolars or bicuspids
4. Molars or tricuspids

Locate the four types of teeth in **Figure 16-5**, *B*, which shows the full set of 32 permanent teeth. Note that the **incisors** have very sharp cutting edges while the **canine** or **cuspid** teeth have more pointed ends well suited for piercing and tearing. The flat **premolars** (**bicuspids**) and **molars** (**tricuspids**) with their two or three grinding "cusps" provide a large surface area to effectively crush ingested food material. Together, the teeth provide for effective chewing or **mastication** of a wide variety and size of ingested food.

In humans, a set of 20 teeth called **deciduous** or *baby teeth* erupt between about 6 to 30 months of age. Although the time frame may vary somewhat, these teeth are generally lost between ages 6 and 13 years old. The first permanent teeth to appear, called the first or "6-year" molars erupt before all of the baby teeth are lost. In the deciduous set of 20 teeth, there are no premolars and only two pairs of molars in each jaw.

When a young adult is somewhere between 17 and 24 years old, the deciduous teeth have all been shed and completely replaced with a full set of 32 **permanent teeth.** The third molars or "wisdom teeth" are the last of the permanent teeth to appear.

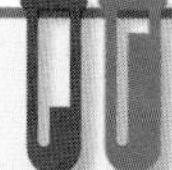

CLINICAL APPLICATION

MALOCCLUSION

Malocclusion of the teeth occurs when missing teeth create wide spaces in the dentition, when teeth overlap, or when malposition of one or more teeth prevents correct alignment of the maxillary and mandibular dental arches (Figures A and B). Malocclusion that results in protrusion of the upper front teeth, causing them to hang over the lower front teeth, is called *overbite* (Figure *A*), whereas the positioning of the lower front teeth outside the upper front teeth is called *underbite* (Figure *B*).

Dental malocclusion may cause significant problems and chronic pain in the functioning of the *temporomandibular joint (TMJ),* contribute to the generation of headaches, or complicate routine mastication of food. Fortunately, even severe malocclusion problems can be corrected by the use of braces and other dental appliances. Orthodontics is that branch of dentistry that deals with the prevention and correction of positioning irregularities of the teeth and malocclusion.

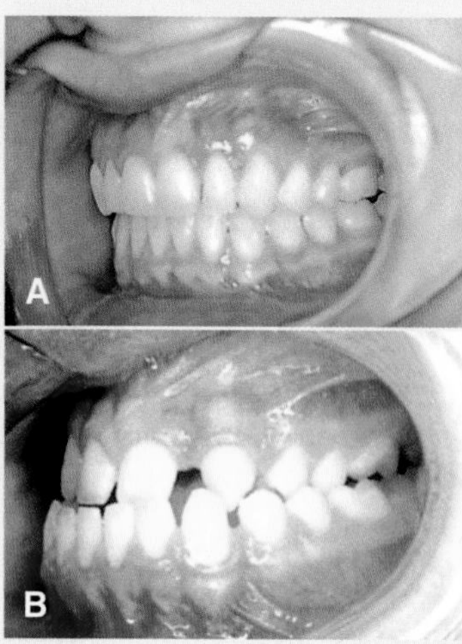

Salivary Glands

Saliva

Three pairs of salivary glands—the parotids, submandibulars, and sublinguals—secrete most (about 1 liter) of the saliva produced each day in the adult. The salivary glands (**Figure 16-7**) are typical of the accessory glands associated with the digestive system. They are located outside of the digestive tube itself and must convey their exocrine secretions by way of ducts into the tract.

Some salivary secretions are said to be **serous** in nature if they are thin, watery, and free of mucus. Serous-type saliva, produced by serous-type secretory cells (see **Figure 16-7**, *B*), contains the digestive enzyme **amylase.** This enzyme begins the chemical digestion of carbohydrates. Another type of saliva is thick and rich in mucus but contains no enzymes. Mucous-type saliva, which is thick and slippery, is produced by mucous-type secretory cells (see **Figure 16-7**, *B*). This type of saliva serves the important function of lubricating food during mastication, thus allowing it to pass with less friction through the esophagus and into the stomach. Some saliva is a mixture of both serous- and mucous-type secretions.

Parotid Glands

The **parotid glands,** the largest of the salivary glands, lie just below and in front of each ear at the angle of the jaw—an interesting anatomical position because it explains why people who have mumps (an infection of the parotid gland) often complain that it hurts when they open their mouths or chew; these movements squeeze the tender, inflamed gland.

To see the openings of the parotid ducts, look in a mirror at the insides of your cheeks opposite the second molar tooth on either side of the upper jaw. The parotids contain only serous-type secretory cells, which produce a watery, or serous, type of saliva containing enzymes but not mucus.

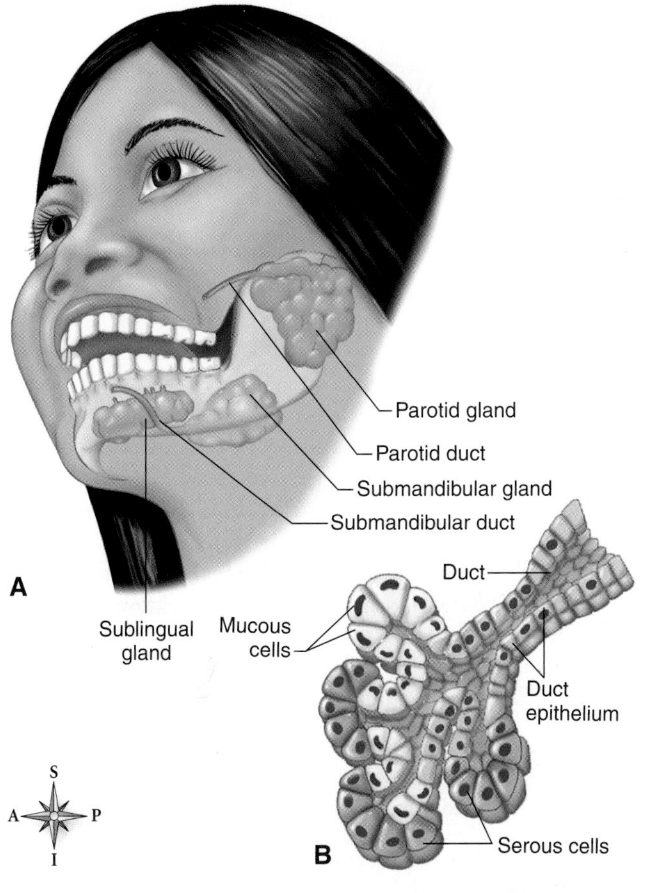

Submandibular Glands

Submandibular glands (see **Figure 16-7**, *A*) are called *mixed* or *compound* salivary glands because they contain both serous (enzyme) and mucus-producing secretory cells (see **Figure 16-7**, *B*). These glands are located just below the mandibular angle, are irregular in form, and are about the size of a walnut. The submandibular ducts open into the mouth on either side of the lingual frenulum.

Sublingual Glands

Sublingual glands are the smallest of the main salivary glands. They lie in front of the submandibular glands, under the mucous membrane covering the floor of the mouth. Each sublingual gland opens via 10 to 15 ducts into the floor of the mouth. Unlike the other salivary glands, the sublingual glands produce only a mucous type of saliva.

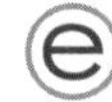
To learn more about the mouth and accessory organs in mechanical digestion, go to AnimationDirect at *evolve.elsevier.com*.

FIGURE 16-7 Salivary glands. A, Location of the salivary glands. **B,** Schematic illustration of the submandibular gland secretory tissue. This mixed- or compound-type gland produces mucus from mucous cells and enzymatic secretion from serous cells.

Pharynx

Structure

The **pharynx** is a tubelike structure made of muscle and lined with mucous membrane. Note its location in **Figure 16-8**. Because of its location behind the nasal cavities and mouth, it functions as part of both the respiratory and digestive systems. Air must pass through the pharynx on its way to the lungs, and food must pass through it on its way to the stomach.

Recall that the pharynx as a whole is subdivided into three anatomical components: **nasopharynx, oropharynx,** and **laryngopharynx.** Also recall that the protective lymphoid ring formed by the three major pairs of *tonsils* in the pharynx help prevent infections of the respiratory and digestive tracts.

Function

Of the three anatomical divisions, the oropharynx is actively and most directly involved in the digestive process because of its important role in a specialized and coordinated type of GI tract motility involved in swallowing. The swallowing of food is called **deglutition.**

First, mastication involves voluntary movements that result in formation of a ball or **bolus** of food in the mouth that is then moved involuntarily through the oropharynx and into the esophagus and, finally, into the stomach.

Swallowing is a complex process requiring the coordination of pharyngeal muscles and other muscles and structures in the head and neck. *Regulation* of voluntary swallowing movements is dependent on nervous impulses originating in the motor cortex of the cerebrum. Involuntary movements are

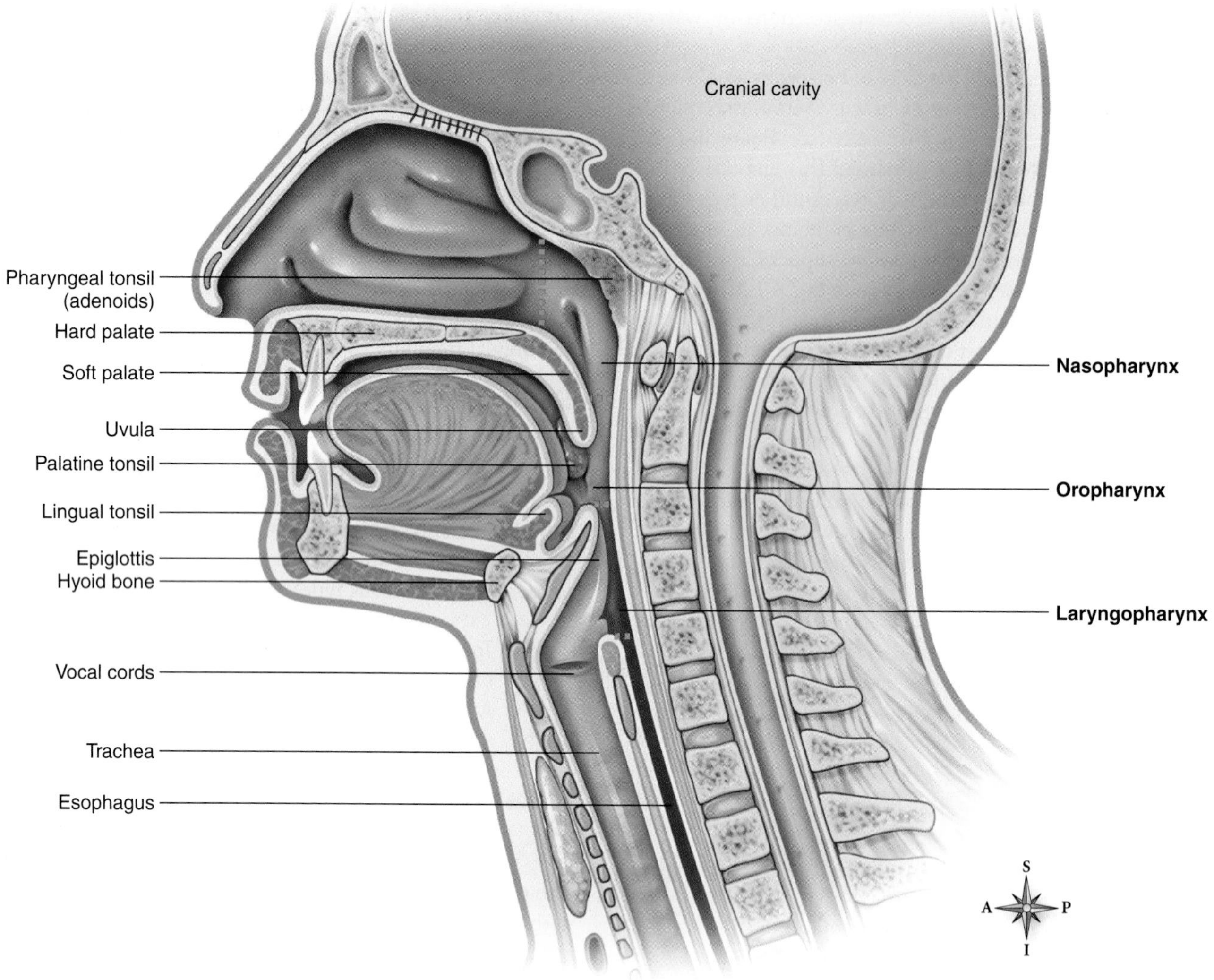

FIGURE 16-8 Pharynx. This midsagittal section of the head and neck shows the pharynx and related structures. The green dotted lines mark the approximate boundaries of the regions of the pharynx. Notice that the esophagus runs inferiorly from the pharynx, behind the trachea.

regulated by impulses originating in the swallowing or "deglutition center" located in the medulla and pons of the brainstem (see **Figure 9-10**).

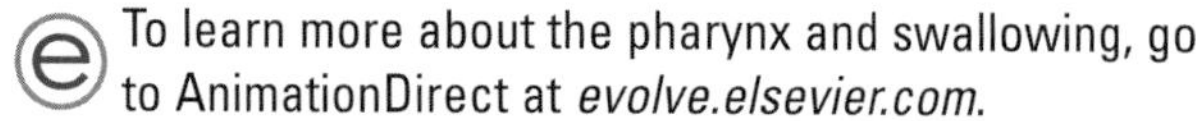

To learn more about the pharynx and swallowing, go to AnimationDirect at *evolve.elsevier.com.*

Esophagus

The **esophagus** is the muscular, mucus-lined tube that connects the pharynx with the stomach. It is about 25 centimeters (10 inches) long. The esophagus serves as a dynamic passageway for food, pushing the food toward the stomach. The production of mucus by glands in the mucosal lining lubricates the tube to permit easier passage of food moving toward the stomach.

Each end of the esophagus is guarded by a muscular **sphincter.** Sphincters are valvelike rings of muscle tissue that often surround tubular structures or body openings. In the GI tract they normally act to keep ingested material moving in one direction down the tube. The **upper esophageal sphincter** (**UES**) helps prevent air from entering the tube during respiration. The **lower esophageal sphincter** (**LES**), or *cardiac sphincter,* normally prevents backflow of acidic stomach contents.

QUICK CHECK

1. What are the four major types of teeth?
2. What digestive enzyme is found in saliva?
3. What roles do the pharynx and esophagus play in the digestive tract?
4. What are the sphincters at each end of the esophagus and what function do they serve in the body?

Stomach

The **stomach** lies in the upper part of the abdominal cavity just under the diaphragm (see Figure 16-1). It serves as a pouch that food enters after it has been chewed, swallowed, and passed through the esophagus.

Structure

The three divisions of the stomach shown in Figure 16-9 are the *fundus, body,* and pylorus. The **fundus** is the enlarged, curving base to the left of and above the opening of the esophagus into the stomach. The **body** is the central part of the stomach, and the **pylorus** is its lower narrow apex section, which joins the first part of the small intestine. The upper right border of the stomach is known as the *lesser curvature,* and the lower left border is called the *greater curvature.*

The stomach looks small when it is empty, not much bigger than a large sausage, but it expands considerably after a large meal. Have you ever felt so uncomfortably full after eating that you could not take a deep breath? If so, it probably meant that your stomach was so full of food that it occupied more space than usual and thus pushed up against the diaphragm. This made it hard for the diaphragm to contract and move downward as much as necessary for you to take a deep breath.

Note in Figure 16-9 that there are three layers of smooth muscle in the stomach wall. The muscle fibers that run lengthwise, around, and obliquely make the stomach one of the strongest internal organs—well able to break up food into tiny particles and to mix them thoroughly with gastric juice to form **chyme.** Stomach muscle contractions result in peristalsis, which propels food down the digestive tract.

Mucous membrane lines the stomach, forming the mucosa. It contains thousands of microscopic **gastric glands** that secrete gastric juice into the stomach. Cells in the stomach also secrete a chemical called *intrinsic factor* that protects vitamin B_{12} and saves it for its later absorption in the distal small intestine. Some individuals may require vitamin B_{12} injections after having had some stomach surgeries.

When the stomach is empty, its mucous lining lies in folds called **rugae.**

Function

After food has entered the stomach by passing through the muscular LES at the lower end of the esophagus, the digestive process continues.

Occasionally, the opening in the diaphragm that permits the passage of the esophagus into the abdomen is enlarged. This may permit a bulging of the end of the esophagus and part or even all of the stomach upward through the diaphragm and into the chest. This displacement is called a **hiatal hernia** and may result in backward movement or reflux of stomach contents into the lower portion of the esophagus. The resulting condition is referred to as **gastroesophageal reflux disease,** or **GERD.**

Contraction of the stomach's muscular walls mixes the food thoroughly with the gastric juice and breaks it down into a semisolid mixture called *chyme.* This liquefaction process is a continuation of the mechanical digestive process that begins in the mouth.

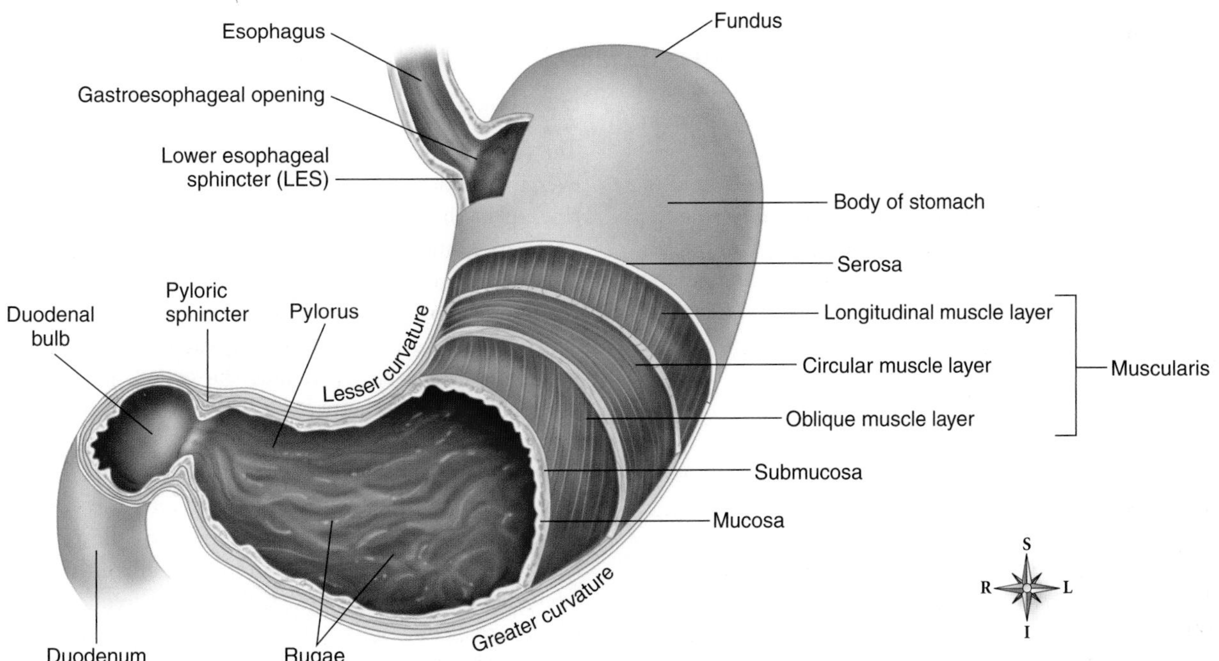

FIGURE 16-9 Stomach. A portion of the anterior wall has been cut away to reveal the three muscle layers of the stomach wall. Notice that the mucosa lining the stomach forms folds called *rugae.*

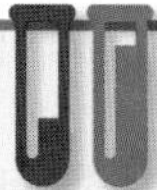

CLINICAL APPLICATION

GASTROESOPHAGEAL REFLUX DISEASE

The terms **heartburn** and *acid indigestion* are often used to describe a number of unpleasant symptoms experienced by more than 60 million Americans each month. Backward flow of stomach acid up into the esophagus causes these symptoms, which typically include burning and pressure behind the breastbone. The term *gastroesophageal reflux disease (GERD)* is now used to better describe this very common and sometimes serious medical condition.

In its simplest form, GERD produces mild symptoms that occur only infrequently (twice a week or less). In these cases, avoiding problem foods or beverages, stopping smoking, or losing weight if needed may solve the problem. Additional treatment with over-the-counter antacids or nonprescription-strength acid-blocking medications may also be used.

More severe and frequent episodes of GERD can trigger asthma attacks, cause severe chest pain (which can mimic the pain of a heart attack), result in bleeding, or promote a narrowing (stricture) or chronic irritation of the esophagus. In these cases, more powerful inhibitors of stomach acid production may be added to the treatment prescribed.

As a last resort, a surgical procedure called *fundoplication* is performed to strengthen the sphincter. The procedure involves wrapping a layer of the upper stomach wall around the sphincter and terminal esophagus to lessen the possibility of acid reflux.

If GERD is left untreated, serious pathological (precancerous) changes in the esophageal lining may develop—a condition called **Barrett esophagus.**

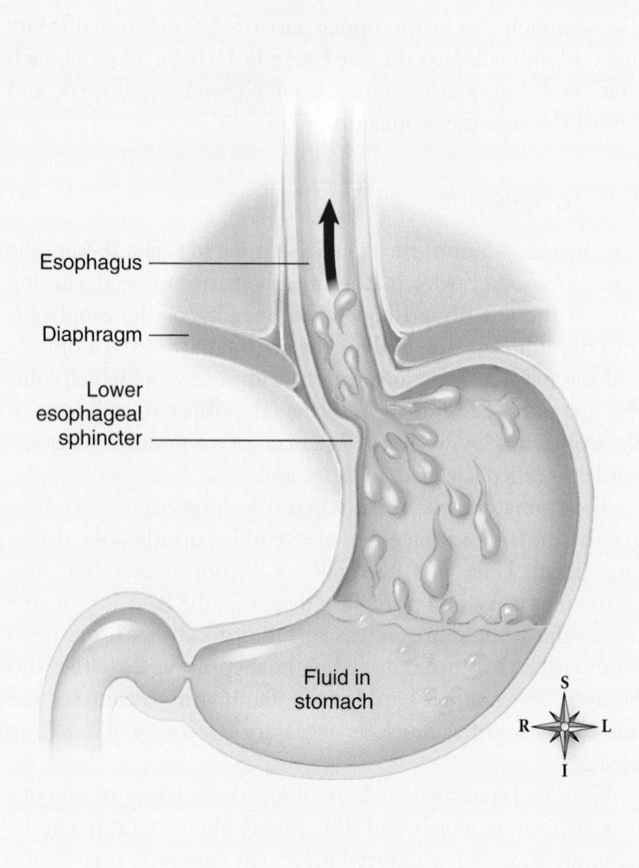

Gastric juice contains hydrochloric acid that unfolds proteins by breaking hydrogen bonds. Then, enzymes in the gastric juice break apart the peptide bonds within protein molecules—all part of chemical digestion.

Partial digestion of proteins occurs after chyme is held in the stomach for some time by the **pyloric sphincter** muscle. The smooth muscle fibers of the sphincter stay contracted most of the time and thereby close off the opening of the pylorus into the small intestine. After food has been mixed in the stomach and protein digestion gets under way, chyme begins its passage through the pyloric sphincter into the first part of the small intestine.

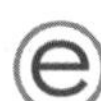

To learn more about the stomach, go to AnimationDirect at *evolve.elsevier.com.*

QUICK CHECK

1. What is chyme?
2. How does the pyloric sphincter muscle help the stomach perform its digestive function?
3. What are the main divisions of the stomach?

Small Intestine

Structure

The **small intestine** is roughly 7 meters (20 feet) long. However, it is noticeably smaller in diameter than the large intestine, so in this respect its name is appropriate (**Figure 16-10**). Different names identify different sections of the small intestine. In the order in which food passes through them, they are the **duodenum, jejunum,** and **ileum.**

To accommodate such a long tube within the relatively short abdominal cavity, it must be coiled into many loops. Thus, a small body cavity can contain a long tube with a large surface area.

Most of the chemical digestion occurs in the first subdivision of the small intestine or duodenum. The duodenum is C-shaped and curves around the head of the pancreas (see **Figure 16-11**). The acid chyme enters the bulb of the duodenum from the stomach. This area is the site of frequent ulceration (duodenal ulcers).

The middle third of the duodenum contains the openings of ducts that empty pancreatic digestive juice and bile from the liver into the small intestine. As you can see in **Figure 16-11**,

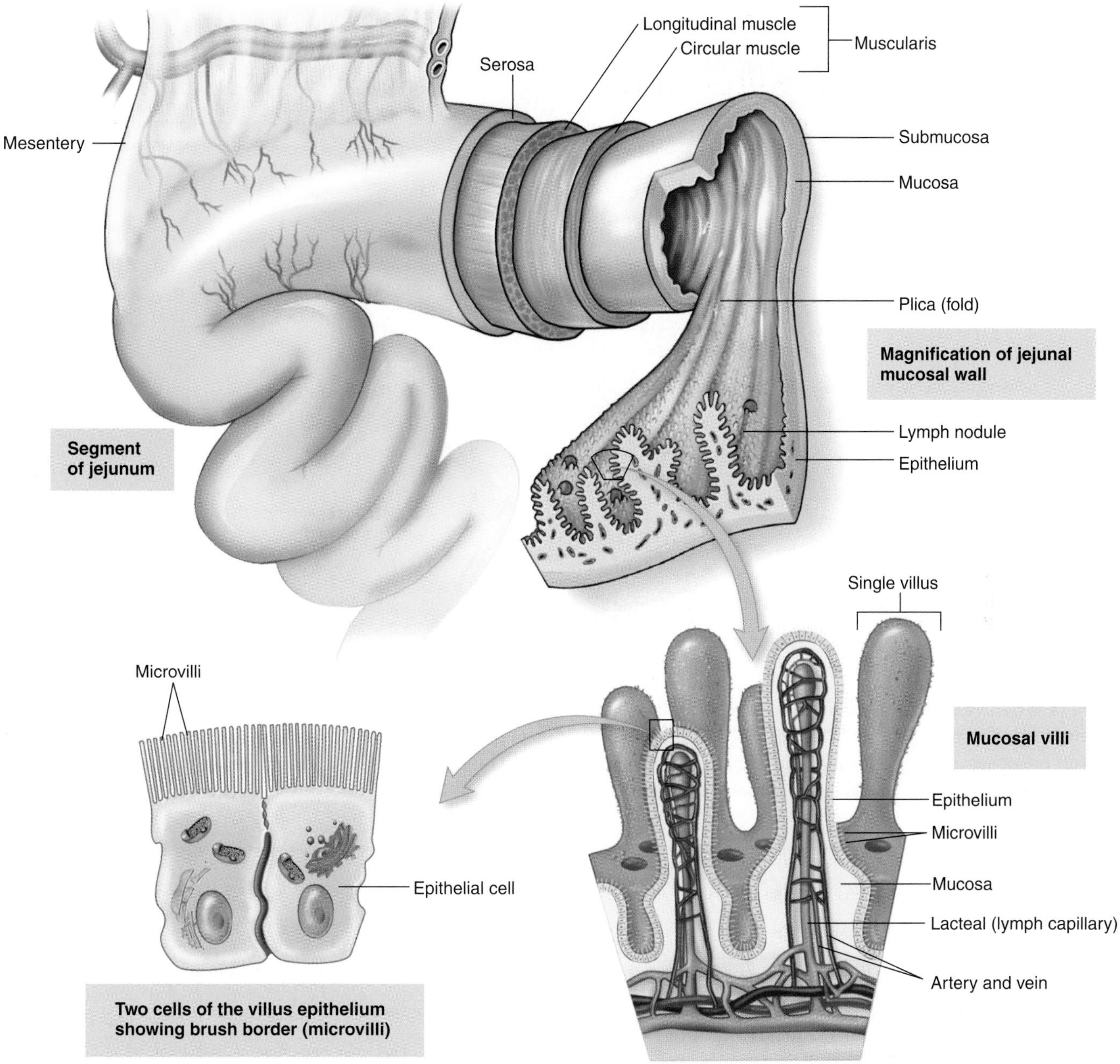

FIGURE 16-10 Small intestine. Note that the folds of mucosa are covered with villi and that each villus is covered with epithelium, which increases the surface area for absorption of food.

the two openings are located at two bumps called the **minor duodenal papilla** and **major duodenal papilla.** Occasionally a gallstone blocks ducts that drain through the major duodenal papilla, causing symptoms such as severe pain, jaundice, and digestive problems.

Function

The main functions of the small intestine are *digestion* and *absorption*. Nearly all the digestion and absorption of the digestive system occurs in the small intestine.

The mucous lining of the small intestine, as with that of the stomach, contains thousands of microscopic glands. These **intestinal glands** secrete the intestinal digestive juice that is rich in a variety of enzymes as well as water and ions. The pancreas excretes bicarbonate into the lumen (hollow interior) of the duodenum to neutralize the stomach acid and also adds enzymes to digest fats, proteins, and carbohydrates that are absorbed in the intestine.

A structural feature of the lining of the small intestine that makes it especially well suited to absorption of food and water is multiple circular folds called **plicae** (see **Figure 16-2** and

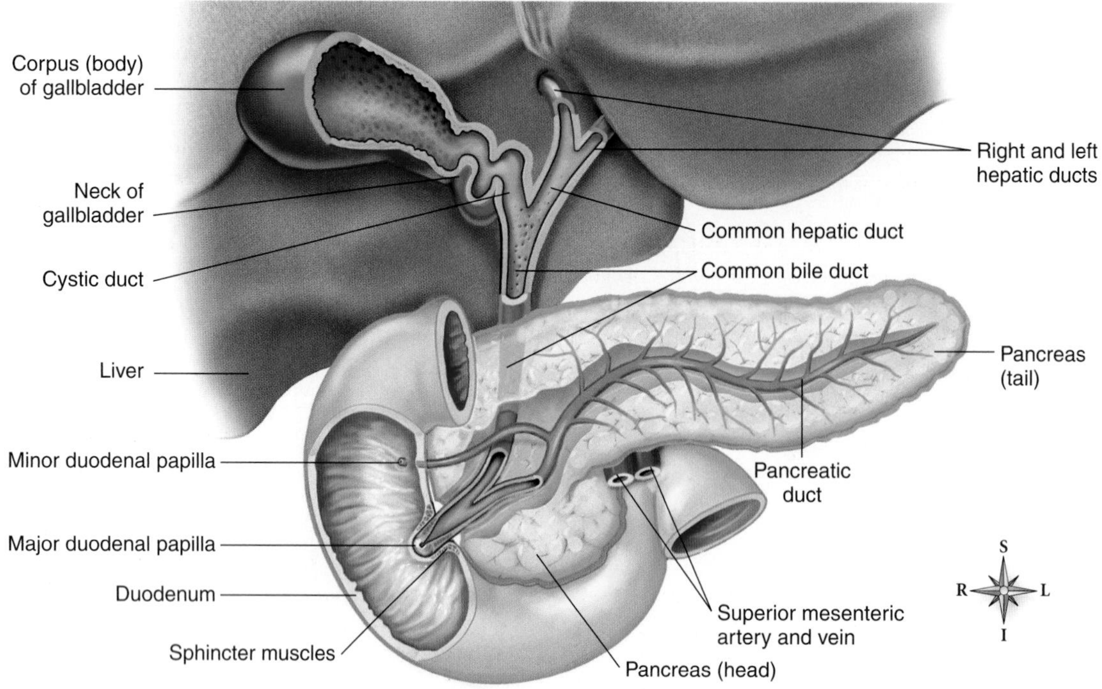

FIGURE 16-11 Gallbladder and bile ducts. Obstruction of the hepatic, or common, bile duct by stone or spasm blocks the exit of bile from the liver, where it is formed, and prevents bile from being ejected into the duodenum.

Figure 16-10). These folds are themselves covered with thousands of tiny "fingers" called **villi.** Under the microscope, the villi can be seen projecting into the lumen of the intestine. Inside each villus lies a rich network of blood capillaries that absorb the products of carbohydrate and protein digestion (sugars and amino acids) and lymph capillaries (**lacteals**) that absorb fats.

Millions and millions of villi jut inward from the mucous lining. This large absorptive surface area allows for faster

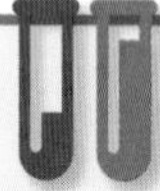

CLINICAL APPLICATION

TREATMENT OF ULCERS

Current statistics show that about 1 in 10 individuals in the United States will suffer from either a gastric (stomach) or duodenal **ulcer** in his or her lifetime. These craterlike lesions, which destroy areas of stomach or intestinal lining, cause gnawing or burning pain and may ultimately result in hemorrhage, perforation, scarring, and other serious medical complications. See the figure.

Long-term use of certain pain medications such as aspirin and ibuprofen, called *nonsteroidal anti-inflammatory agents* (NSAIDs), can cause ulcers. However, we now know that most gastric and duodenal ulcers result from infection with the ***Helicobacter pylori (H. pylori)*** bacterium. This is especially so if the infected individual has a genetic predisposition to ulcer development. *H. pylori* infection is diagnosed by biopsy, breath, or blood antibody tests.

Knowing that most ulcers are caused by a bacterial organism led to the development of a number of treatment programs that were designed to eradicate the bacteria by use of antibiotics while simultaneously blocking or reducing stomach acid secretion. Currently, the standard antibiotic-based treatment used most frequently to both heal ulcers and prevent recurrences is called *triple therapy.* It is successful in 80% to 95% of cases and requires that three medications be taken concurrently for 2 weeks. Triple therapy combines bismuth subsalicylate (Pepto-Bismol) with two antibiotics. The same types of antisecretory drugs used to reduce stomach acid in GERD are also used in ulcer therapy.

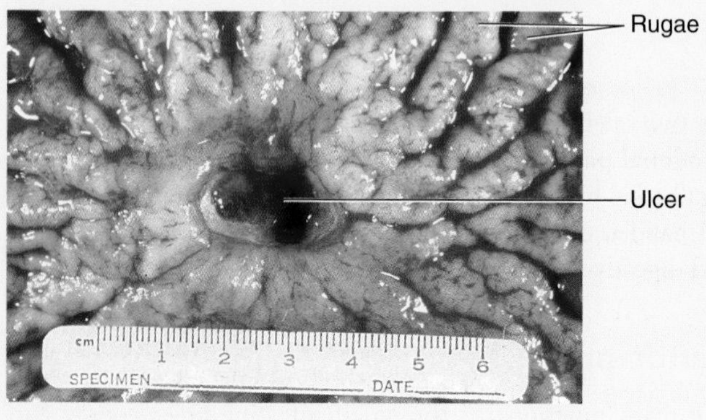

Gastric ulcer.

absorption of nutrients from the intestine into the blood and lymph—yet another case of *form fits function.*

In addition to the millions of villi that increase surface area in the small intestine, each villus is itself covered by epithelial cells, which have a brushlike border composed of **microvilli.** The microvilli further increase the surface area of each villus for absorption of nutrients.

Smooth muscle in the wall of the small intestine contracts to produce peristalsis, the wavelike contraction that moves food through the intestinal tract and to the large intestine (see **Figure 16-3** on p. 370). Segmentation activity helps mix the digestive juices with chyme and also makes absorption more efficient (see **Figure 16-4** on p. 370).

Liver and Gallbladder

Structure

The **liver** is so large that it fills the entire upper right section of the abdominal cavity and even extends partway into the left side. Because its cells secrete a substance called **bile** into ducts, the liver is classified as an exocrine gland. In fact, it is the largest gland in the body. Bile contains a mixture of substances, some of which have direct digestive functions described in the next section.

The liver also removes yellowish bile pigments formed by the breakdown of hemoglobin from old RBCs and puts them into the bile for elimination from the body. The liver also has a wide variety of metabolic functions that are discussed in Chapter 17.

Look again at **Figure 16-11**. First, identify the *hepatic ducts.* They drain bile out of the liver, a fact suggested by the name "hepatic," which comes from the Greek word for liver *(hepar).* Next, notice the duct that drains bile into the small intestine (duodenum), the *common bile duct.*

The liver continuously secretes bile. If there is no chyme in the duodenum, then circular sphincter muscles within the duodenal papillae remain closed—and the bile backs up the common bile duct into the *cystic duct* that leads to the **gallbladder.** The folded lining of the gallbladder allows it to expand and thus act as an overflow reservoir for bile. The gallbladder also concentrates stored bile by reabsorbing water from bile back into the blood.

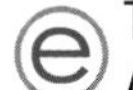
To learn more about bile ducts, go to AnimationDirect at *evolve.elsevier.com.*

Function

Chemically, bile contains significant quantities of cholesterol and substances *(bile salts)* that act as detergents to mechanically break up, or **emulsify,** fats. Because fats form large globules, they must be broken down, or emulsified, into smaller particles to increase the surface area to aid digestion.

In addition to emulsification of fats, bile that is eliminated from the body in the feces serves as a mechanism for excreting cholesterol from the body. Both emulsification of fats and elimination of cholesterol from the body are primary functions of bile.

When chyme containing lipid or fat enters the duodenum, it initiates a mechanism that contracts the gallbladder and forces bile into the small intestine. Fats in chyme trigger the secretion of the hormone **cholecystokinin (CCK)** from the intestinal mucosa of the duodenum. This hormone then travels through the bloodstream and promotes contraction of the gallbladder—and consequently bile flows into the duodenum. Secretion of CCK is a good example of a hormone acting to regulate GI motility.

Visualize a gallstone blocking the common bile duct shown in **Figure 16-11**. Bile could not then drain into the duodenum. Feces would then appear gray-white because the pigments from bile give feces its characteristic color.

If liver secretions slow down as a result of the back-up, bile pigments would not be removed from the blood. A yellowish skin discoloration called **jaundice** would result from increased bile pigment content in the blood. Likewise, obstruction of the common hepatic duct also leads to jaundice.

CLINICAL APPLICATION

GALLSTONES

Gallstones are solid clumps of material (mostly cholesterol) that form in the gallbladder of 1 in 10 Americans (see figure). Some gallstones never cause problems and are called *silent gallstones,* whereas others produce painful symptoms or other medical complications and are called *symptomatic gallstones.*

Gallstones often form when the cholesterol concentration in bile becomes excessive, causing crystallization or precipitation to occur. Stone formation is much more likely to occur if the gallbladder does not empty regularly and chemically imbalanced or cholesterol-laden bile remains in the gallbladder for long periods.

Gallstones can sometimes be treated (dissolved) over time or prevented from developing in at-risk individuals by oral administration of a naturally occurring bile constituent called *ursodeoxycholic acid.* Symptomatic gallstone formation may require surgery—a procedure called **cholecystectomy.**

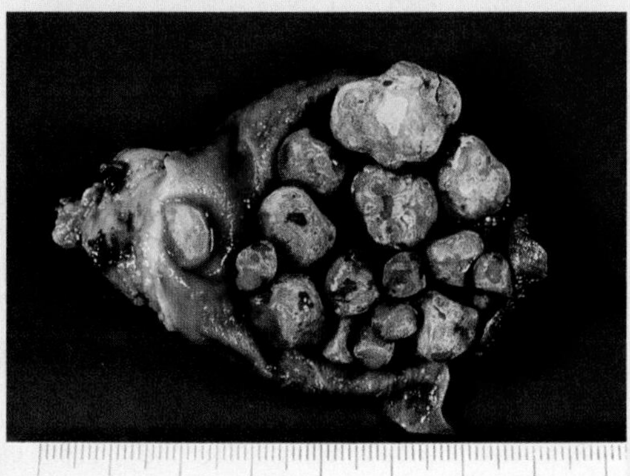

Because bile pigments are not removed from the blood by the gallbladder, no jaundice occurs if only the cystic duct is blocked.

Pancreas

The pancreas lies behind the stomach in the concavity produced by the C shape of the duodenum. The pancreas is both an exocrine gland that secretes pancreatic juice into ducts and an endocrine gland that secretes hormones into the blood. Locate the pancreas and nearby structures in the diagram in **Figure 16-11** and the cadaver dissection in **Figure 16-12**.

Pancreatic juice is the most important digestive juice. It contains enzymes that digest all three major kinds of nutrients—carbohydrates, proteins, and lipids. It also contains sodium bicarbonate, an alkaline substance that neutralizes the hydrochloric acid in the gastric juice that enters the intestines.

Pancreatic juice enters the duodenum of the small intestine at the same place that bile enters. As you can see in **Figure 16-11**, the common bile and pancreatic ducts open into the duodenum at the major duodenal papilla.

Between the cells that secrete pancreatic juice into ducts lie clusters of cells that have no contact with any ducts. These are the **pancreatic islets,** or *islets of Langerhans,* which contain the endocrine cells that secrete the hormones of the pancreas—mainly *insulin* and *glucagon*—described in Chapter 11 (see **Figure 11-11** on p. 251).

QUICK CHECK

1. What are the main divisions of the small intestine?
2. What is bile and where does it come from?
3. What is the function of the gallbladder?
4. Why is the pancreas considered both an endocrine and exocrine gland?

Large Intestine

Structure

The **large intestine** is only about 1.5 meters (5 feet) in length. As the name implies, however, it has a much larger diameter than the small intestine. It forms the lower or terminal portion of the digestive tract.

Chyme containing undigested and unabsorbed food material enters the large intestine after passing through a sphincter called the **ileocecal valve** (**Figure 16-13**). Chyme, which has the consistency of soup, changes to the more solid consistency of fecal matter as water and salts are reabsorbed during its passage through the small intestine. It is this

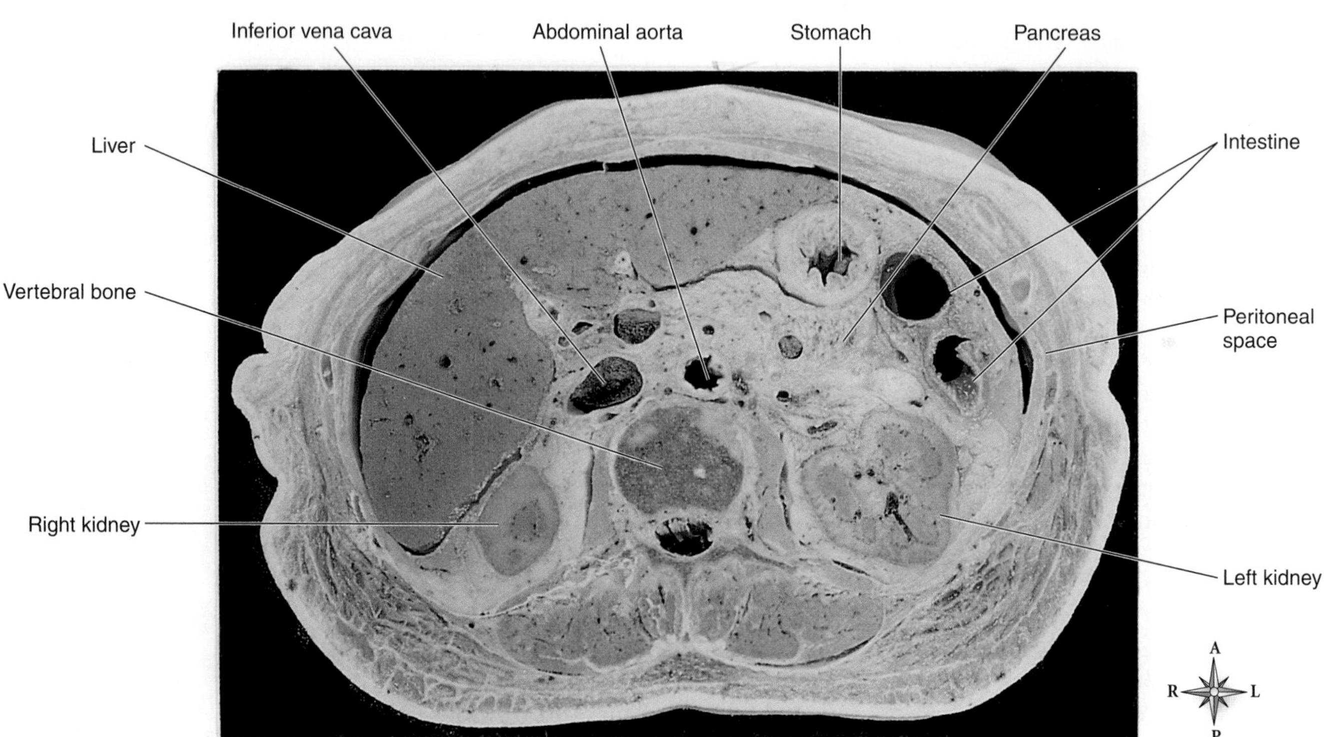

FIGURE 16-12 Horizontal (transverse) section of the abdomen. This inferior view of a cadaver section shows the relative position of some of the major digestive organs of the abdomen. Such a view is typical in images obtained by methods such as computed tomography (CT) scanning and magnetic resonance imaging (MRI).

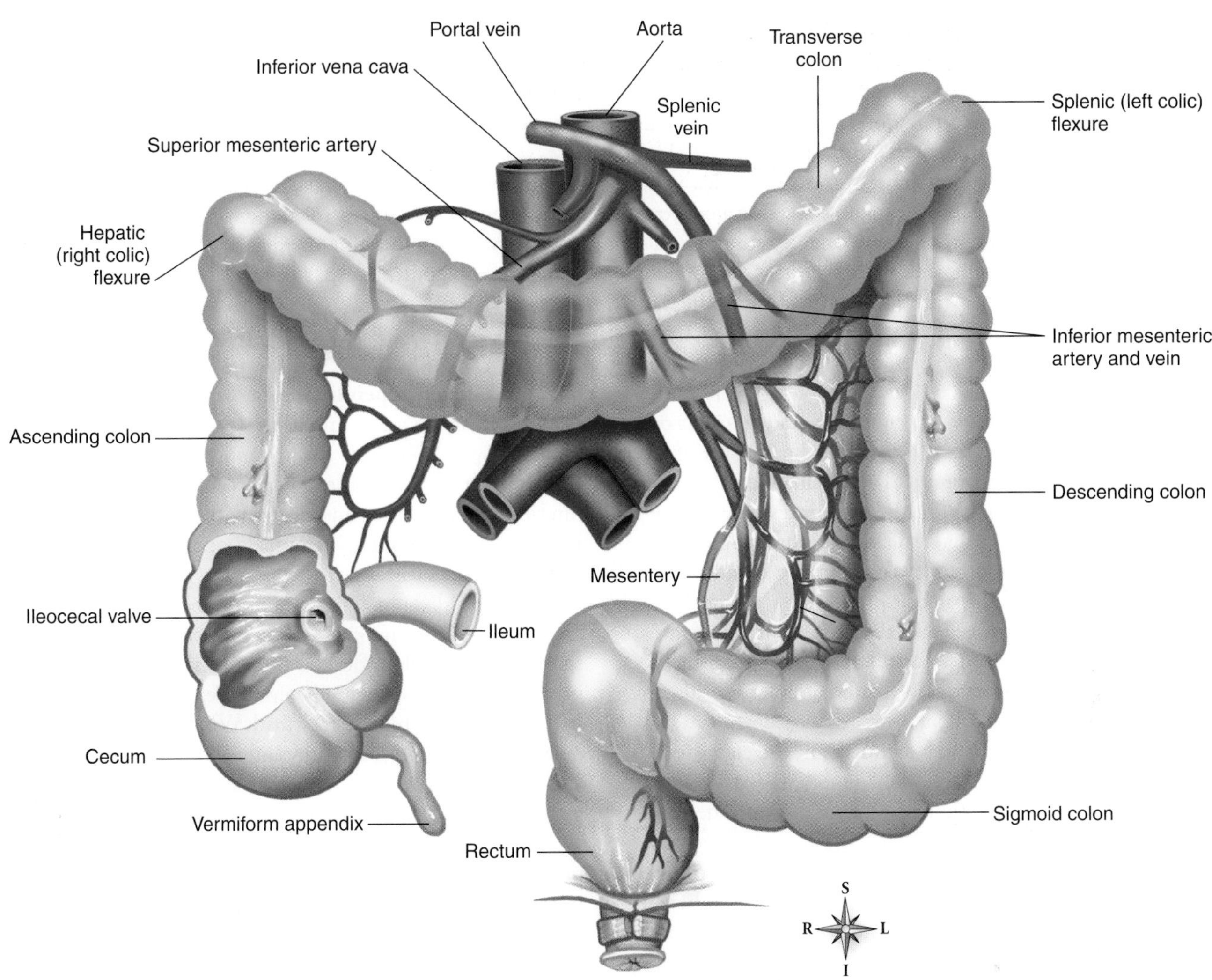

FIGURE 16-13 Divisions of the large intestine.

pastelike material that passes through the valve into the large intestine.

The subdivisions of the large intestine are listed below in the order in which food material or feces passes through them.

1. Cecum
2. Ascending colon
3. Transverse colon
4. Descending colon
5. Sigmoid colon
6. Rectum
7. Anal canal

Note in **Figure 16-13** that the ileocecal valve opens into a pouchlike area called the **cecum.** The opening itself is about 5 or 6 cm (2 inches) above the beginning of the large intestine. Material in the cecum flows upward to a region of the large intestine called the *colon.* Technically the colon does not include the entire large intestine, but often the terms *colon* and *large intestine* are used interchangeably. The colon is divided into three segments: ascending, transverse, and descending colon.

Material moves into the colon on the right side of the body—into the **ascending colon.** The **hepatic flexure** or **right colic flexure** is the bend between the ascending colon and the **transverse colon,** which extends across the front of the abdomen from right to left. The **splenic flexure** or **left colic flexure** marks the point where the **descending colon** turns downward on the left side of the abdomen. The **sigmoid colon** is the S-shaped segment that terminates in the **rectum.** The terminal portion of the rectum is called the **anal canal,** which ends at the external opening, or **anus.**

Function

During its movement through the large intestine, material that escaped digestion in the small intestine is acted on by beneficial bacterial communities called the intestinal **microbiome** or *flora.* As a result of bacterial action, additional nutrients may be released from cellulose and other fibers and absorbed.

In addition to their digestive role, bacteria in the large intestine have other important functions. They are responsible for the synthesis of vitamin K needed for normal blood clotting and for the production of some of the B-complex vitamins. After they are formed, these vitamins are absorbed from the large intestine and enter the blood. The intestinal microbiome also has immune functions that protect us from many intestinal diseases, some of which may be life-threatening.

Some bacteria also produce gases that escape from the colon through the anus—a phenomenon called flatulence or *flatus.*

Although some absorption of water, salts, and vitamins occurs in the large intestine, this segment of the digestive tube is not as well suited for absorption as is the small intestine. No villi are present in the mucosa of the large intestine. As a result, much less surface area is available for absorption. Salts, especially sodium, are absorbed by active transport, and water is moved into the blood by osmosis.

The efficiency and speed of absorption of substances through the wall of the large intestine are lower than in the small intestine. Normal passage of material along the lumen of the large intestine takes about 3 to 5 days.

If the rate of passage of material quickens, the consistency of the stools or fecal material becomes more and more fluid, and **diarrhea** results. If the time of passage through the large intestine is prolonged beyond 5 days, the feces lose volume and become more solid because of excessive water absorption. This reduction of volume decreases stimulation of the bowel emptying reflex, resulting in retention of feces, a condition called **constipation.**

Two sphincter muscles stay contracted to keep the anus closed except during **defecation**—the elimination of feces. Smooth or involuntary muscle composes the *inner anal sphincter,* but striated, or voluntary, muscle composes the *outer anal sphincter.* This anatomical fact sometimes becomes highly important from a practical standpoint. For example, often after a person has had a stroke, the voluntary anal sphincter at first becomes paralyzed. This means, of course, that the individual has no control at that time over bowel movements.

Appendix

The **vermiform appendix** (from *vermis* "worm" and *form* "shape") is, as the name implies, a wormlike, tubular structure. Note in Figure 16-13 that the appendix is directly attached to the back of the cecum. The appendix contains a blind, tubelike interior lumen that communicates with the lumen of the large intestine 3 cm (1 inch) below the opening of the ileocecal valve into the cecum.

The appendix serves as a sort of incubator or "breeding ground" for the nonpathogenic intestinal bacteria found throughout the colon. Besides the normal functions, maintaining a normal intestinal microbiome helps prevent pathogenic bacteria from becoming established. When the normal microbiome of the gut is disrupted by infection or antibiotics, for example, beneficial bacteria hidden away in the appendix can migrate into the colon to restore the normal ecological balance.

Inflammation of the appendix, or **appendicitis,** is a common and potentially very serious medical problem. A site on the surface of the anterior abdominal wall is often used to help in the diagnosis of appendicitis and to estimate the location of the appendix internally. It is called the *McBurney point*

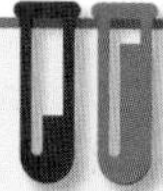

CLINICAL APPLICATION
COLOSTOMY

Colostomy is a surgical procedure in which an artificial anus is created on the abdominal wall by cutting the colon and bringing the cut end or ends out to the surface to form an opening called a *stoma* (see figure). This may be done during a surgery to remove a tumor or a section of the colon. After healing of the colon, the colostomy may be surgically reversed (removed).

Home health care workers help colostomy patients learn to accept the change in body image, which may cause emotional discomfort. The patient or caregiver is also trained in the regular changing of the disposable bag, including how to clean the stoma and how to prevent irritation, chapping, or infection. Irrigation of the colon with isotonic solutions is sometimes necessary. Deodorants may be added to the fresh bag to prevent unpleasant odors.

Patients are also taught to manage their diet to include low-residue food and to avoid foods that produce gas or cause diarrhea. Fluid intake after colostomy is also carefully managed.

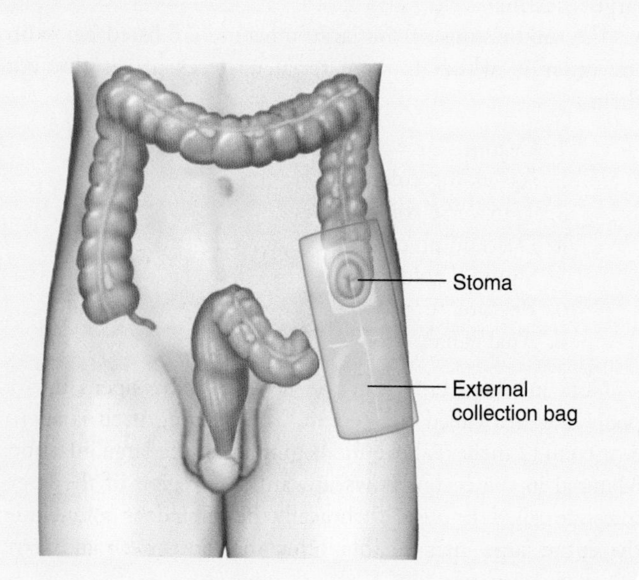

and is located in the right lower quadrant of the abdomen about a third of the way along a line from the right anterior superior iliac spine to the umbilicus. Extreme sensitivity and pain are common when the abdomen of persons with acute appendicitis is palpated over this point.

Peritoneum

Location

The **peritoneum** is a large, moist, slippery sheet of serous membrane that lines the abdominal cavity and covers the organs located in it, including most of the digestive organs. The parietal layer of the peritoneum lines the abdominal cavity. The visceral layer of the peritoneum forms the outer, or covering, layer of each abdominal organ.

The small space between the parietal and visceral layers is called the **peritoneal space.** It contains just enough peritoneal fluid to keep both layers of the peritoneum moist and able to slide freely against each other during breathing and digestive movements (Figure 16-14).

Organs outside of the parietal peritoneum are said to be **retroperitoneal.**

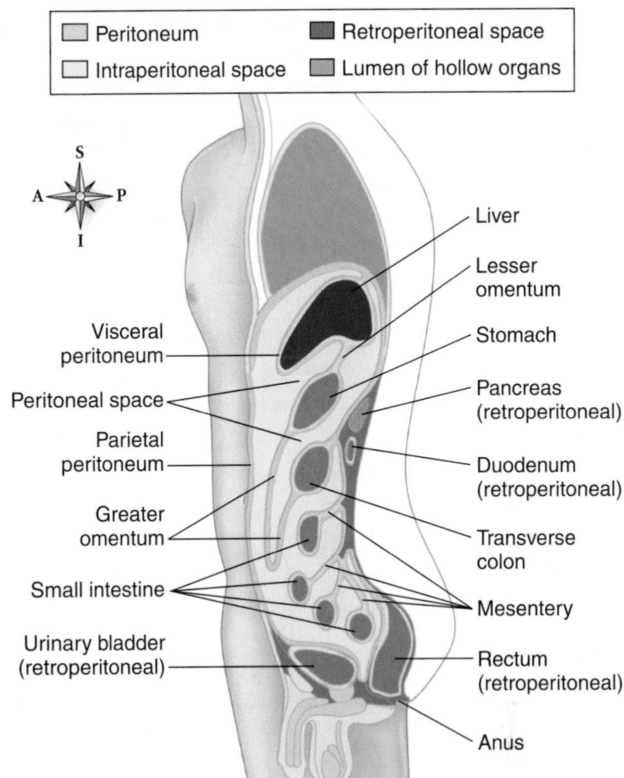

FIGURE 16-14 Peritoneum. The parietal layer of the peritoneum lines the abdominopelvic cavity and then extends in a continuous sheet as a series of mesenteries to form the visceral layer that covers abdominal organs.

Extensions

The two most prominent extensions of the peritoneum are the mesentery and the greater omentum. The **mesentery,** an extension between the parietal and visceral layers of the peritoneum, is shaped like a giant, pleated fan. Its smaller edge attaches to the lumbar region of the posterior abdominal wall, and its long, loose outer edge encloses most of the small intestine, anchoring it to the posterior abdominal wall.

The **greater omentum** is a pouchlike extension of the visceral peritoneum from the lower edge of the stomach, part of the duodenum, and the transverse colon. Shaped like a large apron, it hangs down over the intestines, and because spotty deposits of fat give it a lacy appearance, it has been nicknamed the *lace apron.* It usually envelops a badly inflamed appendix, walling the appendix off from the rest of the abdominal organs.

QUICK CHECK

1. What is the function of the large intestine?
2. Name the divisions of the large intestine.
3. What is the function of the appendix and where is it located in the body?
4. What are two prominent extensions of the peritoneum?

Digestion

Overview of Digestion

Digestion, a complex process that occurs in the alimentary canal, consists of physical and chemical changes that prepare nutrients for absorption.

Mechanical digestion breaks food into tiny particles, mixes them with digestive juices, moves them along the alimentary canal, and finally eliminates the digestive wastes from the body. Note that most types of GI motility such as chewing (mastication), swallowing (deglutition), peristalsis (see Figure 16-3), segmentation (see Figure 16-4), or defecation are considered processes of mechanical digestion.

Chemical digestion breaks down large, nonabsorbable food molecules into smaller, absorbable nutrient molecules that are able to pass through the intestinal mucosa into blood and lymph (Figure 16-15). Chemical digestion consists of numerous chemical reactions catalyzed by enzymes in saliva, gastric juice, pancreatic juice, and intestinal juice.

Enzymes and Chemical Digestion

Enzymes are protein molecules that act as **catalysts.** That is, they speed up specific chemical reactions without themselves being changed or consumed during the reaction process.

During chemical digestion, certain enzymes very selectively speed up the breakdown of specific nutrient molecules and no others. Enzymes responsible for speeding up the breakdown of fats, for example, have no effect on carbohydrates or proteins.

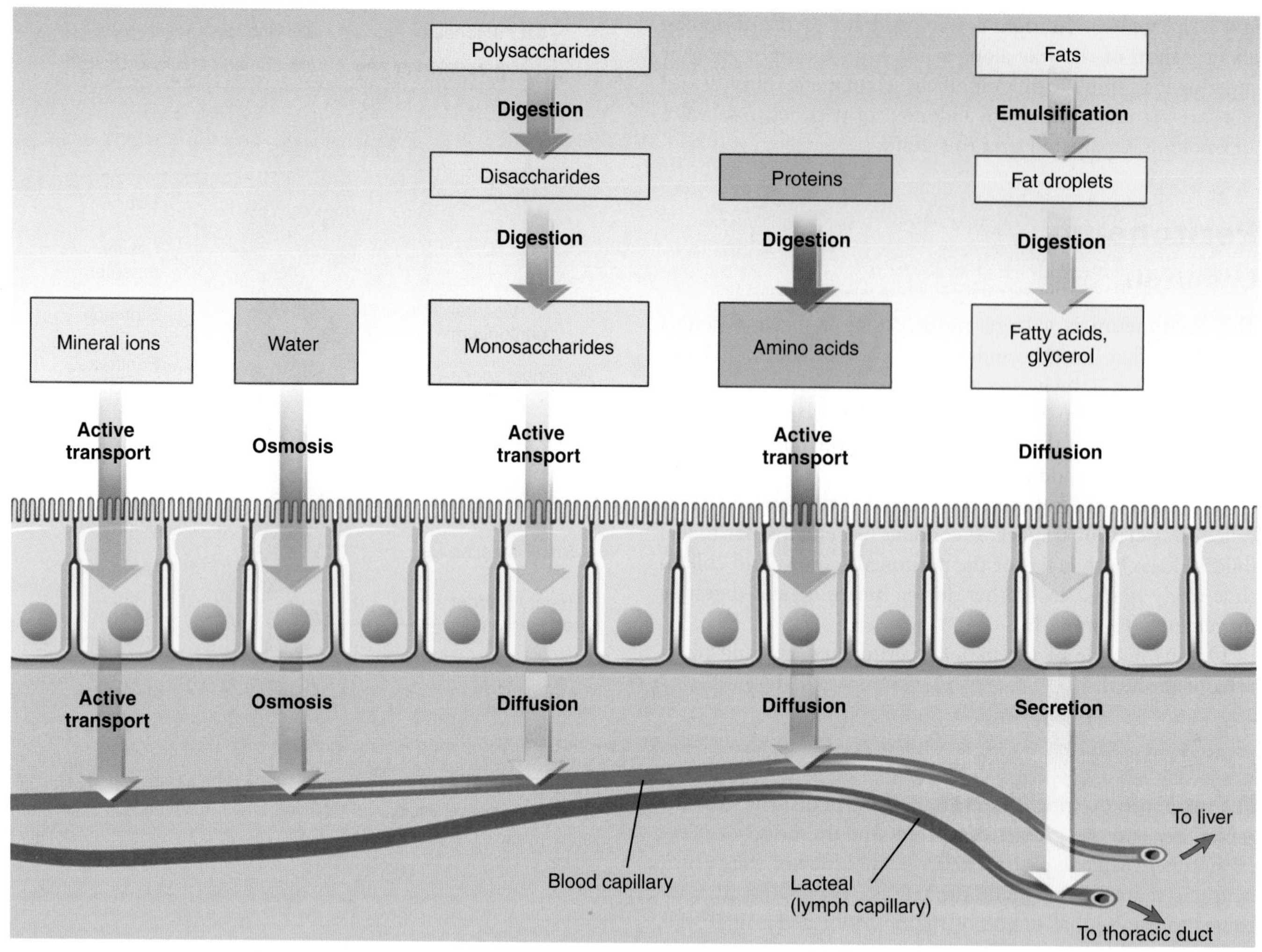

FIGURE 16-15 Digestion and absorption of nutrients, minerals, and water.

The breakdown process is called **hydrolysis**—an important type of chemical reaction first discussed in Chapter 2. Recall that during hydrolysis, enzymes speed up reactions that add water (*hydro*) to chemically break up or split (*lysis*) larger molecules into smaller molecules (see **Figure 2-6** on p. 27).

The names of many enzymes end with the suffix *-ase* combined with the word that describes the type of substance involved in the chemical reaction. *Lipase,* for example, is a fat-digesting enzyme that acts on lipids (fats) and *protease* enzymes serve to break down protein nutrients into smaller molecules. All the digestive enzymes can be classified as *hydrolases* because they catalyze hydrolysis reactions.

Carbohydrate Digestion

Very little digestion of carbohydrates (starches and sugars) occurs before food material reaches the small intestine. Salivary amylase usually has little time to do its work because so many of us swallow our food so fast. Gastric juice contains no carbohydrate-digesting enzymes.

After the food reaches the small intestine, pancreatic and intestinal juice enzymes digest the starches and double sugars. A pancreatic enzyme (amylase) starts the process by breaking down polysaccharides such as starches into disaccharides (double sugars).

Three intestinal enzymes—maltase, sucrase, and lactase—digest disaccharides by changing them into monosaccharides (simple sugars). Maltase digests maltose (malt sugar), sucrase digests sucrose (ordinary cane sugar), and lactase digests lactose (milk sugar).

The end products of carbohydrate digestion are the monosaccharides, the most abundant of which is glucose.

Protein Digestion

Protein digestion starts in the stomach. Hydrochloric acid in gastric juice helps unfold the large, complex protein shapes so digestive enzymes can reach the peptide bonds that hold the amino acids together. **Pepsin,** an enzyme in the gastric juice, then begins breaking peptide bonds to form shorter and shorter chains of amino acids. *Pepsinogen,* a component of gastric juice, is converted into active pepsin enzyme by hydrochloric acid (also in gastric juice).

In the intestine, other enzymes (trypsin in pancreatic juice and peptidases in intestinal juice) finish the job of protein digestion.

TABLE 16-3 Chemical Digestion

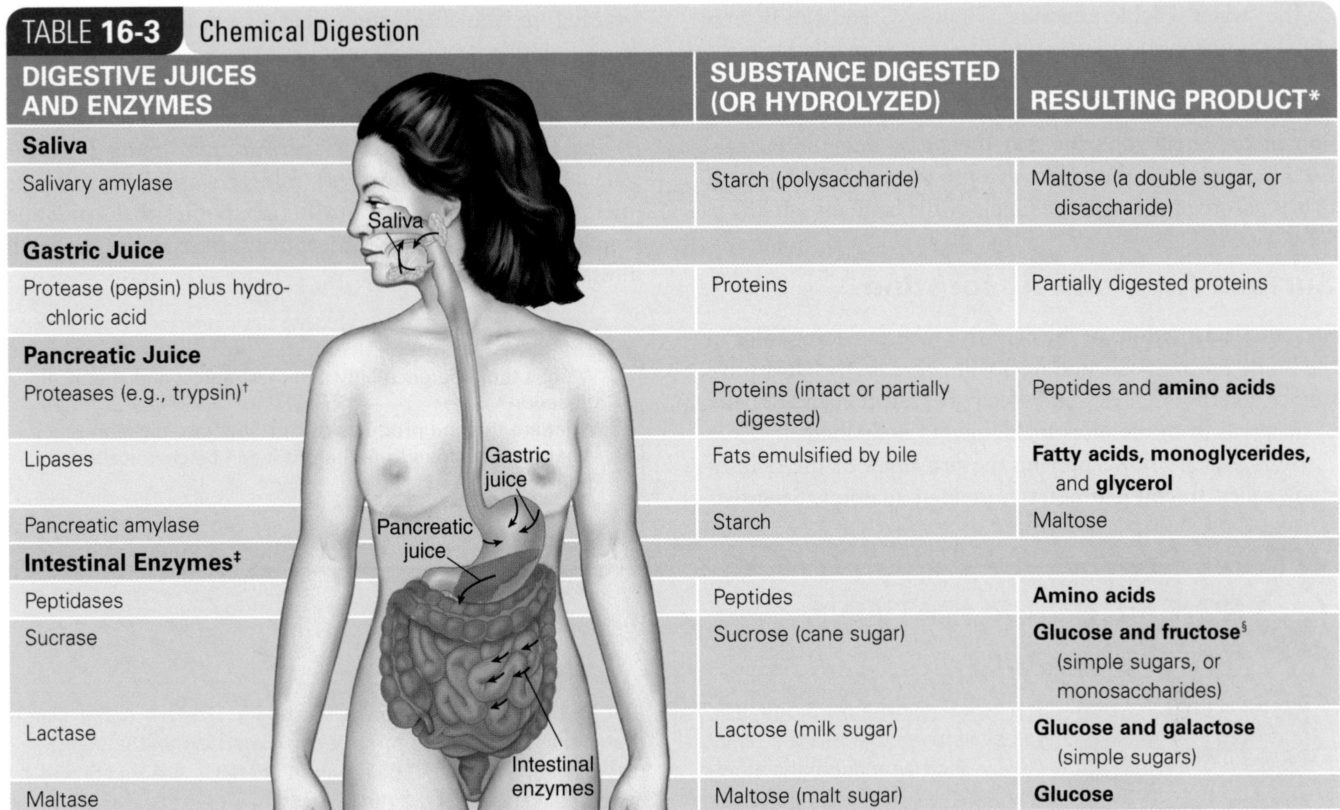

DIGESTIVE JUICES AND ENZYMES	SUBSTANCE DIGESTED (OR HYDROLYZED)	RESULTING PRODUCT*
Saliva		
Salivary amylase	Starch (polysaccharide)	Maltose (a double sugar, or disaccharide)
Gastric Juice		
Protease (pepsin) plus hydrochloric acid	Proteins	Partially digested proteins
Pancreatic Juice		
Proteases (e.g., trypsin)†	Proteins (intact or partially digested)	Peptides and **amino acids**
Lipases	Fats emulsified by bile	**Fatty acids, monoglycerides,** and **glycerol**
Pancreatic amylase	Starch	Maltose
Intestinal Enzymes‡		
Peptidases	Peptides	**Amino acids**
Sucrase	Sucrose (cane sugar)	**Glucose and fructose§** (simple sugars, or monosaccharides)
Lactase	Lactose (milk sugar)	**Glucose and galactose** (simple sugars)
Maltase	Maltose (malt sugar)	**Glucose**

*Substances in boldface type are end products of digestion (that is, completely digested nutrients ready for absorption).
†Secreted in inactive form (trypsinogen); activated by enterokinase, an enzyme in the intestinal brush border.
‡Brush-border enzymes.
§Glucose is also called *dextrose;* fructose is also called *levulose.*

When the protease enzymes have finally split up the large protein molecule into its separate amino acids, protein digestion is completed. Hence the end product of protein digestion is amino acids.

Fat Digestion

Very little fat digestion occurs before food reaches the small intestine. Most fats are undigested until after emulsification into tiny droplets by bile in the duodenum. After this takes place, pancreatic lipase splits up the triglycerides and other large fat molecules into fatty acids and glycerol (glycerin).

The end products of fat digestion, then, are fatty acids and glycerol.

End Products of Digestion

Table 16-3 summarizes the main facts about chemical digestion. When carbohydrate digestion has been completed, starches (polysaccharides) and double sugars (disaccharides) have been changed mainly to glucose, a simple sugar (monosaccharide). The end products of protein digestion, on the other hand, are amino acids. Fatty acid and glycerol are the end products of fat digestion.

Absorption

Mechanisms of Absorption

After food is digested, the resulting nutrients are absorbed and move through the mucous membrane lining of the small intestine into the blood and lymph (see **Figure 16-15**). In other words, nutrient **absorption** is the process by which molecules of amino acids, glucose, fatty acids, and glycerol go from the inside of the intestines into the circulating fluids of the body.

Absorption of nutrients is just as essential as digestion of foods. The reason is fairly obvious. As long as food stays in the intestines, it cannot nourish the millions of cells that compose all other parts of the body. Their lives depend on the absorption of digested food and its transportation to them by the circulating blood.

Many important minerals, such as sodium, are actively transported through the intestinal mucosa. Water follows by osmosis. Other nutrients, such as monosaccharides and amino acids, are also actively transported through the intestinal mucosa and diffuse into the blood of capillaries in the intestinal villi. Fatty acids and glycerol diffuse into the absorptive cells of the GI tract and then are secreted into the lymphatic vessels or lacteals found in intestinal villi.

The "water-soluble vitamins" (vitamin C and the B vitamins) are dissolved in water and absorbed primarily from the small intestine. The "fat-soluble vitamins" (vitamins A, D, E, and K) are absorbed along with the end products of fat digestion in the small intestine and then pass into the lacteals. Bacterial action in the colon also produces some vitamin K that is absorbed through the lining of the large intestine.

Surface Area and Absorption

Structural adaptations of the digestive tube, including folds in the lining mucosa, villi, and microvilli, increase the absorptive surface and the efficiency and speed of absorption and transfer of materials from the intestinal lumen to body fluids.

Biologists are now applying the principles of the field of study called **fractal geometry** to human anatomy. Scientists working in this field study surfaces—called "fractal surfaces"—with a seemingly infinite area, such as the lining of the small intestine. Fractal surfaces have bumps that have bumps that have bumps, and so on.

The fractal-like nature of the intestinal lining is represented in **Figure 16-10**. The plicae (folds) have villi, the villi have microvilli, and even the microvilli have bumps that cannot be seen in the figure. Thus the absorptive surface area of the small intestine is almost limitless.

QUICK CHECK

1. What is the difference between mechanical and chemical digestion?
2. What are the end products of carbohydrate digestion?
3. What must happen to fat before it can be chemically digested?

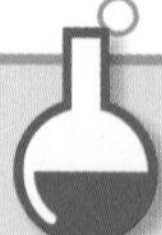

SCIENCE APPLICATIONS

GASTROENTEROLOGY

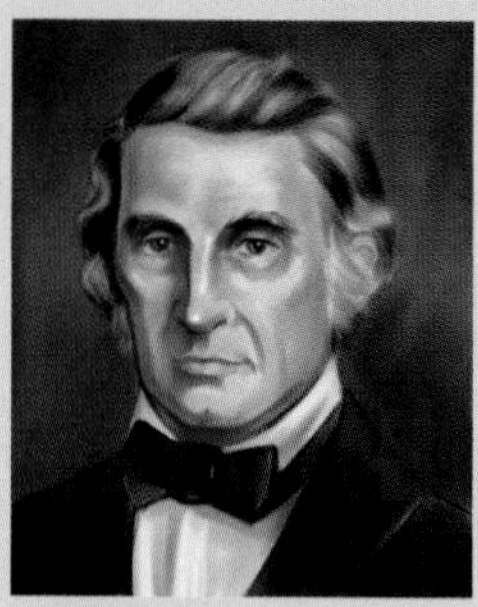

William Beaumont (1785–1853)

The word **gastroenterology** tells you by its parts that it is the study *(-ology)* and treatment of the stomach *(gastro-)* and the intestines *(-entero-)*.

One of the pioneering gastroenterologists was the American physician William Beaumont. In 1822, the young Québécois trapper Alexis St. Martin was shot with a musket near the Army hospital in Michigan where Beaumont was working. Beaumont treated his wound—although expecting St. Martin to die from the injury. However, St. Martin recovered and lived a long life even though the wound did not heal properly. For his entire life thereafter, an open hole remained in his abdomen that led directly into the stomach. Being grateful for his spared life and in need of income, St. Martin reluctantly allowed Beaumont to study gastric secretion through the opening.

Over many years, Beaumont made careful observations about how the stomach works. Many of his conclusions are still valid and serve as the foundation for modern gastroenterology.

Many *physicians* and *nurses* specialize in gastroenterology today. However, many health care providers such as **patient care technicians** and **nursing assistants** still need a basic knowledge of digestive structure and function in order to care for patients effectively. Even workers in the fields of *dietetics, nutrition,* and *food service* benefit from knowledge of the principles of digestion.

LANGUAGE OF SCIENCE AND MEDICINE *(continued from p. 367)*

canine
(KAY-nyne tooth)
[*can-* **dog,** *-ine* **relating to**]

catalyst
(KAT-ah-list)
[*cata-* **lower,** *-lys-* **loosen,** *-ist* **agent**]

cecum
(SEE-kum)
[*cec-* **blind or hidden,** *-um* **thing**]

cementum
(see-MEN-tum)
[*cement-* **mortar,** *-um* **thing or substance**]

cholecystectomy
(kohl-eh-sis-TEK-toh-mee)
[*chole-* **bile,** *-cyst-* **bag,** *-ec-* **out,** *-tom-* **cut,** *-y* **action**]

cholecystokinin (CCK)
(koh-lee-sis-toh-KYE-nin)
[*chole-* **bile,** *-cyst-* **bag,** *-kin-* **movement,** *-in* **substance**]

chyme
(kyme)
[*chym-* **juice**]

colic flexure
(KOHL-ik FLEK-shur)
[*col-* **colon,** *-ic* **pertaining to,** *flex-* **bend,** *-ure* **action**]

colostomy
(kah-LAH-stoh-mee)
[*colo-* **large intestine,** *-stom-* **mouth (opening),** *-y* **activity**]

constipation
(kon-stih-PAY-shun)
[*constipa-* **crowd together,** *-ation* **process**]

crown
(krown)

cuspid
(KUS-pid)
[*cusp-* **point,** *-id* **characterized by**]

deciduous
(deh-SID-yoo-us)
[*decid-* **fall off,** *-ous* **relating to**]

defecation
(def-eh-KAY-shun)
[*de-* **remove,** *-feca-* **waste (feces),** *-tion* **process**]

deglutition
(deg-loo-TISH-un)
[*deglut-* **swallow,** *-tion* **process**]

dental caries
(DENT-al KAYR-ees)
[*dent-* **tooth,** *-al* **relating to,** *caries* **decay**]

dentin
(DEN-tin)
[*dent-* **tooth,** *-in* **substance**]

descending colon
(dih-SEND-ing KOH-lon)
[*de-* **down,** *-scend-* **climb,** *colon* **large intestine**]

diarrhea
(dye-ah-REE-ah)
[*dia-* **through,** *-rrhea* **flow**]

digestion
(dye-JES-chun)
[*digest-* **break apart,** *-tion* **process**]

digestive system
(dye-JES-tiv SIS-tem)
[*digest-* **break apart,** *-tive* **relating to**]

duodenum
(doo-oh-DEE-num)
[*duodenum* **12 fingers,** shortened from *intestinum duodenum digitorum* intestine of 12 finger-widths]

elimination
(eh-lim-uh-NAY-shun)
[*e-* **out,** *-limen-* **threshold,** *-ation* **process**]

emulsify
(eh-MUL-seh-fye)
[*e-* **out,** *-muls-* **milk,** *-i-* **combining vowel,** *-fy* **process**]

enamel
(ih-NA-mel)
[*en-* **in,** *-amel* **melt**]

enzyme
(EN-zyme)
[*en-* **in,** *-zyme* **ferment**]

esophagus
(eh-SOF-ah-gus)
[*eso-* **carry,** *-phagus* **food**]

feces
(FEE-seez)
[*feces* **waste**]

fractal geometry
(FRAK-tal jee-OM-eh-tree)
[*fract-* **break,** *-al* **relating to,** *geo-* **land,** *-metr-* **measure,** *-y* **activity**]

frenulum
(FREN-yoo-lum)
[*fren-* **bridle,** *-ul-* **little,** *-um* **thing**]

fundus
(FUN-dus)
[*fundus* **bottom**]

gallbladder
(GAWL-blad-er)
[*gall-* **bile**]

gallstone
(GAWL-stohn)
[*gall-* **bile**]

gastric gland
(GAS-trik gland)
[*gastr-* **stomach,** *-ic* **relating to,** *gland* **acorn**]

gastroenterology
(gas-troh-en-ter-OL-uh-jee)
[*gastr-* **stomach,** *-entero-* **intestine,** *-o-* **combining vowel,** *-log-* **words (study of),** *-y* **activity**]

gastroesophageal reflux disease (GERD)
(gas-troh-eh-sof-eh-JEE-all REE-fluks dih-ZEEZ)
[*gastro-* **stomach,** *-eso-* **carry,** *-phag-* **food (eat),** *-al* **relating to,** *re-* **again or back,** *-flux* **flow,** *dis-* **opposite of,** *-ease* **comfort**]

gastrointestinal (GI) tract
(gas-troh-in-TES-tih-nul trakt)
[*gastr-* **stomach,** *-intestin-* **intestine,** *-al* **relating to,** *tract* **trail**]

gingiva
(JIN-jih-vah)
[*gingiva* **gum**]

gingivitis
(jin-jih-VYE-tis)
[*gingiv-* **gum,** *-itis* **inflammation**]

greater omentum
(GRAYT-er oh-MEN-tum)
[*omentum* **membrane covering intestines**]

hard palate
(PAL-et)

heartburn
(hart burn)

Helicobacter pylori
(HEEL-ih-koh-BAK-ter pye-LOH-ree)
[*Helic-* **helix,** *-bacter* **rod (bacterium),** *pyl-* **gate,** *-or-* **guard,** *-i* **of the**]

hepatic flexure
(heh-PAT-ik FLEK-sher)
[*hepa-* **liver,** *-ic* **relating to,** *flex-* **that may be bent,** *ure* **action**]

hiatal hernia
(hye-AY-tal HER-nee-ah)
[*hiat-* **gap,** *-al* **relating to,** *hernia* **rupture**]

hydrolysis
(hye-DROL-ih-sis)
[*hydro-* **water,** *-lysis* **loosening**]

ileocecal valve
(il-ee-oh-SEE-kal valv)
[*ileum* **groin or flank,** *cec-* **blind or hidden,** *-al* **relating to**]

ileum
(IL-ee-um)
[*ileum* **groin or flank**]

incisor
(in-SYE-zer)
[*in-* **into,** *-cis-* **cut,** *-or* **agent**]

ingestion
(in-JES-chun)
[*in-* **within,** *-gest-* **carry,** *-tion* **process**]

intestinal gland
(in-TES-tih-nal gland)
[*intestin-* **intestine,** *-al* **relating to,** *gland* **acorn**]

jaundice
(JAWN-dis)
[*jaun-* **yellow,** *-ice* **state**]

jejunum
(jeh-JOO-num)
[*jejun-* **empty,** *-um* **thing**]

lacteal
(LAK-tee-al)
[*lact-* **milk,** *-al* **relating to**]

large intestine
(larj in-TES-tin)

laryngopharynx
(lah-ring-go-FAYR-inks)
[*laryng-* **voice box (larynx),** *-pharynx* **throat**]

liver

lower esophageal sphincter (LES)
(LOH-er eh-SOF-eh-JEE-ul SFINGK-ter)
[*eso-* **carry,** *-phag-* **food,** *-al* **relating to,** *sphinc-* **bind tight,** *-er* **agent**]

lumen
(LOO-men)
[*lumen* **light or window**]

major duodenal papilla
(MAY-jer doo-oh-DEE-nul [or doo-AH-de-nul] pah-PIL-ah)
[*major* **larger,** *duoden-* **12 fingers, shortened from *intestinum duodenum digitorum* intestine of 12 finger-widths,** *-al* **relating to,** *papilla* **nipple**]

malocclusion
(mal-oh-KLOO-zhun)
[*mal-* **bad,** *-oc-* **against,** *-clu-* **shut or close,** *-sion* **state**]

mastication
(mass-tih-KAY-shun)
[*mastica-* **chew,** *-ation* **process**]

mesentery
(MEZ-en-tayr-ee)
[*mes-* **middle,** *-enter-* **intestine,** *-y* **thing**]

microbiome
(my-kroh-BYE-ohm)
[*micro-* **small,** *-bio-* **life,** *-ome* **entire collection**]

microvilli
(my-kroh-VIL-ee)
sing., microvillus
(my-kroh-VIL-us)
[*micro-* **small,** *-villi* **shaggy hairs**]

minor duodenal papilla
(MYE-ner doo-oh-DEE-nul [or doo-AH-de-nul] pah-PIL-ah)
[*minor* **smaller,** *duoden-* **12 fingers, shortened from *intestinum duodenum digitorum* intestine of 12 finger-widths,** *-al* **relating to,** *papilla* **nipple**]

molar
(MOHL-ar)
[*mol-* **millstone,** *-ar* **relating to]**

motility
(moh-TIL-ih-tee)
[*mot-* **move,** *-il-* **relating to,** *-ity* **state]**

mouth

mucosa
(myoo-KOH-sah)
pl., mucosae
(myoo-KOH-see)
[*muc-* **slime,** *-os-* **relating to,** *-a* **thing]**

muscularis
(mus-kyoo-LAYR-is)
[*mus-* **mouse,** *-cul-* **little,** *-ar-* **relating to,** *-is* **thing]**

nasopharynx
(nay-zoh-FAYR-inks)
[*naso-* **nose,** *-pharynx* **throat]**

neck

nursing assistant
(NURS-ing ah-SIS-tent)
[*nurs-* **nourish or nurture,** *assist-* **help,** *-ant* **agent]**

oral cavity
(OR-al KAV-ih-tee)
[*or-* **mouth,** *-al* **relating to,** *cav-* **hollow,** *-ity* **state]**

oropharynx
(or-oh-FAYR-inks)
[*oro-* **mouth,** *-pharynx* **throat]**

pancreatic islet (islet of Langerhans)
(pan-kree-AT-ik eye-let) (EYE-let of LAHN-ger-hans)
[*pan-* **all,** *-creat-* **flesh,** *-ic* **relating to,** *isl-* **island,** *-et* **little]** [*Paul Langerhans* **German pathologist]**

parotid gland
(peh-RAH-tid gland)
[*par-* **beside,** *-ot-* **ear,** *-id* **relating to,** *gland* **acorn]**

patient care technician
(PAY-shent kayr tek-NISH-en)
[*techn-* **art or skill,** *-ic* **relating to,** *-ian* **practitioner]**

pepsin
(PEP-sin)
[*peps-* **digestion,** *-in* **substance]**

periodontal membrane
(payr-ee-oh-DON-tull MEM-brayn)
[*peri-* **around,** *-dont-* **tooth,** *-al* **relating to,** *membrane* **thin skin]**

periodontitis
(payr-ee-oh-don-TYE-tis)
[*peri-* **around,** *-odont-* **tooth,** *-itis* **inflammation]**

peristalsis
(payr-ih-STAL-sis)
[*peri-* **around,** *-stalsis* **contraction]**

peritoneal space
(payr-ih-toh-NEE-al)
[*peri-* **around,** *-tone-* **stretched,** *-al* **relating to]**

peritoneum
(payr-ih-toh-NEE-um)
[*peri-* **around,** *-tone-* **stretched,** *-um* **thing]**

permanent teeth

pharynx
(FAYR-inks)
[*pharynx* **throat]**

plica
(PLYE-kah)
pl., plicae
(PLYE-kee)
[*plica* **fold]**

premolar
(pree-MOHL-ar)
[*pre-* **before,** *-mola-* **millstone,** *-ar* **relating to]**

pyloric sphincter
(pye-LOR-ik SFINGK-ter)
[*pyl-* **gate,** *-or-* **to guard,** *-ic* **relating to,** *sphinc-* **bind tight,** *-er* **agent]**

pylorus
(pye-LOR-us)
[*pyl-* **gate,** *-orus* **guard]**

rectum
(REK-tum)
[*rect-* **straight,** *-um* **thing]**

regulation
(reg-yoo-LAY-shun)
[*regula-* **rule,** *-tion* **process]**

retroperitoneal
(reh-troh-pair-ih-toh-NEE-al)
[*retro-* **backward,** *peri-* **around,** *-tone-* **stretched,** *-al* **relating to]**

root

rugae
(ROO-gee)
sing., ruga
[*ruga* **wrinkle]**

secretion
(seh-KREE-shun)
[*secret-* **separate,** *-tion* **process]**

segmentation
(seg-men-TAY-shun)
[*segment-* **cut section,** *-ation* **process]**

serosa
(see-ROH-sah)
[*ser-* **watery fluid,** *-os-* **relating to,** *-a* **thing]**

serous
(SEE-rus)
[*ser-* **watery fluid,** *-ous* **relating to]**

sigmoid colon
(SIG-moyd KOH-lon)
[*sigm-* **sigma (Σ or σ) 18th letter of Greek alphabet (Roman S),** *-oid* **like,** *colon* **large intestine]**

small intestine
(smahl in-TEST-in)

soft palate
(PAL-et)
[*palat-* **roof of mouth]**

sphincter
(SFINGK-ter)
[*sphinc-* **bind tight,** *-er* **agent]**

splenic flexure
(SPLEN-ik FLEK-shur)
[*splen-* **spleen,** *-ic* **pertaining to,** *flex-* **bend,** *-ure* **action]**

stomach
(STUM-uk)
[*stomach* **mouth]**

sublingual gland
(sub-LING-gwall gland)
[*sub-* **under,** *-lingua-* **tongue,** *-al* **relating to,** *gland* **acorn]**

submandibular gland
(sub-man-DIB-yoo-lar gland)
[*sub-* **under,** *-mandibul-* **chew (mandible or jawbone),** *-ar* **relating to,** *gland* **acorn]**

submucosa
(sub-myoo-KOH-sah)
[*sub-* **under,** *-muc-* **slime,** *-os-* **relating to,** *-a* **thing]**

transverse colon
(tranz-VERS KOH-len)
[*trans-* **across,** *-vers-* **turn,** *colon* **large intestine]**

tricuspid
(try-KUS-pid)
[*tri-* **three,** *-cusp-* **point,** *-id* **characterized by]**

ulcer
(UL-ser)
[*ulcer* **sore]**

upper esophageal sphincter (UES)
(UP-er eh-SOF-ah-JEE-ul SFINGK-ter)
[*eso-* **carry,** *-phag-* **food (eat),** *-al* **relating to,** *sphinc-* **bind tight,** *-er* **agent]**

uvula
(YOO-vyoo-lah)
[*uva-* **grape (or bunch of grapes),** *-ula* **little]**

vermiform appendix
(VERM-ih-form ah-PEN-diks)
[*vermi-* **worm,** *-form* **shape,** *append-* **hang upon,** *-ix* **thing]**

villus
(VIL-us)
pl., villi
(VIL-aye)
[*villus* **shaggy hair]**

❑ OUTLINE SUMMARY

To download a digital audio version of the chapter summary for use with your device, access the ***Audio Chapter Summaries*** *online at evolve.elsevier.com.*

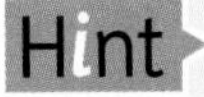

Scan this summary after reading the chapter to help you reinforce the key concepts. Later, use the summary as a quick review before your class or before a test.

Overview of Digestion

A. Irregular tube called *alimentary canal* or *gastrointestinal (GI) tract* and accessory organs of digestion (see **Figure 16-1** and **Table 16-1**)

B. Food must first be digested and absorbed

Primary Mechanisms of the Digestive System

A. The digestive system uses many mechanisms (see **Table 16-2**)

B. Ingestion — complex foods taken into the GI tract

C. Digestion — group of processes that break complex nutrients into simpler ones
   1. Mechanical digestion — breakup of large chunks of food into smaller bits
   2. Chemical digestion — breaks large molecules into smaller ones

D. Motility — a number of GI movements resulting from muscular contraction

E. Secretion — release of digestive juices and hormones that facilitate digestion

F. Absorption — movement of digested nutrients into the internal environment of the body

G. Elimination — movement of residues of digestion out of alimentary canal

H. Regulation — neural, hormonal, and other mechanisms that regulate digestive activity

Wall of the Digestive Tract

A. Digestive tract described as tube that extends from mouth to anus; the inner hollow space is called the *lumen*

B. Wall of the digestive tube is formed by four layers (see **Figure 16-2**)
   1. Mucosa — type varies depending on GI location (tough and stratified or delicate and simple epithelium); mucous production
   2. Submucosa — connective tissue layer
   3. Muscularis — circular, longitudinal, and oblique (in stomach) layers of muscle important in GI motility
      a. Peristalsis — "wavelike" movement pushes food down the tract (see **Figure 16-3**)
      b. Segmentation — "back-and-forth" mixing movement (see **Figure 16-4**)
   4. Serosa — serous membrane that covers the outside of abdominal organs; it attaches the digestive tract to the wall of the abdominopelvic cavity by forming folds called *mesenteries*

Mouth

A. Structure of oral cavity
   1. Roof — formed by hard palate (parts of maxillary and palatine bones) and soft palate, an arch-shaped muscle separating mouth from pharynx; uvula, a downward projection of soft palate helps in speech and swallowing (deglutition)
   2. Floor — formed by tongue and its muscles, lingual frenulum (fold of mucosa that helps anchor tongue) (see **Figure 16-5**)

B. Teeth
   1. Typical tooth (see **Figure 16-6**)
      a. Three main parts — crown, neck, and root
      b. Enamel, which covers the crown, is hardest tissue in body
   2. Types of teeth — incisors, canines (cuspids), premolars (bicuspids), and molars (tricuspids)
   3. Twenty teeth in deciduous or baby set; average age for cutting first tooth about 6 months; set complete at about 30 months of age
   4. Thirty-two teeth in permanent set; 6 years about average age for starting to cut first permanent tooth; set complete usually between ages of 17 and 24 years (see **Figure 16-5**)

C. Salivary glands (see **Figure 16-7**)
   1. Saliva — exocrine gland secretion flows into ducts
      a. Serous type — watery and contains enzymes (salivary amylase) but no mucus
         (1) Produced by serous-type secretory cells (see **Figure 16-7**, *B*)
      b. Mucous type — thick, slippery, and contains mucus but no enzymes
         (1) Lubricates food during mastication
         (2) Produced by mucous-type secretory cells (see **Figure 16-7**, *B*)
   2. Parotid glands (see **Figure 16-7**, *A*)
      a. Largest salivary glands
      b. Produces serous-type saliva
      c. Mumps — infection of parotids
   3. Submandibular glands (see **Figure 16-7**, *A*)
      a. Mixed-gland — produces both serous- and mucous-type saliva (see **Figure 16-7**, *B*)
      b. Located below mandibular angle
      c. Ducts open on either side of lingual frenulum
   4. Sublingual glands (see **Figure 16-7**, *A*)
      a. Produce only mucous-type saliva
      b. Multiple ducts open into floor of mouth

Pharynx

A. Structure
   1. Three divisions: nasopharynx, oropharynx, laryngopharynx (see **Figure 16-8**)
   2. Tonsils form lymphoid ring that prevents digestive tract infection
B. Function — deglutition (swallowing)
   1. Oropharynx is most involved pharyngeal segment in deglutition
   2. Regulation of deglutition movements via motor cortex of cerebrum (voluntary) and "deglutition center" of brainstem (involuntary)

Esophagus

A. Connects pharynx to stomach
B. Dynamic passageway for food
C. Sphincters at each end of esophagus help keep ingested material moving in one direction down the tube
   1. Upper esophageal sphincter (UES)
   2. Lower esophageal sphincter (LES), also called cardiac sphincter

Stomach

A. Structure
   1. Divisions — fundus (outpouched base), body (main part), pylorus (apex)
   2. Size — expands after large meal; about size of large sausage when empty (see **Figure 16-9**)
   3. Muscularis — many smooth muscle fibers in three layers; contractions produce churning movements (peristalsis)
   4. Mucosa
      a. Many microscopic gastric glands secrete gastric juice containing enzymes, hydrochloric acid, and intrinsic factor into stomach
      b. Mucous membrane lies in folds (rugae) when stomach is empty
   5. Pyloric sphincter muscle closes opening between pylorus (lower part of stomach) and duodenum
B. Function
   1. Food enters stomach through LES and digestive process continues
   2. Partial digestion of proteins occurs after chyme is held in the stomach for some time by the muscle
   3. Hiatal hernia occurs when the stomach pushed through an opening in the diaphragm, which may cause gastroesophageal reflux disease (GERD)

Small Intestine

A. Structure
   1. Size — about 7 meters (20 feet) long but only 2 cm or so in diameter (see **Figure 16-10**)
   2. Divisions
      a. Duodenum
      b. Jejunum
      c. Ileum
   3. Many coiled loops accommodate a long tube within the short abdominal cavity
   4. Duodenum is site of much chemical digestion
      a. Ducts from pancreas and liver enter tract here
      b. Major and minor duodenal papillae are bumps where the secretions enter
B. Function
   1. Main functions — digestion and absorption; small intestine does most of these functions for the digestive system
   2. Intestinal secretions and digestions
      a. Intestinal glands — many microscopic glands secrete intestinal juice (water, enzymes, ions)
      b. Pancreatic and liver secretions
      c. Most digestion occurs in duodenum
   3. Absorption
      a. Huge absorptive surface area
         (1) Circular folds (plicae)
         (2) Intestinal villi — microscopic finger-shaped projections
         (3) Blood capillaries absorb carbohydrate and protein products (sugars; amino acids)
         (4) Lacteals (lymph capillaries) absorb fats
   4. Motility — smooth muscle fibers contract to produce movements
      a. Peristalsis pushes chyme along, toward large intestine
      b. Segmentation mixes digestive juices with chyme and helps with absorption

Liver and Gallbladder

A. Structure
   1. Liver
      a. Largest exocrine gland
      b. Fills upper right section of abdominal cavity and extends over into left side (see **Figure 16-12**)
      c. Secretes bile, a mixture of substances
      d. Removes yellowish bile pigments from blood (from breakdown of old RBCs)
      e. Other metabolic functions (discussed in Chapter 17)
   2. Gallbladder
      a. Location — undersurface of the liver, sac with folded interior
      b. Function — concentrates and stores bile produced in the liver
   3. Ducts (see **Figure 16-11**)
      a. Hepatic — drains bile from liver
      b. Cystic — duct by which bile enters and leaves gallbladder
      c. Common bile — formed by union of hepatic and cystic ducts; drains bile from hepatic or cystic ducts into duodenum

B. Function
   1. Bile contains bile salts that emulsify the fats in chyme
   2. Bile contains cholesterol that can be eliminated from the body
   3. CCK (cholecystokinin) is a hormone triggered by fat in chyme; it causes the gallbladder to contract and push stored bile into ducts leading to duodenum
   4. Gallstones can block ducts and possibly cause discolored stool and accumulation of yellow bile pigments in blood and throughout body — a condition called jaundice

Pancreas

A. Exocrine *and* endocrine gland that lies behind stomach
B. Pancreatic cells secrete pancreatic juice
   1. Most important digestive juice, containing enzymes to digest carbohydrates, proteins, lipids; contains sodium bicarbonate that neutralizes stomach acid in chyme
   2. Secreted into pancreatic ducts; main duct empties into duodenum
C. Pancreatic islets (of Langerhans) — endocrine cells not connected with pancreatic ducts; secrete hormones glucagon and insulin into the blood

Large Intestine

A. Structure (see **Figure 16-13**)
   1. Cecum — blind-end pouch at beginning of large intestine; chyme enters cecum through ileocecal valve
   2. Colon — ascending, transverse, descending, and sigmoid segments
   3. Rectum — empties feces through anal canal and external opening called anus
B. Function
   1. Microbiome (flora) — helps digest nutrients, produce vitamins, and support immune protection; produce gases (flatulence or flatus)
   2. Absorption of water, salts, vitamins
   3. Increased motility may produce diarrhea and decreased motility may result in constipation
   4. Defecation — elimination of feces; regulated by voluntary and involuntary anal sphincters

Appendix

A. Blind, worm-shaped tube off cecum
B. Functions as an incubator for bacteria of the intestinal microbiome
C. Appendicitis — inflammation of the appendix

Peritoneum

A. Location and description — continuous serous membrane lining abdominal cavity and covering abdominal organs (see **Figure 16-14**)
   1. Parietal layer of peritoneum lines abdominal cavity
   2. Visceral layer of peritoneum covers abdominal organs
   3. Peritoneal space — lies between parietal and visceral layers; produces lubricating peritoneal (serous) fluid
   4. Retroperitoneal—describes structures outside the parietal peritoneum
B. Extensions — largest are the mesentery and greater omentum
   1. Mesentery is extension of parietal peritoneum, which attaches most of small intestine to posterior abdominal wall
   2. Greater omentum, or "lace apron," hangs down from lower edge of stomach and transverse colon over intestines

Digestion

A. Overview of digestion — transforms foods into nutrient substances that can be absorbed and used by cells (see **Table 16-3**)
   1. Mechanical digestion — chewing (mastication), swallowing (deglutition), and peristalsis break food into tiny particles, mix them well with digestive juices, and move them along the digestive tract
   2. Chemical digestion — breaks up large nutrient molecules into compounds that have smaller molecules; brought about by digestive enzymes (see **Figure 16-15**)
B. Enzymes and chemical digestion
   1. Enzymes are protein molecules that act as catalysts
   2. Breakdown process called hydrolysis
   3. Enzyme names often end in *-ase*
C. Carbohydrate digestion — mainly in small intestine
   1. Pancreatic amylase — breaks polysaccharides down to disaccharides
   2. Intestinal juice enzymes
      a. Maltase — changes maltose to glucose
      b. Sucrase — changes sucrose to glucose
      c. Lactase — changes lactose to glucose
D. Protein digestion — starts in stomach; completed in small intestine
   1. *Hydrochloric acid* in gastric juice unfolds large proteins and converts pepsinogen to active pepsin
   2. Gastric juice enzyme *pepsin* partially digests proteins
   3. Pancreatic enzyme, *trypsin,* continues digestion of proteins
   4. Intestinal enzymes, *peptidases,* complete digestion of partially digested proteins and convert them to amino acids
E. Fat digestion — mainly in small intestine
   1. Bile contains no enzymes but emulsifies fats (breaks fat droplets into very small droplets)
   2. Pancreatic lipase changes emulsified fats to fatty acids and glycerol in small intestine
F. End products of digestion (see **Figure 16-15**)

Absorption

A. Mechanisms of absorption
   1. Definition — process by which digested nutrients move from intestine into blood or lymph
   2. Mechanisms include diffusion, osmosis, and active transport (see **Figure 16-15**)
   3. Nutrients and most water, minerals, and vitamins are absorbed from small intestine; some water and vitamin K also absorbed from large intestine

B. Surface area and absorption
   1. Structural adaptations increase absorptive surface area
   2. Fractal geometry — study of irregular "fragmented" geometric shapes such as those in lining of intestine that have almost unlimited surface area

❑ ACTIVE LEARNING

STUDY TIPS

Hint *Use these tips to achieve success in meeting your learning goals.*

To make the study of the digestive system more efficient, we suggest these tips:

1. Before studying Chapter 16, review coverage of carbohydrates, fats, proteins, enzymes, and hydrolysis in Chapter 2, the nature of smooth muscle in Chapter 4, the synopsis of the digestive system in Chapter 5, and mucous membranes in Chapter 6.
2. Structure of the digestive system involves component parts of the tube itself and accessory organs not in the tube. Create flash cards to use as you learn, and then review the names, locations, and functions of each component. Trace the passage of ingested food through the gastrointestinal (GI) tract, and use your growing deck of flash cards to correlate specific nutrients with the GI segment in which they are absorbed.
3. Learn the names of the layers of the GI tract wall, how they differ in various locations along the tube, and how the lining of the tube increases the efficiency of the absorption of nutrients. Remember that structure and function are related. If you remember this general rule, learning a great deal about both digestive system anatomy and physiology will become easier. As you study this chapter—and every chapter—make a list of examples that demonstrate this relationship.
4. Digestion involves both physical and chemical changes to ingested food that must occur before nutrients can be absorbed and reach body cells. Learn to associate the changes that occur in intestinal contents in each segment of the tract with the differing structure and functions of each segment and related accessory structures.
5. Create your own table or study list that "connects" each digestive enzyme with the major nutrient it breaks down and the names of the resulting smaller, absorbable end products of digestion. Compare your list with **Table 16-2**.
6. In your study group, review the Quick Check questions and questions in the back of the chapter, and discuss possible test questions.

Review Questions

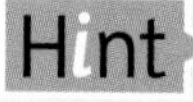

Write out the answers to these questions after reading the chapter and reviewing the Chapter Summary. If you simply think through the answer without writing it down, you won't retain much of your new learning.

1. Name and describe the four layers of the wall of the GI tract.
2. Name the function of the uvula and soft palate.
3. Explain the function of the different types of teeth.
4. Describe the three main parts of a tooth.
5. Name the three pairs of salivary glands and describe where the duct from each enters the mouth.
6. Name the functions of the cardiac and pyloric sphincter muscles.
7. Define *peristalsis.*
8. Explain how bile from the liver and gallbladder reaches the small intestine. What is the function of cholecystokinin?
9. List what is contained in pancreatic juice.
10. Describe what the bacteria in the large intestine contribute to the body.
11. List the seven subdivisions of the large intestine.
12. Describe the mesentery and the greater omentum.
13. Differentiate between mechanical digestion and chemical digestion.
14. Briefly describe the process of carbohydrate digestion.
15. Briefly describe the process of fat digestion.
16. Briefly describe the process of protein digestion.
17. Explain the process of absorption and briefly describe what function the lacteals have in absorption.

Critical Thinking

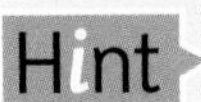

After finishing the Review Questions, write out the answers to these more in-depth questions to help you apply your new knowledge. Go back to sections of the chapter that relate to concepts that you find difficult.

18. What structures in the small intestine increase the internal surface area? What advantage is gained by this increase in surface area?
19. Bile does not cause a chemical change; what is the effect of bile on fat and why does this make fat digestion more efficient?
20. Some people are lactose intolerant. This means they are unable to digest lactose sugar. What enzyme is probably not functioning properly and what types of food should these people try to avoid?
21. Christy had her gallbladder removed and is wondering how this will affect her fat digestion. What could you tell her?

Chapter Test

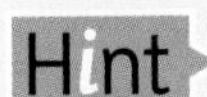

After studying the chapter, test your mastery by responding to these items. Try to answer them without looking up the answers. Then, verify the answers using the key in Appendix C at the back of this book.

1. Food undergoes three kinds of processing in the body. All cells perform metabolism, but absorption and digestion are performed by the digestive system.
2. The muscularis layer of the wall of the GI tract produces peristalsis.
3. The sub-mucosa layer of the wall of the GI tract contains blood vessels and nerves.
4. mucosa is the innermost layer of the wall of the GI tract.
5. serosa is the outermost layer of the wall of the GI tract.
6. The uvula and soft palette prevent food and liquid from entering the nasal cavity above the mouth when food is swallowed.
7. The three main parts of a tooth are crown, root, and neck.
8. The names of the three pairs of salivary glands are the parotid, the sublingual, and the submandibular
9. The tube connecting the pharynx and the stomach is the esophagus
10. The three divisions of the stomach are the fundus, the body, and the pylorus.
11. The three divisions of the small intestine are the duodenum, the jejunum, and the ileum.
12. The tiny, fingerlike projections covering the plicae of the small intestine are called villi.
13. The lymphatic vessel in the villi is called the lacteal.
14. The common bile duct is formed by the union of the Hepatic duct from the liver and the cystic duct from the gallbladder.
15. The part of the large intestine between the ascending and descending colon is the transverse colon
16. The part of the large intestine between the descending colon and the rectum is called the sigmoid colon
17. The two most prominent extensions of the peritoneum are the mesentary and the greater omentum
18. The process by which digested food is moved from the digestive system to the circulating fluids is called absorption

Match each statement in Column B with its corresponding term in Column A.

Column A	Column B
19. e emulsification	a. This enzyme is made in the pancreas and digests fat.
20. i amylase	b. This enzyme is made in the small intestine and digests protein.
21. j pepsin	c. This gland produces bile.
22. k cholecystokinin	d. This is the final end product of protein digestion.
23. b peptidase	e. Bile has this effect on fat droplets.
24. l cystic	f. This enzyme is made in an inactive form in the pancreas and digests protein.
25. f trypsin	g. This is the final end product of carbohydrate digestion.
26. g simple sugars	h. This is one of the final end products of fat digestion.
27. d amino acids	i. This enzyme is made in both the salivary gland and the pancreas and digests starch.
28. c liver	j. This enzyme is made in the stomach in an inactive form and digests protein.
29. a lipase	k. This hormone stimulates the contraction of the gallbladder.
30. h glycerol	l. This duct connects the gallbladder to the common bile duct.

Nutrition and Metabolism

OUTLINE

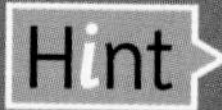

Scan this outline before you begin to read the chapter, as a preview of how the concepts are organized.

OBJECTIVES

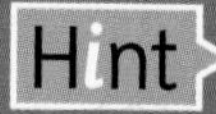

Before reading the chapter, review these goals for your learning.

After you have completed this chapter, you should be able to:

1. Explain metabolism, and define and contrast catabolism and anabolism.
2. Describe the metabolic roles of carbohydrates, fats, proteins, vitamins, and minerals.
3. Define basal metabolic rate and list some factors that affect it.
4. Discuss the physiological mechanisms that regulate body temperature.

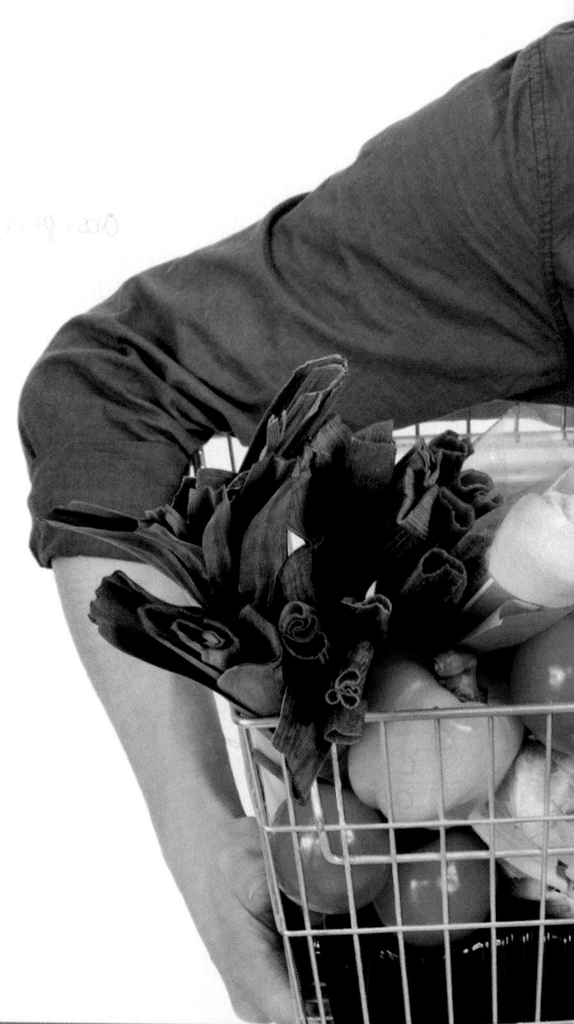

CHAPTER 17

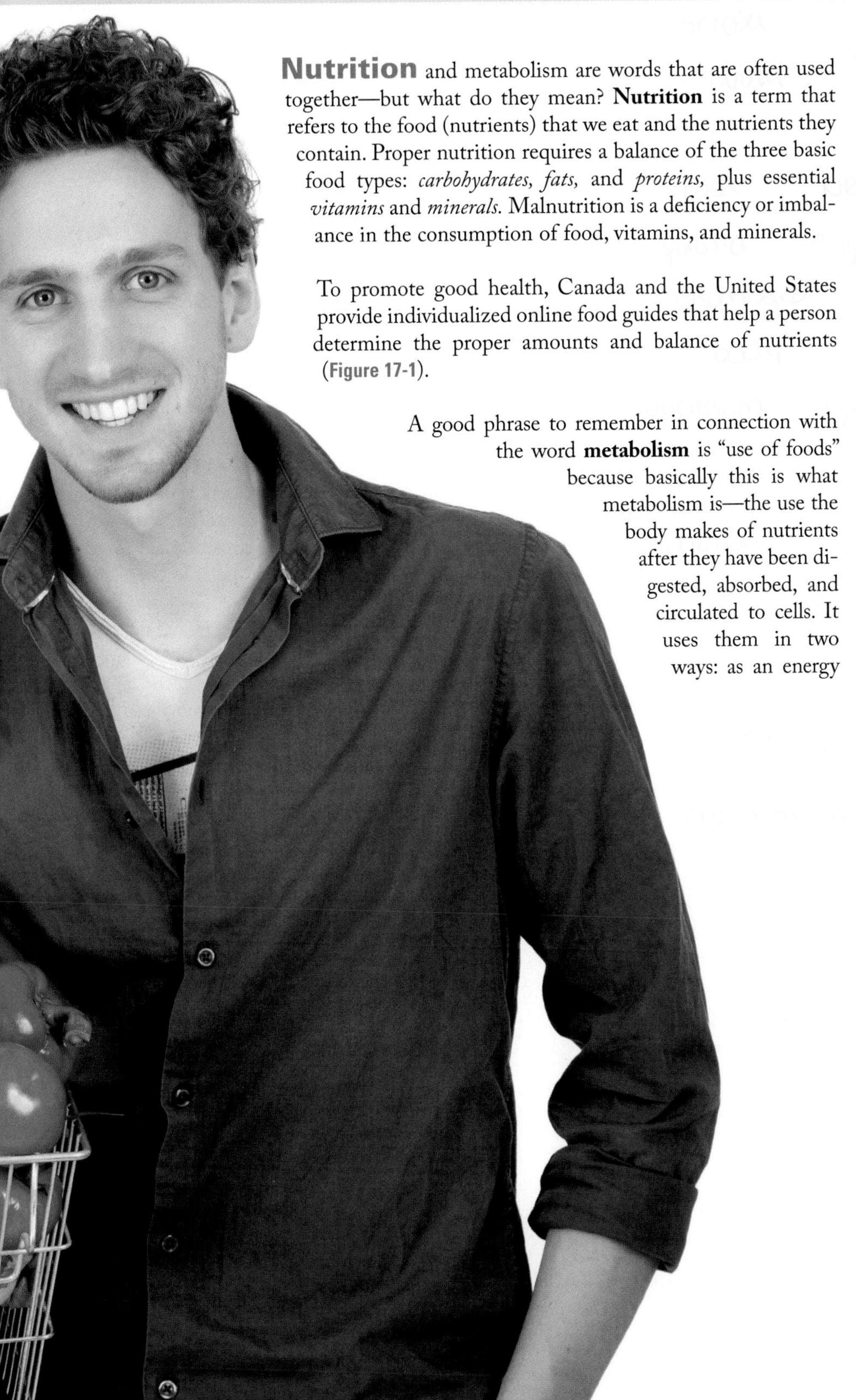

Nutrition and metabolism are words that are often used together—but what do they mean? **Nutrition** is a term that refers to the food (nutrients) that we eat and the nutrients they contain. Proper nutrition requires a balance of the three basic food types: *carbohydrates, fats,* and *proteins,* plus essential *vitamins* and *minerals.* Malnutrition is a deficiency or imbalance in the consumption of food, vitamins, and minerals.

To promote good health, Canada and the United States provide individualized online food guides that help a person determine the proper amounts and balance of nutrients (**Figure 17-1**).

A good phrase to remember in connection with the word **metabolism** is "use of foods" because basically this is what metabolism is—the use the body makes of nutrients after they have been digested, absorbed, and circulated to cells. It uses them in two ways: as an energy

LANGUAGE OF **SCIENCE** AND **MEDICINE**

Hint **Before reading the chapter, say each of these terms out loud. This will help you to avoid stumbling over them as you read.**

aerobic
(ayr-OH-bik)
[*aer-* **air,** *-bi-* **life,** *-ic* **relating to**]

agricultural scientist
(ag-rih-KUL-cher-al SYE-en-tist)
[*agr-* **field,** *-cultur-* **tilling,** *-al* **relating to,** *scien-* **knowledge,** *-ist* **agent**]

amino acid
(ah-MEE-no AS-id)
[*amino* **NH_2,** *acid* **sour**]

anabolism
(ah-NAB-oh-liz-em)
[*ana-* **up,** *-bol-* **throw (build),** *-ism* **action**]

anaerobic
(an-ayr-OH-bik)
[*an-* **without,** *-aer-* **air,** *-bi-* **life,** *-ic* **relating to**]

antioxidant
(an-tee-OK-seh-dent)
[*anti-* **against,** *-oxi-* **sharp (oxygen),** *-ant* **agent**]

appetite center
(AP-ah-tyte SEN-ter)
[*a(d)-* **toward,** *-pet-* **seek out,** *-ite* **relating to**]

assimilation
(ah-sim-ih-LAY-shun)
[*assimila-* **make alike,** *-tion* **process**]

avitaminosis
(ay-vye-tah-mih-NO-sis)
[*a-* **without,** *-vita-* **life,** *-amin-* **ammonia compound,** *-osis* **condition**]

basal metabolic rate (BMR)
(BAY-sal met-ah-BAHL-ik rayt)
[*bas-* **basis,** *-al* **relating to,** *meta-* **over,** *-bol-* **throw,** *-ic* **relating to**]

Continued on p. 404

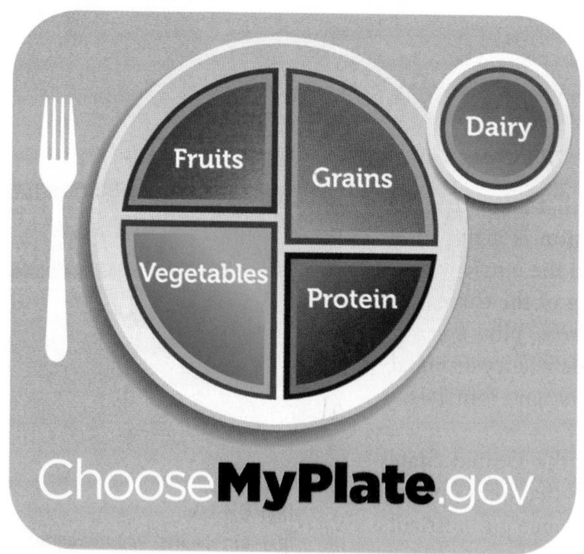

FIGURE 17-1 Food guide. Canada, the United States, and many other countries provide online, individualized food guides that help people determine proper amounts and a healthy balance of nutrients. The website www.ChooseMyPlate.gov is hosted by the United States Department of Agriculture (USDA).

source and as building blocks for making complex chemical compounds.

Before they can be used in these two ways, nutrients have to be *assimilated.* **Assimilation** occurs when nutrient molecules enter cells and undergo many chemical changes there. All the chemical reactions that release energy from nutrient molecules make up the process of **catabolism,** a vital process because it is the only way that the body has of supplying itself with energy for doing any work. Catabolism breaks nutrient molecules down into smaller molecules and releases energy in the process. The many chemical reactions that build nutrient molecules into more complex chemical compounds constitute the process of **anabolism.** Catabolism and anabolism together make up the processes of metabolism.

This chapter explores many of the basic ideas about why certain nutrients are necessary for survival and how they are used by the body.

Metabolic Function of the Liver

As we discussed in Chapter 16, the liver plays an important role in mechanical digestion of lipids because it secretes *bile.* As you recall, bile breaks large fat globules into smaller droplets of fat that are more easily broken down.

In addition, the liver performs other functions necessary for healthy survival. The liver plays a major role in the metabolism of all three main types of nutrients.

For example, the liver helps maintain a normal blood glucose concentration for a few hours after a meal by storing glucose when it is overly abundant, then releasing the glucose into the blood as needed. Many complex chemical reactions, regulated by many different hormones, assist in these storage and release processes.

Liver cells carry on the first steps of protein and fat metabolism. Liver cells also synthesize several kinds of protein compounds. These proteins, when released into the blood, are called the *blood proteins* or **plasma proteins.** Prothrombin and fibrinogen, two of the plasma proteins formed by liver cells, play essential parts in blood clotting (see p. 273). Another protein made by liver cells, albumin, helps maintain normal blood volume.

TABLE 17-1 Major Macronutrients

NUTRIENT	DIETARY SOURCES	FUNCTIONS
Carbohydrate		
Monosaccharide (glucose, galactose, fructose)	Fruit, honey, corn syrup	Used as a source of energy; used to build other carbohydrates
Disaccharide (sucrose, lactose, maltose)	Sugar, fruit, dairy, malted grain products	Source of monosaccharides (for energy)
Polysaccharide (starch, dietary fiber)	Grains, vegetables, nuts, fruits	Source of monosaccharides (for energy); dietary fiber promotes efficient digestive function
Fat (lipid)		
Triglyceride (absorbed as fatty acids, glycerol)	Meat, vegetable oils	Provide energy Structural padding
Cholesterol	Meat, eggs, dairy	Transports lipids; stabilizes cell membranes; is basis of steroid hormones
Protein		
Many types (absorbed as individual amino acids)	Meat, eggs, dairy, vegetables, nuts	Form structures of the body (fibers such as keratin and collagen) Facilitate chemical reactions (enzymes) Send signals and regulate functions (neurotransmitters, nonsteroid hormones) Produce movement (myofilaments) May be used for energy

The liver can detoxify toxic substances such as bacterial products and certain drugs. The liver can also store several useful substances, notably iron and vitamins A and D.

The liver is assisted by an interesting structural feature of the blood vessels that supply it. As you may recall from Chapter 13, the hepatic portal vein delivers blood directly from the gastrointestinal tract to the liver (see **Figure 13-19**). This arrangement allows blood that has just absorbed nutrients and other substances to be processed by the liver before being distributed throughout the body. Thus excess nutrients and vitamins can be stored and toxins can be efficiently removed from the bloodstream before the blood reaches other areas of the body.

QUICK CHECK

1. What are the three basic nutrient types?
2. What is metabolism?
3. What are the functions of the liver?

Macronutrients

Dietary Sources of Nutrients

Put simply, the components of foods that are digested and absorbed by the body are called *nutrients*. The "big three" nutrients in our diets are carbohydrates ("carbs"), fats (lipids), and proteins. Because they form the bulk of our diet, these three nutrients are called **macronutrients**. Vitamins and minerals, by contrast, are called **micronutrients** because they are needed in only very small quantities in our diet.

Table 17-1 summarizes the three macronutrients, their principal sources in our food, and their main functions in our body. The following sections explore some of these functions more deeply.

Carbohydrate Metabolism

Carbohydrates are the preferred energy nutrient of the body. The larger carbohydrate molecules are composed of smaller "building blocks," primarily *glucose* (see Chapter 2). Human cells catabolize (break down) glucose rather than other substances as long as enough glucose enters them to supply their energy needs.

Glucose Catabolism

Three series of chemical reactions, occurring in a precise sequence, make up the process of glucose catabolism. **Glycolysis** is the first series of reactions, **citric acid cycle** (or *Krebs cycle*) is the second series, and **electron transport system (ETS)** is the third.

Glycolysis, the first step of glucose catabolism, occurs in the cytoplasm of each cell of the body. As **Figure 17-2** shows, glycolysis breaks down glucose (a 6-carbon molecule) into two *pyruvic acids* (3-carbon molecules). Glycolysis releases a small amount of energy—enough to generate two ATP molecules—but requires no oxygen to do so. We thus say that it is an **anaerobic** process.

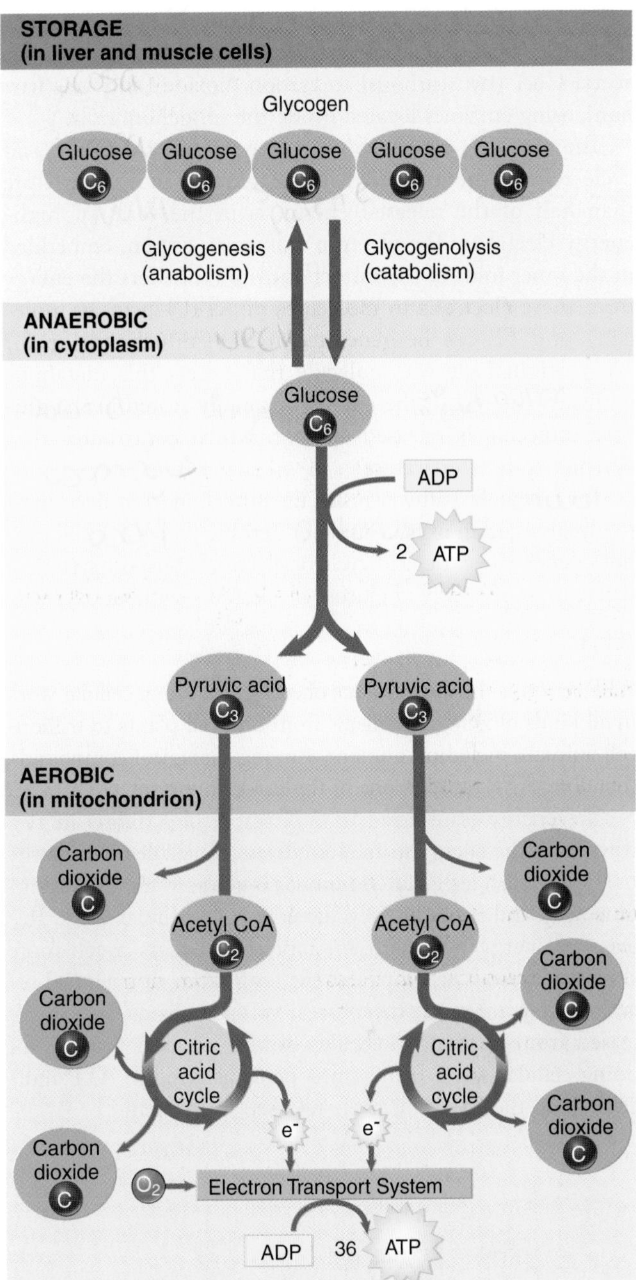

FIGURE 17-2 Metabolism of glucose. Glucose can be stored as subunits of glycogen in liver and muscle cells until needed to make adenosine triphosphate (ATP). After glycogen is split apart, each glucose molecule undergoes glycolysis in the cytoplasm. Glycolysis splits one molecule of glucose (six carbon atoms) into two molecules of pyruvic acid (three carbon atoms each) and produces enough energy to generate two ATPs. Each pyruvic acid is converted to the two-carbon acetyl molecule, which is escorted by coenzyme A (CoA) into the citric acid cycle in the mitochondrion. The citric acid cycle breaks apart each pyruvic acid molecule into three carbon dioxide molecules (one carbon atom each) and many high-energy electrons. The electron transport system (also in the mitochondrion) uses energy from these electrons to generate up to 36 ATPs in the presence of oxygen (O_2).

Each pyruvic acid molecule may then move into a mitochondrion—one of the cell's tiny "battery chargers" that transfers much more of the nutrient energy to ATP. After pyruvic acid is broken down into the 2-carbon acetyl molecule, *coenzyme A (CoA)* escorts it into the citric acid cycle. The citric acid cycle releases high-energy electrons as it breaks down the acetyl CoA (two carbons) to carbon dioxide (only one carbon), using enzymes located inside the mitochondrion.

The chemical reactions of glycolysis and the citric acid cycle release energy stored in the glucose molecule. More than half of the released energy is in the form of high-energy electrons. The electron transport system, embedded in the inner folds of the mitochondrion, transfers the energy from these electrons to molecules of ATP. Up to 36 molecules of ATP can be generated in the mitochondrion for every original glucose molecule that enters this metabolic pathway. The rest of the energy originally stored in the glucose molecule is released as heat, which contributes to a person's body temperature.

The metabolic pathway inside the mitochondrion, in contrast to glycolysis, is an oxygen-using or **aerobic** process. A cell cannot operate the citric acid cycle or electron transport system—where most of energy of glucose is released—without oxygen.

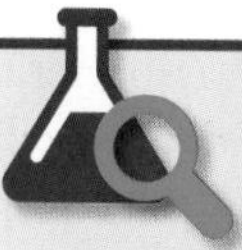

RESEARCH, ISSUES, AND TRENDS

MEASURING ENERGY

Scientists studying metabolism must be able to express a quantity of energy in mathematical terms. The unit of energy measurement most often used is the calorie (cal). A **calorie** is the amount of energy needed to raise the temperature of 1 gram of water 1° C. Because scientists often deal with very large amounts of energy, the larger unit, **kilocalorie** (kcal), or *Calorie* (notice the uppercase C), is used. There are 1000 cal in 1 kcal, or Calorie. Nutritionists prefer to use **Calorie** when they express the amount of energy stored in a nutrient.

Most physiologists in the United States—and most nutritionists outside the United States—prefer to use the metric unit *joule (J)* or *kilojoule (kJ)* instead of calorie-based units. A simple way to convert kilocalories to kilojoules is kcal × 4.2 = kJ.

ATP

ATP serves as the direct source of energy for doing cellular work in all kinds of living organisms from one-cell plants to trillion-cell animals, including humans. Among biological compounds, therefore, ATP ranks as one of the most important.

The energy transferred to ATP molecules differs in two ways from the energy stored in nutrient molecules: the energy in ATP molecules is not stored but is released almost instantaneously, and it can be used directly to do cellular work. Release of energy from nutrient molecules occurs much more slowly because it accompanies the long series of chemical reactions that make up the process of catabolism. Energy released from nutrient molecules cannot be used directly for doing cellular work. It must first be transferred to ATP molecules and then be explosively released from them.

As **Figure 17-3** shows, ATP is made up of an adenosine group and three phosphate groups. The capacity of ATP to release large amounts of energy is found in the high-energy bonds that hold the phosphate groups together, illustrated as curvy lines. When a phosphate group breaks off of the molecule, an adenosine diphosphate (ADP) molecule and free phosphate group result. Energy that had been holding the phosphate bond together is freed to do cellular work (muscle fiber contractions, for example).

As you can see in **Figure 17-3**, the ADP and phosphate are reunited by the energy produced by carbohydrate catabolism, making ATP a reusable energy-storage molecule. Only enough ATP for immediate cellular requirements is made at any one time. New ATP is constantly being made to meet cellular demands. Glucose that is not needed immediately for ATP production is built up (by anabolic processes) into larger molecules that are stored for later use.

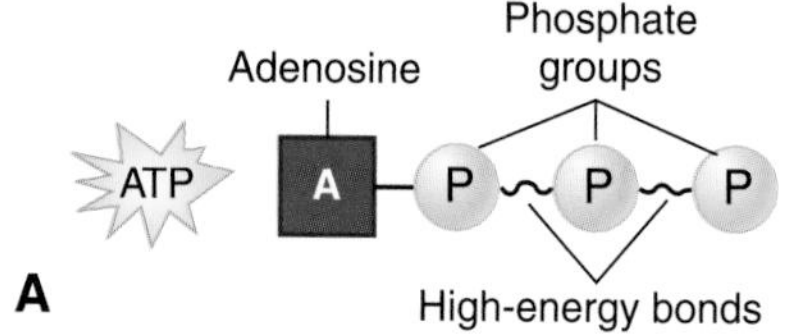

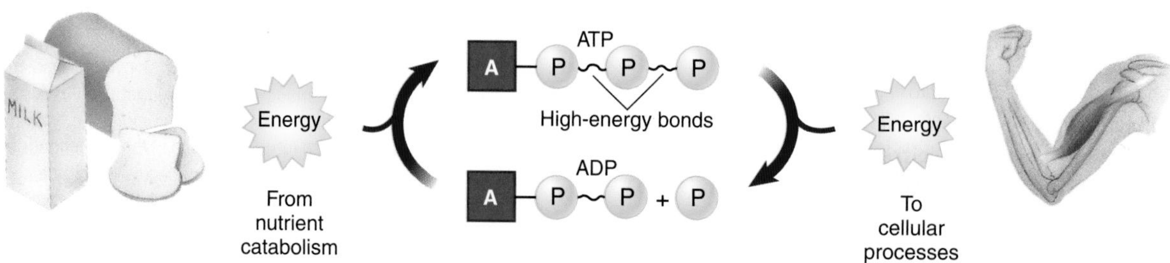

FIGURE 17-3 Adenosine triphosphate (ATP). A, The structure of adenosine triphosphate (ATP). A single adenosine group *(A)* has three attached phosphate groups *(P)*. The high-energy bonds between the phosphate groups can release chemical energy to do cellular work. **B,** ATP energy cycle. ATP stores energy in its last high-energy phosphate bond. When that bond is later broken, energy is released to do cellular work. The adenosine diphosphate (ADP) and phosphate groups that result can be resynthesized into ATP, capturing additional energy from nutrient catabolism.

Glucose Anabolism

Glucose anabolism is called **glycogenesis.** Carried on chiefly by liver and muscle cells, glycogenesis consists of a series of reactions that join glucose molecules together, like many beads in a necklace, to form *glycogen,* a compound sometimes called *animal starch.*

Later, when the glucose stored as glycogen is needed to make ATP, a process called **glycogenolysis** breaks down glycogen chains in the liver or muscle cells to release individual glucose molecules. Glycogenolysis is an example of catabolism.

Regulation of Carbohydrate Metabolism

Something worth noting is that the amount of glucose and other nutrients in the blood normally does not change very much, not even when we go without food for many hours, when we exercise and use a lot of nutrients for energy, or when we sleep and use few nutrients for energy. The amount of glucose in our blood, for example, usually stays at about 80 to 110 milligrams (mg) in 100 milliliters (mL) of blood when we are "fasting" between meals.

Several hormones help regulate carbohydrate metabolism to keep blood glucose at a normal level. **Insulin** is one of the most important of these. Although the exact details of its mechanism of action are still being worked out, insulin is known to accelerate glucose transport through cell membranes. As insulin secretion increases, more glucose leaves the blood and enters the cells. The amount of glucose in the blood therefore decreases as the rate of glucose metabolism in cells increases (see p. 250).

Too little insulin secretion or resistance to insulin effects, such as occurs in people with various forms of *diabetes mellitus (DM),* produces the opposite effects. Less glucose leaves the blood and enters the cells. More glucose therefore remains in the blood, and less glucose is metabolized by cells. In other words, high blood glucose (hyperglycemia) and a low rate of glucose metabolism characterize insulin deficiency.

HEALTH AND WELL-BEING

CARBOHYDRATE LOADING

A number of athletes and others who must occasionally sustain endurance exercise for a significant period practice **carbohydrate loading,** or **glycogen loading.** As with liver cells, some skeletal muscle fibers can take up and store glucose in the form of glycogen. By ceasing intense exercise and switching to a diet high in carbohydrates 2 or 3 days before an endurance event, an athlete can cause the skeletal muscles to store almost twice as much glycogen as usual. This allows the muscles to sustain aerobic exercise for up to 50% longer than usual. The concept of carbohydrate loading has been used to promote the use of "energy bar" sport snacks and some sports or "energy" drinks.

Insulin is the only hormone that significantly lowers the blood glucose level. Several other hormones, on the other hand, can increase it. Growth hormone secreted by the anterior pituitary gland, hydrocortisone secreted by the adrenal cortex, epinephrine secreted by the adrenal medulla, and glucagon secreted by the pancreatic islets are four of the most important hormones that increase blood glucose. More information about these hormones appears in Chapter 11.

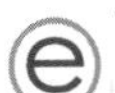

To learn more about the citric acid cycle, go to AnimationDirect at *evolve.elsevier.com.*

Fat Metabolism

Fats, like carbohydrates, are primarily energy nutrients. As cells begin to run low on adequate amounts of glucose to catabolize a few hours after a meal, they immediately shift to the catabolism of fats for energy.

Fats are broken down into fatty acids and glycerol, and then each of these is converted into a chemical form that can enter the citric acid cycle. This happens normally when a person goes without carbohydrates for a few hours. It happens abnormally in individuals with untreated DM. Because of an insulin deficiency, too little glucose enters the cells of a diabetic person to supply all energy needs. The result is that the cells catabolize fats to make up the difference (**Figure 17-4**).

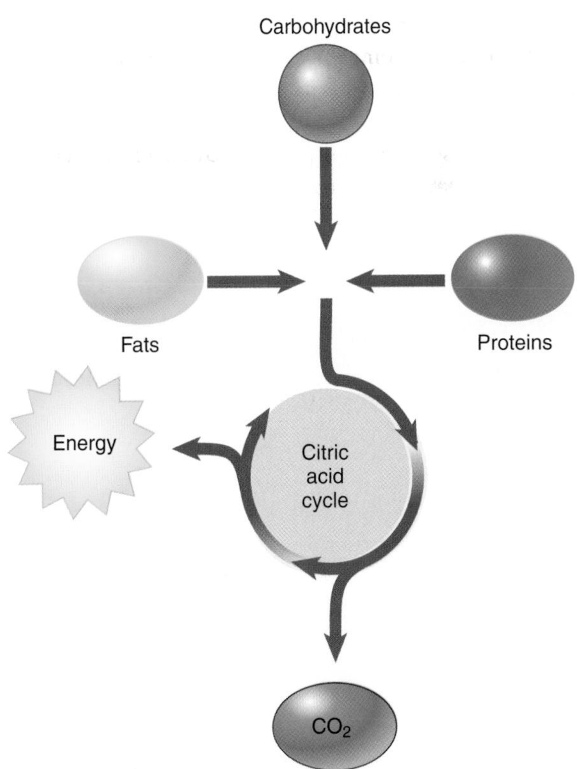

FIGURE 17-4 Catabolism of nutrients. Fats, carbohydrates, and proteins can be converted to products that enter the citric acid cycle to yield energy.

In all persons, fats not needed for catabolism are instead anabolized (built up) to form triglycerides and stored in adipose tissue.

Protein Metabolism

In a healthy person, proteins are catabolized to release energy only to a very small extent. When fat reserves are low, as they are in the starvation that accompanies certain eating disorders such as anorexia nervosa, the body can start to use its protein molecules as an energy source.

Specifically, the amino acids that make up proteins are each broken apart to yield an amine group that is converted to a form of glucose that can enter the citric acid cycle. This process is called **gluconeogenesis** and, as discussed in Chapter 11, it is performed mainly in liver cells.

After a shift to reliance on protein catabolism as a major energy source occurs, death may quickly follow because vital proteins in the muscles and nerves are catabolized (see **Figure 17-4**).

A more common situation in normal bodies is protein anabolism, the process by which the body builds **amino acids** into complex protein compounds (for example, enzymes and proteins that form the structure of the cell). Proteins are assembled from a pool of 20 different kinds of amino acids. If any one type of amino acid is deficient, vital proteins cannot be synthesized—a serious health threat.

One way your body maintains a constant supply of amino acids is by making them from other compounds already present in the body. Only about half of the required 20 types of amino acids can be made by the body, however. The remaining types of amino acids must be supplied in the diet. *Essential amino acids* are those that must be in the diet. *Nonessential amino acids* can be missing from the diet because they can be made by the body (**Table 17-2**).

TABLE 17-2 Amino Acids

ESSENTIAL (INDISPENSABLE)	NONESSENTIAL (DISPENSABLE)
Histidine*	Alanine
Isoleucine	Arginine
Leucine	Asparagine
Lysine	Aspartic acid
Methionine	Cysteine
Phenylalanine	Glutamic acid
Threonine	Glutamine
Tryptophan	Glycine
Valine	Proline
	Serine
	Tyrosine†

*Essential in infants and, perhaps, adult males.
†Can be synthesized from phenylalanine and therefore is nonessential as long as phenylalanine is in the diet.

QUICK CHECK

1. How do aerobic and anaerobic processes differ? How are they alike?
2. How is energy transferred from glucose to ATP?
3. What three processes are responsible for carbohydrate metabolism?
4. How are proteins used once they are absorbed into the body?
5. What are essential amino acids?

Micronutrients

Vitamins

One glance at the label of any packaged food product reveals the importance we place on vitamins and minerals. We know that carbohydrates, fats, and proteins are used by our bodies to build important molecules and to provide energy. So why do we need vitamins and minerals?

First, let us discuss the importance of vitamins. **Vitamins** are organic molecules needed in small quantities for normal metabolism throughout the body. Most vitamin molecules attach to enzymes or *coenzymes* (molecules that assist enzymes) and help them work properly. Many enzymes are totally useless without the appropriate vitamins to activate them. Some vitamins play other important roles in the body. For example, a form of vitamin A plays an important role in detecting light in the sensory cells of the retina. Vitamin D can be converted to a hormone that helps regulate calcium homeostasis in the body. And vitamin E acts as an **antioxidant** that prevents highly reactive oxygen molecules called *free radicals* from damaging DNA and molecules in cell membranes.

Most vitamins cannot be made by the body, so we must eat them in our food. The body can store fat-soluble vitamins—A, D, E, and K—in the liver for later use. Because the body cannot store water-soluble vitamins such as B vitamins and vitamin C, they must be continually supplied in the diet. Vitamin deficiencies can lead to severe metabolic problems. **Table 17-3**

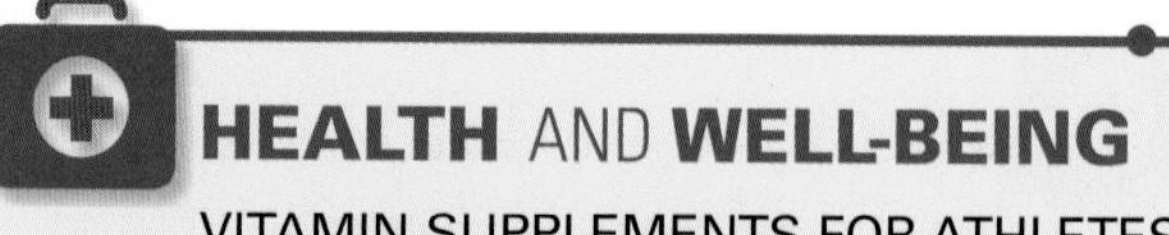

VITAMIN SUPPLEMENTS FOR ATHLETES

Because a deficiency of vitamins (**avitaminosis**) can cause poor athletic performance, many athletes regularly consume vitamin supplements. However, research suggests that vitamin supplementation has little or no effect on athletic performance. A reasonably well-balanced diet supplies more than enough vitamins for even the elite athlete. The use of vitamin supplements therefore has fueled some controversy among exercise experts. Opponents of vitamin supplements cite the cost and the possibility of liver damage associated with some forms of **hypervitaminosis,** whereas supporters cite the benefit of protecting against vitamin deficiency.

TABLE 17-3 Major Vitamins

VITAMIN	DIETARY SOURCE	FUNCTIONS	CONSEQUENCES OF DEFICIENCY
Vitamin A	Green and yellow vegetables, dairy products, and liver	Maintains epithelial tissue and produces visual pigments	Night blindness, dry eye possibly leading to blindness, and flaking skin
B-complex vitamins			
B_1 (thiamine)	Grains, meat, and legumes	Helps enzymes in the citric acid cycle	Nerve problems (beriberi), heart muscle weakness, and edema (B_1 deficiency common in alcoholism)
B_2 (riboflavin)	Green vegetables, organ meats, eggs, and dairy products	Helps enzymes in the citric acid cycle	Inflammation of skin and mucous membranes (including irritation around mouth and eyes)
B_3 (niacin)	Meat and grains	Helps enzymes in the citric acid cycle	Pellagra (scaly dermatitis and mental disturbances), nervous disorders, and diarrhea
B_5 (pantothenic acid)	Organ meat, eggs, and liver	Helps enzymes that connect fat and carbohydrate metabolism	Loss of coordination, decreased peristalsis (rare)
B_6 (pyridoxine)	Vegetables, meats, and grains	Helps enzymes that catabolize amino acids	Convulsions, irritability, and anemia
B_9 (folic acid)	Vegetables	Helps enzymes in amino acid catabolism and blood production	Digestive disorders, anemia, prenatal neural tube defects (NTDs)
B_{12} (cyanocobalamin)	Meat and dairy products	Involved in blood production and other processes	Pernicious anemia
Biotin (vitamin H)	Vegetables, meat, and eggs	Helps enzymes in amino acid catabolism and fat and glycogen synthesis	Mental and muscle problems (rare)
Vitamin C (ascorbic acid)	Fruits and green vegetables	Helps in manufacture of collagen fibers	Scurvy and degeneration of skin, bone, and blood vessels
Vitamin D (calciferol)	Dairy products and fish liver oil	Helps in calcium absorption	Rickets and skeletal deformity
Vitamin E (tocopherol)	Green vegetables and seeds	Protects cell membranes from being catabolized	Muscle and reproductive disorders (rare)
Vitamins K_1, K_2	Intestinal bacteria (synthetic form is K_3)	Helps in blood clotting, bone metabolism	Blood clotting disorders, bone loss

lists some of the better known vitamins, their sources, functions, and consequences of deficiency.

Minerals

Minerals are just as important as vitamins. Minerals are inorganic elements or salts found naturally in the earth. As with vitamins, mineral ions can attach to enzymes and help them work. Minerals also function in a variety of other vital chemical reactions. For example, sodium, calcium, and other minerals are required for nerve conduction and for contraction in muscle fibers. Without these minerals, the brain, heart, and respiratory tract would cease to function. Information about some of the more important minerals is summarized in **Table 17-4**.

Regulating Food Intake

Mechanisms for regulating food intake are still not clearly understood. That the *hypothalamus* in the diencephalon of the brain plays a part in these mechanisms, however, seems certain. There appears to be both an **appetite center** that promotes the feeling of hunger and a **satiety center** that promotes the feeling that we are satisfied or "full" in the hypothalamus. The balance of activity between these two centers appears to be the central mechanism that regulates food intake.

There are many factors that influence these hypothalamic centers and therefore influence the regulation of food intake. Among the many factors identified in affecting appetite are hormones, neurotransmitters, emotions, environmental cues, food sensations, habits, and more. Some examples of factors that affect the appetite-regulating centers of the hypothalamus are listed in **Table 17-5**. It is not important to memorize all these factors, but reading through them will help you understand the complexity of our body's regulation of food intake.

Metabolic Rates

The **basal metabolic rate (BMR)** is the rate at which nutrients are catabolized under basal conditions (that is, when the individual is resting but awake, is not digesting food, and is

TABLE 17-4 Major Minerals

MINERAL	DIETARY SOURCE	FUNCTIONS	SYMPTOMS OF DEFICIENCY
Calcium (Ca)	Dairy products, legumes, and vegetables	Helps blood clotting, bone formation, and nerve and muscle function	Bone degeneration and nerve and muscle malfunction
Chlorine (Cl)	Salty foods	Helps in stomach acid production and acid-base balance	Acid-base imbalance
Cobalt (Co)	Meat	Helps vitamin B_{12} in blood cell production	Pernicious anemia
Copper (Cu)	Seafood, organ meats, and legumes	Involved in extracting energy from the citric acid cycle and in blood production	Fatigue and anemia
Iodine (I)	Seafood and iodized salt	Needed for thyroid hormone synthesis	Goiter (thyroid enlargement) and decrease of metabolic rate
Iron (Fe)	Meat, eggs, vegetables, and legumes	Involved in extracting energy from the citric acid cycle and needed for red blood cell production	Fatigue and anemia
Magnesium (Mg)	Vegetables and grains	Helps many enzymes	Nerve disorders, blood vessel dilation, and heart rhythm problems
Manganese (Mn)	Vegetables, legumes, and grains	Helps many enzymes	Muscle and nerve disorders
Phosphorus (P)	Dairy products and meat	Helps in bone formation and is used to make ATP, DNA, RNA, and phospholipids	Bone degeneration and metabolic problems
Potassium (K)	Seafood, milk, fruit, and meats	Helps muscle and nerve function	Muscle weakness, heart problems, and nerve problems
Sodium (Na)	Salty foods	Helps in muscle and nerve function and fluid balance	Weakness and digestive upset
Zinc (Zn)	Many foods	Helps many enzymes	Metabolic problems, diarrhea

not adjusting to a cold external temperature). Or, stated differently, the BMR is the number of calories of heat that must be produced per hour by catabolism just to keep the body alive, awake, and comfortably warm. To provide energy for muscular work and digestion and absorption of food, an additional amount of nutrient must be catabolized. The amount of additional nutrient depends mainly on how much work the individual does. The more active he or she is, the more

TABLE 17-5 Factors That Influence Appetite*

FACTORS THAT STIMULATE APPETITE	FACTORS THAT INHIBIT APPETITE	SOURCE
Endogenous opioid peptides (EOP) Gamma-aminobutyric acid (GABA) Neuropeptide Y (NPY) Norepinephrine (NE) Orexins	Alpha-melanocyte–stimulating hormone (α-MSH) Cocaine- and amphetamine-regulated transcript (CART) Corticotropin-releasing hormone (CRH)	Hypothalamus
Emotions Environmental stimuli Food sensations (e.g., taste, smell, texture) Internal stimuli (e.g., blood temperature, glucose) Lifestyle choices and habits	Emotions Environmental stimuli Food sensations (e.g., taste, smell) Internal stimuli (e.g., blood temperature, glucose) Lifestyle choices and habits	Nervous system (outside hypothalamus)
Cortisol		Adrenal cortex
Ghrelin (GHRL)	Cholecystokinin (CCK) Glucagon-like peptide-1 (GLP-1)	GI tract
	Leptin Interleukin 18 (IL-18)	Adipose tissue
	Glucose	Liver
	Insulin Pancreatic polypeptide (PP)	Pancreas

*Factors that affect appetite-regulating centers in the hypothalamus.

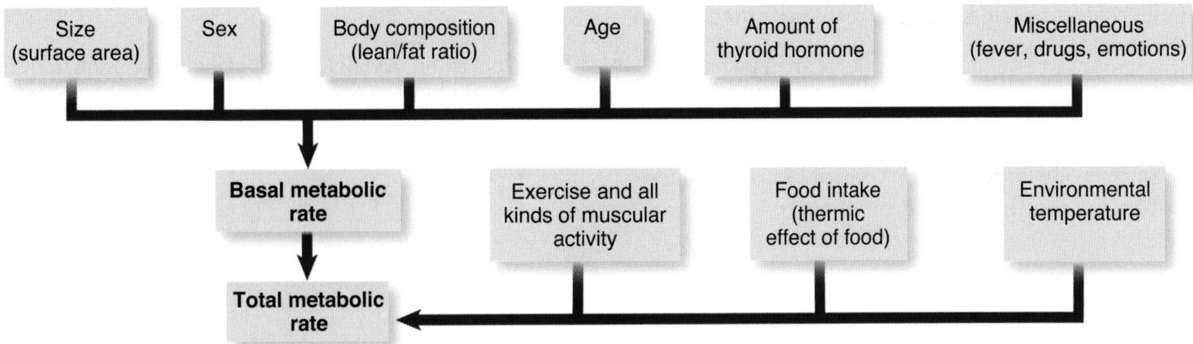

FIGURE 17-5 Factors that determine the basal and total metabolic rates.

nutrient the body must catabolize and the higher the total metabolic rate will be. The **total metabolic rate (TMR)** is the total amount of energy used by the body per day (**Figure 17-5**).

When the number of calories in your food intake equals your TMR, your weight remains constant (except for possible variations resulting from water retention or water loss). When your food intake provides more calories than your TMR, you gain weight; when your food intake provides fewer calories than your TMR, you lose weight. These weight control principles rarely fail to operate. Nature does not forget to count calories. Reducing diets make use of this knowledge. They contain fewer calories than the TMR of the individual eating the diet. See Appendix A for information on the *body mass index (BMI)* and its relationship to body weight.

Body Temperature

Considering the fact that more than 60% of the energy released from nutrient molecules during catabolism is converted to heat rather than being transferred to ATP, it is no wonder that maintaining a constant body temperature is a challenge. Maintaining homeostasis of body temperature, or **thermoregulation,** is the function of the hypothalamus. The hypothalamus operates a variety of negative-feedback mechanisms that keep body temperature in its normal range (36.2° to 37.6° C or 97° to 100° F).

The skin is often involved in negative-feedback loops that maintain body temperature. When the body is overheated, blood flow to the skin increases. Warm blood from the body's core can then be cooled by the skin, which acts as a radiator. At the skin, heat can be lost from blood by the following mechanisms, which are also illustrated in **Figure 17-6**:

1. **Radiation**—flow of heat waves from the blood and skin
2. **Conduction**—transfer of heat energy to the skin and then to cooler external environment
3. **Convection**—transfer of heat energy to cooler air that is continually flowing away from the skin
4. **Evaporation**—absorption of heat from blood and skin by water (sweat) vaporization

When necessary, heat can be conserved by reducing blood flow in the skin, as illustrated in Chapter 6 (see the box on p. 111). Heat can also be conserved by reducing any of the four mechanisms described. For example, warm clothing can totally or partially block any of these mechanisms.

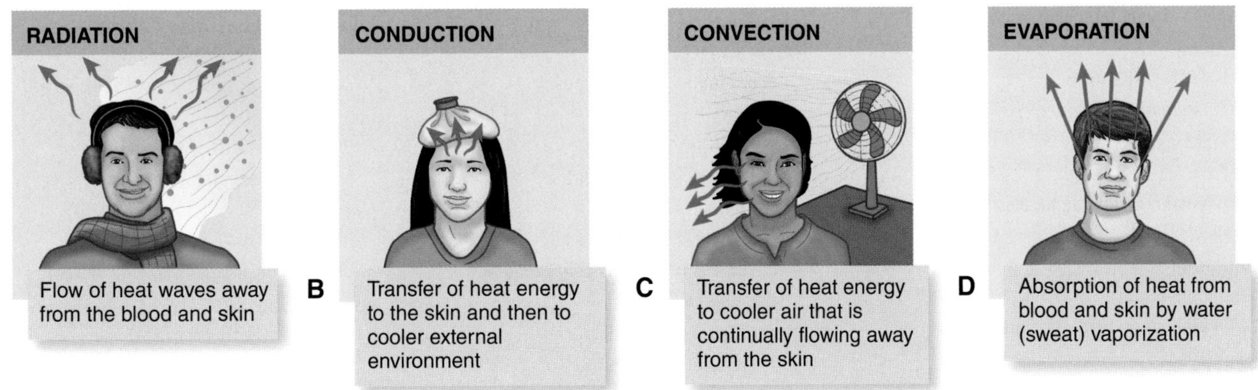

FIGURE 17-6 Mechanisms of heat loss. Heat can be lost from the blood and skin by means of radiation, conduction, convection, and evaporation. Heat can be conserved by altering blood flow in the skin or wearing warm clothing to block the mechanisms shown here.

A number of other mechanisms can be called on to help maintain the homeostasis of body temperature. Heat-generating muscle activities such as shivering and secretion of metabolism-regulating hormones are two of the body's processes that can be altered to adjust the body's temperature. The concept of using feedback control loops in homeostatic mechanisms was introduced in Chapter 1.

QUICK CHECK

1. What is the overall function of vitamins in the body?
2. What is the name for the rate at which nutrients are catabolized under resting conditions?
3. How do calories consumed relate to a person's body weight?
4. What are the four main ways that heat leaves the body?

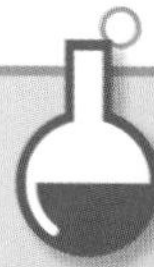

SCIENCE APPLICATIONS

FOOD SCIENCE

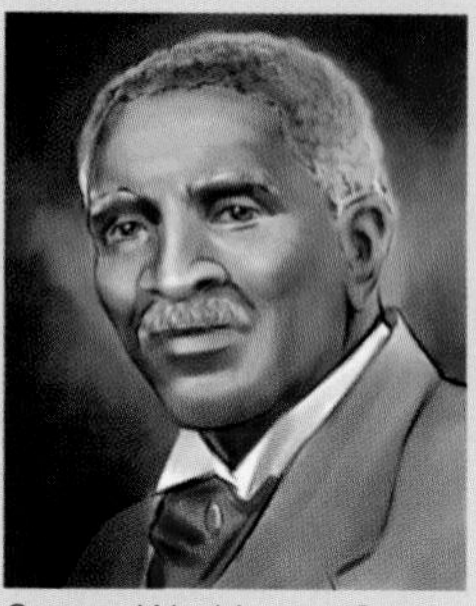

George Washington Carver (1864–1943)

At the dawn of the twentieth century, one figure loomed large in the world of **food science**—George Washington Carver. Born a slave on a Missouri plantation during the Civil War, Carver overcame great obstacles to become one of the most admired American scientists in history. Although talented in music and art, it was his knack for agriculture that led him to a long and successful career as a professor, researcher, and inventor in the agriculture department of Alabama's Tuskegee Institute.

At Tuskegee, his work resulted in the creation of 325 products made from peanuts, nearly 200 products from yams (sweet potatoes), and hundreds more from other plants native to the southern United States. Development of these new products helped poor farmers survive by allowing them to make money from a variety of crops that thrived on their land.

Today, breakthroughs continue to be made in the world of *agriculture* and food science. *Farmers* and *ranchers* work closely with **agricultural scientists** and *technicians* to improve food crops and to improve methods of raising livestock. As did Carver, they strive to work in ways that benefit the land and people. Of course, *nutritionists, dietitians, chefs,* and *food preparers* all play a role in getting these crops to our table in a healthy and appetizing way. *Food scientists* and other *industrial scientists* work to develop technologies and methods for preparing, preserving, storing, and packaging foods.

LANGUAGE OF **SCIENCE** AND **MEDICINE** *(continued from p. 395)*

calorie
(KAL-or-ee)
[*calor-* **heat,** *-ie* **full of**]

carbohydrate loading (glycogen loading)
(kar-boh-HYE-drayt LOHD-ing [GLY-koh-jen])
[*carbo-* **carbon,** *-hydr-* **hydrogen,** *-ate* **oxygen** (*glyco-* **sweet (glucose),** *-gen* **produce**)]

catabolism
(kah-TAB-oh-liz-em)
[*cata-* **against,** *-bol-* **throw,** *-ism* **condition**]

citric acid cycle
(SIT-rik AS-id SYE-kul)
[*citr-* **lemon,** *-ic* **relating to,** *acid* **sour,** *cycle* **circle**]

conduction
(kon-DUK-shun)
[*con-* **with,** *duct-* **lead,** *-tion* **process**]

convection
(kon-VEK-shun)
[*con-* **together,** *-vect-* **carry,** *-tion* **process**]

electron transport system (ETS)
(eh-LEK-tron TRANZ-port SIS-tem)
[*electr-* **electricity,** *-on* **subatomic particle,** *trans-* **across,** *-port* **carry**]

evaporation
(ee-vap-oh-RAY-shun)
[*e-* **out from,** *-vapor* **steam,** *-ation* **process**]

food science
(food SYE-ens)
[*scienc-* **knowledge**]

gluconeogenesis
(gloo-koh-nee-oh-JEN-eh-sis)
[*gluco-* **sweet (glucose),** *-neo-* **new,** *-gen-* **produce,** *-esis* **process**]

glycogen loading
(GLYE-koh-jen LOHD-ing)
[*glyco-* **sweet,** *-gen* **produce**]

glycogenesis
(glye-koh-JEN-eh-sis)
[*glyco-* **sweet (glucose),** *-gen-* **produce,** *-esis* **process**]

glycogenolysis
(glye-koh-jeh-NOL-ih-sis)
[*glyco-* **sweet (glucose),** *-gen-* **produce,** *-o-* **combining form,** *-lysis* **loosening**]

glycolysis
(glye- KAHL-ih-sis)
[*glyco-* **sweet (glucose),** *-o-* **combining form,** *-lysis* **loosening**]

hypervitaminosis
(hye-per-vye-tah-mih-NO-sis)
[*hyper-* **excessive,** *-vita-* **life,** *-amin-* **ammonia compound,** *-osis* **condition**]

insulin
(IN-suh-lin)
[*insul-* **island,** *-in* **substance**]

kilocalorie (kcal, *also* Calorie)
(KIL-oh-kal-oh-ree)
[*kilo-* **one thousand,** *-calor-* **heat,** *-ie* **full of**]

macronutrient
(MAK-roh-NOO-tree-ent)
[*macro-* **large,** *-nutri-* **nourish,** *-ent* **agent**]

metabolism
(meh-TAB-oh-liz-em)
[*meta-* **over,** *-bol-* **throw,** *-ism* **action**]

micronutrient
(MY-kroh-NOO-tree-ent)
[*micro-* **small,** *-nutri-* **nourish,** *-ent* **agent**]

nutrition
(noo-TRIH-shun)
[*nutri-* **nourish,** *-tion* **process**]

plasma protein
(PLAZ-mah PRO-teen)
[*plasma* **substance,** *prote-* **primary,** *-in* **substance]**

radiation
(ray-dee-AY-shun)
[*radiat-* **send out rays,** *-ion* **process]**

satiety center
(sah-TYE-eh-tee SEN-ter)
[*sati-* **enough or full,** *-ety* **state]**

thermoregulation
(ther-moh-reg-yoo-LAY-shun)
[*therm-* **heat,** *-o-* **combining form,** *-regula-* **rule,** *-ation* **process]**

total metabolic rate (TMR)
(TOH-tal met-ah-BOL-ik rayt)
[*meta-* **over,** *-bol-* **throw,** *-ic* **relating to]**

vitamin
(VYE-tah-min)
[*vita-* **life,** *-amin* **ammonia compound]**

❑ OUTLINE SUMMARY

To download a digital audio version of the chapter summary for use with your device, access the ***Audio Chapter Summaries*** *online at evolve.elsevier.com.*

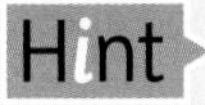

Scan this summary after reading the chapter to help you reinforce the key concepts. Later, use the summary as a quick review before your class or before a test.

Definitions

A. Nutrition — food, vitamins, and minerals that are ingested and assimilated into the body (see **Figure 17-1**)
B. Assimilation — process of getting nutrient molecules into the cells of the body and chemically preparing them for use in the chemical reactions of the body
C. Metabolism — process of using nutrient molecules as energy sources and as building blocks for our own molecules
D. Catabolism — breaks nutrient molecules down, releasing their stored energy; oxygen used in catabolism
E. Anabolism — builds nutrient molecules into complex substances

Metabolic Function of the Liver

A. Secretes bile, which breaks down large fat globules
B. Helps maintain normal blood glucose level
C. Helps metabolize carbohydrates, fats, and proteins; synthesizes several kinds of protein compounds
D. Removes toxins from the blood
E. Stores useful substances

Macronutrients

A. Dietary sources of nutrients
   1. Nutrients — food components digested and absorbed by the body
   2. Macronutrients — nutrients needed in large daily quantities (carbohydrates, fats, proteins) (see **Table 17-1**)
   3. Micronutrients — nutrients needed in tiny daily quantities (vitamins and minerals)

B. Carbohydrates — preferred energy nutrient of the body
   1. Three series of chemical reactions in glucose metabolism
      a. Glycolysis
         (1) Changes glucose to pyruvic acid
         (2) Anaerobic (uses no oxygen)
         (3) Yields small amount of energy, generating two ATPs
         (4) Occurs in cytoplasm
      b. Citric acid cycle (Krebs cycle)
         (1) Changes pyruvic acid to carbon dioxide
         (2) Aerobic (requires oxygen)
         (3) Yields large amount of energy (mostly as high-energy electrons)
         (4) Occurs in mitochondria
      c. Electron transport system (ETS)
         (1) Transfers energy from high-energy electrons (from citric acid cycle) to ATP molecules
         (2) Located in mitochondria
   2. The mitochondrial part of the pathway (citric acid cycle and electron transport system) is aerobic (requires oxygen) and generates up to 36 ATP molecules per original glucose molecule
   3. Carbohydrates are primarily catabolized for energy (see **Figure 17-2**)
   4. Adenosine triphosphate (ATP) — molecule in which energy obtained from breakdown of nutrients is stored; serves as a direct source of energy for cellular work (see **Figure 17-3**)
   5. Anabolism and storage of glucose
      a. Glucose that is not needed immediately for making ATP is stored as glycogen (a long chain of glucose subunits) in liver and muscle cells
      b. Glycogenesis — anabolic process of joining glucose molecules together in a chain to form glycogen (to store glucose for later use)
      c. Glycogenolysis — catabolic process of breaking apart glycogen chains, releasing individual glucose molecules for use in making ATP
   6. Blood glucose (imprecisely, *blood sugar*) — normally stays between about 80 and 110 mg per 100 mL of blood during fasting; insulin accelerates the movement of glucose out of the blood into cells, therefore decreasing blood glucose and increasing glucose catabolism

C. Fats — catabolized to yield energy and anabolized to form adipose tissue (see **Figure 17-4**)

D. Proteins — primarily anabolized and secondarily catabolized
   1. Use of amines from protein in the glucose pathway for energy is called gluconeogenesis
   2. *Essential amino acids* are those that must be in the diet because the body cannot make them (see **Table 17-2**)

Micronutrients

A. Vitamins — organic molecules that are needed in small amounts for normal metabolism (see **Table 17-3**)
B. Minerals — inorganic molecules found naturally in the earth, required by the body for normal function (see **Table 17-4**)

Regulating Food Intake

A. Regulatory centers in the hypothalamus play a primary role in controlling food intake
   1. Appetite center — produces feelings of hunger
   2. Satiety center — produces feelings of satisfaction
B. Food intake regulation results from balance between hypothalamic control centers
C. Many diverse factors influence the hypothalamic control centers (see **Table 17-5**)

Metabolic Rates

A. Basal metabolic rate (BMR) — rate of metabolism when a person is lying down but awake and not digesting food and when the environment is comfortably warm
B. Total metabolic rate (TMR) — the total amount of energy, expressed in calories, used by the body per day (see **Figure 17-5**)

Body Temperature

A. Hypothalamus — regulates the homeostasis of body temperature (thermoregulation) through a variety of processes
B. Skin — can cool the body by losing heat from the blood through four processes: radiation, conduction, convection, evaporation
C. Mechanisms of heat loss (see **Figure 17-6**)
   1. Radiation — flow of heat waves from the blood and skin
   2. Conduction — transfer of heat energy to the skin and then to cooler external environment
   3. Convection — transfer of heat energy to cooler air that is continually flowing away from the skin
   4. Evaporation — absorption of heat from blood and skin by water (sweat) vaporization
D. Other mechanisms can generate heat to maintain homeostasis when necessary

❑ ACTIVE LEARNING

STUDY TIPS

Hint *Use these tips to achieve success in meeting your learning goals.*

To make the study of nutrition and metabolism more efficient, we suggest these tips:

1. This chapter begins with an explanation of the functions of the liver and the importance of the hepatic portal system, both of which were discussed previously in Chapters 13 and 16, so review that material before beginning this chapter.
2. The process of metabolism refers to the body's use of macronutrients. Fats and carbohydrates are used primarily for energy. Proteins can be used for energy, but are mainly used to make other proteins.
3. Carbohydrate metabolism begins with glycolysis. *Glyco-* refers to carbohydrates and *-lysis* means "a breaking"—and the process does exactly that by "breaking" glucose. The end products of glycolysis enter the citric acid cycle, which produces many high-energy molecules. The electron transfer system transfers energy from these molecules to adenosine triphosphate (ATP) for use by cellular processes.
4. ATP is the only energy source your body cells can use directly. The energy is temporarily stored in the bonds between the phosphates in the molecule, and these phosphates break off to release energy to cellular processes.
5. Fat and protein components can be modified so they can also enter the citric acid cycle.
6. The term *nonessential amino acids* is somewhat misleading; it does not mean your body doesn't need them—it means that they can be made from other amino acids your body has available.
7. Vitamins and minerals assist in enzyme function. You can learn the names and functions of the vitamins and minerals from flash cards. In your study group, go over the flash cards for vitamins and minerals.
8. Metabolic rates describe how quickly the nutrients are used. Basal metabolic rate (BMR) is the amount of nutrients you use just to stay alive and awake. The total metabolic rate (TMR) depends on how active you are. Check out this website that allows you to calculate your BMR *bmi-calculator.net/bmr-calculator/*
9. Discuss the ways heat can be lost from the body.
10. Try to understand the "big picture" of metabolism summarized in the study tips before trying to understand the details.
11. Go over the questions in the back of the chapter and discuss possible test questions.

Review Questions

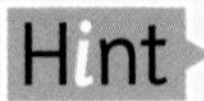

Write out the answers to these questions after reading the chapter and reviewing the Chapter Summary. If you simply think through the answer without writing it down, you won't retain much of your new learning.

1. Define *anabolism* and *catabolism.*
2. Explain the function of the liver.
3. List the macronutrients and micronutrients of the body.
4. Briefly explain the process of glycolysis.
5. Briefly explain the citric acid cycle.
6. Name the function of the electron transfer system.
7. Explain the ways in which energy stored in ATP is different than the energy stored in food molecules.
8. List the hormones that tend to increase the amount of sugar in the blood.
9. Describe when fat catabolism usually occurs.
10. Describe when protein catabolism usually occurs.
11. Describe the function of amino acids.
12. Explain what is meant by a nonessential amino acid.
13. Name three water-soluble and three fat-soluble vitamins.
14. Name three minerals needed by the body.
15. List the functions of vitamins and minerals in the body.
16. Differentiate between basal and total metabolic rate.
17. Name and explain three ways heat can be lost by the skin.

Critical Thinking

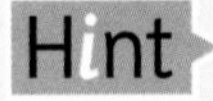

After finishing the Review Questions, write out the answers to these more in-depth questions to help you apply your new knowledge. Go back to sections of the chapter that relate to concepts that you find difficult.

18. Differentiate between absorption and assimilation.
19. Explain the advantage the body gains by having the blood go to the liver through the hepatic portal system.
20. Diagram the ATP-ADP cycle. Include where the energy is added and where it is released.
21. A man went on a 10-day vacation. His total metabolic rate was 2600 calories a day. His calorie intake was 3300 calories a day. He began his trip weighing 178 pounds. What did he weigh by the end of his vacation? (3500 excess calories = 1 pound)

Chapter Test

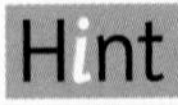

After studying the chapter, test your mastery by responding to these items. Try to answer them without looking up the answers. Then, verify the answers using the key in Appendix C at the back of this book.

1. The process of ________ occurs when nutrient molecules enter the cells and undergo chemical changes.
2. ________ is the term used to describe all the chemical processes that release energy from nutrients.
3. ________ is the term used to describe all the chemical processes that build nutrient molecules into larger compounds.
4. The plasma proteins ________ are made by the liver and are important in blood clot formation.
5. The vitamins ________ can be stored in the liver.
6. The B vitamins are ________ soluble, whereas vitamins K and E are ________ soluble.
7. ________ is the total amount of energy used by the body per day.
8. ________ is the number of calories that must be used just to keep the body alive, awake, and comfortably warm.
9. To lose weight, your total caloric intake must be less than your ________.
10. One way heat can be lost by the skin is ________, which is the transfer of heat to the air that is continually flowing away from the skin.
11. One way heat can be lost by the skin is ________, which is the absorption of heat by water (sweat) vaporization.
12. ________ is the process used by the body as its second choice of energy metabolism. People with diabetes frequently must use this process.
13. In a healthy body, ________ is used almost exclusively for anabolism rather than catabolism.
14. ________ are amino acids needed by the body, but they can be made from other amino acids if they are not supplied by the diet.
15. ________ is the only energy source your body cells can use directly.
16. The "big three" nutrients in our diets are ________.

Match each phrase in Column B with the correct corresponding term in Column A.

Column A	Column B
17. ________ glycolysis	a. part of the cell in which glycolysis occurs
18. ________ citric acid cycle	b. step in carbohydrate metabolism that does not require oxygen
19. ________ electron transport system	c. process that converts high-energy molecules from citric acid to ATP
20. ________ mitochondria	d. step in carbohydrate metabolism that requires oxygen
21. ________ cytoplasm	e. direct source of energy for the body
22. ________ ATP	f. molecule produced when adenosine triphosphate loses a phosphate group
23. ________ glycogenesis	g. the part of the cell in which the citric acid cycle takes place
24. ________ ADP	h. glucose anabolism
25. ________ protein	i. macronutrient

Urinary System

OUTLINE

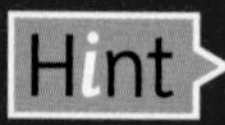

Scan this outline before you begin to read the chapter, as a preview of how the concepts are organized.

OBJECTIVES

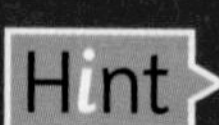

Before reading the chapter, review these goals for your learning.

After you have completed this chapter, you should be able to:

1. Identify the major organs of the urinary system and give the generalized function of each.
2. Name the parts of a nephron and describe the role each component plays in the formation of urine.
3. Explain how the kidneys act as vital organs in maintaining homeostasis.
4. Explain the importance of filtration, reabsorption, and secretion in urine formation.
5. Discuss the mechanisms that control urine volume, including the normal amount and composition of urine.
6. Explain the process of urine elimination.

CHAPTER 18

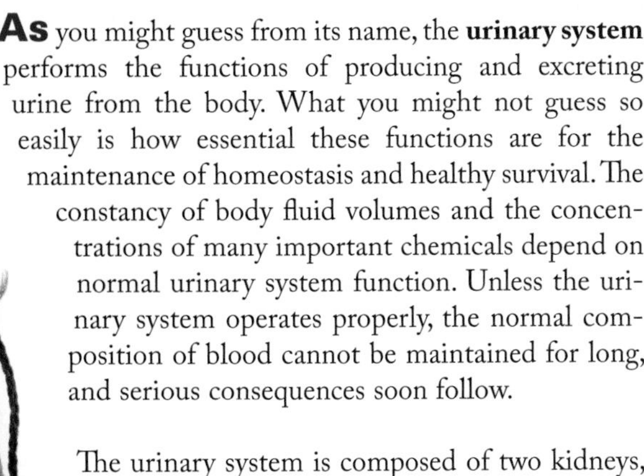

As you might guess from its name, the **urinary system** performs the functions of producing and excreting urine from the body. What you might not guess so easily is how essential these functions are for the maintenance of homeostasis and healthy survival. The constancy of body fluid volumes and the concentrations of many important chemicals depend on normal urinary system function. Unless the urinary system operates properly, the normal composition of blood cannot be maintained for long, and serious consequences soon follow.

The urinary system is composed of two kidneys, two ureters, one bladder, and one urethra (**Figure 18-1**). We begin our discussion with the kidneys. The kidneys "clear" or clean the blood of the many waste products continually produced as a result of metabolism of nutrients in the body cells. As amino acids from protein nutrients are catabolized for energy, the waste products produced must be removed from the blood, or they quickly accumulate to toxic levels—a condition called **uremia** or **uremic poisoning.**

The kidneys also play a vital role in maintaining electrolyte, water, and acid-base balances in the body. In this chapter, we discuss the structure and function of each organ of the urinary system—including the central "blood balancing" role of the kidneys. In the following chapters, we continue the story by exploring fluid and electrolyte balance in Chapter 19 and acid-base balance in Chapter 20.

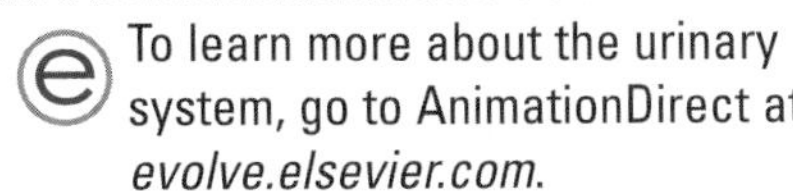

To learn more about the urinary system, go to AnimationDirect at *evolve.elsevier.com.*

LANGUAGE OF **SCIENCE** AND **MEDICINE**

Hint Before reading the chapter, say each of these terms out loud. This will help you to avoid stumbling over them as you read.

aldosterone
(AL-doh-steh-rohn *or* al-DAH-stayr-ohn)
[*aldo-* **aldehyde,** *-stero-* **solid or steroid derivative,** *-one* **chemical**]

antidiuretic hormone (ADH)
(an-tee-dye-yoo-RET-ik HOR-mohn)
[*anti-* **against,** *-dia-* **through,** *-uret-* **urination,** *-ic* **relating to,** *hormon-* **excite**]

anuria
(ah-NOO-ree-ah)
[*a-* **not,** *-ur-* **urine,** *-ia* **condition**]

atrial natriuretic hormone (ANH)
(AY-tree-al nay-tree-yoo-RET-ik HOR-mohn)
[*atria-* **entrance courtyard (atrium of heart),** *-al* **relating to,** *natri-* **natrium (sodium),** *-uret-* **urination,** *-ic* **relating to,** *hormon-* **excite**]

Bowman capsule
(BOH-men KAP-sul)
[*William Bowman* **English anatomist,** *caps-* **box,** *-ule* **little**]

calyx
(KAY-liks)
pl., calyces
(KAY-lih-seez)
[*calyx* **seed pod or cup**]

collecting duct (CD)
(koh-LEK-ting dukt)
[*duct* **a leading**]

Continued on p. 423

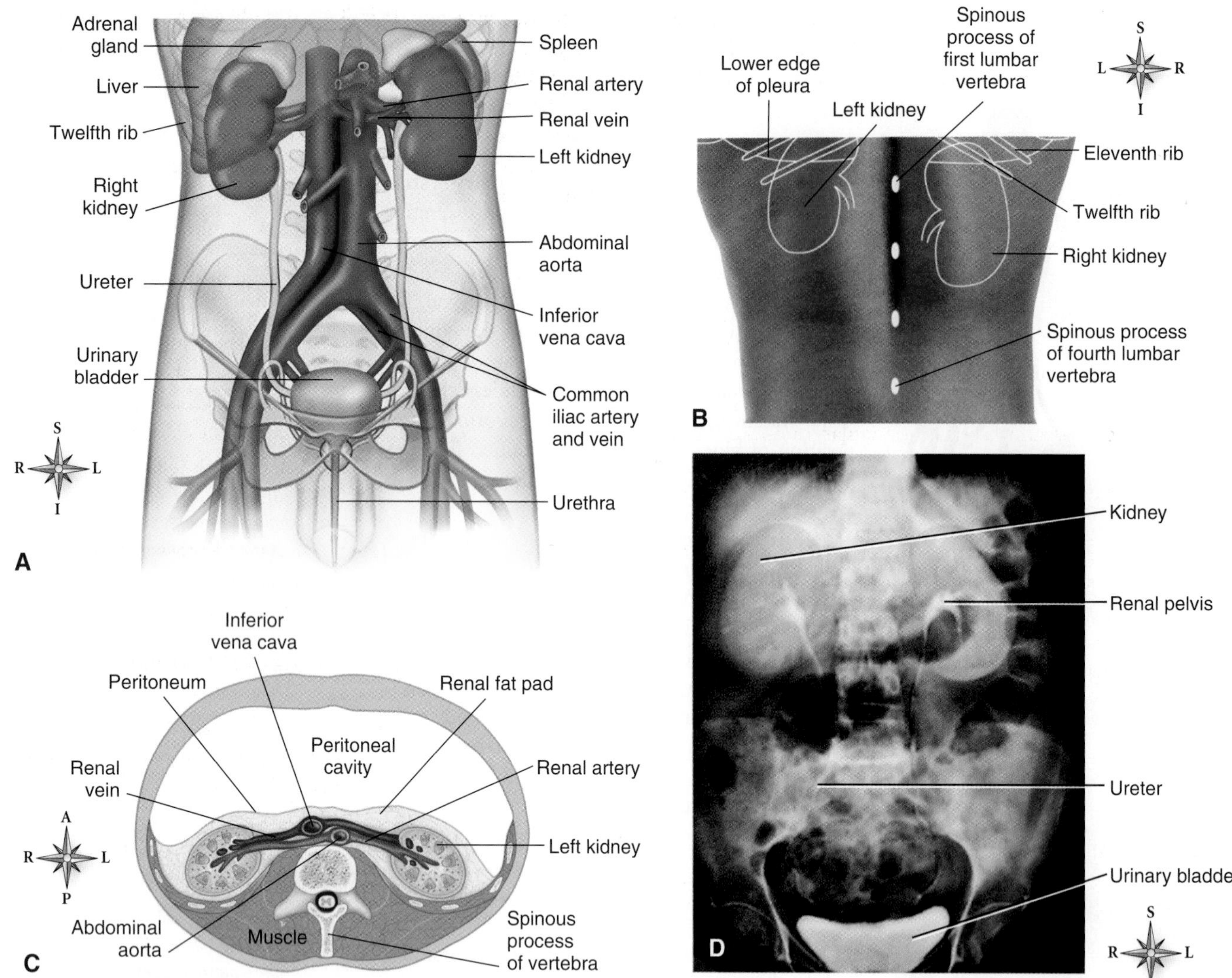

FIGURE 18-1 Urinary system. **A,** Anterior view of urinary organs. **B,** Surface markings of the kidneys, eleventh and twelfth ribs, spinous processes of L1 to L4, and lower edge of pleura viewed from behind. **C,** Horizontal (transverse) section of the abdomen showing the retroperitoneal position of the kidneys. **D,** X-ray film of the urinary organs.

Kidneys

Location of the Kidneys

To locate the kidneys on your own body, stand erect and put your hands on your hips with your thumbs meeting over your backbone. When you are in this position, your kidneys lie above your thumbs on either side of your spinal column, but their placement is higher than you might think. Note in **Figure 18-1** that the right kidney, which touches the liver, is lower than the left.

Both kidneys are protected a bit by the lower rib cage and are located under the muscles of the back and *behind* the parietal peritoneum—the membrane that lines the abdominal cavity (see **Figure 18-1**, *C*). Because of this **retroperitoneal** location, a surgeon can operate on a kidney from behind without cutting through the parietal peritoneum. Once the peritoneum has been cut or opened, the potential for spread of infection throughout the entire abdominal cavity increases.

A heavy cushion of fat—the *renal fat pad*—normally encases each kidney and helps hold it in place.

Note the relatively large diameter of the renal arteries in **Figure 18-1**, *A*. Normally, a little more than 20% of the total blood pumped by the heart each minute enters the kidneys. The rate of blood flow through this organ is among the highest in the body. This is understandable because one of the main functions of the kidney is to remove waste products from the blood. Maintenance of a high rate of blood flow and normal blood pressure in the kidneys is essential for the formation of urine.

Gross Structure of the Kidney

External Anatomy

The kidneys resemble lima beans in shape, that is, roughly oval with a medial indentation (see **Figure 18-1**, *A*). The medial indentation, called the **hilum**, is where vessels, nerves, and the ureter connect with the kidney. An average-sized kidney measures approximately 11 × 7 × 3 cm (4.3 × 2.7 × 1.2 in).

There is a tough fibrous *capsule* that forms the exterior wall of the kidney.

Internal Anatomy

If you were to slice through a kidney from side to side and open it like the pages of a book (called a *coronal section*), you would see the structures shown in Figure 18-2. Identify each of the following parts:

1. **Renal cortex**—the outer part of the kidney (the word *cortex* comes from the Latin word for "bark," so the cortex of an organ is its outer layer).
2. **Renal medulla**—the inner portion of the kidney.
3. **Renal pyramids**—the triangular divisions of the medulla of the kidney. Extensions of cortical tissue that dip down into the medulla between the renal pyramids are called **renal columns.**
4. **Renal papilla** (pl. *papillae*)—narrow, innermost end of a pyramid.
5. **Renal pelvis**—(also called the *kidney pelvis*) an expansion of the upper end of a ureter (the tube that drains urine into the bladder).
6. **Calyx** (pl. *calyces*)—a division of the renal pelvis (the papilla of a pyramid opens into each calyx).

Microscopic Structure

More than a million microscopic units called **nephrons** make up each kidney's interior (Figure 18-3). The shape of a nephron is unique, unmistakable, and admirably suited to its function of producing urine. It looks a little like a tiny funnel with a very long stem, but it is an unusual stem in that it is highly convoluted—that is, it has many bends in it.

The nephron is composed of two principal components: the *renal corpuscle* and the *renal tubule.* The renal corpuscle can be subdivided still further into two parts and the renal tubule into four regions or segments. Identify each part of the renal corpuscle and renal tubule described in Figure 18-4 and Figure 18-5.

A. **Renal corpuscle**
   1. **Bowman capsule**—the cup-shaped top of a nephron. The hollow, saclike Bowman capsule surrounds the glomerulus.
   2. **Glomerulus**—a network of blood capillaries tucked into the Bowman capsule. Note in Figure 18-4, *B* that the small artery (*afferent arteriole*) that delivers blood to the glomerulus is larger in diameter than the *efferent arteriole* that drains blood from it and that it is relatively short. This explains the high blood pressure that exists in the glomerular capillaries. This high pressure is required to filter wastes from the blood.

B. **Renal tubule**
   1. **Proximal convoluted tubule (PCT)**—the first segment of a renal tubule. The PCT is called *proximal* because it lies nearest the tubule's origin from the Bowman capsule, and it is called *convoluted* because it has several bends.
   2. **Nephron loop (Henle loop)**—the extension of the proximal tubule. Observe that the nephron loop consists of a straight *descending limb*, a hairpin turn, and a straight *ascending limb.*

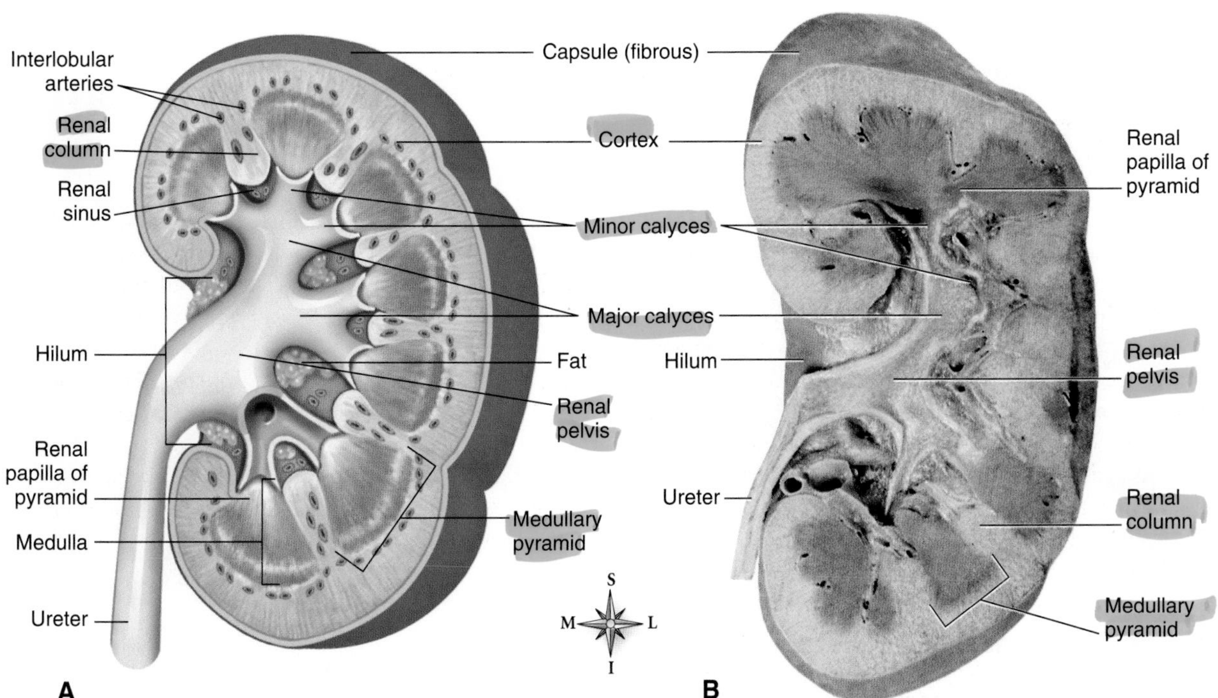

FIGURE 18-2 Internal structure of the kidney. A, Artist's rendering of a coronal section of the kidney. **B,** Photograph of coronal section of a preserved human kidney.

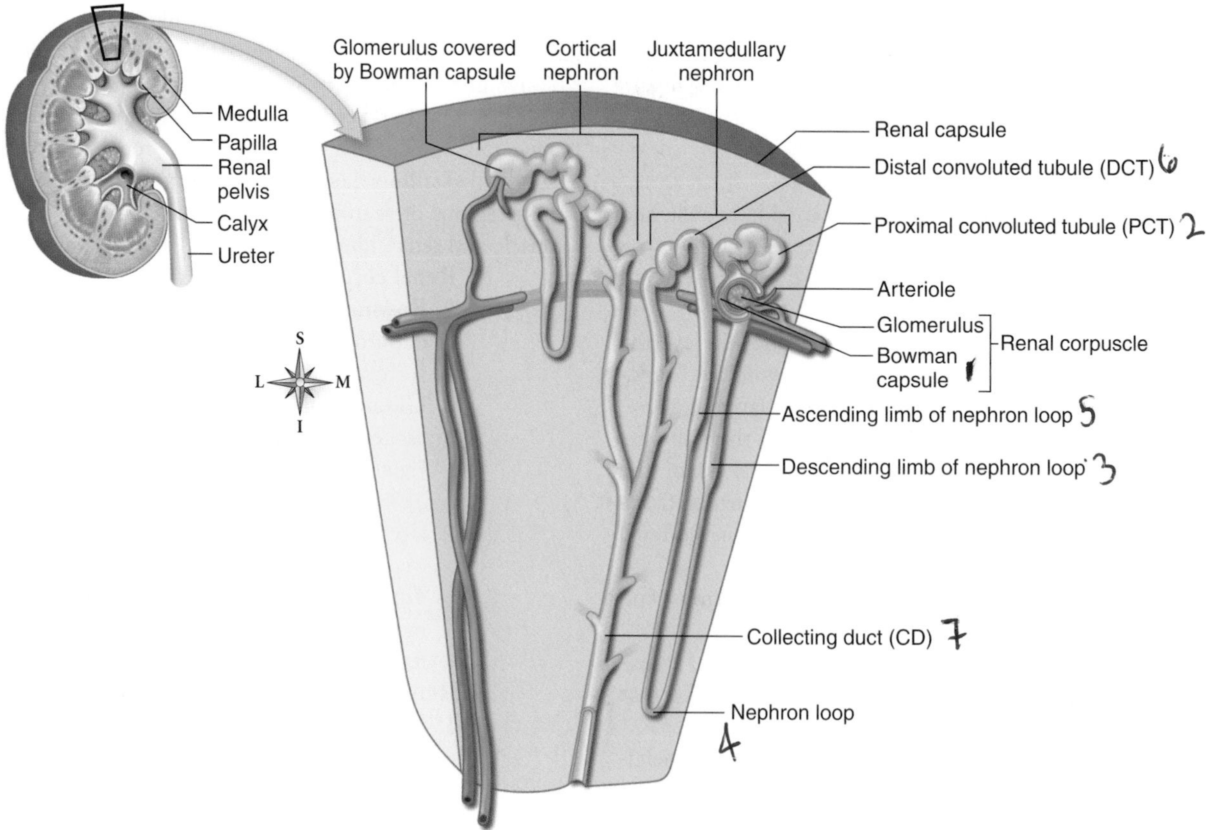

FIGURE 18-3 Location of nephrons. Magnified wedge cut from a renal pyramid shows an example of a cortical nephron and a juxtamedullary nephron.

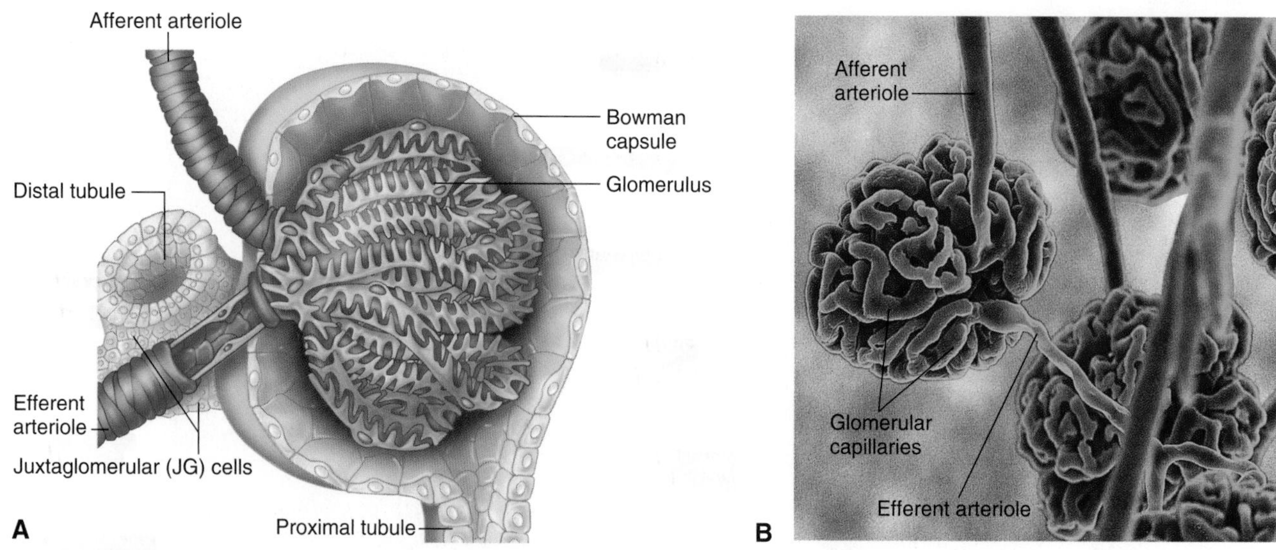

FIGURE 18-4 Renal corpuscle. A, Schematic showing relationship of glomerulus to Bowman capsule (together called the *renal corpuscle*) and adjacent structures. **B,** Scanning electron micrograph showing several glomeruli and their associated blood vessels. The difference in diameters of afferent and efferent arterioles is clearly visible.

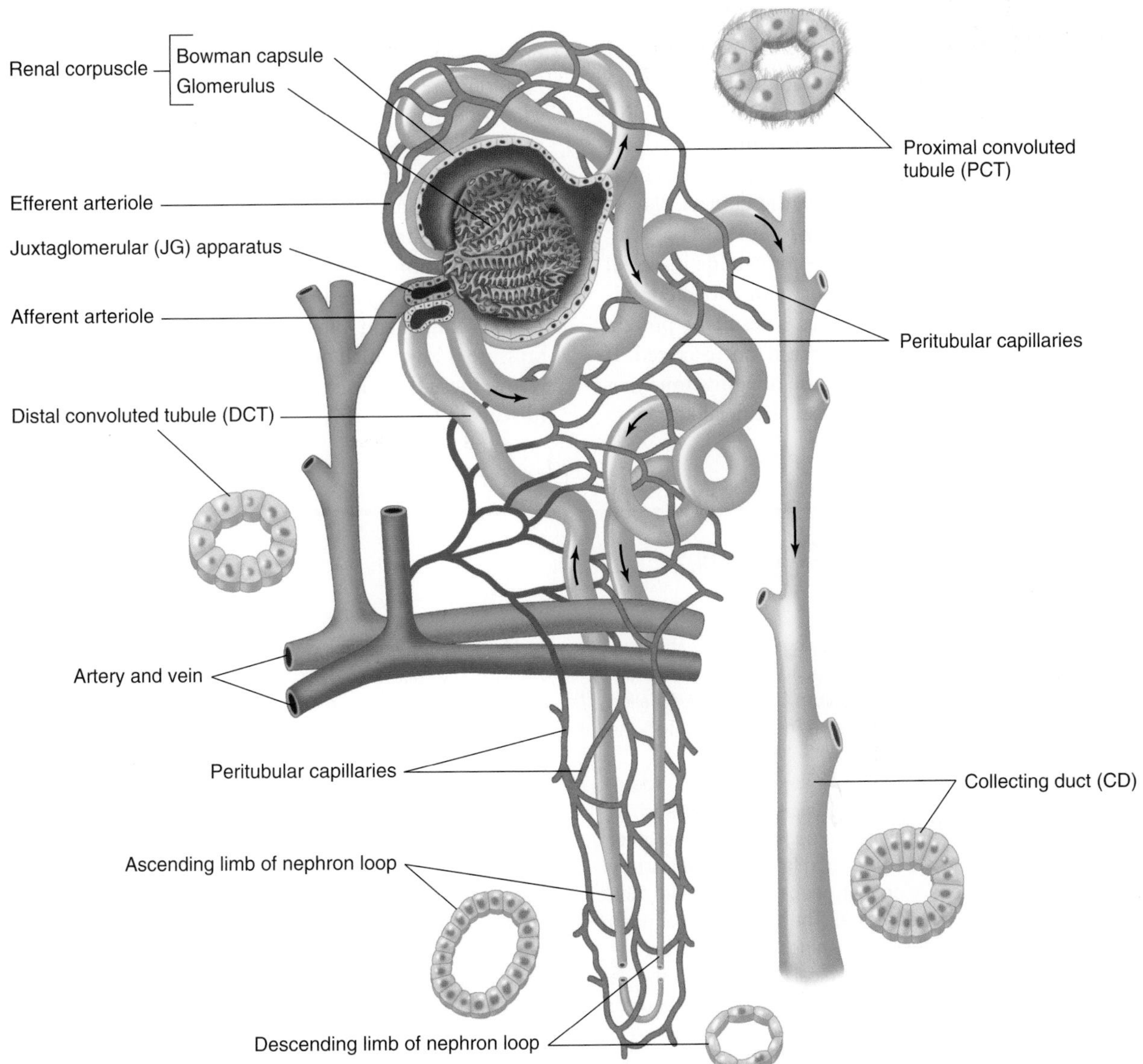

FIGURE 18-5 Nephron structure. Cross sections from the four segments of the renal tubule are shown. The differences in appearance in tubular cells seen in a cross section reflect the differing functions of each nephron segment. A gap in the nephron loop represents additional length that cannot be shown in the allotted space.

3. **Distal convoluted tubule (DCT)**—the part of the tubule distal to the ascending limb of the nephron loop. The DCT is the extension of the ascending limb.
4. **Collecting duct (CD)**—a straight (that is, not convoluted) part of a renal tubule. Distal tubules of several nephrons join to form a single collecting duct.

Urine from the collecting ducts exits from the pyramid through the papilla and enters the calyx and renal pelvis before flowing into the ureter.

Look again at **Figure 18-3**. Notice the differing locations of the two nephrons in the illustration. One is located high in the cortex and is typical of about 85% of all nephrons. Nephrons in this group are located almost entirely in the renal cortex and are called **cortical nephrons.** The remainder, called **juxtamedullary nephrons,** have their renal corpuscles near the junction (juxta) between cortex and medullary layers. These nephrons have nephron loops that dip far into the medulla. Juxtamedullary nephrons have an important role in concentrating urine.

Overview of Kidney Function

The kidneys are vital organs. The function they perform, that of forming urine, is essential for homeostasis and maintenance of life. Early in the process of urine formation, fluid, electrolytes, and wastes from metabolism are filtered from the blood and enter the nephron. Additional wastes may be secreted into the tubules of the nephron as substances useful to the body are reabsorbed into the blood.

Normally the kidneys balance the amount of many substances entering and leaving the blood over time so that normal concentrations can be maintained. In short, the kidneys adjust their output to equal the intake of the body. By eliminating wastes and adjusting fluid balance, the kidneys play an essential part in maintaining homeostasis.

Homeostasis cannot be maintained—nor can life itself—if the kidneys fail and the condition is not soon corrected. Nitrogenous waste products accumulate as a result of protein breakdown and quickly reach toxic levels if not excreted. If kidney function is greatly reduced because of aging, injury, or disease, life can be maintained by using an artificial kidney to cleanse the blood of wastes.

Excretion of toxins and of nitrogen-containing waste products such as urea and ammonia represents only one of the important responsibilities of the kidney. The kidney also plays a key role in regulating the levels of many chemical substances in the blood such as chloride, sodium, potassium, and bicarbonate. The kidneys also regulate the proper balance between body water content and salt by selectively retaining or excreting both substances as requirements demand.

In addition, the cells of the **juxtaglomerular (JG) apparatus** (see **Figure 18-4**, *A*, and **Figure 18-5**) also function in blood volume and blood pressure regulation. When blood pressure is low, which often occurs when blood plasma volume is low, these JG cells secrete an enzyme that triggers a system (discussed later in this chapter) to restore normal blood volume and pressure.

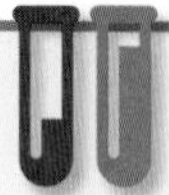

CLINICAL APPLICATION

ARTIFICIAL KIDNEY

The artificial kidney is a mechanical device that uses the principle of dialysis to remove or separate waste products from the blood. In the event of kidney failure, the process called **hemodialysis** can provide a reprieve from death for the patient.

During a hemodialysis treatment, a semipermeable membrane is used to separate large (nondiffusible) particles such as blood cells from small (diffusible) ones such as urea and other wastes. Part *A* of the figure shows blood from the radial artery passing through a porous (semipermeable) cellophane tube that is housed in a tanklike container. The tube is surrounded by a bath, or dialysis solution, containing varying concentrations of electrolytes and other chemicals. The pores in the membrane are small and allow only very small molecules, such as urea, to escape into the surrounding fluid. Larger molecules and blood cells cannot escape and are returned through the tube to reenter the patient via a wrist or leg vein.

By constantly replacing the bath solution in the dialysis tank with freshly mixed solution, levels of waste materials can be kept at low levels. As a result, wastes such as urea in the blood rapidly pass into the surrounding wash solution.

For a patient with complete kidney failure, two or three hemodialysis treatments a week are required. New dialysis methods are now being developed, and dramatic advances in treatment are expected in the next few years.

Another technique used in the treatment of *renal failure* is called **continuous ambulatory peritoneal dialysis (CAPD)**. In this procedure, 1 to 3 L of sterile dialysis fluid is introduced directly into the peritoneal cavity through an opening in the abdominal wall (part *B* of the figure). Peritoneal membranes in the abdominal cavity transfer waste products from blood into the dialysis fluid, which is then drained back into a plastic container after about 2 hours. This technique is less expensive than hemodialysis and does not require the use of complex equipment.

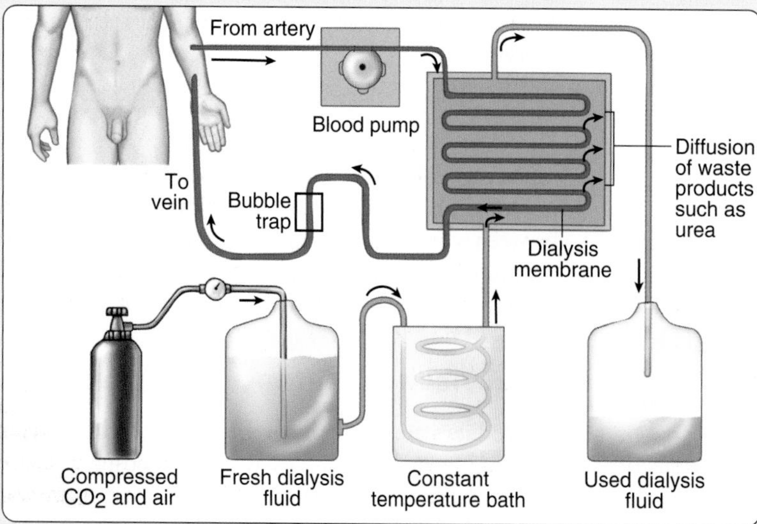

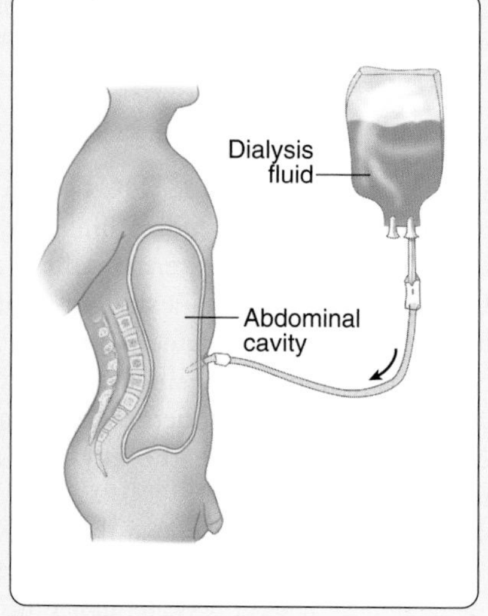

Hemodialysis.

Yet another important function of the kidney is the secretion of the hormone **erythropoietin (EPO)**. During *hypoxia*, a deficiency of oxygen in the body, the erythropoietin is released into the bloodstream. EPO travels in the bloodstream to the red bone marrow, where it stimulates the production of additional erythrocytes (red blood cells). The additional erythrocytes increase the ability of the blood to absorb and transport oxygen to oxygen-starved tissues.

EPO is sometimes used as a drug (one brand is Procrit) to treat anemia caused by critical illness such as cancer. EPO is sometimes abused by athletes attempting to improve their athletic performance by boosting hematocrit—thus increasing the oxygen-carrying capacity of their blood. (See *Blood Doping* on p. 268.)

As you probably guessed, kidney disease can cause anemia by reducing the body's ability to produce EPO when needed.

With all these vital functions, it is easy to understand why the kidneys are often considered to be the most important homeostatic organs in the body.

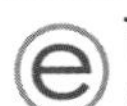 To learn more about the kidney, go to AnimationDirect at *evolve.elsevier.com*.

QUICK CHECK

1. What are the main regions of the kidney?
2. What are the primary structures of a nephron?
3. What is the relationship of the Bowman capsule when discussing the segments of the renal tubule and the directional terms "proximal" and "distal?"
4. What is the role of filtration in the kidney?

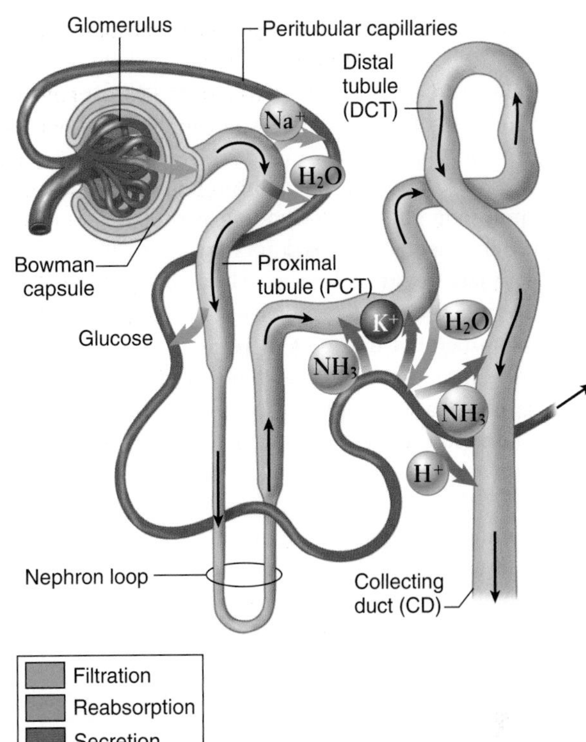

FIGURE 18-6 Formation of urine. Diagram shows examples of the steps in urine formation in successive parts of a nephron: filtration, reabsorption, and secretion.

Formation of Urine

The kidneys' 2 million or more nephrons balance the composition of the blood plasma, thus helping maintain a homeostatic constancy for the entire internal environment of the body. In performing this critical function, the kidneys' nephrons must flush out excess or waste molecules by excreting urine. The nephrons form urine by way of a combination of three blood-balancing processes:

1. Filtration
2. Reabsorption
3. Secretion

Figure 18-6 summarizes these three processes.

Filtration

Urine formation begins with the process of **filtration,** which goes on continually in the renal corpuscles (Bowman capsules plus their encased glomeruli). Blood flowing through the glomeruli exerts pressure, and this glomerular blood pressure is high enough to push water and dissolved substances out of the glomeruli into the Bowman capsule. Briefly, glomerular blood pressure causes filtration through the glomerular-capsular membrane. If the glomerular blood pressure drops below a certain level, filtration and urine formation cease. Hemorrhage, for example, may cause a precipitous drop in blood pressure followed by kidney failure.

Glomerular filtration normally occurs at the rate of 125 mL per minute. As a result, about 180 L (nearly 50 gallons) of **glomerular filtrate** is produced by the kidneys every day.

Obviously no one ever excretes anywhere near 180 L of urine per day. Why? Because most of the fluid that leaves the blood by glomerular filtration, the first process in urine formation, returns to the blood by the second process—*reabsorption*.

Reabsorption

Reabsorption is the movement of substances out of the renal tubules into the blood capillaries located around the tubules (peritubular capillaries). Water, glucose, and other nutrients, as well as sodium and other ions, are substances that are reabsorbed. Reabsorption begins in the proximal convoluted tubules and continues in the nephron loop, distal convoluted tubules, and collecting ducts.

Large amounts of water—approximately 178 L per day—are reabsorbed by osmosis from the proximal tubules. In other words, nearly 99% of the 180 L of water that leaves the blood each day by glomerular filtration returns to the blood by proximal tubule reabsorption. Smaller amounts of water also are reabsorbed in the nephron loops, distal tubules, and collecting ducts.

Common table salt (NaCl) consumed in the diet or introduced by intravenous (IV) infusion of normal saline (0.9%

NaCl) or other NaCl-containing fluids, provides the body with sodium ions (Na^+) and chloride ions (Cl^-). For the most part, sodium ions are actively transported back into blood from the tubular fluid in all segments of the kidney tubule except the collecting ducts.

Sodium reabsorption in the nephron loop is a special case. The nephron loop and its surrounding peritubular capillaries dip far into the medulla and back up in what is called *countercurrent* flow (see **Figure 18-5** on p. 413). This countercurrent flow—flow in opposite directions—of filtrate back up the nephron loop permits transport of large amounts of sodium and chloride into the interstitial fluid of the medulla. This makes the medulla very salty—or *hypertonic*. The countercurrent flow of blood in the peritubular capillaries surrounding the nephron loop fails to remove all of the excess sodium and chloride. Together, these **countercurrent mechanisms** maintain hypertonic conditions in the medulla. By maintaining a hypertonic medulla, the kidney is able to concentrate the urine by reabsorbing more water than otherwise possible. How the kidney thus regulates urine volume is covered below.

The amount of sodium reabsorbed depends largely on the body's intake. In general the greater the amount of sodium intake, the less the amount reabsorbed and the greater the amount excreted in the urine. Also, the less sodium intake, the greater the reabsorption from kidney tubules and the less excreted in the urine.

Rather than being actively reabsorbed from renal tubules as are sodium ions (Na^+), chloride ions (Cl^-) passively move into blood because they carry a negative electrical charge. The positively charged sodium ions that have been reabsorbed and moved into the blood "attract" the negatively charged chloride ions from the tubule fluid into the peritubular capillaries.

Figure 18-7 explains the details of how sodium, chloride, and water are reabsorbed across the tubule wall and into the peritubular blood. Take a few minutes to review each step in the diagram.

All of the filtered glucose is normally reabsorbed from the proximal tubules into peritubular capillary blood. None of this valuable nutrient is wasted by being lost in the urine. **Figure 18-8** shows how sodium-glucose carriers in the tubule wall allow glucose molecules to passively "tag along" as sodium is actively reabsorbed back into the blood.

However, sometimes not all the glucose in the tubule filtrate is recovered by the blood. For example, in *diabetes mellitus (DM),* if blood glucose concentration increases above a certain level, called the **renal threshold,** the tubular filtrate then contains more glucose than kidney tubule cells can reabsorb. There are not enough sodium-glucose transporters to handle the excess glucose immediately. Some of the glucose

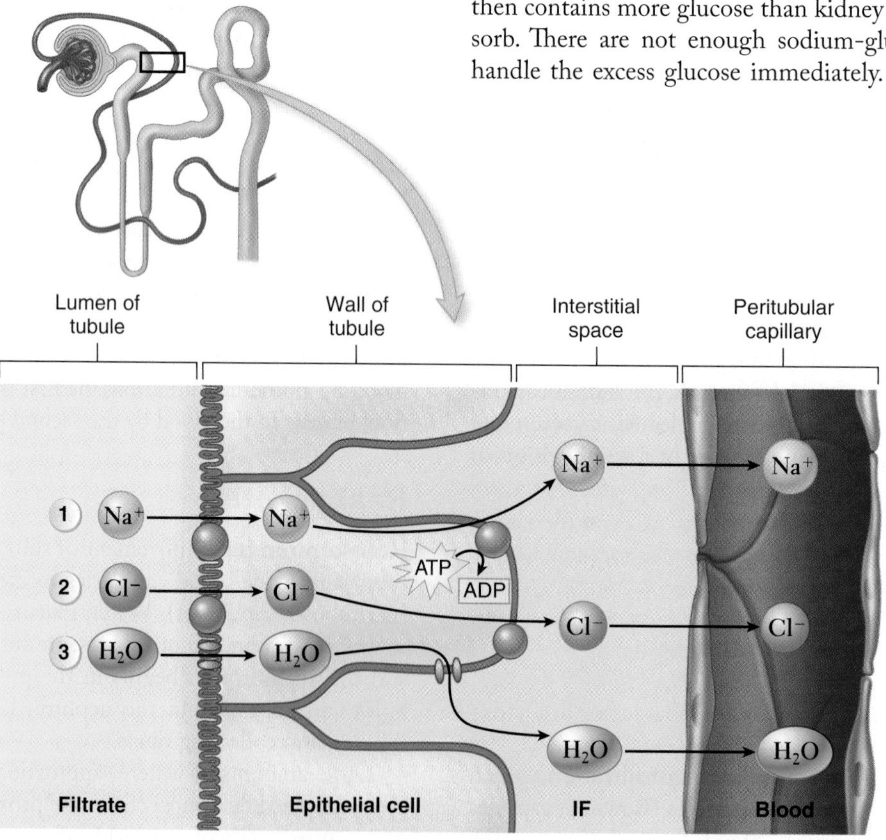

FIGURE 18-7 Reabsorption of ions and water. ①, Sodium ions (Na^+) are pumped from the tubule cell to interstitial fluid (IF), thereby increasing the interstitial Na^+ concentration to a level that drives diffusion of Na^+ into blood. As Na^+ is pumped out of the cell, more Na^+ passively diffuses in from the filtrate to maintain an equilibrium of concentration. Enough Na^+ moves out of the tubule and into blood that an electrical gradient is established (blood is positive relative to the filtrate). ②, Electrical attraction between oppositely charged particles drives diffusion of negative ions in the filtrate, such as chloride (Cl^-), into blood. ③, When the ion concentration in blood increases, osmosis of water from the tubule occurs. Thus active transport of sodium creates a situation that promotes passive transport of negative ions and water.

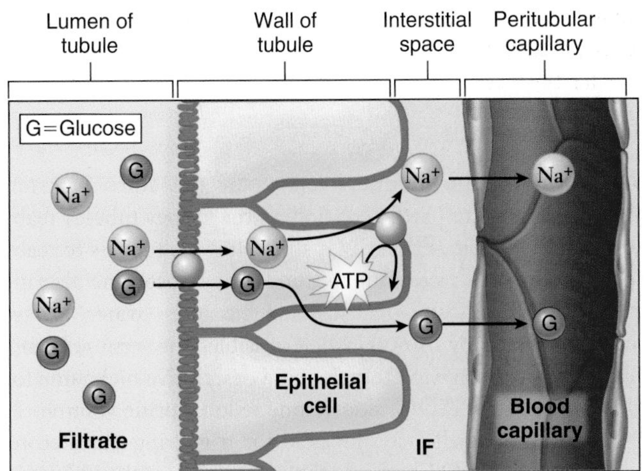

FIGURE 18-8 Reabsorption of glucose. The presence of sodium-glucose transporters provides a way for the active transport of sodium to also passively transport glucose across tubule cells and eventually back into the blood. The availability of these transporters may limit how much glucose can be reabsorbed at one time.

therefore remains behind in the urine. Glucose in the urine—**glycosuria**—is a well-known sign of diabetes mellitus.

The *transport maximum* (T_{max})—the largest amount of any substance that can be reabsorbed at one time—is determined mainly by the number of available transporters of that substance. The transport maximum of any substance helps determine the *renal threshold*—the amount of substance in the blood above which the kidney removes the excess substance from the blood.

Secretion

Secretion is the process by which substances move into urine in the distal and collecting ducts from blood in the capillaries around these tubules. In this respect, secretion is reabsorption in reverse. Whereas reabsorption moves substances out of the urine into the blood, secretion moves substances out of the blood into the urine.

Tubular secretion serves an important function by removing or "clearing" the blood of excess potassium and hydrogen ions, certain drugs including penicillin and phenobarbital, and numerous wastes such as urea, uric acid, and creatinine.

Most substances that are secreted from peritubular blood enter the filtrate primarily in the proximal tubule and, to a lesser extent, the distal convoluted tubule and collecting ducts.

The major exception to this "rule of thumb" is potassium ion, which is secreted primarily into the collecting ducts in an exchange with sodium. Urine volume of potassium ions (K^+) varies greatly with diet. Some **diuretic drugs,** which stimulate the production of urine (see the box on p. 438), are said to be "potassium wasting" because they increase *secretion* of potassium into tubular fluid and thus its excretion in the urine.

In the distal convoluted tubules and collecting ducts, sodium secretion is dependent on hormones also important in regulating urine volume, as discussed below. Ammonia is secreted passively by diffusion.

Kidney tubule secretion plays a crucial role in maintaining the body's fluid, electrolyte, and acid-base balance discussed in Chapters 19 and 20.

Summary of Urine Formation

In summary, the following processes occurring in successive portions of the nephron accomplish the function of urine formation (**Table 18-1**):

1. **Filtration**—of water and dissolved substances out of the blood in the glomeruli into the Bowman capsule.
2. **Reabsorption**—of water and dissolved substances out of kidney tubules back into blood. This prevents substances needed by the body from being lost in urine. Usually, up to 99% of water, sodium, and chloride filtered out of glomerular blood is retrieved from tubules—along with 100% of glucose.
3. **Secretion**—of hydrogen ions, potassium ions, and certain drugs from blood into kidney tubules.

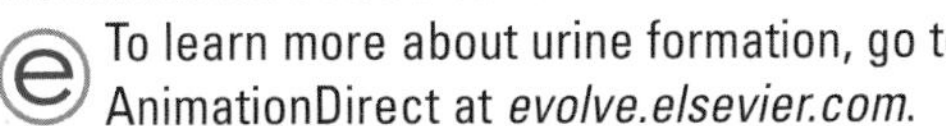

To learn more about urine formation, go to AnimationDirect at *evolve.elsevier.com*.

QUICK CHECK

1. What are the three basic processes that occur in the nephron?
2. Where does filtration occur in the nephron?
3. Where does reabsorption occur in the nephron?

TABLE 18-1 Functions of Parts of Nephron in Urine Formation

PART OF NEPHRON	PROCESS IN URINE FORMATION	SUBSTANCES MOVED
Glomerulus and Bowman capsule	Filtration	Water and solutes (for example, sodium and other ions, glucose and other nutrients filtering out of glomeruli into Bowman capsules)
Proximal tubule	Reabsorption Secretion	Water and solutes (glucose, amino acids, Na^+) Nitrogenous wastes, some drugs
Nephron loop	Reabsorption	Sodium and chloride ions
Distal and collecting tubules	Reabsorption Secretion	Water, sodium, and chloride ions Ammonia, potassium ions, hydrogen ions, and some drugs

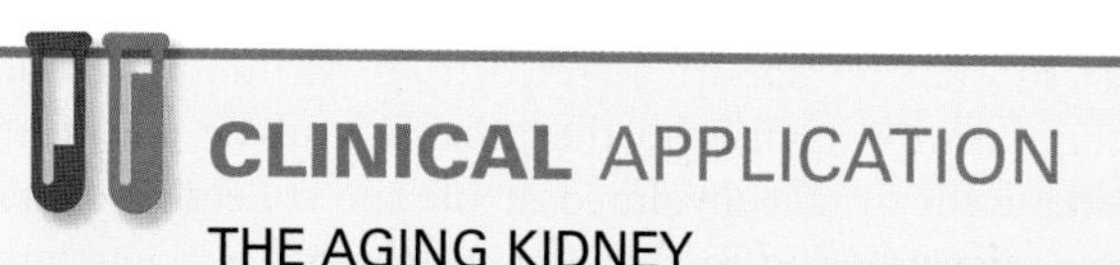

CLINICAL APPLICATION

THE AGING KIDNEY

As with other body organs, the kidneys undergo both age-related structural changes and decreasing functional capacity. Adults older than 35 years of age gradually lose functional nephron units, and kidney weight actually decreases. By approximately 80 to 85 years of age, most individuals will have experienced a 30% reduction in total kidney mass. In spite of a numerical reduction in actual kidney nephron units and a decrease in the metabolic activity of remaining tubular cells, most of these individuals continue to exhibit normal kidney function. This is possible because older persons generally have a lower overall lean body mass and therefore a reduced production of waste products that must be excreted from the body. However, the "margin of safety" is reduced, and any stress on the remaining functional nephrons, such as a systemic infection or a reduction in kidney blood flow, can produce almost immediate symptoms of kidney failure. Marginal kidney function in old age may make it difficult to excrete drugs that are easily cleared from the blood of younger persons, and dosages of many medications have to be adjusted accordingly for older patients.

Control of Urine Volume

The body has ways to control the amount and composition of the urine that it excretes. It does this mainly by controlling the amount of water and dissolved substances that are reabsorbed by the kidney tubules.

Antidiuretic Hormone

An example of regulating water reabsorption in kidney tubules involves a hormone called **antidiuretic hormone (ADH)** secreted from the posterior pituitary gland. ADH decreases the amount of urine by making collecting ducts permeable to water. If no ADH is present, the tubules are practically impermeable to water, so little or no water is reabsorbed from them. When ADH is present in the blood, collecting ducts are permeable to water and water is reabsorbed from them. As a result, less water is lost from the body as urine, or more water is retained from the tubules—whichever way you wish to say it. At any rate, for this reason ADH is accurately described as the "water-retaining hormone." You might also think of it as the "urine-decreasing hormone."

Recall that the countercurrent mechanisms of the nephron loop and its capillaries maintain a hypertonic (salty) medulla. When filtrate moves down the collecting ducts, the action of ADH allows osmosis of water to equilibrate with the hypertonic interstitial fluid of the medulla—thus removing more water from the filtrate than would otherwise be possible. Maintaining a hypertonic medulla thus allows ADH to have a greater effect in concentrating urine, thereby conserving the body's valuable water.

Aldosterone

The hormone **aldosterone,** secreted by the adrenal cortex, plays an important part in controlling the kidney tubules' reabsorption of sodium. Primarily, it stimulates the tubules to reabsorb sodium at a faster rate. Secondarily, aldosterone also increases tubular water reabsorption because "water always follows sodium" by osmosis when possible. The term *salt- and water-retaining hormone* therefore is a descriptive nickname for aldosterone. Like ADH, aldosterone reduces urine volume.

The kidney itself is responsible for triggering aldosterone secretion, a fact that illustrates the importance of the kidney in regulating overall fluid volume and blood pressure in the body. When blood volume and pressure drop below normal, this is sensed by cells in the JG apparatus. JG cells then release an enzyme called **renin** that initiates the **renin-angiotensin-aldosterone system (RAAS)**. The RAAS eventually produces constriction of blood vessels and thus raises blood pressure. The RAAS also triggers adrenal gland secretion of aldosterone, which promotes water retention and thus increases total blood volume—also contributing to a rise in blood pressure. **Figure 18-9** illustrates the main events of the RAAS and how it acts to restore normal plasma volume and blood pressure. Aldosterone mechanisms are also discussed in the next chapter.

Atrial Natriuretic Hormone

Another hormone, **atrial natriuretic hormone (ANH)** secreted from the heart's atrial wall, has the opposite effect of aldosterone. ANH is the primary *atrial natriuretic peptide (ANP)* hormone in humans. ANH stimulates kidney tubules to secrete more sodium and thus lose more water. ANH is a *salt- and water-losing hormone.* Thus ANH increases urine volume.

The body secretes ADH, aldosterone, and ANH in different amounts, depending on the homeostatic balance of body fluids at any particular moment.

Abnormalities of Urine Volume

Sometimes the kidneys do not excrete normal amounts of urine as a result of kidney disease, endocrine imbalances, cardiovascular disease, stress, or a variety of other conditions. Here are some terms associated with abnormal amounts of urine:

1. **Anuria**—absence of urine
2. **Oliguria**—scanty amount of urine
3. **Polyuria**—unusually large amount of urine

Because a change in urine volume or output is a significant indicator in many types of fluid alterations and diseases, measurement of both fluid intake and fluid output (urine volume) over a specified period of time, often abbreviated as **I & O,** is a common practice in clinical medicine. The normal adult urine output is about 1500 to 1600 mL per day.

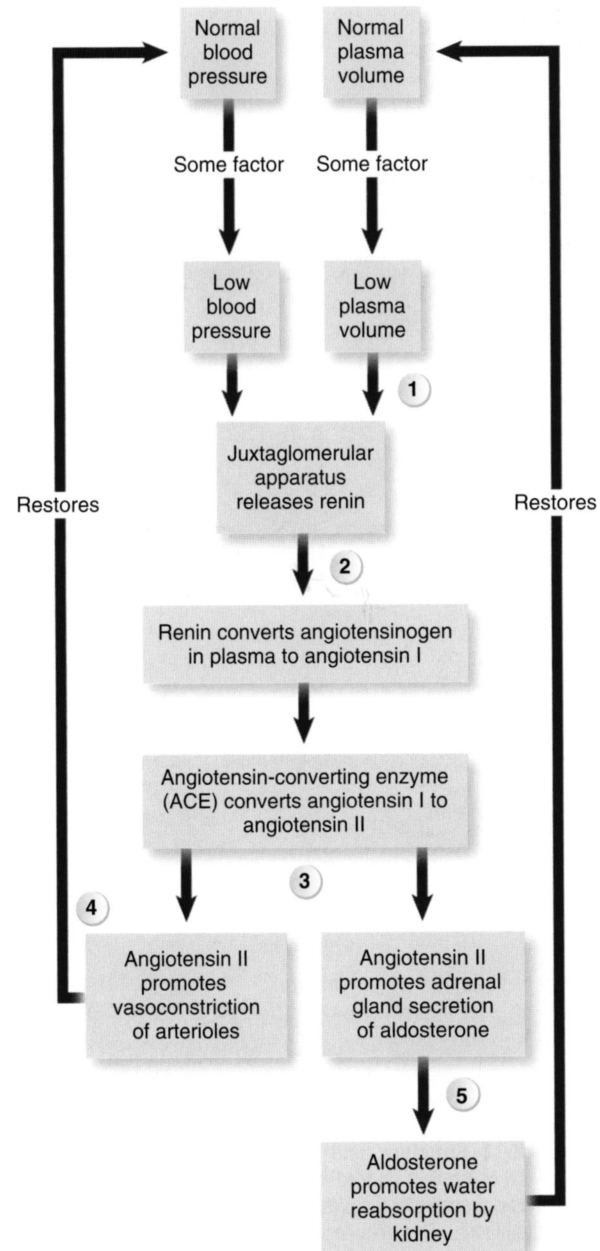

FIGURE 18-9 Renin-angiotensin-aldosterone system (RAAS).
1, Low plasma volume reduces blood pressure below normal, which is detected by juxtaglomerular (JG) cells in the juxtaglomerular apparatus of the kidney.
2, This triggers the release of renin, which converts angiotensinogen into angiotensin I.
3, The enzyme ACE then converts angiotensin I to angiotensin II.
4, Angiotensin II stimulates constriction of arteriolar smooth muscles and thus increases blood pressure back toward normal.
5, Angiotensin II also triggers adrenal gland secretion of aldosterone, which promotes water retention by the kidney and thus restoration of normal blood volume and pressure.

QUICK CHECK

1. What is the function of ANH?
2. How do ADH and aldosterone affect urine output?
3. How do anuria and polyuria differ?

CLINICAL APPLICATION

REMOVAL OF KIDNEY STONES USING ULTRASOUND

Statistics suggest that approximately 1 in every 1000 adults in the United States suffers from kidney stones, or **renal calculi,** at some point in his or her life. Although symptoms of excruciating pain are common, many kidney stones are small enough to pass out of the urinary system spontaneously. If this is possible, no therapy is required other than treatment for pain and antibiotics if the calculi are associated with infection. Larger stones, however, may obstruct the flow of urine and are much more serious and difficult to treat.

Until recently, only traditional surgical procedures were effective in removing relatively large stones that formed in the calyces and renal pelvis of the kidney. In addition to the risks that always accompany major medical procedures, surgical removal of stones from the kidneys frequently required rather extensive hospital and home recovery periods, lasting 6 weeks or more.

A technique that uses ultrasound to pulverize the stones so that they can be flushed out of the urinary tract without surgery is now used in hospitals across the United States. The specially designed ultrasound generator required for the procedure is called a **lithotriptor.** Using a lithotriptor, physicians break up the stones with ultrasound waves, in a process called **lithotripsy,** without making an incision. Recovery time is minimal; patient risk and costs are reduced. One of the original ultrasound lithotripsy techniques requires placement of the individual in a tub of water or in contact with a water cushion to transfer and focus the shock wave, which is generated outside the body and called an "extracorporeal shock wave," on the kidney stone. A number of other lithotripsy techniques are also in use. They use various types of controlled energy, such as pulsed dye lasers, high voltage spark, electromagnetic impulse generators, and direct contact pneumatic pressure probes to fragment kidney stones.

Elimination of Urine

Once urine is formed by the kidneys, it must be eliminated from the body. Our discussion now returns to a focus on anatomy as we discuss the "plumbing" needed to drain the urine away.

Ureters

Urine drains out of the collecting tubules of each kidney into the renal pelvis and down the ureter into the urinary bladder (see **Figure 18-1**). The **renal pelvis** is the basinlike upper end of the ureter located inside the kidney. **Ureters** are narrow tubes less than 6 millimeters (mm) (¼ inch) wide and 25 to 30 centimeters (cm) (10 to 12 inches) long.

Mucous membranes featuring easily stretchable *transitional epithelium* line both ureters and each renal pelvis. Note in **Figure 18-10** that the ureter has a thick, muscular wall. Contraction of the muscular coat produces peristaltic-type movements

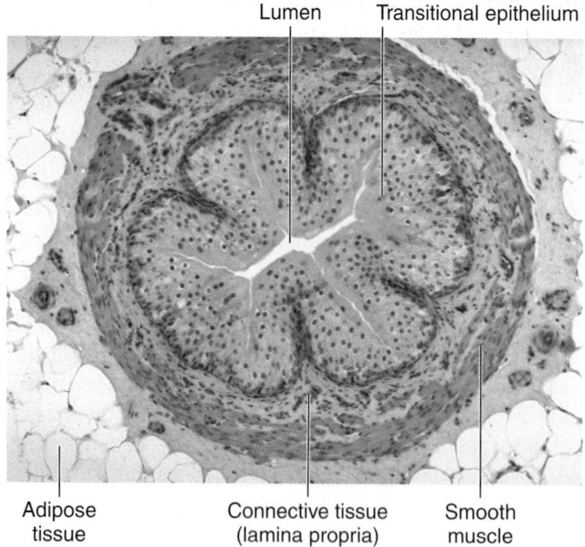

FIGURE 18-10 Ureter cross section. Note the many folds of the mucous lining (transitional epithelium) that permit stretching as urine passes through the tube. A thick muscular layer of smooth muscle helps "pump" urine toward the bladder. On its outer surface the ureter is covered by a tough fibrous connective tissue coat.

that assist in moving urine down the ureters into the bladder. The lining membrane of the ureters is richly supplied with sensory nerve endings.

Episodes of **renal colic**—pain caused by the passage of a kidney stone—have been described in medical writings since antiquity. Kidney stones cause intense pain if they have sharp edges or are large enough to distend the walls or cut the lining of the ureters or urethra as they pass from the kidneys to the exterior of the body. Some of the pain is caused by tearing or stretching of the urinary lining—along with the accompanying inflammation. However, much of the pain is associated with cramping of muscles that attempt to push a kidney stone forward. The term "colic" is used because of its similarity to painful cramps sometimes experienced in the muscle layers of the colon.

Urinary Bladder

The empty urinary bladder lies in the pelvis just behind the pubic symphysis. When full of urine, it projects upward into the lower portion of the abdominal cavity. In women it sits in front of the uterus, whereas in men, it rests on the prostate.

Elastic fibers and involuntary muscle fibers in the wall of the urinary bladder make it well suited for expanding to hold variable amounts of urine and then contracting to empty itself. Mucous membrane containing transitional epithelium lines the urinary bladder (**Figure 18-11**). The lining is loosely attached to the deeper muscular layer so that the bladder is very wrinkled and lies in folds called **rugae** when it is empty. When the bladder is filled, its inner surface may stretch until it is smooth.

Note in **Figure 18-11**, *A,* that one triangular area on the back or posterior surface of the bladder is free of rugae. This area, called the **trigone,** is always smooth. There, the lining membrane is tightly fixed to the deeper muscle coat. The

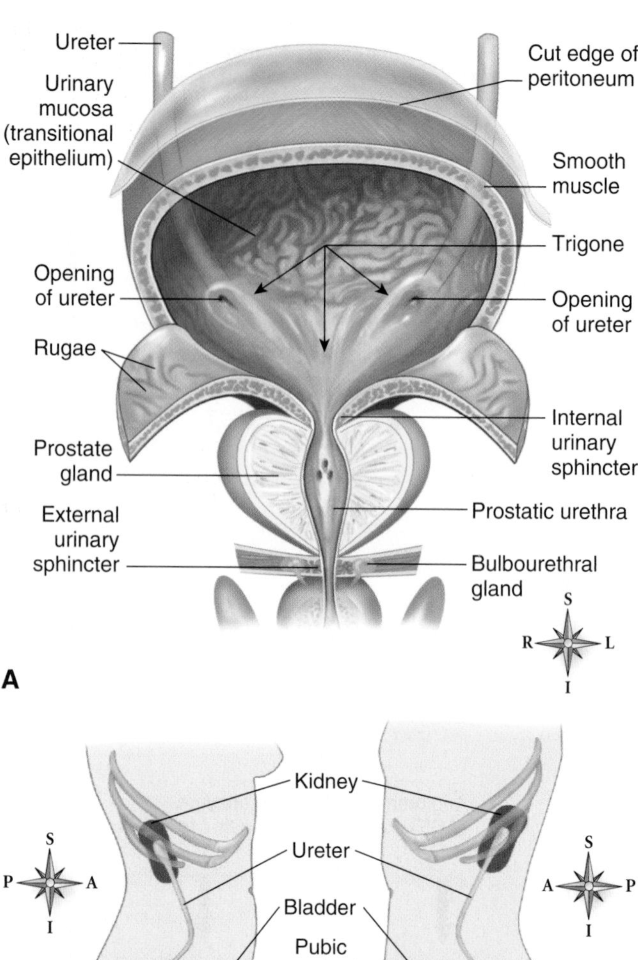

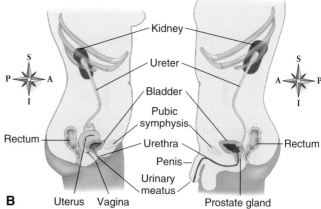

FIGURE 18-11 Structure and location of the urinary bladder. A, Frontal view of a fully distended male bladder dissected to show the interior. Note the relationship of the prostate gland, which surrounds the urethra as it exits the bladder. This relationship is discussed in Chapter 21. **B,** Sagittal section of the female urinary system *(left)* and the male urinary system *(right)* showing relationship of the bladder to other anatomical structures.

trigone extends between the openings of the two ureters above and the point of exit of the urethra below.

Urethra

To leave the body, urine passes from the bladder, down the **urethra,** and out of its external opening, the **urinary meatus.** In other words, the urethra is the lowest part of the urinary tract.

The same sheet of mucous membrane that lines each renal pelvis, the ureters, and the bladder extends down into the urethra, too. It is worth noting the continuity of the urinary mucous lining because it accounts for the fact that an infection of the urethra may spread upward through the urinary tract to cause **cystitis** (bladder infection).

The urethra is a narrow tube; it is only about 4 cm (1½ inches) long in a woman, but it is about 20 cm (8 inches) long in a man. In a man, the urethra has two functions: (1) it is the terminal portion of the urinary tract, and (2) it is the passageway for movement of the reproductive fluid (semen) from the body. In a woman, the urethra is a part of only the urinary tract.

Micturition

The terms **micturition, urination,** and **voiding** all refer to the passage of urine from the body or the emptying of the bladder.

Two **sphincters** (rings of muscle tissue) act as valves that guard the pathway leading from the bladder. The *internal urethral sphincter* is located at the bladder exit, and the *external urethral sphincter* circles the urethra just below the neck of the bladder (see **Figure 18-11**). When contracted, both sphincters seal off the bladder and allow urine to accumulate without leaking to the exterior. The internal urethral sphincter is involuntary, and the external urethral sphincter is composed of striated muscle and is under voluntary control.

The muscular wall of the bladder permits this organ to accommodate a considerable volume of urine with very little increase in pressure until a volume of 300 to 400 mL is reached. As the volume of urine increases, the need to void may be noticed at volumes of 150 mL, but micturition in adults does not normally occur much below volumes of 350 mL.

As the bladder wall stretches, nerve impulses are transmitted to the second, third, and fourth sacral segments of the spinal cord, and an **emptying reflex** is initiated. The reflex causes contraction of the muscle of the bladder wall and relaxation of the internal sphincter. Urine then enters the urethra. If the external sphincter, which is under voluntary control, is relaxed, micturition occurs. Voluntary contraction of the external sphincter suppresses the emptying reflex until the bladder is filled to capacity with urine and loss of control occurs. Contraction of this powerful sphincter also abruptly terminates urination voluntarily.

Higher centers in the brain also function in micturition by integrating bladder contraction and internal and external sphincter relaxation, with the cooperative contraction of pelvic and abdominal muscles. **Urinary retention** is a condition in which no urine is voided. The kidneys produce urine, but the bladder, for one reason or another, cannot empty itself. In **urinary suppression** the opposite is true. The kidneys do not produce any urine, but the bladder retains the ability to empty itself.

Micturition is a complex body function. It requires control and integration of both voluntary and involuntary nervous system components acting on a variety of anatomic structures. Unfortunately, homeostatic control problems occur quite frequently in this complex system. In addition to the 15% to 20% of children who experience some degree of enuresis, voiding dysfunction affects nearly 15 million adult Americans. People over 60 are especially at risk, with elderly women affected almost twice as often as men.

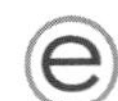

To learn more about the flow of urine through the body, go to AnimationDirect at *evolve.elsevier.com*.

Urinary incontinence or **enuresis** refers to involuntary voiding or loss of urine in an older child or adult. *Urge incontinence* is associated with smooth muscle overactivity in the bladder wall. The term *stress incontinence* is often used to describe the type of urine loss associated with laughing, coughing, or heavy lifting. It is a common problem in women with weakened pelvic floor muscles following pregnancy. So-called *overflow incontinence* is characterized by intermittent dribbling of urine. It results from urinary retention and an overdistended bladder—a common problem in men with an enlarged prostate gland (see Chapter 21).

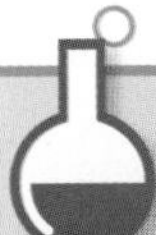

SCIENCE APPLICATIONS

FIGHTING INFECTION

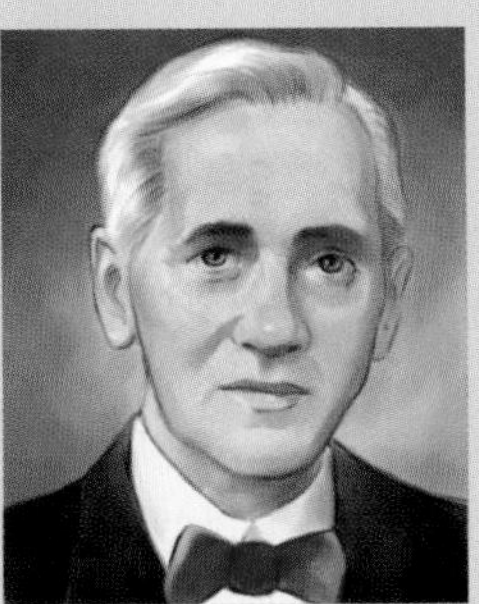

Alexander Fleming (1881-1955)

Unfortunately, the structure of the urinary tract puts it at risk for infection by bacteria and other microorganisms. Because it is open to the external environment, bacteria can enter easily. In women, the short length of the urethra and its location close to the anus may further increase the risk of bacteria getting to the urinary bladder.

A breakthrough in the treatment of *urinary tract infections (UTIs)* came in 1928 in the laboratory of Scots researcher Alexander Fleming. Some mold spores accidentally contaminated one of the dishes in which Fleming was growing bacteria. He marveled at the fact that no bacteria could grow near the mold growth. He isolated a substance from the mold responsible for this antibacterial effect and named it *penicillin.* Fleming subsequently showed that penicillin was effective against a variety of bacteria that cause serious infections in humans. Penicillin became the first "miracle drug" and rapidly became the tool of choice in fighting bacteria.

Although forms of penicillin and other antibiotics derived from natural sources are still the weapon of choice in battling many infections, the infectious bacteria are evolving into strains that resist common antibiotics. UTIs and other types of infections now require more powerful antibiotics and other special techniques to stop them. Some scientists fear that the era of simple antibiotic therapy may be nearing an end.

Many professions are involved directly in the fight against infection, and others continue in the quest to find newer and better treatments for UTIs and other infections that threaten human health. For example, **infection control** managers help hospitals and clinics prevent the spread of infection within facilities, **epidemiologists** prevent or respond to regional outbreaks of infection, and **microbiologists** work to understand the nature of infectious organisms and which therapies may be effective.

Reflex incontinence occurs in the absence of any sensory warning or awareness. It is common in nervous system disorders such as stroke, parkinsonism, or spinal cord injury. If totally cut off from spinal innervation, the bladder musculature acquires some automatic action, and periodic but unpredictable voiding occurs—a condition called **neurogenic bladder.**

Bed wetting at night *(nocturnal enuresis)* often occurs in a child who is beyond the age when voluntary bladder control is expected. Incidence is higher in boys than in girls and is often due to maturational delay of the complex urinary reflexes needed for voluntary control of micturition.

QUICK CHECK

1. Through what tube does urine leave the kidney?
2. What structural characteristics of the bladder allow it to expand to hold urine?
3. Through what structure does urine pass from the bladder to the outside of the body?
4. What is *overflow incontinence?*

TABLE 18-2 Characteristics of Urine

	NORMAL CHARACTERISTICS	ABNORMAL CHARACTERISTICS
Color and Clarity	Normal urine should be clear; color varies with specific gravity Dilute urine: transparent straw color Concentrated urine: deep yellow amber (Occasionally, normal urine may be cloudy because of high dietary levels of fat or phosphate)	Abnormally colored urine may result from (1) pathological conditions, (2) certain foods, and (3) numerous drugs 1. Pathological conditions (examples): Kidney cancer or kidney stones (hemorrhage)—red (RBCs) Bile duct obstruction (gallstones)—orange/yellow (bilirubin) *Pseudomonas* infection—green (bacterial toxins) 2. Foods (examples): Beets—red Rhubarb—brown Carrots—dark yellow Vitamin supplements—bright yellow 3. Drugs (examples): Pyridium (urinary tract analgesic)—orange Dilantin (anticonvulsant)—pink/red brown Dyrenium (diuretic)—pale blue Rifampin (anti-tuberculosis)—red/orange Cloudy urine may result from (examples): (1) bacteria—active infection of urinary system organs (2) blood cells RBCs—hemorrhage from kidney cancer WBCs—pus from urinary tract infection (UTI) (3) casts—various types of tubelike clumps (blood cell, epithelial, hyaline, waxy, etc.) that form in diseased renal tubes (4) proteinuria—(protein—usually albumin) in urine (5) crystals—usually uric acid or phosphate/calcium oxalate in concentrated urine
Compounds	Mineral ions (for example, Na^+, Cl^-, K^+) Nitrogenous wastes: ammonia, creatinine, urea, uric acid Urine pigment: urochrome (product of bilirubin metabolism)	Ketones—generally acetone Protein—generally albumin Glucose Crystals—generally uric acid and phosphate or calcium oxalate Pigments—abnormal levels of bilirubin metabolites
Odor	Slight aromatic Some foods produce a characteristic odor (asparagus) Ammonia-like odor on standing may result from decomposition in stored urine	Strong, sweet, fruity (acetone) odor—uncontrolled diabetes mellitus Foul odor—UTIs Musty odor—phenylketonuria Maple syrup odor—congenital defect in protein metabolism
pH	4.6 to 8.0 (average 6.0) Toward low normal: some foods (meat and cranberries) and drugs (chlorothiazide diuretics) Toward high normal: some foods (citrus fruits, dairy products) and drugs (bicarbonate antacids)	High in alkalosis (kidneys compensate by excreting excess base) Low in acidosis (kidneys compensate by excreting excess H^+)
Specific Gravity	Adult: 1.005 to 1.030 (usually 1.010 to 1.025) Elderly: values decrease with age Newborn: 1.001 to 1.020	Above normal limits: glycosuria, proteinuria, dehydration, high solute load (may result in precipitation of solutes and kidney stone formation) Below normal limits: chronic renal diseases (inability to concentrate urine), overhydration

Urinalysis

The physical, chemical, and microscopic examination of urine is termed **urinalysis**. Like blood, urine is a fluid that reveals much about the function of the body. Changes in the normal characteristics of urine or the appearance of abnormal urine characteristics may be a sign of disease. Table 18-2 lists both the normal and abnormal characteristics of urine.

In clinical and laboratory situations, a standard urinalysis is often referred to as a "routine and microscopic" urinalysis, or simply an "R and M." The "routine" portion is a series of physical and chemical tests, whereas the "microscopic" part refers to the study of urine sediment with a microscope. This series of laboratory tests provides the variety of information often necessary for a physician to make a diagnosis.

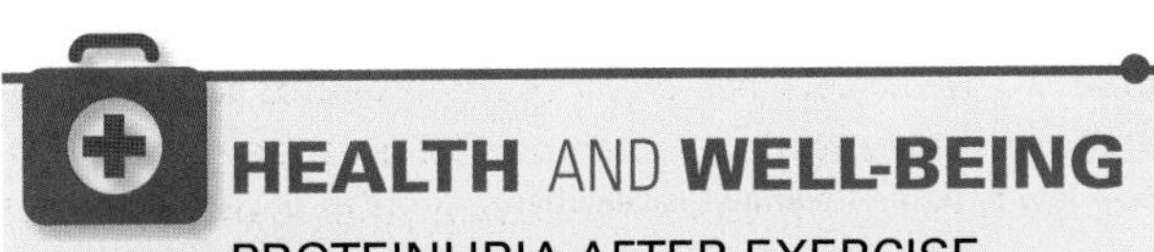

HEALTH AND WELL-BEING

PROTEINURIA AFTER EXERCISE

Proteinuria is the presence of plasma proteins in the urine. Proteinuria is probably the most important indicator of renal disease (**nephropathy**) because only damaged nephrons consistently allow plasma protein molecules to leave the blood. However, intense exercise causes temporary proteinuria in many individuals. Some exercise physiologists believed that intense athletic activities cause kidney damage, but subsequent research has ruled out that explanation. One current hypothesis is that hormonal changes during strenuous exercise increase the permeability of the nephron's filtration membrane, allowing some plasma proteins to enter the filtrate. Some postexercise proteinuria is usually considered normal.

LANGUAGE OF SCIENCE AND MEDICINE *(continued from p. 409)*

continuous ambulatory peritoneal dialysis (CAPD)
(kon-TIN-yoo-us AM-byoo-lah-tor-ee payr-ih-toh-NEE-al dye-AL-ih-sis)
[*ambulat-* **walk,** *-ory* **relating to,** *peritone-* **peritoneum,** *-al* **relating to,** *dia-* **through,** *-lysis* **loosening**]

cortical nephron
(KOHR-tih-kal NEF-ron)
[*cortic-* **bark (cortex),** *-al* **relating to,** *nephro-* **kidney,** *-on* **unit**]

countercurrent mechanism
(KOWN-ter-ker-rent MEK-a-niz-em)
[*counter-* **against,** *-current* **flow**]

cystitis
(sis-TYE-tis)
[*cyst-* **bag,** *-itis* **inflammation**]

distal convoluted tubule (DCT)
(DIS-tal KON-voh-LOO-ted TOO-byool)
[*dist-* **distance,** *-al* **relating to,** *con-* **together,** *-volut-* **roll,** *tub-* **tube,** *-ule* **little**]

diuretic drug
(dye-yoo-RET-ik drug)
[*dia-* **through,** *-ure-* **urine,** *-ic* **relating to**]

emptying reflex
(EMP-tee-ing REE-fleks)
[*re-* **again,** *-flex* **bend**]

enuresis
(en-yoo-REE-sis)
[*en-* **in,** *-uresis* **urinate**]

epidemiologist
(ep-ih-dee-mee-OL-uh-jist)
[*epi-* **upon,** *-dem-* **people,** *-log-* **words (study of),** *-ist* **agent**]

erythropoietin (EPO)
(eh-RITH-roh-POY-eh-tin)
[*erythro-* **red,** *-poiet-* **make,** *-in* **substance**]

filtration
(fil-TRAY-shun)
[*filtr-* **strain,** *-ation* **process**]

glomerular filtrate
(gloh-MAYR-yoo-lar fil-TRAYT)
[*glomer-* **ball,** *-ul-* **little,** *-ar* **relating to,** *filtr-* **strain,** *-ate* **result**]

glomerulus
(gloh-MAYR-yoo-lus)
pl., glomeruli
(gloh-MAYR-yoo-lye)
[*glomer-* **ball,** *-ul-* **little,** *-us* **thing**]

glycosuria
(glye-koh-SOO-ree-ah)
[*glyco-* **sweet (glucose),** *-ur-* **urine,** *-ia* **condition**]

hemodialysis
(hee-moh-dye-AL-ih-sis)
[*hemo-* **blood,** *-dia-* **through or between,** *-lysis* **loosening**]

Henle loop
(HEN-lee loop)
[*Friederich Gustave Henle* **German anatomist**]

hilum
(HYE-lum)
pl., hila
(HYE-lah)
[*hilum* **least bit**]

I & O
(aye and oh)
[*I* **input,** *&* **and,** *O* **output**]

infection control
(in-FEK-shun KON-trol)
[*infect-* **stain,** *-ion* **state**]

juxtaglomerular (JG) apparatus
(juks-tah-gloh-MER-yoo-lar app-ah-RAT-us)
[*juxta-* **near or adjoining,** *-glomer-* **ball,** *-ul-* **little,** *-ar* **relating to,** *apparatus* **tool**]

juxtamedullary nephron
(jux-tah-MED-oo-layr-ee NEF-ron)
[*juxta-* **near or adjoining,** *-medulla-* **middle,** *-ary* **relating to,** *nephro-* **kidney,** *-on* **unit**]

lithotripsy
(LITH-oh-trip-see)
[*litho-* **stone,** *-trips-* **pound,** *-y* **action**]

lithotriptor
(LITH-oh-trip-tor)
[*litho-* **stone,** *-trip-* **pound,** *-or* **agent**]

microbiologist
(my-kroh-bye-OL-uh-jist)
[*micro-* **small,** *-bio-* **life,** *-log-* **words (study of),** *-ist* **agent**]

micturition
(mik-too-RISH-un)
[*mictur-* **urinate,** *-tion* **process**]

nephron
(NEF-ron)
[*nephro-* **kidney,** *-on* **unit**]

nephron loop
(NEF-ron loop)
[*nephro-* **kidney,** *-on* **unit**]

nephropathy
(nef-ROP-ah-thee)
[*nephro-* **kidney,** *-path-* **disease,** *-y* **state**]

neurogenic bladder
(noor-oh-JEN-ik BLAD-der)
[*neuro-* **nerves,** *-gen-* **produce,** *-ic* **relating to,** *bladder* **pimple**]

oliguria
(ol-ih-GYOO-ree-ah)
[*olig-* **few or little,** *-ur-* **urine,** *-ia* **condition**]

polyuria
(pahl-ee-YOO-ree-ah)
[*poly-* **many,** *-ur-* **urine,** *-ia* **condition**]

proteinuria
(pro-teen-YOO-ree-ah)
[*prote-* **first rank,** *-in-* **substance,** *-ur-* **urine,** *-ia* **condition**]

proximal convoluted tubule (PCT)
(PROK-sih-mal KON-voh-LOO-ted TOO-byool)
[*proxima-* **near,** *-al* **relating to,** *con-* **together,** *-volut-* **roll,** *tub-* **tube,** *-ule* **little**]

reabsorption
(ree-ab-SORP-shun)
[*re-* **back again,** *-ab-* **from,** *-sorp-* **suck,** *-tion* **process**]

renal calculi
(REE-nal KAL-kyoo-lye)
sing., calculus
(KAL-kyoo-lus)
[*ren-* **kidney,** *-al* **relating to,** *calc-* **limestone,** *-ul-* **little,** *-i* **things**]

renal colic
(REE-nal KOL-ik)
[*ren-* **kidney,** *-al* **relating to,** *col-* **colon,** *-ic* **relating to**]

renal column
(REE-nall KOL-um)
[*ren-* **kidney,** *-al* **relating to**]

renal corpuscle
(REE-nal KOR-pus-ul)
[*ren-* **kidney,** *-al* **relating to,** *corpus-* **body,** *-cle* **little**]

renal cortex
(REE-nal KOR-teks)
[*ren-* **kidney,** *-al* **relating to,** *cortex* **bark**]

renal medulla
(REE-nal meh-DUL-ah)
[*ren-* **kidney,** *-al* **relating to,** *medulla* **middle**]

renal papilla
(REE-nal pah-PIL-uh)
pl., papillae
(pah-PIL-ee)
[*ren-* **kidney,** *-al* **relating to,** *papilla* **nipple**]

renal pelvis
(REE-nal PEL-vis)
pl., pelves
(PEL-veez)
[*ren-* **kidney,** *-al* **relating to,** *pelvis* **basin**]

renal pyramid
(REE-nal PIR-ah-mid)
[*ren-* **kidney,** *-al* **relating to**]

renal threshold
(REE-nal THRESH-old)
[*ren-* **kidney,** *-al* **relating to**]

renal tubule
(REE-nal TOOB-yool)
[*ren-* **kidney,** *-al* **relating to,** *tub-* **pipe,** *-ule* **small**]

renin
(REE-nin)
[*ren-* **kidney,** *-in* **substance**]

renin-angiotensin-aldosterone system (RAAS)
(REE-nin–an-jee-oh-TEN-sin–al-DAH-stayr-ohn SYS-tem)
[*ren-* **kidney,** *-in* **substance,** *angio-* **vessel,** *-tens-* **pressure or stretch,** *-in* **substance,** *aldo-* **aldehyde,** *-stero-* **solid or steroid derivative,** *-one* **chemical**]

retroperitoneal
(reh-troh-payr-ih-toh-NEE-al)
[*retro-* **backward,** *-peri-* **around,** *-tone-* **stretched,** *-al* **relating to**]

rugae
(ROO-gee)
sing., ruga
[*ruga* **wrinkle**]

secretion
(seh-KREE-shun)
[*secret-* **separate,** *-tion* **process**]

sphincter
(SFINGK-ter)
[*sphinc-* **bind tight,** *-er* **agent**]

trigone
(TRY-gohn)
[*tri-* **three,** *-gon-* **corner**]

uremia (uremic poisoning)
(yoo-REE-mee-ah)
[*ur-* **urine,** *-emia* **blood condition**]

ureter
(YOOR-eh-ter)
[*ure-* **urine,** *-ter* **agent or channel**]

urethra
(yoo-REE-thrah)
[*ure-* **urine,** *-thr-* **agent or channel**]

urinalysis
(yoor-in-AL-is-is)
[*ur-* **urine,** *-in-* **chemical,** *-(an)a-* **apart,** *-lysis* **loosen or break**]

urinary incontinence
(YOOR-ih-nayr-ee in-KON-tih-nens)
[*urin-* **urine,** *-ary* **relating to,** *in-* **without,** *contin-* **contain,** *-ence* **ability**]

urinary meatus
(YOOR-ih-nayr-ee mee-AY-tus)
[*urin-* **urine,** *-ary* **relating to,** *meatus* **passage**]

urinary retention
(YOOR-in-ayr-ee ree-TEN-shun)
[*urin-* **urine,** *-ary* **relating to,** *re-* **back,** *-tenn-* **hold,** *-tion* **condition**]

urinary suppression
(YOOR-in-ayr-ee sup-PRESH-un)
[*urin-* **urine,** *-ary* **relating to,** *sup- (sub-)* **down,** *-press-* **press,** *-ion* **condition**]

urinary system
(YOOR-ih-nayr-ee SYS-tem)
[*urin-* **urine,** *-ary* **relating to**]

urination
(yoor-ih-NAY-shun)
[*urin-* **urine,** *-ation* **process**]

voiding
(VOYD-ing)
[*void-* **empty,** *-ing* **action**]

❑ OUTLINE SUMMARY

To download a digital audio version of the chapter summary for use with your device, access the ***Audio Chapter Summaries*** *online at evolve.elsevier.com.*

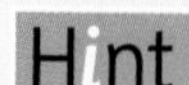

Scan this summary after reading the chapter to help you reinforce the key concepts. Later, use the summary as a quick review before your class or before a test.

Kidneys

A. Location — under back muscles, behind parietal peritoneum, just above waistline; right kidney usually a little lower than left (see **Figure 18-1**)
B. Gross structure (see **Figure 18-2**)
   1. External anatomy
      a. Kidney resembles a lima bean that is 11 cm × 7 cm × 3 cm

b. Hilum — medial indentation where vessels, nerves, ureter connect
c. Capsule — fibrous outer wall
2. Internal anatomy
a. Cortex — outer layer of kidney substance
b. Medulla — inner portion of kidney
c. Pyramids — triangular divisions of medulla
d. Papilla — narrow, innermost end of pyramid
e. Pelvis — expansion of upper end of ureter; lies inside kidney
f. Calyces — divisions of renal pelvis

C. Microscopic structure of the kidney
1. Interior of kidney composed of more than 1 million microscopic nephron units (see **Figure 18-3**)
a. Unique shape of nephron well suited to function
b. Principal components are renal corpuscle and renal tubule
2. Renal corpuscle (see **Figure 18-4**)
a. Bowman capsule — cup-shaped top of nephron
b. Glomerulus — network of blood capillaries surrounded by Bowman capsule
3. Renal tubule (see **Figure 18-5**)
a. Proximal convoluted tubule (PCT) — first segment
b. Nephron loop (Henle loop) — extension of proximal tubule; consists of descending limb, loop, and ascending limb
c. Distal convoluted tubule (DCT) — extension of ascending limb of nephron loop
d. Collecting duct (CD) — straight extension of distal tubule
4. Location of nephrons
a. Cortical nephrons — 85% of total; located mostly in renal cortex
b. Juxtamedullary nephrons — have important role in concentrating urine; located near junction between cortex and medullary layers

D. Kidney function
1. Excrete toxins and nitrogenous wastes
2. Regulate levels of many chemicals in blood
3. Maintain water balance
4. Help regulate blood pressure and volume
5. Regulate red blood cell production by secreting erythropoietin (EPO)

Formation of Urine

A. Millions of nephrons balance blood and flush the excess/wastes as urine in a process that includes three functions: filtration, reabsorption, and secretion (see **Figure 18-6** and **Table 18-1**)

B. Filtration
1. Goes on continually in renal corpuscles
2. Glomerular blood pressure causes water and dissolved substances to filter out of glomeruli into the Bowman capsule
3. Normal glomerular filtration rate 125 mL per minute

C. Reabsorption
1. Movement of substances out of renal tubules into blood in peritubular capillaries
2. Water, nutrients, and ions are reabsorbed (see **Figure 18-7**)
3. Water is reabsorbed by osmosis from proximal tubules
4. Countercurrent mechanisms in the nephron loop and surrounding peritubular capillaries concentrate sodium and chloride to make the renal medulla hypertonic, which helps concentrate urine (see *Control of Urine Volume* below).
5. All glucose is reabsorbed along with sodium, assuming there are enough sodium-glucose transporters to accommodate all the glucose (see **Figure 18-8**)
6. Transport maximum — largest amount of substance that can be reabsorbed at one time
a. Determined by the number of available transporters of the substance
b. Determines the renal threshold — the amount of substance above which the kidney removes the substance from the blood

D. Secretion
1. Movement of substances into urine in the distal and collecting ducts from blood in peritubular capillaries
2. Hydrogen ions, potassium ions, and certain drugs are secreted by active transport
3. Ammonia is secreted by diffusion

Control of Urine Volume

A. Antidiuretic hormone (ADH) — secreted by posterior pituitary; promotes water reabsorption by collecting ducts; reduces urine volume

B. Hypertonic (salty) medulla helps ADH concentrate urine and thus conserve the body's water

C. Aldosterone — secreted by adrenal gland, triggered by the renin-angiotensin-aldosterone system (RAAS) process; promotes sodium and water reabsorption in nephron; reduces urine volume (see **Figure 18-9**)

D. Atrial natriuretic hormone (ANH) — one of the peptide hormones (ANPs) secreted by atrial cells in heart; promotes loss of sodium and water into kidney tubules; increases urine volume

E. Abnormalities of urine volume
1. Anuria — absence of urine
2. Oliguria — scanty amount of urine
3. Polyuria — unusually large amount of urine

Elimination of Urine

A. Ureters (see **Figure 18-10**)
1. Structure — narrow, long tubes with expanded upper end (renal pelvis) located inside kidney and lined with mucous membrane
2. Function — drain urine from renal pelvis to urinary bladder

B. Bladder
  1. Structure (see **Figure 18-11**)
    a. Elastic muscular organ, capable of great expansion
    b. Lined with mucous membrane arranged in rugae, as is stomach mucosa
  2. Functions
    a. Storage of urine before voiding
    b. Voiding
  3. Cystitis — bladder infection
C. Urethra
  1. Structure (see **Figure 18-11**)
    a. Narrow tube from urinary bladder to exterior
    b. Lined with mucous membrane
    c. Opening of urethra to the exterior called *urinary meatus*
  2. Functions
    a. Passage of urine from bladder to exterior of the body
    b. Passage of male reproductive fluid (semen) from the body
D. Micturition
  1. Passage of urine from body (also called *urination* or *voiding*)
  2. Regulatory sphincters
    a. Internal urethral sphincter (involuntary)
    b. External urethral sphincter (voluntary)
  3. Bladder wall permits storage of urine with little increase in pressure
  4. Emptying reflex
    a. Initiated by stretch reflex in bladder wall
    b. Bladder wall contracts
    c. Internal sphincter relaxes
    d. External sphincter relaxes and urination occurs
    e. Enuresis — involuntary urination in young child
  5. Urinary retention — urine produced but not voided
  6. Urinary suppression — no urine produced but bladder is normal
  7. Urinary incontinence (enuresis) — urine is voided involuntarily
    a. Urge incontinence — associated with smooth muscle overactivity in the bladder wall
    b. Stress incontinence — associated with weakened pelvic floor muscles
    c. Overflow incontinence — associated with urinary retention and overdistended bladder
    d. Reflex incontinence occurs in absence of any sensory warning or awareness — common following a stroke or spinal cord injury
    e. Nocturnal enuresis — nighttime bed wetting
    f. Neurogenic bladder — periodic but unpredictable voiding; related to paralysis or abnormal function of the bladder

Urinalysis

A. Examination of the physical, chemical, and microscopic characteristics of urine (see **Table 18-2**)
B. May help determine the presence and nature of a pathologic condition

❑ ACTIVE LEARNING

STUDY TIPS

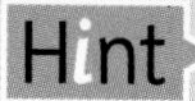

Use these tips to achieve success in meeting your learning goals.

To make the study of the urinary system more efficient, we suggest these tips:

1. Before studying Chapter 18, review filtration in Chapter 3, transitional epithelium in Chapter 4, and the synopsis of the urinary system in Chapter 5.
2. Think of the urinary system as a key homeostatic regulatory system involving formation and excretion of urine, regulation of body fluids, electrolytes, pH, blood pressure, and red blood cell (RBC) formation.
3. Use flash cards to learn the names, locations, and functions of the organs and internal structures of the kidney and the microscopic structures of the nephron. Refer often to appropriate text illustrations.
4. In discussing the segments of the renal tubule, remember that the directional terms *proximal* and *distal* refer to how far away these structures are from the Bowman capsule.
5. The formation of urine involves three processes: filtration, reabsorption, and secretion. It begins with filtration of water and solutes from blood plasma resulting in formation of glomerular filtrate, which then passes through the tubular portion of the nephron to become urine. Reabsorption means taking material out of the tubular fluid and returning it to the blood. Secretion means taking material out of the blood and putting it into the urine.
6. In your study group, discuss how urine volume is controlled by three hormones, each produced in a different organ and regulating volume in a different way. Use flash cards with the name of the hormone, where it is made, its mechanism of action, and its effect on urine volume. Review the process of micturition.
7. Always answer Quick Check questions. Go over the questions at the back of the chapter and discuss possible test questions in your study group.

Review Questions

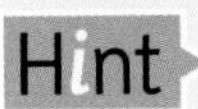

Write out the answers to these questions after reading the chapter and reviewing the Chapter Summary. If you simply think through the answer without writing it down, you won't retain much of your new learning.

1. Describe the location of the kidneys.
2. Name and describe the internal structures of the kidneys.
3. Define *filtration, reabsorption,* and *secretion* as they apply to kidney function.
4. Briefly explain the formation of urine.
5. Name several substances eliminated or regulated by the kidney.
6. Explain the function of the juxtaglomerular apparatus.
7. Describe the structure of the ureters.
8. Describe the structure of the bladder and include the area of the trigone.
9. Describe the structure of the urethra.
10. Briefly describe the process of micturition.
11. Differentiate between retention and suppression of urine.
12. Define incontinence and describe three types of incontinence.

Critical Thinking

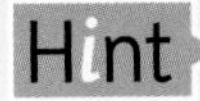

After finishing the Review Questions, write out the answers to these more in-depth questions to help you apply your new knowledge. Go back to sections of the chapter that relate to concepts that you find difficult.

13. Explain how salt and water balance are maintained by aldosterone and ADH.
14. Explain why proper blood pressure is necessary for proper kidney function.
15. If a person were doing strenuous work on a hot day and perspiring heavily, would there be a great deal of ADH in the blood or very little? Explain your answer.

Chapter Test

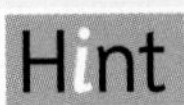

After studying the chapter, test your mastery by responding to these items. Try to answer them without looking up the answers. Then, verify the answers using the key in Appendix C at the back of this book.

1. The kidneys receive about ______% of the total amount of blood pumped by the heart each minute.
2. The renal corpuscle is made up of two structures: ______
3. The two parts of the renal tubules that extend into the medulla of the kidney are the ______
4. The two parts of the renal tubules that are in the cortex of the kidney are the ______
5. The process of ______ is the movement of substances out of the renal tubules and into the blood capillaries.
6. The process of ______ causes substances in the blood to be pushed into the Bowman capsule as a result of blood pressure in the glomerulus.
7. The process of ______ is the movement of substances from the blood into the distal tubule or the collecting tube.
8. The hormone ______ is released from the posterior pituitary gland and reduces the amount of water lost in the urine.
9. The hormone ______ is made by the heart and stimulates the tubules to secrete sodium.
10. The hormone ______ is made in the adrenal cortex and causes the tubules to absorb sodium.
11. The involuntary muscle ______ is at the exit of the bladder.
12. ______ is a condition in which the bladder is able to empty itself but no urine is being produced by the kidneys.
13. ______ is a condition in which a person voids urine involuntarily.
14. ______ is a condition in which the bladder is full and the kidney is producing urine but the bladder is unable to empty itself.

Match each descriptive phrase in Column B with its corresponding term in Column A.

Column A	Column B
15. ______ cortex	a. inner layer of the kidney
16. ______ medulla	b. expansion of the ureter in the kidney
17. ______ pyramids	c. cup-shaped part of the nephron that catches the filtrate
18. ______ renal pelvis	d. tube leading from the bladder to outside the body
19. ______ urethra	e. network of capillaries in the Bowman capsule
20. ______ bladder	f. saclike structure used to hold urine until it is voided
21. ______ ureter	g. outer part of the kidney
22. ______ trigone	h. an area of the bladder that has openings for the two ureters and the urethra
23. ______ Bowman capsule	i. the part of the renal tubules that is located between the proximal and distal tubules
24. ______ glomerulus	j. tube connecting the kidney and bladder
25. ______ nephron loop	k. the triangular divisions in the medulla of the kidney

Fluid and Electrolyte Balance

OUTLINE

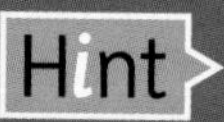

Scan this outline before you begin to read the chapter, as a preview of how the concepts are organized.

OBJECTIVES

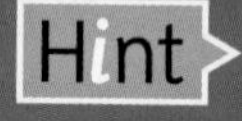

Before reading the chapter, review these goals for your learning.

After you have completed this chapter, you should be able to:

1. List, describe, and compare the body fluid compartments and their subdivisions.
2. Discuss avenues by which water enters and leaves the body and the forces that move fluids into and out of the blood.
3. Explain the mechanisms used by the body to maintain fluid balance.
4. Discuss the nature and importance of electrolytes in body fluids.
5. Describe examples of common fluid and electrolyte imbalances.

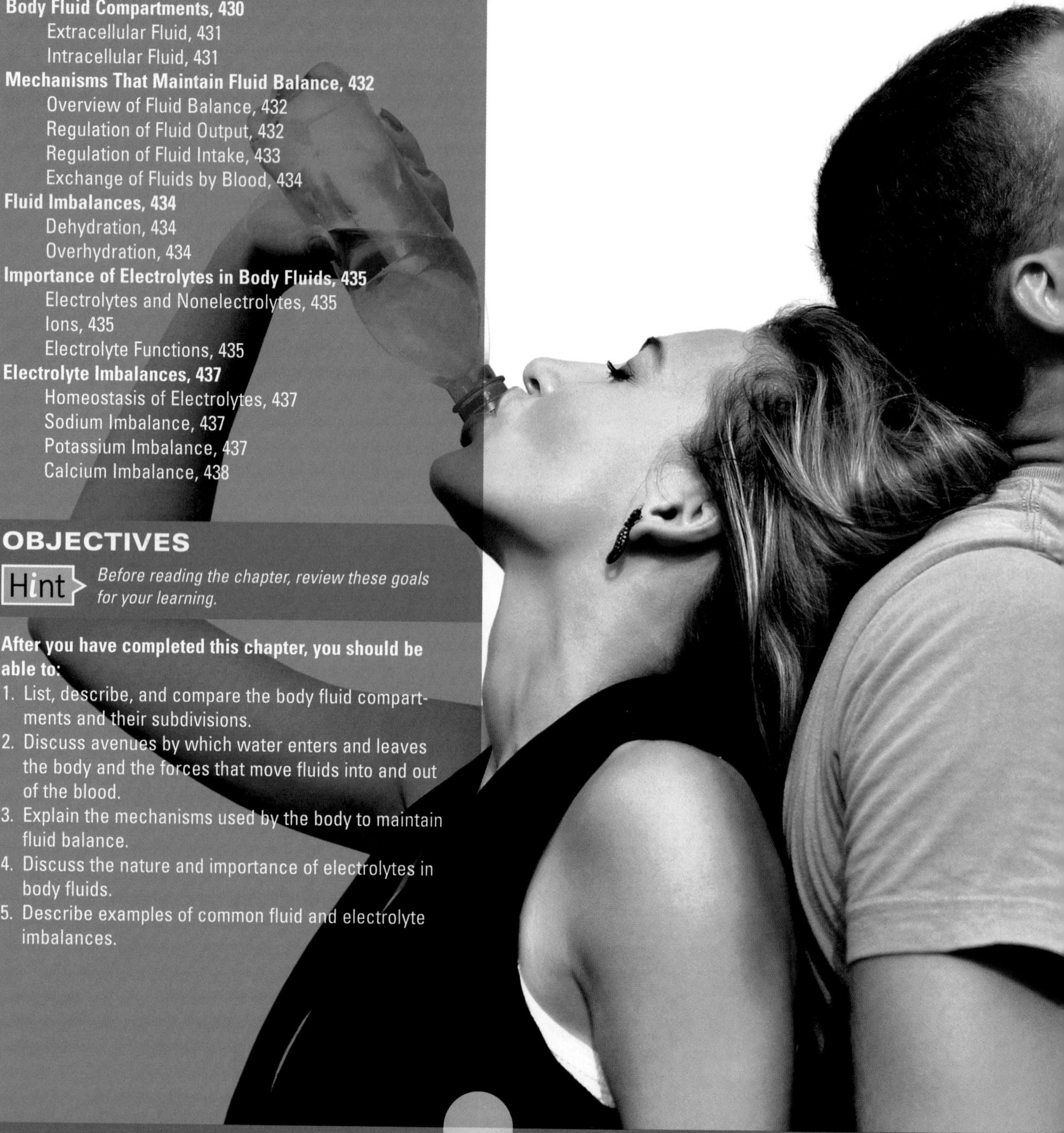

CHAPTER 19

Have you ever wondered why you sometimes excrete great volumes of urine and at other times excrete almost none at all? Why sometimes you feel so thirsty that you can hardly get enough to drink and other times you want no liquids at all? These conditions and many more relate to one of the body's most important functions—that of maintaining its *fluid and electrolyte balance.*

The phrase **fluid balance** implies homeostasis, or relative constancy of body fluid levels—a condition required for healthy survival. It means that both the total volume and distribution of water in the body remain normal and relatively constant. Body "input" or intake of water must be balanced by "output." If water in excess of requirements enters the body, it must be eliminated, and, if excess losses occur, prompt replacement is critical. Because fluid balance refers to normal homeostasis, *fluid imbalance* means that the total volume of water in the body or the amounts in one or more of its fluid compartments have increased or decreased beyond normal limits.

Electrolytes are substances such as salts that dissolve or break apart in water solution to form electrically charged atoms (or groups of atoms) called **ions. Electrolyte balance** refers to homeostasis or relative constancy of normal electrolyte levels in the body fluids. The various types of body fluids serve differing functions in different areas of the body. To do so, each type of body fluid must maintain differing levels and types of electrolytes within a very narrow range of normal. For example, blood, lymph, intracellular fluid, interstitial fluid, cerebrospinal fluid, and joint and eye fluids all depend on complex homeostatic mechanisms to adjust and maintain normal levels of appropriate electrolytes required for that particular type of body fluid to function as it should.

LANGUAGE OF **SCIENCE** AND **MEDICINE**

Hint Before reading the chapter, say each of these terms out loud. This will help you to avoid stumbling over them as you read.

anion
(AN-aye-on)
[*ana-* **up,** *-ion* **to go (ion)**]

cation
(KAT-aye-on)
[*cat-* **down,** *-ion* **to go (ion)**]

dehydration
(dee-hye-DRAY-shun)
[*de-* **remove,** *-hydro* **water,** *-ation* **process**]

dissociate
(dih-SOH-see-ayt)
[*dis-* **apart,** *-socia-* **unite,** *-ate* **action**]

diuretic
(dye-yoo-RET-ik)
[*dia-* **through,** *-ure-* **urine,** *-ic* **relating to**]

edema
(eh-DEE-mah)
[*edema* **a swelling**]

electrolyte
(eh-LEK-troh-lyte)
[*electro-* **electricity,** *-lyt-* **loosening**]

electrolyte balance
(eh-LEK-troh-lyte BAL-ans)
[*electro-* **electricity,** *-lyt-* **loosening**]

extracellular fluid (ECF)
(eks-trah-SELL-yoo-lar FLOO-id)
[*extra-* **outside,** *-cell-* **storeroom,** *-ular* **relating to**]

fluid balance
(FLOO-id BAL-ans)

fluid compartment
(FLOO-id kom-PART-ment)

hypercalcemia
(hye-per-kal-SEE-mee-ah)
[*hyper-* **excessive,** *-calc-* **lime (calcium),** *-emia* **blood condition**]

Continued on p. 439

Health and sometimes even survival itself depend on maintaining the proper volume and distribution of body water and the appropriate levels and types of electrolytes within it.

In this chapter you will find a discussion of body fluids and electrolytes, their normal values, the mechanisms that operate to keep them normal, and some of the more common types of fluid and electrolyte imbalances.

Body Fluid Volumes

Of the hundreds of compounds present in your body, the most abundant is water. Medical reference tables often refer to "average" fluid volumes based on healthy nonobese young adults. In such tables, males weighing 70 kg (154 pounds) will have on average about 60% of their body weight, nearly 40 L, as water (**Figure 19-1**). Young females average about 50% water.

The reason fluid volume values in reference tables are based on nonobese individuals is that adipose, or fat tissue, contains the least amount of water of any body tissue. The more fat present in the body, the less the total water content per kilogram of body weight. Therefore, regardless of age, obese individuals, with their high body fat content, have less body water per kilogram of weight than slender people.

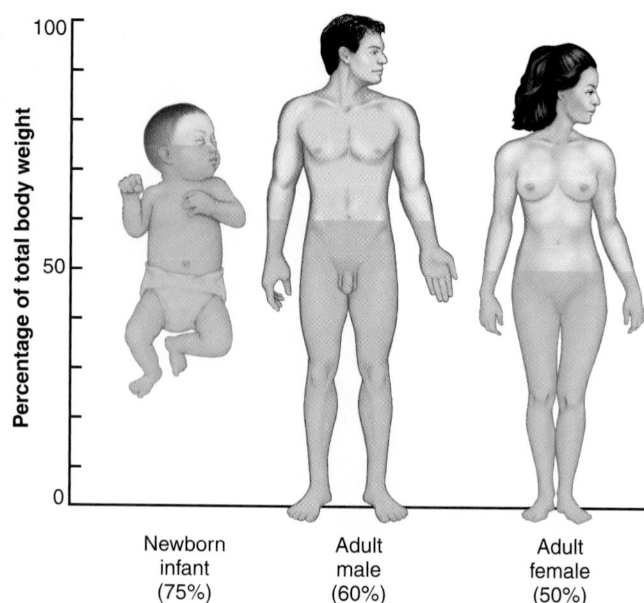

FIGURE 19-2 Water in the body. Proportion of body weight typically made up of water in infants, adult males, and adult females.

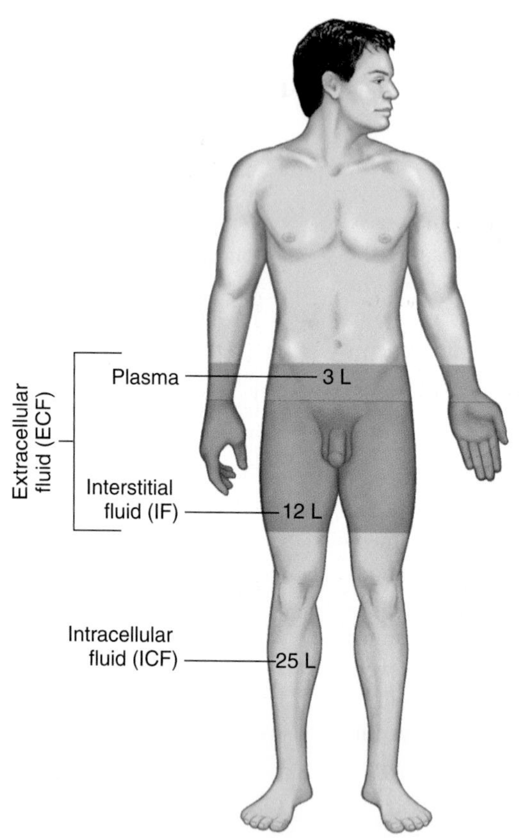

FIGURE 19-1 Relative volumes of three body fluids. Values represent typical fluid distribution in a young adult male.

Although a nonobese male body typically consists of about 60% water, an obese male may consist of only 50% water or even less. The female body contains slightly less water per kilogram of weight because on average it contains slightly more fat than the male body.

Note in **Figure 19-2** that age, as well as gender, influences the amount of water in the body. Remember that body fluids are not all in a single, continuous space in the body—but often function as if they are.

Infants have more water as compared with body weight than adults of either sex. In a newborn, water may account for up to 80% of total body weight. The percentage of water is even higher in premature infants. The need for a high water content in the early stages of life is the reason fluid imbalances in infants caused by diarrhea, for example, can be so serious.

The percentage of body water decreases rapidly during the first 10 years of life. By adolescence, adult values are reached and gender differences, which account for about a 10% variation in body fluid volumes between the sexes, have developed.

In elderly individuals, the amount of water per kilogram of body weight decreases. One reason is that old age is often accompanied by a decrease in muscle mass (65% water) and an increase in fat (20% water). Certain drugs or toxins may have more potent effects in the elderly because they become more concentrated in the smaller volume of water present in the bodies of some elderly people. Of course, such drugs or toxins may have a reduced effect when diluted in the relatively larger amount of water in a young person's body. In both cases, the key factor is the percentage of body weight represented by water.

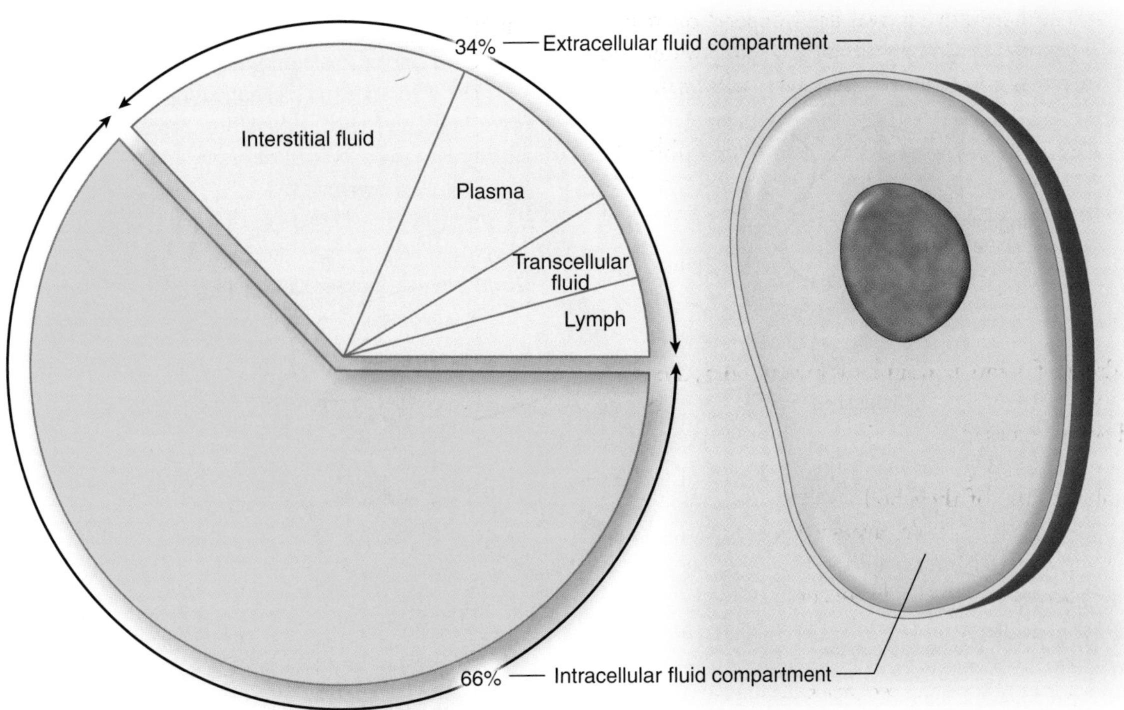

FIGURE 19-3 Distribution of total body water. The fluids of the body are separated by membranes into functional "compartments" of the body. The intracellular fluid (ICF) compartment includes all the fluids inside all the cells of the body. The extracellular fluid (ECF) compartment includes the interstitial fluid (IF) between cells of most tissues and the plasma of the blood tissue. ECF also includes lymph and transcellular fluids.

Body Fluid Compartments

For the sake of discussion, the fluids of the body are thought of as being contained in theoretical "compartments." Each of these **fluid compartments** is actually a group of separated spaces in the body that in many ways function as if they are all in one compartment. Using this concept, total body fluid can be subdivided into two major fluid compartments called the *extracellular* and the *intracellular* fluid compartments. You can see the major fluid compartments illustrated in **Figure 19-3**.

TABLE **19-1** Volumes of Body Fluid Compartments*

BODY FLUID	INFANT	ADULT MALE	ADULT FEMALE
Extracellular Fluid			
Plasma	4	4	4
Interstitial fluid, lymph, and transcellular fluids	26	16	11
Intracellular Fluid	45	40	35
Total	75	60	50

*Percentage of body weight. Compare with volume in liters in **Figure 19-1** and percentage of total body water in **Figure 19-3**.

Extracellular Fluid

Extracellular fluid (ECF) consists mainly of the liquid part of whole blood called the **plasma,** found in the blood vessels, and the **interstitial fluid** (IF) that surrounds the cells.

In addition, a smaller volume of *lymph* and **transcellular fluids** are part of the extracellular fluid compartment. Transcellular fluids include cerebrospinal fluid (CSF), fluids of the eyeball, and the synovial joint fluids.

Table 19-1 lists typical percentage of body weight values for the extracellular fluid compartments. **Figure 19-3** shows the distribution of fluids in the extracellular fluid compartment as a percentage of total body water.

Intracellular Fluid

The term **intracellular fluid** (ICF) refers to the largest volume of body fluid by far. It is located inside all the cells of the body. Water has many functions inside the cell but mainly serves as a solvent in which important chemical reactions of the cell can occur.

QUICK CHECK

1. What are electrolytes?
2. What are the two main fluid compartments of the body?
3. What is meant by the term *fluid balance?*

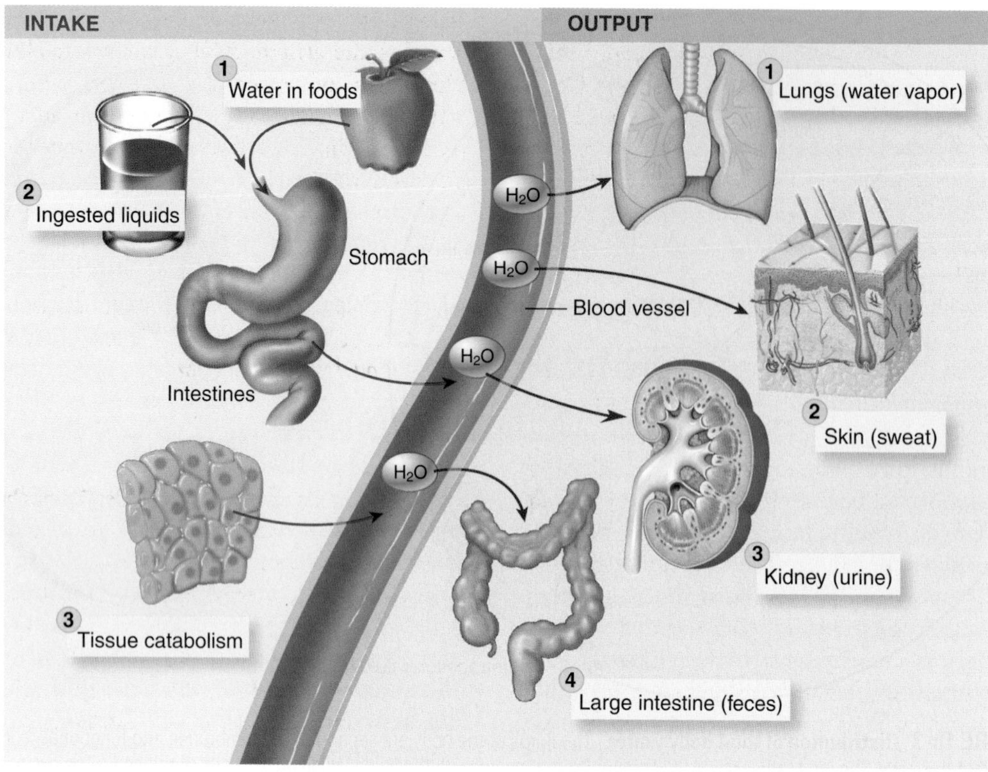

FIGURE 19-4 Fluid balance. Primary mechanisms of fluid intake and fluid output by the body.

Mechanisms That Maintain Fluid Balance

Overview of Fluid Balance

Under normal conditions, homeostasis of the total volume of water in the body is maintained or restored primarily by devices that adjust output (by adjusting urine volume) to intake and secondarily by mechanisms that adjust fluid intake. There is no question about which of the two mechanisms is more important—the body's chief mechanism, by far, for maintaining fluid balance is that of adjusting its fluid output so that it equals its fluid intake.

Obviously, as long as output and intake are equal, the total amount of water in the body does not change. **Figure 19-4** shows the three main sources of fluid intake:

1. Liquids we drink
2. Water in the foods we eat
3. Water formed by catabolism of nutrients (cellular respiration)

We also see in **Figure 19-4** the main avenues of water output by the body:

1. Water vapor lost when we exhale
2. Sweat that evaporates from the skin
3. Urine output by the kidney
4. Water lost in the feces

Table 19-2 gives the normal volumes of each avenue of water intake and output. However, these can vary a great deal and still be considered normal.

A number of factors act as mechanisms for balancing plasma, IF, and ICF volumes. The three main factors are as follows:

1. Regulating fluid output
2. Regulating fluid intake
3. Exchanging fluids between compartments and from place to place within the body

Regulation of Fluid Output

Table 19-2 also indicates that fluid output from the body occurs through four organs: the kidneys, lungs, skin, and intestines.

The fluid output that fluctuates the most is that excreted from the kidneys. The body maintains fluid balance mainly by

TABLE 19-2 Typical Daily Water Intake and Output

INTAKE	AMOUNT*	OUTPUT	AMOUNT*
Water in foods	700 mL	Lungs (water in expired air)	350 mL
Ingested liquids	1500 mL	Skin	
Water formed by catabolism	200 mL	By diffusion	350 mL
		By sweat	100 mL
		Kidneys (urine)	1400 mL
		Intestines (in feces)	200 mL
Typical Daily Totals	**2400 mL**		**2400 mL**

*Amounts vary widely.

changing the volume of urine excreted to match changes in the volume of fluid intake. Everyone knows this from experience. The more liquid one drinks, the more urine one excretes. Conversely, the less the fluid intake, the less the urine volume. How changes in urine volume come about was discussed on p. 418. This would be a good time to review those paragraphs.

It is important to remember from your study of the urinary system that the rate of water and salt reabsorption from the renal tubules is the most important factor in determining urine volume. Urine volume is regulated chiefly by hormones that affect kidney tubule function.

Antidiuretic hormone (ADH) release from the posterior pituitary increases as the ECF volume of the body decreases below normal. In Chapter 11, we learned that ADH promotes water reabsorption from the kidney tubule back into the blood. This reduces urine volume by retaining more water in the body. Thus, ADH reduces water output from the body.

Aldosterone from the adrenal cortex works with ADH to reduce water output even further. Aldosterone increases Na^+ reabsorption from the kidney tubules. Because water follows sodium, water reabsorption into the blood also increases. Thus the body retains water that would otherwise be lost in the urine. Thus we see that ADH and aldosterone are water-conserving hormones.

Figure 19-5 traces the aldosterone mechanism in more detail. Begin in the upper right of the diagram and follow, in sequence, each step to see how the aldosterone mechanism helps maintain a constant volume of ECF in the body.

Atrial natriuretic hormone (ANH) from the atrial wall of the heart, on the other hand, increases urine volume. ANH is released when blood volume is higher than normal, which stretches the atrium. ANH promotes sodium loss from the blood into kidney tubules. Because water follows sodium, water is also lost from the blood—thus increasing loss of water in the urine. Therefore, ANH is a water-loss hormone—or *diuretic* hormone.

Please review hormonal control of urine volume in Chapter 18 (p. 418).

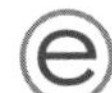
To learn more about the aldosterone regulation mechanism, go to AnimationDirect at *evolve.elsevier.com*.

Regulation of Fluid Intake

Physiologists disagree about the details of the mechanism for controlling and regulating fluid intake to compensate for factors that would lead to dehydration.

In general the mechanism for regulating fluid intake appears to operate in the following ways. When dehydration starts to develop—that is, when fluid loss from the body exceeds fluid intake—changes occur in the ECF. The ECF volume decreases and the solute concentration (osmotic pressure) of the ECF increases.

Sensory receptors in the brain and elsewhere in the body detect the change in the volume and concentration of extracellular fluids caused by dehydration. They relay this information to the thirst centers of the hypothalamus. Signals from the hypothalamus cause water conservation throughout the body, including a decrease in salivary secretion. Decreased salivation produces a "dry-mouth feeling" that enhances a feeling of thirst. The dry mouth causes a person to "feel thirsty" and to drink water. Drinking water increases fluid intake and thereby compensates for previous fluid losses. This tends to restore fluid balance (**Figure 19-6**).

If an individual takes nothing by mouth for days, can his fluid output decrease to zero? The answer—no—becomes obvious after reviewing the information in **Table 19-2**. Despite every effort of homeostatic mechanisms to compensate for zero intake, some output (loss) of fluid occurs as

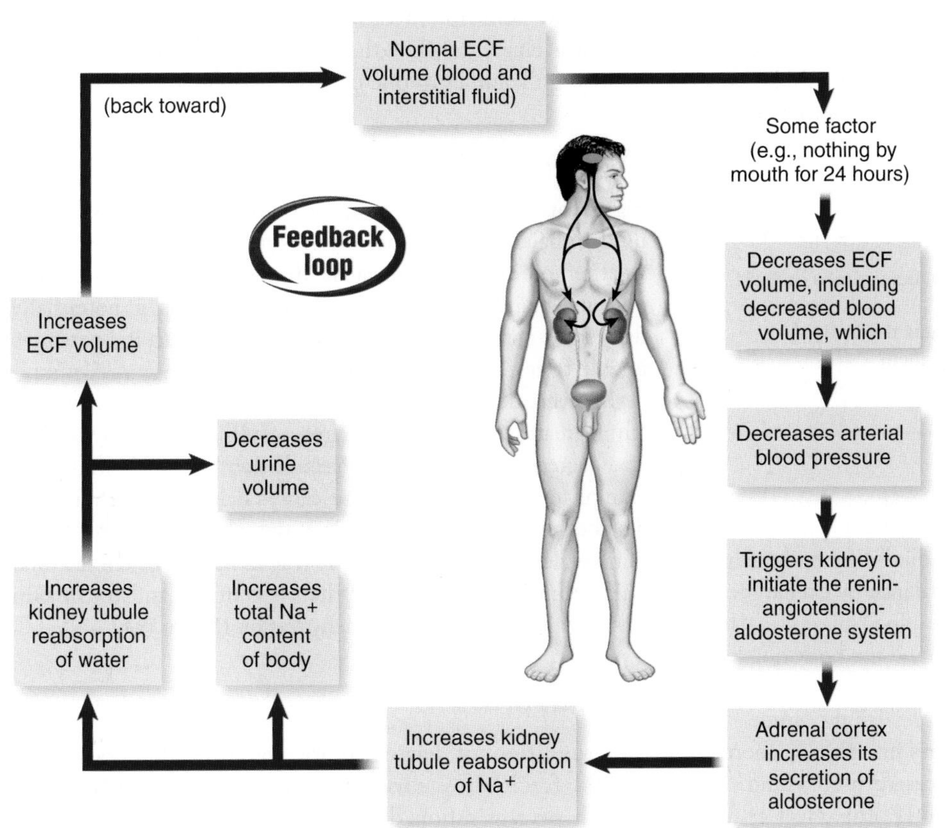

FIGURE 19-5 Aldosterone mechanism. Aldosterone restores normal extracellular fluid (ECF) volume when such levels decrease below normal. Excess aldosterone, however, leads to excess ECF volume—that is, excess blood volume (hypervolemia) and excess interstitial fluid volume (edema)—and also leads to an excess of the total Na^+ content of the body.

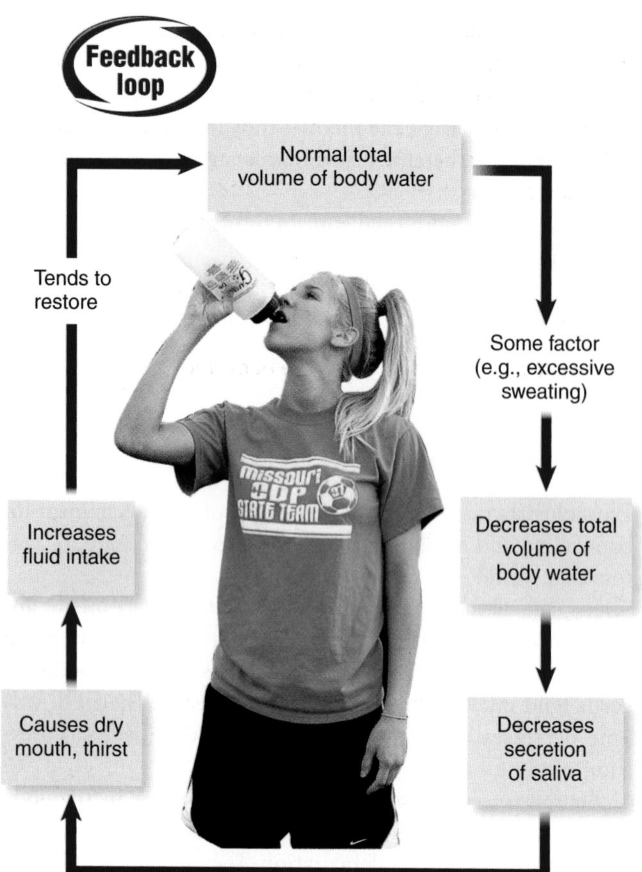

Feedback loop
Normal total volume of body water
Some factor (e.g., excessive sweating)
Decreases total volume of body water
Decreases secretion of saliva
Causes dry mouth, thirst
Increases fluid intake
Tends to restore

FIGURE 19-6 Homeostasis of the total volume of body water. A basic mechanism for adjusting intake to compensate for excess output of body fluid is diagrammed here.

long as life continues. Water is continually lost from the body through expired air and diffusion through skin.

Although the body adjusts fluid intake, factors that adjust fluid output, such as electrolytes and blood proteins, are far more important.

QUICK CHECK

1. Which does the body primarily adjust, fluid *intake* or fluid *output?*
2. What are the chief ways that fluid leaves the body?
3. How does the body maintain fluid balance?
4. What hormones regulate urine volume?
5. What mechanism regulates fluid intake?

Exchange of Fluids by Blood

Besides regulating intake and output of fluids, the body helps maintain a constancy of internal fluid balance by exchanging fluids between fluid compartments. The blood plasma is the mobile medium that can move fluids around the body quickly to "even out" any local fluid imbalances.

Capillary blood pressure is a "water-pushing" force. It pushes fluid out of the blood in capillaries into the IF. Therefore if capillary blood pressure increases, more fluid is pushed—filtered—out of blood into the IF. The effect of an increase in capillary blood pressure, then, is to transfer fluid from blood to IF. In turn, this *fluid shift,* as it is called, changes blood and IF volumes. It decreases blood volume by increasing IF volume. If, on the other hand, capillary blood pressure decreases, less fluid filters out of blood into IF.

Water continually moves in both directions through the membranous walls of capillaries. The amount that moves out of capillary blood into IF depends largely on capillary blood pressure, a water-pushing force. The amount that moves in the opposite direction (that is, into blood from IF) depends largely on the concentration of proteins in blood plasma. Review Figure 13-15 on p. 296 to refresh your knowledge of these forces.

Plasma proteins contribute to osmotic pressure and thereby act as a water-pulling or water-holding force. They hold water in the blood and can pull additional water into the blood from IF. If, for example, the concentration of proteins in blood decreases appreciably—as in protein deficiency—less water moves into blood from IF by osmosis (see Figure 3-8 on p. 50). As a result, blood volume decreases and IF volume increases—causing edema.

Of the three main body fluids, IF volume varies the most. Plasma volume usually fluctuates only slightly and briefly. If a pronounced change in its volume occurs, adequate circulation cannot be maintained.

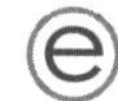
To learn more about fluid shift, go to AnimationDirect at *evolve.elsevier.com.*

Fluid Imbalances

Fluid imbalances are common ailments. They take several forms and stem from a variety of causes, but they all share a common characteristic—that of abnormally low or abnormally high volumes of one or more body fluids.

Dehydration

Significant loss of water from the body, or **dehydration,** is the fluid imbalance seen most often. Figure 19-7 shows how hot weather or exercise can cause dramatic increases in water output—mainly by sweating. Dehydration is a potentially dangerous condition that can soon lead to death if a person is unable to restore the body's fluid volume.

In severe dehydration, IF volume decreases first, but eventually, if treatment has not been given, ICF and plasma volumes also decrease below normal levels. Either too small a fluid intake or too large a fluid output causes dehydration. Prolonged diarrhea or vomiting may result in dehydration due to the loss of body fluids. This is particularly true in infants where the total fluid volume is much smaller than it is in adults. Loss of skin elasticity is a clinical sign of dehydration (Figure 19-8).

Overhydration

The condition of having more water in the body than needed for healthy survival is called **overhydration.** Although overhydration does occur, it is less common than

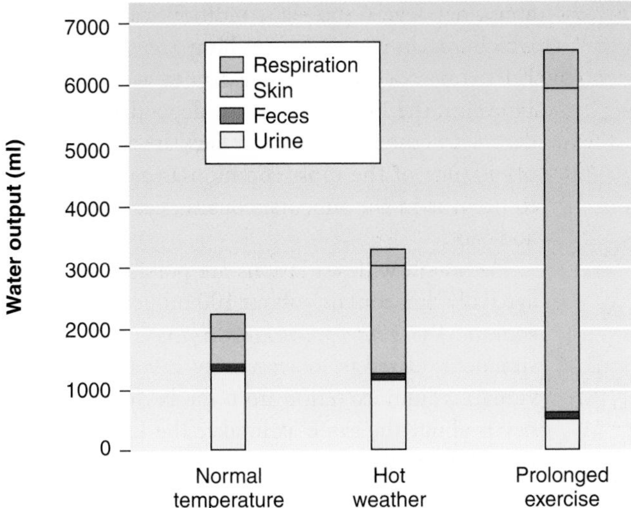

FIGURE 19-7 Water output by the body under varying conditions. Note that water loss from sweating (from the skin) increases total water loss by the body when the weather is hot and during prolonged exercise.

dehydration—and is usually counteracted by a rapid loss of water in the urine.

One grave danger of giving intravenous fluids too rapidly or in too large of an amount is overhydration, which can put too heavy a burden on the heart by increasing the volume of blood to be pumped.

Water intoxication may result from rapidly drinking large volumes of water or giving hypotonic solutions to persons unable to dilute and excrete urine normally. This may occur in patients with kidney insufficiency or abnormal "thirst" mechanisms resulting from neurological disorders. Water content is elevated, and plasma sodium levels are diluted. Development of mental changes such as confusion and lethargy occur. If intoxication is severe, stupor, seizures, and coma may result. Correction of the neurological impairment along with water restriction can reverse the symptoms.

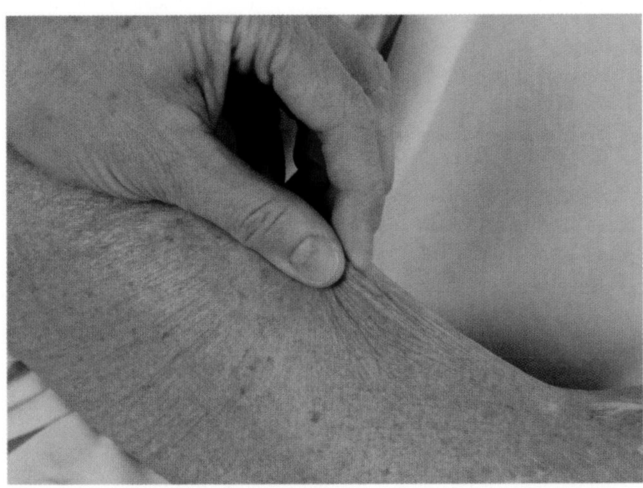

FIGURE 19-8 Testing for dehydration. Loss of skin elasticity is a sign of dehydration. Skin that does not return quickly to its normal shape after being pinched (or tented) indicates interstitial water loss.

Water intoxication can happen in normal individuals if water intake is so rapid that the urinary mechanisms of water loss cannot keep up. Although this is unusual, it can happen—as witnessed by millions a few years ago when a radio station held a "water drinking race" on the air and a contestant died from the effects of severe water intoxication.

QUICK CHECK

1. How does an increase in capillary blood pressure cause fluid to move into the IF?
2. How do plasma proteins affect fluid balance?
3. What conditions might produce dehydration?

Importance of Electrolytes in Body Fluids

Electrolytes and Nonelectrolytes

The bonds that hold together the molecules of certain organic substances such as glucose are such that they do not permit the compound to break up, or **dissociate,** in water solution. Such compounds are called **nonelectrolytes.** Crystals such as ordinary table salt (sodium chloride, NaCl) that have *ionic bonds* permitting them to break up, or dissociate, in water solution into separate particles (Na^+ and Cl^-) are **electrolytes.**

Ions

The dissociated particles of an electrolyte are called **ions** and carry either a positive or negative electrical charge. As a group, all positively charged ions, such as Na^+, are called **cations.** All negatively charged ions, such as Cl^-, are called **anions.** Each of the body fluid compartments contains differing levels of many important ions—both positively charged cations and negatively charged anions. The dissociated ions are themselves often called *electrolytes.*

Important cations include sodium (Na^+), calcium (Ca^{++}), potassium (K^+), and magnesium (Mg^{++}). Important anions include chloride (Cl^-), bicarbonate (HCO_3^-), phosphates ($H_2PO_4^-$ and $HPO_4^=$), and many proteins. Proteins can be anionic when they contain negatively charged amino acids—amino acid side groups that have gained electrons to give them an electrical charge.

Figure 19-9 shows that although ECF contains a number of important ions, by far the most abundant are sodium (positive) and chloride (negative). However, in the ICF, we find mostly potassium (positive) and anionic proteins (negative).

Electrolyte Functions

A variety of electrolytes have important nutrient or regulatory roles in the body. Many ions are major or important "trace" elements in the body. Iron, for example, is required for hemoglobin production, and iodine must be available for synthesis of thyroid hormones. Electrolytes also are required for many cellular activities such as nerve conduction and muscle contraction.

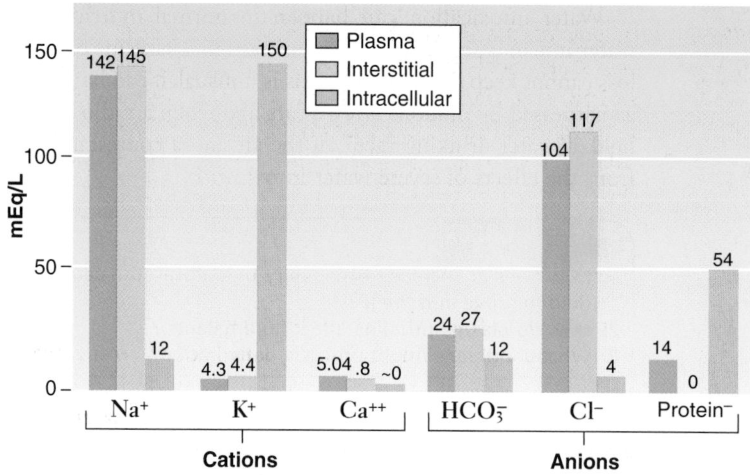

FIGURE 19-9 Electrolytes found in fluid compartments of the body. Note that sodium (Na^+) is the dominant positive ion and chloride (Cl^-) is the dominant negative ion in the extracellular fluid compartments (plasma and interstitial fluid). However, in the intracellular fluid compartment, potassium (K^+) and anionic (negative) proteins dominate. *mEq/L,* milliequivalent per liter.

In addition, electrolytes influence the movement of water among the fluid compartments of the body. To remember how ECF electrolyte concentration affects fluid volumes, remember this one short sentence: *Where sodium goes, water soon follows.*

If, for example, the concentration of sodium in interstitial fluid spaces rises above normal, the volume of IF soon reaches abnormal levels too—a condition called **edema,** which results in tissue swelling (see box below). Edema may occur in any organ or tissue of the body. However, the lungs, brain, and dependent body areas such as the legs and lower back are affected most often. One of the most common areas for swelling to occur is in the subcutaneous tissues of the ankle and foot.

Although wide variations are possible, the average daily diet contains about 100 milliequivalents of sodium. The *milliequivalent (mEq)* is a unit of measurement related to ion reactivity. In a healthy individual, sodium excretion from the body by the kidney is about the same as intake. The kidney acts as the chief regulator of sodium levels in body fluids. It is important to know that many electrolytes such as sodium not only pass into and out of the body but also move back and forth between a number of body fluids during each 24-hour period.

Figure 19-10 shows the large volumes of sodium-containing internal secretions produced each day. During a 24-hour period, more than 8 liters of fluid containing 1000 to 1300 mEq of sodium are poured into the digestive system as part of saliva, gastric secretions, bile, pancreatic juice, and IF secretions. This sodium, along with most of that contained in the diet, is almost completely reabsorbed in the large intestine. Very little sodium is lost in the feces.

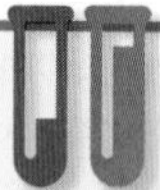

CLINICAL APPLICATION

EDEMA

Edema may be defined as the presence of abnormally large amounts of fluid in the interstitial tissue spaces of the body. The term **pitting edema** is used to describe depressions in swollen subcutaneous tissue that do not rapidly refill after an examiner has exerted finger pressure (see photo). This type of edema is often a symptom in those with congestive heart failure.

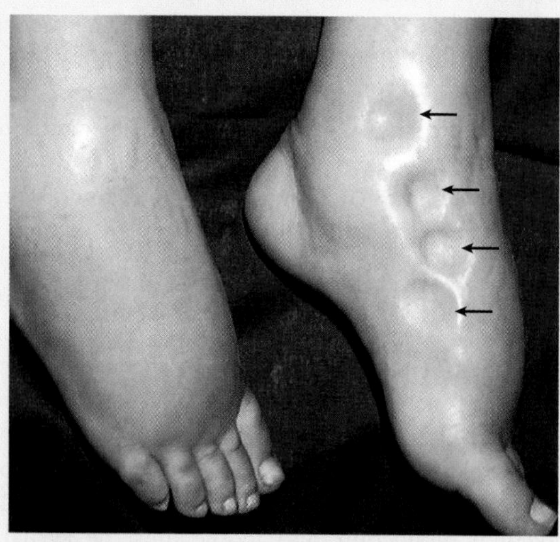

Pitting edema. Note the fingertip-shaped depressions *(arrows)* that do not rapidly refill after an examiner has exerted pressure.

The condition is a classic example of fluid imbalance and may be caused by disturbances in any factor that governs the interchange between blood plasma and IF compartments. Examples include the following:

1. **Retention of electrolytes (especially Na^+) in the interstitial fluid.** This can result from increased aldosterone secretion or can occur after serious kidney disease.
2. **An increase in capillary blood pressure.** Normally, fluid is drawn from the tissue spaces into the venous end of a tissue capillary because of the low venous pressure and the relatively high water-pulling force of the plasma proteins. This balance is upset by anything that increases the capillary hydrostatic pressure. The generalized venous congestion of heart failure is the most common cause of widespread edema. In patients with this condition, blood cannot flow freely through the capillary beds, and therefore the pressure will increase until venous return of blood improves.
3. **A decrease in the concentration of plasma proteins.** This decrease can be caused by "leakage" into the interstitial spaces of proteins normally retained in the blood. This may occur as a result of increased capillary permeability caused by infection, burns, or shock.

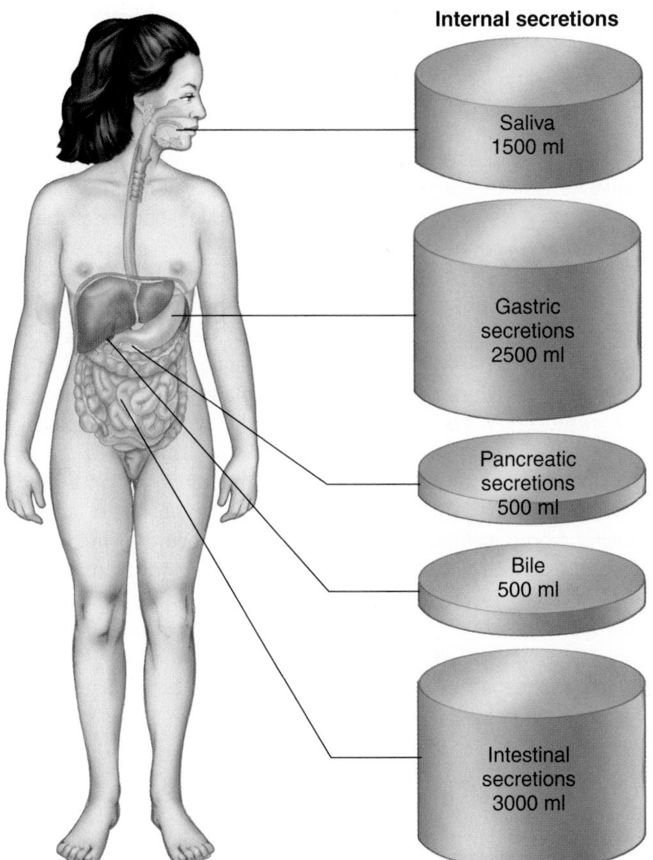

FIGURE 19-10 Sodium-containing internal secretions. The total volume of these secretions may reach 8000 mL or more in 24 hours.

Precise regulation and control of sodium levels are required for survival.

QUICK CHECK

1. What is the difference between an *electrolyte* and a *nonelectrolyte?*
2. What are some of the major roles of ions in the body?
3. Identify the functions of electrolytes in the body.

Electrolyte Imbalances

Homeostasis of Electrolytes

Electrolyte balance, like fluid balance, is related to "intake" and "output" of specific electrolytes. Also important is the absorption of electrolytes that are ingested, their final distribution in the body fluids, and their "availability" for use by the body cells.

ECF normally contains differing levels of some electrolytes than does ICF. In order to maintain different concentrations of electrolytes in the various body fluids, differing homeostatic mechanisms that influence intake, absorption, distribution, and excretion of these electrolytes are needed.

Any disruption in a homeostatic mechanism that controls the level or normal chemical activity of a particular electrolyte in any of the different body fluids produces an *electrolyte imbalance.* Such imbalances are widespread and often very serious, even sometimes fatal, manifestations of disease.

Electrolyte imbalances involving sodium, potassium, and calcium are common in clinical medicine and are described in the following sections.

Sodium Imbalance

The term *natrium* is the Latin word for sodium. The prefixes *hyper-* and *hypo-* refer to "above" and "below," respectively. Knowing this makes the terms *hypernatremia* and *hyponatremia* easier to understand and remember. **Hypernatremia** is used to describe a blood sodium level of more than 145 mEq/L. **Hyponatremia** occurs when blood sodium level is below 136 mEq/L.

Hypernatremia may result from overuse of salt tablets, dehydration, or prolonged diarrhea. Regardless of cause, the condition is characterized by a relative deficit of water to salt in the ECF. Hyponatremia occurs when there is relatively too much water in the ECF compartment for the amount of sodium present. This can occur if excessive antidiuretic hormone is produced or after massive infusion of IV fluids, such as 5% dextrose in water, that do not contain sodium.

Hyponatremia also may be caused by excessive salt loss resulting from burns or certain diuretics. Both of these conditions affect central nervous system (CNS) functioning and are characterized by headache; confusion; seizures; and, in the most severe cases, coma and death.

Potassium Imbalance

The normal range for potassium in blood is 3.5 to 5.1 mEq/L. Although most of the total body potassium is inside the cells, fluctuations or imbalance in the relatively small amounts present in the ECF will cause serious illness.

Hyperkalemia is the clinical term used to describe blood potassium levels of more than 5.1 mEq/L. (*Kalium* is the Latin word for potassium.) Elevation of potassium may be related to increased intake, a shift from the intracellular fluid into the blood—caused by tissue trauma or burns, or in cases of renal failure, by an inability of the kidneys to excrete excess potassium.

Many of the clinical manifestations of hyperkalemia are related to muscle malfunction. As potassium levels increase, skeletal muscles weaken and paralysis develops. Severe hyperkalemia results in cardiac arrest.

Hypokalemia refers to a low blood potassium level (below 3.5 mEq/L). It may be caused by fasting; fad diets low in dietary potassium; abuse of laxatives and certain diuretics in extreme weight loss programs; or by loss of potassium because of diarrhea, vomiting, or gastric suction. As with hyperkalemia, low potassium levels cause skeletal muscle weakness and cardiac problems. **Figure 19-11** shows the effects of low potassium (2.2 mEq/L) in reducing ventricular muscle function and thus causing a prolonged ST segment in the electrocardiogram (ECG).

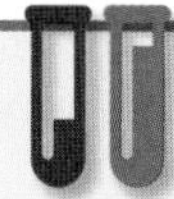

CLINICAL APPLICATION

DIURETICS

The word **diuretic** is from the Greek word *diouretikos* meaning "causing urine." By definition a *diuretic drug* is a substance that promotes or stimulates the production of urine. Recall that an increase in urine volume represents a loss of water from the body.

As a group, diuretics are among the most commonly used drugs in medicine. They are used because of their role in influencing water and electrolyte balance, especially sodium, in the body. Diuretics have their effect on tubular function in the nephron. The various types of diuretics are often classified according to their major site of action in the kidney tubule. Examples would include (1) *proximal tubule diuretics* such as acetazolamide (Diamox), (2) *nephron (Henle) loop diuretics* such as ethacrynic acid (Edecrin) or furosemide (Lasix), and (3) *distal tubule diuretics* such as chlorothiazide (Diuril). Caffeine produces its mildly diuretic effects by inhibiting water reabsorption in the proximal tubule of the nephron.

Classification of diuretic drugs also can be made according to the effect the drug has on the level or concentration of sodium (Na^+), chloride (Cl^-), potassium (K^+), and bicarbonate (HCO_3^-) ions in the tubular fluid.

Alcohol is also a diuretic. It reduces secretion of ADH, which is a water-conserving hormone. Thus water that would have otherwise been conserved by the body is lost under the influence of alcohol.

Diuretics are sometimes used by athletes to quickly reduce their weight just before an event or "weigh-in." Loss of water from the body does in fact reduce a person's weight, but it also reduces his or her athletic ability by creating the condition of dehydration. Diuretics (except for legitimate therapeutic use) are included on the Prohibited List by the World Anti-Doping Agency.

Nursing implications for caregivers monitoring patients receiving diuretics both in hospitals and in home health care environments include (1) keeping a careful record of fluid intake and output and (2) assessing the patient for signs and symptoms of electrolyte and water imbalance. For example, diuretic-induced dehydration resulting in a loss of only 6% of initial body weight will cause tingling in the extremities, stumbling gait, headache, fever, and an increase in both pulse and respiratory rates.

In addition, smooth muscle in the gastrointestinal tract does not contract properly, causing abdominal distention and diminished rate of passage of intestinal contents.

Calcium Imbalance

Calcium is the most abundant mineral in the body. It serves as a basic structural building block in bone and teeth. It is also essential for the maintenance of a normal heartbeat, for functioning of nerves and muscles, cellular metabolism, blood coagulation, and in many enzymatic reactions. Failure of homeostatic mechanisms that regulate levels of this important electrolyte can result in catastrophic illness.

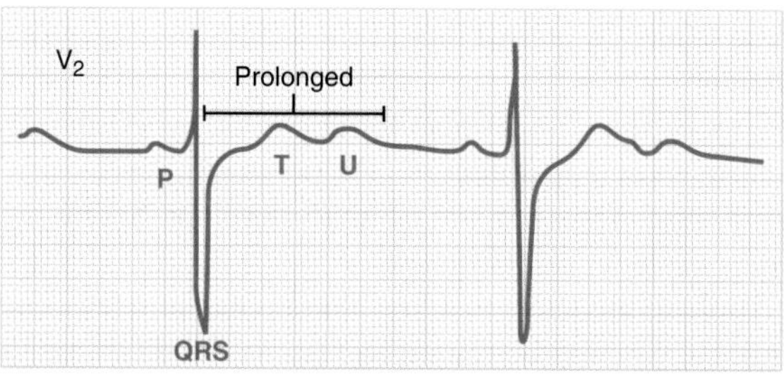

FIGURE 19-11 Effects of hypokalemia on heart function. Low potassium levels (hypokalemia) can cause changes in heart function, including a prolonged ST segment caused by the presence of an extra wave called the *U wave*. Compare with the normal ECG (electrocardiogram) in **Figure 13-10** on pp. 292-293.

The normal range for serum calcium is 8.4 to 10.5 mg/dL. **Hypercalcemia** occurs when blood calcium levels rise above normal limits. The condition may be caused by excessive intake or by increased absorption that may occur following an overdose of vitamin D. Elevated levels also can result from shifts of calcium from bone into the ECF caused by various bone diseases such as bone tumors, or hyperparathyroidism blood levels that will also increase if the kidney cannot normally excrete excess calcium in the urine—a side effect of certain diuretics. Regardless of cause, hypercalcemia decreases neuromuscular irritability resulting in fatigue, muscle weakness, diminished reflexes, and delayed atrioventricular conduction in the heart.

Hypocalcemia may result from dietary calcium deficiency, decreased absorption or availability, and as a result of increased calcium excretion. Diseases such as pancreatitis, hypoparathyroidism, rickets, and osteomalacia and chronic renal insufficiency all lower blood calcium levels. Clinical signs of hypocalcemia involve *increased* neuromuscular irritability, cramping and twitching of muscles, hyperactive reflexes, and abnormal cardiac rhythms characterized by impairment of myocardial contractility.

QUICK CHECK

1. What are the causes of hyponatremia and hypernatremia?
2. Hypokalemia may be responsible for what conditions?
3. Why is calcium a significant mineral in our body?

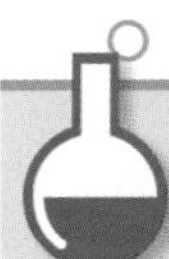

SCIENCE APPLICATIONS

THE CONSTANCY OF THE BODY

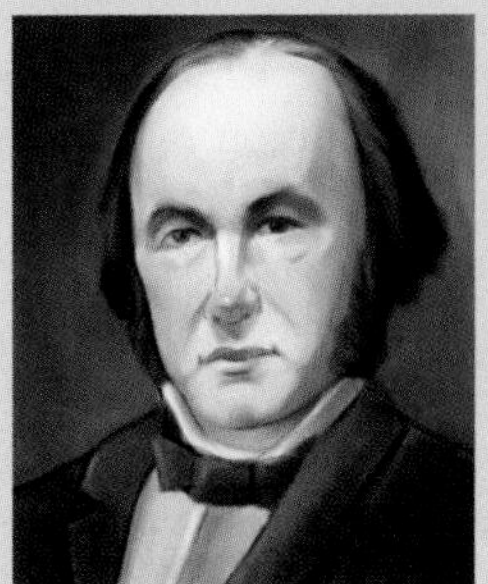

Claude Bernard (1813-1877)

In 1834, a young Claude Bernard left what he thought of at the time as his "boring job" as an apprentice apothecary (druggist) in Lyon, France, to make his fortune as a playwright in Paris. His plays were not appreciated in Paris, but he took a medical course while there and found that many of the doctors appreciated his research skills. Bernard went on to become one of the most important figures in the study of human physiology.

Bernard made groundbreaking discoveries in the functions of the pancreas and the liver, discovered the existence of muscles that control blood vessel dilation, and wrote a manual on experimental medicine that set the standard in research practice for a century. However, one of the most fundamental contributions he made to human physiology is the idea that the body is made up of cells living in an internal fluid environment.

Bernard stated that the internal fluid environment of the body is maintained in a relatively constant state—and that's what ensures the survival of the cells and therefore also ensures the survival of the whole body. Recall from Chapter 1 that we now call this concept *homeostasis* (see pp. 12-16). It was Bernard who showed that the actions of hormones and other control mechanisms maintain constant conditions in the body's internal fluid environment. Bernard also showed that nearly every function of the body somehow relates to the success of keeping body fluids constant.

Today, nearly every health care professional uses concepts based on Bernard's original idea to assess the fluid and electrolyte balance of patients and possibly administer therapies to bring their fluids back into balance. For example, **IV technicians** and others provide fluid and electrolyte therapy through intravenous solutions. Maintaining a healthy fluid and electrolyte balance is one of the key elements to successful patient care in the modern hospital and clinic.

LANGUAGE OF SCIENCE AND MEDICINE *(continued from p. 429)*

hyperkalemia
(hy-per-kal-EE-mee-ah)
[*hyper-* **excessive,** *-kal-* **kalium (potassium),** *-emia* **blood condition]**

hypernatremia
(hy-per-nah-TREE-mee-ah)
[*hyper-* **excessive,** *-natri-* **natrium (sodium),** *-emia* **blood condition]**

hypocalcemia
(hye-poh-kal-SEE-mee-ah)
[*hypo-* **under or below,** *-calc-* **lime (calcium),** *-emia* **blood condition]**

hypokalemia
(hye-poh-kal-EE-mee-ah)
[*hypo-* **under or below,** *-kal-* **kalium (potassium),** *-emia* **blood condition]**

hyponatremia
(hye-poh-nah-TREE-mee-ah)
[*hypo-* **under or below,** *-natri-* **natrium (sodium),** *-emia* **blood condition]**

interstitial fluid (IF)
(in-ter-STISH-al FLOO-id)
[*inter-* **between,** *-stit-* **stand,** *-al* **relating to]**

intracellular fluid (ICF)
(in-trah-SEL-yoo-lar FLOO-id)
[*intra-* **occurring within,** *-cell-* **storeroom,** *-ular* **relating to]**

ion
(AYE-on)
[*ion* **to go]**

IV (intravenous) technician
(aye-vee [in-trah-VEE-nus] tek-NISH-en)
[*intra-* **within,** *-ven-* **vein,** *-ous* **relating to,** *techn-* **art or skill,** *-ic* **relating to,** *-ian* **practitioner]**

nonelectrolyte
(non-ee-LEK-troh-lyte)
[*non-* **not,** *-electro-* **electricity,** *-lyt-* **loosening]**

overhydration
(oh-ver-hye-DRAY-shun)
[*over-* **above,** *-hydr-* **water,** *-ation* **process]**

pitting edema
(pit-ing eh-DEE-mah)
[*edema* **swelling]**

plasma
(PLAZ-mah)
[*plasma* **substance]**

transcellular fluid
(tranz-SEL-yoo-lar)
[*trans-* **across,** *-cell-* **storeroom,** *-ular* **relating to]**

water intoxication
(WAH-ter in-TOK-sih-kay-shen)
[*in-* **in,** *-toxic-* **poison,** *-ation* **process]**

❑ OUTLINE SUMMARY

*To download a digital audio version of the chapter summary for use with your device, access the **Audio Chapter Summaries** online at evolve.elsevier.com.*

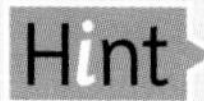

Scan this summary after reading the chapter to help you reinforce the key concepts. Later, use the summary as a quick review before your class or before a test.

Body Fluid Volumes

A. Water is the most abundant body compound
  1. References to "average" body water volume in reference tables are based on a healthy, nonobese, 70-kg male
  2. Volume averages 40 L in a 70-kg male (see **Figure 19-1**)
    a. Plasma (3 L)
    b. Interstitial fluid (12 L)
    c. Intracellular fluid (25 L)
  3. Water is 80% of body weight in newborn infants; 60% in adult males; 50% in adult females (see **Figure 19-2**)
  4. Total body water
    a. Distributed among compartments (see **Figure 19-3**)
    b. Total volume is related to:
      (1) Total body weight of individual
      (2) Fat content of body — the more fat in the body the less the total water content per kilogram of body weight (adipose tissue is low in water content)
      (3) Gender — female body has about 10% less than male body (see **Figure 19-2**)
      (4) Age — in a newborn infant, water may account for 80% of total body weight. In the elderly, water per kilogram of weight decreases (muscle tissue — high in water — replaced by fat which is lower in water)

Body Fluid Compartments

A. The fluids of the body are contained within different "compartments" of the body (see **Figure 19-1** and **Table 19-1**)
B. Extracellular fluid (ECF) — called internal environment of body; surrounds cells and transports substances to and from them
  1. Plasma — liquid part of whole blood
  2. Interstitial fluid (IF) — surrounds the cells
  3. Transcellular — lymph; joint fluids; cerebrospinal fluid; eye humors
C. Intracellular fluid (ICF) — largest fluid compartment
  1. Located inside cells
  2. Serves as solvent to facilitate intracellular chemical reactions

Mechanisms That Maintain Fluid Balance

A. Sources of fluid intake (see **Figure 19-4** and **Table 19-2**)
  1. Liquids we drink
  2. Water in food we eat
  3. Metabolic water (from cellular respiration)
B. Sources of fluid output (see **Figure 19-4** and **Table 19-2**)
  1. Water vapor (during respiration)
  2. Sweating (from skin)
  3. Urine (from kidney)
  4. Water lost in the feces
C. Three main factors affect plasma, IF, and ICF volumes
  1. Regulating fluid output
  2. Regulating fluid intake
  3. Exchanging fluid among compartments and around body
D. Regulation of fluid output
  1. Organs responsible for fluid output — lungs, skin, kidneys, and large intestine
  2. Fluid output, mainly urine volume, adjusts to fluid intake
  3. Antidiuretic hormone (ADH)
    a. ADH released from posterior pituitary gland when ECF volume is low
    b. ADH promotes water reabsorption from kidney tubules into blood.
    c. Water is thus retained by body and less fluid is lost in urine.
  4. Aldosterone mechanism (see **Figure 19-5**)
    a. Aldosterone released from adrenal cortex.
    b. Aldosterone increases kidney tubule reabsorption of sodium from kidney tubules
    c. Water follows sodium from tubules into blood
    d. Water is retained by ECF (and total body fluid) by decreasing urine volume
  5. Atrial natriuretic hormone (ANH)
    a. ANH is released from heart's atrial wall in response to high blood volume
    b. ANH promotes sodium loss from blood into kidney tubules
    c. Water follows sodium from blood, thus increasing loss of water in urine
E. Regulation of fluid intake (see **Figure 19-6**)
  1. Sensory receptors detect change in volume and ECF concentration and send signals to the hypothalamus
  2. Signals from hypothalamus cause feeling of thirst, which triggers drinking of fluids to restore balance
F. Exchange of fluids by blood
  1. Constancy of internal fluid balance also maintained by exchanging fluids between fluid compartments
  2. Increased capillary blood pressure transfers fluid from blood plasma to IF — a fluid shift
  3. Blood plasma protein concentration contributes to osmotic pressure, thus attracting water and holding it in the plasma

Fluid Imbalances

A. Dehydration — total volume of body fluids smaller than normal
   1. IF volume shrinks first, and then if treatment is not given, ICF volume and plasma volume decrease
   2. Dehydration occurs when fluid output exceeds intake for an extended period (see **Figure 19-7** and **Figure 19-8**)

B. Overhydration — total volume of body fluids larger than normal
   1. Fluid intake exceeds output
   2. Excess volume burdens pumping action of heart

C. Water intoxication — possibly life-threatening neurological impairment caused by severe overhydration and accompanying electrolyte imbalance

Importance of Electrolytes in Body Fluids

A. Electrolytes
   1. Nonelectrolytes — organic substances that do not break up or dissociate when placed in water solution (e.g., glucose)
   2. Electrolytes — compounds that break up or dissociate in water solution into separate particles called ions (e.g., ordinary table salt or sodium chloride)

B. Ions — the dissociated particles of an electrolyte that carry an electrical charge
   1. Cations are positively charged ions (e.g., potassium [K^+] and sodium [Na^+])
   2. Anions are negatively charged ions (e.g., chloride [Cl^-], bicarbonate [HCO_3^-], anionic proteins)

C. Electrolyte composition of body fluids (see **Figure 19-9**)
   1. ECF dominated by sodium (positive) and chloride (negative)
   2. ICF dominated by potassium (positive) and anionic proteins (negative)

D. Edema — swelling caused by high IF volume

E. Sodium-containing internal secretions (see **Figure 19-10**)

Electrolyte Imbalances

A. Homeostasis of electrolytes — related to "intake" and "output" of electrolytes and also absorption and distribution of electrolytes in body fluids and availability for use by body cells

B. Sodium imbalance
   1. Hypernatremia — blood sodium more than 145 mEq/L
      a. Characterized by relative deficit of water to salt in ECF
      b. Causes include overuse of salt tablets; dehydration; and prolonged diarrhea
   2. Hyponatremia — blood sodium less than 136 mEq/L
      a. Results when there is relatively too much water in the ECF for the amount of sodium present
      b. Causes include excessive secretion of antidiuretic hormone, massive infusion of sodium-free IV solution, burns, and prolonged use of certain diuretics
      c. Symptoms of both hypernatremia and hyponatremia are related to CNS malfunction and include headache, confusion, seizures, and coma

C. Potassium imbalance
   1. Hyperkalemia — blood potassium more than 5.1 mEq/L
      a. Causes include increased intake, shift of potassium from ICF to blood caused by tissue trauma and burns, renal failure
      b. Clinical signs of hyperkalemia are related to muscle malfunction and include skeletal muscle weakness, paralysis, and cardiac arrest
   2. Hypokalemia — blood potassium less than 3.5 mEq/L
      a. Causes include fasting, diets low in potassium, abuse of laxatives and certain diuretics, diarrhea, vomiting, and gastric suction
      b. Clinical signs include skeletal muscle and cardiac problems; smooth muscle weakness causing abdominal distention, and slow rate of passage of GI contents (see **Figure 19-11**)

D. Calcium imbalance
   1. Hypercalcemia — blood calcium levels more than 10.5 mg/dL
      a. Caused by excessive intake, increased absorption, shifts of calcium from bone to ECF, Paget disease and other bone tumors, hyperparathyroidism
      b. Clinical signs related to decreased neuromuscular activity — fatigue, muscle weakness, diminished reflexes, cardiac problems
   2. Hypocalcemia — blood calcium levels less than 8.4 mg/dL
      a. Caused by dietary deficiency, decreased absorption or availability, increased excretion, pancreatitis, hypoparathyroidism, rickets, osteomalacia, and renal insufficiency
      b. Clinical signs related to increased neuromuscular irritability — cramping, muscle twitching, hyperactive reflexes, and abnormal cardiac rhythms

❑ ACTIVE LEARNING

STUDY TIPS

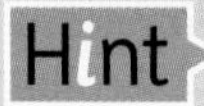

Use these tips to achieve success in meeting your learning goals.

To make the study of fluid and electrolyte balance more efficient, we suggest these tips:

1. Chapter 19 expands on some of the material from Chapter 18. A quick review of Chapter 18 will better prepare you for this chapter.
2. Make flash cards and check online resources to help you learn the terms in this chapter. For a better understanding of the terms in this chapter, review the Language of Science and Medicine section.
3. Electrolytes are charged particles or ions. One of the functions of ions is to control water movement. The body cannot directly control water movement so it must move electrolytes and water will then follow.
4. The capillary pressure and blood protein mechanism regulates the movement of water between the blood and interstitial fluid. Blood pressure determines the amount of plasma that is pushed out into the interstitial fluid, and plasma proteins determine the amount of water that gets pulled back into the blood.
5. In your study group, review the flash cards with the terms. Discuss how electrolytes function in regulating water movement. Go over the aldosterone mechanism (see **Figure 19-5**). Discuss the plasma protein and capillary blood pressure mechanism for regulating the balance between blood plasma and interstitial fluid. Review the questions and chapter outline summary at the end of the chapter and discuss possible test questions.

Review Questions

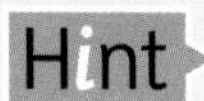

Write out the answers to these questions after reading the chapter and reviewing the Chapter Summary. If you simply think through the answer without writing it down, you won't retain much of your new learning.

1. Name and locate the three main fluid compartments of the body. Identify which of these compartments make up the ECF.
2. List and explain the effect of each factor that influences the percentage of water in the body.
3. List the three sources of water for the body.
4. Identify the main factors that act as mechanisms for balancing plasma, IF, and ICF volumes.
5. List the four organs from which fluid output occurs.
6. Explain how aldosterone influences water movement between the kidney tubules and the blood.
7. Explain why the body is unable to reduce its fluid output to zero.
8. Explain the role of capillary blood pressure in water movement between the plasma and interstitial fluid.
9. Explain the role of plasma proteins in water movement between the plasma and interstitial fluid.
10. Define dehydration and give a possible cause.
11. Define overhydration and give a possible cause.
12. Differentiate between an electrolyte and a nonelectrolyte.
13. Name three important anions.
14. Name three important cations.
15. Describe the clinical manifestations of hyperkalemia.

Critical Thinking

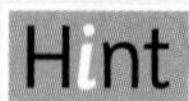

After finishing the Review Questions, write out the answers to these more in-depth questions to help you apply your new knowledge. Go back to sections of the chapter that relate to concepts that you find difficult.

16. Name the three hormones that regulate the urine volume. State where each hormone is made and the specific effect on urine volume.
17. Atrial natriuretic hormone has the opposite effect of aldosterone. Explain its effect on water movement between the kidney tubules and the blood.
18. Regarding fluid and electrolyte balance, what would be the consequences of a large loss of skin (e.g., third-degree burns or scraping injuries)?
19. If a person rapidly drank a liter of distilled water, how would their ICF be affected?

Chapter Test

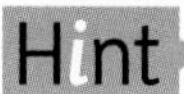

After studying the chapter, test your mastery by responding to these items. Try to answer them without looking up the answers. Then, verify the answers using the key in Appendix C at the back of this book.

1. The extracellular fluid compartment is composed of ________.
2. The largest volume of water is in this fluid compartment: ________.

Fill in the blanks in questions 3, 4, and 5 with either "more" or "less" as appropriate.

3. In general, an obese person has ________ water per pound of body weight than a slim person.
4. In general, a man has ________ water per pound of body weight than a woman.
5. In general, an infant has ________ water per pound of body weight than an adult.
6. The body's chief mechanism for maintaining fluid balance is that of adjusting its ________.
7. The body has three sources of fluid intake: the liquids we drink, the water in the food we eat, and ________.
8. The four organs from which fluid output occurs are the ________.
9. Urine volume is regulated by three hormones: ADH released from the pituitary gland, ________ released from the adrenal cortex, and ________ released from the heart.
10. When electrolytes dissociate in water, they form charged particles called ________.
11. The most abundant negatively charged particle in the blood is ________.
12. The most abundant positively charged particle in the blood is ________.
13. When the blood level of aldosterone increases:
    a. sodium is moved from the blood to the kidney tubules
    b. sodium is moved from the kidney tubules to the blood
    c. more urine is formed
    d. ANH is released
14. Aldosterone causes:
    a. an increase in intracellular fluid
    b. a decrease in intracellular fluid
    c. an increase in extracellular fluid
    d. a decrease in extracellular fluid
15. Increased capillary pressure:
    a. moves fluid from the intracellular to the extracellular compartment
    b. moves fluid from the plasma to the interstitial fluid
    c. moves fluid from the interstitial fluid to the plasma
    d. has no effect on fluid movement
16. Blood plasma proteins act to:
    a. move interstitial fluid into the plasma
    b. move plasma into the interstitial fluid
    c. move extracellular fluid into the intracellular fluid
    d. move interstitial fluid into the extracellular fluid

Acid-Base Balance

OUTLINE

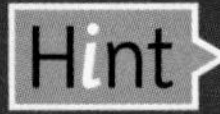

Scan this outline before you begin to read the chapter, as a preview of how the concepts are organized.

OBJECTIVES

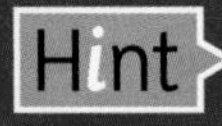

Before reading the chapter, review these goals for your learning.

After you have completed this chapter, you should be able to:

1. Define the term *acid-base balance* and discuss the concept of pH.
2. Define the terms *buffer* and *buffer pair* and contrast strong and weak acids and bases.
3. Contrast the respiratory and urinary mechanisms of pH control.
4. Define acidosis and alkalosis, and compare and contrast metabolic and respiratory types of pH imbalances.
5. Discuss compensatory mechanisms that may help return blood pH to near-normal levels in cases of pH imbalances.

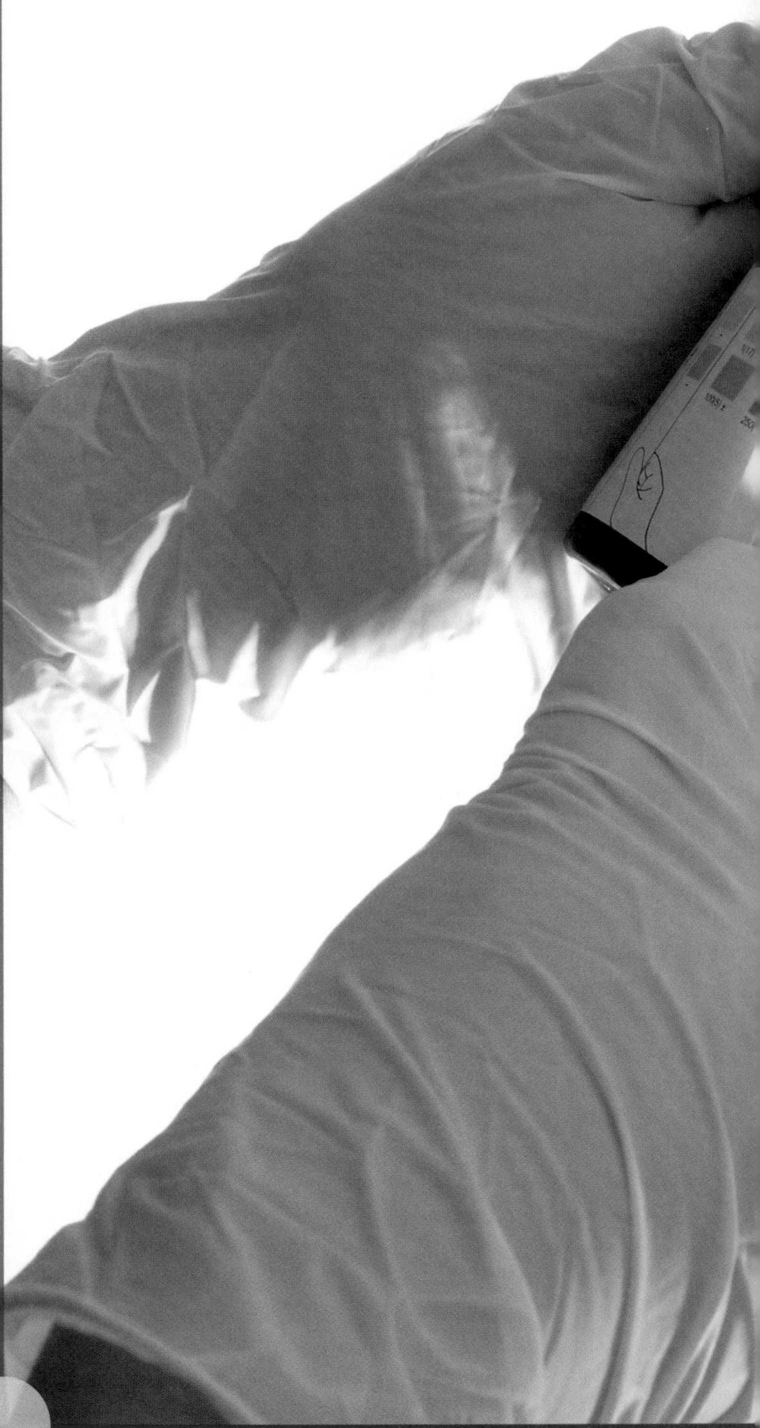

CHAPTER 20

Acid-base balance is one of the most important of the body's homeostatic mechanisms. Maintaining acid-base balance means keeping the concentration of hydrogen ions in body fluids relatively constant. Effective functioning of many important body proteins, such as cellular enzymes and hemoglobin, closely depends on maintaining precise regulation of hydrogen ion concentration. This is of vital importance. If the hydrogen ion concentration veers away from normal even slightly, serious illness or even death may occur. Healthy survival depends on the ability of the body to maintain, or quickly restore, the acid-base balance of its fluids if imbalances occur.

Acid-base regulation requires a series of coordinated homeostatic mechanisms that involve the blood and other body fluids, the lungs, and the kidneys. Ultimately, all of these mechanisms are based on chemical processes. Recall that many important chemical principles related to the life process were covered in Chapter 2. You may wish to refer back to those principles of biochemistry as you study how the body so precisely regulates its acid-base balance in this chapter.

pH of Body Fluids

Water and all water solutions contain **hydrogen ions** (**H^+**) and **hydroxide ions** (**OH^-**). pH is an acronym for "power of H^+." The term **pH** followed by a number indicates a solution's hydrogen ion concentration compared with hydroxide concentration.

Using the pH Scale

At pH 7.0 a solution contains an equal concentration of hydrogen and hydroxide ions. Therefore pH 7.0 also indicates that a fluid is **neutral** in reaction (that is, neither acid nor alkaline) (**Figure 20-1**). The pH of pure water, for example, is 7.0.

A pH higher than 7.0 indicates an **alkaline** solution (that is, one with a lower concentration of hydrogen than hydroxide ions). The more alkaline a solution, the higher is its pH value. Alkaline solutions are also called *basic* solutions.

A pH lower than 7.0 indicates an **acid** solution (that is, one with a higher hydrogen ion concentration than hydroxide ion concentration). The higher the hydrogen ion concentration, the lower the pH and the more acidic a solution is.

LANGUAGE OF SCIENCE AND MEDICINE

Hint Before reading the chapter, say each of these terms out loud. This will help you to avoid stumbling over them as you read.

acid
(AS-id)
[*acid* **sour**]

acid-base balance
(AS-id bays BAL-ans)
[*acid* **sour,** *bas-* **foundation,** *bal-* **twice,** *-lanc* **dish (two scales)**]

acidosis
(as-ih-DOH-sis)
[*acid-* **sour,** *-osis* **condition**]

alkaline
(AL-kah-lin)
[*alkal-* **ashes,** *-ine* **relating to**]

alkalosis
(al-kah-LOH-sis)
[*alkal-* **ashes,** *-osis* **condition**]

arterial blood gas (ABG)
(ar-TEER-ee-al blud gas)
[*arteri-* **airpipe (artery),** *-al* **relating to**]

bicarbonate loading
(bye-KAR-boh-net LOHD-ing)
[*bi-* **two,** *-carbon-* **coal (carbon),** *-ate* **oxygen**]

buffer
(BUFF-er)
[*buffe-* **cushion,** *-er* **agent**]

buffer pair
(BUFF-er payr)
[*buffe-* **cushion,** *-er* **agent**]

carbonic anhydrase (CA)
(kar-BON-ik an-HYE-drayz)
[*carbo-* **coal,** *-ic* **relating to,** *an-* **without,** *-hydr-* **water,** *-ase* **enzyme**]

compensation
(kom-pen-SAY-shun)
[*compens-* **balance,** *-tion* **process**]

Continued on p. 454

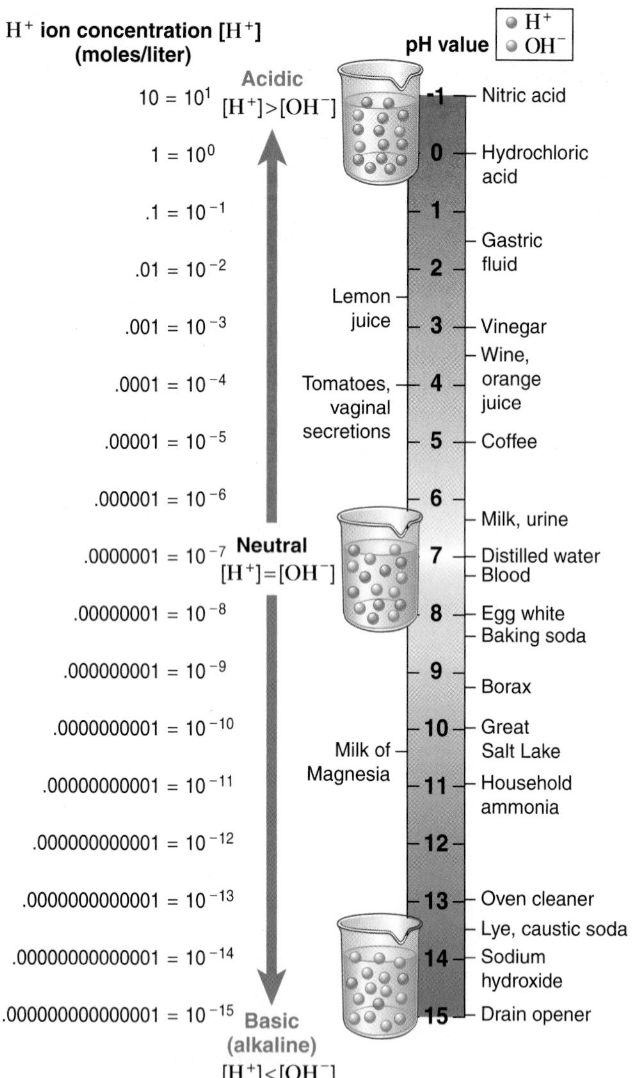

FIGURE 20-1 The pH range. The overall pH range is expressed numerically on what is called a logarithmic scale of 1 to 14. This means that a change of 1 pH unit represents a tenfold difference in actual concentration of hydrogen ions. Note that as the concentration of H^+ ions increases, the solution becomes increasingly acidic and the pH value decreases. As OH^- concentration increases, the pH value also increases, and the solution becomes more and more basic, or alkaline. A pH of 7 is neutral, a pH of 2 is very acidic, and a pH of 13 is very basic.

With a pH as low as 1.6, gastric juice is the most acid substance in the body. Saliva often has a pH of 7.7, on the alkaline side. Normally, the pH of systemic arterial blood is about 7.45, and the pH of systemic venous blood is about 7.35.

By applying the information given in the previous paragraph, you can deduce the answers to the following questions. Is systemic arterial blood slightly acid or slightly alkaline? Is systemic venous blood slightly acid or slightly alkaline?

Systemic arterial and venous blood are both slightly alkaline because both have a pH slightly higher than 7.0. Systemic venous blood, however, is less alkaline than systemic arterial blood because systemic venous blood's pH of about 7.35 is slightly lower than systemic arterial blood's pH of 7.45.

The pH Unit

The pH unit is based on exponents of 10 from one unit to the next. That means that on the pH scale moving from one unit to the next multiplies the relative H^+ concentration by 10 times. Thus the difference between pH 7 and pH 6 is a *tenfold* increase in H^+. Moving from pH 7 to pH 5 is a *hundredfold* increase in H^+ concentration.

This tenfold difference between pH units is important to remember when we look at the normal pH range of blood plasma—a key fluid compartment of the body. What may seem like a small change in acidity at first glance is really 10 times bigger than it looks!

QUICK CHECK

1. What does pH measure?
2. What does a pH of "neutral" indicate?
3. What does it mean when a solution's pH increases?

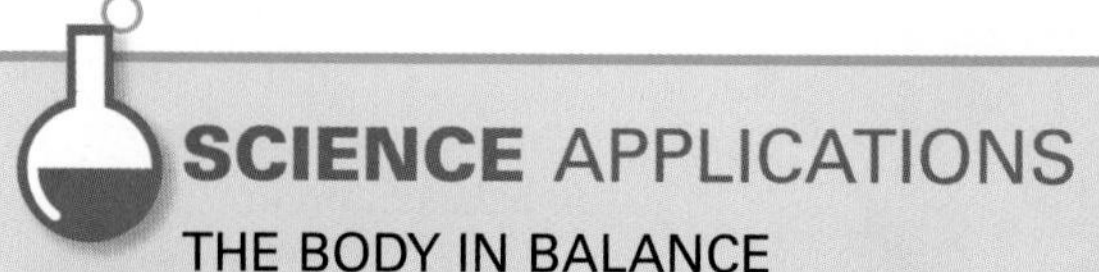

SCIENCE APPLICATIONS

THE BODY IN BALANCE

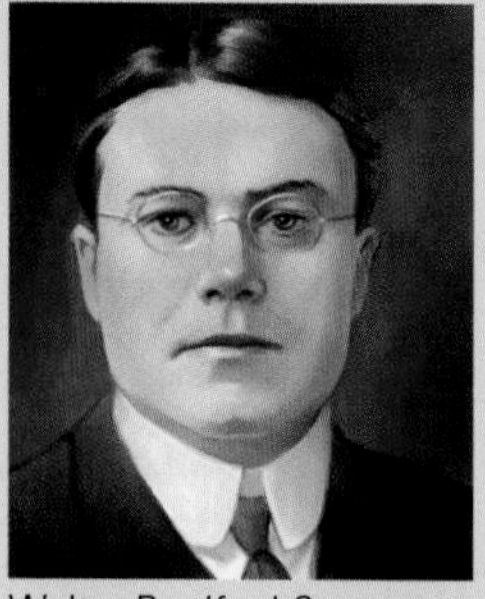

Walter Bradford Cannon (1871-1945)

Keeping the pH of the body stable is but one aspect of maintaining health. The American physiologist Walter Cannon gave us a name for the principle of balance, or constancy, of the internal fluid environment of the body—*homeostasis.* In 1932, his popular book *The Wisdom of the Body* finally gave a name to the concept first explained by Claude Bernard seven decades earlier (see p. 439). However, Cannon did more than name the concept. In his book, Cannon explained the incredibly complex set of mechanisms that allows our bodies to adjust to tremendous internal and external fluctuations that would otherwise kill us.

Much of Cannon's thought came from his groundbreaking discoveries in how the body copes with stress. In examining the fight-or-flight response, the effects of emotional stimuli, the mechanisms of cardiovascular shock, and in developing the "case study" approach to learning about human health and disease, Walter Cannon developed a clear understanding of the interactive nature of the organs of the body. It was Cannon who led scientists to look at their work in this new framework that explains the "big picture" of human body function.

Cannon's explanation of homeostasis revolutionized the way we look at the body—and how we look at patient care. As with fluid and electrolyte balance, knowledge of the mechanisms of acid-base balance is critical in direct patient care. Therefore *many physicians, nurses, respiratory therapists, IV technicians, first responders* (for example, *emergency medical technicians* and *paramedics*), and others need a basic knowledge of how the body maintains a constancy of pH in the blood.

Mechanisms That Control pH of Body Fluids

Overview of pH Control Mechanisms

The body has three mechanisms for regulating the pH of its fluids. They are

1. Buffer mechanism in blood
2. Respiratory mechanism
3. Urinary mechanism

Together, the listed processes constitute the complex pH homeostatic mechanism—the machinery that normally keeps blood slightly alkaline, with a pH that stays remarkably constant. Its usual limits are very narrow, about 7.35 to 7.45.

The slightly lower pH of systemic venous blood compared with systemic arterial blood results primarily from carbon dioxide (CO_2) entering venous blood as a waste product of cellular metabolism. As carbon dioxide enters the blood, some of it combines with water (H_2O) and is converted into carbonic acid by **carbonic anhydrase (CA)**, an enzyme found in red blood cells. The following chemical equation represents this reaction. If you need to review chemical formulas and equations, please refer to Chapter 2.

$$CO_2 + H_2O \xrightarrow{\text{carbonic anhydrase}} H_2CO_3$$

The lungs remove the equivalent of more than 30 L of carbonic acid each day from the venous blood by elimination of CO_2. This almost unbelievable quantity of acid is so well buffered that a liter of venous blood contains only about 1/100,000,000 grams more H^+ than does 1 liter of arterial blood. What incredible constancy! The pH homeostatic mechanism does indeed control effectively—astonishingly so.

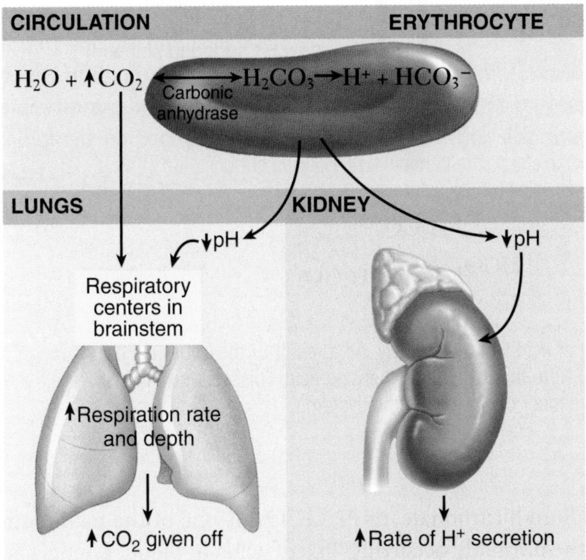

FIGURE 20-2 Integration of pH control mechanisms. Elevated CO_2 levels result in increased formation of carbonic acid in red blood cells. The resulting increase in hydrogen ions, coupled with elevated CO_2 levels, causes an increase in respiratory rate and secretion of hydrogen ions by the kidneys, thus helping to regulate the pH of body fluids.

Integration of pH Control

Integration of the three homeostatic mechanisms that act to maintain the pH of body fluids is illustrated in Figure 20-2.

Think of the circulating blood and RBCs as providing a *chemical pH control mechanism*, which is based on buffers (discussed below), and which acts immediately to help prevent harmful swings in pH when added acids or bases enter body fluids. If this immediate-acting chemical control mechanism is unable to stabilize the pH, the lungs and kidneys can both provide a *physiological pH control mechanism* to halt and reverse harmful pH shifts. The lungs respond in 1 to 2 minutes when the brainstem adjusts the respiratory rate (see Figure 15-14 on p. 355) and thus the adjustment of CO_2 is accomplished.

If the respiratory mechanism is unable to stop the pH shift, powerful but slower-acting renal mechanisms will be initiated within 24 hours. Details of each mechanism are discussed in the paragraphs that follow.

Buffers

Buffers are chemical substances that prevent a sharp change in the pH of a fluid when an acid or base is added to it. Strong acids and bases, if added to blood, would "dissociate" almost completely and release large quantities of H^+ or OH^- ions. The result would be drastic changes in blood pH. Survival itself depends on protecting the body from such drastic pH changes.

More acids than bases are usually added to body fluids. This is because catabolism, a process that goes on continually in every cell of the body, produces acids that enter blood as it flows through tissue capillaries. Almost immediately, one of the salts present in blood—a buffer, that is—reacts with these relatively strong acids to change them into weaker acids. The weaker acids decrease blood pH only slightly, whereas the stronger acids formed by catabolism would have decreased it greatly if they were not buffered.

Buffers consist of two kinds of substances and are therefore often called **buffer pairs.** One of the main blood buffer pairs is ordinary baking soda (sodium bicarbonate, or $NaHCO_3$) and carbonic acid (H_2CO_3).

Let us consider, as a specific example of buffer action, how the $NaHCO_3$–H_2CO_3 system works with a strong acid or base.

If a strong base, such as sodium hydroxide (NaOH), were added to this buffer system, the reaction shown in Figure 20-3 would take place. The H^+ of H_2CO_3 ($H \cdot HCO_3$), the weak acid of the buffer pair, combines with the OH^- of the strong base NaOH to form H_2O. Note what this accomplishes. It decreases the number of OH^- ions added to the solution, and this in turn prevents the drastic rise in pH that would occur without buffering.

Figure 20-4 shows how a buffer system works with a strong acid. Although useful in demonstrating the principles of buffer action, HCl or similar strong acids are never introduced directly into body fluids under normal circumstances. Instead, the $NaHCO_3$ buffer system is most often called on to buffer a number of weaker acids produced during catabolism. Lactic acid is a good example. As a weak acid, it does not "dissociate" as completely as HCl. Incomplete dissociation of lactic acid

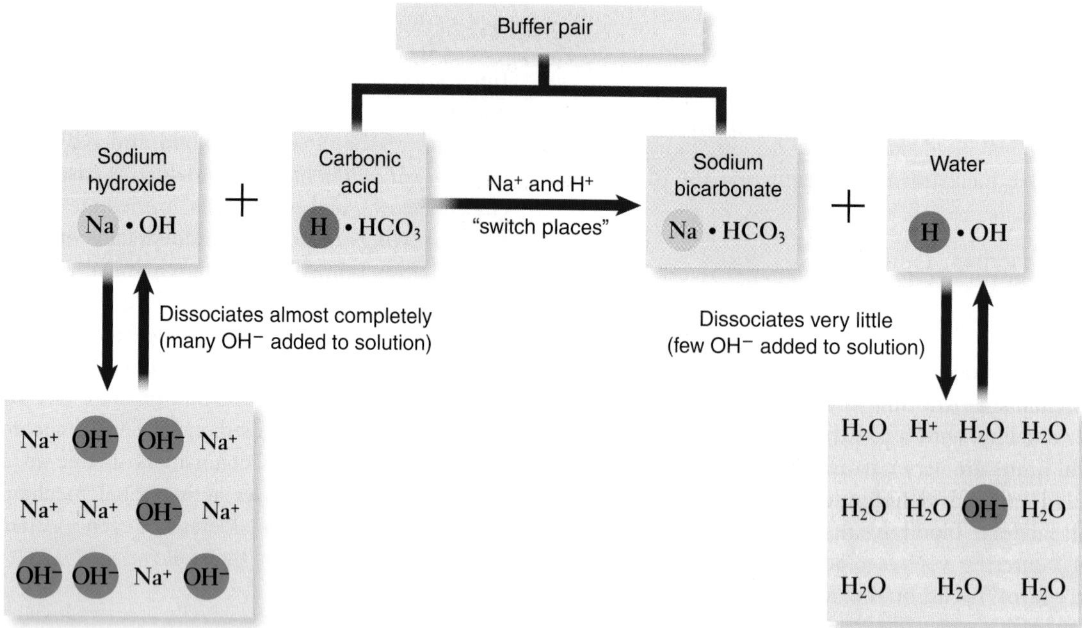

FIGURE 20-3 Buffering action of carbonic acid. Buffering of base NaOH by H_2CO_3. As a result of buffer action, the strong base (NaOH) is replaced by $NaHCO_3$ and H_2O. As a strong base, NaOH "dissociates" almost completely and releases large quantities of OH^-. Dissociation of H_2O is minimal. Buffering decreases the number of OH^- ions in the system.

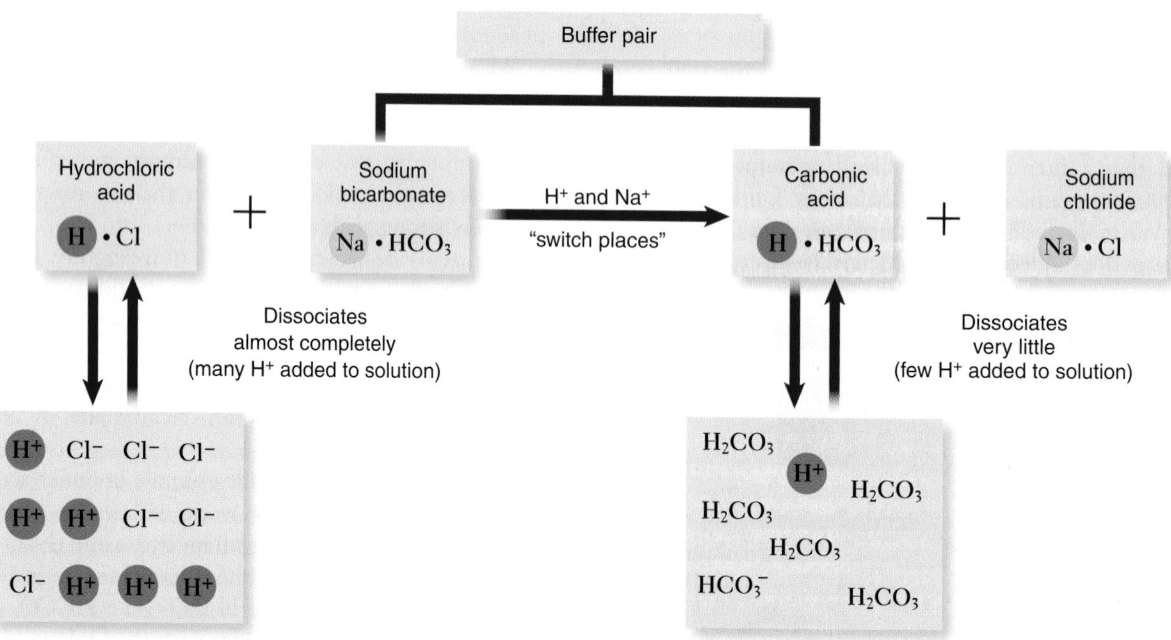

FIGURE 20-4 Buffering action of sodium bicarbonate. Buffering of acid HCl by $NaHCO_3$. As a result of the buffer action, the strong acid (HCl) is replaced by the weaker carbonic acid (H • HCO_3). Note that HCl, being a strong acid, "dissociates" almost completely and releases more H^+ than H_2CO_3. Buffering decreases the number of H^+ ions in the system.

results in fewer hydrogen ions being added to the blood and a less drastic lowering of blood pH than would occur if HCl were added in an equal amount.

Without buffering, however, lactic acid buildup results in significant H^+ accumulation over time. The resulting decrease of pH can produce serious acidosis. Ordinary baking soda (sodium bicarbonate, or $NaHCO_3$) is one of the main buffers of the normally occurring "fixed" acids in blood. Lactic acid is one of the most abundant of the "fixed" acids (acids that do not break down to form a gas).

Figure 20-5 shows the compounds formed by buffering of lactic acid (a "fixed" acid), produced by normal catabolism. The

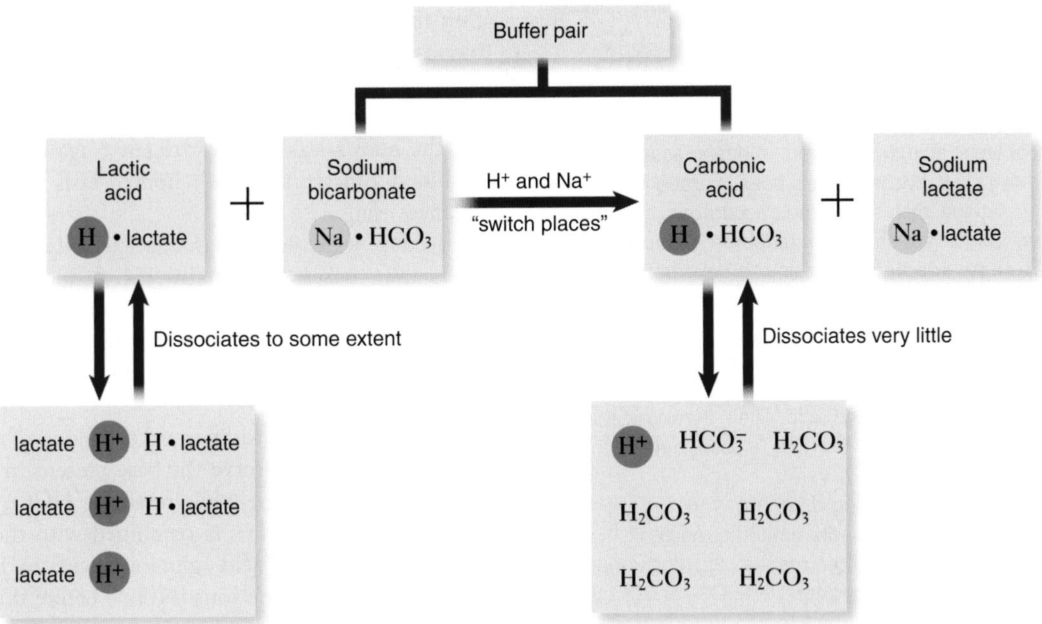

FIGURE 20-5 Lactic acid buffered by sodium bicarbonate. Lactic acid (H • lactate) and other "fixed" acids are buffered by $NaHCO_3$ in the blood. Carbonic acid (H • HCO_3, or H_2CO_3, a weaker acid than lactic acid) replaces lactic acid. As a result, fewer H^+ ions are added to blood than would be added if lactic acid were not buffered.

following changes in blood result from buffering of fixed acids in tissue capillaries:

1. The amount of H_2CO_3 in blood increases slightly because an acid (such as lactic acid) is converted to H_2CO_3.
2. The amount of bicarbonate in blood (mainly $NaHCO_3$) decreases because bicarbonate ions become part of the newly formed H_2CO_3. Normal systemic arterial blood with a pH of 7.45 contains 20 times more $NaHCO_3$ than H_2CO_3. If this ratio decreases, blood pH decreases below 7.45.
3. The H^+ concentration of blood increases slightly. H_2CO_3 adds hydrogen ions to blood, but it adds fewer of them than lactic acid would have because it is a weaker acid than lactic acid. In other words, the buffering mechanisms do not totally prevent blood hydrogen ion concentration from increasing. It simply minimizes the increase.
4. Blood pH decreases slightly because of the small increase in blood H^+ concentration.

H_2CO_3 is the most abundant acid in body fluids because it is formed by the buffering of fixed acids and also because CO_2 forms it by combining with H_2O. Large amounts of CO_2, an end product of catabolism, continually pour into tissue capillary blood from cells. Much of the H_2CO_3 formed in blood diffuses into red blood cells where it is buffered by the potassium salt of hemoglobin.

Some of the H_2CO_3 breaks down to form the gas CO_2 and water (H_2O). This takes place in the blood as it moves through the lung capillaries. The next part of our discussion explains how this affects blood pH.

QUICK CHECK

1. What three mechanisms does the body have for regulating pH of body fluids?
2. What are buffers?

Respiratory Mechanism of pH Control

Respirations play a vital part in controlling pH. With every expiration, CO_2 and H_2O leave the body in the expired air. The CO_2 has diffused out of the pulmonary blood as it moves through the lung capillaries. Less CO_2 therefore remains in the blood leaving the lung capillaries, so less of it is available for combining with water to form H_2CO_3. Hence after expiration the blood contains less H_2CO_3, has fewer hydrogen ions, and has a higher pH (7.45) than does the deoxygenated blood entering the pulmonary circulation (pH 7.35).

Let us consider now how a change in respirations can alter blood pH. Suppose you were to pinch your nose shut and hold your breath for a full minute or a little longer. Obviously, no CO_2 would leave your body by way of expired air during that time, and the blood's CO_2 content would consequently increase. This would increase the amount of H_2CO_3 and the hydrogen-ion concentration of blood, which in turn would decrease blood pH.

However, this situation would not last for long. The respiratory control centers in your brainstem detect the dropping pH and rising CO_2 in your blood and respond strongly by forcing you to inhale (see Chapter 15, p. 355). This survival mechanism explains why a person cannot hold his or her breath indefinitely. It also explains why during exercise, a drop in pH caused by increased muscle production of CO_2 triggers

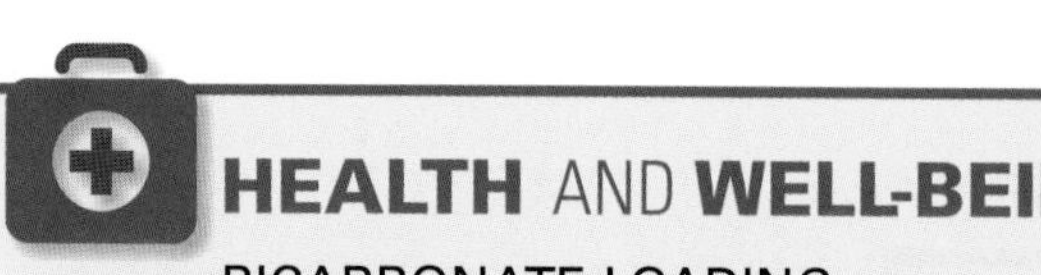

HEALTH AND WELL-BEING

BICARBONATE LOADING

The buildup of lactic acid in the blood, released as a waste product from working muscles, has been blamed for the soreness and fatigue that sometimes accompany strenuous exercise. Some athletes have adopted a technique called **bicarbonate loading,** ingesting large amounts of sodium bicarbonate ($NaHCO_3$) to counteract the effects of lactic acid buildup.

This practice is most popular in sports involving brief powerful muscle contractions that rely on aerobic respiration that quickly produces lactic acid. Their theory is that fatigue is avoided because the $NaHCO_3$, a base, buffers the lactic acid.

However, bicarbonate loading does not work for everyone. When it does, it is only under limited conditions. Unfortunately, the diarrhea that often results can trigger fluid and electrolyte imbalances. Long-term $NaHCO_3$ abuse can lead to disruption of acid-base balance and its disastrous effects.

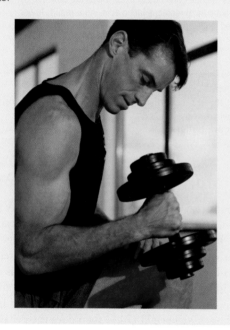

an increase in breathing rate. Of course, the opposite is true as well—when blood pH increases to or above normal, then the rate of breathing slows.

Here then are two useful facts to remember. Any factor that causes an appreciable decrease in respirations may in time produce **acidosis.** Conversely, any factor that causes an excessive increase in respirations may in time produce **alkalosis.**

Urinary Mechanism of pH Control

Most people know that the kidneys are vital organs and that life soon ebbs away if they stop functioning. One reason is that the kidneys are the body's most effective regulators of blood pH. They can eliminate much larger amounts of acid than can the lungs and, if it becomes necessary, they also can excrete excess base. The lungs cannot. In short, the kidneys are the body's last and best defense against wide variations in blood pH. If they fail, homeostasis of pH—acid-base balance—fails.

Because more acids than bases usually enter blood, more acids than bases are usually excreted by the kidneys. In other words, most of the time the kidneys acidify urine—that is, they excrete enough acid to give urine an acid pH, frequently as low as 4.8. (How does this compare with normal blood pH?)

The tubules of the kidneys rid the blood of excess acid and at the same time conserve the base present in it by secreting H^+ ions into the urine while retaining HCO_3^- in the blood. Much of the excess H^+ is combined with the amine group (NH_2) of an amino acid (glutamic acid) to form ammonia (NH_3) and ammonium ions (NH_4^+) before it is secreted into urine.

QUICK CHECK

1. How can breathing affect the pH of the blood?
2. By what mechanism can the kidney change the pH of the blood?
3. What is the body's last and best defense against wide variations in blood pH?

pH Imbalances

Acidosis and Alkalosis

Acidosis and **alkalosis** are the two kinds of pH or acid-base imbalance. Although any pH value above 7.0 is considered chemically basic, in clinical medicine the term *acidosis* is used to describe an arterial blood pH of less than 7.35, and *alkalosis* is used to describe an arterial blood pH greater than 7.45.

In acidosis the blood pH falls as H^+ ion concentration increases or bases are lost. Only rarely does it fall as low as 7.0 (neutrality), and almost never does it become even slightly acidic, because death usually intervenes before the pH drops this much. In alkalosis, which develops less often than acidosis, the blood pH is higher than normal because of a loss of acids or an accumulation of bases.

From a clinical standpoint, disturbances in acid-base balance can be considered dependent on the relative quantities (ratio) of H_2CO_3 and $NaHCO_3$ in the blood. Components of this important buffer pair must be maintained at the proper ratio (20 times more $NaHCO_3$ than H_2CO_3) if acid-base balance is to remain normal. It is fortunate that the body can regulate both chemicals in the $NaHCO_3$–H_2CO_3 buffer system. Blood levels of $NaHCO_3$ can be regulated by the kidneys and H_2CO_3 levels by the respiratory system (lungs).

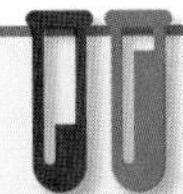

CLINICAL APPLICATION

DIABETIC KETOACIDOSIS

An important part of home care for people with diabetes involves monitoring the level of glucose in the blood and, especially for patients taking insulin, carefully watching for the appearance of **ketone bodies** in the urine. Accumulation of these acidic substances in the blood results from the excessive metabolism of fats found most often in uncontrolled type 1 diabetics. These individuals have trouble metabolizing carbohydrates and instead burn fat as a primary energy source.

The accumulation of ketone bodies results in a condition called **diabetic ketoacidosis** that causes the blood to become dangerously acidic. The body attempts to correct or "compensate" for the acidosis by rapid breathing to "blow off" CO_2 and thus decrease blood carbonic acid levels. As blood levels of ketones increase, they "spill over" into the urine and can be detected by use of appropriate reagent strips. Ketones also may give a "fruity" odor to the breath and urine. As the body compensates for the acidosis, rapid breathing may occur.

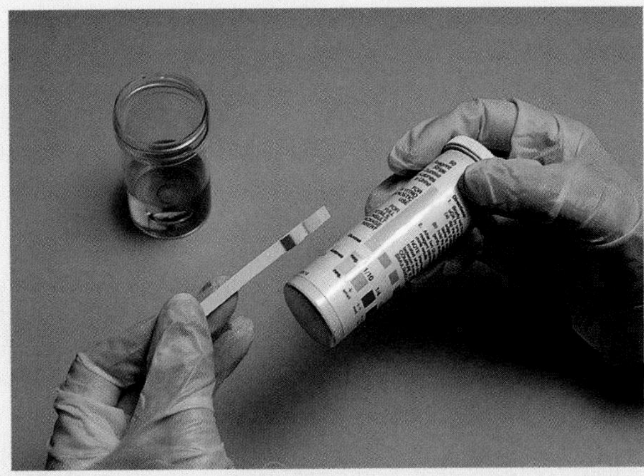

Ketonuria. Using a reagent strip to check for the presence of ketone bodies in the urine of a diabetic patient.

Metabolic and Respiratory Disturbances

Two types of disturbances, metabolic and respiratory, can alter the proper ratio of these components. Metabolic disturbances affect the bicarbonate ($NaHCO_3$) element of the buffer pair, and respiratory disturbances affect the H_2CO_3 element, as follows:

1. **Metabolic disturbances**
   a. **Metabolic acidosis** (bicarbonate deficit). Patients in metabolic acidosis with a bicarbonate deficit often suffer from renal disease, uncontrolled diabetes, prolonged diarrhea, or have ingested toxic chemicals such as antifreeze (ethylene glycol) or wood alcohol (methanol).
   b. **Metabolic alkalosis** (bicarbonate excess). The bicarbonate excess in metabolic alkalosis can result from diuretic therapy, loss of acid-containing gastric fluid caused by vomiting or suction, or from certain diseases such as Cushing syndrome.
2. **Respiratory disturbances**
   a. **Respiratory acidosis** (H_2CO_3 excess). The increase in H_2CO_3 characteristic of respiratory acidosis is caused most frequently by slow breathing (hypoventilation), which results in excess CO_2 in the systemic arterial blood. Causes include depression of the respiratory center by drugs or anesthesia or by pulmonary diseases such as emphysema and pneumonia. Serious respiratory acidosis also follows recovery from cardiac arrest.
   b. **Respiratory alkalosis** (H_2CO_3 deficit). Hyperventilation leads to a H_2CO_3 deficit caused by excessive loss of CO_2 in expired air. The result is respiratory alkalosis. Anxiety (hyperventilation syndrome), overventilation of patients on ventilators, or hepatic coma can all reduce H_2CO_3 and CO_2 to dangerously low levels.

Compensation for pH Imbalances

When acidosis or alkalosis occurs in the body, our various pH-balancing mechanisms—buffers and the respiratory and urinary mechanisms—try to restore balance as soon as possible. We often use the term **compensation** for this set of processes because the body is using means that "compensate" for the abnormal shift in pH.

Compensation is a clinically important concept. Because compensation mechanisms in the body can quickly counteract an abnormal shift in blood pH, a person may have a serious, ongoing medical condition and yet temporarily have what appears to be a normal blood pH.

For example, a person could have a metabolic disease such as diabetes that causes acidosis, but is hyperventilating to compensate for the drop in pH. Such a patient could have a normal arterial blood pH. The underlying condition, however, has not been resolved. This case would be labeled *compensated metabolic acidosis*. If the respiratory system had not yet compensated for the drop in pH resulting from the metabolic condition, then we would label it a case of *uncompensated metabolic acidosis*.

QUICK CHECK

1. What is acidosis? What is alkalosis?
2. What factors may cause a metabolic disturbance in pH?
3. What situations may cause a respiratory disturbance in pH?
4. What does the term "compensate" mean when referring to pH imbalances?

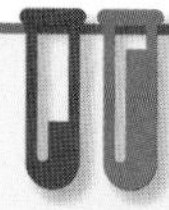

CLINICAL APPLICATION

VOMITING

Vomiting, sometimes referred to as **emesis**, is the forcible emptying or expulsion of gastric and occasionally intestinal contents through the mouth. It can occur as a result of various stimuli, including foul odors or tastes, irritation of the stomach or intestinal mucosa caused by food poisoning, certain bacterial or viral infections, and alcohol intoxication.

A "vomiting center" in the brainstem regulates the many coordinated, but primarily involuntary, steps involved (see illustration). The pernicious vomiting of pregnancy, the severe and repetitive (cyclic) vomiting that sometimes occurs in childhood (especially with pyloric obstruction in infants) can be life threatening because of the fluid, electrolyte, and acid-base imbalances that may result.

One of the most frequent and serious complications of repetitive vomiting that continues over time is **metabolic alkalosis.** The bicarbonate excess of metabolic alkalosis results indirectly because of the massive loss of chloride. The lost chloride, which is a component of hydrochloric acid (HCl) in gastric secretions, is replaced by bicarbonate in the extracellular fluid. The result is metabolic alkalosis (see illustration).

The body "compensates" for the imbalance by suppressing respirations to increase blood CO_2 levels and, ultimately, levels of H_2CO_3 in the extracellular fluid. The kidneys also assist in the compensation process by conserving H^+ and eliminating additional HCO_3^- in an alkaline urine.

Therapy to actually *restore* the buffer pair ratio ($NaHCO_3$ to H_2CO_3) to normal includes intravenous administration of chloride-containing solutions such as **normal saline** (0.9% NaCl). The chloride ions of the solution replace the bicarbonate ions and thus help relieve the bicarbonate excess that is responsible for the imbalance.

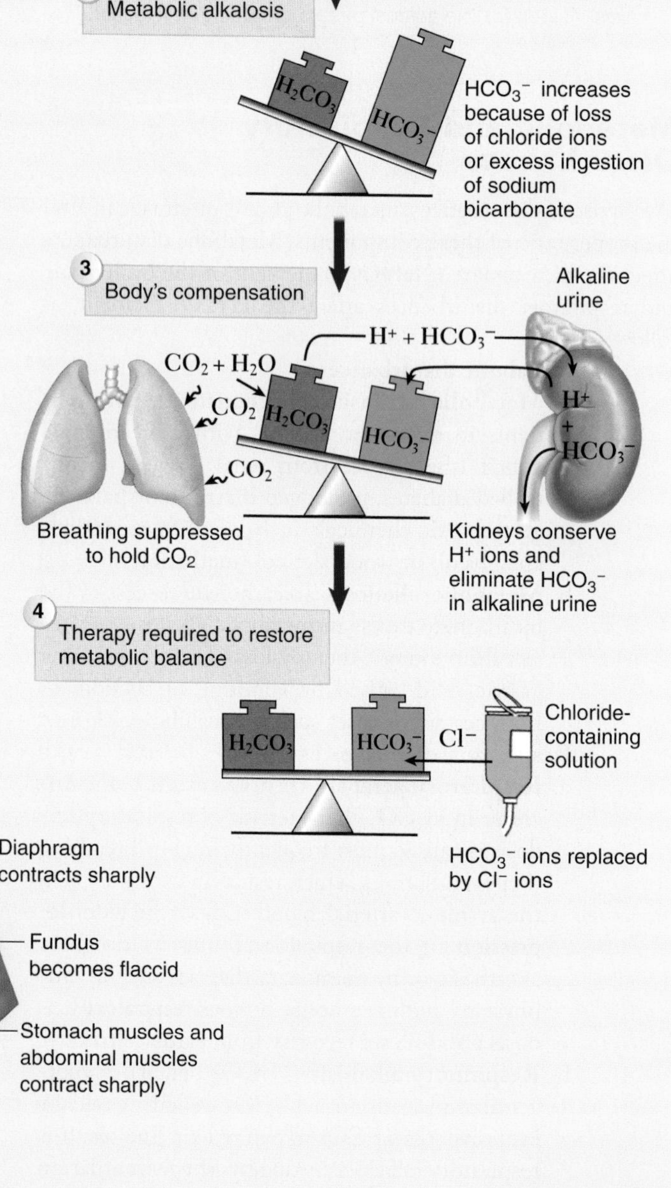

Soft palate rises

Hypersalivation occurs

Epiglottis closes

Larynx and hyoid bone are drawn forward

Diaphragm contracts sharply

Fundus becomes flaccid

Cardiac sphincter relaxes

Stomach muscles and abdominal muscles contract sharply

CLINICAL APPLICATION

CARDIAC ARREST AND RESPIRATORY ACIDOSIS

A cascade of rapid-fire catastrophic homeostatic failures follows *cardiac arrest*—the sudden cessation of blood pumping by the heart. One such failure involves almost immediate development of respiratory acidosis (carbonic acid excess) caused by retention of CO_2 in the body when respiration ceases and blood flow through the lung capillaries stops. Even if emergency CPR (cardiopulmonary resuscitation) measures can restore breathing and start the heart beating again, respiratory acidosis must be successfully treated and normal blood pH levels restored quickly in order to sustain life.

As in other types of pH imbalances, absolute changes in the amount or ratio of the bicarbonate-carbonic acid buffer pair components is the first line of defense to prevent massive changes in blood pH. Then, the body initiates both respiratory and renal compensatory mechanisms to help deal with the carbonic acid excess in severe respiratory acidosis.

The most important respiratory compensatory mechanism—increased breathing rate—does "blow off" some additional CO_2 but cannot significantly lower the very elevated carbonic acid buildup that follows cardiac arrest and remains after the blood buffers have been overwhelmed.

Finally, renal compensatory mechanisms that stabilize blood pH and help control many forms of respiratory acidosis are initiated after cardiac arrest. They include (1) decreasing the elimination of bicarbonate ions (HCO_3^-) and (2) increasing the elimination of hydrogen ions (H^+) in acidic urine. Although helpful in controlling chronic forms of respiratory acidosis that develop slowly over time, these slow-acting homeostatic compensatory mechanisms are unable to adequately address the serious, acute-onset acidosis that follows cardiac arrest. Medical intervention is required.

In the past, immediate intravenous (IV) infusion of bicarbonate- or lactate-containing solutions (lactate is converted to bicarbonate ions in the liver) was considered the emergency treatment of choice in treating respiratory acidosis after cardiac arrest—and these solutions are still used for that purpose. However, clinical studies have shown that aggressive treatment employing controlled ventilation to dramatically increase CO_2 elimination from the body may, in many cases, be more effective in restoring pH balance.

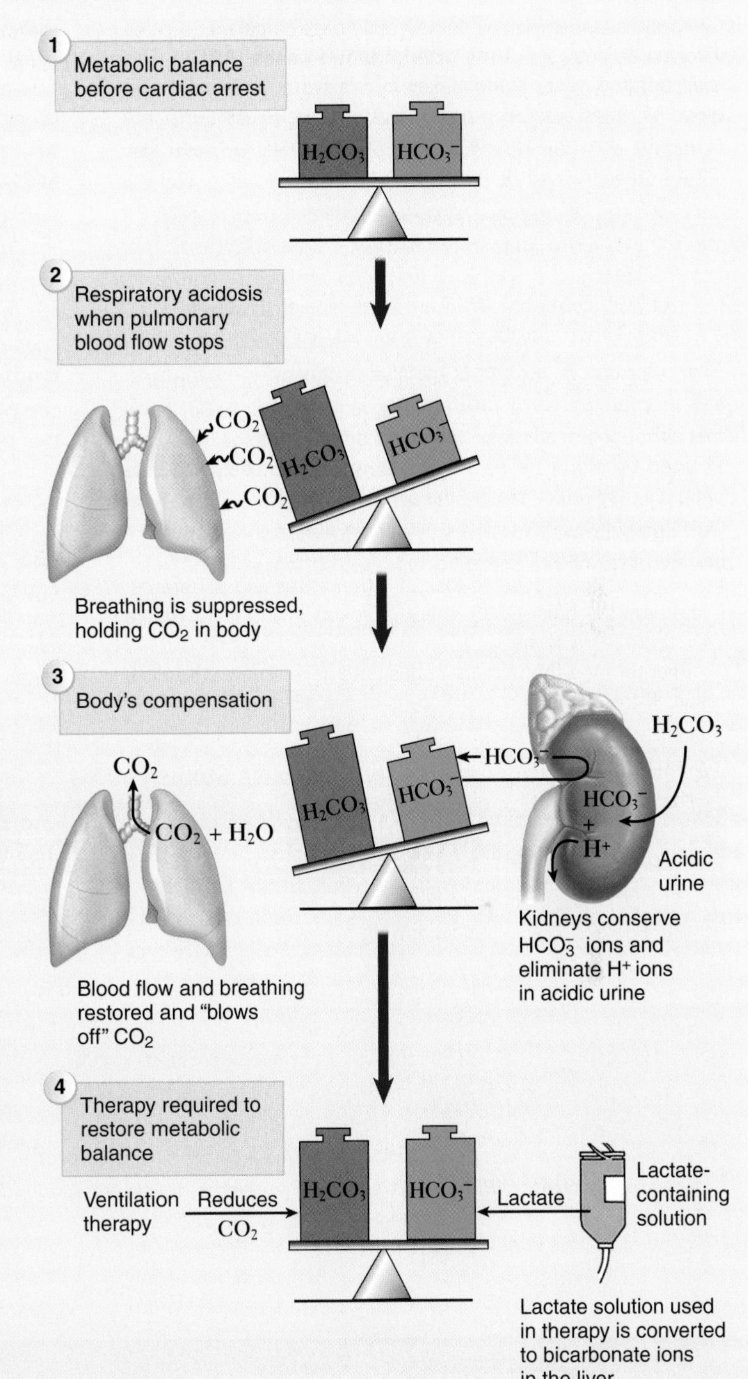

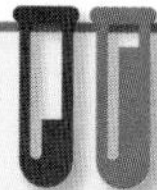

CLINICAL APPLICATION

ARTERIAL BLOOD GAS ANALYSIS

Clinically, assessment of primary acid-base imbalances often involves an analysis of the **arterial blood gases (ABGs)**. This is a laboratory test of blood taken from a systemic artery (most blood samples are taken from a systemic vein). As the name suggests, this test shows the key characteristics of blood related to respiratory function:

1. Oxygen partial pressure or Po_2
2. Oxygen saturation of hemoglobin or $\%SO_2$
3. pH
4. Concentration of bicarbonate ions or $[HCO_3^-]$
5. Carbon dioxide partial pressure or Pco_2

Sometimes these values are labeled with an "a" to emphasize that these are "arterial" values, as in Pao_2 or $Paco_2$. Note that although not all these values are actually "gases," they are affected by blood gases. ABG test results not only reveal a patient's respiratory status, the pH, Pco_2, and $[HCO_3^-]$ components can also give key information about status of acid-base homeostasis (see the table).

pH is the first result to look at when assessing pH status. If the result is below 7.35, there is *acidosis*, and if it's above 7.45, there is *alkalosis*.

To determine the primary status, one next looks at the Pco_2 result. If the pH is low and Pco_2 is above 45 mm Hg, the primary status is *respiratory* acidosis and if pH is high and Pco_2 is below 35 mm Hg the status is *respiratory* alkalosis.

Next, look at the $[HCO_3^-]$ result. If pH is low and $[HCO_3^-]$ is below 22 mEq/L, the primary status is *metabolic* acidosis. If the pH is high and the $[HCO_3^-]$ is above 26 mEq/L, the primary status is *metabolic* alkalosis.

One may then try to determine whether compensation is occurring in the body. This can be done by looking at the pH-balancing mechanism *not* directly involved in determining the primary status to see if has changed in a way that counterbalances—or *compensates* for—the primary problem. For example, if the arterial pH is low (acidotic) and the Pco_2 (acid) is high, as in respiratory acidosis, the body may compensate by increasing the $[HCO_3^-]$ (base). Likewise, if the arterial pH is high (alkalotic) and the $[HCO_3^-]$ (base) is high, as in metabolic alkalosis, the body may compensate by increasing the Pco_2 (acid).

Many students have used this memory aid when learning ABG interpretation: *ROME (Respiratory Opposite, Metabolic Equal).* If you look at the table, you can see that in respiratory disorders the pH and Pco_2 move in opposite directions. However, in metabolic disorders, the pH and Pco_2 move in the same (equal) direction.

Arterial Blood Gas Analysis for Acid-Base Status

ABG COMPONENT	NORMAL VALUES	ACIDOSIS		ALKALOSIS	
		RESPIRATORY	METABOLIC	RESPIRATORY	METABOLIC
pH	7.35-7.45	↓ < 7.35	↓ < 7.35	↑ > 7.45	↑ > 7.45
Pco_2	35-45 mm Hg	↑ > 45	Uncompensated: = 35-45 Compensated: ↓ < 35	↓ < 35	Uncompensated: = 35-45 Compensated: ↑ > 45
$[HCO_3^-]$	22-26 mEq/L	Uncompensated: = 22-26 Compensated: ↑ > 26	↓ < 22	Uncompensated: = 22-26 Compensated: ↓ < 22	↑ > 26

↓, decrease; ↑, increase; *ABG*, arterial blood gas; *Pco_2*, carbon dioxide pressure; *$[HCO_3^-]$*, bicarbonate concentration

LANGUAGE OF SCIENCE AND MEDICINE *(continued from p. 445)*

diabetic ketoacidosis
(dye-ah-BET-ik kee-toh-as-ih-DOH-sis)
[*diabet-* **siphon (diabetes mellitus),** *-ic* **relating to,** *keto-* **acetone,** *-acid-* **sour,** *-osis* **condition]**

emesis
(EM-eh-sis)
[*emesis* **vomiting]**

hydrogen ion (H^+)
(HYE-droh-jen AYE-on)
[*hydro-* **water,** *-gen* **produce,** *ion* **to go]**

hydroxide ion (OH^-)
(hye-DROK-syde aye-on)
[*hydr-* **water (hydrogen),** *-ox-* **sharp (oxygen),** *-ide* **chemical,** *ion* **to go]**

ketone body
(KEE-tohn BOD-ee)
[*keto-* **acetone,** *-one* **chemical]**

metabolic acidosis
(met-ah-BOL-ik as-ih-DOH-sis)
[*meta-* **over,** *-bol-* **throw,** *-ic* **relating to,** *-ic* **relating to,** *acid-* **sour,** *-osis* **condition]**

metabolic alkalosis
(met-ah-BOL-ik al-kah-LOH-sis)
[*meta-* **over,** *-bol-* **throw,** *-ic* **relating to,** *alkal-* **ashes,** *-osis* **condition**]

neutral
(NOO-trel)
[*neutr-* **neither,** *-al* **relating to**]

normal saline
(NOR-mall SAY-leen)
[*sal-* **salt,** *-ine* **relating to**]

pH
[abbreviation for *potenz* **power,** *hydrogen* **hydrogen**]

respiratory acidosis
(RES-pih-rah-tor-ee as-ih-DOH-sis)
[*re-* **again,** *-spir-* **breathe,** *-tory* **relating to,** *acid-* **sour,** *-osis* **condition**]

respiratory alkalosis
(RES-pih-rah-tor-ee al-kah-LOH-sis)
[*re-* **again,** *-spir-* **breathe,** *-tory* **relating to,** *alkal-* **ashes,** *-osis* **condition**]

❑ OUTLINE SUMMARY

To download a digital audio version of the chapter summary for use with your device, access the ***Audio Chapter Summaries*** *online at evolve.elsevier.com.*

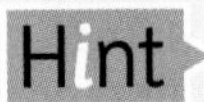

Scan this summary after reading the chapter to help you reinforce the key concepts. Later, use the summary as a quick review before your class or before a test.

pH of Body Fluids

A. pH — a number that indicates the relative hydrogen ion (H^+) concentration (compared with OH^-) of a fluid (see Figure 20-1)
   1. pH 7.0 indicates neutrality (neutral solution)
   2. pH higher than 7.0 indicates alkalinity (alkaline or basic solution; base)
   3. pH less than 7.0 indicates acidity (acid solution)
B. Normal range of blood pH is approximately 7.35 to 7.45
   1. Systemic arterial blood pH — about 7.45
   2. Systemic venous blood pH — about 7.35
C. pH scale based on multiples of 10
   1. H^+ concentration changes by 10 times for each pH unit
   2. Large pH fluctuations may appear small

Mechanisms That Control pH of Body Fluids

A. pH homeostatic mechanism — three coordinated homeostatic mechanisms act to maintain the normal pH of body fluids and prevent pH swings when excess acids or bases are present (see Figure 20-2)
   1. Chemical pH control mechanism — based on buffers in blood/RBCs/and body fluids — act immediately
   2. Physiological pH control mechanisms
      a. Changes in pH regulated by changes in respiratory rate that result in changes in blood CO_2 — act within minutes
      b. Changes in pH regulated by altered renal activity — act within hours
B. Buffers
   1. Definition — chemical substances that prevent a sharp change in the pH of a fluid when an acid or base is added to it (Figures 20-3 and 20-4)
   2. Buffers usually include two different chemicals — called a buffer pair
   3. "Fixed" acids are buffered mainly by sodium bicarbonate ($NaHCO_3$)
   4. Changes in blood produced by buffering of "fixed" acids in the tissue capillaries (see Figure 20-5)
      a. Amount of carbonic acid (H_2CO_3) in blood increases slightly
      b. Amount of $NaHCO_3$ in blood decreases; ratio of amount of $NaHCO_3$ to the amount of H_2CO_3 does not normally change; normal ratio is 20:1
      c. H^+ concentration of blood increases slightly
      d. Blood pH decreases slightly below arterial level
C. Respiratory mechanism of pH control
   1. Respirations remove some CO_2 from blood as blood flows through lung capillaries
   2. Amount of H_2CO_3 in blood is decreased and thereby its H^+ concentration is decreased; this in turn increases blood pH
   3. Respiratory control centers in brainstem react to dropping pH and promote increased respirations; when pH increases, then breathing slows
D. Urinary mechanism of pH control
   1. Kidneys are the body's most effective regulator of blood pH
   2. Usually urine is acidified by way of the distal tubules secreting hydrogen ions into the urine from blood in exchange for HCO_3^- being retained in the blood; much of the excess H^+ is secreted as ammonia (NH_3) and ammonium ions (NH_4^+)

pH Imbalances

A. Acidosis and alkalosis are the two kinds of pH, or acid-base, imbalances
   1. Disturbances in acid-base balance depend on relative quantities of $NaHCO_3$ and H_2CO_3 in the blood
   2. Body can regulate both of the components of the $NaHCO_3$–H_2CO_3 buffer system
      a. Blood levels of $NaHCO_3$ are regulated by kidneys
      b. H_2CO_3 levels are regulated by lungs

B. Metabolic and respiratory disturbances — both can alter the normal 20:1 ratio of $NaHCO_3$ to H_2CO_3 in blood
  1. Metabolic disturbances affect the $NaHCO_3$ levels in blood
     a. Metabolic acidosis — bicarbonate ($NaHCO_3$) deficit
     b. Metabolic alkalosis — bicarbonate ($NaHCO_3$) excess; complication of severe vomiting (see box, p. 452)
  2. Respiratory disturbances affect the H_2CO_3 levels in blood
     a. Respiratory acidosis (H_2CO_3 excess)
     b. Respiratory alkalosis (H_2CO_3 deficit)

C. Compensation for pH imbalances
  1. Compensated acidosis or alkalosis — occurs when the body's pH-balancing mechanisms temporarily counteract an abnormal shift in pH
  2. Uncompensated acidosis or alkalosis — occurs when the body's mechanisms have not yet normalized the pH

❑ ACTIVE LEARNING

STUDY TIPS

Hint *Use these tips to achieve success in meeting your learning goals.*

To make the study of acid-base balance more efficient, we suggest these tips:

1. Before studying Chapter 20, go back and review initial coverage of the pH scale, acids, and bases in Chapter 2. Review also respiratory function in Chapter 15 and urinary function in Chapter 18.
2. Think of the pH scale as a "shortcut" to express long numbers containing multiple zeros with a simple number between 0 and 14. A solution with a pH of 0 has 1.0 grams of hydrogen ions (H^+) per liter (10^0) while a solution with a pH of 14 contains only 0.00000000000001 (10^{-14}) grams of hydrogen ions. Each increase or decrease of one pH unit represents a tenfold difference in hydrogen ion concentration.
3. Understanding the concept of pH and the pH scale is based on understanding the relationship between the concentration of acidic hydrogen ions (H^+) and basic hydroxide ions (OH^-) in the solution. A solution with a pH of 7 contains equal numbers of H^+ and OH^- ions and is said to be neutral. It is neither acid nor alkaline. Solutions with a pH between 0 and 6.9 are acidic. Basic (alkaline) solutions have a pH between 7.1 and 14.
4. Buffer systems can be thought of as hydrogen or hydroxide ion sponges. They remove those ions so they will have less of an effect on the pH of a solution, in this case, the blood. In the $NaHCO_3$–H_2CO_3 buffer system, the sodium bicarbonate can absorb hydrogen ions by having the hydrogen replace the sodium. The carbonic acid can give up one of its hydrogen atoms, which bonds with a hydroxide ion to form water. In both cases the pH of the buffered solution will change very little.
5. Blood carries carbon dioxide as carbonic acid. When the lungs exhale carbon dioxide, there is less carbonic acid in the blood and so the pH of the blood rises. The kidneys use a similar buffer system to secrete hydrogen ions.
6. The buffer system in the blood usually works well, but it can be overwhelmed. Acidosis is a condition in which the blood becomes too acidic, and alkalosis is a condition in which the blood becomes too basic. Develop a concept map of the respiratory and urinary mechanisms of control involved in maintaining normal pH of body fluids.
7. If you have difficulty with the chemistry in this chapter, discuss it in your study group. Someone in the group may have a stronger chemistry background. Review the Language of Science and Medicine section. Discuss the pH system. Carefully go over the diagrams of the blood and kidney buffer systems. Review the types of acidosis and alkalosis and what causes each of them. Go over the questions and the chapter outline summary at the end of the chapter and discuss possible test questions.

Review Questions

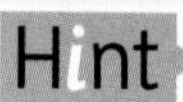

Write out the answers to these questions after reading the chapter and reviewing the Chapter Summary. If you simply think through the answer without writing it down, you won't retain much of your new learning.

1. Explain the relationship between pH and the relative concentration of hydrogen and hydroxide ions in a solution.
2. Write out the chemical reaction that converts carbon dioxide and water to carbonic acid. Name the enzyme that catalyzes this reaction.
3. Describe buffers and the role that they play in the pH of body fluids.
4. Explain how a buffer pair would react if more hydrogen ions were added to the blood.

5. Explain how a buffer pair would react if more hydroxide ions were added to the blood.
6. Explain the four changes that occur in the blood as the result of buffering fixed acids.
7. Explain the respiratory mechanism of pH control.
8. Explain how changes in the respiration rate affect blood pH.
9. Explain how the kidney handles H^+ and HCO_3^- to remove excess acid from the blood.
10. Define *acidosis* and *alkalosis.*
11. Explain metabolic disturbances of the buffer pair.
12. Explain respiratory disturbances of the buffer pair.

Critical Thinking

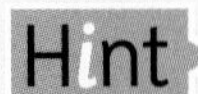

After finishing the Review Questions, write out the answers to these more in-depth questions to help you apply your new knowledge. Go back to sections of the chapter that relate to concepts that you find difficult.

13. Explain how excessive vomiting causes metabolic alkalosis and explain why normal saline can be used to correct it.
14. What is the proper ratio of $NaHCO_3$ and H_2CO_3 in a buffer pair? Explain how the body can use this ratio to correct uncompensated metabolic acidosis.
15. Liam had a sudden heart attack and was transported by ambulance to the hospital. Explain why one of the immediate concerns was respiratory acidosis and what compensatory mechanisms in the body would be initiated to deal with the acidosis.

Chapter Test

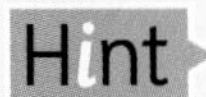

After studying the chapter, test your mastery by responding to these items. Try to answer them without looking up the answers. Then, verify the answers using the key in Appendix C at the back of this book.

1. The enzyme that converts carbon dioxide and water into carbonic acid is ________.
2. ________ are chemical substances that prevent sharp changes in pH when an acid or base is added to it.
3. If a strong acid such as HCl were added to the buffer pair $NaHCO_3$ and H_2CO_3, the $NaHCO_3$ would become ________.
4. If a strong base such as NaOH were added to the buffer pair in question 3, the H_2CO_3 would become ________.
5. The part of the nephron that is important in regulation of blood pH is the ________.
6. When NH_2 (amine) is used by the kidney to remove hydrogen ions from the blood, the end products that leave the body in the urine are NH_3 and ________.
7. When the kidney removes hydrogen ions from the blood, the pH of urine will ________.
8. The kidney is more effective in pH regulation than the lung because it can remove ________, which the lung cannot do.
9. The condition in which the blood pH is higher than normal is called ________.
10. The condition in which the blood pH is lower than normal is called ________.
11. For the buffer pair to function properly, the concentration of $NaHCO_3$ must be ________ times greater than the concentration of H_2CO_3.
12. Metabolic disturbances usually have an effect on the ________ part of the buffer pair.
13. Respiratory disturbances usually have an effect on the ________ part of the buffer pair.
14. Severe vomiting is a metabolic disturbance that can cause metabolic ________.
15. An acid solution has:
    a. a pH greater than 7.0
    b. a pH less than 7.0
    c. more hydroxide ions than hydrogen ions
    d. both a and c
16. An alkaline solution has:
    a. a pH greater than 7.0
    b. a pH less than 7.0
    c. more hydrogen ions than hydroxide ions
    d. both b and c
17. Which of the following statements is true?
    a. A solution with a pH of 5 has more hydrogen ions than a solution with a pH of 2
    b. A solution with a pH of 9 is a base
    c. The pH value increases as the number of hydrogen ions increase
    d. Both a and c are true
18. Systemic arterial blood has a pH of 7.45, and systemic venous blood has a pH of 7.35; therefore:
    a. arterial blood is slightly more acid than venous blood
    b. arterial blood is slightly more alkaline than venous blood
    c. venous blood is slightly more alkaline than arterial blood
    d. both a and c

For questions 19 through 24, fill in the blank with either "increases" or "decreases" as appropriate.

19. When a fixed acid is buffered in the blood, the amount of $NaHCO_3$ in the blood ________.
20. When a fixed acid is buffered in the blood, the amount of hydrogen ions in the blood ________.
21. When a fixed acid is buffered in the blood, the amount of H_2CO_3 in the blood ________.
22. When a fixed acid is buffered in the blood, the pH of the blood ________.
23. Anything that causes an excessive increase in the respiration rate ________ the pH of the blood.
24. Anything that causes an appreciable decrease in the respiration rate ________ the pH of the blood.

Reproductive Systems

OUTLINE

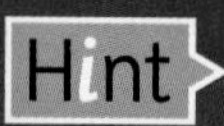

Scan this outline before you begin to read the chapter, as a preview of how the concepts are organized.

OBJECTIVES

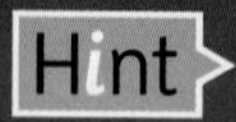

Before reading the chapter, review these goals for your learning.

After you have completed this chapter, you should be able to:

1. List the essential and accessory organs of the male and female reproductive systems and give the general function of each.
2. Describe the gross and microscopic structure of the gonads in both sexes and explain the developmental steps in spermatogenesis and oogenesis.
3. Discuss the primary functions of the sex hormones and identify the cell type or structure responsible for their secretion.
4. Identify and describe the structures that constitute the external genitals in both sexes.
5. Identify and discuss the phases of the endometrial or menstrual cycle and correlate each phase with its occurrence in a typical 28-day cycle.

CHAPTER 21

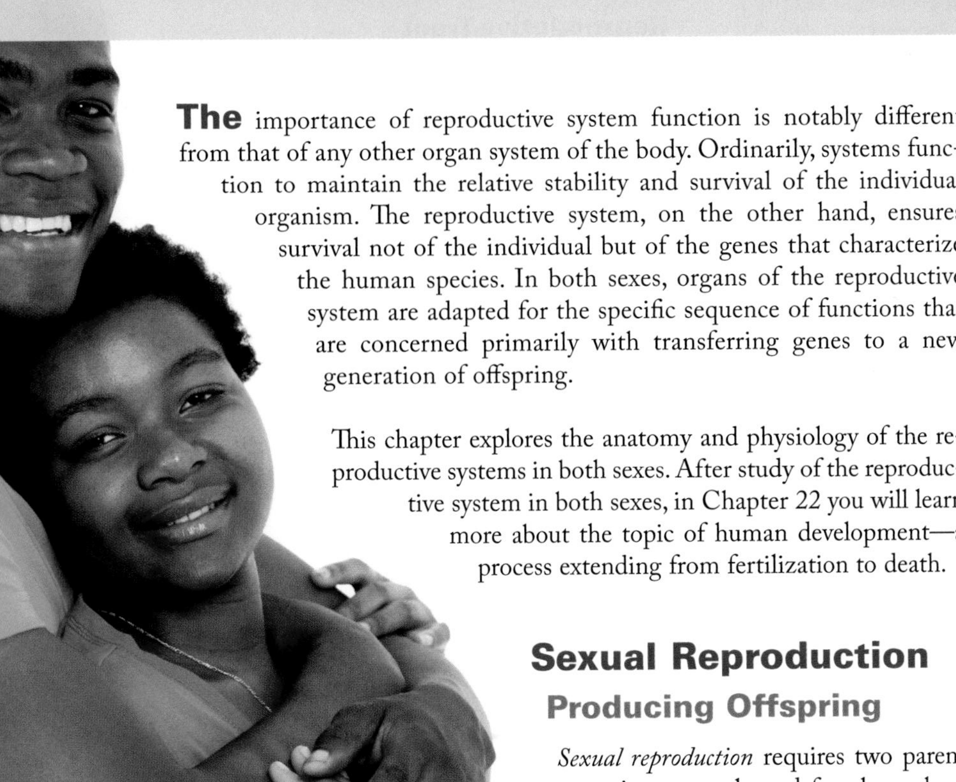

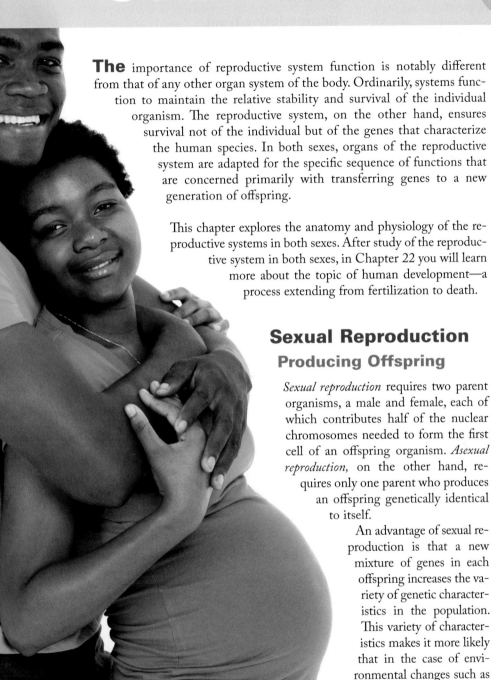

The importance of reproductive system function is notably different from that of any other organ system of the body. Ordinarily, systems function to maintain the relative stability and survival of the individual organism. The reproductive system, on the other hand, ensures survival not of the individual but of the genes that characterize the human species. In both sexes, organs of the reproductive system are adapted for the specific sequence of functions that are concerned primarily with transferring genes to a new generation of offspring.

This chapter explores the anatomy and physiology of the reproductive systems in both sexes. After study of the reproductive system in both sexes, in Chapter 22 you will learn more about the topic of human development—a process extending from fertilization to death.

Sexual Reproduction

Producing Offspring

Sexual reproduction requires two parent organisms, a male and female, each of which contributes half of the nuclear chromosomes needed to form the first cell of an offspring organism. *Asexual reproduction,* on the other hand, requires only one parent who produces an offspring genetically identical to itself.

An advantage of sexual reproduction is that a new mixture of genes in each offspring increases the variety of genetic characteristics in the population. This variety of characteristics makes it more likely that in the case of environmental changes such as disease, natural disaster, or shifting climatic conditions, there will be at least some individuals likely to survive and carry on the reproductive line.

The reproductive system of each parent produces the sex or reproductive cells called **gametes** needed to form the

LANGUAGE OF **SCIENCE** AND **MEDICINE**

Hint Before reading the chapter, say each of these terms out loud. This will help you to avoid stumbling over them as you read.

accessory organ
(ak-SES-oh-ree OR-gun)
[*access-* **extra,** *-ory* **relating to,** *organ* **instrument**]

acrosome
(AK-roh-sohm)
[*acro-* **top or tip,** *-some* **body**]

amenorrhea
(ah-men-oh-REE-ah)
[*a-* **without,** *-men-* **month,** *-rrhea* **flow**]

antrum
(AN-trum)
[*antrum* **cave**]

areola
(ah-REE-oh-lah)
[*are-* **area or space,** *-ola* **little**]

benign prostatic hypertrophy (BPH)
(be-NYNE pro-STAT-ik hye-PER-troh-fee)
[*benign* **kind,** *pro-* **before,** *-stat-* **set or place,** *-ic* **relating to,** *hyper-* **excessive or above,** *-troph-* **nourishment,** *-y* **state**]

breast
(brest)

bulbourethral gland (Cowper gland)
(BUL-boh-yoo-REE-thral gland [KOW-per])
[*bulb-* **swollen root,** *-ure-* **urine,** *-thr-* **agent or channel (urethra),** *-al* **relating to,** *gland* **acorn** (*William Cowper* **English anatomist**)]

cervix
(SER-viks)
pl., cervices or cervixes
(SER-vis-eez or SER-viks-ez)
[*cervix* **neck**]

circumcision
(ser-kum-SIH-zhun)
[*circum-* **around,** *-cision* **cutting**]

Continued on p. 476

offspring. These gametes, called an **ovum** (from the female parent) and a **sperm** (from the male parent), fuse during the process of fertilization. The new offspring cell that results is called the **zygote.** After many complicated and amazing developmental stages, the zygote ultimately develops into a new individual organism.

Each reproductive system also produces hormones that regulate development of the secondary sex characteristics that promote successful reproduction. For example, hormones create structural and behavioral differences in the sexes that permit adults to recognize and form sexual attractions with the opposite sex. Reproductive hormones and other regulatory mechanisms give us the urge to have sex, which is often reinforced with the pleasant sensations that sexual activity can produce. This sex drive is essential to success in producing offspring.

Sexual maturity and the ability to reproduce occur at puberty. The male reproductive system consists of organs whose functions are to produce, transfer, and ultimately introduce mature sperm into the female reproductive tract, where the nuclear chromosomes from each parent can unite to form a new offspring.

Male and Female Systems

Although the organs and specific functions of the male and female reproductive systems are discussed separately, it is important to understand that a common general structure and function can be identified between the systems in both sexes and that both sexes contribute in uniquely important ways to overall reproductive success.

In both men and women, the organs of the reproductive system are adapted for the specific sequence of functions that permit development of sperm or ova followed by successful fertilization and then the normal development and birth of a baby. In addition, production of hormones that permit development of secondary sex characteristics, such as breast development in women and beard growth in men, occurs as a result of normal reproductive system activity.

As you study the specifics of each system, keep in mind that the male organs function to produce, store, and ultimately introduce mature sperm into the female reproductive tract and that the female system is structured to produce ova, receive the sperm, and permit fertilization. In addition, the female reproductive system permits the fertilized ovum to develop and mature until birth.

The complex and cyclic control of reproductive functions in both men and women is particularly crucial to overall reproductive success in humans. The production of sex hormones is required not only for development of the secondary sexual characteristics but also for normal reproductive functions in both sexes. This chapter ends with a table that compares the reproductive structures and functions in women and men.

QUICK CHECK

1. What are gametes?
2. What is the ultimate function of the reproductive systems?

Male Reproductive System

Structural Plan

Reproductive Tract

You may recall from Chapter 18 (see p. 421) that in males the urethra has a dual function. It serves as a passageway for *both* urine and semen from the body. The term *urogenital tract* is sometimes used in place of *reproductive tract* to describe this dual urinary and reproductive function.

So many organs make up the male reproductive system that we need to look first at the structural plan of the system as a whole. Reproductive organs can be classified as *essential* or *accessory*.

Essential Organs

The **essential organs** of reproduction in men and women are called the **gonads.** The gonads of men consist of a pair of main sex glands called the **testes.** The testes produce the male sex cells—the *sperm* or **spermatozoa.** The testes also produce the hormone testosterone.

Accessory Organs

The **accessory organs** of reproduction in men consist of the following structures:

1. A series of passageways or ducts that carry the sperm from the testes to the exterior
2. Additional sex glands that provide secretions that protect and nurture sperm
3. The external reproductive organs called the *external genitals*

Table 21-1 lists the names of the essential and accessory organs of reproduction in men, and **Figure 21-1** shows the location of most of them. The table and the illustration are included very early in the chapter to provide a preliminary but important overview. Refer back to this table and illustration frequently as you learn about each organ in the pages that follow.

Testes

Structure and Location

The paired **testes** are the gonads of men. They are located in the pouchlike **scrotum,** which is suspended outside of the body cavity below the penis (see **Figure 21-1**). This exposed

TABLE 21-1 Male Reproductive Organs

ESSENTIAL ORGANS	ACCESSORY ORGANS
Gonads: testes (right testis and left testis)	Ducts: epididymis (two), vas deferens (two), ejaculatory duct (two), and urethra Supportive sex glands: seminal vesicle (two), bulbourethral or Cowper gland (two), and prostate gland External genitals: scrotum and penis

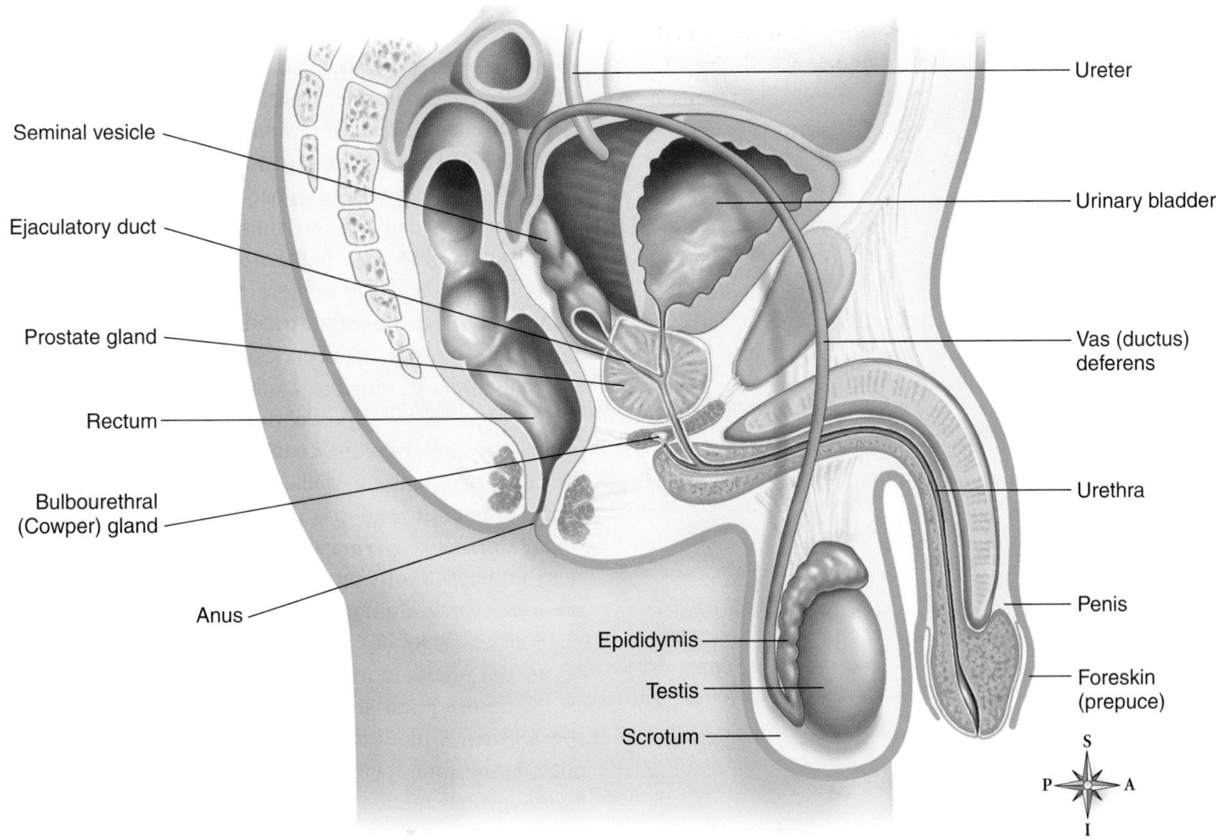

FIGURE 21-1 Organization of the male reproductive organs.

location provides an environment about 1° to 3° C cooler than normal body temperature, an important requirement for the normal production and survival of sperm.

Each testis is a small, oval gland about 3.8 cm (1.5 inches) long and 2.5 cm (1 inch) wide. The testis is shaped like an egg that has been flattened slightly from side to side. Note in **Figure 21-2** that each testis is surrounded by a tough, whitish membrane called the **tunica albuginea.** This membrane covers the testicle and then enters the gland to form the many septa that divide it into sections or lobules.

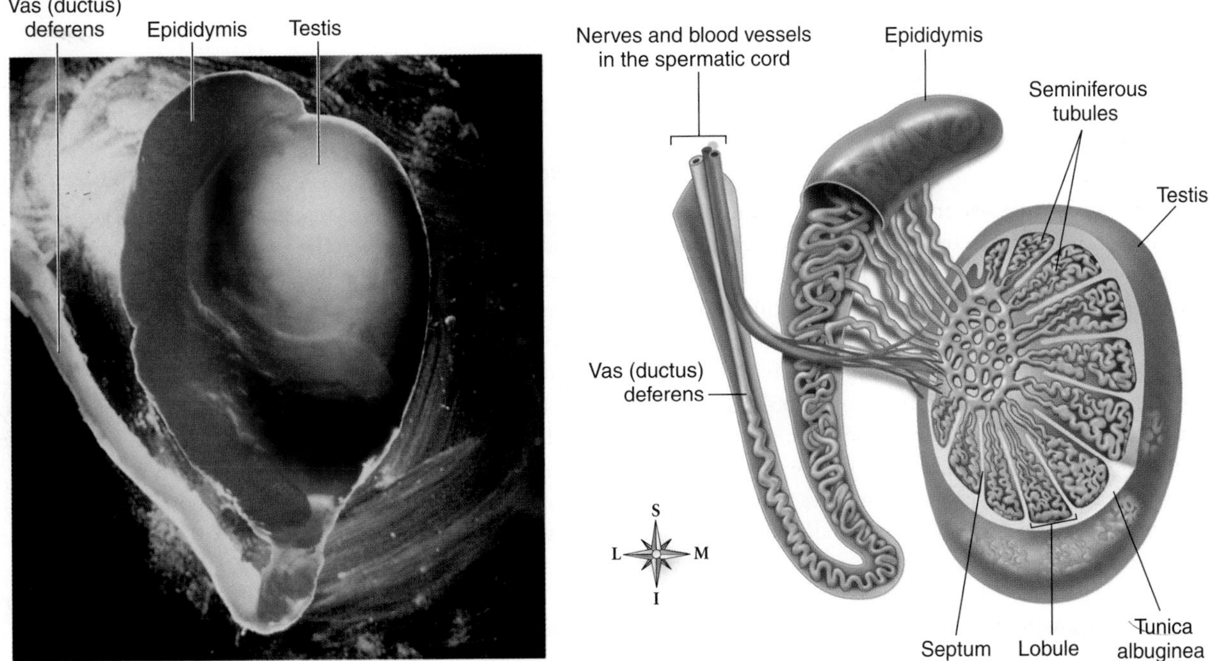

FIGURE 21-2 Tubules of the testis and epididymis. The ducts and tubules are exaggerated in size. In the photograph, the testicle is the darker sphere in the center.

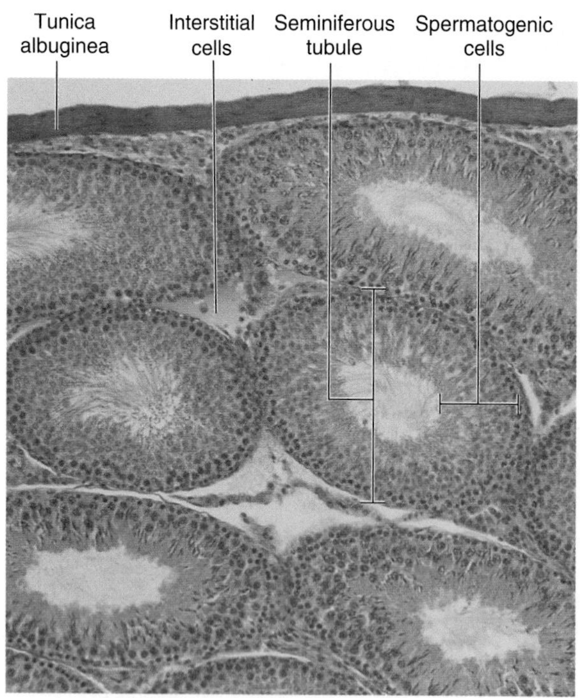

FIGURE 21-3 Testis tissue. Several seminiferous tubules surrounded by septa containing interstitial cells are shown.

As you can see in Figure 21-2, each lobule consists of a narrow but long and coiled **seminiferous tubule.** These coiled structures form the bulk of the testicular tissue mass. Small endocrine cells lying near the septa that separate the lobules can be seen in Figure 21-3. These are the **interstitial cells** of the testes that secrete the male sex hormone **testosterone.**

Each seminiferous tubule is a long duct with a central lumen or passageway (see Figure 21-3). Sperm develop in the walls of the tubule and are then released into the lumen and begin their journey to the exterior of the body (see Figure 21-5, *B*).

To learn more about testes, go to AnimationDirect at *evolve.elsevier.com.*

Testis Functions

Spermatogenesis

Sperm production is called **spermatogenesis.** From puberty on, the seminiferous tubules continuously form spermatozoa (sperm). Although the number of sperm produced each day diminishes with increasing age, most men continue to produce significant numbers throughout life.

The testes prepare for sperm production before puberty by increasing the numbers of sperm precursor (stem) cells called **spermatogonia.** These cells are located near the outer edge of each seminiferous tubule (Figure 21-4, *A*). Before puberty, spermatogonia increase in number by the process of mitotic cell division, which was described in Chapter 3. Recall that mitosis results in the division of a "parent" cell into two "daughter" cells, each identical to the parent and each containing a complete copy of the genetic material represented in the normal number of 46 chromosomes.

The hypothalamus is a small but functionally important structure located near the base of the brain. One of its many functions, in both males and females, is to secrete **gonadotropin-releasing hormone (GnRH)**, which then stimulates the anterior pituitary to secrete the gonadotropins **follicle-stimulating hormone (FSH)** and **luteinizing hormone (LH)**. A gonadotropin is a hormone that has a stimulating effect on the gonads—the testes and ovaries.

You may want to review these roles of the hypothalamus and pituitary gland in Chapters 9 and 11. Also, peek ahead to Figure 21-15, where you will see the hypothalamus and pituitary depicted at the top of the diagram.

When a boy enters puberty, circulating levels of FSH cause spermatogonia to undergo a unique series of cell divisions to produce sperm cells. When the spermatogonium undergoes mitosis and cell division occurs under the influence of FSH, it produces two daughter cells. One of these cells remains as a spermatogonium and the other forms another type of cell called a **primary spermatocyte.** These primary spermatocytes then undergo another type of cell division characterized by **meiosis,** which ultimately results in sperm formation.

Note in Figure 21-4, *B*, that in meiosis, two cell divisions occur (not one as in mitosis) and four daughter cells (not two as in mitosis) are formed. The daughter cells are called **spermatids.** Unlike the two daughter cells that result from mitosis, the four spermatids each have only half the genetic material in its nucleus and half of the nuclear chromosomes (23 instead of 46) of other body cells. These spermatids then develop into spermatozoa.

Look again at the diagram of meiosis in Figure 21-4, *B*. It shows that each primary spermatocyte ultimately produces four sperm cells. Note that, in the portion of a seminiferous tubule shown in Figure 21-4, *B*, spermatogonia are found at the outer surface of the tubule, primary and secondary spermatocytes lie deeper in the tubule wall, and mature but immotile sperm are seen about to enter the lumen of the tube and begin their journey through the reproductive ducts to the exterior of the body.

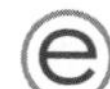
To learn more about spermatogenesis, go to AnimationDirect at *evolve.elsevier.com.*

Sperm

Sperm are among the smallest and most unusual cells in the body (Figure 21-5, *A*). The term sperm comes from Latin *spermatozoan* meaning "seed animal." This is because, somewhat like a seed, each sperm cell is part of the reproductive process. And each sperm cell has a tail and moves independently somewhat like a microscopic animal.

All of the characteristics that a baby will inherit from its father at fertilization are contained in the nuclear chromosomes found in each sperm head. However, this genetic information from the father will unite with chromosomes contained in the mother's ovum only if successful fertilization occurs.

The forceful ejection of fluid containing sperm, or **ejaculation,** of sperm into the female vagina during sexual intercourse is only one step in the long journey that these sex cells must make before they can meet and fertilize an ovum. To accomplish their task, these tiny packages of genetic

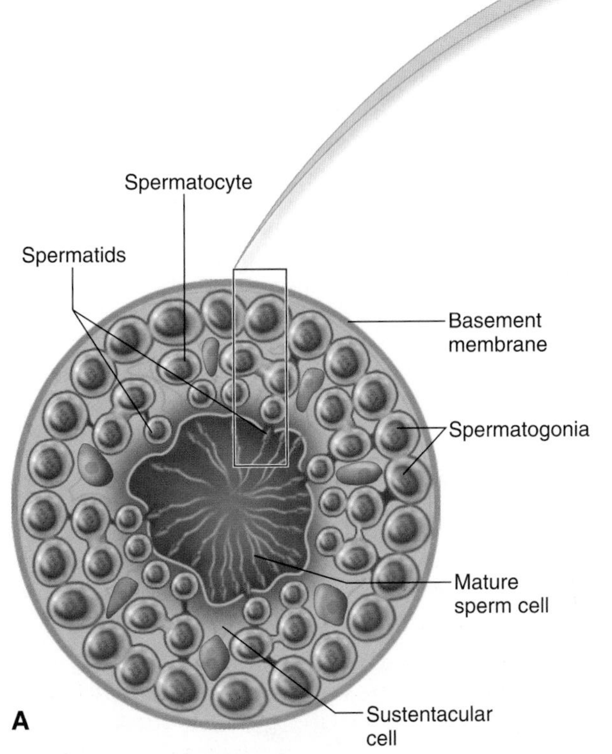

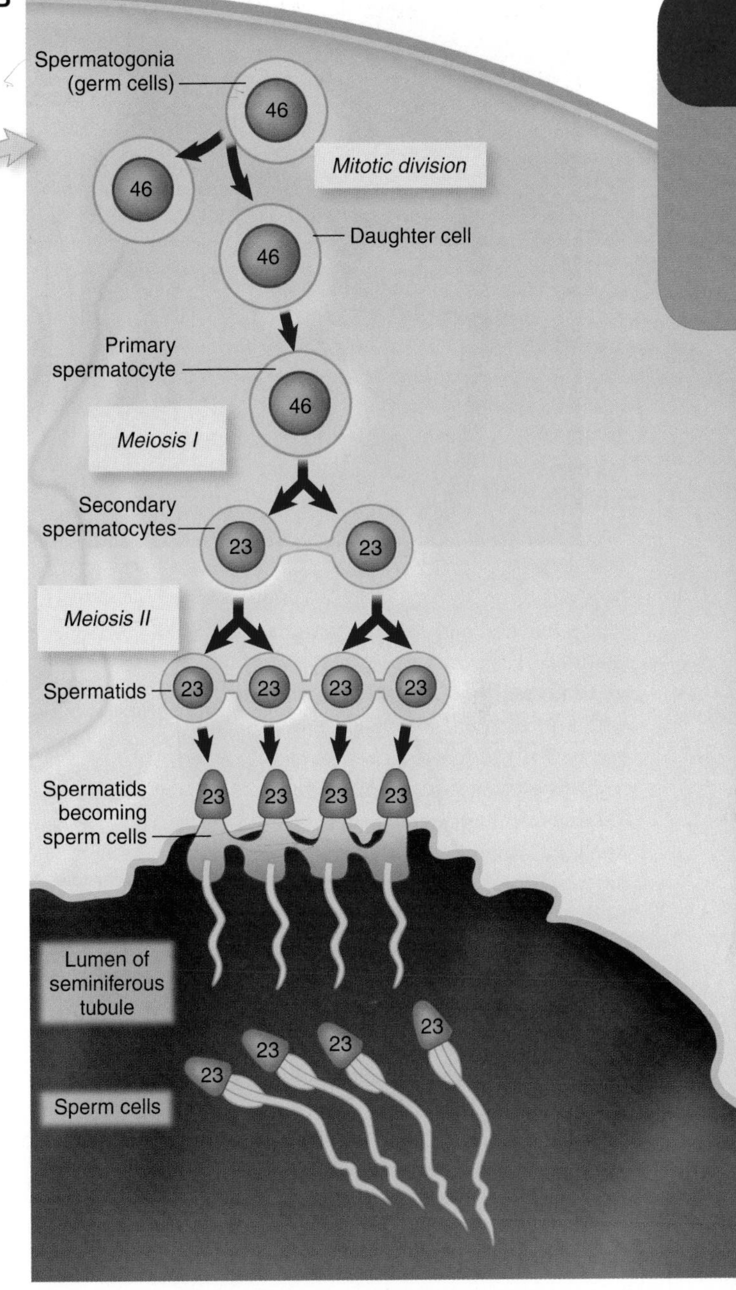

FIGURE 21-4 Spermatogenesis. A, Cross section of seminiferous tubule shows layers of cells undergoing the process of spermatogenesis. **B,** Steps of spermatogenesis, including the role of meiosis in producing daughter sperm cells with half the number of nuclear chromosomes found in typical body cells.

information are equipped with tails for motility and enzymes to penetrate the outer membrane of the ovum when contact occurs with it.

The structure of a mature sperm is diagrammed in **Figure 21-5**, *B*. Note the sperm *head* containing the nucleus with its genetic material from the father. The sperm head is covered by the **acrosome**—a caplike structure containing enzymes that enable the sperm to break down the covering of the ovum and permit entry if contact occurs.

In addition to the head with its covering of acrosome, each sperm has a *midpiece* and an elongated *tail*. Mitochondria in the midpiece release adenosine triphosphate (ATP) to provide an energy source for the tail movements required to propel the sperm and allow them to swim for relatively long distances through the female reproductive ducts. The tail is actually a flagellum, previously described in Chapter 3—see **Figure 3-4** (p. 46) and **Figure 3-5** (p. 47).

Production of Testosterone

In addition to spermatogenesis, the other function of the testes is to secrete the male hormone, **testosterone.** This function is carried out by the **interstitial cells** of the testes, not by their seminiferous tubules. Hypothalamic secretion of GnRH causes the anterior pituitary to secrete LH, which stimulates the interstitial cells to secrete testosterone.

Testosterone serves the following general functions:

1. Testosterone masculinizes. The various characteristics that we think of as "male" develop because of testosterone's influence. For instance, when a young boy's voice changes, it is testosterone that brings this about.
2. Testosterone promotes and maintains the development of the male accessory organs (prostate gland, seminal vesicles, and so on).
3. Testosterone has a stimulating effect on protein anabolism—it is an *anabolic steroid* hormone. Testosterone thus is responsible for the greater muscular development and strength of the male.

A good way to remember testosterone's functions is to think of it as "the masculinizing hormone" and the "anabolic

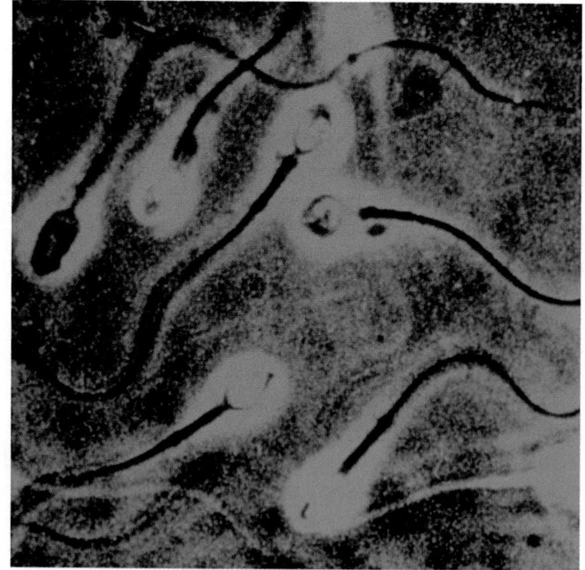

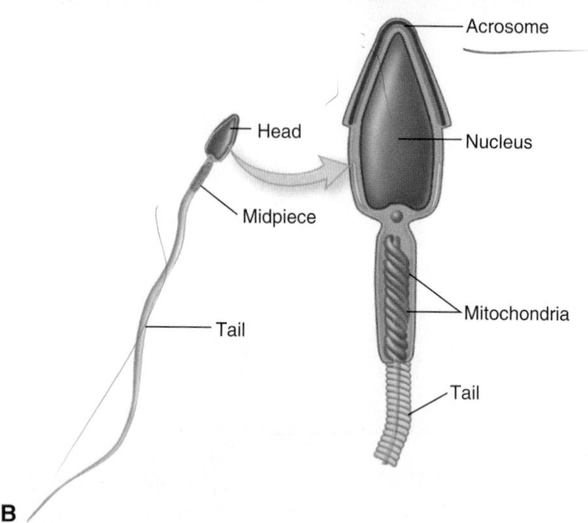

FIGURE 21-5 Human sperm. **A,** Micrograph shows the heads and long, slender tails of several spermatozoa. **B,** Illustration shows the components of a mature sperm cell and an enlargement of a sperm head and midpiece.

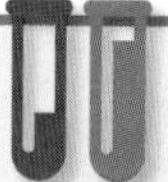

CLINICAL APPLICATION

CRYPTORCHIDISM

Early in fetal life the testes are located in the abdominal cavity but normally descend into the scrotum about 2 months before birth. Occasionally a baby is born with undescended testes, a condition called **cryptorchidism,** which is readily observed by palpation of the scrotum at delivery. The word *cryptorchidism* is from the Greek words *kryptikos* (hidden) and *orchis* (testis).

Failure of the testes to descend may be caused by hormonal imbalances in the developing fetus or by a physical deficiency or obstruction. Regardless of cause, in the cryptorchid infant the testes remain "hidden" in the abdominal cavity. Because the higher temperature inside the body cavity inhibits spermatogenesis, measures must be taken to bring the testes down into the scrotum to prevent permanent sterility.

Early treatment of this condition by surgery or by injection of testosterone, which stimulates the testes to descend, may result in normal testicular and sexual development.

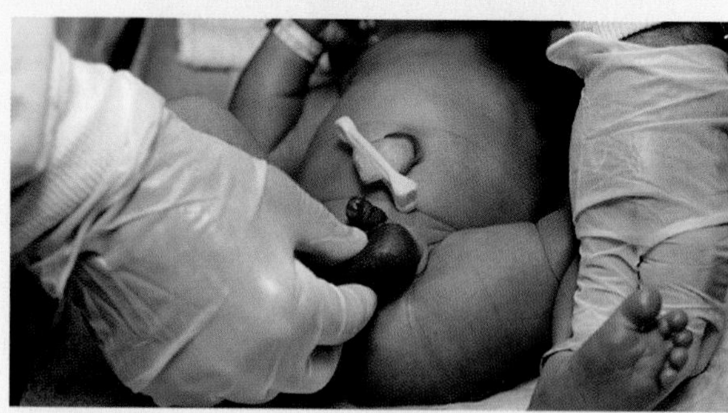

Screening for cryptorchidism in newborn infant. Properly descended testicles can be palpated easily in the scrotal sac.

hormone." Go back and review *Enhancing Muscle Strength* in Chapter 8 (p. 163), which discusses the abuse of anabolic steroids by some athletes.

QUICK CHECK

1. What is the name of the male gonad?
2. What specific structure of the gonad is responsible for sperm production?
3. What hormone is produced in the male gonad?

Reproductive Ducts

The ducts through which sperm must pass after exiting from the testes until they reach the exterior of the body are important components of the accessory reproductive structures. The other two components included in the listing of accessory organs of reproduction in the male—the supportive sex glands and external genitals—are discussed separately.

Sperm are formed within the walls of the seminiferous tubules of the testes. When they exit from these tubules within the testis, they enter and then pass, in sequence, through the epididymis, vas deferens (ductus deferens), ejaculatory duct, and the urethra on their journey out of the body.

Epididymis

Each **epididymis** consists of a single and very tightly coiled tube about 6 meters (20 feet) in length. It is a comma-shaped structure (see **Figure 21-2**) that lies along the top and behind the testes inside the scrotum. Sperm mature and develop their ability to move or swim as they are temporarily stored in the epididymis.

Specialized cells lining the epididymis secrete nutrients for developing sperm and also remove substantial amounts of excess testicular fluid as the developing sex cells enter and eventually pass through the lumen of this highly coiled tube.

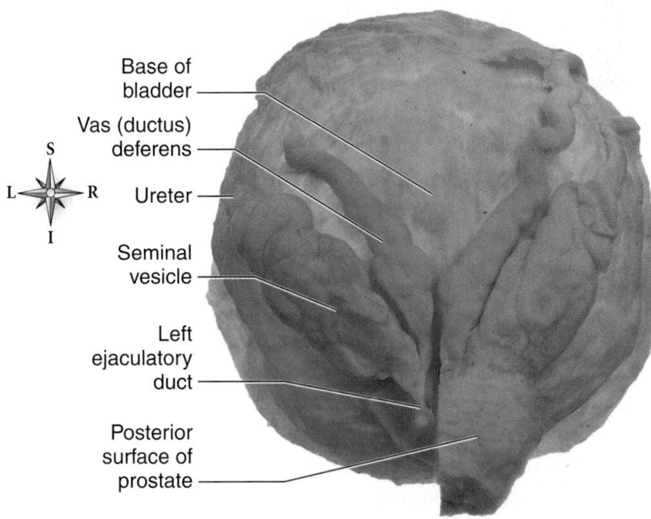

FIGURE 21-6 Male accessory glands. Dissection photo showing bladder, prostate, vas deferens, left ejaculatory duct, and seminal vesicles from behind.

Vas Deferens

The **vas deferens,** or *ductus deferens,* is the tube that permits sperm to exit from the epididymis and pass from the scrotal sac upward into the abdominal cavity.

Each vas deferens is a thick, smooth, very muscular, and movable tube that can easily be felt or "palpated" through the thin skin of the scrotal wall. It passes through the inguinal canal into the abdominal cavity as part of the *spermatic cord,* a connective tissue sheath that also encloses blood vessels and nerves.

Ejaculatory Duct and Urethra

Once in the abdominal cavity, the vas deferens extends over the top and down the posterior surface of the bladder, where it joins the duct from the seminal vesicle to form the **ejaculatory duct** (Figure 21-6).

Note in Figure 21-1 and Figure 21-6 that the ejaculatory duct passes through the substance of the prostate gland and permits sperm to empty into the **urethra,** which eventually passes through the penis and opens to the exterior at the external urinary meatus.

Accessory Glands

The term **semen,** or **seminal fluid,** is used to describe the mixture of sex cells, or sperm, produced by the testes and the secretions of the accessory, or supportive, sex glands. The accessory glands, which contribute more than 95% of the secretions to the gelatinous fluid part of the semen, include the two seminal vesicles, one prostate gland, and two bulbourethral (Cowper) glands. In addition to the production of sperm, the seminiferous tubules of the testes contribute somewhat less than 5% of the seminal fluid volume.

Usually 3 to 5 milliliters (mL) (about 1 teaspoon) of semen is ejaculated at one time, and each milliliter normally contains about 100 million sperm. These numbers vary considerably in healthy men, even from day to day. Semen is slightly alkaline and protects sperm from the acidic environment of the female reproductive tract.

Seminal Vesicles

The paired **seminal vesicles** are pouchlike glands that contribute about 60% of the seminal fluid volume. Their secretions are yellowish, thick, and rich in the sugar fructose. This fraction of the seminal fluid helps provide a source of energy for the highly motile sperm.

Prostate Gland

The **prostate gland** lies just below the bladder and is shaped like a doughnut. The urethra passes through the center of the prostate before traversing the penis to end at the external urinary orifice.

The prostate secretes a thin, milk-colored fluid that constitutes about 30% of the total seminal fluid volume. This fraction of the ejaculate helps activate the sperm and maintain their motility.

Bulbourethral Glands

Each of the two **bulbourethral glands** (also called *Cowper glands*) resembles a pea in size and shape. They are located just below the prostate gland and empty their secretions into the penile portion of the urethra. Because the bulbourethral

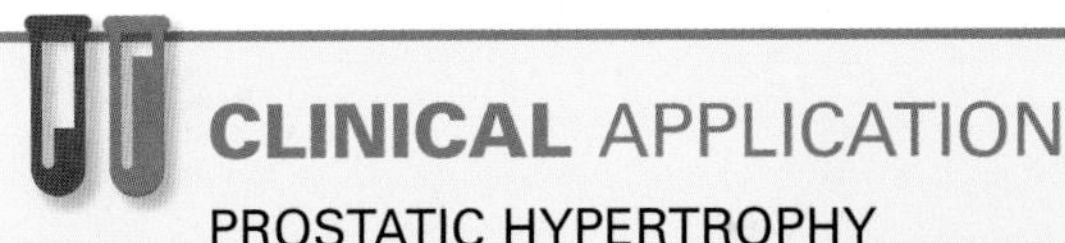

CLINICAL APPLICATION

PROSTATIC HYPERTROPHY

A noncancerous condition called **benign prostatic hypertrophy (BPH)** is a common problem in older men. The condition is characterized by an enlargement or hypertrophy of the prostate gland.

That the urethra passes through the center of the prostate after exiting from the bladder is a matter of considerable clinical significance in this condition. As the prostate enlarges, it squeezes the urethra, frequently closing it so completely that urination becomes very difficult or even impossible.

In some cases, drugs (Avodart, Flomax, others) may be used to improve urine flow and reduce symptoms of BPH. Surgical removal of part or all of the gland, a procedure called **prostatectomy** is also a treatment option.

Prostate cancer also causes hypertrophy of the gland and restricted or obstructed urine flow caused by malignant tumor growth. In addition to surgery, cancerous prostatic growths may also be treated using systemic chemotherapy, cryotherapy (freezing) of prostatic tissue, microwave (heat) therapy, hormonal therapy, inserting radioactive "seeds" directly into the tumor, and the use of various types of external-beam radiation.

In addition to enlargement of the prostate, adult men often develop inflammation of the gland, a condition called **prostatitis.**

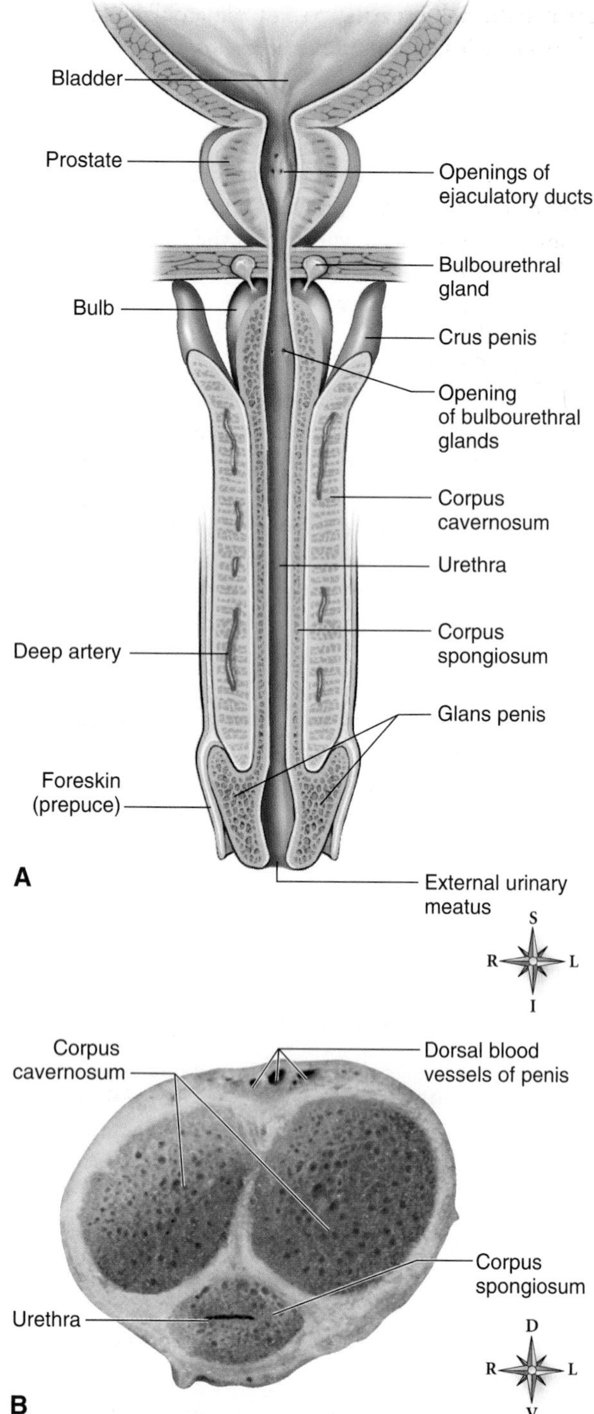

FIGURE 21-7 Penis. A, In this sagittal section of the penis viewed from above, the urethra is exposed throughout its length and can be seen exiting from the bladder and passing through the prostate gland before entering the penis to end at the external urethral orifice. **B,** Photograph of a cross section of the shaft of the penis. Note the urethra within the substance of the corpus spongiosum.

secretion is often released just before most of the rest of the semen is ejaculated, it is sometimes called the "pre-ejaculate."

The mucuslike secretions of the bulbourethral glands serve several functions. They neutralize any residue of sperm-damaging acidic urine in the urethra. They also lubricate the urethra to protect sperm from friction damage and add to the external lubrication of the penis needed for intercourse.

The bulbourethral glands contribute less than 5% of the seminal fluid volume ejaculated from the urethra.

External Genitals

The penis and scrotum constitute the external male reproductive organs—sometime called the **genitals** or **genitalia.**

The **penis** (Figure 21-7) is the organ that, when made stiff and erect by the filling of its spongy or erectile tissue components with blood during sexual arousal, can enter and deposit sperm in the vagina during intercourse. The penis has three separate columns of erectile tissue in its shaft: one column of **corpus spongiosum,** which surrounds the urethra, and two columns of **corpora cavernosa,** which lie dorsally. The spongy nature of erectile tissue is apparent in Figure 21-7.

At the distal end of the shaft of the penis is the enlarged *glans penis*, or more simply, **glans.** The external urinary meatus is the opening of the urethra at the tip of the glans.

The sensitive skin of the distal end of the penis is folded doubly to form a loose-fitting retractable collar around the glans called the **foreskin,** or **prepuce.**

If the foreskin fits too tightly about the glans, a **circumcision,** or surgical removal of the foreskin shortly after birth is usually performed to prevent irritation. Although recommended by some authorities for other medical reasons such as reduction in the spread of acquired immunodeficiency syndrome (AIDS) and other sexually transmitted infections (STIs) later in life, most circumcisions are "elective" and are performed at the discretion of the parents for religious or cultural reasons.

The **scrotum** is a skin-covered pouch suspended from the groin. Internally, it is divided into two sacs by a septum; each sac contains a testis, epididymis, the lower part of the vas deferens, and the beginning of the spermatic cord.

QUICK CHECK

1. What duct leads from the epididymis?
2. Which organs produce the fluid in semen?
3. What is the function of erectile tissues?
4. What is the glans penis?

Female Reproductive System

Structural Plan

The structural plan of the reproductive system in both sexes is similar in that organs are characterized as *essential* or *accessory.*

Essential Organs

The essential organs of reproduction in women, the **gonads,** are the paired **ovaries.** The female sex cells, or **ova,** are

TABLE 21-2 Female Reproductive Organs

ESSENTIAL ORGANS	ACCESSORY ORGANS
Gonads: ovaries (right ovary and left ovary)	Ducts: uterine tubes (two), uterus, vagina Accessory sex glands: greater vestibular glands (two), lesser vestibular glands (two), breasts (two) External genitals: vulva

produced in the ovaries. The ovaries also produce the hormones estrogen and progesterone.

Accessory Organs

The accessory organs of reproduction in women consist of the following structures:

1. A series of ducts or modified duct structures that extend from near the ovaries to the exterior
2. Additional sex glands, including the mammary glands, which have an important reproductive function only in women
3. The external reproductive organs, or external genitals

Table 21-2 lists the names of the essential and accessory female organs of reproduction, and Figure 21-8 shows the location of most of them. Refer back to this table and illustration as you read about each structure in the pages that follow.

Ovaries

Structure and Location

The paired **ovaries** are the gonads of women. They have a puckered, uneven surface; each weighs about 3 grams. The ovaries resemble large almonds in size and shape. They are attached to ligaments in the pelvic cavity on each side of the uterus.

Embedded in a connective tissue matrix just below the outer layer of each ovary in a newborn baby girl are about 1 million **ovarian follicles.** Each follicle contains an **oocyte,** an immature stage of the female sex cell. By the time a girl reaches puberty, however, further development has resulted in the formation of a reduced number (about 400,000) of what are now called **primary follicles.** Each primary follicle has a layer of **granulosa cells** around the oocyte.

The progression of development from primary follicle to ovulation is shown in Figure 21-9. As the thickness of the granulosa cell layer around the oocyte increases, a hollow chamber called an **antrum** appears, and a *secondary follicle* is formed.

During the reproductive lifetime of most women, only about 350 to 500 of the primary follicles fully develop into *mature follicles.* It is the mature follicle that releases an ovum for potential fertilization—a process called **ovulation.**

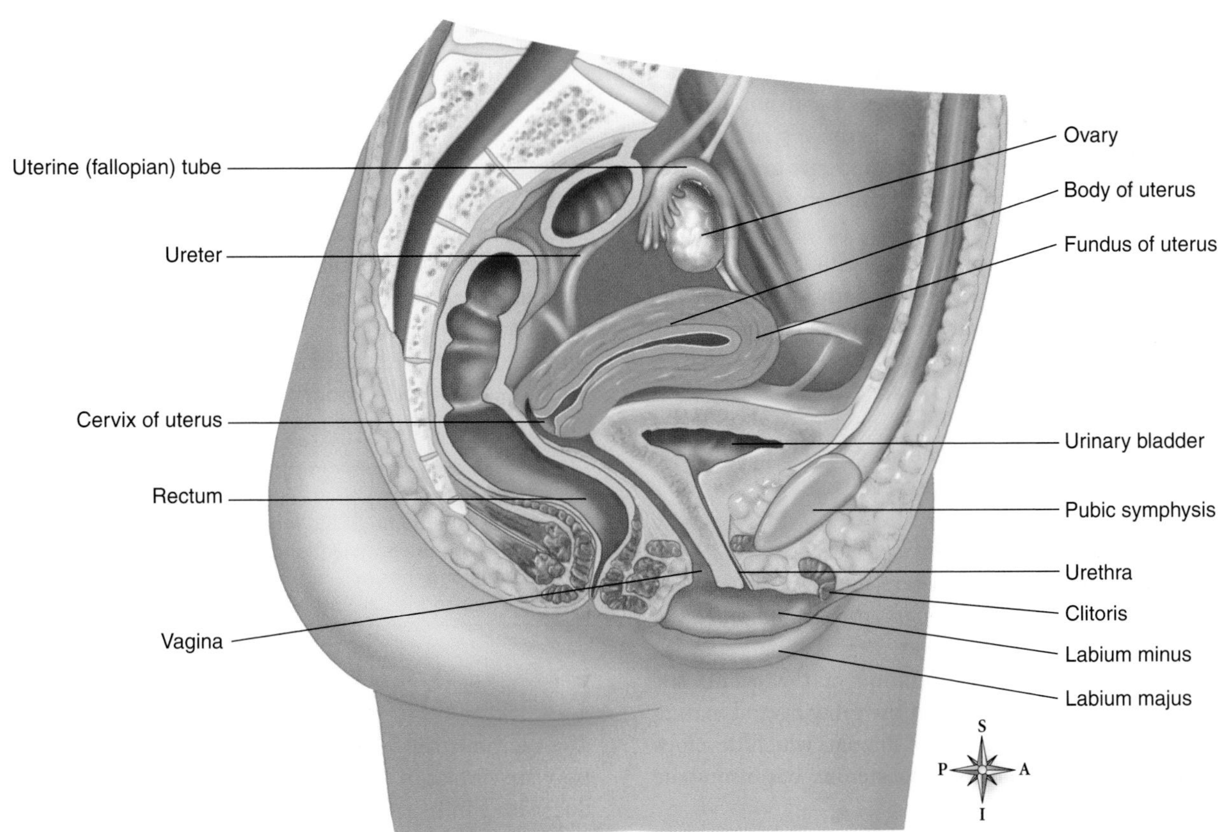

FIGURE 21-8 Organization of the female reproductive organs.

Follicles that do not mature degenerate and are reabsorbed into the ovarian tissue.

The mature ovarian follicle is often called a **graafian follicle,** in honor of the Dutch anatomist Regnier de Graaf who discovered it some 300 years ago.

After ovulation, the ruptured follicle is transformed into a hormone-secreting glandular structure called the **corpus luteum,** which is described later. *Corpus luteum* is a Latin phrase meaning "yellow body"—an appropriate name to describe the yellow appearance of this glandular structure.

To learn more about the ovaries, go to AnimationDirect at *evolve.elsevier.com.*

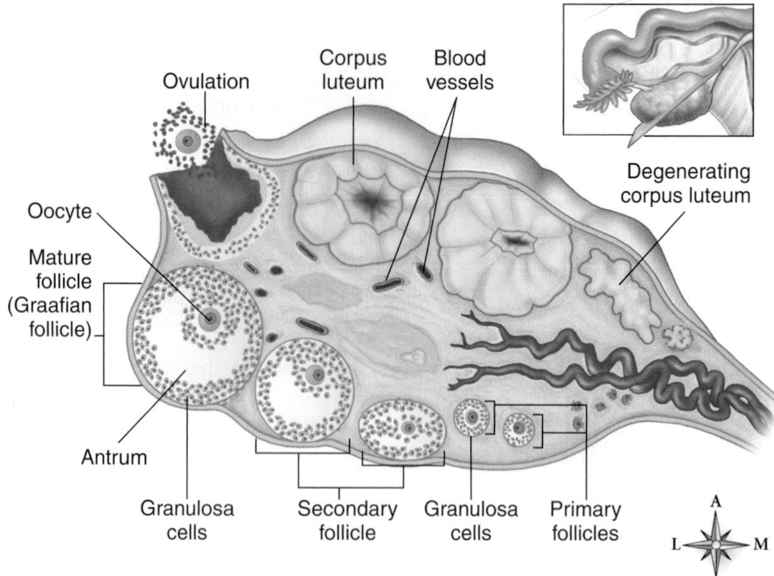

FIGURE 21-9 Ovary. Cross section of ovary shows successive stages of ovarian follicle development. Begin with the first stage (primary follicle) and follow around clockwise to the final state (degenerating corpus luteum).

Ovary Functions

Oogenesis

The production of female gametes, or sex cells, is called **oogenesis.**

The unusual form of cell division that results in sperm formation, *meiosis,* is also responsible for development of ova. During the developmental phases experienced by the female sex cell from its earliest stage to just after fertilization, two meiotic divisions occur. As a result of meiosis in the female sex cell, the number of chromosomes is reduced equally in each daughter cell to half the number (23) found in other body cells (46).

However, the amount of cytoplasm is divided unequally among the daughter oocytes, as you can see in **Figure 21-10**. The result is formation of one large ovum and small daughter cells called **polar bodies** that degenerate. The ovum, with its large supply of cytoplasm, is one of the body's largest cells and is uniquely structured to provide nutrients for rapid development of the embryo until implantation in the uterus occurs.

At fertilization, the final phase of meiotic cell division in the ovum completes and the last polar body is released. The sex cells from both parents unite fully and the normal chromosome number (46) is achieved in the zygote that is formed.

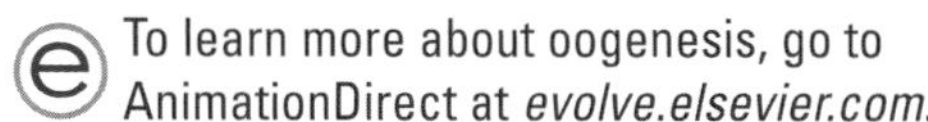
To learn more about oogenesis, go to AnimationDirect at *evolve.elsevier.com.*

Production of Estrogen and Progesterone

The second major function of the ovary, in addition to oogenesis, is secretion of the sex hormones, *estrogen* and *progesterone.* Hormone production in the ovary begins at puberty with the cyclic development and maturation of the ovum. The granulosa cells around the oocyte in the growing and mature follicle secrete estrogen. The corpus luteum, which develops after ovulation, chiefly secretes progesterone but also some estrogen.

Estrogen is the sex hormone that causes the development and maintenance of the female secondary sex characteristics and stimulates growth of the epithelial cells lining the uterus. Some of the actions of estrogen include the following:

1. Development and maturation of female reproductive organs, including the external genitals
2. Appearance of pubic hair and breast development
3. Development of female body contours by deposition of fat below the skin surface and in the breasts and hip region
4. Initiation of the first menstrual cycle

Progesterone is produced by the corpus luteum, which is a glandular structure that develops from a follicle that has just released an ovum. If stimulated by the appropriate anterior pituitary hormone, the corpus luteum produces progesterone for about 11 days after ovulation. Progesterone stimulates proliferation and vascularization of the epithelial lining of the uterus and acts with estrogen to initiate the menstrual cycle in girls entering puberty.

QUICK CHECK

1. What is the name of the female gonads?
2. Where are the female glands located?
3. What is oogenesis?
4. What hormones are produced by the female gonads?

Reproductive Ducts

The reproductive ducts in the male and female reproductive tract are similar in some fundamental ways. First, both sets of ducts lead from each of the paired gonads, then join into a single passage that leads out of the body. Second, both male and female ducts carry gametes away from the gonads.

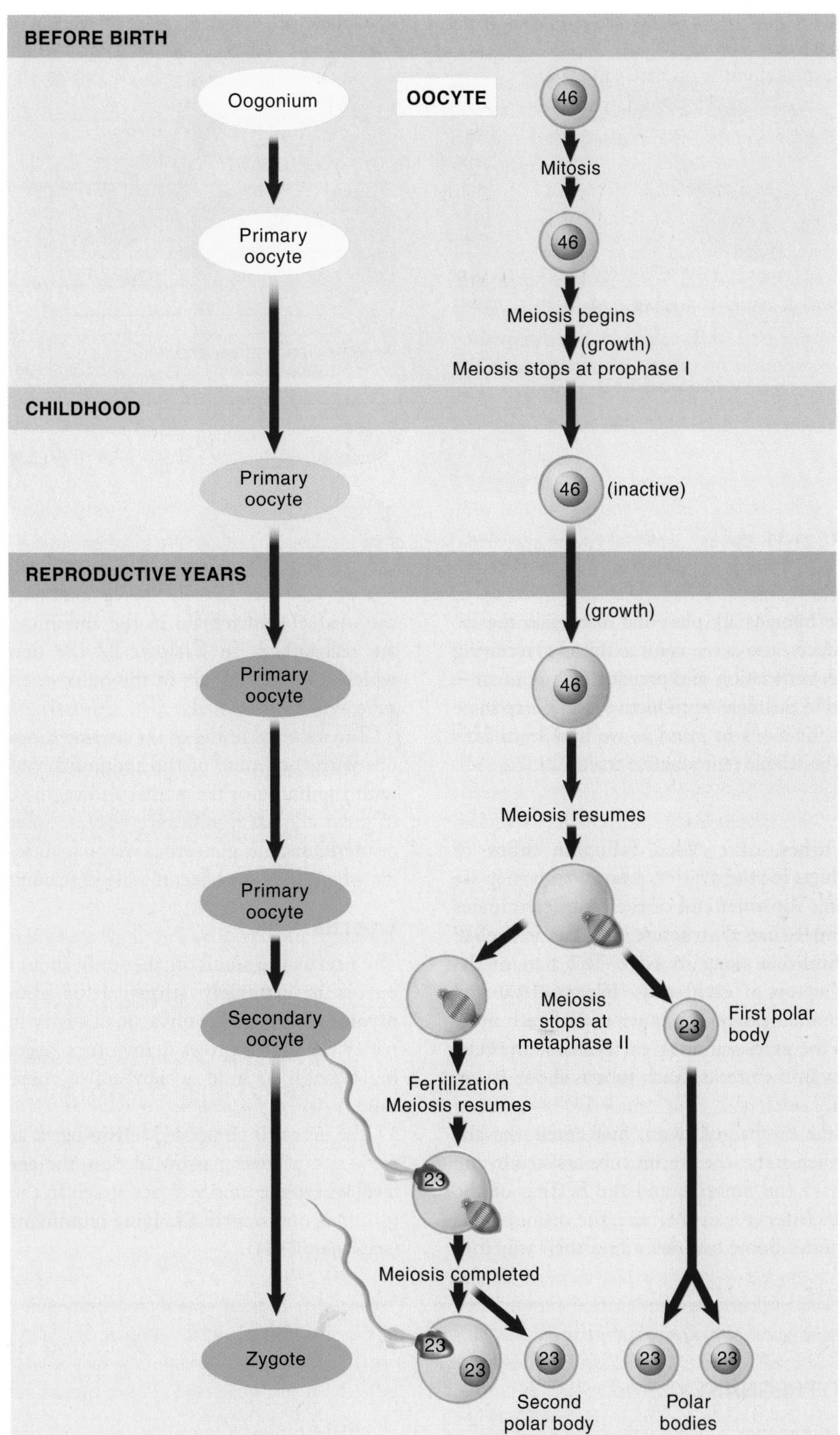

FIGURE 21-10 Oogenesis. Production of a mature ovum and subsequent fertilization are shown as a series of cell divisions. Notice that meiosis pauses in meiosis I before birth, then resumes in some primary oocytes beginning at puberty. Meiosis II does not complete until fertilization occurs.

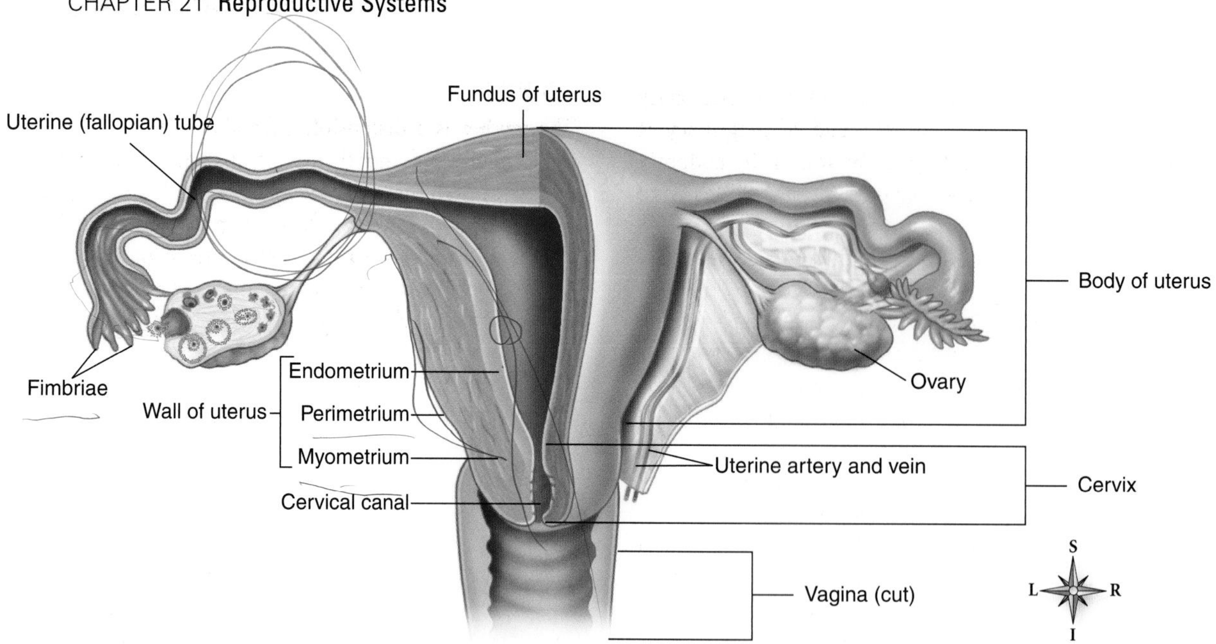

FIGURE 21-11 Uterus. Sectioned view shows muscle layers of the uterus and its relationship to the ovaries and vagina.

However, because humans are placental mammals, the female reproductive ducts also have central roles in receiving sperm from the male, fertilization, and prenatal development—functions not needed in the male reproductive tract. Keep these unique reproductive functions in mind as we now learn how *form fits function* in the female reproductive tract.

Uterine Tubes

The two **uterine tubes,** also called **fallopian tubes** or **oviducts,** serve as ducts for the ovaries, even though they are not attached to them. The outer end of each tube terminates in an expanded, funnel-shaped structure that has fringelike projections called **fimbriae** along its edge. This part of the tube curves over the top of each ovary (Figure 21-11) and opens into the abdominal cavity. The inner end of each uterine tube attaches to the uterus, and the cavity inside the tube opens into the cavity in the uterus. Each tube is about 10 cm (4 inches) in length.

After ovulation the discharged ovum first enters the abdominal cavity and then enters the uterine tube assisted by the wavelike movement of the fimbriae and the beating of the cilia on their surface. After it is in the tube, the ovum begins its journey to the uterus. Some ova never find their way into the oviduct and remain in the abdominal cavity where they are reabsorbed. In Chapter 22 the details of fertilization, which normally occurs in the outer one third of the uterine tube, will be discussed.

The mucosal lining of the uterine tubes is directly continuous with the lining of the abdominal cavity on one end and with the lining of the uterus and vagina on the other. This is of great clinical significance because infections of the vagina or uterus such as gonorrhea may pass into the abdominal cavity, where they may become life-threatening.

Uterus

The **uterus** is a small organ—only about the size of a pear—but it is extremely strong. It is almost all muscle, or **myometrium,** with only a small cavity inside. During pregnancy the uterus grows many times larger so that it becomes big enough to hold a baby and a considerable amount of fluid.

The uterus is composed of two parts: an upper portion, the *body,* and a lower narrow section, the **cervix.** Just above the level where the uterine tubes attach to the body of the uterus, it rounds out to form a bulging prominence called the **fundus** (see Figure 21-11).

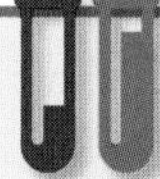

CLINICAL APPLICATION

ECTOPIC PREGNANCY

The term **ectopic pregnancy** is used to describe a pregnancy resulting from the implantation of a fertilized ovum in any location other than the uterus. Occasionally, because the outer ends of the uterine tubes open into the pelvic cavity and are not actually connected to the ovaries, an ovum does not enter an oviduct but becomes fertilized and remains in the abdominal cavity.

Although rare, if implantation occurs on the surface of an abdominal organ or on one of the mesenteries, development may continue to term. In such cases, delivery by cesarean section is required. Most ectopic pregnancies involve implantation in the uterine tube and are therefore called *tubal pregnancies.* They result in fetal death and, if not treated, tubal rupture.

Except during pregnancy, the uterus lies in the pelvic cavity just behind the urinary bladder. By the end of pregnancy, it becomes large enough to extend up to the top of the abdominal cavity. It then pushes the liver against the underside of the diaphragm—a fact that explains a comment such as "I can't seem to take a deep breath since I've gotten so big," made by many women late in their pregnancies.

The uterus functions in three processes—menstruation, pregnancy, and labor. The corpus luteum stops secreting progesterone and decreases its secretion of estrogens about 11 days after ovulation. About 3 days later, when the progesterone and estrogen concentrations in the blood are at their lowest, menstruation starts. Small pieces of the mucous membrane lining of the uterus, or the **endometrium,** pull loose, leaving torn blood vessels underneath. Blood and bits of endometrium trickle out of the uterus into the vagina and out of the body.

Immediately after menstruation the endometrium starts to repair itself. It again grows thick and becomes lavishly supplied with blood in preparation for pregnancy.

If fertilization does not take place, the uterus again sheds the lining made ready for a pregnancy that did not occur. Because these changes in the uterine lining continue to repeat themselves, they are spoken of as the **menstrual cycle** (see p. 473).

If fertilization occurs, pregnancy begins, and the endometrium remains intact. The events of pregnancy are discussed in Chapter 22.

Menstruation first occurs at puberty, often around the age of 11 to 12 years. Normally the cycle repeats about every 28 days or 13 times a year for some 30 to 40 years before it ceases at **menopause,** when a woman is somewhere around the age of 50 years.

CLINICAL APPLICATION

HYSTERECTOMY

The word **hysterectomy** comes from the combination of two Greek words: *hystera,* meaning "uterus," and *ektome,* meaning "to cut out." By definition it is the surgical removal of the uterus.

Hysterectomy is a term that is often misused, however, by incorrectly expanding its definition to include the removal of the ovaries or other reproductive structures. Only the uterus is removed in a hysterectomy. If the total uterus, including the cervix, is removed, the terms *total hysterectomy* or *panhysterectomy* may be used. If the cervical portion of the uterus is left in place and only the body of the organ is removed, the term *subtotal hysterectomy* is appropriate.

The actual removal of the uterus may be performed through an incision made in the abdominal wall—*abdominal hysterectomy*—or through the vagina—*vaginal hysterectomy.* The term **oophorectomy** is used to describe removal of the ovaries. Although the two surgical procedures may take place during the same operation—for a woman with uterine or ovarian cancer, for example—the terms used to describe them should not be used interchangeably.

Vagina

The **vagina** is a distensible tube about 10 cm (4 inches) long, made mainly of smooth muscle and lined with mucous membrane. It lies in the pelvic cavity between the urinary bladder and the rectum (see **Figure 21-8**). As the part of the female reproductive tract that opens to the exterior, the vagina is the organ that sperm enter during their journey to meet an ovum, and it is also the organ from which a baby emerges to meet its new world.

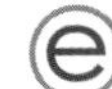

To learn more about female reproductive ducts, go to AnimationDirect at *evolve.elsevier.com.*

Accessory Glands

Vestibular Glands

Two pairs of exocrine glands lie imbedded in tissue to the left and right of the vaginal outlet and release mucous fluid into the vestibule of the *vulva* (described later in **Figure 21-13**).

One pair of these small glands are called the **greater vestibular glands** and the other pair are called the **lesser vestibular glands.** The greater vestibular glands are also called *Bartholin glands* and the lesser vestibular glands may be called *Skene glands* or *female prostate.*

Mucus from these glands may contribute to lubrication during sexual intercourse. The vestibular glands have clinical importance because they may become infected. For example, the bacteria that cause *gonorrhea* are often hard to eliminate once they infect a vestibular gland.

Breasts

The **breasts** lie over the pectoral muscles and are attached to them by *fibrous suspensory ligaments (Cooper ligaments).* Breast size is determined more by the amount of fat around the glandular (milk-secreting) tissue than by the amount of glandular tissue itself. Hence the size of the breast has little to do with its ability to secrete adequate amounts of milk after the birth of a baby.

Each breast consists of 15 to 20 divisions or lobes that are arranged radially (**Figure 21-12**). Each lobe consists of several lobules, and each lobule consists of milk-secreting glandular cells. The milk-secreting cells are arranged in grapelike clusters of small chambers called *alveoli* (**Figure 21-12**, *inset*). Small contractile cells surround the alveoli and push milk into ducts when stimulated by *oxytocin (OT)* released from the posterior pituitary gland—an event called "milk let-down."

Small **lactiferous ducts** drain the alveoli and converge toward the nipple like the spokes of a wheel. Only one lactiferous duct leads from each lobe to an opening in the nipple. Each lactiferous duct widens into a *lactiferous sinus* just before reaching the nipple. Each sinus acts like the bulb at the end of an eyedropper, pumping milk out of the nipple as an infant rhythmically squeezes its jaws as it nurses.

The colored surface area around the nipple is the **areola.** It contains many tiny bumps called *areolar glands.* Areolar glands are large sebaceous glands that secrete skin oils that condition the skin while nursing an infant. The areola also has a network of smooth muscles that contract to cause the nipple

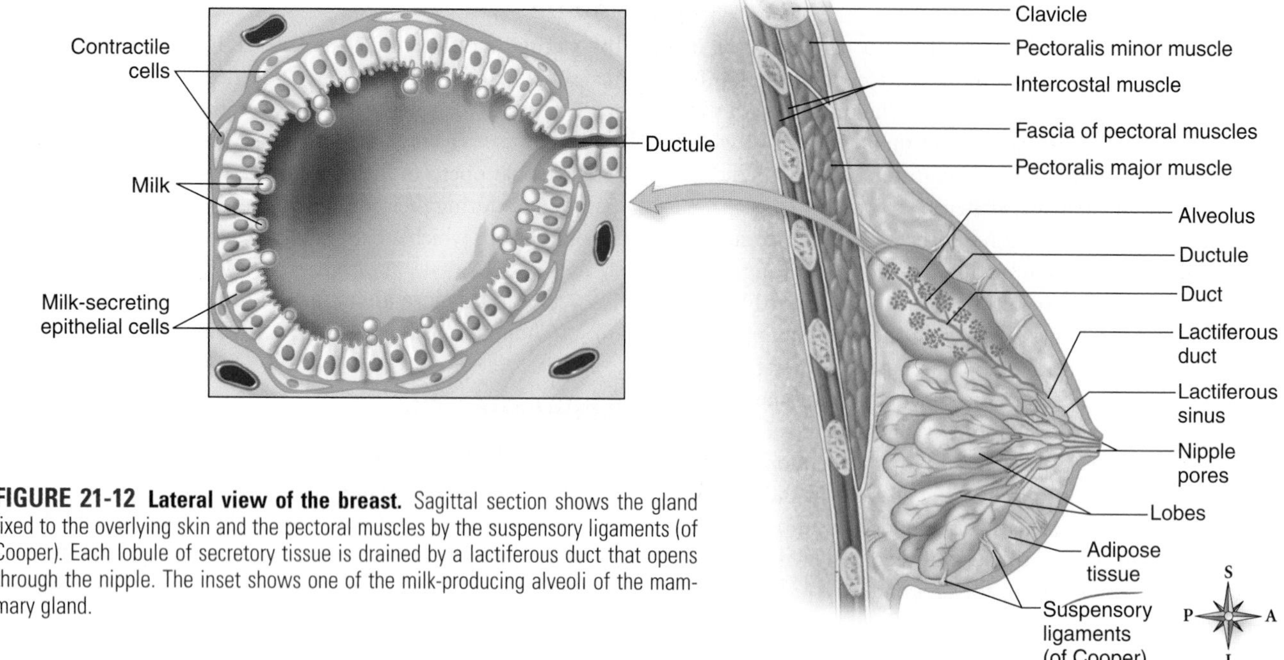

FIGURE 21-12 Lateral view of the breast. Sagittal section shows the gland fixed to the overlying skin and the pectoral muscles by the suspensory ligaments (of Cooper). Each lobule of secretory tissue is drained by a lactiferous duct that opens through the nipple. The inset shows one of the milk-producing alveoli of the mammary gland.

to become erect—which often helps an infant latch on to the breast at the most efficient location.

Knowledge of the lymphatic drainage of the breast is important because cancerous cells from breast tumors often spread to other areas of the body through the lymphatic system. This lymphatic drainage is discussed in Chapter 14 (see **Figure 14-4**).

 To learn more about breast structure, go to AnimationDirect at *evolve.elsevier.com*.

QUICK CHECK

1. What is another name for the uterine tubes?
2. What three major functions does the uterus perform?
3. What substance is conducted through lactiferous ducts?
4. How are the ducts of the male and female reproductive tract similar and how do they differ?

External Genitals

The **external genitalia** of women consist of several structures collectively called the **vulva.** These include:

1. Mons pubis
2. Clitoris
3. External urinary meatus
4. Labia minora
5. Hymen
6. Openings of vestibular gland ducts
7. Orifice (opening) of vagina
8. Labia majora

The **mons pubis** is a skin-covered pad of fat over the symphysis pubis. Pubic hair appears on this mound of fat at puberty and persists throughout life.

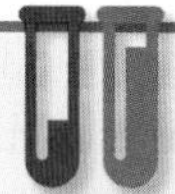

CLINICAL APPLICATION

PELVIC INFLAMMATORY DISEASE

Pelvic inflammatory disease (PID) is a common disorder that affects more than 800,000 women each year in the United States. It is characterized by pelvic pain, fever, and vaginal discharge. PID occurs as either an acute or a chronic inflammatory condition that can be caused by several different types of pathogens. Organisms that cause a number of *sexually transmitted infections (STIs)*, especially chlamydia, continue as a common cause of PID.

As the infection spreads upward from the vagina, it often involves the uterus, uterine tubes, ovaries, and other pelvic organs—frequently resulting in the development of scar tissue and adhesions. Some STIs that ultimately result in serious complications, such as PID, do not initially cause symptoms and are said to be "asymptomatic." Chlamydia, the most common cause of PID, is often asymptomatic for extended periods of time. In addition, developing PID caused by the chlamydia infection may also remain asymptomatic until significant damage has occurred. In these cases, women may be unaware that an infection is under way and causing serious problems.

Infertility is one of the most commonly feared consequences of long-standing or chronic PID and is a serious complication of chlamydia, gonorrhea, and other STI infections. Direct laparoscopic examination is often used to determine the severity of the PID infection and the reproductive organs involved.

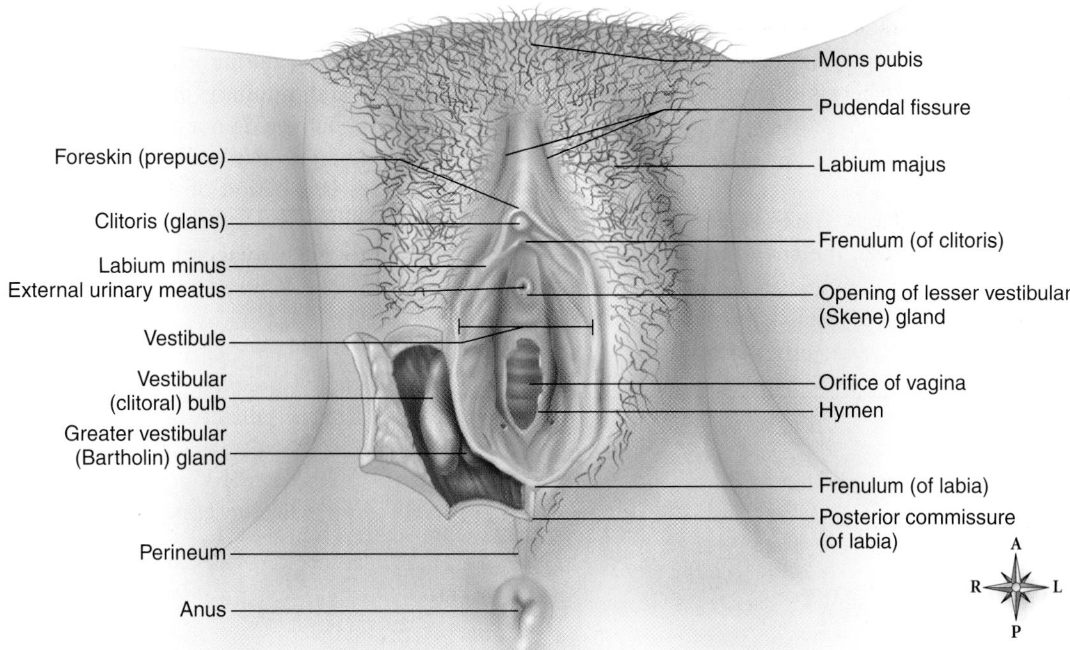

FIGURE 21-13 External genitals of the female.

Extending downward from the elevated mons pubis are the **labia majora,** literally "large lips." These elongated folds, which are composed mainly of fat and glands, are covered with pigmented skin and pubic hair on the outer surface and are smooth and free from hair on the inner surface. The **labia minora**—literally "small lips"—are nestled medially between the labia majora and are covered with thin skin. These two small lips join anteriorly at the midline.

The space between the labia minora is the **vestibule** (**Figure 21-13**). Several genital structures are located in the vestibule. The glans or head of the **clitoris,** which is composed of erectile tissue similar to that found in the penis, is located just behind the anterior junction of the labia minora. The deeper erectile tissue of the clitoris branches into two bulbs, one of which can be seen under a labium majus in the cut-away on right side of the specimen in **Figure 21-13**.

Situated between the glans clitoris and the vaginal opening is the *external urethral meatus.*

The vaginal orifice is bordered by a thin fold of mucous membrane called the **hymen.** Sometimes, the hymen partially blocks the vaginal opening. The ducts of the vestibular glands open on either side of the vaginal orifice, medial to the labia minora.

The term **perineum** is used to describe the area between the vaginal opening and anus. This area is sometimes cut in a surgical procedure called an **episiotomy** to prevent tearing of tissue during childbirth.

Menstrual Cycle

Overview

The menstrual cycle consists of many changes in the uterus, ovaries, vagina, and breasts and in the anterior pituitary gland's secretion of hormones (**Figure 21-14**). In the majority of women, these changes occur with regularity throughout their reproductive years. The first indication of changes comes with the first menstrual period. The first **menses,** or menstrual flow, is referred to as the **menarche.**

A typical menstrual cycle covers a period of about 28 days. However, the length of the cycle varies among women. Some women, for example, may have a regular cycle that covers

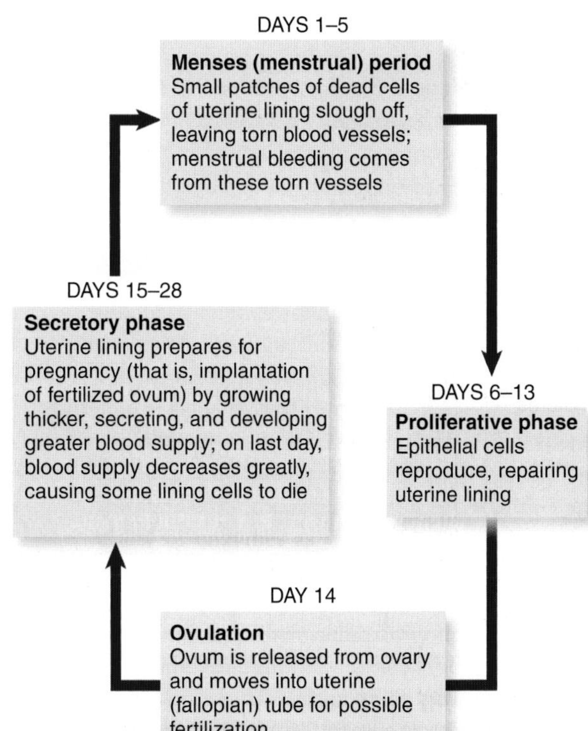

FIGURE 21-14 A 28-day menstrual cycle.

about 24 days. The length of the cycle also varies within one woman. Some women, for example, may have irregular cycles that range from 21 to 28 days, whereas others may have cycles that are 2 to 3 months long.

Phases

Each cycle consists of three phases. The three periods of time in each cycle are called the *menses,* the *proliferative phase,* and the *secretory phase.* Refer often to **Figure 21-15** as you read about the events occurring during each phase of the cycle in the hypothalamus and pituitary gland, the ovary, and in the uterus. Be sure that you do not overlook the event that occurs around day 14 of a 28-day cycle.

The **menses** is a period of 4 or 5 days characterized by menstrual bleeding. The first day of menstrual flow is considered day 1 of the menstrual cycle.

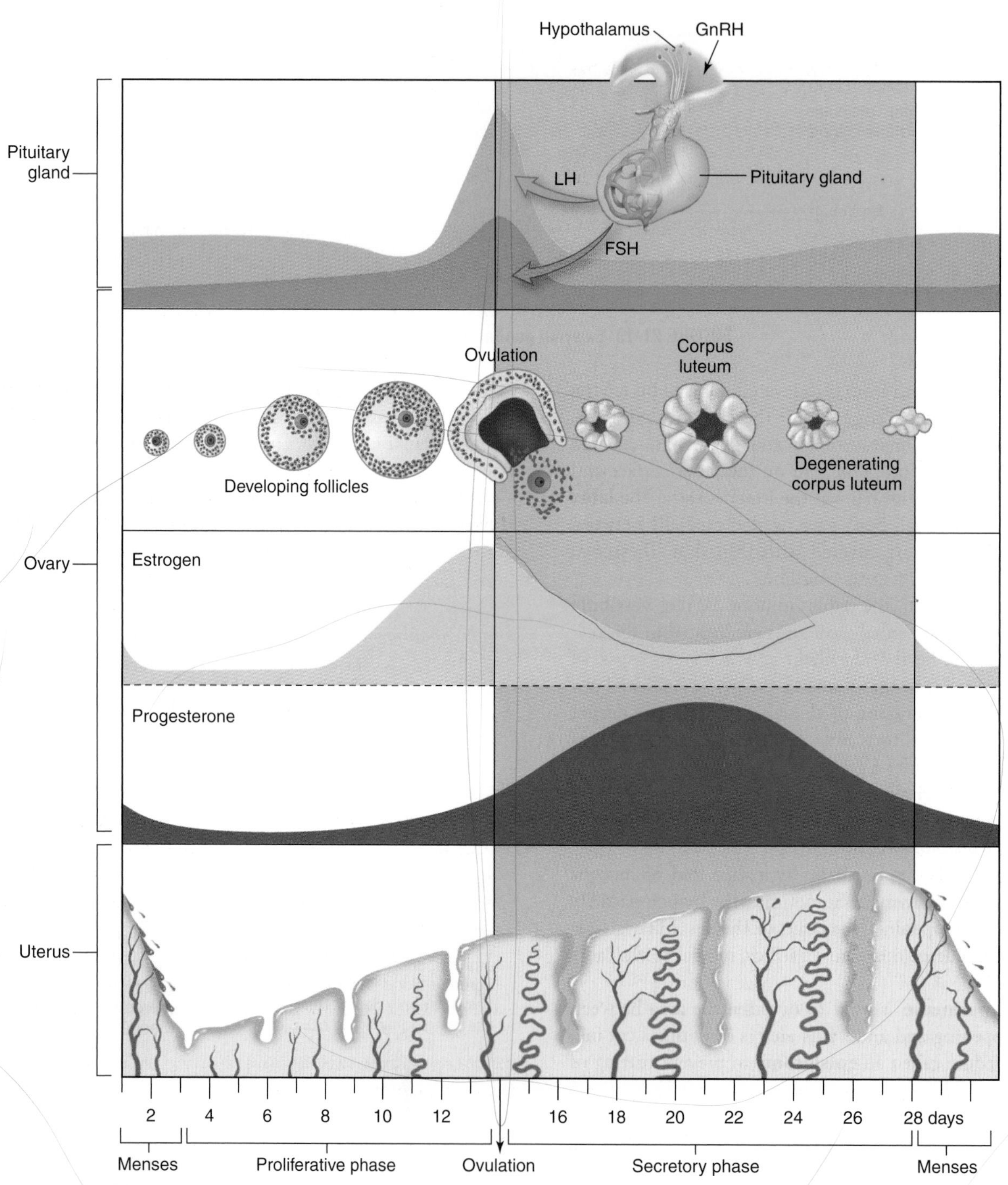

FIGURE 21-15 Human menstrual cycle. Diagram illustrates the interrelationship of pituitary, ovarian, and uterine functions throughout a typical 28-day cycle. A sharp increase in luteinizing hormone (LH) levels causes ovulation, whereas menstruation (sloughing off of the endometrial lining) is initiated by lower levels of progesterone.

The **proliferative phase** begins after the menstrual flow ends and lasts until ovulation. During this period the follicles mature, the uterine lining thickens (proliferates), and estrogen secretion increases to its highest level.

The **secretory phase** of the menstrual cycle begins at ovulation and lasts until the next menses begins. It is during this phase of the menstrual cycle that the uterine lining reaches its greatest thickness and the ovary secretes its highest levels of progesterone.

Ovulation

As a general rule, during the 30 or 40 years that a woman has periods, only one ovum matures each month. However, there are exceptions to this rule. Some months, more than one matures, and some months, no ovum matures.

Ovulation occurs 14 days before the next menses begins. In a 28-day cycle, this means that ovulation occurs around day 14 of the cycle, as shown in **Figure 21-14**. (Recall that the first day of the menses is considered the first day of the cycle.) In a 30-day cycle, however, ovulation would not occur on the 14th cycle day, but instead on the 16th. And in a 25-day cycle, ovulation would occur on the 11th cycle day.

The time of ovulation has great practical importance because the possibility of fertilization—the fusion of a sperm and egg—can occur only during a short period of time during each menstrual cycle. Although a few "super" sperm may remain viable for up to 5 days, most sperm retain their fertilizing power for only 24 to 72 hours after being deposited in the female reproductive tract following ejaculation. The oocyte remains viable and capable of being fertilized for only about 12 to 24 hours after ovulation. A woman's fertile period therefore lasts only a few days each month—from between 3 to 5 days before, and no later than 24 hours after, ovulation.

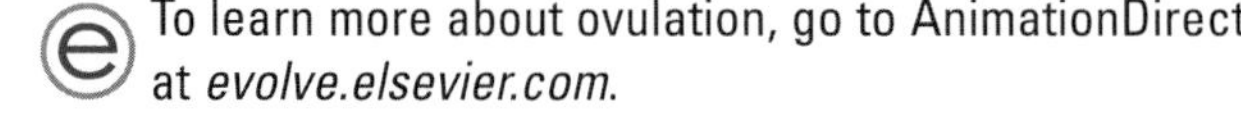

To learn more about ovulation, go to AnimationDirect at *evolve.elsevier.com*.

Control of the Menstrual Cycle

The anterior pituitary gland plays a critical role in regulating the cyclic changes that characterize the functions of the female reproductive system (see Chapter 11). As noted earlier, secretion of GnRH from the hypothalamus stimulates the anterior pituitary gland to secrete both FSH and LH. From day 1 to about day 7 of the menstrual cycle, GnRH selectively stimulates the anterior pituitary gland to secrete increasing amounts of FSH. A high blood concentration of FSH stimulates several immature ovarian follicles to start growing and secreting estrogen (see **Figure 21-15**).

Working together, increasing levels of estrogen and GnRH in the blood stimulate the anterior pituitary gland to release increasing amounts of LH. LH causes maturing of a follicle and its ovum, ovulation (rupturing of mature follicle with ejection of ovum), and luteinization (formation of a yellow body, the corpus luteum, from the ruptured follicle).

Which hormone—FSH or LH—would you call the "ovulating hormone"? Do you think ovulation could occur if the blood concentration of FSH remained low throughout the menstrual cycle? If you answered LH to the first question and no to the second, you answered both questions correctly. Ovulation cannot occur if the blood level of FSH stays low because a high concentration of this hormone is essential to stimulation of ovarian follicle growth and maturation. With a low level of FSH, no follicles start to grow, and therefore none become ripe enough to ovulate. Ovulation is caused by the combined actions of FSH and LH. Birth control pills that contain estrogen substances suppress FSH secretion. This indirectly prevents ovulation.

Ovulation occurs, as we have said, because of the combined actions of the two anterior pituitary hormones, FSH and LH. The next question is, what causes menstruation? A brief answer is this: a sudden, sharp decrease in estrogen and progesterone secretion toward the end of the secretory phase causes the uterine lining to break down and another menstrual period to begin.

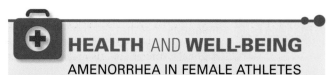

HEALTH AND WELL-BEING

AMENORRHEA IN FEMALE ATHLETES

Failure to have a menstrual period is called **amenorrhea.** Amenorrhea occurs in some female athletes, probably resulting from a body fat composition that is too low to sustain normal reproductive function. Although it keeps the hematocrit (red blood cell level) higher than during menstruation, it is not considered a desirable condition. Besides infertility, amenorrhea may cause other problems. For example, the low blood levels of estrogen associated with long-term amenorrhea may cause osteoporosis (loss of bone mass).

Summary of the Reproductive Systems

The reproductive systems in both sexes revolve around the production of reproductive cells, or gametes (sperm and ova), as well as mechanisms that ensure union of these two cells; the fusion of these cells enables transfer of parental genetic information to the next generation.

Table 21-3 compares several analogous components of the reproductive systems in both sexes. You can see that men and women have similar structures to accomplish complementary functions. In addition, the female reproductive system permits development and birth of the offspring—the first subject of our next chapter.

QUICK CHECK

1. Which female structure is made of erectile tissue?
2. What is another term for *menses?*
3. Which hormone reaches a high peak just before ovulation?

TABLE 21-3 Analogous* Features of the Reproductive Systems

FEATURES	FEMALE	MALE
Essential organs	Ovaries	Testes
Sex cells	Ova (eggs)	Sperm
Hormones	Estrogen and progesterone	Testosterone
Hormone-producing cells	Granulosa cells and corpus luteum	Interstitial cells
Duct systems	Uterine (fallopian) tubes, uterus, and vagina	Vas deferens, urethra, and epididymis
External genitals	Clitoris and vulva	Penis and scrotum

*Resembling or similar in some respects

SCIENCE APPLICATIONS

REPRODUCTIVE SCIENCES

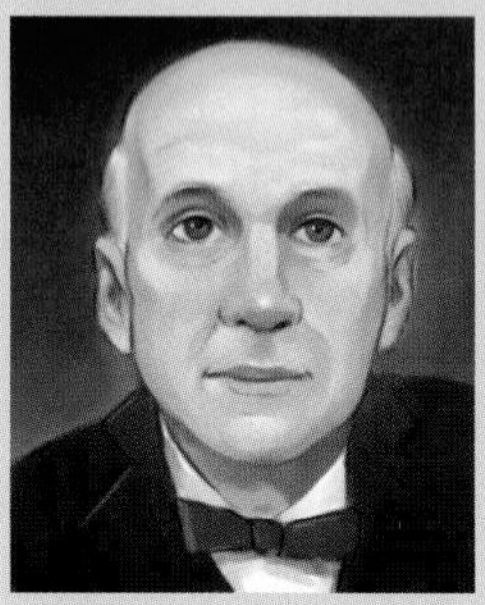

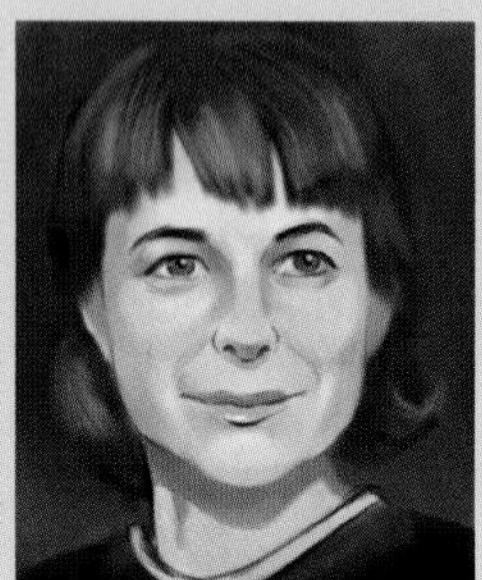

William Masters (1915–2001) and Virginia Johnson (1925-2013)

The study of human reproduction, and especially sexual function, has many cultural implications. So it is no wonder that American researchers William Masters and Virginia Johnson encountered a great deal of controversy during their decades of pioneering work in the field of human sex and reproduction. They were the first to study human sexual physiology in the laboratory. William Masters was a **gynecologist** (physician specializing in women's health) and Virginia Johnson was trained in psychology. In 1966, their book *Human Sexual Response* clearly explained the physiology of sex for the first time. Besides making discoveries in the physiology of human sex and reproduction, they also developed therapies for treating sex-related conditions, and they trained *therapists* from around the world.

In addition to the broad fields of *biology, medicine, psychology,* and the *behavioral sciences,* the pioneering work of Masters and Johnson paved the way for advances in such diverse and specialized areas of knowledge as *comparative neuroscience* and *social dynamics.*

Today, there are many opportunities to apply knowledge of reproductive science in a variety of professions. *Reproductive health nurses, gynecologists,* and **urologists** often provide primary reproductive care to adult men and women. Reproductive medicine clinical staff help couples improve fertility. *Psychologists* and *counselors* help patients struggling with various sexual concerns.

LANGUAGE OF SCIENCE AND MEDICINE (continued from p. 459)

clitoris
(KLIT-oh-ris)
[*clitoris* **small key or latch**]

corpora cavernosa
(KOHR-pohr-ah kav-er-NO-sah)
sing., corpus cavernosum
(KOHR-pus kav-er-NO-sum)
[*corpus* **body,** *cavern-* **large hollow,** *-os-* **relating to,** *-um* **thing**]

corpus luteum
(KOHR-pus LOO-tee-um)
pl., corpora lutea
(KOHR-pohr-ah LOO-tee-ah)
[*corpus* **body,** *lute-* **yellow,** *-um* **thing**]

corpus spongiosum
(KOHR-pus spun-jee-OH-sum)
[*corpus* **body,** *spong-* **sponge,** *-os-* **relating to,** *-um* **thing**]

cryptorchidism
(krip-TOR-kih-diz-em)
[*crypt-* **hidden,** *-orchid-* **testis,** *-ism* **condition**]

ectopic pregnancy
(ek-TOP-ik PREG-nan-see)
[*ec-* **out of,** *-top-* **place,** *-ic* **relating to**]

ejaculation
(ee-jak-yoo-LAY-shun)
[*e-* **out or away,** *-jacula-* **throw,** *-ation* **process**]

ejaculatory duct
(ee-JAK-yoo-lah-toh-ree dukt)
[*e-* **out or away,** *-jacula-* **throw,** *-ory* **relating to,** *duct* **a leading or path**]

endometrium
(en-doh-MEE-tree-um)
[*endo-* **within,** *-metr-* **womb,** *-um* **thing**]

epididymis
(ep-ih-DID-ih-miss)
[*epi-* **upon,** *-didymis* **pair**]

episiotomy
(eh-piz-ee-OT-oh-mee)
[*episio-* **pubic region,** *-tom-* **cut,** *-y* **action**]

essential organ
(eh-SEN-shul OR-gun)
[*organ* **instrument**]

estrogen
(ES-troh-jen)
[*estro-* **frenzy,** *-gen* **produce**]

fallopian tube
(fal-LOH-pee-an toob)
[*Gabriele Fallopio* **Italian anatomist**]

fimbria
(FIM-bree-ah)
pl., fimbriae
(FIM-bree-yee)
[*fimbria* **fringe**]

follicle-stimulating hormone (FSH)
(FOL-lih-kul-STIM-yoo-lay-ting HOR-mohn)
[*foll-* **bag,** *-icle* **little,** *stimul-* **excite,** *-at-* **process,** *-ing* **action,** *hormon-* **excite**]

foreskin (prepuce)
(FORE-skin)
[*fore-* **front,** *-skin* **a hide**]

fundus
(FUN-dus)
[*fundus* **bottom**]

gamete
(GAM-eet)
[*gamet-* **sexual union or marriage partner**]

genital
(JEN-ih-tal)
pl., genitalia
(jen-ih-TAIL-yah)
[*gen-* **produce,** *-al* **relating to**]

glans
(glanz)
[*glans* **acorn**]

gonad
(GO-nad)
[*gon-* **offspring,** *-ad* **relating to**]

gonadotropin-releasing hormone (GnRH)
(go-nah-doh-TROH-pin ree-LEEZ-ing HOR-mohn)
[*gon-* **offspring,** *-ad-* **relating to,** *-trop-* **nourish,** *-in* **substance,** *hormon-* **excite**]

graafian follicle
(GRAH-fee-en FOL-lih-kul)
[*Reijnier de Graaf* **Dutch physician,** *-an* **relating to,** *foll-* **bag,** *-icle* **little**]

granulosa cell
(gran-yoo-LOH-sah sel)
[*gran-* **grain,** *-ul-* **little,** *-osa* **relating to,** *cell* **storeroom**]

greater vestibular gland (Bartholin gland)
(GRAYT-er ves-TIB-yoo-lar gland)
[*vestibul-* **entrance hall,** *-ar* **relating to,** *gland* **acorn** (*Bartholin* **Caspar Bartholin, Danish physician**)]

gynecologist
(gye-neh-KOL-oh-jist)
[*gyneco-* **woman or female gender,** *-log-* **words (study of),** *-ist* **agent**]

hymen
(HYE-men)
[*hymen* **membrane**]

hysterectomy
(his-teh-REK-toh-mee)
[*hyster-* **uterus,** *-ec-* **out,** *-tom-* **cut,** *-y* **action**]

interstitial cell
(in-ter-STISH-al sell)
[*inter-* **between,** *-stit-* **stand,** *-al* **relating to,** *cell* **storeroom**]

labia majora
(LAY-bee-ah mah-JOH-rah)
sing., labium majus
(LAY-bee-um MAY-jus)
[*labia* **lips,** *majora* **large**]

labia minora
(LAY-bee-ah mih-NO-rah)
sing., labium minus)
(LAY-bee-um MYE-nus)
[*labia* **lips,** *minora* **small**]

lactiferous duct
(lak-TIF-er-us dukt)
[*lact-* **milk,** *-fer-* **bear or carry,** *-ous* **having to do with,** *duct* **a leading or path**]

lesser vestibular gland (Skene gland)
(LESS-er ves-TIB-yoo-lar gland)
[*vestibul-* **entrance hall,** *-ar* **relating to,** *gland* **acorn** (*Alexander Johnston Chalmers Skene* **American gynecologist**)]

luteinizing hormone (LH)
(loo-tee-in-EYE-zing HOR-mohn)
[*lute-* **yellow,** *-izing* **process,** *hormon-* **excite**]

meiosis
(my-OH-sis)
[*mei-* **smaller,** *-osis* **process**]

menarche
(meh-NAR-kee)
[*men-* **month,** *-arche* **beginning**]

menopause
(MEN-oh-pawz)
[*men-* **month,** *-paus-* **cease**]

menses
(MEN-seez)
[*menses* **months**]

menstrual cycle
(MEN-stroo-al SYE-kul)
[*mens-* **month,** *-al* **relating to,** *cycle* **circle**]

mons pubis
(monz PYOO-bis)
[*mons* **mountain,** *pubis* **groin**]

myometrium
(my-oh-MEE-tree-um)
[*myo-* **muscle,** *-metr-* **womb,** *-um* **thing**]

oocyte
(OH-oh-syte)
[*oo-* **egg,** *-cyte* **cell**]

oogenesis
(oh-oh-JEN-eh-sis)
[*oo-* **egg,** *-gen-* **produce,** *-esis* **process**]

oophorectomy
(oh-off-eh-REK-toh-mee)
[*oophoro-* **ovary,** *-ec-* **out,** *-tom-* **cut,** *-y* **action**]

ovarian follicle
(oh-VAYR-ee-an FOL-ih-kul)
[*ov-* **egg,** *-arian* **relating to,** *foll-* **bag,** *-icle* **little**]

ovary
(OH-var-ee)
[*ov-* **egg,** *-ar-* **relating to,** *-y* **location of process**]

oviduct
(OH-vih-dukt)
[*ovi-* **egg,** *- duct* **a leading or path**]

ovulation
(ov-yoo-LAY-shun)
[*ov-* **egg,** *-ation* **process**]

ovum
(OH-vum)
pl., ova
(OH-vah)
[*ovum* **egg**]

pelvic inflammatory disease (PID)
(PEL-vik in-FLAM-ah-tor-ee dih-ZEEZ)
[*pelv-* **basin,** *-ic* **relating to,** *inflam-* **set afire,** *-ory* **relating to,** *dis-* **opposite of,** *-ease* **comfort**]

penis
(PEE-nis)
pl., penes or penises
[*penis* **male sex organ**]

perineum
(payr-ih-NEE-um)
[*peri-* **around or near,** *-ine-* **excrete or evacuate,** *-um* **thing**]

polar body
(POH-lar BOD-ee)
[*pol-* **pole,** *-ar* **relating to**]

primary follicle
(PRY-mair-ee FOL-ih-kul)
[*prim-* **first,** *-ary* **state,** *folli-* **bag,** *-cle* **small**]

primary spermatocyte
(PRYE-mayr-ee SPER-mah-toh-syte)
[*prim-* **first,** *-ary* **state,** *sperm-* **seed,** *-cyte* **cell**]

progesterone
(proh-JES-ter-ohn)
[*pro-* **provide for,** *-gester-* **bearing (pregnancy),** *-stero-* **solid or steroid derivative,** *-one* **chemical**]

proliferative phase
(PROH-lif-er-eh-tiv fayz)
[*proli-* **offspring,** *-fer-* **bear or carry,** *-at-* **process,** *-ive* **relating to**]

prostate cancer
(PROS-tayt KAN-ser)
[*pro-* **before,** *-stat-* **set or place,** *cancer* **crab or malignant tumor**]

prostate gland
(PROS-tayt gland)
[*pro-* **before,** *-stat-* **set or place,** *gland* **acorn**]

prostatectomy
(pros-tah-TEK-toh-mee)
[*pro-* **before,** *-stat-* **set or place (prostate gland),** *-ec-* **out,** *-tom-* **cut,** *-y* **action**]

prostatitis
(pros-tah-TYE-tis)
[*pro-* **before,** *-stat-* **set or place,** *-itis* **inflammation**]

scrotum
(SKROH-tum)
[*scrotum* **bag**]

secretory phase
(SEEK-reh-toh-ree fayz)
[*secret-* **separate,** *-ory* **relating to**]

semen (seminal fluid)
(SEE-men)
[*semen* **seed**]

seminal fluid

seminal vesicle
(SEM-ih-nal VES-ih-kul)
[*semin-* **seed,** *-al* **relating to,** *vesic-* **blister,** *-cle* **little**]

seminiferous tubule
(seh-mih-NIF-er-us TOOB-yool)
[*semin-* **seed,** *-fer-* **bear or carry,** *-ous* **relating to,** *tub-* **tube,** *-ul-* **little**]

sperm
(sperm)
pl., sperm
[*sperm* **seed**]

spermatid
(SPER-mah-tid)
[*sperm-* **seed,** *-id* **relating or belonging to**]

spermatogenesis
(sper-mah-toh-JEN-eh-sis)
[*sperm-* **seed,** *-gen-* **produce,** *-esis* **process**]

spermatogonia
(sper-mah-toh-GO-nee-ah)
[*sperm-* **seed,** *-gonia* **offspring**]

spermatozoon
(sper-mah-tah-ZOH-on)
pl., spermatozoa
(sper-mah-tah-ZOH-ah)
[*sperm-* **seed,** *-zoon* **animal**]

testis
(TES-tis)
pl., testes
(TES-teez)
[*testis* **witness (male gonad)**]

testosterone
(tes-TOS-teh-rohn)
[*testo-* **witness (testis),** *-stero-* **solid or steroid derivative,** *-one* **chemical**]

tunica albuginea
(TOO-nih-kah al-byoo-JIN-ee-ah)
[*tunica* **tunic or coat,** *albuginea* **white**]

urethra
(yoo-REE-thrah)
[*ure-* **urine,** *-thr-* **agent or channel**]

urologist
(yoo-ROL-uh-jist)
[*uro-* **urine,** *-log-* **words (study of),** *-ist* **agent**]

uterine tube
(YOO-ter-in toob)
[*uter-* **womb,** *-ine* **relating to**]

uterus
(YOO-ter-us)
[*uterus* **womb**]

vagina
(vah-JYE-nah)
[*vagina* **sheath**]

vas deferens (ductus deferens)
(vas DEF-er-enz [DUK-tus])
[*vas* **duct or vessel,** *de-* **away from,** *-fer-* **bear or carry,** (*ductus* **duct**)]

vestibule
(VES-tih-byool)
[*vestibul-* **entrance hall**]

vulva
(VUL-vah)
[*vulva* **wrapper**]

zygote
(ZYE-goht)
[*zygot-* **union or yoke**]

❑ OUTLINE SUMMARY

To download a digital audio version of the chapter summary for use with your device, access the ***Audio Chapter Summaries*** *online at evolve.elsevier.com.*

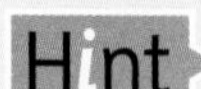

Scan this summary after reading the chapter to help you reinforce the key concepts. Later, use the summary as a quick review before your class or before a test.

Sexual Reproduction

A. Producing offspring
   1. Sexual reproduction involves two parents (unlike one-parent asexual reproduction); increases variation of genetic traits among offspring of same parents
   2. Gametes—sex cells that fuse at fertilization to form a one-celled zygote, the first cell of the offspring
      a. Sperm—gamete from the male parent
      b. Ovum—gamete from the female parent
   3. Reproductive hormones regulate sexual characteristics that promote successful reproduction
   4. Ability to reproduce begins at puberty

B. Male and female systems
   1. Common general structure and function can be identified between the systems in both sexes
   2. Systems adapted for development of sperm or ova followed by successful fertilization, development, and birth of offspring
   3. Sex hormones in both sexes are important in development of secondary sexual characteristics and normal reproductive system activity

Male Reproductive System

A. Structural plan of the reproductive tract (also called *uro-genital tract*)
   1. Organs classified as *essential* or *accessory* (see **Table 21-1**)
   2. Essential organs of reproduction are the gonads (testes), which produce sex cells (sperm or spermatozoa)
   3. Accessory organs of reproduction
      a. Ducts — passageways that carry sperm from testes to exterior
      b. Sex glands — produce protective and nutrient solution for sperm
      c. External genitals

B. Testes — the gonads of men
   1. Structure and location (see **Figure 21-1** and **Figure 21-2**)
      a. Testes in scrotum — lower temperature
      b. Covered by tunica albuginea, which divides testis into lobules containing seminiferous tubules
      c. Interstitial cells produce testosterone (see **Figure 21-3**)
   2. Functions
      a. Spermatogenesis is process of sperm production (see **Figure 21-4**)
         (1) Sperm precursor cells called *spermatogonia*
         (2) Meiosis produces primary spermatocyte, which forms four spermatids with 23 chromosomes
         (3) Spermatozoa — small, mobile cells (see **Figure 21-5**)
            (a) Head contains genetic material
            (b) Acrosome contains enzymes to assist sperm in penetration of ovum
            (c) Mitochondria in midpiece provide energy for movement
      b. Production of testosterone by interstitial cells
         (1) Testosterone "masculinizes" and promotes development of male accessory organs
         (2) Promotes and maintains development of male accessory organs
         (3) Stimulates protein anabolism and development of muscle strength

C. Reproductive ducts — ducts through which sperm pass after exiting testes until they exit from the body
   1. Epididymis — single, coiled tube about 6 meters in length; lies along the top and behind each testis in the scrotum
      a. Sperm mature and develop the capacity for motility as they pass through epididymis
   2. Vas deferens — also called *ductus deferens*
      a. Receives sperm from the epididymis and transports them from scrotal sac through the abdominal cavity
      b. Passes through inguinal canal and then joins duct of seminal vesicle to form the ejaculatory duct (see **Figure 21-6**)

D. Accessory glands — produce components of semen
   1. Semen — also called seminal fluid
      a. Mixture of sperm and secretions of accessory sex glands
      b. Averages 3 to 5 mL per ejaculation, with each milliliter containing about 100 million sperm (but is highly variable, even day to day)
   2. Seminal vesicles
      a. Pouchlike glands that produce about 60% of seminal fluid volume
      b. Secretion is yellowish, thick, and rich in fructose to provide energy needed by sperm for motility
   3. Prostate gland
      a. Shaped like a doughnut and located below bladder
      b. Urethra passes through the gland
      c. Secretion represents 30% of seminal fluid volume — is thin and milk-colored
      d. Activates sperm and is needed for ongoing sperm motility
   4. Bulbourethral (Cowper) glands
      a. Resemble peas in size and shape
      b. Secrete mucus-like fluid constituting less than 5% of seminal fluid volume

E. External genitals (also called *genitalia*)
   1. Penis and scrotum (see **Figure 21-7**)
   2. Penis has three columns of erectile tissue — two dorsal columns called *corpora cavernosa* and one ventral column surrounding urethra called *corpus spongiosum*
   3. Glans penis covered by foreskin (prepuce)
   4. Surgical removal of foreskin called *circumcision*

Female Reproductive System

A. Structural plan — organs classified as essential or accessory (see **Table 21-2** and **Figure 21-8**)
   1. Essential organs are gonads (ovaries), which produce sex cells (ova)
   2. Accessory organs of reproduction
      a. Ducts or modified ducts — including oviducts, uterus, and vagina
      b. Sex glands — including the breasts
      c. External genitals

B. Ovaries
   1. Structure and location
      a. Paired glands weighing about 3 grams each
      b. Resemble large almonds
      c. Attached to ligaments in pelvic cavity on each side of uterus
      d. Microscopic structure (see **Figure 21-9**)
         (1) Ovarian follicles — contain an oocyte, which is an immature sex cell (about 1 million at birth)
         (2) Primary follicles — about 400,000 at puberty are covered with granulosa cells

(3) About 350 to 500 mature follicles ovulate during the reproductive lifetime of most women — sometimes called *graafian follicles*
(4) Secondary follicles have a hollow chamber called the *antrum*
(5) Corpus luteum forms after ovulation

2. Functions
   a. Oogenesis (see **Figure 21-10**)
      (1) Involves meiotic cell division that produces daughter cells with equal chromosome numbers (23) but unequal cytoplasm.
      (2) Ovum is large; polar bodies are small and degenerate
   b. Production of estrogen and progesterone
      (1) Granulosa cells surrounding the oocyte in the mature and growing follicles produce estrogen
      (2) Corpus luteum produces progesterone
      (3) Estrogen causes development and maintenance of secondary sex characteristics
      (4) Progesterone stimulates secretory activity of uterine epithelium and assists estrogen in initiating menses

C. Reproductive ducts
1. Both male and female reproductive ducts carry gametes from each (of two) gonads, join into a single passage, and exit the body
2. Only the female ducts also function in receiving sperm, fertilization, and prenatal development
3. Uterine (fallopian) tubes (oviducts)
   a. Extend about 10 cm from uterus into abdominal cavity
   b. Expanded distal end surrounded by fimbriae
   c. Mucosal lining of tube is directly continuous with lining of abdominal cavity
4. Uterus — composed of body, fundus, and cervix (see **Figure 21-11**)
   a. Lies in pelvic cavity just behind urinary bladder
   b. Myometrium is muscle layer
   c. Endometrium lost in menstruation
   d. Menopause — end of repetitive menstrual cycles (about 45 to 50 years of age)
5. Vagina
   a. Distensible tube about 10 cm long
   b. Located between urinary bladder and rectum in the pelvis
   c. Receives penis during sexual intercourse and is birth canal for normal delivery of baby at end of term of pregnancy

D. Accessory glands
1. Greater and lesser vestibular glands
   a. Secrete mucous fluid that may lubricate during sexual intercourse
   b. Ducts open between labia minora
   c. Clinically important when they become infected (as in gonorrhea)
2. Breasts (see **Figure 21-12**)
   a. Located over pectoral muscles of thorax
   b. Size determined by fat quantity more than amount of glandular (milk-secreting) tissue
   c. Lactiferous ducts drain at nipple, which is surrounded by pigmented areola
   d. Lymphatic drainage important in spread of cancer cells to other body areas

E. External genitals (see **Figure 21-13**)
1. Vulva includes mons pubis, clitoris, external urinary meatus, openings of vestibular glands, vagina, labia minora and majora, and hymen
2. Perineum — area between vaginal opening and anus
   a. Surgical cut during childbirth called *episiotomy*

F. Menstrual cycle — involves many changes in the uterus, ovaries, vagina, and breasts (see **Figure 21-14** and **Figure 21-15**)
1. Length — about 28 days, varies from month to month among individuals and in the same individual
2. Phases
   a. Menses — about the first 4 or 5 days of the cycle, varies somewhat
      (1) Characterized by sloughing of bits of endometrium (uterine lining) with bleeding
      (2) First day of flow is day 1 of menstrual cycle
   b. Proliferative phase — days between the end of menses and secretory phase; varies in length
      (1) The shorter the cycle, the shorter the proliferative phase; the longer the cycle, the longer the proliferative phase
      (2) Characterized by proliferation of endometrium
   c. Secretory phase — days between ovulation and beginning of next menses; secretory about 14 days before next menses
      (1) Characterized by further thickening of endometrium
      (2) Secretion by its glands in preparation for implantation of fertilized ovum
3. Ovulation — typically one ovum released per cycle, 14 days before next menses; timing of ovulation is useful in timing sexual intercourse to maximize fertility
4. Control — combined actions of the anterior pituitary hormones FSH and LH cause ovulation; sudden sharp decrease in estrogens and progesterone brings on menstruation if pregnancy does not occur

Summary of the Reproductive Systems

A. In men and women the organs of the reproductive system are adapted for the specific sequence of functions that permit development of sperm or ova after the successful fertilization and then the normal development and birth of offspring

B. The male organs produce, store, and ultimately introduce mature sperm into the female reproductive tract
C. The female system produces ova, receives the sperm, and permits fertilization followed by fetal development and birth, with lactation afterward
D. Men and women have analogous reproductive structures (see **Table 21-3**)
E. Production of sex hormones is required for development of secondary sex characteristics and for normal reproductive functions in both sexes

❑ ACTIVE LEARNING

STUDY TIPS

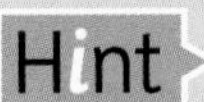

Use these tips to achieve success in meeting your learning goals.

To make the study of the reproductive systems more efficient, we suggest these tips:

1. Before studying Chapter 21, review the synopsis of the male and female reproductive systems in Chapter 5, endocrine glands and hormones in Chapter 11, and coverage of the male urethra in Chapter 18.
2. Sexual reproduction in humans requires production of gametes or sex cells: sperm cells in males and egg cells, or ova, in females.
3. One sperm cell and one ovum come together during the process of fertilization to produce a cell called the *zygote,* which ultimately develops into the offspring.
4. Create flash cards to help (1) review the essential and accessory organs of reproduction and their functions in both males and females (see **Table 21-1** and **Table 21-2**); (2) outline the cell types and steps—including changes in chromosome numbers—that characterize spermatogenesis and oogenesis; and (3) list and compare the origin and functions of the sex hormones in both males and females.
5. In your study group construct concept maps as you discuss (1) the phases and events of the menstrual cycle, referring often to **Figure 21-14** and **Figure 21-15**; and (2) the analogous features of the male and female reproductive systems (see **Table 21-3**).
6. Always be able to correctly answer each set of Quick Check questions before proceeding further in the text, and discuss questions at the end of the chapter in addition to possible test questions in your study group.

Review Questions

Hint *Write out the answers to these questions after reading the chapter and reviewing the Chapter Summary. If you simply think through the answer without writing it down, you won't retain much of your new learning.*

1. Describe the structure and location of the testes.
2. Describe the structure of the spermatozoa.
3. List the functions of testosterone.
4. List and briefly describe the reproductive ducts of the male reproductive system.
5. List and briefly describe the glands of the male reproductive system and what each gland contributes to seminal fluid.
6. Describe the structure and location of the ovaries.
7. Explain the development of an ovarian follicle from the primary follicle to the corpus luteum.
8. List the functions of estrogen.
9. List the functions of progesterone.
10. Describe the structure of the uterine tubes.
11. Describe the structure of the uterus.
12. Describe the structure of the vagina.
13. Describe the structure of the breasts.
14. Explain "milk let-down."
15. Explain what occurs during the proliferative phase of the reproductive cycle.
16. Explain what occurs during the secretory phase of the reproductive cycle.
17. List, locate, and briefly describe the function of the four hormones involved in the regulation of the reproductive cycle.

Critical Thinking

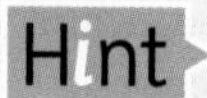
After finishing the Review Questions, write out the answers to these more in-depth questions to help you apply your new knowledge. Go back to sections of the chapter that relate to concepts that you find difficult.

18. Differentiate between spermatogenesis and oogenesis. How do these differences relate to the role of the male and female in reproduction?
19. Why are the testes located outside the body cavity in the scrotum?
20. What is unique about the chromosome content of the gametes? Why is this important?
21. Maddie is on a birth control pill. Her doctor told her that it would "shut her reproductive system off" and thus prevent pregnancy. Maddie wonders about her female hormones. Will estrogen and progesterone be "shut off" too?

Chapter Test

Hint *After studying the chapter, test your mastery by responding to these items. Try to answer them without looking up the answers. Then, verify the answers using the key in Appendix C at the back of this book.*

1. The essential organs of the male reproductive system are the testes.
2. The pouchlike sac where the male gonads are located is called the Scrotum
3. The membrane that covers the testicle and also divides the interior into lobes is called the tunica albuginea
4. The ________ is a long duct in the testicle where sperm develop. Seminefor us tubile
5. The ________ are the cells in the testes that secrete testosterone. intersitial cells
6. The primary spermatocyte develops from a cell called the spermatogensis
7. The primary spermatocyte forms sperm cells by undergoing a specialized type of cell division called meiosis.
8. The sperm cell contains an acrosome which contains an enzyme that can digest the covering of the ovum.
9. The epdidyms is a reproductive duct that consists of a tightly coiled tube that lies along the top and behind the testes.
10. The vas deferens is a reproductive duct that permits the sperm to move out of the scrotum upward into the abdominal cavity.
11. The prostate gland is a gland that secretes a thin, milk-colored fluid that makes up about 20% of the seminal fluid.
12. The seminal vesicle are a pair of glands that produce a thick, yellowish, fructose-rich fluid that makes up about 60% of the seminal fluid.
13. The penis is composed of three columns of erectile tissue: one is called the corpus spongiosum, and the other two are called the corpora cavernosa
14. The essential organs of the female reproductive system are the ovaries.
15. Another name for a mature ovarian follicle is a graafin follicle.
16. The process that produces the female gamete is called oogenesis
17. Meiosis in the female produces one large ovum and three small daughter cells called polar bodies, which degenerate.
18. The uterine tubes are the reproductive tubes connecting the ovary and the uterus.
19. The muscle layer of the uterus is called the myometrium
20. The uterus is composed of two parts: the upper part, called the body, and the narrow lower part, called the cervix.
21. The innermost layer of the uterus, which is shed during menstruation, is called the endometrium.
22. The vagina is the part of the female reproductive system that opens to the exterior.
23. The ________ glands are glands that secrete a mucuslike lubricating fluid into the vestibule. greater vestibular
24. The milk-secreting glandular cells of the breast are arranged in grapelike structures called alveioli. These drain into lactiferous ducts that converge toward the nipple.

Match each phrase in Column B with the correct corresponding term in Column A.

Column A	Column B
25. H FSH	a. what the egg follicle becomes after ovulation
26. C menstruation	b. ovarian hormone that reaches its highest concentration in the proliferative phase
27. A corpus luteum	c. caused by the rapid drop of blood levels of estrogen and progesterone
28. B estrogen	d. phase of the reproductive cycle that begins after ovulation
29. D secretory phase	e. ovarian hormone that reaches its highest concentration during the secretory phase
30. E progesterone	f. term used to describe the egg being released from the ovary
31. I LH	g. the uterine wall begins to thicken during this phase of the reproductive cycle
32. G proliferative phase	h. pituitary hormone that stimulates the formation of an egg follicle
33. F ovulation	i. pituitary hormone that can be called the ovulating hormone

Growth, Development, and Aging

OUTLINE

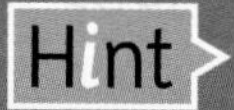

Scan this outline before you begin to read the chapter, as a preview of how the concepts are organized.

OBJECTIVES

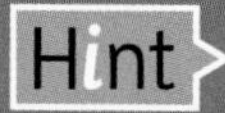

Before reading the chapter, review these goals for your learning.

After you have completed this chapter, you should be able to:

1. Discuss the concept of development as a biological process characterized by continuous modification and change.
2. Discuss the major developmental changes characteristic of the prenatal stage of life from fertilization to birth.
3. Identify the three primary germ layers and several derivatives in the adult body that develop from each layer.
4. Discuss the three stages of labor that characterize a normal vaginal birth.
5. List and discuss the major developmental changes characteristic of the four postnatal periods of life.
6. Discuss effects of aging on the major organ systems.

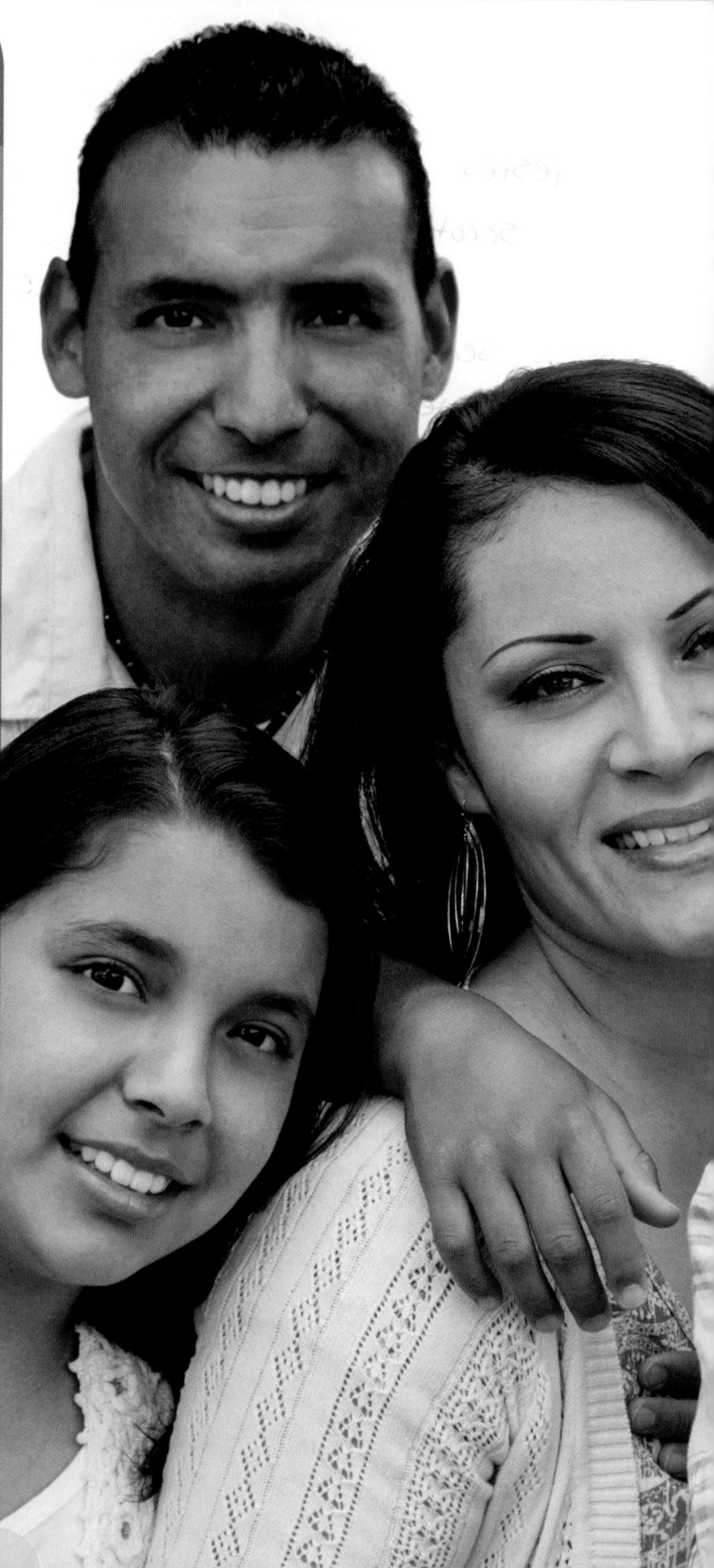

CHAPTER 22

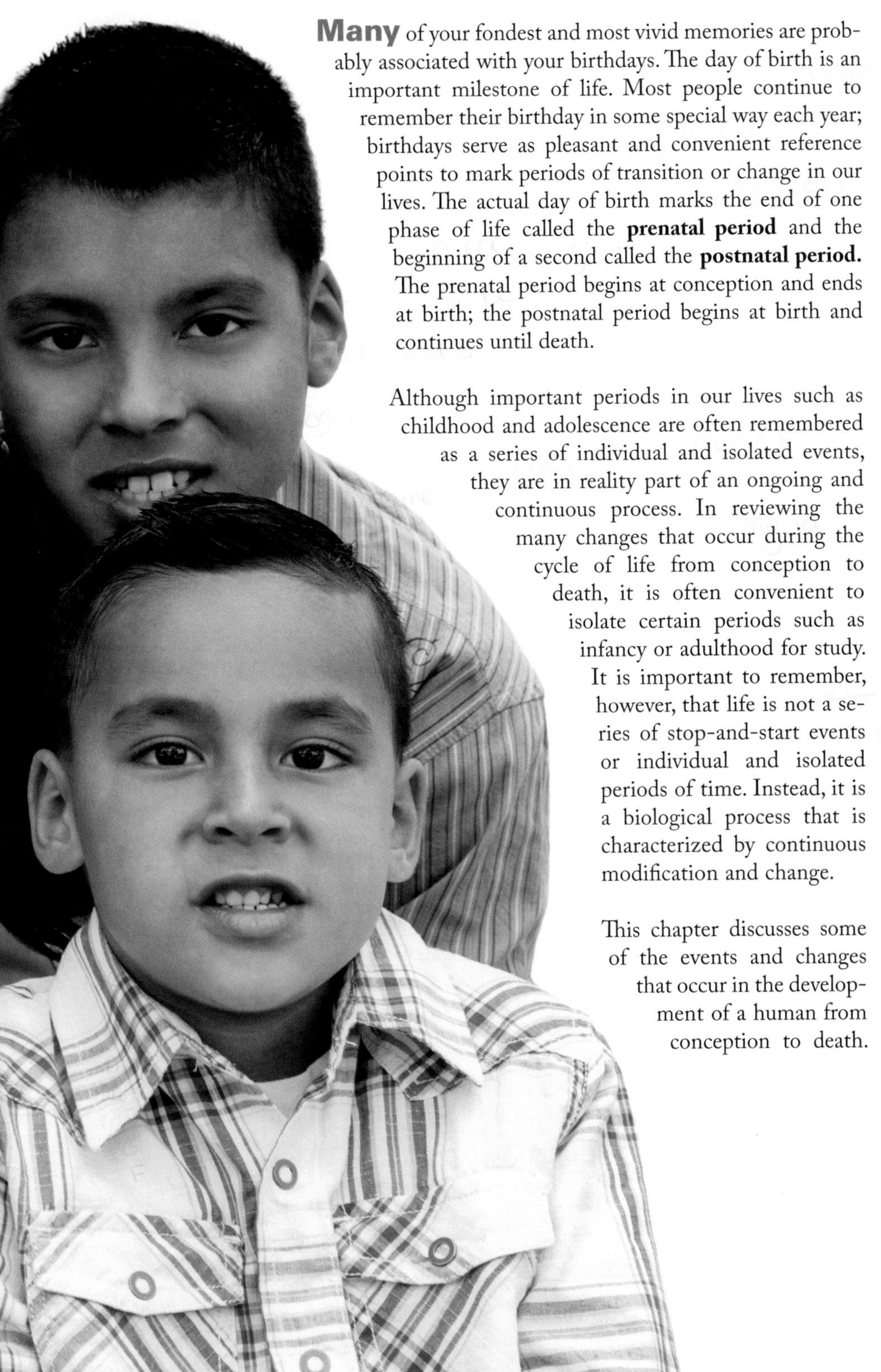

Many of your fondest and most vivid memories are probably associated with your birthdays. The day of birth is an important milestone of life. Most people continue to remember their birthday in some special way each year; birthdays serve as pleasant and convenient reference points to mark periods of transition or change in our lives. The actual day of birth marks the end of one phase of life called the **prenatal period** and the beginning of a second called the **postnatal period.** The prenatal period begins at conception and ends at birth; the postnatal period begins at birth and continues until death.

Although important periods in our lives such as childhood and adolescence are often remembered as a series of individual and isolated events, they are in reality part of an ongoing and continuous process. In reviewing the many changes that occur during the cycle of life from conception to death, it is often convenient to isolate certain periods such as infancy or adulthood for study. It is important to remember, however, that life is not a series of stop-and-start events or individual and isolated periods of time. Instead, it is a biological process that is characterized by continuous modification and change.

This chapter discusses some of the events and changes that occur in the development of a human from conception to death.

LANGUAGE OF SCIENCE AND MEDICINE

Hint Before reading the chapter, say each of these terms out loud. This will help you to avoid stumbling over them as you read.

adolescence
(ad-oh-LES-ens)
[*adolesc-* **grow up,** *-ence* **state**]

adulthood
(ah-DULT-hood)

amniotic cavity
(am-nee-OT-ik KAV-ih-tee)
[*amnio-* **fetal membrane,** *-ic* **relating to,** *cav-* **hollow,** *-ity* **state**]

antenatal medicine
(an-tee-NAY-tal MED-ih-sin)
[*ante-* **before,** *-nat-* **birth,** *-al* **relating to**]

Apgar score
(AP-gar skohr)
[*Virginia Apgar* **American physician**]

arteriosclerosis
(ar-tee-ree-oh-skleh-ROH-sis)
[*arteri-* **vessel (artery),** *-sclero-* **harden,** *-osis* **condition**]

atherosclerosis
(ath-er-oh-skleh-ROH-sis)
[*ather-* **porridge,** *-sclero-* **harden,** *-osis* **condition**]

birth defect
(berth DEE-fekt)

blastocyst
(BLAS-toh-sist)
[*blasto-* **bud,** *-cyst* **pouch**]

cataract
(KAT-ah-rakt)
[*cataract* **broken water**]

cesarean section
(seh-SAYR-ee-an SEK-shun)
[*Julius Caesar* **Roman emperor,** *-ean* **relating to,** *sect-* **cut,** *-ion* **condition**]

childhood
(CHILD-hood)

Continued on p. 499

Study of development during the prenatal period is followed by a discussion of the birth process and a review of changes that occur during infancy and adulthood. Finally, some important changes that occur in the individual organ systems of the body as a result of aging are discussed.

Prenatal Period

The *prenatal stage of development* begins at the time of conception, or **fertilization** (that is, at the moment the female ovum and the male sperm cells unite) (Figure 22-1). The period of prenatal development continues until the birth of the child about 39 weeks later. The science of the development of the offspring before birth is called **embryology.** It is a story of biological marvels, describing the means by which a new human life is started and the steps by which a single microscopic cell is transformed into a complex human being.

Fertilization to Implantation

After ovulation the discharged ovum first enters the abdominal cavity and then finds its way into a uterine (fallopian) tube.

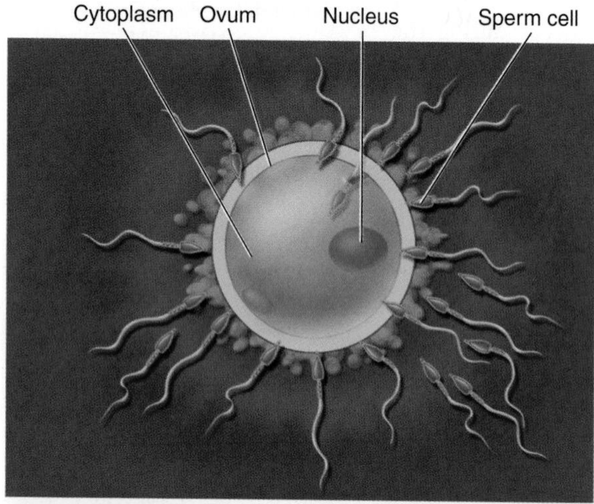

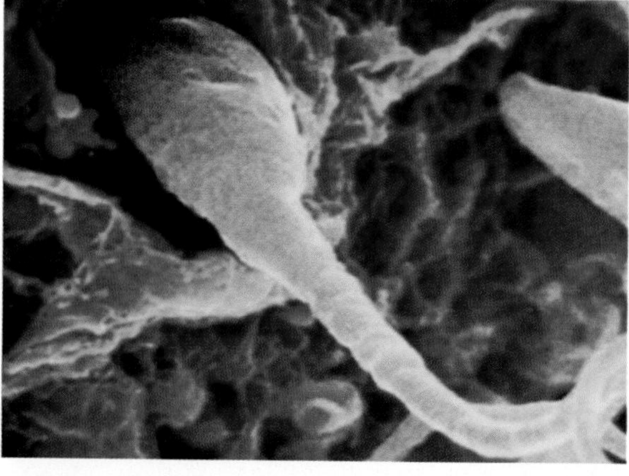

FIGURE 22-1 Fertilization. Fertilization is a specific biological event. It occurs when the male and female sex cells fuse. After union between a sperm cell and the ovum has occurred, the cycle of life begins. The scanning electron micrograph shows spermatozoa attaching themselves to the surface of an ovum. Only one will penetrate and fertilize the ovum.

Sperm cells swim up the uterine tubes toward the ovum. Look at the relationship of the ovary, the two uterine tubes, and the uterus in Figure 22-2. Recall from Chapter 21 that each uterine tube extends outward from the uterus for about 10 centimeters (cm). It then ends in the abdominal cavity near the ovary, as you can see in Figure 22-2, in an opening surrounded by fringelike processes, the *fimbriae.*

Sperm cells that are deposited in the vagina must enter and swim through the uterus and through the uterine tube to meet the ovum. **Fertilization** most often occurs in the outer one third of the oviduct, as shown in Figure 22-2.

The fertilized ovum, or **zygote,** is genetically complete—it is a new single-celled offspring. Time and nourishment are all that is needed for expression of characteristics such as sex, body build, and skin color that were determined at the time of fertilization. As you can see in the figure, the zygote immediately begins mitotic division, and in about 3 days a solid mass of cells called a **morula** is formed (see Figure 22-2). The cells of the morula continue to divide, and by the time the developing embryo reaches the uterus, it is a hollow ball of cells called a **blastocyst.**

During the 10 days from the time of fertilization to the time when the blastocyst completes **implantation** in the uterine lining, few nutrients from the mother are available. The rapid cell division taking place up to the blastocyst stage occurs with no significant increase in total mass compared with the zygote (Figure 22-3). One of the specializations of the ovum is its incredible store of nutrients that help support this embryonic development until implantation has occurred.

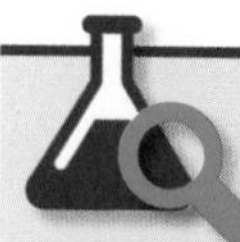

RESEARCH, ISSUES, AND TRENDS

IN VITRO FERTILIZATION

The Latin term *in vitro* means, literally, "within a glass." In the case of in vitro fertilization, it refers to the glass laboratory dish where an ovum and sperm are mixed and where fertilization occurs.

In the classic technique, the ovum is obtained from the woman by first inserting a fiber-optic viewing instrument called a **laparoscope** through a very small incision in her abdomen. After it is in the abdominal cavity, the device allows the physician to view the ovary, puncture it, and "suck up" an ovum from a mature follicle. Over the years refinements to this technique have been made, and less invasive procedures are currently being used.

After fertilization in a laboratory dish and about 2.5 days' growth in a temperature-controlled environment, the developing zygote (which by then has reached the 8- or 16-cell stage) is placed by the physician into the mother's uterus. If implantation is successful, growth will continue and the subsequent pregnancy will progress. In the most successful fertility clinics in the United States, a normal term birth will occur in about 30% of in vitro fertilization attempts.

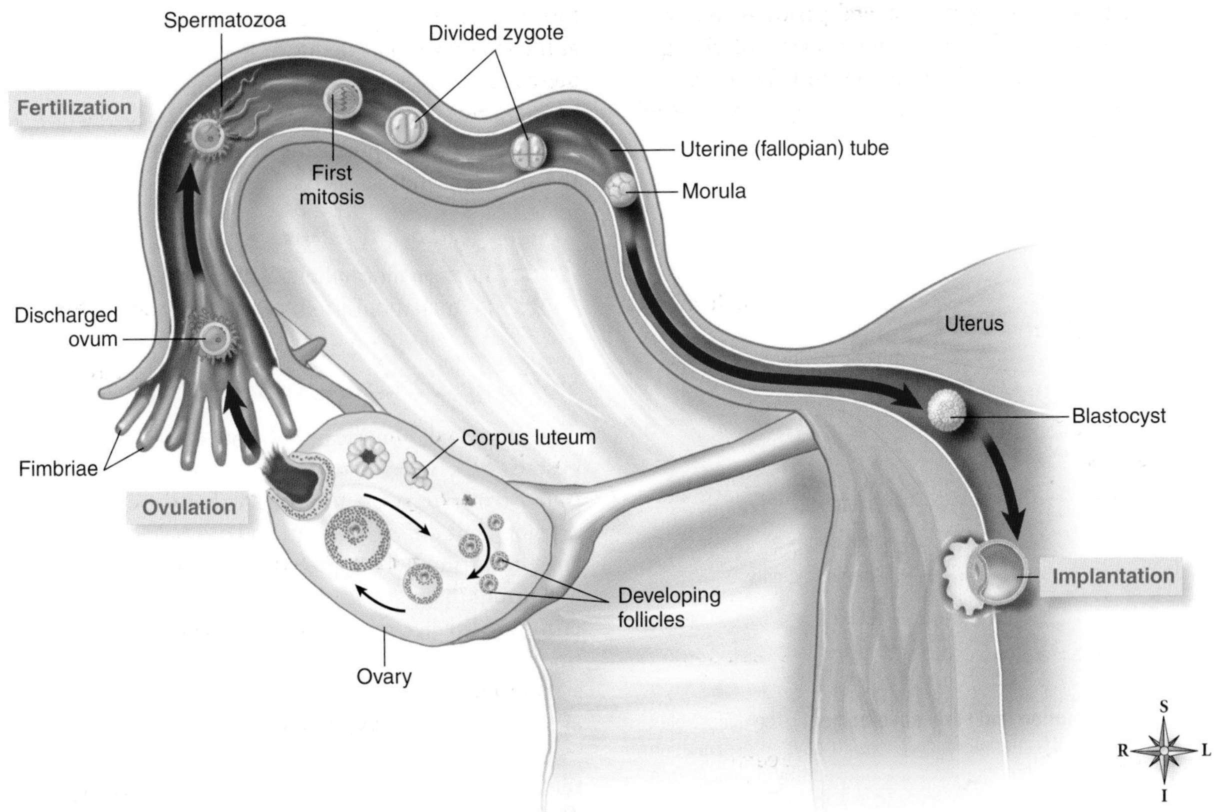

FIGURE 22-2 Fertilization and implantation. At ovulation, an ovum is released from the ovary and begins its journey through the uterine tube. While in the tube, the ovum is fertilized by a sperm to form the single-celled zygote. After a few days of rapid mitotic division, a ball of cells called a *morula* is formed. After the morula develops into a hollow ball called a *blastocyst,* implantation occurs.

Amniotic Cavity and Placenta

Note in Figure 22-4 that the blastocyst consists of an outer layer of cells and an inner cell mass. As the blastocyst develops, it forms a structure with two cavities, the **yolk sac** and **amniotic cavity.** The yolk sac is most important in animals, such as birds, that depend heavily on yolk as the sole source of nutrients for the developing embryo. In these animals, the yolk sac digests the yolk and provides the resulting nutrients to the embryo. Because uterine fluids provide nutrients to the developing human embryo until the placenta develops, the function of the yolk sac is not a nutritive one. Instead, it has other functions—including production of blood cells.

The amniotic cavity becomes a fluid-filled, shock-absorbing sac, sometimes called the *bag of waters,* in which the embryo floats during development. The **chorion,** shown in Figure 22-4 and Figure 22-5, develops into an important fetal membrane in the **placenta.** The **chorionic villi,** shown in Figure 22-5, connect the blood vessels of the chorion to the rest of the placenta. The placenta (see Figure 22-5) anchors the developing fetus to the uterus and provides a "bridge" for the exchange of nutrients and waste products between mother and baby.

The *placenta* is a unique structure that has a temporary but very important series of functions during pregnancy. It is composed of tissues from mother and child and functions not

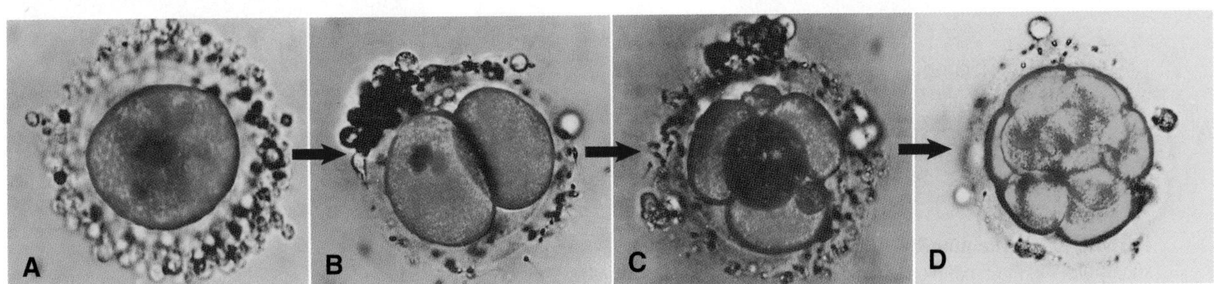

FIGURE 22-3 Early stages of human development. A, Fertilized ovum or zygote. **B** to **D,** Early cell divisions produce more and more cells. The solid mass of cells shown in **D** forms the morula—an early stage in embryonic development.

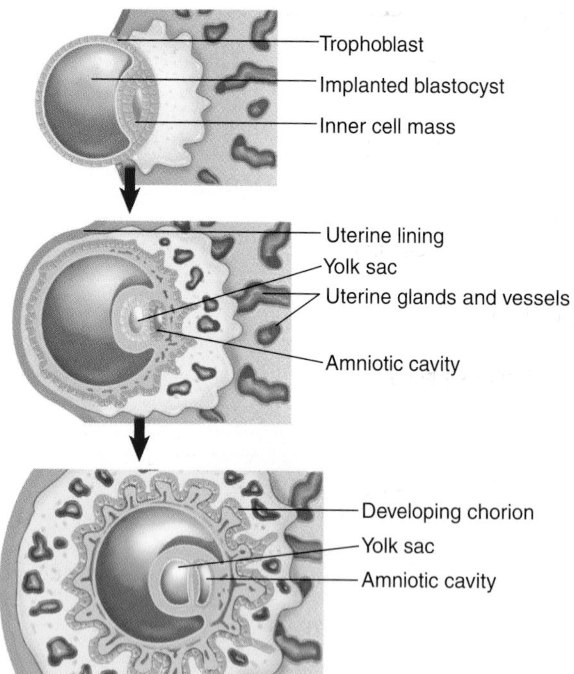

FIGURE 22-4 Implantation and early development. The hollow blastocyst implants itself in the uterine lining about 10 days after ovulation. Until the placenta is functional, nutrients are obtained by diffusion from uterine fluids. Notice the developing chorion and how the blastocyst eventually forms a yolk sac and amniotic cavity.

only as a structural "anchor" and nutritive bridge but also as an excretory, respiratory, and endocrine organ (see Figure 22-5).

Placental tissue normally separates the maternal blood, which fills the lacunae of the placenta, from the fetal blood so that no intermixing occurs. The very thin layer of placental tissue that separates maternal and fetal blood also serves as an effective "barrier" that can protect the developing baby from many harmful substances that may enter the mother's bloodstream. Unfortunately, toxic substances such as alcohol and some infectious organisms may nonetheless penetrate this protective placental barrier and injure the developing baby. The virus responsible for *cytomegalovirus (CMV)* or the bacterium that causes syphilis, for example, can easily pass through the placenta and cause tragic developmental defects in the fetus.

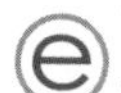

To learn more about fertilization and implantation, go to AnimationDirect at *evolve.elsevier.com.*

Periods of Development

The length of pregnancy (about 39 weeks)—called the **gestation period**—is divided into three 3-month segments called **trimesters.** A number of terms are used to describe development during these periods, known as the first, second, and third trimesters of pregnancy.

During the first trimester or 3 months of pregnancy, many terms are used. *Zygote* describes the ovum just after fertilization by a sperm cell. After about 3 days of constant cell division, the solid mass of cells, identified earlier as the *morula,* enters the uterus. Continued development transforms the morula into the hollow *blastocyst,* which then implants into the uterine wall.

The **embryonic phase** of development extends from the third week after fertilization until the end of week 8 of **gestation.** During this period in the first trimester, the term **embryo** is used to describe the developing offspring. By day 35 of gestation (Figure 22-6, *A*), the heart is beating. Although the embryo is only 8 millimeters (mm) (about ⅜ inch) long at this stage, the eyes and *limb buds,* which ultimately form the arms and legs, are clearly visible.

The period of development extending from week 9 to week 39 is termed the **fetal phase.** During this period, the term *embryo* is replaced by **fetus.** Figure 22-6, *C,* shows the stage of

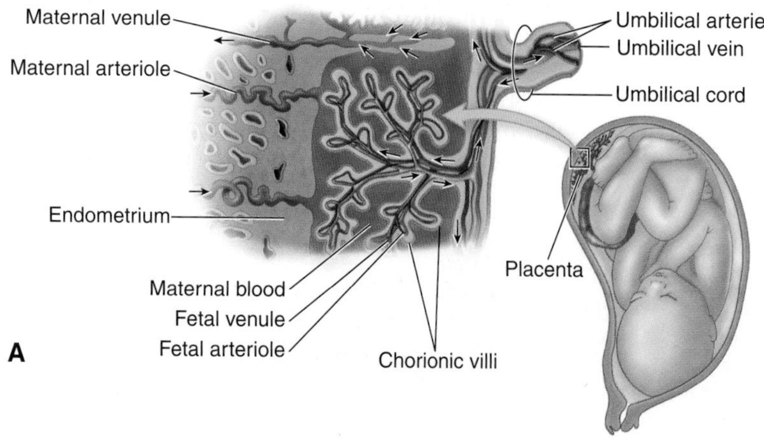

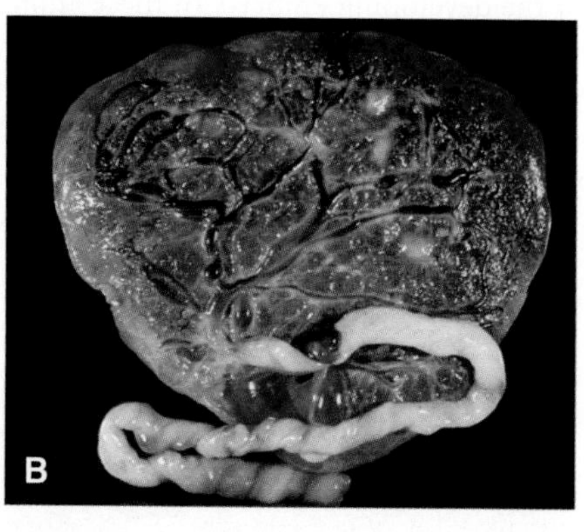

FIGURE 22-5 The placenta. Relationship of uterus, developing infant, and placenta. The close placement of the fetal blood supply and the maternal blood in the lacunae of the placenta permits diffusion of nutrients and other substances. It also forms a thin barrier to prevent diffusion of most harmful substances. No mixing of fetal and maternal blood occurs. **A,** Diagram showing a cross-section of the placental structure. **B,** Photograph of a normal, full-term placenta (fetal side) showing the branching of the placental blood vessels.

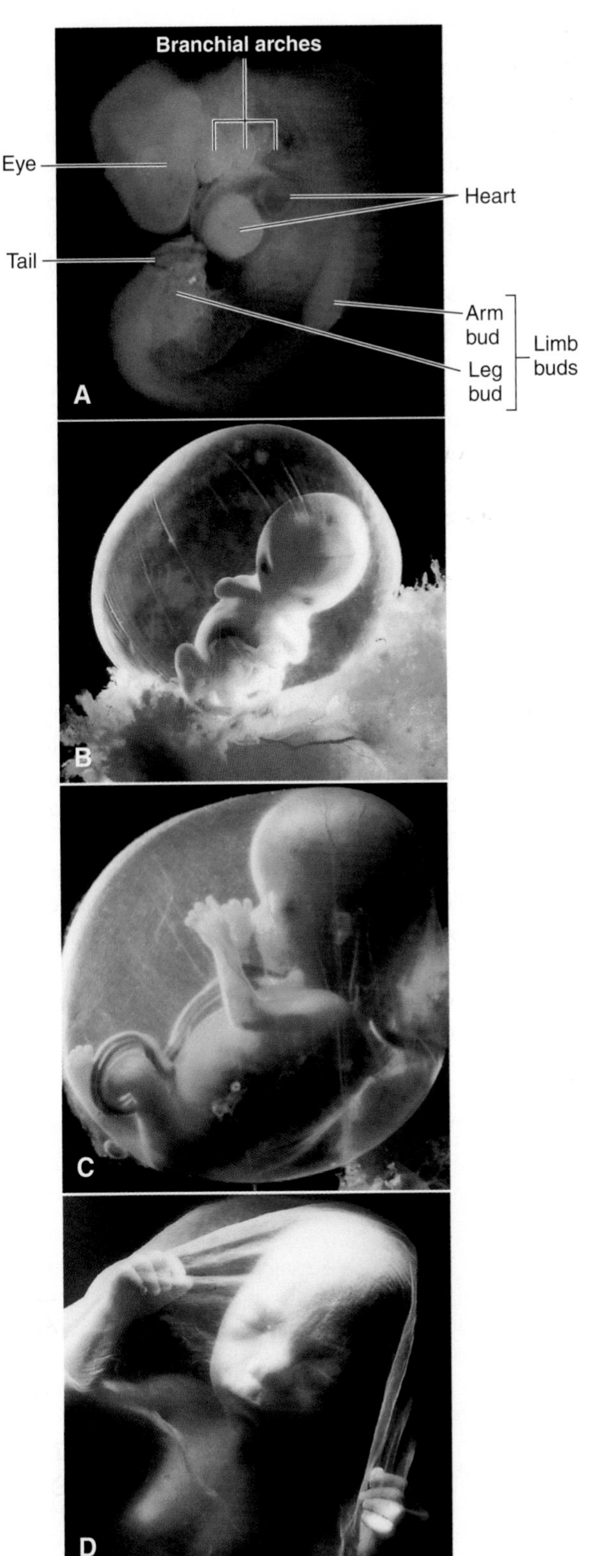

FIGURE 22-6 Human embryos and fetuses. A, At 35 days. **B,** At 49 days. **C,** At the end of the first trimester. **D,** At 4 months.

development of the fetus at the end of the first trimester of gestation. Body size is about 7 to 8 cm (3.2 inches) long. The facial features of the fetus are apparent, the limbs are complete, and gender can be identified. By month 4 (see Figure 22-6, *D*) all organ systems are complete and in place.

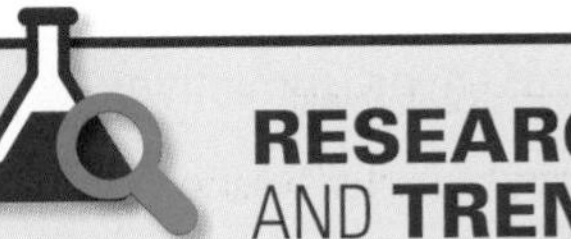

RESEARCH, ISSUES, AND TRENDS

HOW LONG DOES PREGNANCY LAST?

This seems like a silly question to most of us—the answer is 9 months, isn't it? Actually, the length of gestation (the amount of time one is pregnant) is defined in different ways in different situations and can vary from one pregnancy to another. The average gestation in humans is 266 days, starting at the day of conception. But physicians instead usually count from the beginning of the woman's last menstrual period, for an average of 280 days. However, these are only averages. What is normal in one case can be different from what is normal in another case. In practice, any pregnancy of less than 37 weeks (259 days) is said to be premature, and any lasting more than 42 weeks (294 days) is said to be postmature. So, as with many statistics regarding human function, what is "normal" can be spoken of only in generalities and averages.

Formation of the Primary Germ Layers

At the very beginning of the embryonic stage, all of the cells are **stem cells.** Stem cells are unspecialized cells that reproduce to form specific lines of specialized cells. At this stage, they have their highest "stemness" or potency—that is, they are capable of producing many different kinds of cells in the body.

Adult stem cells remain after early development, but can only produce a few specialized kinds of cells in a particular tissue. We have already encountered these adult stem cells when we discussed hematopoiesis—formation of RBCs, WBCs, and platelets—in bone marrow. Other stem cells are found in the skin, many glands, muscles, nerve tissue, bone, and the gastrointestinal (GI) tract. Adult stem cells replace the specialized cells in a tissue and thus ensure stable, functional populations of the cell types needed for survival.

Early in the first trimester of pregnancy, three layers of stem cells develop that embryologists call the **primary germ layers** (Table 22-1). Each layer gives rise to definite structures such as the skin, nervous tissue, muscles, or digestive organs. Table 22-1 lists a number of structures derived from each of the three primary germ layers:

1. **Endoderm**—inside layer
2. **Mesoderm**—middle layer
3. **Ectoderm**—outside layer

Histogenesis and Organogenesis

The process of how the primary germ layers develop into many different kinds of tissues is called **histogenesis.** The way in which those tissues arrange themselves into organs is called **organogenesis.**

TABLE 22-1 Primary Germ Layer Derivatives

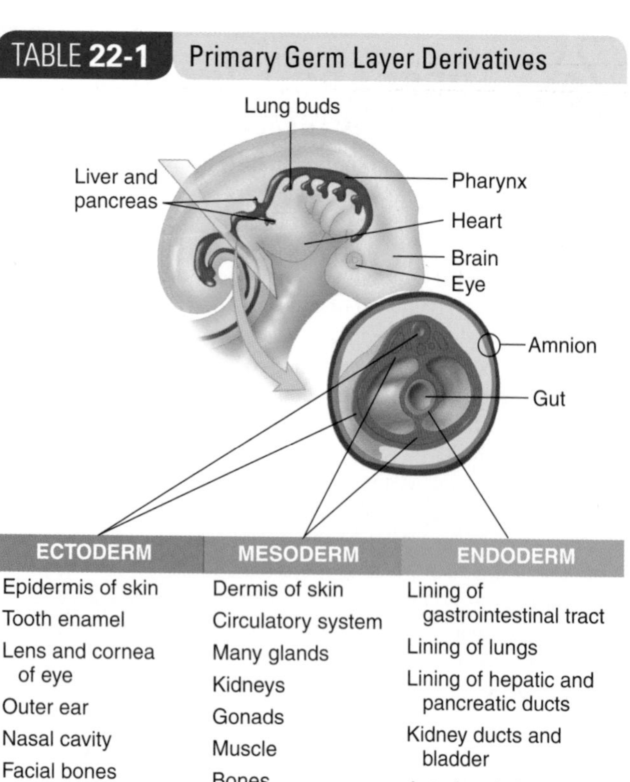

ECTODERM	MESODERM	ENDODERM
Epidermis of skin	Dermis of skin	Lining of gastrointestinal tract
Tooth enamel	Circulatory system	Lining of lungs
Lens and cornea of eye	Many glands	Lining of hepatic and pancreatic ducts
Outer ear	Kidneys	Kidney ducts and bladder
Nasal cavity	Gonads	Anterior pituitary gland (adenohypophysis)
Facial bones	Muscle	Thymus gland
Skeletal muscles in head	Bones (except facial)	Thyroid gland
Brain and spinal cord		Parathyroid gland
Sensory neurons		Tonsils
		Adrenal medulla

The fascinating story of histogenesis and organogenesis in human development is long and complicated—its telling belongs to the science of *embryology.* But for the beginning student of anatomy and physiology, it seems sufficient to appreciate that human development begins when two sex cells unite to form a single-celled zygote. It is also necessary to understand that the offspring's body evolves by a series of processes that consist of cell differentiation, multiplication, growth, and rearrangement, all of which take place in a definite, orderly sequence (**Figure 22-7**).

Development of structure and function go hand in hand, and from 4 months of gestation, when every organ system is complete and in place, until term (about 280 days), fetal development is mainly a matter of growth. **Figure 22-8**, *step 1,* shows the normal intrauterine placement of a fetus just before birth in a full-term pregnancy.

Birth Defects

Developmental problems present at birth are often called **birth defects.** Such abnormalities may be structural or functional, perhaps even involving behavior and personality.

Birth defects may be caused by genetic factors such as abnormal genes or inheritance of an abnormal number of chromosomes. Birth defects also may be caused by exposure to environmental factors called **teratogens.** Teratogens include radiation (for example, x rays), chemicals (for example, drugs, cigarettes, or alcohol), and infections in the mother (for example, herpes or rubella). Some teratogens are also mutagens because they do their damage by changing the genetic code in cells of the developing embryo. Nutritional deficiencies during pregnancy also can lead to birth defects.

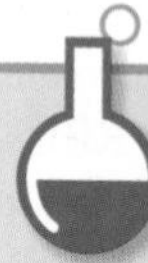

SCIENCE APPLICATIONS

EMBRYOLOGY

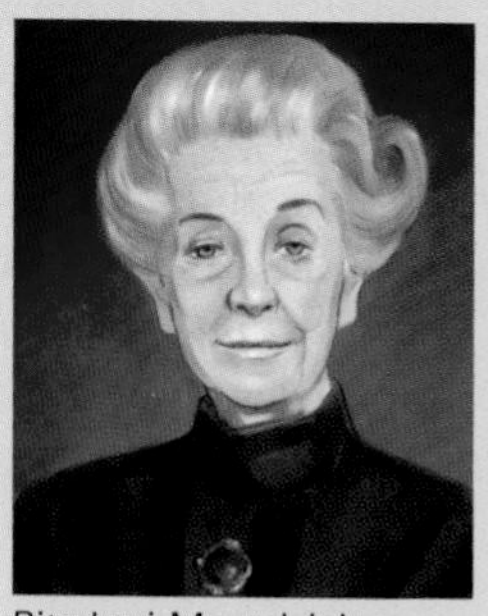

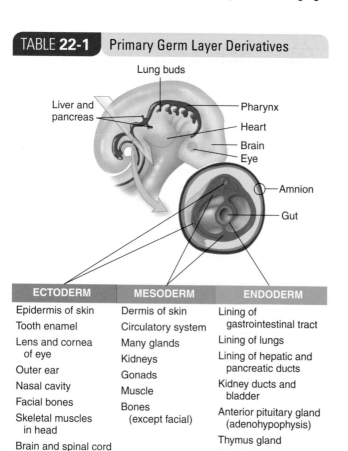

Rita Levi-Montalcini (1909-2012)

Rita Levi-Montalcini had just finished a medical degree in her native Italy when in 1938 the Fascist government under Mussolini barred all "non-Aryans" from working in academic and professional careers. Being Jewish, Levi-Montalcini was forced to move to Belgium to work. But when Belgium was about to be invaded by the Nazis, she decided to return home to Italy and work in secret.

Her home laboratory was very crude, but in it she made some important discoveries about how the nervous system develops during embryonic development. After World War II, she was invited to Washington University in St. Louis to work. There, she discovered the existence of *nerve growth factor (NGF),* for which she later won the 1986 Nobel Prize. Her discovery of a chemical that regulates the growth of new nerves during early brain development has led to many different paths of investigation. For example, by learning more about growth regulators, we now know more about how the nervous system develops, as well as other tissues, organs, and systems of the body.

Today, many professions make use of the discoveries of **embryology**—the study of early development. Not only are these discoveries important for health professionals such as **obstetricians, obstetric nurses,** and others involved in *prenatal health care,* but they are also important in understanding adult medicine more fully. In fact, even **gerontology** (study of aging) and **geriatrics** (treatment of the aged) have benefited from embryological research. How? By providing insights on how tissue development is regulated in the embryo, scientists can better understand how to possibly stimulate damaged tissue in older adults to repair or regenerate itself.

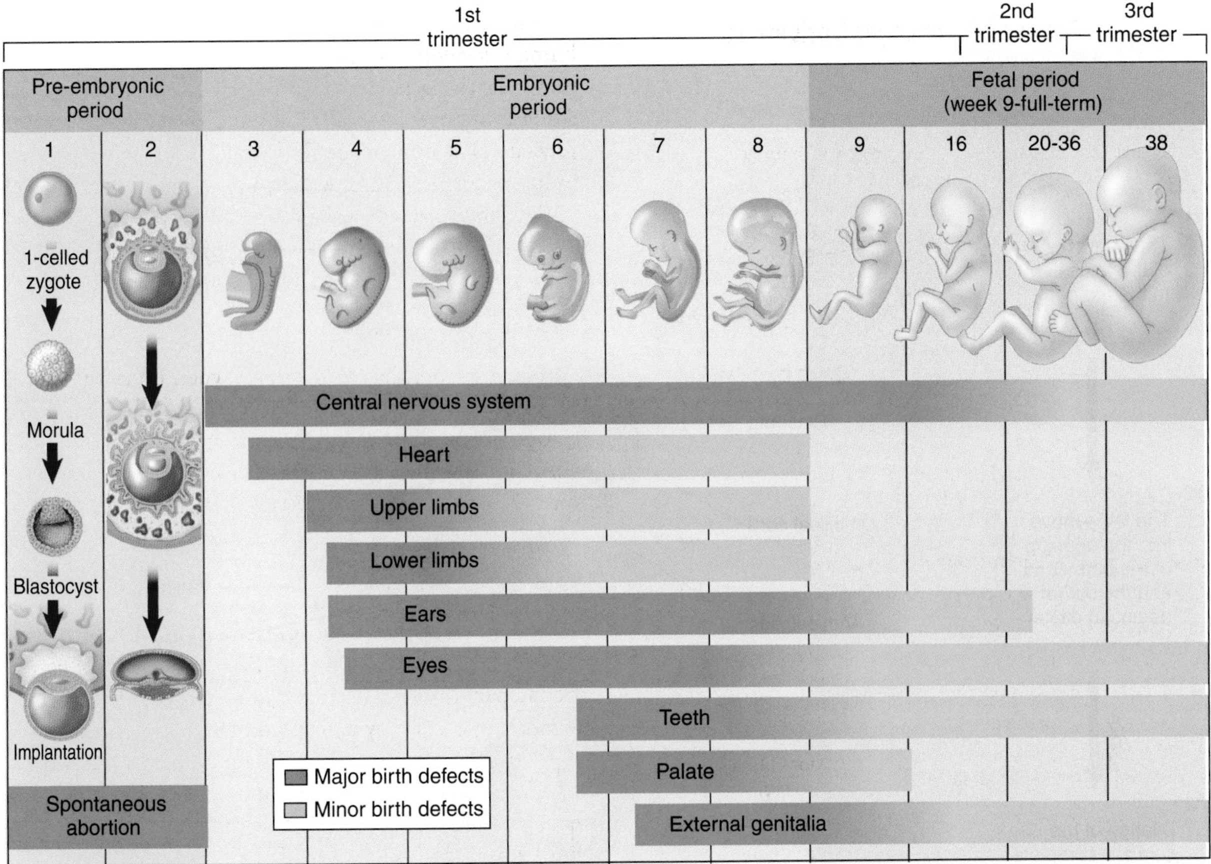

FIGURE 22-7 Critical periods of neonatal development. The red areas show when teratogens are most likely to cause major birth defects, and the yellow areas show when minor defects are more likely to arise. Numbers refer to weeks of gestation.

As **Figure 22-7** shows, the period during the first trimester when the tissues are beginning to differentiate and the organs are just starting to develop is the time that teratogens are most likely to cause damage. In fact, teratogens can cause spontaneous abortion (miscarriage) if significant damage occurs during the pre-embryonic stage.

QUICK CHECK

1. What is the prenatal period? What is the postnatal period?
2. What is a zygote? How is it different from a morula or blastocyst?
3. What are germ layers?
4. What is meant by the term *organogenesis?*

Birth

Parturition

The process of birth—sometimes called **parturition**—is the point of transition between the prenatal and postnatal periods of life.

As pregnancy draws to a close, the uterus becomes "irritable" and, ultimately, muscular contractions begin and cause the cervix to dilate or open, thus permitting the fetus to move from the uterus through the vagina, or "birth canal," to the exterior. When contractions occur, the amniotic sac, or "bag of waters," ruptures, and labor begins.

The process normally begins with the fetus taking a head-down position against the cervix (see **Figure 22-8**, *step 1*). A *breech birth* is one in which the fetus fails to turn head downward and consequently the feet are born first. This condition usually requires the baby to be born by **cesarean section.** Often called simply a *C-section,* it is a surgical procedure in which the newborn is delivered through an incision in the abdomen and uterine wall. The procedure may be done when abnormal conditions of the mother or fetus (or both) make normal vaginal delivery hazardous or impossible.

Stages of Labor

Labor is the process that results in the birth of a baby. It has three stages (see **Figure 22-8**, *steps 2 to 5*):

1. Stage 1—period from onset of uterine contractions until dilation of the cervix is complete
2. Stage 2—period from the time of maximal cervical dilation until the baby exits through the vagina
3. Stage 3—process of expulsion of the placenta through the vagina

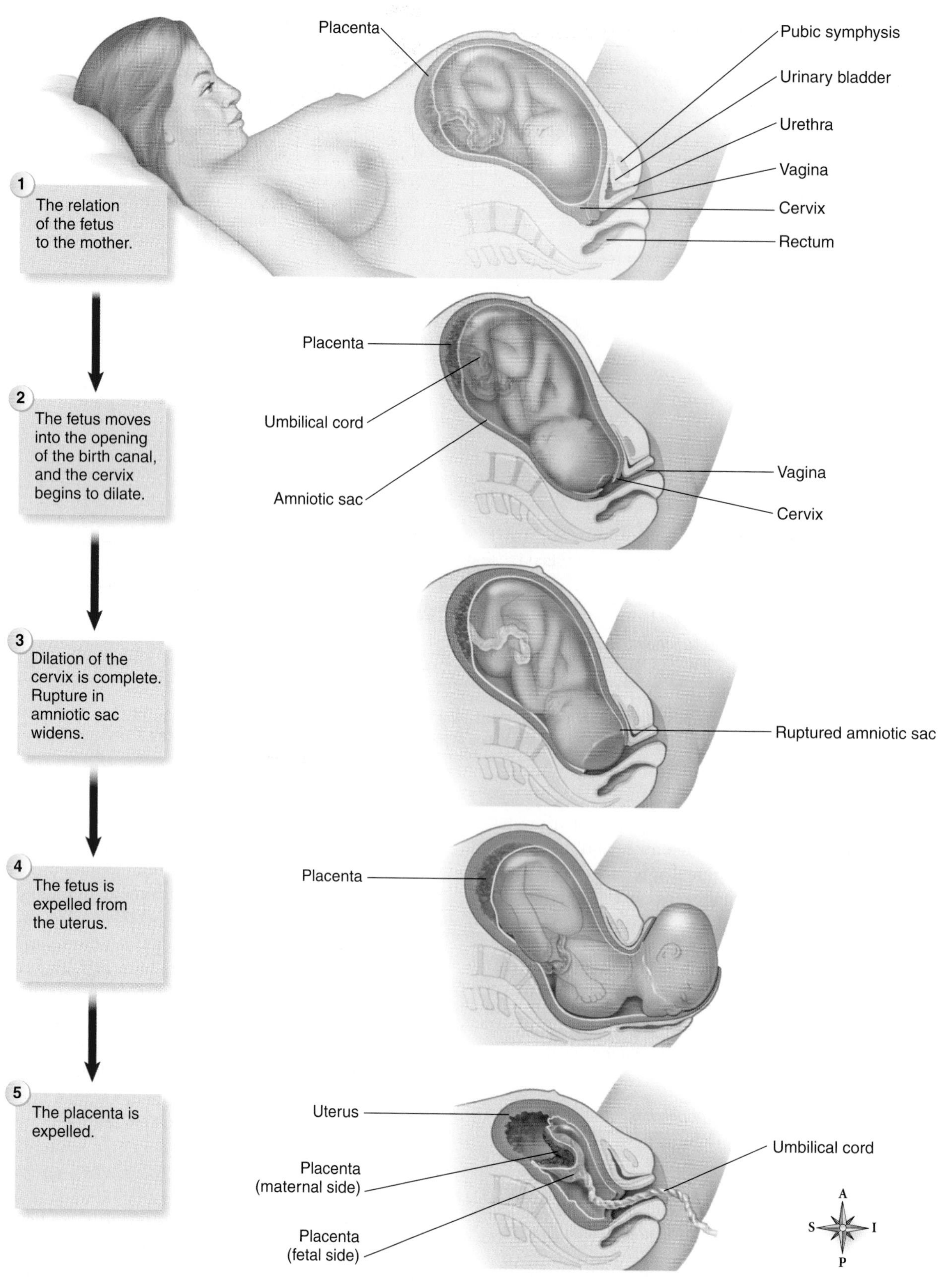

FIGURE 22-8 Parturition.

The time required for normal vaginal birth varies widely and may be influenced by many variables, including whether the woman has previously had a child. In most cases, stage 1 of labor lasts from 6 to 24 hours, and stage 2 lasts from a few minutes to an hour. Delivery of the placenta (stage 3) normally occurs within 15 minutes after the birth of the baby.

Figure 1-12 on p. 15 illustrates the role of oxytocin (OT) in promoting rapid delivery. A synthetic version of OT is sometimes given therapeutically if labor becomes dangerously slow.

To assess the general condition of a newborn, a system that scores five health criteria is often used. The criteria are heart rate (HR), respiration, muscle tone, skin color, and response to stimuli. Each aspect is scored as 0, 1, or 2—depending on the condition of the infant. The resulting total score is called the **Apgar score.** The Apgar score in a completely healthy newborn is 10.

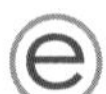

To learn more about the three stages of birth, go to AnimationDirect at *evolve.elsevier.com*.

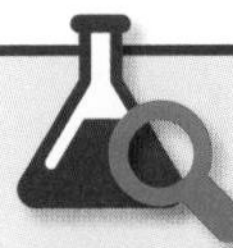

RESEARCH, ISSUES, AND TRENDS

FREEZING UMBILICAL CORD BLOOD

The concept of development of blood cells from red bone marrow, a process called **hematopoiesis,** was introduced in Chapter 12. Ultimately, the presence of "stem cells" is required for bone marrow to produce blood cells. The fact that umbilical cord blood is rich in these stem cells has great clinical significance.

In the past, if the stem cells in the bone marrow of a child were destroyed as a result of leukemia or by chemotherapy, death would result unless a bone marrow transplant was possible. Infusion of stored umbilical cord blood obtained from the child at the time of birth is an attractive alternative. The blood is rich in stem cells and can be obtained without risk; this procedure is much more cost-effective than a bone marrow transplant.

Removing and freezing umbilical cord blood at the time of birth may become a type of biological insurance against some types of leukemia that may affect a child later in life. Cord blood is readily available at birth and is a better source of stem cells than is bone marrow.

When the umbilical cord is cut after birth, the blood that remains in the cord is simply drained into a sterile bag (see photo), frozen, and then stored in liquid nitrogen in one of about a dozen cord-blood centers in the United States.

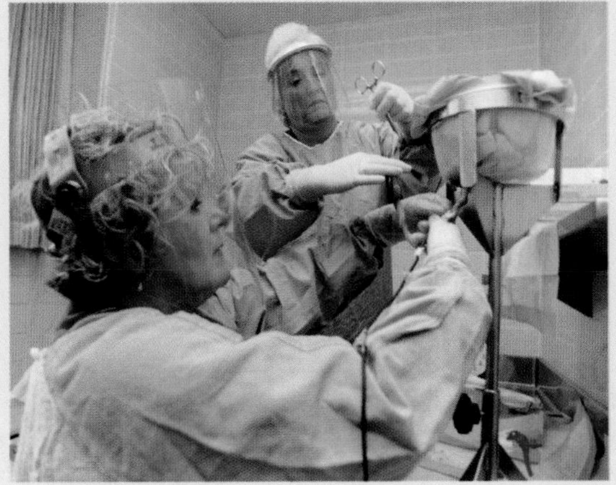

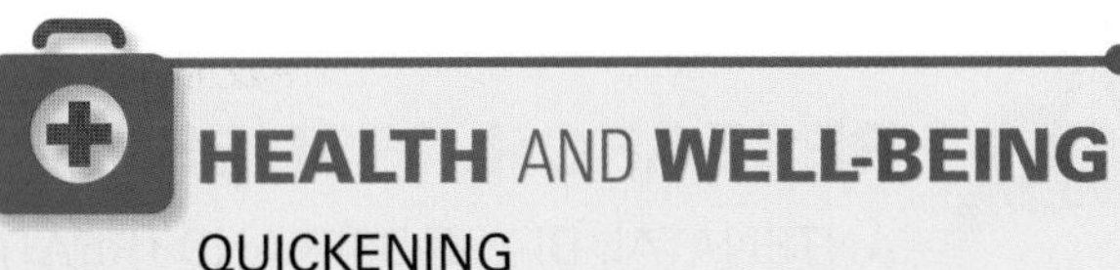

HEALTH AND WELL-BEING

QUICKENING

Pregnant women usually notice fetal movement for the first time between weeks 16 and 18 of pregnancy. The term **quickening** has been used for generations to describe these first recognizable movements of the fetus. From an occasional "kick" during months 4 and 5 of pregnancy, the frequency of fetal movements steadily increases as gestation progresses. The frequency of fetal movements is an excellent indicator of the unborn baby's health.

Recent studies have shown that simply by recording the number of fetal movements each day after week 28 of pregnancy, a woman can provide her physician with extremely useful information about the health of her unborn child. Ten or more movements during a daily measurement period are considered normal.

Educating pregnant women about fetal movements and how to monitor their frequency is but one example of expanded interest in prenatal home care. Assisting pregnant women with making informed judgments about nutrition, exercise, lifestyle adjustments, and birthing options before they enter the hospital for delivery of their babies is an important and growing part of home health care services.

QUICK CHECK

1. What is meant by the term *parturition?*
2. What are the three stages of labor?
3. What is an Apgar score?

Postnatal Period

Growth, Development, and Aging

The **postnatal period** begins at birth and lasts until death. Although it is often divided into major periods for study, we need to understand and appreciate that growth, development, and aging are continuous processes that occur throughout the life cycle.

Gradual changes in the physical appearance of the body as a whole and in the relative proportions of the head, trunk, and limbs are quite noticeable between birth and adolescence. Note in **Figure 22-9** the obvious changes in the size of bones and in the proportionate sizes between different bones and body areas. The head, for example, becomes proportionately smaller. Whereas the infant head is approximately one fourth of the total height of the body, the adult head is only about one eighth of the total height. The facial bones also show several changes between infancy and adulthood. In an infant the face is one eighth of the skull surface, but in an adult the face is half of the skull surface.

Another change in proportion involves the trunk and lower extremities. The legs become proportionately longer and the trunk proportionately shorter. In addition, the thoracic and abdominal contours change, roughly speaking, from round to elliptical.

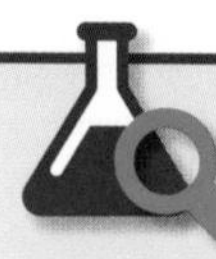

RESEARCH, ISSUES, AND TRENDS

ANTENATAL DIAGNOSIS AND TREATMENT

Advances in **antenatal** (from the Latin *ante,* "before," *natus,* "birth") **medicine** now permit extensive diagnosis and treatment of disease in the fetus much like that in any other patient. This new dimension in medicine began with techniques by which Rh-positive babies could be given transfusions before birth.

Current procedures using images provided by ultrasound equipment (Figures *A* and *B*) allow physicians to prepare for and perform, before the birth of a baby, corrective surgical procedures such as bladder repair. These procedures also allow physicians to monitor the progress of other types of treatment on a developing fetus. Figure *A* shows placement of the ultrasound transducer on the abdominal wall. The resulting image (see Figure *B*), called an **ultrasonogram,** shows a 22-week embryo.

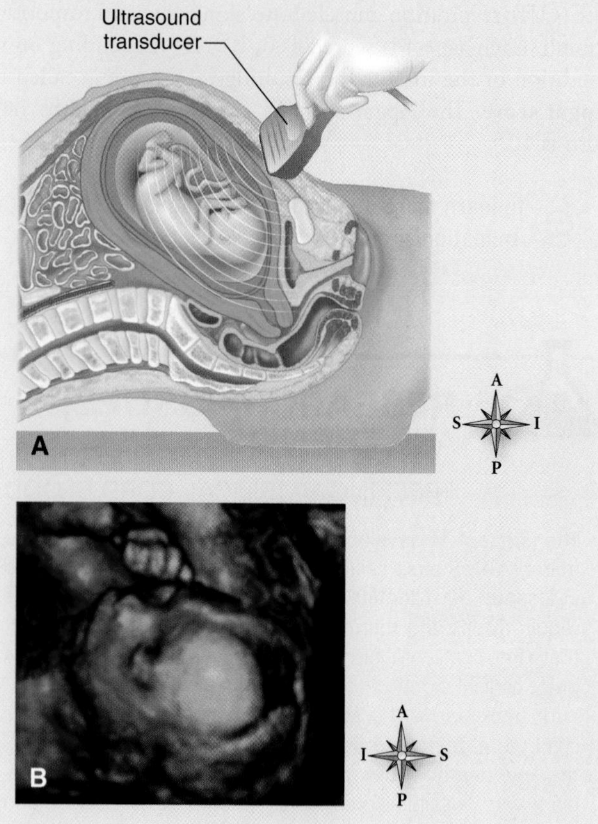

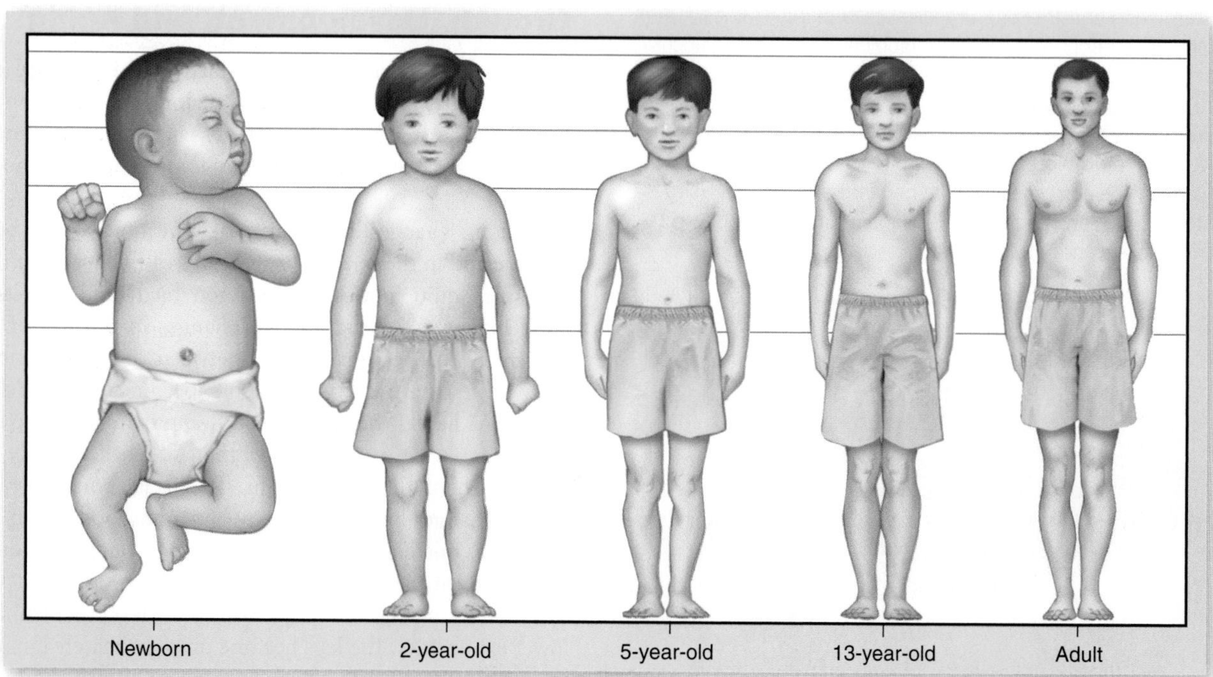

FIGURE 22-9 Changes in the proportions of body parts from birth to maturity. Note the dramatic differences in head proportion.

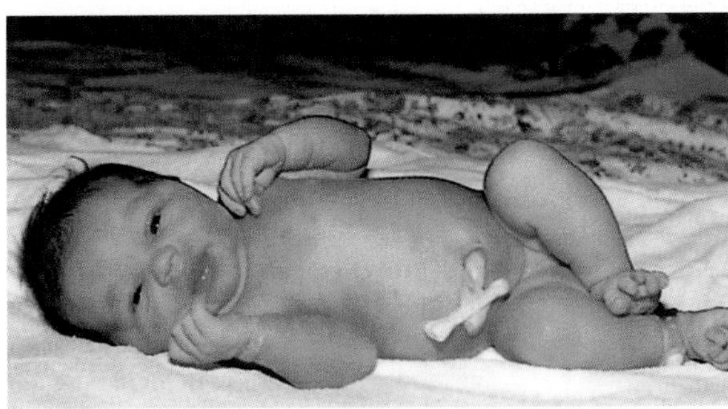

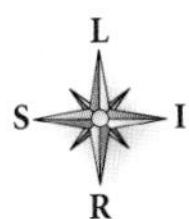

FIGURE 22-10 The neonate infant. The umbilical cord has been cut.

Such changes are good examples of the ever-changing and ongoing nature of growth, development, and aging. It is unfortunate that many of the changes that occur in the later years of life do not result in increased function. These degenerative changes are certainly important, however, and are discussed later in this chapter. The following are the most common postnatal periods: (1) *infancy,* (2) *childhood,* (3) *adolescence,* (4) *adulthood,* and (5) *older adulthood.*

Infancy

The period of **infancy** begins abruptly at birth and lasts about 18 months. The first 4 weeks of infancy are often referred to as the **neonatal period** (Figure 22-10). The baby is referred to as a **neonate.** Dramatic changes occur at a rapid rate during this short but critical period. **Neonatology** is the medical and nursing specialty concerned with the diagnosis and treatment of disorders of the newborn. Advances in this area have resulted in dramatically reduced infant mortality.

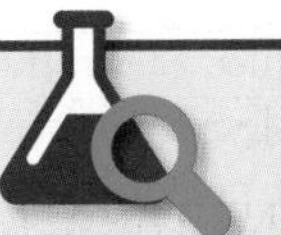

RESEARCH, ISSUES, AND TRENDS

FETAL ALCOHOL SYNDROME

Consumption of alcohol by a woman during her pregnancy can have tragic effects on a developing fetus. Educational efforts to inform pregnant women about the dangers of alcohol use continue to receive national attention. Even very limited consumption of alcohol during pregnancy poses significant hazards to the developing baby because alcohol can easily cross the placental barrier and enter the fetal bloodstream.

When alcohol enters the fetal blood, the potential result, called **fetal alcohol syndrome (FAS)**, can cause tragic congenital abnormalities such as "small head," or **microcephaly,** low birth weight, developmental disabilities such as mental retardation, and even fetal death.

Many of the changes that occur in the cardiovascular and respiratory systems at birth are necessary for survival. Whereas the fetus totally depends on the mother for life support, the newborn infant must become totally self-supporting in terms of blood circulation and respiration immediately after birth. A baby's first breath is deep and forceful. The stimulus to breathe results primarily from the increasing amounts of carbon dioxide (CO_2) that accumulate in the blood after the umbilical cord is cut following delivery.

Many developmental changes occur between the end of the neonatal period and 18 months of age. Birth weight doubles during the first 4 months and then triples by 1 year. The baby also increases in length by 50% by the 12th month. The "baby fat" that accumulated under the skin during the first year begins to decrease, and the plump infant becomes leaner.

Early in infancy the baby has only one spinal curvature (Figure 22-11, *A*). The lumbar curvature appears between 12 and 18 months, and the once-helpless infant becomes a toddler who can stand (see Figure 22-11, *B*). One of the most striking changes to occur during infancy is the rapid development of the nervous and muscular systems. This permits the infant to follow a moving object with the eyes (2 months); lift the head and raise the chest (3 months); sit when well supported (4 months); crawl (10 months); stand alone (12 months); and run, although a bit stiffly (18 months).

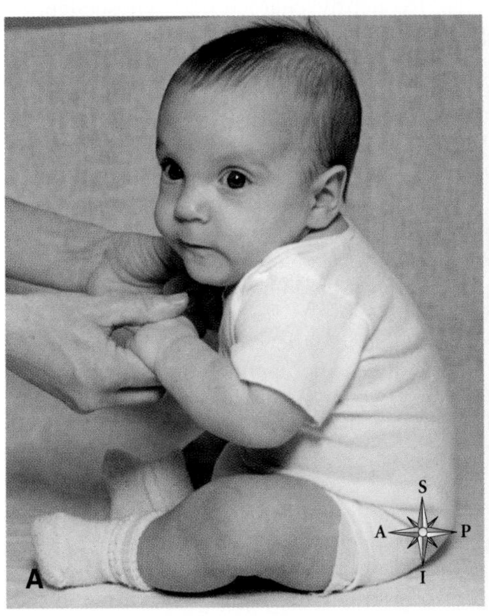

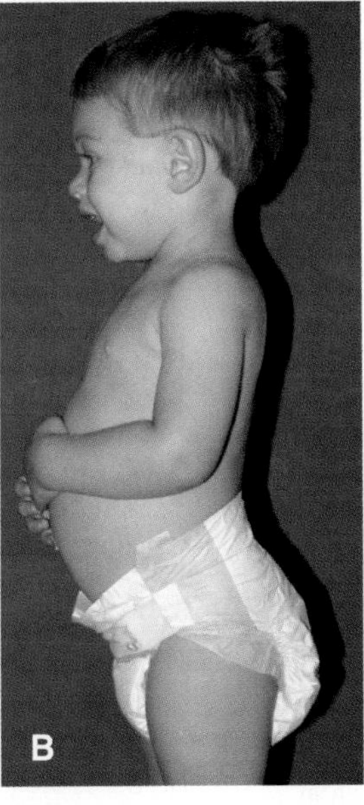

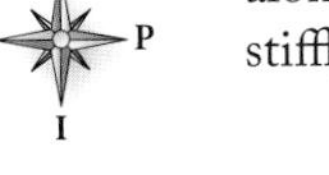

FIGURE 22-11 Spinal curvatures. A, Normal rounded curvature of the vertebral column in an infant. **B,** Normal vertebral curvature in a toddler. The dark shadow emphasizes the distinct lumbar curvature that develops with the ability to walk. (See Figure 7-13 on p. 134 to compare to the adult curvatures.)

Childhood

Childhood extends from the end of infancy to sexual maturity or puberty—12 to 14 years in girls and 14 to 16 years in boys.

Overall, growth during early childhood continues at a rather rapid pace, but month-to-month gains become less consistent. By the age of 6, the child appears more like a preadolescent than an infant or toddler. The child becomes less chubby, the potbelly becomes flatter, and the face loses its babyish look.

The nervous and muscular systems continue to develop rapidly during the middle years of childhood; by 10 years of age, the child has developed numerous motor and coordination skills.

The *deciduous teeth,* which began to appear at about 6 months of age, are lost during childhood, beginning at about 6 years of age. The permanent teeth, with the possible exception of the third molars (or wisdom teeth), all erupt by age 14.

Adolescence

The average age range of **adolescence** varies, but generally the teenage years (13 to 19) are called the adolescent years. This period is marked by rapid and intense physical growth, which ultimately results in sexual maturity.

Many of the developmental changes that occur during this period are controlled by the secretion of sex hormones and are classified as **secondary sex characteristics.** Breast development is often the first sign of approaching puberty in girls, beginning about age 10. Most girls begin to menstruate at 12 to 13 years of age, which is about 3 years earlier than a century ago. In boys the first sign of puberty is often enlargement of the testicles, which begins between 10 and 13 years of age. Both sexes show a spurt in height during adolescence (**Figure 22-12**). In girls the spurt in height begins between the ages of 10 and 12 and is nearly complete by 14 or 15 years. In boys the period of rapid growth begins between 12 and 13 and is generally complete by 16.

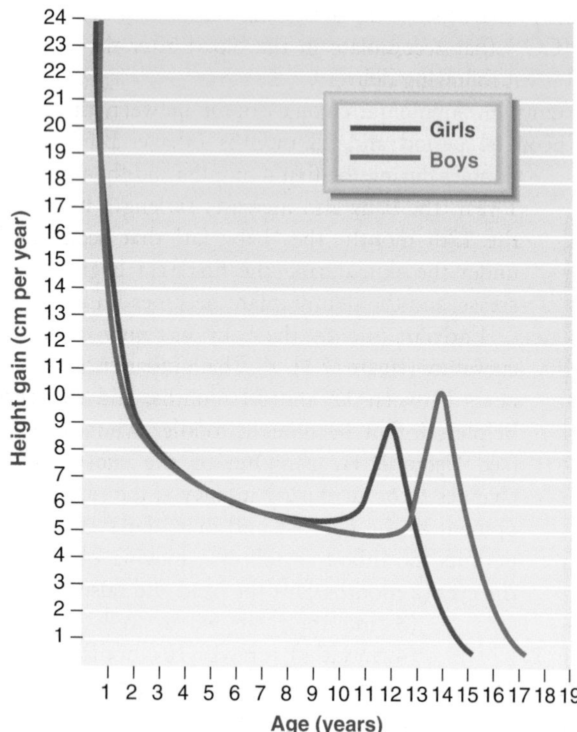

FIGURE 22-12 Growth in height. The figure shows typical patterns of gain in height until adulthood for girls and boys. Notice the rapid gain in height during the first few years, a period of slower growth, then another burst of growth during adolescence—finally ending at the beginning of adulthood.

Adulthood

Many developmental changes that began early in childhood are not completed until the early or middle years of **adulthood.** Examples include the maturation of bone, resulting in the full closure of the growth plates, as well as changes in the size and placement of other body components such as the sinuses. Many body traits do not become apparent for years after birth. Normal balding patterns, for example, are determined at the time of fertilization by heredity but do not appear until maturity.

As a general rule, adulthood is characterized by maintenance of existing body tissues. With the passage of years the ongoing effort to maintain and repair body tissues becomes more and more difficult. As a result, degeneration begins. It is the process of aging, and it culminates in death.

Older Adulthood

Most body systems are in peak condition and function at a high level of efficiency during the early years of adulthood. As a person grows older, a gradual but certain decline takes place in the functioning of every major organ system in the body. The study of aging is called **gerontology.** The remainder of this chapter deals with a number of the more common degenerative changes that frequently characterize **senescence,** or **older adulthood.**

Many of the biological changes associated with advancing age are shown in **Figure 22-13.** The illustration highlights the proportion of remaining function in a number of organs in an older adult as compared with a 20-year-old person.

QUICK CHECK

1. How do the proportions of the human body change during postnatal development?
2. What is the neonatal period of development? Senescence?
3. During which phase of development do the deciduous teeth appear?
4. What biological changes happen during puberty?

Effects of Aging

Aging is an imperfectly understood process. Although advanced age brings with it the higher risk of many disorders, it also brings some biological advantages. We explore just a few of the changes associated with aging here.

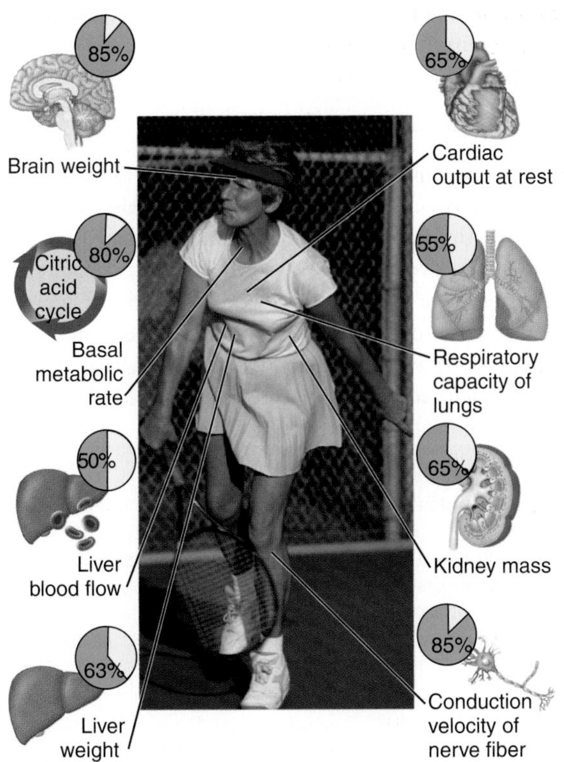

FIGURE 22-13 Some biological changes associated with maturity and aging. *Insets* show proportion of remaining function in the organs of a person in late adulthood compared with that of a 20-year-old. These are average numbers, so many individuals experience far different situations.

Integumentary System (Skin)

With advancing age the skin becomes dry, thin, and inelastic. It "sags" on the body because of increased wrinkling and skinfolds. Pigmentation changes and the thinning or loss of hair are also common problems associated with the aging process.

Skeletal System

In older adulthood, bones undergo changes in texture, degree of calcification, and shape. Instead of clean-cut margins, older bones develop indistinct and shaggy-appearing margins with spurs—a process called *lipping*. This type of degenerative change restricts movement because of the piling up of bone tissue around the joints.

With advancing age, changes in calcification may result in reduction of bone size and in bones that are porous and subject to fracture. The lower cervical and thoracic vertebrae are the sites of frequent fractures. The result is curvature of the spine and the shortened stature so typical of late adulthood. Degenerative joint diseases such as **osteoarthritis** are also common in elderly adults.

However, many of the aging effects seen in the skeleton can be lessened by physical activity—especially if exercise starts earlier in life. Loss of bone mass and reduced mobility can be avoided or reduced by an ongoing program of physical activity coupled with good nutrition.

Central Nervous System

Advancing age brings with it the risk of **dementia**—the loss of memory and other functions of conscious thinking—and other degenerative conditions that affect the central nervous system. For most of us, however, our memories remain mostly intact and have helped us develop a mature ability to reason and make decisions. Although some elderly individuals suffer from depression, especially when they become ill or separated from family, the average elderly person is happier than during early and middle adulthood.

Special Senses

The sense organs, as a group, all show a gradual decline in performance and capacity as a person ages. Most people are farsighted by age 65 because eye lenses become hardened and lose elasticity; the lenses cannot be curved to accommodate for near vision. This hardening of the lens is called **presbyopia,** which means "old eye." Many individuals first notice the change at about 40 or 45 years of age, when it becomes difficult to do close-up work or read without holding printed material at arm's length. This explains the increased need, with advancing age, for bifocals (glasses that incorporate two lenses) to assist the eye in accommodating for near and distant vision.

Loss of transparency of the lens or its covering capsule is another common age-related eye change. If the lens actually becomes cloudy and significantly impairs vision, it is called a **cataract** and must be removed surgically.

The incidence of **glaucoma,** the most serious age-related eye disorder, increases with age. Glaucoma causes an increase in the pressure within the eyeball and, unless treated, often results in blindness. The risk of retinal degeneration or detachment also increases with age.

In many elderly people, a very significant loss of hair cells in the organ of Corti (inner ear) causes a serious decline in the ability to hear certain frequencies. In addition, the eardrum and attached ossicles become more fixed and less able to transmit mechanical sound waves. Some degree of hearing impairment is universally present in the older adult.

The senses of smell and taste are also decreased. The resulting loss of appetite may be caused partly by the replacement of taste buds with connective tissue cells. Only about 40% of the taste buds present at age 30 remain in an individual at age 75.

Cardiovascular System

Degenerative heart and blood vessel disease are among the most common and serious effects of aging. Fatty deposits build up in blood vessel walls and narrow the passageway for the movement of blood, much as the build-up of scale in a water pipe decreases flow and pressure. The resulting condition, called **atherosclerosis,** often leads to eventual blockage of the coronary arteries and a "heart attack" (myocardial infarction [MI]).

If fatty accumulations or other substances in blood vessels calcify, actual hardening of the arteries, or **arteriosclerosis,** occurs. Rupture of a hardened vessel in the brain (stroke or cerebrovascular accident [CVA]) is a frequent cause of serious disability or death in the older adult.

Hypertension (**HTN**), or high blood pressure, is also more common.

Respiratory System

In older adulthood the costal cartilages that connect the ribs to the sternum become hardened or calcified. This makes it difficult for the rib cage to expand and contract as it normally does during inspiration and expiration. In time the ribs gradually become "fixed" to the sternum, and chest movements become difficult. When this occurs, the rib cage remains in a more expanded position, respiratory efficiency decreases, and a condition called "barrel chest" results.

With advancing years a generalized atrophy or wasting of muscle tissue takes place as the contractile muscle cells are replaced by connective tissue. This loss of muscle cells decreases the strength of the muscles associated with inspiration and expiration.

Urinary System

The number of nephron units in the kidney decreases by almost 50% between the ages of 30 and 75. Also, because less blood flows through the kidneys as an individual ages, there is a reduction in overall function and excretory capacity or the ability to produce urine. In the bladder, significant age-related problems often occur because of diminished muscle tone. Muscle atrophy (wasting) in the bladder wall results in decreased capacity and inability to empty or void completely.

QUICK CHECK

1. What changes occur in the skeleton as one ages? Are they avoidable?
2. What changes occur in eyesight during older adulthood?
3. What changes occur in the cardiovascular system during older adulthood?
4. How is kidney function affected during older adulthood?

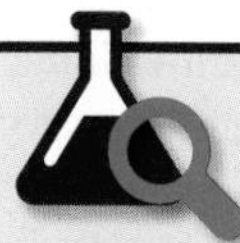

RESEARCH, ISSUES, AND TRENDS

EXTENDING THE HUMAN LIFE SPAN

When reviewing a previous edition of this textbook, a colleague of ours said that ending with the depressing topic of "degeneration associated with aging" was not appropriate to the overall upbeat tone of our book. At first we thought our ending was better than the most obvious and technically accurate ending: "then you die." But it occurred to us that we could take this opportunity to point out one of the most remarkable and important areas of achievement in modern medical research—extending the length, and improving the quality, of life.

In the past few decades, the increased availability of better food, safer surroundings, and advanced medical care has extended quality living for many around the world. But even simple changes in lifestyle, regardless of modern medical wonders, can keep the effects of aging from creeping up too soon. Perhaps the three most important "low-tech" methods for improving the quality of life as you age are healthy diet, exercise, and stress management.

A well-balanced diet is not available to some individuals, but it is available to many of us. We are learning more every day about what kind of diet is best, even to the point of being able to manage specific diseases through diet. Exercise performed on a regular basis, even if light or moderate, can not only keep our skeletal and muscular systems more fit but also decrease aging's effects on the nervous system, endocrine system, digestive system, and immune system—the list seems endless. And lastly, even ancient and simple techniques of stress management such as meditation, tai chi, and yoga have been shown to help reduce the effects of aging and the diseases that often accompany aging, such as heart disease and stroke.

So to end this chapter, and this book, we say: you can stay young much longer if you *eat right, exercise,* and *relax.* And keep studying human structure and function so you'll know that you are doing it right!

LANGUAGE OF **SCIENCE** AND **MEDICINE** *(continued from p. 485)*

chorion
(KOH-ree-on)
[*chorion* **skin**]

chorionic villi
(koh-ree-ON-ik VIL-aye)
[*chorion-* **skin,** *-ic* **relating to**]

dementia
(deh-MEN-shah)
[*de-* **off,** *-mens-* **mind,** *-ia* **condition of**]

ectoderm
(EK-toh-derm)
[*ecto-* **outside,** *-derm* **skin**]

embryo
(EM-bree-oh)
[*em-* **in,** *-bryo* **fill to bursting**]

embryology
(em-bree-OL-uh-gee)
[*em-* **in,** *-bryo-* **fill to bursting,** *-log-* **words (study of),** *-y* **activity**]

embryonic phase
(em-bree-ON-ik fayz)
[*em-* **in,** *bryo* **fill to bursting,** *-ic* **relating to**]

endoderm
(EN-doh-derm)
[*endo-* **within,** *-derm* **skin**]

fertilization
(FER-tih-lih-ZAY-shun)
[*fertil-* **fruitful,** *-ization* **process**]

fetal alcohol syndrome (FAS)
(FEE-tal AL-koh-hol SIN-drohm)
[*fet-* **offspring,** *-al* **relating to,** *syn-* **together,** *-drome* **running or (race) course**]

fetal phase
(FEE-tal fayz)
[*fet-* **offspring,** *-al* **relating to**]

fetus
(FEE-tus)
[*fetus* **offspring**]

geriatrics
(jayr-ee-A-triks)
[*ger-* **old,** *-iatr-* **treatment,** *-ic* **relating to**]

gerontology
(jayr-on-TOL-uh-jee)
[*ger-* **old,** *-onto-* **age,** *-log-* **words (study of),** *-y* **activity**]

gestation period
(jes-TAY-shun PEER-ee-id)
[*gesta-* **bear,** *-tion* **process**]

glaucoma
(glaw-KOH-mah)
[*glauco-* **gray or silver,** *-oma* **tumor (growth)**]

hematopoiesis
(hee-mat-oh-poy-EE-sis)
[*hemo-* **blood,** *-poiesis* **making**]

histogenesis
(hiss-toh-JEN-eh-sis)
[*histo-* **tissue,** *-gen-* **produce,** *-esis* **process**]

hypertension (HTN)
(hye-per-TEN-shun)
[*hyper-* **excessive,** *-tens-* **stretch or pull tight,** *-sion* **state**]

implantation
(im-plan-TAY-shun)
[*im-* **in,** *-plant-* **set or place,** *-ation* **process**]

infancy
(IN-fan-see)
[*in-* **not,** *-fanc-* **speak,** *-y* **state**]

laparoscope
(LAP-ah-roh-skohp)
[*laparo-* **abdomen,** *-scop-* **see**]

mesoderm
(MEZ-oh-derm)
[*meso-* **middle,** *-derm* **skin**]

microcephaly
(my-kroh-SEF-ah-lee)
[*micro-* **small,** *-ceph-* **head,** *-al* **relating to,** *-y* **state**]

morula
(MOR-yoo-lah)
[*mor-* **mulberry,** *-ula* **little**]

neonatal period
(nee-oh-NAY-tal PEER-ee-id)
[*neo-* **new,** *-nat-* **birth,** *-al* **relating to**]

neonate
(NEE-oh-nayt)
[*neo-* **new,** *-nat-* **born**]

neonatology
(nee-oh-nay-TOL-oh-jee)
[*neo-* **new,** *-nat-* **born,** *-log-* **words (study of),** *-y* **activity**]

obstetric nurse
(ob-STET-rik nurs)
[*ob-* **in front,** *-stet-* **stand,** *-tric(s)* **female agent,** *nurs-* **nourish or nurture**]

obstetrician
(ob-steh-TRISH-an)
[*ob-* **in front,** *-stet-* **stand,** *-tric(s)* **female agent,** *-ian* **practitioner**]

older adulthood
(OLD-er ah-DULT-hood)

organogenesis
(or-gah-no-JEN-eh-sis)
[*organ-* **instrument (organ),** *-gen-* **produce,** *-esis* **process**]

osteoarthritis
(os-tee-oh-ar-THRY-tis)
[*osteo-* **bone,** *-arthr-* **joint,** *-itis* **inflammation**]

parturition
(pahr-too-RIH-shun)
[*parturi-* **give birth,** *-tion* **process**]

placenta
(plah-SEN-tah)
[*placenta* **flat cake**]

postnatal period
(POST-nay-tal PEER-ee-id)
[*post-* **after,** *-nat-* **birth,** *-al* **relating to**]

prenatal period
(PREE-nay-tal PEER-ee-id)
[*pre-* **before,** *-nat-* **birth,** *-al* **relating to**]

presbyopia
(pres-bee-OH-pee-ah)
[*presby-* **aging,** *-op-* **vision,** *-ia* **condition**]

primary germ layer
(PRYE-mayr-ee jerm LAY-er)
[*prim-* **first,** *-ary* **state,** *germ* **sprout**]

quickening
(KWIK-en-ing)

secondary sex characteristic
(SEK-on-dayr-ee seks kayr-ak-ter-ISS-tik)
[*second-* **second,** *-ary* **relating to**]

senescence
(seh-NES-enz)
[*senesc-* **grow old,** *-ence* **state**]

stem cell
(stem sel)
[*stem* **stem of plant,** *cell* **storeroom**]

teratogen
(TER-ah-toh-jen)
[*terato-* **monster,** *-gen* **produce**]

trimester
(TRY-mes-ter)
[*tri-* **three,** *-me(n)s-* **month,** *-ster* **thing**]

ultrasonogram
(ul-trah-SON-uh-gram)
[*ultra-* **beyond,** *-sono-* **sound,** *-gram* **drawing**]

yolk sac
(yohk sak)
[*yolk* **yellow part**]

zygote
(ZYE-goht)
[*zygot-* **union or yoke**]

❑ OUTLINE SUMMARY

To download a digital audio version of the chapter summary for use with your device, access the ***Audio Chapter Summaries*** *online at evolve.elsevier.com.*

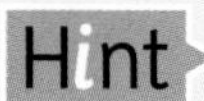

Scan this summary after reading the chapter to help you reinforce the key concepts. Later, use the summary as a quick review before your class or before a test.

Prenatal Period

A. Prenatal period begins at conception and continues until birth (about 39 weeks) (see **Figure 22-1**)
B. Science of fetal growth and development called *embryology*
C. Fertilization to implantation requires about 10 days
   1. Fertilization normally occurs in outer third of oviduct (see **Figure 22-2**)
   2. Fertilized ovum called a *zygote;* zygote is genetically complete — all that is needed for expression of hereditary traits is time and nourishment
   3. After 3 days of cell division, the zygote has developed into a solid cell mass called a *morula* (see **Figure 22-3**)
   4. Continued cell divisions of the morula produce a hollow ball of cells called a *blastocyst*
   5. Blastocyst implants in the uterine wall about 10 days after fertilization
   6. Blastocyst forms the amniotic cavity and chorion of the placenta (see **Figure 22-4**)
   7. Placenta provides for exchange of nutrients between the mother and fetus (see **Figure 22-5**)
D. Periods of development
   1. Length of pregnancy, or gestation period, is about 39 weeks
   2. Embryonic phase extends from the third week after fertilization to the end of week 8 of gestation
   3. Fetal phase extends from week 8 to week 39 of gestation
   4. All organ systems are formed and functioning by month 4 of gestation (see **Figure 22-6**)
E. Stem cells — unspecialized cells that reproduce to form specific lines of specialized cells
F. Three primary germ layers appear in the developing embryo after implantation of the blastocyst (see **Table 22-1**):
   1. Endoderm — inside layer
   2. Ectoderm — outside layer
   3. Mesoderm — middle layer
G. Histogenesis and organogenesis
   1. Formation of new organs (organogenesis) and tissues (histogenesis) occurs from specific development of the primary germ layers
   2. Each primary germ layer gives rise to definite structures such as the skin and muscles
   3. Growth processes include cell differentiation, multiplication, growth, and rearrangement
   4. From 4 months of gestation until delivery, the development of the baby is mainly a matter of growth
H. Birth defects
   1. Any structural or functional abnormality present at birth
   2. May be caused by genetic factors
      a. Abnormal genes
      b. Abnormal number of chromosomes
   3. May be caused by environmental factors
      a. Environmental factors are called *teratogens*
      b. Include radiation, chemicals, and infections
      c. Especially harmful during the first trimester (see **Figure 22-7**)

Birth or Parturition

A. Process of birth called *parturition* (see **Figure 22-8**)
   1. At the end of week 39 of gestation, the uterus becomes "irritable"
   2. Fetus takes head-down position against the cervix
   3. Muscular contractions begin, and labor is initiated
   4. Amniotic sac ("bag of waters") ruptures
   5. Cervix dilates
   6. Fetus moves through vagina to exterior
B. Stages of labor
   1. Stage 1 — period from onset of uterine contractions until dilation of the cervix is complete
   2. Stage 2 — period from the time of maximal cervical dilation until the baby exits through the vagina
   3. Stage 3 — process of expulsion of the placenta through the vagina

Postnatal Period

A. Postnatal period begins at birth and lasts until death
B. Divisions of postnatal period into isolated time frames can be misleading; life is a continuous process; growth, development, and aging are continuous
C. Obvious changes in the physical appearance of the body — in whole and in proportion — occur between birth and maturity (see **Figure 22-9**)
D. Divisions of postnatal period
   1. Infancy
   2. Childhood
   3. Adolescence
   4. Adulthood
   5. Older adulthood
E. Infancy
   1. First 4 weeks called *neonatal period* (see **Figure 22-10**)
   2. Neonatology — medical and nursing specialty concerned with the diagnosis and treatment of disorders of the newborn

3. Many cardiovascular changes occur at the time of birth; fetus is totally dependent on mother, whereas the newborn must immediately become totally self-supporting (in respect to respiration and circulation)
4. Respiratory changes at birth include a deep and forceful first breath
5. Developmental changes between the neonatal period and 18 months include:
   a. Doubling of birth weight by 4 months and tripling by 1 year
   b. Fifty-percent increase in body length by 12 months
   c. Development of normal spinal curvature by 15 months (see **Figure 22-11**)
   d. Ability to raise head by 3 months
   e. Ability to crawl by 10 months
   f. Ability to stand alone by 12 months
   g. Ability to run by 18 months

F. Childhood
1. Extends from end of infancy to puberty — 13 years in girls and 15 in boys
2. Overall rate of growth remains rapid but decelerates
3. Continuing development of motor and coordination skills
4. Loss of deciduous (baby) teeth and eruption of permanent teeth

G. Adolescence
1. Average age range of adolescence varies; usually considered to be from 13 to 19 years
2. Period of rapid growth resulting in sexual maturity (adolescence)
3. Appearance of secondary sex characteristics regulated by secretion of sex hormones
4. Growth spurt typical of adolescence; begins in girls at about 10 and in boys at about 12 (see **Figure 22-12**)

H. Adulthood
1. Growth plates fully close in adult; other structures such as the sinuses assume adult placement
2. Adulthood characterized by maintenance of existing body tissues
3. Degeneration of body tissue begins in adulthood

I. Older adulthood (see **Figure 22-13**)
1. Degenerative changes characterize older adulthood (also called *senescence*)
2. Every organ system of the body undergoes degenerative changes
3. Senescence culminates in death

Effects of Aging

A. Integumentary system (skin)
1. With age, skin "sags" and becomes thin, dry, wrinkled
2. Pigmentation problems are common
3. Frequently thinning or loss of hair occurs

B. Skeletal system
1. Aging causes changes in the texture, calcification, and shape of bones
2. Bone spurs develop around joints
3. Bones become porous and fracture easily
4. Degenerative joint diseases such as osteoarthritis are common
5. Physical activity can reduce loss of bone mass and mobility

C. Central nervous system
1. Increased risk of dementia
2. Mature reasoning ability

D. Special senses
1. All sense organs show a gradual decline in performance with age
2. Eye lenses become hard and cannot accommodate for near vision; result is farsightedness in many people by age 45 (presbyopia, or "old eye")
3. Loss of transparency of lens or cornea is common (cataract)
4. Glaucoma (increase in pressure in eyeball) is often the cause of blindness in older adulthood
5. Increased risk of retinal degeneration or detachment
6. Loss of hair cells in inner ear produces frequency deafness in many older people
7. Decreased transmission of sound waves caused by loss of elasticity of eardrum and fixing of the bony ear ossicles is common in older adulthood
8. Some degree of hearing impairment is universally present in the aged
9. Smell and taste may be reduced — only about 40% of the taste buds present at age 30 remain at age 75

E. Cardiovascular system
1. Degenerative heart and blood vessel disease is among the most common and serious effects of aging
2. Fat deposits in blood vessels (atherosclerosis) decrease blood flow to the heart and may cause complete blockage of the coronary arteries
3. Hardening of arteries (arteriosclerosis) may result in rupture of blood vessels, especially in the brain (stroke)
4. Hypertension or high blood pressure is common in older adulthood

F. Respiratory system
1. Calcification of costal cartilages causes rib cage to remain in expanded position — barrel chest
2. Wasting of respiratory muscles decreases respiratory efficiency
3. Respiratory membrane thickens; movement of oxygen from alveoli to blood is slowed

G. Urinary system
1. Nephron units decrease in number by 50% between ages 30 and 75
2. Blood flow to kidney decreases and therefore ability to form urine decreases
3. Bladder problems such as inability to void completely are caused by muscle wasting in the bladder wall

❑ ACTIVE LEARNING

STUDY TIPS

Hint *Use these tips to achieve success in meeting your learning goals.*

To make the study of human growth, development, and aging more efficient, we suggest these tips:

1. Review the concepts of human reproduction from the previous chapter.
2. The term *germ* in primary *germ layer* refers to "germinate." All the structures of the body come from one of these layers. They are named based on their location in the developing embryo. *Endoderm* means inner skin, *mesoderm* means middle skin, and *ectoderm* means outer skin.
3. *Genesis* means to create. *Histogenesis* means to create tissues, and *organogenesis* means to create organs.
4. The early developmental stages can be put on flash cards. You might also want to include on the flash card where, in the developmental sequence, the particular stage is—in other words, from what it developed. Remember to include the functions of the amnion, chorion, and placenta. In your study group, go over the flash cards concerning the stages of development, making sure you know the proper sequence.
5. Use flash cards to match the primary germ layers and the structures that come from each of them.
6. The stages of labor, the important events in the postnatal periods, and the effects of aging on various organ systems can also be put on flash cards. Review them in your study group.
7. Study the questions at the end of the chapter and discuss possible test questions.

Review Questions

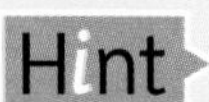

Write out the answers to these questions after reading the chapter and reviewing the Chapter Summary. If you simply think through the answer without writing it down, you won't retain much of your new learning.

1. Explain the concept of development as a biological process characterized by continuous modification and change.
2. Explain what occurs between ovulation and the implantation of the fertilized egg into the uterus.
3. Explain the function of the chorion and placenta.
4. Name the three primary germ layers, and name three structures that develop from each layer.
5. Define *histogenesis* and *organogenesis*.
6. Describe and give the approximate length of the three stages of labor.
7. What is the stimulus for the baby's first breath?
8. Name three developmental changes that occur during infancy.
9. Briefly explain what developmental changes occur during childhood.
10. Briefly explain what developmental changes occur during adolescence.
11. Briefly explain what developmental changes occur during adulthood.
12. Explain the effects of aging on the skeletal system.
13. Explain the effects of aging on the respiratory system.
14. Explain the effects of aging on the cardiovascular system.
15. Explain the effects of aging on vision.

Critical Thinking

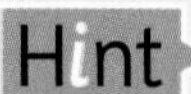

After finishing the Review Questions, write out the answers to these more in-depth questions to help you apply your new knowledge. Go back to sections of the chapter that relate to concepts that you find difficult.

16. Where do the nutrients used by the zygote from fertilization to implantation come from?
17. Explain the evolution of the function of the yolk sac.
18. What hormones are produced by the placenta? What is their function?
19. Baby Adams's mother was unable to make it to the hospital and he was born at home under emergency conditions. The EMS personnel were there within minutes and while in transport to the hospital, his mother heard them say "(Appearance) Color is pink but hands and feet are blue; (Pulse) Pulse is normal; (Grimace) Reflex irritability is good; (Activity) Activity is good; (Respirations) Respirations are normal. Remembering that a perfect score is 10 on an Apgar, what Apgar score do you think the EMS personnel will assign to Baby Adams?

Chapter Test

Hint *After studying the chapter, test your mastery by responding to these items. Try to answer them without looking up the answers. Then, verify the answers using the key in Appendix C at the back of this book.*

1. The fertilized ovum is called a ________.
2. After about 3 days of mitosis, the fertilized ovum forms a solid mass of cells called the ________.
3. Mitosis continues, and by the time the developing egg reaches the uterus, it has become a hollow ball of cells called the ________.
4. The ________ anchors the developing fetus to the uterus and provides a bridge for exchanging of substances between mother and baby.
5. The ________ period lasts about 39 weeks and is divided into trimesters.
6. The three primary germ layers are the ________.
7. The process by which the primary germ layers develop into tissues is called ________.
8. The process by which tissues develop into organs is called ________.
9. The process of birth is called ________.
10. The first 4 weeks of infancy is referred to as the ________ period.
11. ________ is a degenerative joint disease that is common in older adults.
12. ________ is another name for "hardening of the arteries."
13. ________ means "old eye" and causes older adults to be farsighted.
14. If the lens of the eye becomes cloudy and impairs vision, the condition is called a ________.
15. ________ causes an increase in pressure within the eyeball.

Match each phrase in Column B with the correct corresponding term in Column A.

Column A	Column B
16. ________ infancy	a. period in which the deciduous teeth are lost
17. ________ childhood	b. period in which closure of the bone growth plates occurs
18. ________ adolescence	c. period that begins at birth
19. ________ adulthood	d. senescence
20. ________ older adulthood	e. period during which the secondary sex characteristics usually begin to develop

APPENDIX A
Body Mass Index

Are you a healthy weight? One way that researchers and health professionals use to determine whether you are overweight is called the *body mass index (BMI)*. Here is how to calculate your BMI:

1. Multiply your height (m*) by itself (that is, square it).
2. Divide your weight (kg*) by your answer in step 1.

An even easier way is to use the diagram shown here. Simply find your weight along the bottom of the graph and go straight up from that point to the horizontal line that is closest to your height. That point is at your BMI. If it is in the 18.5 to 25 range, you are a healthy weight, according to current research. If it is in the 25 to 30 range, you are considered to be "overweight" and at a greater than normal risk for health problems such as heart disease, diabetes, and certain types of cancer. In the range higher than 30, you are considered to be "obese" and at a very high risk for health problems.

The use of BMI is not universal and it has its critics among health professionals. Because it does not take into account the proportion of lean tissue (muscle) and fat in a person's body, it's not a complete picture of a person's health risks. However, for many it continues to be useful as a quick and easy "snapshot" that may serve as an important warning sign for overweight people.

*kg is kilograms (to find your weight in kilograms, divide your weight in pounds by 2.2); *m* is meters (to find your height in meters, divide your height in inches by 39.4).

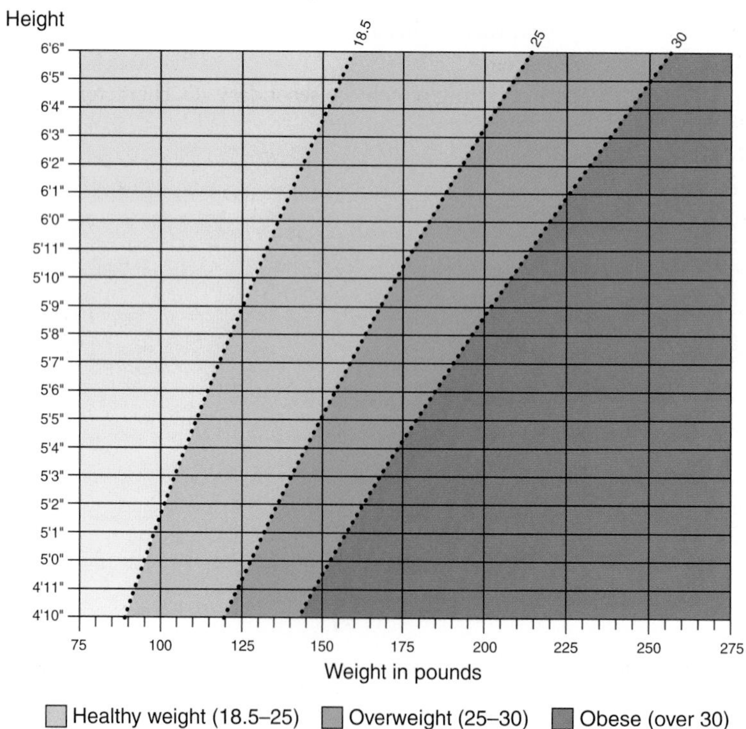

Body mass index chart. (Adapted from the Report of the Dietary Guidelines Advisory Committee on the Dietary Guidelines for Americans, 2000.)

APPENDIX B
Common Medical Abbreviations, Prefixes, and Suffixes

Abbreviations and Acronyms

aa	of each
ā.c̄.	before meals
ad lib.	as much as desired
alb.	albumin
am	before noon
amt.	amount
ante	before
aq.	water
AV.	average
AZT ♦	azidothymidine
Ba	barium
b.i.d.	twice a day
b.m.	bowel movement
BMR	basal metabolic rate
BP	blood pressure
BRP	bathroom privileges
BUN	blood urea nitrogen
c̄	with
CBC	complete blood cell count
cc ♦	cubic centimeter
CCU	coronary care unit
CHF	congestive heart failure
CNS	central nervous system
Co	cobalt
CVA	cerebrovascular accident, stroke
D&C	dilation and curettage
d/c ♦	discontinue
DOA	dead on arrival
Dx	diagnosis
ECG	electrocardiogram
EDC	expected date of confinement
EEG	electroencephalogram
EENT	ear, eye, nose, throat
EKG	electrocardiogram
ER	emergency room
FUO	fever of undetermined origin
GI	gastrointestinal
GP	general practitioner
GU	genitourinary
h.	hour
Hb	hemoglobin
HCT	hematocrit
h.s.	at bedtime
H_2O	water
ICU	intensive care unit
IU ♦♦	International Unit
KUB	kidney, ureter, and bladder
MI	myocardial infarction
non rep.	do not repeat
NPO	nothing by mouth
NSAID	nonsteroidal anti-inflammatory drug
OR	operating room
p.c.	after meals
per	by
PH	past history
PI	previous illness
pm	after noon
p.r.n.	as needed
q.	every
q.d. ♦	every day
q.h.	every hour
q.i.d.	four times a day
q.n.s.	quantity not sufficient
q.o.d. ♦♦	every other day
q.s.	quantity required or sufficient
RBC	red blood cell
Rx	prescription
s̄	without
sp. gr.	specific gravity
SQ ♦	subcutaneous
ss. ♦	one half or sliding scale
SSRI ♦	serotonin-specific reuptake inhibitor
stat.	at once, immediately
T & A	tonsillectomy and adenoidectomy
T.B.	tuberculosis
t.i.d.	three times a day
TPR	temperature, pulse, respiration
TUR	transurethral resection
WBC	white blood cell

ALERT! Items marked with ♦ are subject to health-threatening errors of interpretation and should no longer be used in clinical settings even though they are still often used in nonclinical or research settings. Items with ♦♦ are banned from use in clinical settings by The Joint Commission (TJC), formerly The Joint Commission on Accreditation of Healthcare Organizations (JCAHO).

Prefixes

A prefix is a word part used at the *beginning* of a term and describes or alters the meaning of the word part(s) that follows the prefix. For example, *an-* means "without," so *anuria* means "without urine," or the condition of having no urine output.

a-	without
ab-	away from
ad-	to, toward
adeno-	glandular
amphi-	on both sides
an-	without
ante-	before, forward
anti-	against
bi-	two, double, twice
circum-	around, about
contra-	opposite, against
de-	away from, from
di-	double
dia-	across, through
dis-	separate from, apart
dys-	difficult
e-	out, away
ecto-	outside
en-	in
endo-	in, inside
epi-	on
eu-	well
ex-	from, out of, away from
exo-	outside
extra-	outside, beyond; in addition
hemi-	half
hyper-	over, excessive, above
hypo-	under, deficient
infra-	underneath, below
inter-	between, among
intra-	within, on the side
intro-	into, within
iso-	equal, like
para-	beside
peri-	around, beyond
post-	after, behind
pre-	before, in front of
pro-	before, in front of
re-	again
retro-	backward, back
semi-	half
sub-	under, beneath
super-	above, over
supra-	above, on the upper side
syn-	with, together
trans-	across, beyond
ultra-	excessive

Suffixes

A suffix is a word part used at the *end* of a term and describes or alters the meaning of the word part(s) that comes before the suffix. For example, *-ectomy* means "cut out," so *appendectomy* means "appendix cut out," or the procedure of surgically removing the appendix.

-algia	pain, painful
-asis	condition
-blast	young cell
-cele	swelling
-centesis	puncture for aspiration
-cide	killer
-cyte	cell
-ectomy	cut out
-emia	blood
-genesis	production, development
-itis	inflammation
-kin	in motion, action
-logy	study of
-megaly	enlargement
-odynia	pain
-oid	resembling
-oma	tumor
-osis	condition
-opathy	disease
-penia	abnormal reduction
-pexy	fixation
-phagia	eating, swallowing
-phasia	speaking condition
-phobia	fear
-plasty	plastic surgery
-plegia	paralysis
-poiesis	formation
-ptosis	downward displacement
-rhaphy	suture
-scope	instrument for examination
-scopy	examination
-stomy	creation of an opening
-tomy	incision
-uria	urine

APPENDIX C
Chapter Test Answers

Chapter 1

1. anatomy
2. physiology
3. theory, law
4. chemical, cell, tissue, organ, organ system
5. prone, supine
6. transverse
7. frontal
8. sagittal
9. midsagittal
10. movements
11. axial
12. appendicular
13. c
14. b
15. d
16. d
17. b
18. d
19. e
20. d
21. a
22. c
23. b

Chapter 2

1. matter
2. atoms
3. protons
4. energy
5. compounds
6. covalent
7. ion
8. electrolyte
9. organic
10. solvent
11. dehydration synthesis
12. acids
13. buffers
14. d
15. f
16. g
17. e
18. a
19. c
20. b
21. c
22. a
23. d
24. b
25. c

Chapter 3

1. phospholipid, cholesterol
2. organelle
3. active transport, passive transport
4. pinocytosis
5. DNA, mRNA
6. translation
7. transcription
8. gene
9. genome
10. ion pumps
11. d
12. c
13. a
14. b
15. c
16. d
17. g
18. c
19. e
20. i
21. b
22. a
23. d
24. f
25. h

Chapter 4

1. connective tissue
2. matrix
3. elastin
4. endocrine
5. goblet
6. matrix
7. areolar tissue
8. brown fat
9. hematopoietic tissue
10. collagen
11. haversian systems, osteons
12. d
13. d
14. b
15. c
16. a
17. b
18. d
19. b
20. d
21. e
22. a
23. d
24. c
25. b

Chapter 5

1. digestive tract
2. skeletal muscle
3. lymphoid
4. nerve impulses
5. hair, nails, glands, sense organs
6. thymus
7. urethra
8. testes, ovaries
9. cartilage, ligament
10. f
11. k
12. a
13. i
14. b
15. g
16. c
17. j
18. d
19. e
20. h

Chapter 6

1. cutaneous, serous, mucous
2. basement membrane
3. parietal pleura
4. visceral peritoneum
5. synovial membrane
6. stratum corneum, stratum germinativum
7. keratin
8. dermal papillae
9. eccrine
10. apocrine
11. sebum
12. protection, sensation, temperature regulation
13. b
14. c
15. a

16. d
17. b
18. d
19. a
20. c

Chapter 7

1. articular cartilage
2. medullary cavity
3. trabeculae
4. haversian systems
5. lacunae
6. central canal
7. osteoblasts
8. endochondral ossification
9. epiphyseal plate
10. axial, appendicular
11. synarthroses, amphiarthroses, diarthroses
12. ligaments
13. c
14. b
15. a
16. d
17. c
18. b
19. a
20. b
21. d
22. d
23. c
24. d
25. c
26. b
27. d
28. b
29. a
30. d
31. a
32. b
33. a
34. b
35. a

Chapter 8

1. muscle fiber
2. heart
3. insertion
4. origin
5. actin
6. myosin
7. sarcomere
8. movement, posture, heat production
9. ATP
10. lactic acid
11. motor unit
12. threshold stimulus
13. isotonic
14. isometric
15. abduction
16. extension
17. supination
18. b
19. d
20. a
21. b
22. d
23. d
24. a
25. c or b
26. c
27. d
28. a
29. c
30. d
31. b

Chapter 9

1. peripheral nervous system
2. central nervous system
3. nerve
4. neurons, glia
5. reflex arc
6. nerve impulse
7. positive, negative
8. sodium
9. synapse
10. neurotransmitters
11. dura mater, arachnoid layer, pia mater
12. 12, 31
13. dermatomes
14. parasympathetic nervous system
15. sympathetic nervous system
16. acetylcholine, norepinephrine
17. acetylcholine, acetylcholine
18. cardiac muscle, smooth muscle, glandular epithelial
19. g
20. c
21. e
22. a
23. b
24. f
25. d
26. k
27. h
28. o
29. m
30. i
31. n
32. l
33. j

Chapter 10

1. chemoreceptors, proprioceptors
2. organ of Corti or spiral organ
3. crista ampullaris
4. taste
5. sweet, sour, bitter, salty, umami, metallic
6. papillae
7. olfactory receptors
8. e
9. i
10. j
11. b
12. a
13. g
14. c
15. f
16. h
17. d
18. k
19. f
20. g
21. a
22. b
23. e
24. c
25. d

Chapter 11

1. exocrine
2. endocrine, hormones
3. nonsteroid, steroid
4. target organ
5. cyclic AMP (cAMP)
6. on the cell membrane, in the nucleus
7. prostaglandins
8. posterior pituitary (neurohypophysis)
9. anterior pituitary (adenohypophysis)
10. posterior pituitary gland, hypothalamus
11. d
12. b
13. c
14. b
15. b

16. a
17. d
18. f
19. i
20. a
21. e
22. c
23. h
24. g
25. b

Chapter 12

1. plasma
2. albumin, globulin, fibrinogen
3. serum
4. red blood cells (erythrocytes), white blood cells (leukocytes), platelets (thrombocytes)
5. myeloid, lymphatic
6. hemoglobin
7. anemia
8. polycythemia
9. neutrophils
10. B lymphocytes
11. calcium
12. fibrinogen, fibrin
13. K
14. thrombus
15. embolus
16. antigen
17. A and B, no (none)
18. B, anti-A
19. O, Rh-negative
20. AB, Rh-positive
21. erythroblastosis fetalis
22. hematocrit
23. Sickle cell anemia
24. Acidosis
25. Leukocytosis

Chapter 13

1. ventricles
2. atria
3. myocardium
4. interventricular septum
5. endocardium
6. epicardium
7. systole
8. diastole
9. tricuspid (right atrioventricular)
10. stroke volume
11. sinoatrial node
12. Subendocardial branches (Purkinje fibers)
13. QRS complex
14. P wave
15. veins
16. arteries
17. capillaries
18. tunica intima
19. tunica adventitia
20. pulmonary circulation
21. foramen ovale, ductus arteriosus
22. blood viscosity, heart rate
23. central venous pressure
24. sphygmomanometer
25.
   a. 7
   b. 2
   c. 3
   d. 6
   e. 10
   f. 8
   g. 9
   h. 5
   i. 1
   j. 4

Chapter 14

1. lymph
2. thoracic duct
3. right lymphatic duct
4. cisterna chyli
5. lymph nodes
6. afferent, efferent
7. T lymphocytes (T cells), thymosin
8. palatine, pharyngeal, lingual
9. spleen
10. inflammation
11. complement cascade
12. monocytes
13. c
14. b
15. d
16. a
17. B
18. B
19. T
20. B
21. T
22. T
23. B
24. T
25. B or T

Chapter 15

1. air distributor, gas exchanger
2. nose, pharynx, larynx
3. trachea, bronchial tree, lungs
4. respiratory membrane
5. respiratory mucosa
6. paranasal sinuses
7. lacrimal
8. conchae or turbinates
9. pharynx
10. larynx
11. trachea
12. primary bronchi, secondary bronchi, bronchioles, alveolar ducts
13. Surfactant
14. 3, 2
15. internal respiration
16. external respiration
17. diaphragm
18. oxyhemoglobin
19. bicarbonate, carbaminohemoglobin
20. medulla
21. stretch receptors
22. chemoreceptors
23. tidal
24. tidal, expiratory reserve, inspiratory reserve
25. residual

Chapter 16

1. digestion, absorption
2. muscularis
3. submucosa
4. mucosa
5. serosa
6. uvula, soft palate
7. crown, neck, root
8. parotid, submandibular, sublingual
9. esophagus
10. fundus, body, pylorus
11. duodenum, jejunum, ileum
12. villi
13. lacteal
14. hepatic duct, cystic duct
15. transverse colon
16. sigmoid colon
17. mesentery, greater omentum
18. absorption
19. e
20. i
21. j
22. k
23. b
24. l
25. f
26. g

27. d
28. c
29. a
30. h

Chapter 17

1. assimilation
2. catabolism
3. anabolism
4. prothrombin, fibrinogen
5. A, D
6. water, fat
7. total metabolic rate
8. basal metabolic rate
9. total metabolic rate
10. convection
11. evaporation
12. fat metabolism
13. protein
14. nonessential amino acids
15. ATP
16. Carbohydrates, fats and proteins
17. b
18. d
19. c
20. g
21. a
22. e
23. h
24. f
25. i

Chapter 18

1. 20
2. Bowman capsule, glomerulus
3. Henle loop, collecting tubule
4. proximal convoluted tubule, distal convoluted tubule
5. reabsorption
6. filtration
7. secretion
8. antidiuretic hormone
9. atrial natriuretic hormone
10. aldosterone
11. internal urethral sphincter
12. suppression
13. urinary incontinence
14. retention
15. g
16. a
17. k
18. b
19. d
20. f
21. j
22. h
23. c
24. e
25. i

Chapter 19

1. interstitial fluid, plasma, and transcellular fluid
2. intracellular fluid
3. less
4. more
5. more
6. fluid output
7. water from catabolism
8. kidneys, skin, lungs, intestines
9. aldosterone, atrial natriuretic hormone
10. ions
11. chloride
12. sodium
13. b
14. c
15. b
16. a

Chapter 20

1. carbonic anhydrase
2. buffers
3. H_2CO_3
4. $NaHCO_3$
5. distal tubule
6. NH_4^+
7. decrease
8. base
9. alkalosis
10. acidosis
11. 20
12. $NaHCO_3$ (bicarbonate)
13. H_2CO_3
14. alkalosis
15. b
16. a
17. b
18. b
19. decreases
20. increases
21. increases
22. decreases
23. increases
24. decreases

Chapter 21

1. testes
2. scrotum
3. tunica albuginea
4. seminiferous tubule
5. interstitial cells
6. spermatogonium
7. meiosis or spermatogenesis
8. acrosome
9. epididymis
10. vas deferens (ductus deferens)
11. prostate gland
12. seminal vesicles
13. corpora cavernosa
14. ovaries
15. graafian
16. oogenesis
17. polar bodies
18. uterine tubes (oviducts, fallopian tubes)
19. myometrium
20. cervix
21. endometrium
22. vagina
23. greater vestibular
24. alveoli, lactiferous
25. h
26. c
27. a
28. b
29. d
30. e
31. i
32. g
33. f

Chapter 22

1. zygote
2. morula
3. blastocyst
4. placenta
5. gestation
6. ectoderm, mesoderm, endoderm
7. histogenesis
8. organogenesis
9. parturition
10. neonatal
11. osteoarthritis
12. arteriosclerosis
13. presbyopia
14. cataract
15. glaucoma
16. c
17. a
18. e
19. b
20. d

Glossary

A

abdomen (AB-doh-men) body area between the diaphragm and pelvis
abdominal (ab-DOM-ih-nal) related to the abdomen (belly)
abdominal cavity (ab-DOM-ih-nal KAV-ih-tee) the cavity containing the abdominal organs
abdominal muscles (ab-DOM-ih-nal MUS-elz) muscles supporting the anterior aspect of the abdomen
abdominal quadrant (ab-DOM-ih-nal KWOD-rant) health professionals divide the abdomen (through the navel) into four areas or quadrants to help locate specific organs
abdominal region (ab-DOM-ih-nal REE-jun) anatomists have divided the abdomen into nine regions to identify the location of organs
abdominopelvic cavity (ab-DOM-ih-noh-PEL-vik KAV-ih-tee) term used to describe the single cavity containing the abdominal and pelvic organs
abduct (ab-DUKT) move away from the center or midline; see **abduction**
abduction (ab-DUK-shun) moving away from the midline of the body; opposite motion of adduction
ABO system (ay bee oh SIS-tem) system of tissue typing that classifies red blood cells by presence of immunological markers designated A and B
absorption (ab-SORP-shun) passage of a substance through a membrane, such as skin or mucosa, into blood
accessory organ (ak-SES-oh-ree OR-gan) an organ that assists other organs in accomplishing their functions
acetabulum (as-eh-TAB-yoo-lum) socket in the hip bone (os coxa or innominate bone) into which the head of the femur fits
acetylcholine (as-ee-til-KOH-leen) chemical neurotransmitter
acid (AS-id) any substance that, when dissolved in water, contributes to an excess of H^- ions (i.e., a *low* pH)
acid-base balance (AS-id bays BAL-ans) maintaining the concentration of hydrogen ions in body fluids
acidosis (as-ih-DOH-sis) condition in which there is an excessive proportion of acid in the blood (and thus an abnormally low blood pH); opposite of alkalosis
acne (AK-nee) a bacterial infection of the skin characterized by red pustules formed when hair follicles become infected
acquired immunity (ah-KWIRED ih-MYOO-nih-tee) immunity that is obtained after birth through the use of injections or exposure to a harmful agent
acquired immunodeficiency syndrome (AIDS) (ah-KWIRED ih-myoo-noh-deh-FISH-en-see SIN-drohm [aydz]) disease in which the HIV virus attacks the T cells, thereby compromising the body's immune system
acromegaly (ak-roh-MEG-ah-lee) condition caused by hypersecretion of growth hormone after puberty, resulting in enlargement of facial features (e.g., jaw, nose), fingers, and toes
acrosome (AK-roh-sohm) structure on the sperm's head containing enzymes that break down the covering of the ovum to allow entry
actin (AK-tin) contractile protein found in the thin myofilaments of skeletal muscle
action potential (AK-shun poh-TEN-shal) nerve impulse
active transport (AK-tiv TRANS-port) movement of a substance into and out of a living cell requiring the use of cellular energy
adaptation (ad-ap-TAY-shun) condition of many sensory receptors in which the magnitude of a receptor potential decreases over a period of time in response to a continuous stimulus
adaptive immunity (ah-DAP-tiv ih-MYOO-nih-tee) another name for **specific immunity**
Addison disease (AD-ih-son dih-ZEEZ) disease of the adrenal gland resulting in low blood sugar, weight loss, and weakness
adduct (ad-DUKT) move toward the center or midline; see **adduction**
adduction (ah-DUK-shun) moving toward the midline of the body; opposite motion of abduction
adductor muscle (ad-DUK-tor MUS-el) any of a group of muscles of the leg that each originate on the pelvic bone and insert on the femur (along the inside thigh) and draw the leg toward the midline of the body (adduction)
adenine (AD-eh-neen) one of the nitrogenous bases of the nucleotides in RNA, DNA, and related molecules; abbreviated *a* or *A*
adenohypophysis (ad-eh-noh-hye-POF-ih-sis) anterior pituitary gland, which has the structure of an endocrine gland
adenoid (AD-eh-noyd) literally, glandlike; adenoids, or pharyngeal tonsils, are paired lymphoid structures in the nasopharynx
adenosine diphosphate (ADP) (ah-DEN-oh-seen dye-FOS-fayt [ay dee pee]) molecule similar to adenosine triphosphate but containing only two phosphate groups
adenosine triphosphate (ATP) (ah-DEN-oh-seen try-FOS-fayt [ay tee pee]) chemical compound that provides energy for use by body cells
adipose (AD-ih-pohs) fat tissue
adolescence (ad-oh-LES-ens) period between puberty and adulthood
adrenal cortex (ah-DREE-nal KOHR-teks) outer portion of adrenal gland that secretes hormones called *corticoids*
adrenal gland (ah-DREE-nal gland) glands that rest on the top of the kidneys, made up of the cortex and medulla
adrenal medulla (ah-DREE-nal meh-DUL-ah) inner portion of adrenal gland that secretes epinephrine and norepinephrine

adrenergic fiber (ad-ren-ER-jik FYE-ber) axon whose terminal releases norepinephrine and epinephrine

adrenocorticotropic hormone (ACTH) (ah-dree-noh-kor-teh-koh-TROH-pic HOHR-mohn [ay see tee aych]) hormone that stimulates the adrenal cortex to secrete larger amounts of hormones

adulthood (ah-DULT-hood) period after adolescence

aerobic (ayr-OH-bik) requiring oxygen

aerobic training (ayr-OH-bik TRAYN-ing) continuous vigorous exercise requiring the body to increase its consumption of oxygen and develop the muscles' ability to sustain activity over a long period

afferent (AF-fer-ent) carrying or conveying toward the center (e.g., an afferent neuron carries nerve impulses toward the central nervous system)

afferent lymphatic vessel (AF-fer-ent limf VES-el) any small lymphatic vessel that carries lymphatic fluid toward a lymph node; compare to **efferent lymphatic vessel**

afferent neuron (AF-fer-ent NOO-ron) neuron that carries impulses toward the central nervous system from the periphery; sensory neuron

agglutinate (ah-GLOO-tin-ayt) antibodies causing antigens to clump or stick together

aging process (AJ-ing PROS-es) the gradual degenerative changes that occur after young adulthood as a person ages

agranular leukocyte (ah-GRAN-yoo-lar LOO-koh-syte) type of white blood cell without cytoplasmic granules when stained

agricultural scientist (ag-rih-KUL-cher-al SYE-en-tist) scientist who studies the growing of crops

AIDS (aydz) see **acquired immunodeficiency syndrome**

AIDS-related complex (ARC) (aydz ree-LAY-ted KOM-pleks [ark or ay ar see]) a more mild form of AIDS that produces fever, weight loss, and swollen lymph nodes

albumin (al-BYOO-min) one of several types of proteins normally found in blood plasma; helps thicken the blood

aldosterone (AL-deh-steh-rohn *or* al-DAH-stayr-ohn) hormone that stimulates the kidney to retain sodium ions and water

alimentary canal (al-ih-MEN-tar-ee kah-NAL) the digestive tract as a whole

alkaline (AL-kah-lin) base; any substance that, when dissolved in water, contributes to an excess of OH^- ions (thus creating a high pH)

alkalosis (al-kah-LOH-sis) condition in which there is an excessive proportion of alkali (base) in the blood, causing an abnormally high blood pH; opposite of acidosis

all or none when stimulated, a muscle fiber will contract fully or not at all; whether a contraction occurs depends on whether the stimulus reaches the required threshold

allergen (AL-er-jen) any substance that produces an allergic reaction

allergy (AL-er-jee) hypersensitivity of the immune system to relatively harmless environmental antigens; a medical specialty that treats disorders involving hyperimmunity

allied health professions (AL-ayed helth proh-FESH-unz) fields of health-care work such as therapists, medical assistants, technicians, and others, who are not physicians or nurses

alpha cell (AL-fah sel) pancreatic cell that secretes glucagon

alveolar duct (al-VEE-oh-lar dukt) airway that branches from the smallest bronchioles; alveolar sacs arise from alveolar ducts

alveolar sac (al-VEE-oh-lar sak) each alveolar duct ends in several sacs that resemble a cluster of grapes

alveolus (al-VEE-oh-lus) (*pl.,* alveoli) literally, a small cavity; alveoli of lungs are microscopic saclike dilations of terminal bronchioles

amenorrhea (ah-men-oh-REE-ah) absence of normal menstruation

amino acid (ah-MEE-no AS-id) category of chemical units from which protein molecules are built; *essential amino acids* are those that must be in the diet but *nonessential amino acids* can be missing from the diet because they can be made by the body

amniotic cavity (am-nee-OT-ik KAV-ih-tee) cavity within the blastocyst that will become a fluid-filled sac in which the embryo will float during development

amphiarthrosis (am-fee-ar-THROH-sis) slightly movable joint such as the joint joining the two pubic bones

amylase (AM-ih-lays) enzyme that digests carbohydrates

anabolic steroid (an-ah-BOL-ik STAYR-oyd) a lipid molecule of the steroid variety that acts as a hormone to stimulate anabolism (specifically protein synthesis) in body tissues such as muscle (e.g., testosterone)

anabolism (ah-NAB-oh-liz-em) cells making complex molecules (e.g., hormones) from simpler compounds (e.g., amino acids); opposite of catabolism

anaerobic (an-ayr-OH-bik) does not require the presence of oxygen

anal canal (AY-nal kah-NAL) terminal portion of the rectum

anaphase (AN-ah-fayz) stage of mitosis; duplicate chromosomes move to poles of dividing cell

anaphylactic shock (an-ah-fih-LAK-tik shock) shock resulting from a severe allergic reaction; may be fatal

anatomical position (an-ah-TOM-ih-kal poh-ZISH-un) the reference position for the body, which gives meaning to directional terms

anatomist (ah-NAT-oh-mist) professional engaged in the study of the structure of an organism and the relationships of its parts

anatomy (ah-NAT-oh-mee) the study of the structure of an organism and the relationships of its parts

androgen (AN-droh-jen) male sex hormone

anemia (ah-NEE-mee-ah) deficient number of red blood cells or deficient hemoglobin

anesthesia (an-es-THEE-zhah) loss of sensation

angina pectoris (an-JYE-nah PECK-tor-is) severe chest pain resulting when the myocardium is deprived of sufficient oxygen

angioplasty (AN-jee-oh-plas-tee) medical procedure in which vessels occluded by arteriosclerosis ("hardening of arteries") are opened (i.e., the channel for blood flow is widened)

angstrom (ANG-strom) unit of length equivalent to 0.0000000001 m (1/10,000,000,000 of a meter or about 1/250,000,000 of an inch)
anion (AN-aye-on) negatively charged particle
anorexia nervosa (an-oh-REK-see-ah ner-VOH-sah) a behavior involving an irrational fear of being overweight, resulting in severe weight loss caused by self-starvation
antagonist muscle (an-TAG-oh-nist MUS-el) those having opposing actions; for example, muscles that flex the arm are antagonists to muscles that extend it
antebrachial (an-tee-BRAY-kee-al) refers to the forearm
antecubital (an-tee-KYOO-bih-tal) refers to the elbow
antenatal medicine (an-tee-NAY-tal MED-ih-sin) prenatal medicine
anterior (an-TEER-ee-or) front or ventral; opposite of posterior or dorsal
anthropology (an-throh-POL-oh-jee) science of human origins, culture, characteristics, society, and beliefs
antibody (AN-tih-bod-ee) substance produced by the body that destroys or inactivates a specific substance (antigen) that has entered the body
antibody-mediated immunity (AN-tih-bod-ee MEE-dee-ayt-ed ih-MYOO-nih-tee) immunity that is produced when antibodies make antigens unable to harm the body
anticoagulant (an-tee-koh-AG-yoo-lant) agent that opposes blood clotting
antidiuretic hormone (ADH) (an-tee-dye-yoo-RET-ik HOHR-mohn [ay dee aych]) hormone produced in the posterior pituitary gland to regulate the balance of water in the body by accelerating the reabsorption of water
antigen (AN-tih-jen) substance that, when introduced into the body, causes formation of antibodies against it
antigen-presenting cell (APC) (AN-tih-jen prih-ZENT-ing sel [ay pee see]) immune cell that presents antigens on their surface and thus allow recognition and reaction by other immune system cells
antioxidant (an-tee-awk-seh-dant) chemical substance that prevents oxidizers such as free radicals from damaging chemical structures of the body
antrum (AN-trum) cavity
anuria (ah-NOO-ree-ah) absence of urine
anus (AY-nus) distal end or outlet of the rectum
aorta (ay-OR-tah) main and largest artery in the body
aortic body (ay-OR-tik BOD-ee) small cluster of chemosensitive cells that respond to carbon dioxide and oxygen levels
aortic semilunar valve (ay-OR-tic sem-ih-LOO-nar valve) valve between the aorta and left ventricle that prevents blood from flowing back into the ventricle
apex (AY-peks) pointed end of a conical structure
Apgar score (AP-gar skor) system of assessing general health of newborn infant, in which heart rate, respiration, muscle tone, skin color, and response to stimuli are scored
aplastic anemia (ay-PLAS-tik ah-NEE-mee-ah) blood disorder characterized by a low red blood cell count; caused by destruction of myeloid tissue in the bone marrow
apnea (AP-nee-ah) temporary cessation of breathing
apocrine sweat gland (AP-oh-krin swet gland) type of sweat gland located in the axilla and genital regions; these glands enlarge and begin to function at puberty
apoptosis (ap-op-TOH-sis) programmed cell death by means of several biochemical processes built into each cell; apoptosis clears space for newer cells, as in early embryonic development or in tissue repair
appendage (ah-PEN-dij) something that is attached
appendicitis (ah-pen-dih-SYE-tis) inflammation of the vermiform appendix
appendicular (ah-pen-DIK-yoo-lar) refers to the upper and lower extremities of the body
appendicular skeleton (ah-pen-DIK-yoo-lar SKEL-eh-ton) the bones of the upper and lower extremities of the body
appetite center (AP-ah-tyte SEN-ter) cluster of neurons in the hypothalamus whose impulses cause an increase in appetite
aqueous humor (AY-kwee-us HYOO-mor) watery fluid that fills the anterior chamber of the eye, in front of the lens
aqueous solution (AY-kwee-us sol-OO-shen) liquid mixture in which water is the solvent; for example, saltwater is an aqueous solution because water is the solvent
arachnoid mater (ah-RAK-noyd MAH-ter) delicate, weblike middle membrane covering the brain; the meninges
areola (ah-REE-oh-lah) small space; the pigmented ring around the nipple
areolar connective tissue (ah-REE-oh-lar, koh-NEK-tiv TISH-yoo) type of connective tissue consisting of fibers and a variety of cells embedded in a loose matrix of soft, sticky gel; also called *loose fibrous connective tissue*
arrector pili (ah-REK-tor PYE-lye) smooth muscles of the skin that are attached to hair follicles; when contraction occurs, the hair stands up, resulting in "goose flesh"
arterial blood gas (ABG) (ar-TEER-ee-al blud gas [ay bee jee]) any of the blood characteristics related to respiratory gases normally measured in a lab analysis of arterial blood (Po_2, Pco_2, $\%SO_2$, pH, $[HCO_3^-]$)
arteriole (ar-TEER-ee-ohl) small branch of an artery
arteriosclerosis (ar-tee-ree-oh-skleh-ROH-sis) hardening of arteries; materials such as lipids (as in atherosclerosis) accumulate in arterial walls, often becoming hardened as calcium is deposited
artery (AR-ter-ee) vessel carrying blood away from the heart
articular cartilage (ar-TIK-yoo-lar KAR-tih-lij) cartilage covering the joint ends of bones
articulation (ar-tik-yoo-LAY-shun) joint
artificial kidney (ar-tih-FISH-al KID-nee) mechanical device that removes wastes from the blood that would normally be removed by the kidney
artificial pacemaker (ar-tih-FISH-al PAYS-may-ker) an electrical device that is implanted into the heart to treat a heart block
ascending colon (ah-SEND-ing KOH-lon) portion of the colon extending from the cecum to the hepatic flexure
asexual (a-SEKS-yoo-al) one-celled plants and bacteria that do not produce specialized sex cells
assimilation (ah-sim-ih-LAY-shun) when food molecules enter the cell and undergo chemical changes

association area (ah-soh-shee-AY-shun AYR-ee-ah) region of the cerebral cortex of the brain that functions to put together or associate information from many parts of the brain to help make sense of or analyze the information
astrocyte (AS-troh-syte) a glial cell
atherosclerosis (ath-er-oh-skleh-ROH-sis) hardening of the arteries; lipid deposits lining the inside of the arteries
athletic trainer (ath-LET-ik TRAY-ner) health care professional who works with a physician and specializes in prevention, diagnosis, and therapy of sports-related injuries
atlas (AT-lis) another name for the first cervical vertebra (C1)
atom (AT-om) smallest particle of a pure substance (element) that still has the chemical properties of that substance; composed of protons, electrons, and neutrons (subatomic particles)
atomic mass (ah-TOM-ik mas) combined total number of protons and neutrons in an atom
atomic number (ah-TOM-ik NUM-ber) total number of protons in an atom's nucleus; atoms of each element have a characteristic atomic number
atrial natriuretic hormone (ANH) (AY-tree-al nah-tree-yoo-RET-ik HOHR-mohn [ay en aych]) hormone secreted by the heart cells that regulates fluid and electrolyte homeostasis
atrioventricular (AV) node (ay-tree-oh-ven-TRIK-yoo-lar nohd) see **AV node**
atrioventricular (AV) valve (ay-tree-oh-ven-TRIK-yoo-lar [ay vee] valv) either of two valves that separate the atrial chambers from the ventricles
atrium (AY-tree-um) chamber or cavity; for example, atrium of each side of the heart
atrophy (AT-roh-fee) wasting away of tissue; decrease in size of a part; sometimes referred to as *disuse atrophy*
audiologist (aw-dee-OL-uh-jist) health-care professional who treats hearing disorders
auditory tube (AW-dih-toh-ree) tube that connects the throat with the middle ear to equalize air pressure on both sides of the tympanum (eardrum); also called **eustachian tube**
auricle (AW-rih-kul) part of the ear attached to the side of the head; earlike appendage of each atrium of the heart
autonomic effector (aw-toh-NOM-ik ef-FEK-tor) tissues to which autonomic neurons conduct impulses
autonomic nervous system (ANS) (aw-toh-NOM-ik NER-vus SIS-tem [ay en es]) division of the human nervous system that regulates involuntary actions
autonomic neuron (aw-toe-NOM-ik NOO-ron) motor neurons that make up the autonomic nervous system
AV bundle (ay-VEE BUN-dul) fibers in the heart that relay a nerve impulse from the AV node to the ventricles; also known as the *bundle of His*
AV node (ay-VEE nohd) a small mass of specialized cardiac muscle tissue; part of the conduction system of the heart; see **atrioventricular (AV) node**
avitaminosis (ay-vye-tah-mih-NOH-sis) vitamin deficiency
axial (AK-see-al) refers to the head, neck, and torso, or trunk of the body
axial skeleton (AK-see-al SKEL-eh-ton) the bones of the head, neck, and torso
axilla (AK-sil-ah) armpit
axillary (AK-sil-layr-ee) relating to the armpit
axis (AK-sis) (*pl.,* axes) central line or structure around which something turns; the second cervical vertebra
axon (AK-son) nerve cell process that transmits impulses away from the cell body

B

B cell (bee sel) a lymphocyte; activated B cells develop into plasma cells, which secrete antibodies into the blood; also called *B lymphocyte*
ball-and-socket joint (bawl and SOK-et joynt) type of synovial joint in which the spherical end of one bone fits into a cuplike socket of another bone or structure
Barrett esophagus (BAHR-ett ee-SOF-ah-guss) condition related to untreated gastroesophageal reflux disease; may develop precancerous changes in the esophageal lining
Bartholin gland (BAR-tuh-lin) either of two glands, each located to the side of the vaginal outlet that secretes mucuslike lubricating fluid; also known as *greater vestibular gland*
basal cell carcinoma (BAY-sal sel car-sin-OH-mah) one of the most common forms of skin cancer, usually occurring on upper face, with low potential for metastasizing
basal ganglion (BAY-sal GANG-lee-on) also known as *basal nucleus;* see **cerebral nucleus**
basal metabolic rate (BMR) (BAY-sal met-ah-BOL-ik [bee em ar]) number of calories of heat that must be produced per hour by catabolism to keep the body alive, awake, and comfortably warm
basal nucleus (BAY-sal NOO-klee-us) see **cerebral nucleus**
base (bays) 1. A chemical that, when dissolved in water, reduces the relative concentration of H^+ ions in the whole solution (sometimes by adding OH^- ions); 2. In the context of nucleic acids (DNA and RNA), *base* or *nitrogen base* refers to one part of a nucleotide (sugar, phosphate, and base) that is the basic building block of nucleic acid molecules; possible bases include adenine, thymine, guanine, cytosine, and uracil
basement membrane (BAYS-ment MEM-brayn) the connective tissue layer of the serous membrane that holds and supports the epithelial cells
basophil (BAY-soh-fil) white blood cell that stains readily with basic dyes
benign prostatic hypertrophy (bee-NYNE pros-TAT-ik hye-PER-troh-fee) a noncancerous enlargement of the prostate in older men
benign tumor (bee-NYNE TOO-mer) a relatively harmless neoplasm
beta cell (BAY-tah) pancreatic islet cell that secretes insulin
bicarbonate ion (bye-KAR-boh-nayt EYE-on) negative ion common in water solutions, including body fluids; HCO_3^-; often acts as a buffer to increase pH (reduce acidity) of a solution

bicarbonate loading (bye-KAR-boh-nayte LOHD-ing) ingesting large amounts of sodium bicarbonate to counteract the effects of lactic acid build-up, thereby reducing fatigue; however, there are potentially dangerous side effects

biceps brachii (BYE-seps BRAY-kee-aye) the primary flexor of the forearm

biceps femoris (BYE-seps FEM-oh-ris) powerful flexor of the leg

bicuspid tooth (bye-KUS-ped tooth) tooth type with a large flat surface and two or three grinding cusps; also called *premolars*

bicuspid valve (bye-KUS-ped valv) one of the two AV valves; located between the left atrium and ventricle and sometimes called the **mitral valve**

bile (byle) substance that reduces large fat globules into smaller droplets of fat that are more easily broken down

bile duct (byle dukt) structure formed by the union of the common hepatic and cystic ducts; drains bile into the small intestine

biochemist (bye-oh-KEM-ist) scientist who works primarily in the field of biochemistry; see **biochemistry**

biochemistry (bye-oh-KEM-is-tree) scientific field that studies the chemical properties and processes of living organisms

biological filtration (bye-oh-LOJ-eh-kal fil-TRAY-shun) process in which cells alter the contents of the filtered fluid

biomechanical engineering (bye-oh-meh-KAN-ik-al en-juh-NEER-ing) discipline of engineering that applies principles of mechanical engineering to biological systems, as in biomedical engineering

biomedical engineering (bye-oh-MED-ik-al en-juh-NEER-ing) field of machine design applied to therapeutic strategies; also called *bioengineering*

birth defect (birth DEE-fekt) any abnormality, whether caused by genetic or environmental factors, that exists at birth; see **teratogen**

blackhead (BLAK-hed) sebum that accumulates, darkens, and enlarges some of the ducts of the sebaceous glands; also known as a *comedo*

bladder (BLAD-der) a sac, usually referring to the urinary bladder

blastocyst (BLAS-toh-sist) postmorula stage of developing embryo that implants in uterine wall; hollow ball of cells plus an inner cell mass

blister (BLIS-ter) a baglike fluid-filled elevation of the skin caused by an irritant such as heat, friction, or a chemical

blood (blud) fluid connective tissue that circulates through the cardiovascular system

blood-brain barrier (BBB) (blud brayn BAYR-ee-er [bee bee bee]) two-ply wall formed by the wall of a capillary and the surrounding extensions of a glial cell called an *astrocyte;* functions to prevent harmful chemicals from entering vital brain tissue

blood doping (blud DOH-ping) reinfusion of red blood cells (RBCs) (or drugs that increase RBC production) into an athlete before competition in an attempt to increase performance levels or stamina by increasing the oxygen-carrying capacity of the blood

blood pressure (blud PRESH-er) pressure of blood exerted on walls of the blood vessels; expressed as systolic pressure over diastolic pressure (e.g., 120/80 mm Hg)

blood pressure gradient (blud PRESH-er GRAY-dee-ent) the difference between two blood pressures in the body

blood type (blud type) any of the different types of blood that are identified by specific antigens in red blood cells (A, B, AB, O, and Rh-negative or Rh-positive)

body (of stomach) (BOD-ee) unified and complex assembly of structurally and functionally interactive components; also, the main part of an organ, cell, or other structure

body composition percentages of the body made of lean tissue and fat tissue

bolus (BOW-lus) a small, rounded mass of masticated food to be swallowed

bond a link; in chemistry, an attractive force that links atoms to each other

bone (bohn) highly adapted connective tissue whose matrix is hard and calcified

bone marrow (bohn MAYR-oh) soft material that fills cavities of the bones; red bone marrow is vital to blood cell formation, yellow bone marrow is inactive fatty tissue

bony labyrinth (BOHN-ee LAB-ih-rinth) the fluid-filled complex maze of three spaces (the vestibule, semicircular canals, and cochlea) in the temporal bone

Bowman capsule (BOH-men KAP-sul) the cup-shaped top of a nephron that surrounds the glomerulus

brachial (BRAY-kee-al) relating to the arm

breast (brest) structure on the anterior aspect of the chest made up of skin, fat, and mammary glands; may produce milk to sustain offspring

bronchi (BRONG-kye) (*sing.,* bronchus) the branches of the trachea

bronchiole (BRONG-kee-ole) small branch of a bronchus

bronchus (BRONG-kus) see **bronchi**

buccal (BUK-al) relating to the cheek

buffer (BUF-er) compound that combines with an acid or with a base to form a weaker acid or base, thereby lessening the change in hydrogen-ion concentration that would occur without the buffer

buffer pair (BUF-er) two kinds of chemical substances that together prevent a sharp change in the pH of a fluid; for example, sodium bicarbonate ($NaHCO_3$) and carbonic acid (H_2CO_3)

buffy coat (BUF-ee koht) thin layer of white blood cells (WBCs) and platelets located between red blood cells (RBCs) and plasma in a centrifuged sample of blood

bulbourethral gland (BUL-boh-yoo-REE-thral gland) small gland located just below the prostate gland whose mucus-like secretions lubricate the terminal portion of the urethra and contribute less than 5% of the seminal fluid volume; also known as *Cowper gland*

bundle of His (BUN-dul ov his) see **AV bundle**

burn (bern) an injury to tissues resulting from contact with heat, chemicals, electricity, friction, or radiant and electromagnetic energy; classified into four categories, depending on the number of tissue layers involved

bursa (BER-sah) (*pl.,* bursae) small, cushionlike sac found alongside joints, cushioning moving bones

bursitis (ber-SYE-tis) inflammation of a bursa

C

calcaneus (kal-KAY-nee-us) heel bone; largest tarsal in the foot

calcitonin (CT) (kal-sih-TOH-nin [see tee]) a hormone secreted by the thyroid that decreases calcium in the blood

calorie (c) (KAL-or-ree) heat unit; the amount of heat needed to raise the temperature of 1 gram of water 1° C

Calorie (C) (KAL-or-ree) heat unit; kilocalorie; the amount of heat needed to raise the temperature of 1 kilogram of water 1° C

calyx (KAY-liks) cup-shaped division of the renal pelvis

canaliculi (kan-ah-LIK-yoo-lye) see **canaliculus**

canaliculus (kan-ah-LIK-yoo-lus) (*pl.,* canaliculi) an extremely narrow tubular passage or channel in compact bone

cancellous bone (KAN-seh-lus bohn) porous bone tissue found inside bone organs; also called *spongy bone* or *trabecular bone*

canine tooth (KAY-nyne) the tooth with the longest crown and the longest root, which is located lateral to the second incisor; also called *cuspids* or *eye teeth*

capillary (KAP-ih-layr-ee) tiny vessels that connect arterioles and venules

capillary blood pressure (KAP-ih-layr-ee) the blood pressure found in the capillary vessels

capsule (KAP-sul) found in diarthrotic joints; holds the bones of joints together while allowing movement; made of fibrous connective tissue lined with a smooth, slippery synovial membrane

carbaminohemoglobin ($HbCO_2$) (karb-am-ee-noh-hee-moh-GLOH-bin) the compound formed by the union of carbon dioxide with hemoglobin

carbohydrate (kar-boh-HYE-drayt) organic compounds containing carbon, hydrogen, and oxygen in certain specific proportions (C, H, O in a 1 : 2 : 1 ratio); for example, sugars, starches, and cellulose

carbohydrate loading (kar-boh-HYE-drayt LOHD-ing) the method used by athletes to increase the stores of muscle glycogen, allowing more sustained aerobic exercise

carbon (C) (KAR-bun) element 6

carbon dioxide (CO_2) (KAR-bun dye-AHK-syde [see oh too]) compound of carbon and oxygen, formed in the body as a waste product of cellular metabolism

carbonic anhydrase (kar-BON-ik an-HYE-drays) the enzyme that converts carbon dioxide into carbonic acid

cardiac (KAR-dee-ak) refers to the heart

cardiac cycle (KAR-dee-ak) each complete heartbeat, including contraction and relaxation of the atria and ventricles

cardiac muscle (KAR-dee-ak) the type of muscle tissue that makes up most of the heart wall

cardiac output (KAR-dee-ak) volume of blood pumped by one ventricle per minute

cardiac sphincter (KAR-dee-ak SFINK-ter) a ring of muscle between the stomach and esophagus that prevents food from re-entering the esophagus when the stomach contracts; also called **gastroesophageal sphincter**

cardiac vein (KAR-dee-ak) any vein that carries blood from the myocardial capillary beds to the coronary sinus

cardiologist (kar-dee-AH-luh-jist) physician specializing in treatment of the heart and heart disease

cardiology (kar-dee-OL-oh-jee) study and treatment of the heart and heart disease

cardiopulmonary resuscitation (CPR) (kar-dee-oh-PUL-moh-nayr-ree ree-sus-ih-TAY-shun [see pee ar]) combined external cardiac (heart) massage and artificial respiration

cardiovascular (kar-dee-oh-VAS-kyoo-lar) relating to the heart and blood vessels

cardiovascular system (kar-dee-oh-VAS-kyoo-lar SIS-tem) organ system that includes the heart and blood vessels

caries (KAYR-eez) decay of teeth or of bone; often called **dental caries**

carotid body (kah-ROT-id) chemoreceptor located in the carotid artery that detects changes in oxygen, carbon dioxide, and blood acid levels

carpal (KAR-pal) relating to the wrist

carpal tunnel syndrome (KAR-pul TUN-el SIN-drohm) muscle weakness, pain, and tingling in the radial side (thumb side) of the wrist, hand, and fingers—perhaps radiating to the forearm and shoulder; caused by compression of the median nerve within the carpal tunnel (a passage along the ventral concavity of the wrist)

cartilage (KAR-tih-lij) a type of fibrous connective tissue that has the consistency of a firm plastic or gristlelike gel

catabolism (kah-TAB-oh-liz-em) breakdown of food compounds or cytoplasm into simpler compounds; opposite of anabolism, the other phase of metabolism

catalyst (KAT-ah-list) chemical that speeds up reactions without being changed itself

cataract (KAT-ah-rakt) opacity of the lens of the eye

catecholamine (kat-eh-KOHL-ah-meen) class of neurotransmitters that includes norepinephrine and epinephrine

catheterization (kath-eh-ter-ih-ZAY-shun) passage of a flexible tube (catheter) into the bladder through the urethra for the withdrawal of urine (urinary catheterization)

cation (KAT-aye-on) positively charged particle

cavity (KAV-ih-tee) hollow place or space in a tooth; see **dental caries**

cecum (SEE-kum) blind pouch; the pouch at the proximal end of the large intestine

cell (sel) the basic biological and structural unit of the body consisting of a nucleus surrounded by cytoplasm and enclosed by a membrane

cell body (sel) the main part of a neuron from which the dendrites and axons extend

cell-mediated immunity (sel MEE-dee-ayt-ed ih-MYOO-nih-tee) resistance to disease organisms resulting from the actions of cells; chiefly sensitized T cells

cellular respiration (SEL-yoo-lar res-pih-RAY-shun) enzymes in the mitochondrial wall and matrix using oxygen to break down glucose and other nutrients to release energy needed for cellular work

cementum (see-MEN-tum) hard dental tissue that covers the root and neck of each tooth

centimeter (SEN-tih-mee-ter) 1/100 of a meter; approximately 2.5 cm equals 1 inch

central canal (SEN-tral kah-NAL) any tubelike passage at the center of a structure, such as the canal running through the center of the spinal cord or through the center of each osteon in compact bone

central nervous system (CNS) (SEN-tral NER-vus SIS-tem [see en es]) portion of the nervous system that includes the brain and spinal cord

central venous pressure (SEN-tral VEE-nus PRESH-ur) venous blood pressure within the right atrium that influences the pressure in the large peripheral veins

centriole (SEN-tree-ol) one of a pair of tiny cylinders in the centrosome of a cell; believed to be involved with the spindle fibers formed during mitosis

centromere (SEN-troh-meer) a beadlike structure that attaches one chromatid to another during the early stages of mitosis

centrosome (SEN-troh-sohm) area of the cytoplasm near the nucleus that coordinates the building and breaking up of microtubules in the cell; contains centrioles

cephalic (seh-FAL-ik) refers to the head

cerebellum (sayr-eh-BELL-um) the second largest part of the human brain that plays an essential role in the production of normal movements

cerebral cortex (seh-REE-bral KOHR-teks) a thin layer of gray matter made up of neuron dendrites and cell bodies that compose the surface of the cerebrum

cerebral nucleus (seh-REE-bral NOO-klee-us) any of a group of islands of gray matter located in the base of the cerebrum that are responsible for automatic movements and postures; also called *basal nucleus;* historically known as *basal ganglion*

cerebrospinal fluid (CSF) (seh-ree-broh-SPY-nal FLOO-id [see es ef]) fluid that fills the subarachnoid space in the brain and spinal cord and in the cerebral ventricles

cerebrovascular accident (CVA) (seh-ree-broh-VAS-kyoo-lar AK-sih-dent [see vee ay]) a hemorrhage or cessation of blood flow through cerebral blood vessels resulting in destruction of neurons; commonly called a *stroke*

cerebrum (seh-REE-brum) the largest and uppermost part of the human brain that controls consciousness, memory, sensations, emotions, and voluntary movements

cerumen (seh-ROO-men) ear wax

ceruminous gland (seh-ROO-mih-nus) gland that produces a waxy substance called cerumen (ear wax)

cervical (SER-vih-kal) relating to the neck

cervix (SER-viks) neck; any necklike structure

cesarean section (seh-SAYR-ee-an SEK-shun) surgical removal of a fetus through an incision of the skin and uterine wall; also called *C-section*

chemical level (KEM-ih-kal LEV-el) level of biological organization that includes chemical particles such as atoms and molecules

chemoreceptor (kee-moh-ree-SEP-tor) any receptor that responds to chemicals, such as those responsible for taste and smell

chemoreflex (kee-moh-REE-fleks) any reaction triggered by a chemical change, as when the heart rate changes in response to shift in oxygen concentration in the blood

chest thorax

Cheyne-Stokes respiration (CSR) (chayn stokes res-pih-RAY-shun [see es ar]) pattern of breathing associated with critical conditions such as brain injury or drug overdose and characterized by cycles of apnea and hyperventilation

childhood (CHILD-hood) from infancy to puberty

chiropractor (KYE-roh-prak-ter) physician specializing in therapy based on principle that alignment of the skeleton promotes healing

cholecystectomy (kohl-eh-sis-TEK-toh-mee) the surgical removal of the gallbladder

cholecystokinin (CCK) (koh-lee-sis-toh-KYE-nin [see see kay]) hormone secreted from the intestinal mucosa of the duodenum that stimulates the contraction of the gallbladder, resulting in bile flowing into the duodenum

cholesterol (koh-LES-ter-ol) steroid lipid found in all body cell membranes and in animal fat present in food

cholinergic fiber (koh-lin-ER-jik FYE-ber) axon whose terminals release acetylcholine

chondrocyte (KON-droh-syte) cartilage cell

chordae tendineae (KOHR-dee ten-DIN-ee) group of stringlike structures that attach the AV valves to the wall of the heart

chorion (KOH-ree-on) develops into an important fetal membrane in the placenta

chorionic gonadotropin (koh-ree-ON-ik goh-na-doh-TROH-pin) hormone secreted by the developing placenta during pregnancy and that has a gonad-stimulating effect

chorionic villus (koh-ree-ON-ik VIL-lus) (*pl.,* villi) tiny fingerlike projections that connect the placental blood vessels of the uterine wall

choroid (KOH-royd) middle layer of the eyeball that contains a dark pigment to prevent the scattering of incoming light rays

choroid plexus (KOH-royd PLEK-sus) a network of brain capillaries that are involved with the production of cerebrospinal fluid

chromatid (KROH-mah-tid) either of two replicated chromatin (DNA) strands within a chromosome of a cell ready to divide

chromatin granule (KROH-mah-tin GRAN-yool) easily stained substance in the nucleus of cells made up of DNA strands wound around spools of protein; condenses into chromosomes during mitosis

chromosome (KROH-moh-sohm) DNA molecule that has coiled to form a compact mass during mitosis or meiosis; each chromosome is composed of regions called *genes,* each of which transmits hereditary information

chronic obstructive pulmonary disease (COPD) (KRON-ik ob-STRUK-tiv PUL-moh-nayr-ee dih-ZEEZ [see oh pee dee]) general term referring to a group of disorders characterized by progressive, irreversible obstruction of airflow in the lungs

chyme (kyme) partially digested food mixture leaving the stomach

cilia (SIL-ee-ah) (*sing.*, cilium) hairlike projections of cells; eyelashes

ciliary escalator (SIL-ee-ayr-ee ES-kuh-lay-ter) process of cilia moving mucus and entrapped particles upward and out of the respiratory tract

ciliary muscle (SIL-ee-ayr-ee MUS-el) smooth muscle in the ciliary body of the eye that suspends the lens and functions in accommodation of focus for near vision

circulatory system (SER-kyoo-lah-tor-ee SIS-tem) the system that supplies transportation for cells of the body

circumcision (ser-kum-SIH-zhun) surgical removal of the foreskin or prepuce

circumduct (sir-kum-DUKT) move the distal end in a circular path; see **circumduction**

circumduction (ser-kum-DUK-shun) the process of moving the distal end of a body part in a circular path; see **circumduct**

circumvallate papilla (ser-kum-VAL-ayt pah-PIL-ah) (*pl.*, papillae) broad, flattened bumps arranged in inverted V pattern at the back of the tongue

cisterna chyli (sis-TER-nah KYE-lye) an enlarged pouch on the thoracic duct that serves as a storage area for lymph moving toward its point of entry into the venous system

citric acid cycle (SIT-rik AS-id sye-kul) the second series of chemical reactions in the process of glucose metabolism; an aerobic process; also called *Krebs cycle*

clavicle (KLAV-ih-kul) collarbone; connects the upper extremity to the axial skeleton

cleavage furrow (KLEEV-ij FUR-oh) depression in the parent cell surface during cell division; appears at the end of anaphase and begins to divide the cell into two daughter cells

clinical laboratory technician (KLIN-ih-kal LAB-rah-tor-ee tek-NISH-en) health-care worker who collects samples and scientifically analyzes tissues, body fluids, and other materials for medical purposes; also called *medical laboratory technologist* or *technician*

clitoris (KLIT-oh-ris) erectile tissue located at the anterior corner of the vestibule of the vagina

clone (klohn) any of a family of many identical cells descended from a single "parent" cell

coccyx (KOK-sis) last bone of the vertebral column, made up of four or five vertebrae that have fused together

cochlea (KOHK-lee-ah) snail shell or structure of similar shape

cochlear duct (KOHK-lee-ar) membranous tube within the bony cochlea

cochlear nerve (KOHK-lee-ar nerv) part of vestibulocochlear nerve (cranial nerve VIII) attached to the cochlea; sensory nerve responsible for hearing

codon (KOH-don) in RNA, a triplet of three base pairs that codes for a particular amino acid; subunit of a protein-coding gene

collagen (KAHL-ah-jen) principal organic constituent of connective tissue

collecting duct (CD) (koh-LEK-ting dukt [see dee]) a straight part of a renal tubule formed by distal tubules of several nephrons joining together

colloid (KOL-oyd) dissolved particles with diameters of 1 to 100 millimicrons (1 millimicron equals about 1/25,000,000 of an inch)

colon (KOH-lon) part of the large intestine

colostomy (koh-LAH-stoh-mee) surgical procedure in which an artificial anus is created on the abdominal wall by cutting the colon and bringing the cut end or ends out to the surface to form an opening called a *stoma*

columnar (koh-LUM-nar) shape in which cells are taller than they are wide

combining site (kom-BYNE-ing syte) antigen-binding site; any of the antigen receptor regions on antibody molecule; shape of each combining site is complementary to shape of a specific antigen

comedo (KOM-ee-doh) inflamed, plugged sebaceous gland duct, common in acne conditions; also called *blackhead*

compact bone (kom-PAKT bohn) dense bone

compensated metabolic acidosis (KOM-pen-say-ted met-ah-BOL-ik as-ih-DOH-sis) condition in which metabolic acidosis has occurred and the body is able to make adjustments to return the blood pH to near-normal levels

compensation (kom-pen-SAY-shun) process by which the body attempts to counteract a shift away from homeostatic balance, thus compensating for the change

complement (KOM-pleh-ment) any of several inactive enzymes normally present in blood, which, when activated, kill foreign cells by dissolving them

complementary base pairing (kom-pleh-MENT-uh-ree bays PAYR-ing) bonding purines and pyridines in DNA; adenine always binds with thymine, and cytosine always binds with guanine

complement-binding site (KOM-pleh-ment BIND-ing syte) part of an antibody molecule that binds with complement proteins during certain immune reponses

complement cascade (KOM-pleh-ment kas-KAYD) rapid-fire series of chemical reactions involving proteins called *complements* (normally present in blood plasma), which are triggered by certain antibody-antigen reactions (and other stimuli), and resulting in the formation of tiny protein rings that create holes in a foreign cell and thus cause its destruction

complement fixation (KOM-pleh-ment fik-SAY-shun) process in which complement proteins promote formation of highly specialized antigen-antibody complexes that can destroy a foreign cell

complete blood cell count (CBC) (kom-PLEET blud sel kownt [see bee see]) clinical blood test that usually includes standard red blood cell, white blood cell, thrombocyte counts, the differential white blood cell count, hematocrit, and hemoglobin content

compound (KOM-pownd) substance whose molecules have more than one kind of element in them

concave (KON-kayv) a rounded, somewhat depressed surface

concentric contraction (kon-SENT-rik kon-TRAK-shen) type of isotonic muscle contraction in which a muscle's length decreases

concentric lamella (kon-SEN-trik lah-MEL-ah) (*pl.*, lamellae) ring of calcified matrix surrounding the haversian canal

conchae (KONG-kee) shell-shaped structure; for example, bony projections into the nasal cavity

conduction (kon-DUK-shun) transfer of heat energy to the skin and then the external environment

condyloid joint (KON-dih-loyd joynt) ellipsoidal joint in which an oval process fits into an oval socket

cone (kohn) receptor cell located in the retina that is stimulated by bright light

conjunctiva (kon-junk-TIH-vah) mucous membrane that lines the eyelids and covers the sclera (white portion)

connective tissue (kon-NEK-tiv TISH-yoo) most abundant and widely distributed tissue in the body; has numerous functions

connective tissue membrane (kon-NEK-tiv TISH-yoo MEM-brayn) one of the two major types of body membranes; composed exclusively of various types of connective tissue

constipation (kon-stih-PAY-shun) retention of feces

contact dermatitis (KON-takt der-mah-TYE-tis) a local skin inflammation lasting a few hours or days after being exposed to an antigen

continuous ambulatory peritoneal dialysis (CAPD) (kon-TIN-yoo-us AM-byoo-lah-tor-ee payr-ih-toh-NEE-al dye-AL-ih-sis [see ay pee dee]) an alternative form of treatment for renal failure rather than the more complex and expensive hemodialysis

contractile unit (kon-TRAK-til YOO-nit) the sarcomere, the basic functional unit of skeletal muscle

contractility (kon-TRAK-til-ih-tee) the ability to contract a muscle

contraction (kon-TRAK-shun) ability of muscle cells to shorten or contract

control center (kon-TROHL SEN-ter) a nervous system structure that acts as an integrating or regulating mechanism

convection (kon-VEK-shun) transfer of heat energy to air that is flowing away from the skin

convex (KON-veks) a rounded, somewhat elevated surface

cornea (KOR-nee-ah) transparent, anterior portion of the sclera

coronal (koh-ROH-nal) literally "like a crown"; a coronal plane divides the body or an organ into anterior and posterior regions

coronary artery (KOHR-oh-nayr-ee AR-ter-ee) the first artery to branch off the aorta; supplies blood to the myocardium (heart muscle)

coronary bypass surgery (KOHR-oh-nayr-ee BYE-pass SER-jer-ee) surgery to relieve severely restricted coronary blood flow; veins are taken from other parts of the body to bypass the partial blockage

coronary circulation (KOHR-oh-nayr-ee ser-kyoo-LAY-shun) delivery of oxygen and removal of waste product from the myocardium (heart muscle)

coronary embolism (KOHR-oh-nayr-ee EM-boh-liz-em) blocking of a coronary blood vessel by a clot

coronary heart disease (KOHR-oh-nayr-ee) disease (blockage or other deformity) of the vessels that supply the myocardium (heart muscle); one of the leading causes of death among adults in the United States

coronary sinus (KOHR-oh-nayr-ee SYE-nus) area that receives deoxygenated blood from the coronary veins and empties into the right atrium

coronary thrombosis (KOHR-oh-nayr-ee throm-BOH-sis) formation of a blood clot in a coronary blood vessel

corpora cavernosa (KOHR-pohr-ah kav-er-NOH-sah) two columns of erectile tissue found in the shaft of the penis

corpus callosum (KOHR-pus kah-LOH-sum) where the right and left cerebral hemispheres are joined

corpus luteum (KOHR-pus LOO-tee-um) a hormone-secreting glandular structure transformed after ovulation from a ruptured follicle; it secretes chiefly progesterone, with some estrogen secreted as well

corpus spongiosum (KOHR-pus spun-jee-OH-sum) a column of erectile tissue surrounding the urethra in the penis

cortex (KOHR-teks) outer part of an internal organ; for example, the outer part of the cerebrum and of the kidneys

cortical nephron (KOHR-tih-kal NEF-ron) nephron located in the renal cortex

corticoid (KOHR-tih-koyd) category of hormones secreted by any of the three cell layers of the adrenal cortex

cortisol (KOHR-tih-sol) hormone secreted by the adrenal cortex to stimulate the availability of glucose in the blood; in large amounts, cortisol can depress immune functions, as when it is used as a drug treatment; see **hydrocortisone**

cosmetic surgery (koz-MET-ik SUR-jeh-ree) surgical medical specialty focused on improving one's appearance

cosmetician (koz-meh-TISH-un) worker who specializes in the manufacture, sale, or application of makeup or other products that affect one's appearance

cotransport (koh-TRANZ-port) active transport process in which two substances are moved together across a cell membrane; for example, sodium and glucose may be transported together across a membrane

countercurrent mechanism (KON-ter-ker-rent MEK-a-niz-em) system in which renal tubule filtrate flows in opposite directions; facilitates concentration of urine excreted from kidney

covalent bond (koh-VAY-lent) chemical bond formed when atoms share electrons by overlapping their energy levels (electron shells)

coxal bone (KOKS-al) the pelvic bone or hipbone (also known as the *os coxae* or the *innominate bone);* formed by fusion of three distinct bones (ilium, ischium, and pubis) during skeletal development

cranial (KRAY-nee-al) toward the head

cranial cavity (KRAY-nee-al KAV-ih-tee) space inside the skull that contains the brain

cranial nerve (KRAY-nee-al nerv) any of 12 pairs of nerves that attach to the undersurface of the brain and conduct impulses between the brain and structures in the head, neck, and thorax

craniosacral (kray-nee-oh-SAY-kral) relating to parasympathetic nerves

cranium (KRAY-nee-um) bony vault made up of eight bones that encase the brain

crenation (kreh-NAY-shun) abnormal notching in an erythrocyte resulting from shrinkage after suspension in a hypertonic solution

cretinism (KREE-tin-iz-em) dwarfism caused by hyposecretion of the thyroid gland

crista ampullaris (KRIS-tah am-pyoo-LAYR-is) a sensory structure located within the semicircular canals that detects head movements

crown (krown) topmost part of an organ or other structure

cruciate ligament (KRU-shee-ayt LIG-a-ment) either of two crossed ligaments inside the knee joint cavity that connect the tibia to the femur; the *anterior cruciate ligament (ACL)* and the *posterior cruciate ligament (PCL)*

crural (KROOR-al) refers to the leg

cryptorchidism (krip-TOR-kih-diz-em) undescended testicles

cubital (KYOO-bih-tal) refers to the elbow or to the forearm

cuboid (KYOO-boyd) resembling a cube

cuboidal (KYOO-boyd-al) cell shape resembling a cube

cupula (KYOO-pyoo-lah) the small cup-shaped, flaplike structure at the base of each semicircular canal of the ear that bends during movement of the head to facilitate the sense of dynamic equilibrium

Cushing syndrome (KOOSH-ing SIN-drohm) condition caused by the hypersecretion of glucocorticoids from the adrenal cortex

cuspid (KUS-ped) tooth that serves to pierce or tear food being eaten; also called **canine tooth**

cutaneous (kyoo-TAYN-ee-us) relating to the skin

cutaneous membrane (kyoo-TAYN-ee-us MEM-brayn) primary organ of the integumentary system; the skin

cuticle (KYOO-tih-kul) skinfold covering the root of the nail

cyanosis (SYE-ah-NOH-sis) bluish appearance of the skin caused by deficient oxygenation of the blood

cyclic AMP (cAMP) (SIK-lik ay em pee [SEE ay em pee]) adenosine monophosphate, one of several second messengers that delivers information inside the cell and thus regulates the cell's activity

cystic duct (SIS-tik dukt) joins with the common hepatic duct to form the common bile duct

cystitis (sis-TYE-tis) inflammation of the urinary bladder

cytokine (SYE-toh-kyne) chemical released from cells to trigger or regulate innate and adaptive immune responses

cytologist (SYE-TOL-uh-jist) scientist who studies cells

cytoplasm (SYE-toh-plaz-em) the gel-like substance of a cell exclusive of the nucleus and other organelles

cytosine (SYE-toh-seen) one of the nitrogenous bases of the nucleotides in RNA, DNA, and related molecules; abbreviated *c* or *C*

cytoskeleton (sye-toh-SKEL-e-ton) cell's internal supporting, moving framework

D

deciduous (deh-SID-yoo-us) temporary; shedding at a certain stage of growth; for example, deciduous teeth that are commonly referred to as baby teeth

deep farther away from the body's surface

defecation (def-eh-KAY-shun) process of expelling feces from the digestive tract

deglutition (deg-loo-TISH-un) swallowing

dehydration (dee-hye-DRAY-shun) excessive loss of body water; the most common fluid imbalance; an abnormally low volume of one or more body fluids

dehydration synthesis (dee-hye-DRAY-shun SIN-theh-sis) chemical reaction in which large molecules are formed by removing water from smaller molecules and joining them together

deltoid (DEL-toyd) triangular; for example, the deltoid muscle

dementia (de-MEN-shah) degenerative disease that can result in destruction of neurons in the brain

dendrite (DEN-dryte) branching or treelike; a nerve cell process that transmits impulses toward the body

dendritic cell (DC) (DEN-drih-tik sel [dee see]) phagocytic cells with numerous branches in the immune system

dense bone (dents bohn) bone with an outer layer that is hard and dense

dense fibrous connective tissue (dents FYE-brus koh-NEK-tiv TISH-yoo) tissue consisting of fibers packed densely in the matrix

dental caries (DEN-tal KAYR-eez) decay of teeth; see **cavity**

dentin (DEN-tin) hard, mineralized connective tissue similar to bone that forms the body of the tooth

deoxyribonucleic acid (DNA) (dee-OK-see-rye-boh-noo-KLEE-ik [dee en ay]) genetic material of the cell that carries the chemical "blueprint" of the body

depolarization (dee-poh-lar-ih-ZAY-shun) the electrical activity that triggers a contraction of the heart muscle

dermal-epidermal junction (DER-mal-EP-ih-der-mal JUNK-shun) junction between the thin epidermal layer of the skin and the dermal layer providing support for the epidermis

dermal papilla (DER-mal pah-PIL-ah) tiny bumps in the upper region of the dermis that forms part of the dermal-epidermal junction and produces the ridges and grooves of fingerprints

dermatology (der-mah-TOL-uh-jee) medical specialty that deals with skin health

dermatome (DER-mah-tohm) any of the skin surface areas supplied by a single spinal nerve

dermis (DER-mis) the deeper of the two major layers of the skin, composed of dense fibrous connective tissue interspersed with glands, nerve endings, and blood vessels; sometimes called the *true skin*

descending colon (dih-SEND-ing KOH-lon) portion of the colon that lies in the vertical position, on the left side of the abdomen; extends from splenic flexure to the sigmoid colon

developmental process (deh-VEL-up-ment-al PROS-es) changes and functions occurring during a human's early years as the body becomes more efficient and more effective

diabetes insipidus (dye-ah-BEE-teez in-SIP-ih-dus) condition resulting from hyposecretion of ADH in which large volumes of urine are formed and, if left untreated, may cause serious health problems

diabetes mellitus (DM) (dye-ah-BEE-teez MELL-ih-tus [dee em]) a condition resulting when the pancreatic islets secrete too little insulin, resulting in increased levels of blood glucose

diabetic ketoacidosis (dye-ah-BET-tik kee-toh-as-ih-DOH-sis) see **ketoacidosis**

dialysis (dye-AL-ih-sis) separation of smaller (diffusible) particles from larger (nondiffusible) particles through a semipermeable membrane

diaphragm (DYE-ah-fram) membrane or partition that separates one thing from another; the flat muscular sheet that separates the thorax and abdomen and is a major muscle of respiration

diaphysis (dye-AF-ih-sis) shaft of a long bone

diarrhea (dye-ah-REE-ah) defecation of liquid feces

diarthrosis (dye-ar-THROH-sis) (*pl.*, diarthroses) freely movable joint

diastole (dye-AS-toh-lee) relaxation of the heart, interposed between its contractions; opposite of systole

diastolic pressure (dye-ah-STOL-ik PRESH-ur) blood pressure in arteries during diastole (relaxation) of the heart

diencephalon (dye-en-SEF-ah-lon) "between" brain; parts of the brain between the cerebral hemispheres and the mesencephalon or midbrain

dietitian (dye-eh-TISH-en) person who works in nutrition science by developing healthful meals and dietary health strategies; also *dietician*

differential WBC count (dif-er-EN-shal DUB-el-yoo bee see kownt) proportion of each type of WBC reported as a percentage of the total WBC count

differentiate (dif-er-EN-shee-ayt) a process by which daughter cells become different in structure and function (by using different genes from the genome all cells of the body share), as when some of the original cells of early developmental stages differentiate to become muscle cells and other cells become nerve cells, and so on (*differentiation* is another form of this term)

diffusion (dih-FYOO-shun) spreading; for example, scattering of dissolved particles

digestion (dih-JEST-chun) the breakdown of food materials either mechanically (i.e., chewing) or chemically (i.e., digestive enzymes)

digestive system (dih-JEST-tiv SIS-tem) organs that work together to ensure proper digestion and absorption of nutrients

digital (DIJ-ih-tal) refers to fingers and toes

diploe (DIP-loh-EE) region of cancellous (spongy) bone within the wall of a flat bone of the cranium; also spelled *diploë*

directional term (dih-REK-shun-al term) a word that signifies or relates to anatomical direction, such as anterior, posterior, superior, inferior

disaccharide (dye-SAK-ah-ryde) double sugar, such as sucrose or lactose; made up of two monosaccharides

discharging chambers (dis-CHARJ-ing CHAM-berz) the two lower chambers of the heart called *ventricles*

dissection (dis-SEK-shun) cutting technique used to separate body parts for study

dissociate (dis-SOH-see-ayt) when a compound breaks apart in solution

dissociation (dis-soh-see-AY-shun) separation of ions as they dissolve in water

distal (DIS-tal) toward the end of a structure; opposite of proximal

distal convoluted tubule (DCT) (DIS-tal KON-voh-loo-ted TOO-byool [dee see tee]) the part of the tubule distal to the ascending limb of the nephron loop in the kidney

disuse atrophy (DIS-yoos AT-roh-fee) when prolonged inactivity results in the muscles getting smaller in size

diuretic (dye-yoo-RET-ik) a substance that promotes or stimulates the production of urine; diuretic drugs are among the most commonly used drugs in medicine

diverticulitis (dye-ver-tik-yoo-LYE-tis) inflammation of diverticula (abnormal outpouchings) of the large intestine, possibly causing constipation

DNA replication (dee en ay rep-lih-KAY-shun) the unique ability of DNA molecules to make copies of themselves

dopamine (DOH-pah-meen) chemical neurotransmitter

dorsal (DOR-sal) referring to the back; opposite of ventral; in humans, the posterior is dorsal

dorsal body cavity (DOR-sal BOD-ee KAV-ih-tee) includes the cranial and spinal cavities

dorsiflex (dor-sih-FLEKS) bend the foot upward

dorsiflexion (dor-sih-FLEK-shun) angular movement when the top of the foot is elevated (brought toward the front of the leg) with the toes pointing upward

double helix (HE-lix) shape of DNA molecules; a double spiral

ductless gland (DUKT-less gland) type of gland that secretes hormones directly into the blood

ductus arteriosus (DUK-tus ar-teer-ee-OH-sus) connects the aorta and the pulmonary artery, allowing most blood to bypass the fetus' developing lungs

ductus deferens (DUK-tus DEF-er-enz) a thick, smooth, muscular tube that allows sperm to exit from the epididymis and pass from the scrotal sac into the abdominal cavity; also known as the **vas deferens**

ductus venosus (DUK-tus veh-NOH-sus) a continuation of the umbilical vein that shunts blood returning from the placenta past the fetus's developing liver directly into the inferior vena cava

duodenal papillae (doo-oh-DEE-nal pah-PIL-ee) ducts located in the middle third of the duodenum that empty pancreatic digestive juices and bile from the liver into the small intestine; there are two ducts, the major duodenal papillae and the minor papillae

duodenum (doo-oh-DEE-num) the first subdivision of the small intestine where most chemical digestion occurs

dura mater (DOO-rah MAH-ter) literally "strong or hard mother"; outermost layer of the meninges

dust cell (dust sel) type of macrophage that ingests particulate matter in the small air sacs of the lungs

dwarfism (DWARF-iz-em) condition of abnormally small stature, sometimes resulting from hyposecretion of growth hormone

dynamic equilibrium (dye-NAM-ik ee-kwih-LIB-ree-um) sense of speed and direction of body movement

dyspnea (DISP-nee-ah) difficult or labored breathing

E

eardrum (EAR-drum) the tympanic membrane that separates the external ear and middle ear

eccentric contraction (ek-SENT-rik kon-TRAK-shun) type of isotonic muscle contraction in which a muscle's length increases under a load

eccrine sweat gland (EK-rin swet gland) any of a group of small sweat glands distributed over the total body surface

ectoderm (EK-toh-derm) the innermost of the primary germ layers that develops early in the first trimester of pregnancy

ectopic pregnancy (ek-TOP-ik PREG-nan-see) a pregnancy in which the fertilized ovum implants some place other than in the uterus

edema (eh-DEE-mah) excessive fluid in the tissues

effector (ef-FEK-tor) responding organ; for example, voluntary and involuntary muscle, the heart, and glands

effector cell (ef-FEK-tor sel) a category of B or T lymphocytes that carries out active immune functions, in contrast to a memory cell that remains immunologically inactive

efferent (EF-fer-ent) carrying from, as neurons that transmit impulses from the central nervous system to the periphery; opposite of afferent

efferent lymphatic vessel (EE-fer-ent limf VES-el) any of the small lymphatic vessels that carry lymphatic fluid away from a lymph node; compare to *afferent lymphatic vessel*

efferent neuron (EF-fer-ent NOO-ron) neuron that transmits impulses from the central nervous system to the periphery; opposite (in direction) of *afferent neuron;* see **efferent**

ejaculation (ee-jak-yoo-LAY-shun) sudden discharge of semen from the body

ejaculatory duct (ee-JAK-yoo-lah-toh-ree dukt) duct formed by the joining of the ductus deferens and the duct from the seminal vesicle that allows sperm to enter the urethra

elastic cartilage (eh-LAS-tik KAR-tih-lij) cartilage with elastic, as well as collagenous, fibers; provides elasticity and firmness, as in, for example, the cartilage of the external ear

elastin (e-LAS-tin) protein found in elastic fiber

electrocardiogram (ECG or EKG) (ee-lek-troh-KAR-dee-oh-gram [ee see jee or ee kay jee]) graphic record of the heart's action potentials

electrocardiograph (ee-lek-troh-KAR-dee-oh-graf) machine that produces electrocardiograms, graphic records of the heart's electrical activity (voltage fluctuations)

electrolyte (eh-LEK-troh-lyte) substance that ionizes (dissociates to form ions) in solution, rendering the solution capable of conducting an electric current

electrolyte balance (eh-LEK-troh-lyte BAL-ans) homeostasis of electrolytes

electron (eh-LEK-tron) negatively charged particle orbiting the nucleus of an atom

electron transport system (ETS) (eh-LEK-tron TRANS-port SIS-tem [ee tee es]) cellular process within mitochondria that transfers energy from high-energy electrons from glycolysis and the citric acid cycle to ATP molecules so that the energy is available to do work in the cell

element (EL-eh-ment) pure substance, composed of only one type of atom

elimination (eh-lim-uh-NAY-shun) moving something out of the body, as in defecation

embolism (EM-boh-liz-em) obstruction of a blood vessel by foreign matter carried in the bloodstream

embolus (EM-boh-lus) a blood clot or other substance (bubble of air) that is moving in the blood and may block a blood vessel

embryo (EM-bree-oh) animal in early stages of intrauterine development; in humans, the first 3 months after conception

embryology (em-bree-OL-oh-jee) study of the development of an individual from conception to birth

embryonic phase (em-bree-ON-ik fayz) the period extending from fertilization until the end of the eighth week of gestation; during this phase the term *embryo* is used

emergency medical technician (e-MER-jen-see MED-ih-kal tek-NISH-en) first responder trained to assess health conditions and administer emergency medical care

emesis (EM-eh-sis) vomiting

emphysema (em-fi-SEE-mah) abnormal condition characterized by trapping of air in alveoli of the lung that causes them to rupture and fuse to other alveoli

emptying reflex (EMP-tee-ing REE-fleks) the reflex that causes the contraction of the bladder wall and relaxation of the internal sphincter to allow urine to enter the urethra, which is followed by urination if the external sphincter is voluntarily relaxed

emulsify (eh-MUL-seh-fye) in digestion, when bile breaks up fats

enamel (ih-NA-mel) hard, mineralized connective tissue, harder than bone, forms hard covering of exposed tooth surfaces; hardest substance in body

endocarditis (en-doh-kar-DYE-tis) inflammation of the lining of the heart

endocardium (en-doh-KAR-dee-um) thin layer of very smooth tissue lining each chamber of the heart

endochondral ossification (en-doh-KON-dral os-ih-fih-KAY-shun) the process in which most bones are formed from cartilage models

endocrine (EN-doh-krin) secreting into the blood or tissue fluid rather than into a duct; opposite of exocrine

endocrine gland (EN-doh-krin gland) any of the ductless glands that are part of the endocrine system and secrete hormones into intercellular spaces, where they diffuse into the bloodstream

endocrine system (EN-doh-krin SIS-tem) the series of ductless glands that are found in the body

endocrinology (en-doh-krin-OL-oh-jee) study and treatment of the endocrine glands, hormones, and their disorders

endoderm (EN-doh-derm) the outermost layer of the primary germ layers that develops early in the first trimester of pregnancy

endolymph (EN-doh-limf) thick, clear fluid that fills the membranous labyrinth of the inner ear

endometrium (en-doh-MEE-tree-um) mucous membrane lining the uterus

endoneurium (en-doh-NOO-ree-um) the thin wrapping of fibrous connective tissue that surrounds each axon in a nerve

endoplasmic reticulum (ER) (en-doh-PLAS-mik reh-TIK-yoo-lum [ee ar]) network of tubules and vesicles in cytoplasm

endorphin (en-DOR-fin) any of a group of chemicals in the central nervous system that influence pain perception; a natural painkiller

endosteum (en-DOS-tee-um) a fibrous membrane that lines the medullary cavity

endothelium (en-doh-THEE-lee-um) squamous epithelial cells that line the inner surface of the entire circulatory system and the vessels of the lymphatic system

endotracheal intubation (en-doh-TRAY-kee-al in-too-BAY-shun) medical procedure in which a hollow tube is placed through the neck and directly into the trachea to allow airflow

endurance training (en-DOO-runts TRAYN-ing) continuous vigorous exercise requiring the body to increase its consumption of oxygen and developing the muscles' ability to sustain activity over a prolonged period

energy level (EN-er-jee LEH-vel) limited region surrounding the nucleus of an atom at a certain distance containing electrons; also called a *shell*

enkephalin (en-KEF-ah-lin) peptide chemical in the central nervous system that acts as a natural painkiller

enuresis (en-yoo-REE-siss) see **urinary incontinence**

enzyme (EN-zyme) a functional protein acting as a biochemical catalyst, allowing chemical reactions to take place in a suitable time frame

eosinophil (ee-oh-SIN-oh-fil) white blood cell that is readily stained by eosin

epicardium (ep-ih-KAR-dee-um) the inner layer of the pericardium that covers the surface of the heart; also called the *visceral pericardium*

epidemiologist (ep-ih-dee-mee-OL-uh-jist) scientist engaged in the study, prevention, and treatment of the occurrence, distribution, and transmission of diseases in human populations

epidermis (ep-ih-DER-mis) "false" skin; outermost layer of the skin

epididymis (ep-ih-DID-ih-mis) tightly coiled tube that lies along the top and behind the testes where sperm mature and develop the ability to swim

epigastric region (ep-ih-GAS-trik REE-jun) superior, center region of nine regions of the abdominopelvic cavity, as identified by a "tic-tac-toe" grid laid out over the abdominopelvic area; found just inferior to the sternum

epiglottis (ep-ih-GLOT-is) lidlike cartilage overhanging the entrance to the larynx

epinephrine (ep-ih-NEF-rin) adrenaline; secretion of the adrenal medulla

epineurium (ep-ih-NOO-ree-um) a tough fibrous sheath that covers the whole nerve

epiphyseal fracture (ep-ih-FEEZ-ee-al FRAK-cher) when the epiphyseal plate is separated from the epiphysis or diaphysis; can disrupt the normal growth of the bone

epiphyseal line (ep-ih-FEEZ-ee-al lyne) faint line remaining after the epiphysis fuses with the diaphysis

epiphyseal plate (ep-ih-FEEZ-ee-al) the cartilage plate that is between the epiphysis and the diaphysis and allows growth to occur; sometimes referred to as a *growth plate*

epiphysis (eh-PIF-ih-sis) (*pl.*, epiphyses) ends of a long bone

episiotomy (eh-piz-ee-OT-oh-mee) a surgical procedure used during birth to prevent a laceration of the mother's perineum or the vagina

epithelial membrane (ep-ih-THEE-lee-al MEM-brayn) membrane composed of epithelial tissue with an underlying layer of connective tissue

epithelial tissue (ep-ih-THEE-lee-al TISH-yoo) covers the body and its parts; lines various parts of the body; forms continuous sheets that contain no blood vessels; classified according to shape and arrangement

ergonomics (er-goh-NOM-iks) applied study of workers and their work environment

erythroblastosis fetalis (eh-rith-roh-blas-TOH-sis feh-TAL-is) a disease that may develop when an Rh-negative mother has anti-Rh antibodies and gives birth to an Rh-positive baby and the antibodies react with the Rh-positive cells of the baby

erythrocyte (eh-RITH-roh-syte) red blood cell

erythropoietin (EPO) (eh-RITH-roh-POY-eh-tin [ee-pee-oh]) hormone secreted to increase red blood cell production in response to oxygen deficiency

esophagus (eh-SOF-ah-gus) the muscular, mucus-lined tube that connects the pharynx with the stomach; also known as the *foodpipe*

essential organ (ee-SEN-shal OR-gan) any reproductive organ that must be present for reproduction to occur and is known as a **gonad**

estrogen (ES-troh-jen) sex hormone secreted by the ovary that causes the development and maintenance of the female secondary sex characteristics and stimulates growth of the epithelial cells lining the uterus

eupnea (YOOP-nee-ah) normal respiration
eustachian tube (yoo-STAY-shun toob) see **auditory tube**
evaporation (ee-vap-oh-RAY-shun) heat being lost from the skin by sweat being vaporized
eversion (ee-VER-zhen) foot movement that turns the ankle so that the sole faces out to the side
evert (ee-VERT) to turn outward
exercise physiologist (EK-ser-syze fiz-ee-OL-uh-jist) scientist who studies the process of muscular exercise and related phenomena
exhalation (eks-hah-LAY-shun) moving air out of the lungs; also known as **expiration**
exocrine (EK-soh-krin) secreting into a duct; opposite of endocrine
exocrine gland (EK-soh-krin gland) glands that secrete their products into ducts that empty onto a surface or into a cavity; for example, sweat glands
experimental control (eks payr-uh-MEN-tul kon-TROHL) any procedure within a scientific experiment that ensures that the test situation itself is not affecting the outcome of the experiment
experimentation (eks-payr-uh-men-TAY-shen) performing an experiment, which is usually a test of a tentative explanation of nature called a **hypothesis**
expiration (eks-pih-RAY-shun) moving air out of the lungs; also known as **exhalation**
expiratory center (eks-PYE-rah-tor-ee) one of the two most important respiratory control centers, located in the medulla
expiratory muscle (eks-PYE-rah-tor-ee) any of the muscles that allow more forceful expiration to increase the rate and depth of ventilation; the internal intercostals and the abdominal muscles
expiratory reserve volume (ERV) (eks-PYE-rah-tor-ee ree-ZURV VOL-yoom [ee ar vee]) the amount of air that can be forcibly exhaled after expiring the tidal volume (TV)
extend (eks-TEND) straighten a bend; see **extension**
extension (ek-STEN-shun) increasing the angle between two bones at a joint
external acoustic canal (eks-TER-nal ak-OOS-tik) a curved tube (approximately 2.5 cm) extending from the auricle into the temporal bone, ending at the tympanic membrane
external auditory canal (eks-TER-nal AW-dih-toh-ree) another name for **external acoustic canal**
external ear (eks-TER-nal eer) the outer part of the ear that is made up of the auricle and the external acoustic canal
external genitalia (eks-TER-nal jen-ih-TAYL-yah) external reproductive organs
external intercostal (eks-TER-nal in-ter-KOS-tal) any of the inspiratory muscles between the ribs that enlarge the thorax, causing the lungs to expand and air to rush in
external nares (eks-TER-nal NAY-reez) nostrils
external oblique (eks-TER-nal oh-BLEEK) the outermost layer of the anterolateral abdominal wall
external otitis (eks-TER-nal oh-TYE-tis) a common infection of the external ear; also known as *swimmer's ear*
external respiration (eks-TER-nal res-pih-RAY-shun) the exchange of gases between air in the lungs and in the blood
extracellular fluid (ECF) (eks-trah-SEL-yoo-lar FLOO-id [ee see ef]) the water found outside of cells located in two compartments between cells (interstitial fluid) and in the blood (plasma)

F

face (fays) anterior aspect of the head or skull
facial (FAY-shal) referring to the face
fallen arch (FALL-en arch) condition in which the tendons and ligaments of the foot weaken, allowing the normally curved arch to flatten out
fallopian tube (fal-LOH-pee-an toob) either of the pair of tubes that conduct the ovum from the ovary to the uterus; also called **uterine tubes**
false rib (fawls rib) member of the eighth, ninth, and tenth pairs of ribs that are attached to the cartilage of the seventh ribs rather than the sternum
fascia (FAY-shah) general name for the fibrous connective tissue masses located throughout the body, surrounding various organs
fascicle (FAS-ih-kul) small bundle of fibers, as in a small bundle of nerve fibers or muscle fibers
fasciculus (fah-SIK-yoo-lus) little bundle
fat one of the three basic food types; primarily a source of energy
fatigue (fah-TEEG) loss of muscle power; weakness
fat tissue (fat TISH-yoo) adipose tissue; specialized to store lipids
fatty acid (FAT-tee AS-id) product of fat digestion; building block of fat molecules
feces (FEE-seez) waste material discharged from the intestines
feedback loop a highly complex and integrated communication control network, classified as negative or positive; negative feedback loops are the most important and most numerous homeostatic control mechanisms
femoral (FEM-or-al) referring to the thigh
femur (FEE-mur) the thigh bone, which is the longest bone in the body
fertilization (FER-tih-lih-ZAY-shun) the moment the female's ovum and the male's sperm cell unite
fetal alcohol syndrome (FAS) (FEE-tal AL-koh-hol SIN-drohm [ef ay es]) a condition that may cause congenital abnormalities in a baby that results from a woman consuming alcohol during pregnancy
fetal phase (FEE-tal fayz) period extending from the eighth to the thirty-ninth week of gestation; during this phase the term *fetus* is used
fetus (FEE-tus) unborn young, especially in the later stages; in human beings, from the third month of the intrauterine period until birth
fever (FEE-ver) a form of inflammatory response characterized by abnormally elevated body temperature
fiber (FYE-ber) threadlike structure; for example, collagen fiber, nerve fiber, or muscle fiber
fibrin (FYE-brin) insoluble protein in clotted blood

fibrinogen (fye-BRIN-oh-jen) soluble blood protein that is converted to insoluble fibrin during clotting

fibrocartilage (fye-broh-KAR-tih-lij) cartilage with the greatest number of collagenous fibers; strongest and most durable type of cartilage

fibrous connective tissue (FYE-brus koh-NEK-tiv) strong, nonstretchable, white collagen fibers that compose tendons

fibula (FIB-yoo-lah) the slender non–weight-bearing bone located on the lateral aspect of the leg

fibularis group (fib-YOO-lay-ris groop) leg muscles that plantar flexes and everts the foot; formerly called **peroneous group**

fight-or-flight response (fyte or flyte reh-SPONTS) the changes produced by increased sympathetic impulses allowing the body to deal with any type of stress

filtration (fil-TRAY-shun) movement of water and solutes through a membrane by a higher hydrostatic pressure on one side

fimbria (FIM-bree-ah [FIM-bree-ee]) (*pl.,* fimbriae) fringe-like appendages that surround the distal ends of the uterine tubes or other structures

first-degree burn (first deh-GREE bern) minor burn with only minimal discomfort and no blistering; epidermis may peel but no dermal injury occurs

flagellum (flah-JEL-um [flah-JEL-ah]) (*pl.,* flagella) single projection extending from the cell surface; only example in humans is the "tail" of the male sperm

flat bone (flat bohn) one of the four types of bone; the frontal bone is an example of a flat bone

flat feet condition in which the tendons and ligaments of the foot weaken, allowing the normally curved arch to flatten out

flex (fleks) bend; see **flexion**

flexion (FLEK-shun) act of bending; decreasing the angle between two bones at the joint

floating rib (FLOHT-ing rib) member of the eleventh and twelfth pairs of ribs, which are attached only to the thoracic vertebrae

fluid balance (FLOO-id BAL-ans) homeostasis of fluids; the volumes of interstitial fluid, intracellular fluid, and plasma and total volume of water remain relatively constant

fluid compartment (FLOO-id kom-PART-ment) any of the areas in the body where the fluid is located; for example, interstitial fluid or intracellular fluid

follicle (FOL-lih-kul) a pocketlike structure, such as the cylindrical pocket from which a hair grows

follicle-stimulating hormone (FSH) (FOL-lih-kul STIM-yoo-lay-ting HOHR-mohn [ef es aych]) hormone present in males and females; in males, FSH stimulates the production of sperm; in females, FSH stimulates the ovarian follicles to mature and follicle cells to secrete estrogen

fontanel (FON-tah-nel) "soft spot" on an infant's head, from which new bone develops; unossified areas in the infant skull

food science (food SYE-ens) study of the characteristics of food and effects of storing, handling, and preparing food

foramen (foh-RAY-men) small opening; for example, the vertebral foramen, which allows the spinal cord to pass through the vertebral canal

foramen ovale (foh-RAY-men oh-VAL-ee) shunts blood from the right atrium directly into the left atrium, allowing most blood to bypass the baby's developing lungs

forensic science (foh-REN-zik SYE-ens) field of scientific investigation applied to legal questions, such as cause of death, crime scene investigation, and related matters

foreskin (FORE-skin) a loose-fitting retractable casing located over the glans of the penis; also known as the **prepuce**

formed element (formd EL-eh-ment) any of the cells of blood tissue

fourth-degree burn (forth deh-GREE bern) a full-thickness burn that destroys both dermis and epidermis and also extends below the subcutaneous tissue to damage underlying tissues such as muscles or bone

fovea centralis (FOH-vee-ah sen-TRAL-iss) small depression in the macula lutea where cones are most densely packed; vision is sharpest where light rays focus on the fovea

fractal geometry (FRAK-tul jee-OM-eh-tree) the study of surfaces with a seemingly infinite area, such as the lining of the small intestine

free nerve ending (free nerv END-ing) type of simple, unencapsulated sensory receptor in the skin that responds to pain

free radical (free RAD-ih-kel) an atom or molecule with one or more unpaired electrons, making it highly reactive and therefore potentially damaging to other molecules in the body

frenulum (FREN-yoo-lum) the thin membrane that attaches the tongue to the floor of the mouth

frontal (FRON-tal) lengthwise plane running from side to side, dividing the body into anterior and posterior portions

frontal muscle (FRON-tal MUS-el) one of the muscles of facial expression; it moves the eyebrows and furrows the skin of the forehead

frontal plane (FRUN-tall playn) lengthwise section or plane running from side to side, dividing the body into anterior and posterior portions; also called *coronal plane*

frontal sinusitis (FRON-tal sye-nyoo-SYE-tis) inflammation in the frontal sinus

fructose (FROOK-tohs) simple sugar (monosaccharide) often found in fruits

full-thickness burn burn that (1) destroys epidermis, dermis, and subcutaneous tissue (see **third-degree burn**); and (2) extends below skin and subcutaneous tissue to reach muscle and bone (see **fourth-degree burn**)

functional protein (FUNK-shen-al PROH-teen) category of proteins that affect the functional operations of a cell; contrast with **structural protein**

fundus (FUN-duss) part of the organ opposite of its main opening; the base of an organ, opposite the apex of the organ

G

galactose (gah-LAK-tohs) simple sugar (monosaccharide) found in lactose (milk sugar)

gallbladder (GAWL-blad-er) hollow sac connected to the common bile duct and that stores and concentrates bile

gallstone (GAWL-stohn) solid concretion or stone, often composed of cholesterol or bile salts, found in the gallbladder or common bile duct

gamete (GAM-eet) either of the two sex cells, sperm cells (spermatozoa) from the male or eggs (ova) from the female

ganglion (GANG-lee-on) (*pl.*, ganglia) a region of gray (unmyelinated) nerve tissue (usually this term is used only for gray matter regions in the PNS)

ganglion cell (GANG-glee-on sel) type of sensory neuron in the retina of the eye that collect information from rods and cones and also act as photoreceptors themselves

gastric gland (GAS-trik gland) any of the many tiny glands in the stomach lining that secrete enzymes, mucus, and hydrochloric acid

gastritis (gas-TRY-tiss) pain and inflammation of the stomach lining

gastrocnemius (GAS-trok-NEE-mee-us) superficial muscle of the calf of the leg, connected (along with the soleus muscle) to the calcaneus bone of the foot by way of the Achilles (calcaneal) tendon; its action is to dorsiflex the foot, bending the toes upward

gastroenterology (gas-troh-en-ter-OL-oh-jee) study and treatment of the stomach and intestines and their diseases

gastroesophageal reflux disease (GERD) (GAS-troh-eh-sof-eh-jee-al REE-fluks [gerd]) also known as GERD, a set of symptoms resulting from a hiatal hernia that allows stomach (gastric) contents to flow back (reflux) into the esophagus; symptoms include heartburn or chest pain and coughing or choking during or just after a meal

gastroesophageal sphincter (GAS-troh-eh-sof-eh-jee-al SFINK-ter) a ring of smooth muscle around the opening of the stomach at the lower end of the esophagus that acts as a valve to allow food to enter the stomach but prevents stomach contents from moving back into the esophagus; also called **cardiac sphincter** or **lower esophageal sphincter (LES)**

gastrointestinal (GI) tract (GAS-troh-in-TES-tih-nul [jee aye] trakt) principal tubelike structure of the digestive system extending from mouth to anus; sometimes called the **alimentary canal**

gene (jean) one of many segments of a chromosome (DNA molecule); each gene contains the genetic code for synthesizing a protein molecule such as an enzyme or hormone

general senses (JEN-er-al SEN-sez) senses detected by simple, microscopic receptors widely distributed throughout the body (skin, muscles, tendons, joints, etc.) involving modes of pain, temperature, touch, pressure, or body position

genetic counselor (jeh-NET-ik KOWN-se-lor) science professional who consults with families regarding genetic diseases

genetic engineer (jeh-NET-ik en-juh-NEER) someone who specializes in manipulating the genetic code

genetics (jeh-NET-iks) the science of heredity and genetic information

genital (JEN-ih-tal) (*pl.*, genitalia or genitals) an external reproductive organ

genome (JEE-nohm) entire set of chromosomes in a cell; the human genome refers to the entire set of human chromosomes

genomics (jeh-NOH-miks) field of endeavor involving the analysis of the genetic code contained in the human or other species' genome

geriatrics (jayr-ee-A-triks) medical speciality that focuses on treatment of the elderly

gerontology (jayr-on-TOL-oh-jee) study of the aging process

gestation period (jes-TAY-shun PEER-ee-ed) the length of pregnancy, approximately 9 months in humans

ghrelin (GRAY-lin) hormone secreted by epithelial cells lining the stomach; boosts appetite, slows metabolism, and reduces fat burning; may be involved in the development of obesity

gigantism (jye-GAN-tiz-em) a condition produced by hypersecretion of growth hormone during the early years of life; results in a child who grows to gigantic size

gingiva (JIN-jih-vah) (*pl.*, gingivae) the gum or membrane of the jaw, around the base of the teeth

gingivitis (jin-jih-VYE-tis) inflammation of the gum (gingiva), often caused by poor oral hygiene

gland secreting structure

glandular epithelium (GLAN-dyoo-lar ep-ih-THEE-lee-um) cells that are specialized for secreting activity

glans (glanz) the sensitive distal end or "head" of the shaft of the penis or the clitoris

glaucoma (glaw-KOH-mah) disorder characterized by elevated pressure in the eye

glia (GLEE-ah) supporting cells of nervous tissue; also called *neuroglia*

gliding joint (GLY-ding joynt) type of diarthrotic joint formed by flat surfaces that glide past each other

glioma (glee-OH-mah) one of the most common types of brain tumors

globulin (GLOB-yoo-lin) a type of plasma protein that includes antibodies

glomerular filtrate (gloh-MER-yoo-lar FIL-trayt) water and dissolved substances forced out of the blood in the glomerular capillaries and into Bowman capsule

glomerulus (gloh-MER-yoo-lus) compact cluster; for example, capillaries in the kidneys

glottis (GLOT-iss) the space between the vocal cords

glucagon (GLOO-kah-gon) hormone secreted by alpha cells of the pancreatic islets

glucocorticoid (GC) (gloo-koh-KOHR-tih-koyd [jee see]) category of hormones that influences food metabolism; secreted by the adrenal cortex

gluconeogenesis (gloo-koh-nee-oh-JEN-eh-sis) formulation of glucose or glycogen from protein or fat compounds

glucose (GLOO-kohs) monosaccharide or simple sugar; the principal blood sugar

gluteal (GLOO-tee-al) of or near the buttocks

gluteus maximus (GLOO-tee-us MAX-ih-mus) major extensor of the thigh and also supports the torso in an erect position

glycerol (GLIS-er-ol) product of fat digestion
glycogen (GLYE-koh-jen) polysaccharide made up of a chain of glucose (monosaccharide) molecules; animal starch
glycogenesis (glye-koh-JEN-eh-sis) formation of glycogen from glucose or from other monosaccharides, fructose, or galactose
glycogen loading (GLYE-koh-jen LOHD-ing) see **carbohydrate loading**
glycogenolysis (glye-koh-jeh-NOL-ih-sis) hydrolysis of glycogen to glucose 6-phosphate or to glucose
glycolysis (glye-KOHL-ih-sis) the first series of chemical reactions in glucose metabolism; changes glucose to pyruvic acid in a series of anaerobic reactions
glycosuria (glye-koh-SOO-ree-ah) glucose in the urine; a sign of diabetes mellitus
goblet cell (GOB-let) specialized cell found in simple columnar epithelium that produces mucus
goiter (GOY-ter) enlargement of the thyroid gland
Golgi apparatus (GOL-jee ap-ah-RAH-tus) small sacs stacked on one another near the nucleus that makes carbohydrate compounds, combines them with protein molecules, and packages the product in a globule
Golgi tendon receptors (GOL-jee TEN-don ree-SEP-torz) sensors that are responsible for proprioception
gonad (GOH-nad) sex gland in which reproductive cells (gametes) are formed
gonadotropin-releasing hormone (GnRH) (goh-nah-doh-TROH-pin ree-LEEZ-ing HOHR-mohn [jee en ar aych]) hormone released by the hypothalamus that triggers the secretion of FSH and LH (gonadotropins) from the anterior pituitary gland
G protein (jee PROH-teen) a protein molecule usually embedded in a cell's plasma membrane that plays an important role in getting a signal from a receptor (also in the plasma membrane) to the inside of the cell
graafian follicle (GRAH-fee-en FOL-lih-kul) a mature ovum in its sac
gradient (GRAY-dee-ent) a slope or difference between two levels; for example, blood pressure gradient is the difference between the blood pressure in two different vessels
gram the unit of measure in the metric system on which mass is based (approximately 454 grams equals 1 pound)
granular leukocyte (GRAN-yoo-lar LOO-koh-syte) leukocyte with granules in cytoplasm when stained
granulosa cell (gran-yoo-LOH-sah sel) cell layer surrounding the oocyte
gray matter tissue comprising cell bodies and unmyelinated axons and dendrites
greater omentum (oh-MEN-tum) a pouchlike extension of the visceral peritoneum
greater vestibular gland (ves-TIB-yoo-lar) either of the glands located on each side of the vaginal outlet; secretes mucuslike lubricating fluid; also known as **Bartholin gland**
growth hormone (HOHR-mohn) hormone secreted by the anterior pituitary gland that controls the rate of skeletal and visceral growth
guanine (GWAH-neen) one of the nitrogenous bases of the nucleotides in RNA, DNA, and related molecules; abbreviated *g* or *G*
gustation (gus-TAY-shun) the process of tasting
gustatory cell (GUS-tah-tor-ee sel) cells of taste; chemoreceptors
gynecologist (gye-neh-KOL-uh-jist) physician specializing in medicine of the female reproductive system
gyrus (JYE-rus) (*pl.,* gyri) ridge

H

hair follicle (hayr FOL-lih-kul) a small tube where hair growth occurs
hair papilla (hayr pah-PIL-ah) a small, cap-shaped cluster of cells located at the base of the follicle where hair growth begins
hamstring muscle (HAM-string MUS-el) any of the powerful flexors of the hip; the hamstring group is made up of the semimembranosus, semitendinosus, and biceps femoris muscles
hard palate (hard PAL-let) hard, bony, anterior portion of roof of mouth formed by parts of palatine and maxillary bones
haversian canal (ha-VER-zhun or HAV-er-zhen kah-NAL) the canal in the haversian system that contains a blood vessel; also called *central canal*
haversian system (hah-VER-zhun or HAV-er-zhen SIS-tem) the circular arrangements of calcified matrix and cells that give bone its characteristic appearance
heart block (hart blok) a blockage of impulse conduction from atria to ventricles so that the heart beats at a slower than normal rate
heartburn (HART-burn) burning sensation characterized by pain and a feeling of fullness beneath the sternum; caused by the esophageal mucosa being irritated by stomach acid
heart rate (HR) (hart rayt [aych ar]) rate (beats per minute) of cardiac cycle
Heimlich maneuver (HIME-lik mah-NOO-ver) lifesaving technique used to free the trachea of objects blocking the airway
Helicobacter pylori (HEEL-ih-koh-BAK-ter pye-LOH-ree) type of bacteria that may cause damage to the stomach lining leading to the formation of ulcers
hematocrit (Hct) (hee-MAT-oh-krit [aych see tee]) volume percent of blood cells in whole blood
hematology (hee-mah-TOL-oh-jee) study or medical treatment of blood and blood disorders
hematopoiesis (hee-MA-toh-poy-EE-sis) blood cell formation
hematopoietic tissue (hee-MAH-toh-poy-EE-tik) type of connective tissue that is responsible for the formation of blood cells and lymphatic system cells; found in red bone marrow, spleen, tonsils, and lymph nodes
heme (HEEM) iron-containing component of hemoglobin molecule

hemodialysis (hee-moh-dye-AL-ih-sis) use of dialysis to separate waste products from the blood
hemodynamics (hee-moh-dye-NAM-iks) study of mechanisms of blood flow
hemoglobin (Hb) (hee-moh-GLOH-bin [aych bee]) iron-containing protein in red blood cells
hemolytic anemia (hee-moh-LIT-ik) inherited blood disorder that is characterized by abnormal types of **hemoglobin**
hemorrhagic anemia (HEM-oh-raj-ick ah-NEE-mee-ah) condition characterized by low oxygen-carrying capacity of blood; caused by decreased red blood cell (RBC) life span and/or increased rate of RBC destruction
hemostasis (hee-moh-STAY-sis) stoppage of blood flow
Henle loop (HEN-lee loop) see **nephron loop**
heparin (HEP-ah-rin) substance obtained from the liver; inhibits blood clotting
hepatic duct (heh-PAT-ik) any of the small tubes that drain bile out of the liver
hepatic flexure (heh-PAT-ik FLEK-sher) the bend between the ascending colon and the transverse colon; also called *hepatic colic flexure* or *right colic flexure*
hepatic portal circulation (heh-PAT-ik POR-tal ser-kyoo-LAY-shun) the route of blood flow through the liver
hepatic portal vein (heh-PAT-ik POR-tal vayn) delivers blood directly from the gastrointestinal tract to the liver
hepatitis (hep-ah-TYE-tis) inflammation of the liver due to viral or bacterial infection, injury, damage from alcohol, drugs, or other toxins, or other factors
herpes zoster (HER-peez ZOS-ter) "shingles," viral infection that affects the skin of a single dermatome
hiatal hernia (hye-AY-tal HER-nee-ah) a bulging out (hernia) of the stomach through the opening (hiatus) of the diaphragm through which the esophagus normally passes; this condition may prevent the valve between the esophagus and stomach from closing, thus allowing stomach contents to flow back into the esophagus; see **gastroesophageal reflux disease**
hiccup (HIK-up) involuntary spasmodic contraction of the diaphragm
hilum (HYE-lum) (*pl.,* hila) small opening on the side of an organ (lung, kidney, lymph node) to allow vessels and nerves to enter/exit
hinge joint (hinj joynt) type of diarthrotic synovial joint that allows movement around a single axis in the manner of a hinge
hip the joint connecting the legs to the trunk; pelvic girdle
histamine (HIS-tah-meen) inflammatory chemical
histogenesis (his-toh-JEN-eh-sis) formation of tissues from primary germ layers of embryo
histologist (hih-STOL-uh-jist) scientist that studies tissue structure and function
homeostasis (hoh-mee-oh-STAY-sis) relative uniformity of the normal body's internal environment
homeostatic mechanism (hoh-mee-oh-STAT-ik MEK-ah-niz-em) a system that maintains a constant environment enabling body cells to function effectively
hormone (HOHR-mohn) substance secreted by an endocrine gland
human immunodeficiency virus (HIV) (HYOO-man ih-myoo-noh-deh-FISH-en-see VYE-rus [aych aye vee]) the retrovirus that causes acquired immunodeficiency syndrome (AIDS)
humerus (HYOO-mer-us) the second longest bone in the body; the long bone of the arm
humoral immunity (HYOO-mor-al ih-MYOO-nih-tee) see **antibody-mediated immunity**
hyaline cartilage (HYE-ah-lin KAR-tih-lij) most common type of cartilage; appears gelatinous and glossy
hybridoma (hye-brid-OH-mah) fused or hybrid cells that continue to produce the same antibody as the original lymphocyte
hydrocephalus (hye-droh-SEF-ah-lus) abnormal accumulation of cerebrospinal fluid; "water on the brain"
hydrocortisone (hye-droh-KOHR-tih-zohn) a hormone secreted by the adrenal cortex; cortisol; compound F
hydrogen (H) (HYE-droh-jen [aych]) element 1
hydrogen bond (HYE-droh-jen) weak chemical bond that occurs between the partial positive charge on a hydrogen atom covalently bound to a nitrogen or oxygen atom and the partial negative charge of another polar molecule
hydrogen ion (HYE-droh-jen eye-on) found in water and water solutions; produces an acidic solution; H^+
hydrolysis (hye-DROL-ih-sis) chemical reaction in which water is added to a large molecule, causing it to break apart into smaller molecules
hydrostatic pressure (hye-droh-STAT-ik) the force of a fluid pushing against some surface
hydroxide ion (hye-DROK-side EYE-on) found in water and water solutions; produces an alkaline solution; chemical notation is OH^-
hymen (HYE-men) Greek for "membrane"; mucous membrane that encircles the distal vagina and that may partially or entirely occlude the vaginal outlet
hyoid bone (HYE-oyd bohn) U-shaped bone of the neck between the mandible and the larynx, not articulating with any other bone
hyperacidity (hye-per-ah-SID-ih-tee) excessive secretion of acid; an important factor in the formation of ulcers
hypercalcemia (hye-per-kal-SEE-mee-ah) a condition in which there is harmful excess of calcium in the blood
hyperglycemia (hye-per-glye-SEE-mee-ah) higher than normal blood glucose concentration
hyperkalemia (hy-per-kal-EE-mee-ah) excessive potassium in the blood
hypernatremia (hy-per-nah-TREE-mee-ah) excessive sodium in the blood
hyperopia (hye-per-OH-pee-ah) farsightedness
hyperplasia (hye-per-PLAY-zee-ah) growth of an abnormally large number of cells at a local site, as in a neoplasm or tumor
hypersecretion (hye-per-seh-KREE-shun) too much of a substance is being secreted

hypertension (HTN) (hye-per-TEN-shun [aych tee en]) abnormally high blood pressure

hyperthyroidism (hye-per-THYE-royd-iz-em) oversecretion of thyroid hormones that increases metabolic rate, resulting in loss of weight, increased appetite, and nervous irritability

hypertonic (hye-per-TON-ik) a solution containing a higher level of salt (NaCl) than is found in a living red blood cell (above 0.9% NaCl)

hypertrophy (hye-PER-troh-fee) increased size of a part caused by an increase in the size of its cells

hyperventilation (hye-per-ven-tih-LAY-shun) very rapid deep respirations

hypervitaminosis (hye-per-vye-tah-mih-NOH-sis) condition caused by excess amounts of vitamins; usually associated with the use of vitamin supplements

hypocalcemia (hye-poh-kal-SEE-mee-ah) abnormally low calcium levels in the blood

hypochondriac regions (hy-poh-KON-dree-ak) far left and right superior corner regions of nine regions of the abdominopelvic cavity, as identified by a "tic-tac-toe" grid laid out over the abdominopelvic area; located partly beneath the cartilage of the lower rib cage

hypodermis (hye-poh-DER-mis) the loose, ordinary (areolar) tissue just under the skin and superficial to the muscles; also called **subcutaneous tissue** or *superficial fascia*

hypogastric region (hye-poh-GAS-trik) inferior, center region of nine regions of the abdominopelvic cavity, as identified by a "tic-tac-toe" grid laid out over the abdominopelvic area; located approximately in the central pelvic area

hypoglycemia (hye-poh-glye-SEE-mee-ah) lower-than-normal blood glucose concentration

hypokalemia (hye-poh-kal-EE-mee-ah) abnormally low blood potassium level

hyponatremia (hye-poh-nah-TREE-mee-ah) abnormally low sodium levels in the blood

hyposecretion (hye-poh-seh-KREE-shun) too little of a substance is being secreted

hypothalamus (hye-poh-THAL-ah-muss) vital neuroendocrine and autonomic control center beneath the thalamus

hypothermia (hye-poh-THER-mee-ah) subnormal core body temperature below 37° C

hypothesis (hye-POTH-eh-sis) (*pl.*, hypotheses) a proposed explanation of an observed phenomenon

hypothyroidism (hye-poh-THY-royd-iz-em) undersecretion of thyroid hormones; early in life results in cretinism; later in life results in myxedema

hypotonic (hye-poh-TON-ik) a solution containing a lower level of salt (NaCl) than is found in a living red blood cell (below 0.9% NaCl)

hypoventilation (hye-poh-ven-tih-LAY-shun) slow and shallow respirations

hypovitaminosis (hye-poh-VYTE-ah-min-oh-sis) condition of having too few vitamin molecules in the body for normal function

hypoxia (hye-POCK-see-ah) abnormally low concentration of oxygen in the blood or tissue fluids

hysterectomy (his-teh-REK-toh-mee) surgical removal of the uterus

I

ileocecal valve (il-ee-oh-SEE-kal) the sphincterlike structure between the end of the small intestine and the beginning of the large intestine

ileum (IL-ee-um) the distal portion of the small intestine

iliac crest (IL-ee-ak krest) the superior edge of the ilium

iliac region (IL-ee-ak REE-jen) either of the far left and right inferior corner regions of nine regions of the abdominopelvic cavity, as identified by a "tic-tac-toe" grid laid out over the abdominopelvic area; located in the right or left pelvic areas

iliopsoas (il-ee-op-SOH-us) a flexor of the thigh and an important stabilizing muscle for posture

ilium (IL-ee-um) one of the three separate bones that forms the os coxa

immune system (ih-MYOON) the body's defense system against disease

immunization (ih-myoo-nih-ZAY-shun) deliberate artificial exposure to disease to produce acquired immunity

immunology (im-yoo-NOL-uh-jee) study of the immune system and its actions; medical specialty that treats disorders of immune function

implantation (im-plan-TAY-shun) when a fertilized ovum implants in the uterus

inborn immunity (IN-born ih-MYOO-nih-tee) immunity to disease that is inherited

incisor (in-SYE-zor) one of the four front teeth in each dental arch; each incisor has a crown that is chisel shaped and has a sharp cutting edge for biting off pieces of tough food; prominent in plant-eating animals

incontinence (in-KON-tih-nens) when an individual voids urine involuntarily

incus (IN-kus) the anvil; the middle ear bone that is shaped like an anvil

infancy (IN-fan-see) from birth to about 18 months of age

infant respiratory distress syndrome (IRDS) (IN-fant RES-per-ah-toh-ree dih-STRESS SIN-drohm [aye ar dee es]) leading cause of death in premature babies, due to a lack of surfactant in the alveolar air sacs

infection control (in-FEK-shun KON-trol) any practice intended to limit the spread of infection in a population

inferior lower; opposite of superior

inferior vena cava (VEE-nah KAY-vah) one of two large veins carrying blood into the right atrium

inflammatory response (in-FLAM-ah-toh-ree) nonspecific immune process produced in response to injury and resulting in redness, pain, heat, and swelling and promoting movement of white blood cells to the affected area

ingestion (in-JES-chun) taking in of complex foods, usually by mouth

inguinal (ING-gwih-nal) of the groin

inhalation (in-hah-LAY-shun) inspiration or breathing in; opposite of exhalation or expiration

inherited immunity (in-HAYR-ih-ted ih-MYOO-nih-tee) inborn immunity

inhibiting hormone (IH) (in-HIB-ih-ting HOHR-mohn [aye aych]) hormone produced by the hypothalamus that slows the release of anterior pituitary hormones

innate immunity (in-AYT ih-MYOON-ih-tee) see **nonspecific immunity**

inorganic compound (in-or-GAN-ik KOM-pownd) compound whose molecules do not contain carbon-carbon or carbon-hydrogen bonds

INR (International Normalized Ratio) (aye-en-ar [in-ter-NASH-un-al NORM-uh-lahyzd RAY-shee-oh]) a mathematical calculation reported as a number (normal 0.8 to 1.2) used to standardize the results of anticoagulation testing

insertion (in-SER-shun) attachment of a muscle to the bone that it moves when contraction occurs (as distinguished from its origin)

inspiration (in-spih-RAY-shun) moving air into the lungs; same as inhalation, opposite of exhalation or expiration

inspiratory center (in-SPY-rah-tor-ee) one of the two most important control centers located in the medulla; the other is the expiratory center

inspiratory muscle (in-SPY-rah-tor-ee MUS-el) the muscles that increase the size of the thorax, including the diaphragm and external intercostals, and allow air to rush into the lungs

inspiratory reserve volume (IRV) (in-SPY-rah-tor-ee ree-ZURV VOL-yoom [aye ar vee]) the amount of air that can be forcibly inspired over and above a normal respiration

insulin (IN-suh-lin) hormone secreted by the pancreatic islets

integument (in-TEG-yoo-ment) the skin

integumentary system (in-teg-yoo-MEN-tar-ee) the skin; the largest and most important organ in the body

interarytenoid notch (IN-ter-ar-ih-tee-noyd notch) the V-shaped groove at the median of the posterior margin of the opening of the larynx, between the two arytenoid cartilages of the larynx

intercalated disk (in-TER-kah-lay-ted) any of the disklike cell connections that exist between cardiac muscle fibers

intercostal muscles (in-ter-KOS-tal MUS-els) the respiratory muscles located between the ribs

interferon (in-ter-FEER-on) small proteins produced by the immune system that inhibit virus multiplication

interleukins (ILs) (in-ter-LOO-kinz) any of several intracellular signals (cytokines) released by white blood cells (leukocytes), usually involved in immune responses

internal oblique (in-TER-nal oh-BLEEK) the middle layer of the anterolateral abdominal walls

internal respiration (in-TER-nal res-pih-RAY-shun) the exchange of gases that occurs between the blood and cells of the body

interneuron (in-ter-NOO-ron) nerve that conducts impulses from sensory neurons to motor neurons; sometimes called a *central* or *connecting neuron*

interphase (IN-ter-fayz) the phase immediately before the visible stages of cell division when the DNA of each chromosome replicates itself

interstitial cell (in-ter-STISH-al) small endocrine cells in the testes that secrete the male sex hormone, testosterone

interstitial cell-stimulating hormone (ICSH) (in-ter-STISH-al sel STIM-yoo-lay-ting HOHR-mohn [aye see es aych]) name by which luteinizing hormone (as produced in males) was previously known; causes testes to develop and secrete testosterone

interstitial fluid (IF) (in-ter-STISH-al FLOO-id [aye ef]) fluid located in the microscopic spaces between the cells

intestinal gland (in-TES-tih-nal gland) any of thousands of glands found in the mucous membrane of the mucosa of the small intestines; secretes intestinal digestive juice

intracellular fluid (ICF) (in-tra-SEL-yoo-lar FLOO-id [aye-see-ef]) a fluid located within the cells; largest fluid compartment

intramembranous ossification (in-trah-MEM-brah-nus os-ih-fih-KAY-shun) process by which most flat bones are formed within connective tissue membranes

intraocular pressure (in-trah-OK-yoo-lar PRESH-ur) fluid pressure within the eyeball

intravenous (IV) technician (in-trah-VEE-nus [aye vee] tek-NISH-en) health-care professional specializing in preparation and administration of therapeutic fluids and medicines into veins

intrinsic factor (in-TRIN-sik FAK-ter) substance that binds to molecules of vitamin B_{12}, protecting them from the acids and enzymes of the stomach; secreted by parietal cells of gastric glands

inversion (in-VER-zhen) foot movement that turns the ankle so that the sole faces inward toward the midline of the body

invert (in-VERT) move the foot so that the sole faces inward toward the midline of the body; any turning inward or back upon itself

in vitro (in VEE-troh) refers to the glass laboratory container in which a mature ovum is fertilized by a sperm

involuntary muscle (in-VOL-un-tayr-ee MUS-el) smooth muscles that are not under conscious control and are found in hollow organs such as the stomach and small intestine

involution (in-voh-LOO-shun) return of an organ to its normal size after an enlargement; also retrograde or degenerative change

I&O (aye and oh) abbreviation used in clinical medicine to indicate the measurement of fluid intake and urine output over a period of time

ion (EYE-on) electrically charged atom or group of atoms

ion pump (EYE-on) a cellular membrane component that moves ions from an area of low concentration to an area of high concentration

ionic bond (eye-ON-ik) chemical bond formed by the positive-negative attraction between two ions

iris (EYE-ris) colored portion of the eye

iron deficiency anemia (EYE-ern deh-FISH-en-see ah-NEE-mee-ah) condition in which there are inadequate levels of iron in the diet so that less hemoglobin is produced; results in extreme fatigue

ischium (IS-kee-um) one of three separate bones that form the os coxa

isometric contraction (eye-soh-MET-rik kon-TRAK-shen) type of muscle contraction in which muscle does not shorten

isotonic (eye-soh-TON-ik) relating to the same pressure or tension; for example, isotonic solutions have the same osmotic pressure

isotonic contraction (eye-soh-TON-ik kon-TRAK-shen) contraction in which the length changes, but the tension seems to be about the same; a mobilizing kind of contraction

IV technician (aye vee tek-NISH-en) see **intravenous (IV) technician**

J

jaundice (JAWN-dis) abnormal yellowing of skin, mucous membranes, and white of eyes

jejunum (jeh-JOO-num) the middle third of the small intestine

joints (joynts) articulation

juxtaglomerular (JG) apparatus (juks-tah-gloh-MER-yoo-lar [jay jee] app-ah-RAT-us) in the nephron, the complex of cells from the distal tubule and the afferent arteriole, which helps regulate blood pressure by secreting renin in response to blood pressure changes in the kidney; located near the glomerulus

juxtamedullary nephron (jux-tah-MED-oo-layr-ee NEF-ron) type of nephron that lies near the junction of the cortical and medullary layers of the kidney and with a nephron loop extending into the medulla

K

Kaposi sarcoma (KS) (KAH-poh-see sar-KOH-mah [kay es]) a malignant neoplasm (cancer) of the skin characterized by purplish spots

keratin (KER-ah-tin) protein substance found in hair, nails, outer skin cells, and horny tissues

keratotomy (kayr-ah-TOT-ah-mee) superficial incisions made on the surface of the cornea, usually to correct vision

ketoacidosis (kee-toh-as-ih-DOH-sis) a condition of abnormally low blood pH (acidity) caused by the presence of an abnormally large number of ketone bodies or "keto acids" that are produced when fats are converted to forms of glucose to be used for cellular respiration; often occurs in diabetes mellitus, when it is more specifically called **diabetic ketoacidosis;** see also **acidosis**

ketone body (KEE-tohn) any of the acidic products of lipid metabolism that may accumulate in blood of individuals with uncontrolled type 1 diabetes

kidney (KID-nee) organ that cleanses the blood of waste products continually produced by metabolism

kilocalorie (Kcal) (KIL-oh-kal-oh-ree [kay kal]) 1000 calories; see **Calorie**

kinesthesia (kin-es-THEE-zee-ah) "muscle sense"; that is, sense of position and movement of body parts

Krause end bulb (KROWZ end bulb) skin receptor that detects sensations of cold

Kupffer cell (KOOP-fer sel) macrophage found in spaces between liver cells

L

labia majora (LAY-bee-ah mah-JOH-rah) (*sing.,* labium majus) "large lips" of the vulva

labia minora (LAY-bee-ah mih-NOH-rah) (*sing.,* labium minus) "small lips" of the vulva

labor (LAY-ber) the process that results in the birth of the baby

laboratory technician (LAB-rah-tor-ee tek-NISH-en) a trained assistant in a medical or scientific laboratory

lacrimal gland (LAK-rih-mal) the glands that produce tears, located in the upper lateral portion of the orbit

lacrimal sac (LAK-rih-mal sak) pouch that collects tears from the eye, and then drains them toward the nasal cavity

lacteal (LAK-tee-al) a lymphatic vessel located in each villus of the intestine; serves to absorb fat materials from the chyme passing through the small intestine

lactiferous duct (lak-TIF-er-us) the duct that drains the grapelike cluster of milk-secreting glands in the breast

lacuna (lah-KOO-nah) (*pl.,* lacunae) space or cavity; for example, lacunae in bone contain bone cells

lambdoidal suture (LAM-doyd-al SOO-chur) the immovable joint formed by the parietal and occipital bones

lamella (lah-MEL-ah) thin layer, as of bone

lamellar corpuscle (lah-MEL-ar KOR-pus-ul) sensory receptor with a layered encapsulation found deep in the dermis that detects pressure on the skin surface; also called *Pacini corpuscle*

lamina propria (LAM-in-ah PROH-pree-ah) fibrous connective tissue underlying the epithelium in mucous membranes

lanugo (lah-NOO-go) the extremely fine and soft hair found on a newborn infant

laparoscope (LAP-ah-roh-skope) medical device that functions as an optical viewing tube for visualizing internal structures

large intestine (larj in-TES-tin) part of GI tract that includes cecum; ascending, transverse, descending, and sigmoid colons; rectum; and anal canal

laryngopharynx (lah-ring-goh-FAYR-inks) the lowest part of the pharynx

larynx (LAYR-inks) the voice box, located just below the pharynx; the largest piece of cartilage making up the larynx is the thyroid cartilage, commonly known as the Adam's apple

LASIK (laser-assisted in situ keratomileusis) (LAY-zer ah-SIS-ted in SYE-too kayr-at-oh-mill-YOO-sis) refractory eye surgery using a microkeratome to cut a corneal cap, which is replaced after an excimer laser is used to vaporize and reshape underlying corneal tissue

lateral (LAT-er-al) of or toward the side; opposite of medial

lateral longitudinal arch (LAT-er-al lawnj-ih-TOOD-in-al arch) outer lengthwise (anteroposterior) support structure of the foot

latissimus dorsi (lah-TIS-ih-muss DOR-sye) an extensor of the arm

law a scientific law is a theory, or explanation of a scientific principle, with an extraordinarily high degree of confidence of scientists based on experimentation

lens (lenz) the refracting mechanism of the eye that is located directly behind the pupil

leptin (LEHP-tin) hormone, secreted by fat-storing cells, that regulates how hungry or full we feel and how fat is metabolized by the body

lesser vestibular gland (Skene gland) (LES-er ves-TIB-yoo-lar gland) tiny mucous gland located near the female's urinary meatus by way of two small ducts; also called *Skene gland*

leukemia (loo-KEE-mee-ah) blood cancer characterized by an increase in white blood cells

leukocyte (LOO-koh-syte) white blood cell

leukocytosis (loo-koh-sye-TOH-sis) abnormally high white blood cell numbers in the blood

leukopenia (loo-koh-PEE-nee-ah) abnormally low white blood cell numbers in the blood

levels of organization (LEV-elz ov or-gan-ih-ZAY-shun) groupings of structural components from microscopic to gross, used as a manner of organizing concepts of biological scale

levodopa (LEV-oh-doh-pah) also called *L-dopa* (el DOH-pah), this chemical is manufactured by the brain cells and then converted to the neurotransmitter dopamine; it has been used to treat disorders involving dopamine deficiencies such as in Parkinson disease

ligament (LIG-ah-ment) bond or band connecting two objects; in anatomy a band of white fibrous tissue connecting bones

limbic system (LIM-bik) a collection of various small regions of the brain that act together to produce emotion and emotional response; sometimes called "the emotional brain"

lingual tonsil (LING-gwal TAHN-sil) mass of lymphoid tissue located in the mucous membrane at the base of the tongue

lipase (LYE-payse) fat-digesting enzymes

lipid (LIP-id) organic molecule usually composed of glycerol and fatty acid units; types include triglycerides, phospholipids, and cholesterol; a fat, wax, or oil

liposuction (LIP-oh-suk-shun or LYE-poh-suk-shun) medical procedure in which adipose tissue is removed from the body by a suction device

lithotripsy (lih-thoh-TRIP-see) use of ultrasound waves to break up kidney stones without making an incision

lithotriptor (LITH-oh-trip-tor) an ultrasound generator that is used to pulverize kidney stones

liver (LIV-er) large, multilobed exocrine gland in the right upper abdominal quadrant, producing bile and having many metabolic functions

liver glycogenolysis (LIV-er glye-koh-jeh-NOL-ih-sis) chemical process by which liver glycogen is converted to glucose

lock-and-key model concept that explains how molecules react when they fit together in a complementary way in the same manner that a key fits into a lock to cause the lock to open or close; the analogy is often used to explain the action of hormones, enzymes, and other biological molecules

longitudinal arch (lon-jih-TOO-dih-nal) two arches, the medial and lateral, that extend lengthwise in the foot

lower esophageal sphincter (LES) (LOH-er eh-SOF-eh-JEE-ul SFINGK-ter [el ee es]) muscle located at the junction between the terminal portion of the esophagus and the stomach; also called *cardiac sphincter*

lower respiratory tract (RES-pih-rah-tor-ee) division of respiratory tract that is within the thorax and is composed of the trachea, all segments of the bronchial tree, and the lungs

lumbar (LUM-bar) lower back, between the ribs and pelvis

lumbar puncture (LUM-bar PUNK-chur) when some cerebrospinal fluid is withdrawn from the subarachnoid space in the lumbar region of the spinal cord

lumbar region (LUM-bar REE-jen) either of the far left and right middle regions of nine regions of the abdominopelvic cavity, as identified by a "tic-tac-toe" grid laid out over the abdominopelvic area; located at approximately the same level as the lumbar vertebrae

lumen (LOO-men) the hollow space within a tube

lung organ of respiration; the right lung has three lobes and the left lung has two lobes

lunula (LOO-nyoo-lah) crescent-shaped white area under the proximal nail bed

luteinization (loo-tee-in-aye-ZAY-shun) the formation of a golden body (corpus luteum) in the ruptured follicle

luteinizing hormone (LH) (LOO-tee-in-AYE-zing HOHR-mohn [el aych]) acts in conjunction with follicle-stimulating hormone (FSH) to stimulate follicle and ovum maturation and release of estrogen and ovulation; known as the *ovulating hormone;* in males, causes testes to develop and secrete testosterone

lymph (limf) watery fluid, formed in the tissue spaces, that returns excess fluid and protein molecules to the blood

lymphatic capillary (lim-FAT-ik CAP-ih-layr-ee) any of the tiny, blind-ended lymph-collecting tubes distributed in the tissue spaces

lymphatic duct (lim-FAT-ik) terminal vessel into which lymphatic vessels empty lymph; the duct then empties the lymph into the circulatory system

lymphatic system (lim-FAT-ik) a system that plays a critical role in the functioning of the immune system; moves fluids and large molecules from the tissue spaces and fat-related nutrients from the digestive system to the blood

lymphatic vessel (lim-FAT-ik VES-el) any of the vessels that carry lymph to its eventual return to the circulatory system

lymph node (limf) performs biological filtration of lymph on its way to the circulatory system
lymphocyte (LIM-foh-syte) type of white blood cell; see **B cell** and **T cell**
lymphoid tissue (LIM-foyd) tissue that is responsible for manufacturing lymphocytes and monocytes; found mostly in the lymph nodes, thymus, and spleen
lyse (lize) disintegration of a cell
lysosome (LYE-soh-sohm) membranous organelles containing various enzymes that can dissolve most cellular compounds; hence called *digestive bags* or *suicide bags* of cells

M

macronutrient (MAK-roh-NOO-tree-ent) nutrient needed in large amounts; carbohydrates, fats, and proteins
macrophage (MAK-roh-fayj) a category of phagocytic cells in the immune system
macula (MAK-yoo-lah) spot of sensory epithelium in the vestibule of the ear; provides information related to head position relative to gravity
macula lutea (MAK-yoo-lah LOOT-ee-ah) yellowish area near center of the retina where cones are densely distributed; also called simply *macula*
malignant (mah-LIG-nant) cancerous growth
major duodenal papilla (MAY-jer doo-oh-DEE-nul [or doo-AH-de-nul] pah-PIL-ah) muscular bump in lining of duodenum where common bile duct enters; also called *greater duodenal papilla*
malleus (MAL-ee-us) hammer; the tiny middle ear bone that is shaped like a hammer
malocclusion (MAL-oh-cloo-zhun) abnormal contact between the teeth of the upper jaw and lower jaw
mammary (MAM-mah-ree) relating to the breast
mammary gland (MAM-mah-ree gland) exocrine gland within the breast; produces milk (lactation)
massage therapy (mah-SAHJ THAYR-ah-pee) pressing, rubbing, or other manipulation of muscle and other soft tissue to prevent or treat a variety of health conditions
masseter (mas-EET-er) large muscle of the cheek, used to lift the lower jaw (mandible) and thus provide chewing movement
mast cell (mast sel) immune system cell to which antibodies become attached in early stages of inflammation
mastication (mas-tih-KAY-shun) chewing
matrix (MAY-triks) the intracellular substance of a tissue; for example, the matrix of bone is calcified, whereas that of blood is liquid
matter any substance that occupies space and has mass
mature follicle (mah-CHUR FOL-lih-kul) see **graafian follicle**
maximum oxygen consumption (VO_{2max}) (MAKS-im-um AHK-si-jen kon-SUMP-shun [vee-oh-too-MAKS]) the maximum amount of oxygen taken up by the lungs, transported to the tissues, and used to do work
mechanoreceptor (mek-an-oh-ree-SEP-tor) receptors that are mechanical in nature; for example, equilibrium and balance sensors in the ears
medial (MEE-dee-al) of or toward the middle; opposite of lateral
medial longitudinal arch (MEE-dee-al lon-jih-TOO-dih-nal arch) inner lengthwise (anteroposterior) support structure of the foot
mediastinum (mee-dee-as-TIH-num) a subdivision in the midportion of the thoracic cavity
medic (MED-ik) member of a military medical corps
medicine (MED-ih-sin) practice of applying scientific principles to the prevention and treatment of health conditions
medulla (meh-DUL-ah) Latin for "marrow"; hence the inner portion of an organ in contrast to the outer portion or cortex
medulla oblongata (meh-DUL-ah ob-long-GAH-tah) the lowest part of the brainstem; an enlarged extension of the spinal cord; the vital centers are located within this area
medullary cavity (MED-yoo-layr-ee KAV-ih-tee) hollow area inside the diaphysis of the bone that contains yellow bone marrow
meiosis (my-OH-sis) nuclear division in which the number of chromosomes is reduced to half the original number; produces gametes
Meissner corpuscle (MYZ-ner KOR-pus-ul) see **tactile corpuscle**
melanin (MEL-ah-nin) brown skin pigment
melanocyte (MEL-ah-noh-syte) specialized cells in the skin that produce the dark brown pigment melanin
melanoma (mel-ah-NOH-mah) a malignant neoplasm (cancer) of the pigment-producing cells of the skin (melanocytes); also called *malignant melanoma*
melatonin (mel-ah-TOH-nin) important hormone produced by the pineal gland that is believed to regulate the onset of puberty and the menstrual cycle; also referred to as the *third eye* because it responds to levels of light and is thought to be involved with the body's internal clock
membrane (MEM-brayn) thin layer or sheet
membranous labyrinth (MEM-brah-nus LAB-ih-rinth) a membranous sac that follows the shape of the bony labyrinth and is filled with endolymph
memory cell (MEM-or-ee sel) cell that remains in reserve in the lymph nodes until its ability to secrete antibodies is needed
menarche (meh-NAR-kee) beginning of the menstrual function
meninges (meh-NIN-jeez) fluid-containing membranes surrounding the brain (*sing.*, meninx) and spinal cord
meniscus (meh-NIS-kus) (*pl.*, menisci) articular cartilage disk
menopause (MEN-oh-pawz) termination of menstrual cycles
menses (MEN-seez) menstrual flow
menstrual cycle (MEN-stroo-al sye-kul) the cyclical changes in the uterine lining
mesentery (MEZ-en-tayr-ee) a large double fold of peritoneal tissue that anchors the loops of the digestive tract to the posterior wall of the abdominal cavity

mesoderm (MEZ-oh-derm) the middle layer of the primary germ layers

messenger RNA (mRNA) (MES-en-jer ar-en-ay [EM-ar-en-ay]) a duplicate copy of a gene sequence on the DNA that passes from the nucleus to the cytoplasm

metabolic acidosis (met-ah-BOL-ik as-ih-DOH-sis) a disturbance affecting the bicarbonate element of the bicarbonate-carbonic acid buffer pair; bicarbonate deficit

metabolic alkalosis (met-ah-BOL-ik al-kah-LOH-sis) disturbance affecting the bicarbonate element of the bicarbonate-carbonic acid buffer pair; bicarbonate excess

metabolic disturbance (met-ah-BOL-ik dih-STUR-buhns) acidosis (low blood pH) or alkalosis (high blood pH) caused by a metabolic dysfunction such as renal disease or diarrhea

metabolism (meh-TAB-oh-liz-em) complex process by which food is used by a living organism

metacarpal (met-ah-KAR-pal) the part of the hand between the wrist and fingers

metallic (meh-TAL-ik) relating to metal

metaphase (MET-ah-fayz) second stage of mitosis, during which the nuclear envelope and nucleolus disappear

metatarsal arch (met-ah-TAR-sal arch) the arch that extends across the ball of the foot; also called the **transverse arch**

metatarsal bone (met-ah-TAR-sal bohn) any of the five bones that form the body of the foot

meter (MEE-ter) a measure of length in the metric system; equal to about 39.5 inches

microbiologist (my-kroh-bye-OL-uh-jist) scientist specializing in the study of microorganisms such as bacteria

microbiome (my-kroh-BYE-ohm) all the interacting ecosystems of microbes (bacteria, fungi, etc.) that live on or in the human body; also called the *human microbiome* or *human microbial system*

microcephaly (my-kroh-SEF-ah-lee) a congenital abnormality in which an infant is born with a small head

microfilaments (my-kroh-FIL-ah-ments) smallest types of fibers in the cytoskeleton of the cell; "cellular muscles"

microglia (my-KROG-lee-ah) one type of connective tissue found in the brain and spinal cord

micron (MY-kron) 1/1000 millimeter; 1/25,000 inch

micronutrient (MY-kroh-NOO-tree-ent) nutrient needed by the body in very small quantity, such as vitamins and minerals

microtubule (my-kroh-TOOB-yool) thick cell fiber (compared to microfilament); hollow tube responsible for movement of substances within the cell or movement of the cell itself

microvilli (my-kroh-VIL-aye) (*sing.*, microvillus) small, moving cell extensions that form the brushlike border made up of epithelial cells found on each villus in the small intestine; increase the surface area for absorption of nutrients

micturition (mik-too-RISH-un) urination, voiding

midbrain (MID-brayn) one of the three parts of the brainstem

middle ear (MID-el eer) a tiny and very thin epithelium-lined cavity in the temporal bone that houses the ossicles; in the middle ear, sound waves are amplified

midsagittal plane (mid-SAJ-ih-tal playn) a cut or plane that divides the body or any of its parts into two equal halves

mineral (MIN-er-al) any of the inorganic elements or salts found naturally in the earth, many of which are vital to the proper functioning of the body

mineralocorticoid (MC) (min-er-al-oh-KOHR-tih-koyd [em see]) hormone that influences mineral salt metabolism; secreted by adrenal cortex; aldosterone is the chief mineralocorticoid

minor duodenal papilla (MYE-ner doo-oh-DEE-nul [or doo-AH-de-nul] pah-PIL-ah) small muscular bump in lining of duodenum where the accessory pancreatic duct enters

mitochondria (my-toh-KON-dree-ah) threadlike structures

mitosis (my-TOH-sis) indirect cell division involving complex changes in the nucleus

mitral valve (MY-tral valve) also known as the **bicuspid valve;** located between the left atrium and ventricle

mode (mohd) category of sensation detected by a sensory receptor; also called *modality*

molar (MOHL-ar) a tricuspid tooth, which is a relatively flat-topped grinding tooth near the posterior of the jaw

molecular motor (moh-LEK-yoo-lar MOH-ter) small structures in the cell made up of one or two molecules and that act as mechanisms of movement

molecule (MOL-eh-kyool) particle of matter composed of one or more smaller units called **atoms**

monoclonal antibody (mon-oh-KLONE-al AN-tih-bod-ee) specific antibody produced from a population of identical cells

monocyte (MON-oh-syte) a phagocyte

monoglyceride (mon-oh-GLIH-seh-ryde) lipid molecule made up of one fatty acid attached to a glycerol group; a product of fat digestion

monosaccharide (mon-oh-SAK-ah-ryde) simple sugar, such as glucose or fructose; building block of carbohydrates

mons pubis (monz PYOO-bis) skin-covered pad of fat over the symphysis pubis in the female

morula (MOR-yoo-lah) a solid mass of cells formed by the divisions of a fertilized egg

motility (moh-TIL-ih-tee) ability to move

motor neuron (NOO-ron) transmits nerve impulses from the brain and spinal cord to muscles and glandular epithelial tissues

motor unit (MOH-ter YOO-nit) a single motor neuron with the muscle cells it innervates

mucocutaneous junction (myoo-koh-kyoo-TAY-nee-us JUNK-shun) the transitional area where the skin and mucous membrane meet

mucosa (myoo-KOH-sah) mucous membrane

mucous membrane (MYOO-kus MEM-brayn) epithelial membranes that line body surfaces opening directly to the exterior and secrete a thick, slippery material called **mucus**

mucus (MYOO-kus) thick, slippery material that is secreted by the mucous membrane and that keeps the membrane moist

multiple sclerosis (MS) (MULT-ih-pul skleh-ROH-sis [em es]) the most common primary disease of the central nervous system; a myelin disorder
muscle fiber any of the specialized contractile cells of muscle tissue
muscle strain (MUS-el strayn) overstretching or tearing skeletal muscle fibers resulting from overexertion or trauma
muscle tone (MUS-el tohn) the tension of muscle or tonic contraction; characteristic of muscle of a normal individual who is awake
muscular system (MUS-kyoo-lar SIS-tem) the muscles of the body
muscularis (mus-kyoo-LAYR-is) two layers of muscle surrounding the digestive tube that produce wavelike, rhythmic contractions, called **peristalsis,** which move food material along the digestive tract
myelin (MY-eh-lin) lipoid substance found in the myelin sheath around some nerve fibers
myelin disorder (MY-eh-lin dis-OR-der) any of several disorders characterized by loss or improper development of the myelin sheath that surrounds many axons of the nervous system
myelinated fiber (MY-eh-lih-nay-ted) axons outside the central nervous system that are surrounded by a segmented wrapping of myelin
myeloid tissue (MY-eh-loyd TISH-yoo) tissue that makes up bone marrow
myocardial infarction (MI) (my-oh-KAR-dee-al in-FARK-shun [em aye]) death of cardiac muscle cells resulting from inadequate blood supply as in coronary thrombosis
myocardium (my-oh-KAR-dee-um) muscle of the heart
myofilament (my-oh-FIL-ah-ment) any of the ultramicroscopic, threadlike protein structures found in cylindrical groupings within each muscle fiber and involved in muscle contraction
myoglobin (my-oh-GLOH-bin) large protein molecule in the cytoplasm of muscle cells that attracts oxygen and holds it temporarily
myometrium (my-oh-MEE-tree-um) muscle layer in the uterus
myopia (my-OH-pee-ah) nearsightedness
myosin (MY-oh-sin) contractile protein found in the thick filaments of skeletal muscle
myxedema (mik-seh-DEE-mah) condition caused by deficiency of thyroid hormone in adults

N

nail body (nayl BOD-ee) the visible part of the nail
nail root (nayl root) the part of the nail that is hidden by the cuticle
nanometer (NAN-oh-mee-ter) a measure of length in the metric system; one billionth of a meter
nares (NAY-reez) nostrils
nasal (NAY-zal) relating to the nose
nasal cavity (NAY-zal KAV-ih-tee) the moist, warm cavities lined by mucosa located just beyond the nostrils; olfactory receptors are located in the mucosa
nasal septum (NAY-zal SEP-tum) a partition that separates the right and left nasal cavities
nasopharynx (nay-zoh-FAYR-inks) the uppermost portion of the tube just behind the nasal cavities
neck (of tooth) narrow portion of tooth that joins crown of tooth to the root
necrosis (neh-KROH-sis) death of cells in a tissue, often resulting from ischemia
negative feedback (NEG-ah-tiv FEED-bak) see **negative feedback loop**
negative feedback loop (NEG-ah-tiv FEED-bak loop) homeostatic control system in which information feeding back to the control center causes the level of a variable to be changed in the direction opposite to that of the initial stimulus; see also **feedback control loop**
neonatal period (nee-oh-NAY-tal PEER-ee-uhd) developmental stage that occurs during the first 4 weeks after birth
neonate (NEE-oh-NAYT) a newborn infant
neonatology (nee-oh-nay-TOL-oh-jee) diagnosis and treatment of disorders of the newborn infant
neoplasm (NEE-oh-plaz-em) an abnormal mass of proliferating cells that may be either benign or malignant
nephritis (neh-FRY-tis) kidney disease; inflammation of the nephrons
nephron (NEF-ron) anatomical and functional unit of the kidney, consisting of the renal corpuscle and the renal tubule
nephron loop (NEF-ron loop) extension of the proximal tubule of the kidney; also known as *loop of Henle* or *Henle loop*
nephropathy (neh-FROP-ah-thee) kidney disease
nerve (nerv) collection of nerve fibers
nerve impulse (nerv IM-puls) signals that carry information along the nerves
nervous system (NER-vus SIS-tem) organ system made up of the brain, spinal cord, and nerves
nervous tissue (NER-vus TISH-yoo) consists of neurons and glia that provide rapid communication and control of body function
neurilemma (noo-rih-LEM-mah) nerve sheath
neurogenic bladder (noor-oh-JEN-ik BLAD-der) disorder of the bladder that results in loss of control of normal voiding; due to disruption of nervous input to the bladder
neurohypophysis (noo-roh-hye-POF-ih-sis) posterior pituitary gland
neurologist (noo-ROL-uh-jist) physician specializing in the treatment of nervous system disorders
neuromuscular junction (NMJ) (noo-roh-MUS-kyoo-lar JUNK-shun [en em jay]) the point of contact between the nerve endings and muscle fibers
neuron (NOO-ron) nerve cell, including its processes (axons and dendrites)
neuroscientist (noo-roh-SYE-en-tist) scientist specializing in research concerning the structure and function of the nervous system
neurotransmitter (noo-roh-tranz-MIT-ter) chemicals by which neurons communicate

neutral (NOO-truhl) relating to a solution that is neither acid nor base, having a pH of 7
neutron (NOO-tron) electrically neutral particle within the nucleus of an atom
neutrophil (NOO-troh-fil) white blood cell that stains readily with neutral dyes
nitric oxide (NO) (NYE-trik OK-side [en oh]) small gas molecule used as a neurotransmitter or paracrine agent
nitrogen (N) (NYE-troh-jen [en]) element 7
Nobel Prize (noh-BEL pryze) international award created by the late Alfred Nobel and awarded each year to up to three recipients in each of several categories such as chemistry, physics, and medicine or physiology (each Nobel laureate [prizewinner] receives a diploma, a medal, and a cash prize at a ceremony in Stockholm, Sweden)
nodes of Ranvier (nohdz ov rahn-vee-AY) indentations that are found between adjacent Schwann cells
nonelectrolyte (non-eh-LEK-troh-lyte) compound that does not dissociate into ions in solution; for example, glucose
nonspecific immunity (non-spih-SIH-fik ih-MYOON-ih-tee) the protective mechanisms that provide immediate, generic protection against any bacteria, toxin, or other injurious particle; also called **innate immunity**
nonsteroid hormone (non-STAYR-oyd HOHR-mohn) general type of hormone that does not have the lipid steroid structure (derived from cholesterol) but is instead a protein or protein derivative; also sometimes called *protein hormone*
norepinephrine (NE) (nor-ep-ih-NEF-rin [en ee]) hormone secreted by adrenal medulla; released by sympathetic nervous system
normal saline (NOR-mall SAY-leen) sodium chloride solution often used intravenously to restore homeostatic balance in the blood
nose (nohz) respiratory organ
nosocomial infection (noh-zoh-KOAM-ee-al) infection that begins in the hospital or clinic
nuclear envelope (NOO-klee-ar EN-veh-lohp [or AHN-veh-lohp]) membrane that surrounds the cell nucleus
nuclear medicine technologist (NOO-klee-ar MED-ih-sin tek-NOL-uh-jist) medical professional who prepares and administers radioactive drugs or other substances
nucleic acid (noo-KLEE-ik AS-id) the two major nucleic acids are ribonucleic acid, abundant in the cytoplasm, and deoxyribonucleic acid, found in the nucleus; made up of units called *nucleotides,* each of which includes a phosphate, a five-carbon sugar, and a nitrogen base
nucleolus (noo-KLEE-oh-lus) critical to protein formation because it "programs" the formation of ribosomes in the nucleus
nucleoplasm (NOO-klee-oh-plaz-em) a special type of cytoplasm found in the nucleus
nucleotide (NOO-klee-oh-tide) chemical subunit made up of three types of chemical groups (sugar, phosphate, nitrogen base) that can act alone or to make up a larger molecule (nucleic acid, such as RNA or DNA)
nucleus (NOO-klee-us) spherical structure within a cell; a group of neuron cell bodies in the brain or spinal cord; central core of the atom, made up of protons and (sometimes) neutrons
nurse (nurs) health-care professional trained to care for the sick and injured
nursing assistant (NURS-ing ah-SIS-tent) health-care worker under the supervision of a nurse to care for patients
nutrition (noo-TRISH-en) food, vitamins, and minerals that are ingested and assimilated into the body
nutritionist (noo-TRISH-en-ist) professional consultant specializing in diet and food

O

oblique plane (oh-BLEEK playn) imagined flat plane that runs diagonally to an axis of the body or one of its parts, producing a slanted, oblique section or cut
obstetric nurse (ob-STET-rik nurs) nurse specializing in pregnancy, labor, and delivery care
obstetrician (ob-steh-TRISH-an) physician specializing in pregnancy, labor, and delivery care
occipital (ok-SIP-it-al) relating to the back of the skull, as in *occipital bone* or *occipital region*
occupational therapist (ak-yoo-PAY-shun-al THAYR-ah-pist) health professional who treats injuries or disorders to develop or recover everyday living skills
older adulthood (OLD-er ah-DULT-hood) see **senescence**
olecranal (oh-LEK-rah-nal) relating to the elbow
olecranon (oh-LEK-rah-nahn) the large bony process of the ulna; commonly referred to as the tip of the elbow; also called *olecranon process*
olecranon fossa (oh-LEK-rah-nahn FOS-ah) a large depression on the posterior surface of the humerus
olfaction (ohl-FAK-shun) sense of smell
olfactory receptor (ol-FAK-tor-ee) chemical receptors responsible for the sense of smell; located in the epithelial tissue in the upper part of the nasal cavity
oligodendrocyte (ohl-ih-goh-DEN-droh-syte) a cell that holds nerve fibers together and produces the myelin sheath around axons in the central nervous system
oliguria (ohl-ih-GYOO-ree-ah) scanty amounts of urine
oocyte (OH-oh-syte) immature stage of the female sex cell
oogenesis (oh-oh-JEN-eh-sis) production of female gametes
oophorectomy (oh-of-eh-REK-toh-mee) surgical procedure to remove the ovaries
ophthalmic (op-THAL-mik) relating to the eye
ophthalmologist (of-thal-MOL-eh-jist) physician specializing in treating disorders of the eye and vision
ophthalmoscope (of-THAL-mah-skohp) instrument used to examine the retinal surface and internal eye structures
opposition (op-uh-ZISH-en) moving the thumb to touch the tips of the fingers; the movement used to hold a pencil to write
optic disk (OP-tic) the area in the retina where the optic nerve fibers exit and there are no rods or cones; also known as a *blind spot*

optometrist (op-TOM-eh-trist) clinical practitioner who examines eyes and vision and prescribes corrective lenses or other treatments; one who practices *optometry*

oral (OR-al) relating to the mouth

oral cavity (OR-al KAV-ih-tee) mouth

orbicularis oculi (or-bik-yoo-LAYR-is OK-yoo-lie) facial muscle that causes a squint

orbicularis oris (or-bik-yoo-LAYR-is OH-ris) facial muscle that puckers the lips

orbital (OR-bih-tal) relating to the eye region or orbit (socket) of the eye; region of an atom inhabited by electrons

organ (OR-gan) group of several tissue types that performs a special function

organelle (or-gah-NELL) cell organ; for example, the ribosome

organism (or-gah-NIZ-em) an individual, living thing

organization (biological levels) (or-gan-ih-ZAY-shun) see **levels of organization**

organ of Corti (OR-gan ov KOHR-tye) the organ of hearing located in the cochlea with ciliated sensory receptor cells; also called *Corti organ* or *spiral organ*

organic compound (or-GAN-ik KOM-pownd) compound whose large molecules contain carbon and that include C—C bonds and/or C—H bonds

organogenesis (or-gah-noh-JEN-eh-sis) formation of organs from the primary germ layers of the embryo

origin (OR-ih-jin) the attachment of a muscle to the bone that does not move when contraction occurs, as distinguished from insertion

oropharynx (oh-roh-FAYR-inks) the portion of the pharynx that is located behind the mouth

orthopedic surgeon (or-thoh-PEE-dik SUR-jen) physician in a medical specialty dealing with surgery to treat skeletal injury and disease

osmosis (os-MOH-sis) type of passive movement of water (only) through a semipermeable membrane

ossicle (OS-sih-kul) little bone; for example, the auditory ossicles found in the ears

osteoarthritis (os-tee-oh-ar-THRY-tis) degenerative joint disease; a noninflammatory disorder of a joint characterized by degeneration of articular cartilage

osteoblast (OS-tee-oh-blast) bone-forming cell

osteoclast (OS-tee-oh-klast) bone-dissolving cell

osteocyte (OS-tee-oh-syte) inactive bone cell

osteon (OS-tee-on) structural unit of compact bone tissue made up of concentric layers (lamellae) of hard bone matrix and bone cells (osteocytes); also called **haversian system**

osteoporosis (os-tee-oh-poh-ROH-sis) a bone disease in which there is an excessive loss of calcified matrix and collagenous fibers from bone

otitis media (oh-TYE-tis MEE-dee-ah) a middle ear infection

otologist (oh-TOL-uh-jist) physician specializing in treating disorders of the ear

otoscope (OH-toh-skohp) lighted instrument used to examine the external ear canal and outer surface of the tympanic membrane

ova (OH-vah) (*sing.*, ovum) female gametes; egg

oval window (OH-vel WIN-doh) a small, membrane-covered opening that separates the middle and inner ear

ovarian follicle (oh-VAYR-ee-an FOL-lih-kul) pockets in the ovaries that contain developing oocytes

ovary (OH-var-ee) either of paired female gonads that produce ova (sex cells)

overactive bladder (oh-ver-AK-tiv BLAD-er) refers to frequent urination characterized by urgency and pain

overhydration (oh-ver-hye-DRAY-shun) too large a fluid input that can put a burden on the heart

oviduct (OH-vih-dukt) uterine or fallopian tube

ovulation (ov-yoo-LAY-shun) release of an egg (ovum) from the ovary

ovum (OH-vum) (*pl.*, ova) female gamete; egg

oxygen (O) (AHK-sih-jen [oh]) element 8

oxygen concentrator (AHK-sih-jen kon-sen-TRAY-ter) a device used in health care that increases the proportion of oxygen gas in the air of the room in which it is placed—it is sometimes used in respiratory and other conditions that produce hypoxia (low oxygen concentration in the blood)

oxygen debt (AHK-sih-jen det) continued increased oxygen consumption that occurs after exercise; also called *excess post-exercise oxygen consumption (EPOC)*

oxygen therapy (AHK-sih-jen THAYR-ah-pee) administration of oxygen gas to individuals suffering from hypoxia (low oxygen concentration in the blood)

oxyhemoglobin (HbO_2) (ahk-see-hee-moh-GLOH-bin) oxygenated form of hemoglobin

oxytocin (OT) (ahk-see-TOH-sin [oh tee]) hormone secreted by the posterior pituitary gland before and after delivering a baby; thought to initiate and maintain labor, it also causes the release of breast milk into ducts for the baby to suck

P

pacemaker (PASE-may-ker) see **sinoatrial (SA) node**

pacinian corpuscle (pah-SIN-ee-an KOR-pus-ul) a receptor found deep in the dermis that detects pressure on the skin surface

pain receptor (payn ree-SEP-tor) sensory neuron that detects painful stimuli; also called *nociceptor*

palate (PAL-let) the roof of the mouth; made up of the hard (anterior portion of the mouth) and soft (posterior portion of the mouth) palates

palatine tonsil (PAL-ah-tine TAHN-sil) either of a pair of lymphoid masses located behind and below the pillars of the fauces

paleontologist (pay-lee-un-TOL-uh-jist) scientist that studies organisms that lived in the ancient past

palmar (PAHL-mar) palm of the hand

palpable (PAL-pah-bul) can be identified by touch, such as bony landmarks located beneath the skin

palpebral fissure (PAL-peh-bral FISH-ur) opening between the two eyelids

pancreas (PAN-kree-as) endocrine gland located in the abdominal cavity; contains pancreatic islets that secrete glucagon and insulin

pancreatic islet (pan-kree-AT-ik eye-LET) endocrine portion of the pancreas; made up of small groupings of alpha and beta cells among others; also known as *islet of Langerhans*

papilla (pah-PIL-ah) (*pl.,* papillae) small, nipple-shaped elevations

paracrine [agent or hormone] (PAYR-ah-krin [AY-jent or HOHR-mohn]) hormone that regulates activity in nearby cells within the same tissue as their source

paralysis (pah-RAL-ih-sis) loss of the power of motion, especially voluntary motion

paramedic (payr-ah-MED-ik) health-care worker trained to assist a physician or to give care in the absence of a physician, often as part of a first-responder team

paranasal sinus (payr-ah-NAY-sal SYE-nus) four pairs of sinuses that have openings into the nose

parasympathetic nervous system (PNS) (par-ah-sim-pah-THET-ik NERV-us SIS-tem) part of the autonomic nervous system; ganglia are connected to the brainstem and the sacral segments of the spinal cord; controls many visceral effectors under normal conditions

parasympathetic postganglionic neuron (payr-ah-sim-pah-THET-ik post-gang-glee-ON-ik NOO-ron) ANS neuron in which dendrites and cell body are in a parasympathetic ganglion, and axon travels to a variety of visceral effectors

parasympathetic preganglionic neuron (payr-ah-sim-pah-THET-ik pree-gang-glee-ON-ik NOO-ron) ANS neuron in which dendrites and cell body are located in the gray matter of the brainstem and sacral cord segments; axon terminates in a parasympathetic ganglion

parathyroid gland (PAYR-ah-THY-royd gland) any of the endocrine glands located in the neck on the posterior aspect of the thyroid gland; secretes parathyroid hormone

parathyroid hormone (PTH) (PAYR-ah-THY-royd HOHR-mohn [pee tee aych]) hormone produced by the parathyroid gland that increases the concentration of calcium in the blood

parietal (pah-RYE-ih-tal) relating to the walls of an organ or cavity

parietal pericardium (pah-RYE-ih-tal payr-ih-KAR-dee-um) outer layer of the serous membrane pericardium surrounding the heart

parietal peritoneum (pah-RYE-ih-tal payr-ih-TOH-nee-um) serous membrane that lines the walls of the abdominopelvic cavity

parietal pleura (pah-RYE-ih-tal PLOO-rah) (*pl.,* plurae) serous membrane that lines the walls of the left and right pleural cavities within the thoracic cavity

parietal layer (pah-RYE-ih-tal LAY-er) portion of the serous membrane that lines the walls of a body cavity

Parkinson disease (PD) (PARK-in-son dih-ZEEZ [pee-dee]) a chronic disease of the nervous system characterized by a set of signs called *parkinsonism* that results from a deficiency of the neurotransmitter dopamine in certain regions of the brain that normally inhibit overstimulation of skeletal muscles; parkinsonism is characterized by muscle rigidity and trembling of the head and extremities, forward tilt of the body, and shuffling manner of walking

parotid gland (pah-ROT-id gland) largest of the salivary glands located just below and in front of each ear at the angle of the jaw

partial pressure (PAR-shal PRESH-er) pressure exerted by any one gas in a mixture of gases or in a liquid; symbol used to designate partial pressure is the capital letter P preceding the chemical symbol for the gas

partial-thickness burn (PAR-shal THIK-nes bern) term used to describe both minor burn injury (see **first-degree burn**) and more severe burns that injure both epidermis and dermis (see **second-degree burn**)

parturition (pahr-too-RIH-shun) act of giving birth

passive transport (PAS-iv TRANZ-port) cellular process in which substances move through a cellular membrane with their own energy

patella (pah-TEL-ah) small, shallow pan; the kneecap

pathologist (pah-THOL-uh-jist) scientist who studies disease processes

patient care technician (PAY-shent kayr tek-NISH-en) health-care worker who provides personal care to patients under the supervision of nurses, physicians, and other professionals

pectoral girdle (PEK-toe-ral GIR-dul) shoulder girdle; the scapula and clavicle

pectoralis major (pek-teh-RAH-liss MAY-jor) major flexor of the arm

pedal (PEED-al) foot

pelvic (PEL-vik) relating to the pelvis (basin formed by coxal bones)

pelvic cavity (PEL-vik KAV-ih-tee) portion of the ventral cavity formed by the basin of the pelvic (hip) girdle; the inferior portion of the abdominopelvic cavity

pelvic girdle (PEL-vik GIR-dul) ring of coxal bones that connects the legs to the trunk; also called *hip girdle*

pelvic inflammatory disease (PID) (PEL-vik in-FLAM-ah-toh-ree dih-ZEEZ [pee-aye-dee]) inflammatory disease of the female reproductive and other pelvic organs caused by a number of different pathogens, including those responsible for many STDs (sexually transmitted diseases) such as gonorrhea

pelvis (PEL-vis) basin or funnel-shaped structure

penis (PEE-nis) forms part of the male genitalia; when sexually aroused, becomes stiff to enable it to enter and deposit sperm in the vagina

pepsin (PEP-sin) protein-digesting enzyme of the stomach

pepsinogen (pep-SIN-oh-jen) component of gastric juice that is converted into pepsin by hydrochloric acid

peptide bond (PEP-tyde bond) covalent bond linking amino acids within a protein molecule

pericarditis (payr-ih-kar-DYE-tis) when the pericardium becomes inflamed

pericardium (payr-ih-KAR-dee-um) membrane that surrounds the heart

perilymph (PAYR-ih-limf) a watery fluid that fills the bony labyrinth of the ear

perineal (payr-ih-NEE-al) refers to the area between the anus and genitals; the perineum

perineum (payr-ih-NEE-um) see **perineal**

perineurium (payr-ih-NOO-ree-um) connective tissue that encircles a bundle of nerve fibers within a nerve

periodontal membrane (payr-ee-oh-DON-tal MEM-brayn) fibrous membrane around the root of a tooth, forming a junction with the jaw bone

periodontitis (payr-ee-oh-don-TYE-tis) inflammation of the periodontal membrane (periodontal ligament) that anchors teeth to jaw bone; common cause of tooth loss among adults

periosteum (payr-ee-OS-tee-um) tough, connective tissue covering the bone

peripheral (peh-RIF-er-al) relating to an outside surface

peripheral nervous system (PNS) (peh-RIF-er-al NERV-us SIS-tem [pee-en-es]) the nerves connecting the brain and spinal cord to other parts of the body

peripheral resistance (PR) (peh-RIF-er-al ree-SIS-tents [pee ar]) resistance (blocked effort) to blood flow encountered in the peripheral arteries (arteries that branch off the aorta and pulmonary arteries)

peristalsis (payr-ih-STAL-sis) wavelike, rhythmic contractions of the stomach and intestines that move food material along the digestive tract

peritoneal (payr-ih-toh-NEE-al) relating to the peritoneum

peritoneal space (payr-ih-toh-NEE-al) small, fluid-filled space between the visceral and parietal layers that allows the layers to slide over each other freely in the abdominopelvic cavity

peritoneum (payr-ih-toh-NEE-um) large, moist, slippery sheet of serous membrane that lines the abdominopelvic cavity (parietal layer) and its organs (visceral layer)

peritonitis (payr-ih-toh-NYE-tis) inflammation of the serous membranes in the abdominopelvic cavity; sometimes a serious complication of an infected appendix

permanent teeth (PER-mah-nent teeth) set of 32 teeth that replaces deciduous teeth; also called *adult teeth*

permeable membrane (PER-mee-ah-bul) a membrane that allows passage of substances

pernicious anemia (per-NISH-us ah-NEE-mee-ah) deficiency of red blood cells resulting from a lack of vitamin B_{12}

peroneal muscle (per-oh-NEE-al MUS-el) any of a group of plantar flexors and evertors of the foot; the peroneus longus forms a support arch for the foot

peroneus group (per-on-EE-uss groop) see **peroneal muscle**

perspiration (per-spih-RAY-shun) transparent, watery liquid released by glands in the skin that eliminates ammonia and uric acid and helps maintain body temperature; also known as **sweat**

pH (pee-AYCH) mathematical expression of relative H^+ concentration (acidity); pH value higher than 7 is basic, pH value less than 7 is acidic, pH value equal to 7 is neutral

phagocyte (FAG-oh-syte) white blood cell that engulfs microbes and digests them

phagocytosis (fag-oh-sye-TOH-sis) ingestion and digestion of particles by a cell

phalanges (fah-LAN-jeez) (*sing.,* phalanx) the bones that make up the fingers and toes

pharmacist (FAR-mah-sist) health-care worker trained to dispense drugs and educate patients in their proper use

pharmacologist (far-mah-KAHL-uh-jist) scientist specializing in the study of drug actions

pharmacy technician (FAR-mah-see tek-NISH-en) health-care worker trained to dispense drugs under the supervision of a pharmacist

pharyngeal tonsil (fah-RIN-jee-al TAHN-sil) tonsil located in the nasopharynx on its posterior wall; when enlarged, referred to as adenoids

pharynx (FAYR-inks) organ of the digestive and respiratory system; commonly called the *throat*

phlebotomist (fleh-BOT-oh-mist) health-care worker specializing in drawing blood from veins for laboratory analysis or donation

phospholipid (fos-foh-LIP-id) phosphate-containing fat molecule found in cell membranes; one end of the molecule is water-soluble and the other end is lipid-soluble

photopigment (foh-toh-PIG-ment) any of the chemicals in retinal cells that are sensitive to light

photoreceptor (FOH-toh-ree-sep-tor) type of sensory nerve cell stimulated by light; for example, rods and cones of the retina

phrenic nerve (FREN-ik nerv) the nerve that stimulates the diaphragm to contract

physical education (FIS-ik-al ed-yoo-KAY-shun) teaching discipline that focuses on health, fitness, and sports

physical therapist (FIS-ik-al THAYR-ah-pist) health professional who helps patients improve body movements and manage pain

physician (fih-ZISH-en) health-care professional, usually holding a doctorate in medicine or related discipline, licensed to provide and supervise medical care

physiology (fiz-ee-OL-oh-jee) the study of body function

pia mater (PEE-ah MAH-ter) the vascular innermost covering (meninx) of the brain and spinal cord

pigment (PIG-ment) colored substance

pineal gland (PIN-ee-al gland) endocrine gland located in the third ventricle of the brain; produces melatonin

pinocytosis (pin-oh-sye-TOH-sis) the active transport mechanism used to transfer fluids or dissolved substances into cells

pitting edema (pitt-ing eh-DEE-mah) condition characterized by easily made depressions in swollen subcutaneous tissue

pituitary gland (pih-TOO-ih-tayr-ee gland) endocrine gland located in the skull; made up of the adenohypophysis and the neurohypophysis

pivot joint (PIV-it joynt) type of diarthrotic synovial joint in which a projection from one bone articulates with a ring or notch in another bone, allowing rotational movement

placenta (plah-SEN-tah) anchors the developing fetus to the uterus and provides a "bridge" for the exchange of nutrients and waste products between the mother and developing baby

plane (playn) flat surface or imagined flat surface

plantar (PLAN-tar) relating to the sole of the foot

plantar flexion (PLAN-tar FLEK-shun) action of the bottom of the foot being directed downward; this motion allows a person to stand on his or her tiptoes

plasma (PLAZ-mah) the liquid part of the blood

plasma cell (PLAZ-mah sel) type of lymphocyte (B lymphocyte) white blood cell that secretes huge amounts of antibody into the blood

plasma membrane (PLAZ-mah MEM-brayn) membrane that separates the contents of a cell from the tissue fluid; encloses the cytoplasm and forms the outer boundary of the cell

plasma protein (PLAZ-mah PROH-teen) any of several proteins normally found in the plasma; includes albumins, globulins, and fibrinogen

platelet (PLAYT-let) see **thrombocyte**

platelet plug (PLAYT-let pluhg) a temporary accumulation of platelets (thrombocytes) at the site of an injury; it precedes the formation of a blood clot

pleura (PLOOR-ah) the serous membrane in the thoracic cavity that lines each pleural cavity and covers the lungs

pleural (PLOOR-al) relating to pleural cavity, a pleural membrane, or the ribs

pleural cavity (PLOOR-al KAV-ih-tee) a lateral subdivision of the thorax where a lung resides

pleural space (PLOOR-al spays) the space between the visceral and parietal pleurae filled with just enough fluid to allow them to glide effortlessly with each breath

pleurisy (PLOOR-ih-see) inflammation of the pleura

plexus (PLEK-sus) (*pl.*, plexuses) literally a braid or network, any structure involving convergence and divergence of pathways, as in each plexus of spinal nerves or the choroid plexus of blood vessels in the brain ventricles

plica (PLYE-kah) (*pl.*, plicae) circular fold

pneumocystosis (noo-moh-sis-TOE-sis) a protozoan infection; most likely to invade the body when the immune system has been compromised

pneumothorax (noo-moh-THOH-raks) accumulation of air in the pleural space, causing collapse of the lung

podiatrist (poh-DYE-a-trist) physician who specializes in health care of the foot, ankle, and leg

polar body (POH-lar BOD-ee) small, nonfunctional cell produced during meiotic divisions in the formation of the female gamete

polycythemia (pol-ee-sye-THEE-mee-ah) an excessive number of red blood cells

polysaccharide (pahl-ee-SAK-ah-ryde) complex sugar or starch, such as glycogen and plant starches; made up of many monosaccharides

polyuria (pol-ee-YOO-ree-ah) unusually large amounts of urine

pons (ponz) the part of the brainstem between the medulla oblongata and the midbrain

popliteal (pop-lih-TEE-al) behind the knee

pore (pohr) pinpoint-size opening on the skin that serves as an outlet of a small duct from the eccrine sweat glands

positive feedback (POZ-ih-tiv FEED-bak) see **positive feedback loop**

positive feedback loop (POZ-ih-tiv FEED-bak loop) homeostatic control system in which information feeding back to the control center causes the level of a variable to be pushed further in the direction of the original deviation, causing an amplification of the original stimulus; ordinarily this mechanism is used by the body to amplify a process and quickly finish it, as in labor contractions and blood clotting; see **feedback control loop**

posterior (pos-TEER-ee-or) located behind; opposite of anterior

posterior pituitary gland (pos-TEER-ee-or pih-TOO-ih-tayr-ee gland) neurohypophysis; hormones produced are ADH and oxytocin

posterior root ganglion (pos-TEER-ee-or root GANG-lee-un) ganglion located near the spinal cord; where the neuron cell body of the dendrites of the sensory neuron is located

postganglionic neuron (post-gang-lee-ON-ik NOO-ron) autonomic neuron that conducts nerve impulses from a ganglion to cardiac or smooth muscle or glandular epithelial tissue

postnatal period (POST-nay-tal PEER-ee-uhd) the period beginning after birth and ending at death

postsynaptic neuron (post-sih-NAP-tik NOO-ron) a neuron situated distal to a synapse

posture (POS-chur) position of the body

precapillary sphincter (pree-CAP-pih-layr-ee SFINK-ter) smooth muscle cell in arteriolar wall that affects blood flow to the capillary

preganglionic neuron (pree-gang-lee-ON-ik NOO-ron) autonomic neuron that conducts nerve impulses between the spinal cord and a ganglion

premolar (pree-MOHL-ar) type of tooth found between the canine and molars; also called a *bicuspid tooth*

prenatal period (PREE-nay-tal PEER-ee-uhd) the period beginning after conception and lasting until birth

prepuce (PREE-pus) loose-fitting, retractable, double fold of skin covering the glans penis; also known as the **foreskin**

presbycusis (pres-bih-KYOO-sis) progressive hearing loss as a result of nerve impairment; common among elderly

presbyopia (pres-bee-OH-pee-ah) farsightedness of old age

presynaptic neuron (pree-sih-NAP-tik NOO-ron) a neuron situated proximal to a synapse

primary bronchi (PRY-mayr-ee BRAHN-kye) first branches of the trachea (right and left primary bronchi)

primary follicle (PRY-mayr-ee FOL-lih-kul) the type of ovarian follicle present at puberty; covered with granulosa cells

primary germ layer (PRY-mayr-ee jerm LAY-er) any of the three layers of developmental cells that give rise to specialized tissues and organs as the embryo develops

primary spermatocyte (PRY-mayr-ee SPER-mah-toh-syte) developmental cell that undergoes meiosis to ultimately form sperm

prime mover (pryme MOOV-er) the muscle responsible for producing a particular movement

product (PROD-ukt) any substance formed as a result of a chemical reaction

progesterone (proh-JES-ter-ohn) hormone produced by the corpus luteum; stimulates secretion of the uterine lining; with estrogen, helps initiate the menstrual cycle in girls entering puberty

prolactin (PRL) (proh-LAK-tin [pee ar el]) hormone secreted by the anterior pituitary gland during pregnancy to stimulate the breast development needed for lactation

proliferative phase (proh-LIF-eh-rah-tiv fayz) phase of menstrual cycle that begins after the menstrual flow ends and lasts until ovulation

pronate (PROH-nayt) to turn the palm downward

pronation (proh-NAY-shen) see **pronate**

prone (prohn) term used to describe the body lying in a horizontal position facing downward

prophase (PROH-fayz) first stage of mitosis during which chromosomes become visible

proprioceptor (proh-pree-oh-SEP-tor) receptor located in the muscles, tendons, and joints; allows the body to recognize its position

prostaglandin (PG) (pros-tah-GLAN-din) any of a group of naturally occurring fatty acids that regulate body functions within a local area; also called *tissue hormones*

prostate cancer (PROS-tayt KAN-ser) malignancy of the prostate gland, an exocrine gland under the male urinary bladder

prostatectomy (pros-tah-TEK-toh-mee) surgical removal of part or all of the prostate gland

prostate gland (PROS-tayt gland) gland that lies just below the bladder; secretes a fluid that constitutes about 30% of the seminal fluid volume; helps activate sperm and helps them maintain motility

prostatitis (pros-tah-TYE-tiss) inflammation of the prostate gland

protease (PROH-tee-ayse) protein-digesting enzyme

protein (PROH-teen) one of the basic nutrients needed by the body; a nitrogen-containing organic compound composed of a folded strand of amino acids

proteinuria (proh-teen-YOO-ree-ah) presence of abnormally high amounts of plasma protein in the urine; usually an indicator of kidney disease

proteoglycan (PROH-tee-oh-GLYE-kan) large molecule made up of a protein strand that forms a backbone to which are attached many carbohydrate molecules

proteome (PROH-tee-ohm) the entire group of proteins encoded by the genome; see **genome**

proteomics (proh-tee-OH-miks) the endeavor that involves the analysis of the proteins encoded by the genome, with the ultimate goal of understanding the role of each protein in the body

prothrombin (proh-THROM-bin) a protein present in normal blood that is required for blood clotting

prothrombin activator (proh-THROM-bin AK-tiv-ayt-or) a protein formed by clotting factors from damaged tissue cells and platelets; converts prothrombin into thrombin, a step essential to forming a blood clot

prothrombin time (PT) (proh-THROM-bin tyme [pee tee]) clinical laboratory test in which the time it takes for clot formation in blood is determined

proton (PROH-ton) positively charged particle within the nucleus of an atom

proximal (PROK-sih-mal) next or nearest; located nearest the center of the body or the point of attachment of a structure

proximal convoluted tubule (PROK-sih-mal kon-voh-LOO-ted TOOB-yool) the first segment of a renal tubule

pseudo (SOO-doh) false

pseudostratified epithelium (SOOD-oh-STRAT-ih-fyed ep-ih-THEE-lee-um) type of tissue similar to simple columnar epithelium; forms a membrane made up of single layer of cells that are tall and narrow but have been squeezed together in a way that pushes the nuclei into two layers and thus gives the appearance that it is stratified

psychiatrist (sye-KYE-a-trist) physician specializing in mental health

psychologist (sye-KOL-uh-jist) someone who studies mental processes or treats mental conditions through counseling or related therapies

pubis (PYOO-bis) joint in the midline between the two pubic bones

pulmonary artery (PUL-moh-nayr-ee AR-ter-ee) artery that carries deoxygenated blood from the right ventricle to the lungs

pulmonary circulation (PUL-moh-nayr-ee ser-kyoo-LAY-shun) venous blood flow from the right atrium to the lung and returning to the left atrium

pulmonary semilunar valve (PUL-moh-nayr-ee sem-ih-LOO-nar) valve located at the beginning of the pulmonary artery

pulmonary vein (PUL-moh-nayr-ee vane) any vein that carries oxygenated blood from the lungs to the left atrium

pulmonary ventilation (PUL-moh-nayr-ee ven-tih-LAY-shun) breathing; process that moves air in and out of the lungs

pulse (puls) alternating expansion and recoil of the arterial walls produced by the alternate contraction and relaxation of the ventricles; travels as a wave away from the heart

pupil (PYOO-pil) the opening in the center of the iris that regulates the amount of light entering the eye

Purkinje fiber (pur-KIN-jee FYE-ber) conductive cardiac muscle cell located in the walls of the ventricles; relays impulses from the AV node to the ventricles, causing them to contract; also called *subendocardial branch*

P wave (pee wayv) deflection on an ECG that occurs with depolarization of the atria

pyloric sphincter (pye-LOR-ik SFINK-ter) sphincter that prevents food from leaving the stomach and entering the duodenum

pylorus (pye-LOR-us) the small narrow section of the stomach that joins the first part of the small intestine

pyramid (PEER-ah-mid) any of the triangular-shaped divisions of the medulla of the kidney; also called *renal pyramid*

Q

QRS complex (kyoo ar es KOM-pleks) deflection on an ECG that occurs as a result of depolarization of the ventricles

quadriceps femoris (KWOD-reh-seps feh-MOR-is) extensor of the leg

quickening (KWIK-en-ing) moment when a pregnant woman first feels recognizable movements of the fetus

R

radiation (ray-dee-AY-shun) flow of energy in the form of waves, as in heat waves that radiate away from the body

radioactive isotope (ray-dee-oh-AK-tiv EYE-soh-tope) unstable isotope that spontaneously emits subatomic particles and electromagnetic radiation

radiography (ray-dee-OG-rah-fee) imaging technique using x-rays that pass through certain tissues more easily than others, allowing an image of tissues to form on a photographic plate; invented by Wilhelm Röntgen in 1895

radiological technologist (ray-dee-oh-LOJ-ih-kul tek-NOL-uh-jist) health-care worker who performs diagnostic imaging procedures, such as x-rays and CT or MRI scans

radiologist (ray-dee-AHL-uh-jist) physician who specializes in diagnosis using medical imaging such as x-rays and CT or MRI scans

radiopaque material (ray-dee-oh-PAYK) substance that does not permit passage of x-rays, such as barium sulfate

radius (RAY-dee-us) one of the two bones in the forearm; located on the thumb side of the forearm

reabsorption (ree-ab-SORP-shun) process of absorbing again that occurs in the kidneys

reactant (ree-AK-tant) any substance entering (and being changed by) a chemical reaction

receiving chamber (ree-SEE-ving CHAME-ber) either atrium of the heart; receives blood from the superior and inferior vena cava (right) or pulmonary veins (left)

receptor (ree-SEP-tor) peripheral beginning of a sensory neuron's dendrite

reconstructive surgery (ree-kon-STRUK-tiv SUR-jeh-ree) surgical medical specialization focusing on rebuilding damaged or dysfunctional body parts

rectum (REK-tum) distal portion of the large intestine

rectus abdominis (REK-tus ab-DOM-ih-nis) muscle that runs down the middle of the abdomen; protects the abdominal viscera and flexes the spinal column

red blood cell (RBC) (red blud sel [ar bee see]) disk-shaped blood cell filled with hemoglobin; also called *erythrocyte*

referred pain (re-FERD payn) pain that originates in a different location in the body from where it is perceived by the brain

reflex (REE-fleks) involuntary action

reflex arc (REE-fleks ark) allows an impulse to travel in only one direction

reflux (REE-fluhks) backflow, as in flow of stomach contents back into esophagus

refraction (ree-FRAK-shun) bending of a ray of light as it passes from a medium of one density to one of a different density

regulation (reg-yoo-LAY-shun) process of control of body functions

releasing hormone (ree-LEE-sing HOHR-mohn) hormone produced by the hypothalamus gland that causes the anterior pituitary gland to release its hormones

renal calculus (REE-nal KAL-kyoo-lus) (*pl.,* calculi) kidney stones

renal colic (REE-nal KOL-ik) pain caused by the passage of a kidney stone

renal column (REE-nall KOL-um) within the kidneys, the cortical tissue in the medulla between the pyramids

renal corpuscle (REE-nal KOR-pus-ul) the part of the nephron located in the cortex of the kidney

renal cortex (REE-nal KOR-teks) outer portion of the kidney

renal medulla (REE-nal meh-DUL-ah) inner portion of the kidney

renal papilla (REE-nal pah-PIL-uh) (*pl.*, papillae) tip of a renal pyramid

renal pelvis (REE-nal PEL-vis) basinlike upper end of the ureter that is located inside the kidney

renal pyramid (REE-nal PIR-ah-mid) any of the distinct triangular wedges that make up most of the medullary tissue in the kidney

renal threshold (REE-nal THRESH-hold) when the amount of a substance that is normally fully reabsorbed from tubular fluid (such as glucose) increases above this "threshold" level, the kidney tubules are unable to reabsorb all of it and the substances "spill over" into the urine

renal tubule (REE-nal TOOB-yool) one of the two principal parts of the nephron

renin (REE-nin) enzyme produced by the juxtaglomerular apparatus of the kidney nephrons that catalyzes the formation of angiotensin, a substance that increases blood pressure

renin-angiotensin-aldosterone system (RAAS) (REE-nin–an-jee-oh-TEN-sin–al-DAH-stayr-ohn SIS-tem) mechanism that causes changes in blood plasma volume mainly by controlling aldosterone secretion

repolarization (ree-poh-lah-rih-ZAY-shun) phase that begins just before the relaxation phase of cardiac muscle activity

reproductive system (ree-proh-DUK-tiv SIS-tem) produces hormones that permit the development of sexual characteristics and the propagation of the species

residual volume (RV) (reh-ZID-yoo-al VOL-yoom [ar vee]) the air that remains in the lungs after the most forceful expiration

respiration (res-pih-RAY-shun) processes that result in the absorption, transport, and utilization or exchange of respiratory gases between an organism and its environment

respiratory acidosis (RES-pih-rah-tor-ee as-ih-DOH-sis) a respiratory disturbance that results in a carbonic acid excess

respiratory alkalosis (RES-pih-rah-tor-ee al-kah-LOH-sis) a respiratory disturbance that results in a carbonic acid deficit

respiratory arrest (RES-pih-rah-tor-ee ah-REST) cessation of breathing without resumption

respiratory control center (RES-pih-rah-tor-ee kon-TROL SEN-ter) any of the centers located in the medulla and pons that regulate the muscles of respiration

respiratory distress syndrome (RDS) (RES-pih-rah-tor-ee dih-STRESS SIN-drohm [ar dee es]) difficulty in breathing caused by absence or failure of the surfactant in fluid lining the alveoli of the lung; IRDS is infant respiratory distress syndrome; ARDS is adult respiratory distress syndrome

respiratory disturbance (RES-pih-rah-tor-ee dih-STUR-buhns) acidosis (low blood pH) or alkalosis (high blood pH) caused by changes in breathing rate and depth

respiratory membrane (RES-pih-rah-tor-ee MEM-brayn) the single layer of cells that makes up the wall of the alveoli

respiratory mucosa (RES-pih-rah-tor-ee myoo-KOH-sah) mucus-covered membrane that lines the tubes of the respiratory tree

respiratory muscle (RES-pih-rah-tor-ee MUS-el) any of the muscles that are responsible for the changing shape of the thoracic cavity that allows air to move in and out of the lungs

respiratory system (RES-pih-rah-tor-ee SIS-tem) the organs that allow the exchange of oxygen from the air with the carbon dioxide from the blood

respiratory therapist (RES-pih-rah-tor-ee THAYR-ah-pist) health professional who helps patients increase respiratory function or overcome or cope with the effects of respiratory conditions

respiratory tract (RES-pih-rah-tor-ee trakt) the two divisions of the respiratory system are the upper and lower respiratory tracts

reticular formation (reh-TIK-yoo-lar for-MAY-shun) located in the medulla where bits of gray and white matter mix intricately

reticular tissue (reh-TIK-yoo-lar TISH-yoo) meshwork of netlike tissue that forms the framework of the spleen, lymph nodes, and bone marrow

retina (RET-ih-nah) innermost layer of the eyeball; contains rods and cones and continues posteriorly with the optic nerve

retroperitoneal (reh-troh-payr-ih-toh-NEE-al) area outside of the peritoneum

Rh system (ar aych SIS-tem) a system of blood typing that identifies the presence or absence of Rhesus (Rh) antigens (also called D antigens) on the surfaces of red blood cells

Rh-negative (ar aych NEG-ah-tiv) red blood cells that do not contain the antigen called Rh factor

RhoGAM (ROH-gam) an injection of a special protein given to an Rh-negative woman who is pregnant to prevent her body from forming anti-Rh antibodies, which may harm an Rh-positive baby in a subsequent pregnancy

Rh-positive (ar aych POZ-ih-tiv) red blood cells that contain an antigen called Rh factor

rib (rib) any of the 24 flat bones forming part of the framework of the thoracic wall

ribonucleic acid (RNA) (rye-boh-noo-KLAY-ik AS-id [ar en ay]) a nucleic acid found in the cytoplasm that is crucial to protein synthesis

ribosomal RNA (rRNA) (rye-boh-SOHM-al ar-en-ay [AR-ar-en-ay]) a form of RNA that makes up most of the structures (subunits) of the ribosome organelle of the cell

ribosome (RYE-boh-sohm) organelle in the cytoplasm of cells that synthesizes proteins; also known as a *protein factory*

right lymphatic duct (ryte lim-FAT-ik dukt) short vessel into which lymphatic vessels from the right upper quadrant of the body empty lymph; the duct then empties the lymph into the circulatory system at the right subclavian vein; compare to **thoracic duct**

rigor mortis (RIG-or MOR-tis) literally "stiffness of death"; the permanent contraction of muscle tissue after death caused by the depletion of ATP

rod receptor located in the retina that is responsible for night vision

root (root) portion of a structure that forms its base, often hidden within a deeper structure; for example, the *root of the tongue*, the *root of the tooth*

rotate (roh-TAYT) move in a circle around a central point

rotation (roh-TAY-shun) movement around a longitudinal axis; for example, shaking your head "no"

rugae (ROO-gee) (*sing.*, ruga) wrinkles or folds

rule of nines (rool ov nynez) a frequently used method to determine the extent of a burn injury; the body is divided into 11 areas of 9% each and 1% to the perineum to help estimate the amount of skin surface burned in an adult

S

sacrum (SAY-krum) bone of the lower vertebral column between the last lumbar vertebra and the coccyx, formed by the fusion of five sacral vertebrae

saddle joint (SAD-el joynt) type of diarthrotic joint formed by two saddle-shaped surfaces, allowing movement in two different axes

sagittal plane (SAJ-ih-tal playn) a longitudinal section or flat cut extending from front to back, dividing body or body part into right and left subdivisions

salivary amylase (SAL-ih-vayr-ee AM-eh-lays) digestive enzyme found in the saliva that begins the chemical digestion of carbohydrates

salt (sawlt) a neutral ionic compound, often formed by combination of acids with bases

saltatory conduction (SAL-tah-tor-ee kon-DUK-shun) when a nerve impulse encounters myelin and "jumps" from one node of Ranvier to the next

sarcomere (SAR-koh-meer) contractile unit of muscle; length of a cylindrical grouping of myofilaments between two Z bands

satiety center (sah-TYE-eh-tee SEN-ter) cluster of cells in the hypothalamus that send impulses to decrease appetite so that an individual feels satisfied

scapula (SKAP-yoo-lah) shoulder blade bone

Schwann cell (shown sel) large nucleated cell that forms a myelin sheath around peripheral neurons

scientific method (sye-en-TIF-ik METH-uhd) any logical and systematic approach to discovering principles of nature, often involving testing of tentative explanations called *hypotheses*

sclera (SKLEH-rah) white portion of the outer fibrous coat of the eyeball

scrotum (SKROH-tum) pouchlike sac that contains the testes

sebaceous gland (seh-BAY-shus gland) oil-producing gland found in the skin

sebum (SEE-bum) secretion of sebaceous glands

secondary bronchi (SEK-on-dayr-ee BRAHN-kye) smaller bronchial branches resulting from division of primary bronchi

secondary sex characteristic (SEK-on-dayr-ee seks kayr-ik-tuh-RIS-tik) any of the sexual characteristics that appear at the onset of puberty, except for the ability to produce gametes (which is a primary characteristic)

second-degree burn (SEK-ond deh-GREE bern) a partial-thickness burn injury that is more severe than a first-degree burn and often involves damage to the dermis

second messenger (SEK-ond MES-en-jer) chemical that provides communication within a hormone's target cell; for example, cyclic AMP

secretion (seh-KREE-shun) release of a substance from a cell

secretory phase (SEEK-reh-toh-ree fayz) phase of menstrual cycle that begins at ovulation and lasts until the next menses begins

section (SEK-shun) process of making a cut; a cutting; a segment of a larger structure

segmentation (seg-men-TAY-shun) occurs when digestive reflexes cause a forward-and-backward movement within a single region of the GI tract

sella turcica (SEL-lah TER-sih-kah) small depression of the sphenoid bone that contains the pituitary gland

semen (SEE-men) male reproductive fluid; also called **seminal fluid**

semicircular canal (sem-ih-SIR-kyoo-lar kah-NAL) any of the curved, fluid-filled tubes located in the inner ear; contain a sensory structure called *crista ampullaris* that generates a nerve impulse on movement of the head

semilunar (SL) valve (sem-ih-LOO-nar [es el] valv) valve located between either the ventricular chamber or the large artery that carries blood away from the heart; SL valves also found in the veins

seminal fluid (SEM-ih-nal FLOO-id) semen

seminal vesicle (SEM-ih-nal VES-ih-kul) paired, pouchlike gland that contributes about 60% of the seminal fluid volume; rich in fructose, which is a source of energy for sperm

seminiferous tubule (seh-mih-NIF-er-us TOOB-yool) long, coiled structure that forms the bulk of the testicular mass

senescence (seh-NES-ens) older adulthood; aging

sense organ (sens OR-gan) structure specializing in the detection of sensory stimuli

sensor (SEN-sor) in a feedback loop, the mechanism that detects changes in the physiological variable being monitored and regulated

sensory neuron (SEN-sor-ee NOO-ron) neuron that transmits impulses to the spinal cord and brain from any of various parts of the body

sensory receptor (SEN-soh-ree ree-sep-tohr) sense organ made up of afferent neurons in the peripheral nervous system that enables the body to respond to stimuli caused by changes in its internal or external environment

serosa (seh-ROH-sah) outermost covering of the digestive tract; composed of the parietal pleura in the abdominal cavity

serotonin (sayr-oh-TOH-nin) a neurotransmitter that belongs to a group of compounds called **catecholamines**

serous (SEE-rus) watery; refers to clear serous fluid or the type of membrane that produces it

serous membrane (SEE-rus MEM-brayn) a two-layered epithelial membrane that lines body cavities and covers the surfaces of organs

serum (SEER-um) blood plasma minus its clotting factors, still contains antibodies

sex hormone (seks HOHR-mohn) any hormone that has a reproductive function

shingles (SHING-ulz) see **herpes zoster**

sickle cell anemia (SIK-ul sel ah-NEE-mee-ah) severe, possibly fatal, hereditary disease caused by an abnormal type of hemoglobin

sickle cell trait (SIK-ul sel trayt) when only one defective gene is inherited and only a small amount of hemoglobin that is less soluble than usual is produced

sigmoid colon (SIG-moyd KOH-lon) S-shaped segment of the large intestine that terminates in the rectum

signal transduction (tranz-DUK-shen) term that refers to the whole process of getting a chemical signal (such as a hormone or neurotransmitter) to the inside of a cell; in a way, signal transduction is really "signal translation" by the cell

simple columnar epithelium (SIM-pel koh-LUM-nar ep-ih-THEE-lee-um) arrangement of columnar (taller than wide) epithelial cells in a single layer

simple cuboidal epithelium (SIM-pel KYOO-boyd-al ep-ih-THEE-lee-um) arrangement of cuboidal (tall as wide) epithelial cells in a single layer

simple epithelium (SIM-pel ep-ih-THEE-lee-um) arrangement of epithelial cells in a single layer

simple goiter (SIM-pel GOY-ter) condition in which the thyroid enlarges because iodine is lacking in the diet

simple squamous epithelium (SIM-pel SKWAY-muss ep-ih-THEE-lee-um) arrangement of squamous (flat) epithelial cells in a single layer

sinoatrial (SA) node (sye-noh-AY-tree-al) the heart's pacemaker; where the impulse conduction of the heart normally starts; located in the wall of the right atrium near the opening of the superior vena cava

sinus (SYE-nus) a space or cavity inside some of the cranial bones

sinusitis (sye-nyoo-SYE-tis) sinus infections

skeletal muscle (SKEL-eh-tal MUSS-el) also known as **voluntary muscle**; muscle under willed or voluntary control

skeletal system (SKEL-eh-tal SIS-tem) the bones, cartilage, and ligaments that provide the body with a rigid framework for support and protection

skull (skuhl) part of the skeleton in the head

sliding filament theory (SLY-ding FILL-ah-ment THEE-ree) concept in muscle physiology describing the contraction of a muscle fiber in terms of the sliding of microscopic protein filaments past each other within the sarcomere in a manner that shortens all the sarcomeres and thus the entire muscle

small intestine (smal in-TEST-in) part of GI tract that includes duodenum, jejunum, and ileum

smooth muscle (smoothe MUS-el) muscle that is not under conscious control; also known as *involuntary* or *visceral muscle;* forms the walls of blood vessels and hollow organs

sodium-potassium pump (SOH-dee-um poh-TAS-ee-um pump) a system of coupled ion pumps that actively transports sodium ions out of a cell and potassium ions into the cell at the same time; found in all living cells; also called *Na-K pump*

soft palate (soft PAL-let) soft, muscular posterior portion of the roof of the mouth

solute (SOL-yoot) substance that dissolves into another substance; for example, in saltwater the salt is the solute dissolved in water

solution (sol-OO-shen) fluid mixture in which one or more solutes is dissolved in a solvent such as water

solvent (SOL-vent) substance in which other substances are dissolved; for example, in saltwater the water is the solvent for salt

somatic nervous system (soh-MAH-tik NER-vus SIS-tem) the motor neurons that control the voluntary actions of skeletal muscles

special senses (SPESH-ul SEN-sez) senses detected by receptors in specific locations associated with complex structures and involve modes of smell, taste, vision, hearing, or equilibrium

specific immunity (ih-MYOON-ih-tee) the protective mechanisms that provide specific protection against certain types of bacteria or toxins

sperm the male spermatozoon; sex cell

spermatid (SPER-mah-tid) resulting daughter cell from the primary spermatocyte undergoing meiosis; spermatid cells have only half the nuclear chromosomes of other body cells

spermatogenesis (sper-mah-toh-JEN-eh-sis) the production of sperm cells

spermatogonia (sper-mah-toh-GOH-nee-ah) sperm precursor cells

spermatozoa (sper-mah-toh-ZOh-ah) (*sing.,* spermatozoon) sperm cells

sphincter (SFINK-ter) ring-shaped muscle, usually acting as a valve

sphygmomanometer (sfig-moh-mah-NAH-meh-ter) device for measuring blood pressure in the arteries of a limb

spinal cavity (SPY-nal KAV-ih-tee) the space inside the spinal column through which the spinal cord passes

spinal nerve (SPY-nal) nerve that connects the spinal cord to peripheral structures such as the skin and skeletal muscles

spinal tract (SPY-nal trakt) any of the white columns of the spinal cord that provide two-way conduction paths to and from the brain; ascending tract carries information to the brain, whereas descending tracts conduct impulses from the brain

spindle fiber (SPIN-dul FYE-ber) a network of tubules formed in the cytoplasm between the centrioles as they are moving away from each other

spiral organ (SPY-rel OR-gun) the organ of hearing located in the cochlea with ciliated sensory receptor cells; also called *organ of Corti*

spirometer (spih-ROM-eh-ter) an instrument used to measure the amount of air exchanged in breathing

spleen largest lymphoid organ; filters blood, destroys worn-out red blood cells, salvages iron from hemoglobin, and serves as a blood reservoir

splenectomy (spleh-NEK-toh-mee) surgical removal of the spleen

splenic flexure (SPLEEN-ik FLEK-shur) point at which the descending colon turns downward on the left side of the abdomen; also called *splenic colic flexure* or *left colic flexure*

spongy bone (SPUN-jee bohn) porous bone found inside bone organs; may be filled with red or yellow marrow; also called *cancellous bone* or *trabecular bone*

sports physician (sports fih-ZISH-un) physician specializing in the prevention and treatment of athletic injury

squamous (SKWAY-muss) scalelike

squamous cell carcinoma (SKWAY-muss sel car-sih-NOH-mah) malignant tumor of the epidermis; slow-growing cancer that is capable of metastasizing; the most common type of skin cancer

squamous suture (SKWAY-muss SOO-chur) the immovable joint between the temporal bone and the sphenoid bone

stapes (STAY-peez) tiny, stirrup-shaped bone in the middle ear

staph (staff) a short form of the term *Staphylococcus,* a category of bacteria that can infect the skin and other organs, sometimes seriously

static equilibrium (STAT-ik ee-kwih-LIB-ree-um) sense of the position of the body relative to gravity

stem cell (stem sel) ancestor cell that has the ability to maintain a constant population of newly differentiating cells

Stensen duct (STEN-sen dukt) the duct of the parotid gland that enters the mouth cavity; also called *parotid duct*

sternoclavicular joint (ster-noh-klah-VIK-yoo-lar joynt) the direct point of attachment between the bones of the upper extremity and the axial skeleton

sternocleidomastoid (stern-oh-klye-doh-MAS-toyd) "strap" muscle located on the anterior aspect of the neck

sternum (STER-num) breastbone

steroid hormones (STEH-royd HOHR-mohnz) lipid-soluble hormones that pass intact through the cell membrane of the target cell and influence cell activity by acting on specific genes

stimulus (STIM-yoo-lus) agent that causes a change in the activity of a structure

stoma (STOH-mah) an opening, such as the opening created in a colostomy procedure

stomach (STUHM-uhk) an expansion of the digestive tract between the esophagus and small intestine

stratified epithelium (STRAT-ih-fyde ep-ih-THEE-lee-um) epithelial cells layered one on another

stratified squamous epithelium (STRAT-ih-fyde SKWAY-muss ep-ih-THEE-lee-um) epithelial cells layered one on another, the most superficial layer being flattened squamous cells

stratified transitional epithelium (STRAT-ih-fyde tran-ZISH-en-al ep-ih-THEE-lee-um) epithelial cells layered one on another, all of varying shape, capable of stretching without injury

stratum corneum (STRAH-tum KOR-nee-um) the tough outer layer of the epidermis; cells are filled with keratin

stratum germinativum (STRAH-tum JER-mih-nah-tiv-um) the innermost of the tightly packed epithelial cells of the epidermis; cells in this layer are able to reproduce themselves

strength training (strayngth TRAYN-ing) contracting muscles against resistance to enhance muscle hypertrophy

stress (stress) an actual or perceived threat, or the reaction of the body to such a threat; pressure

striated muscle (STRYE-ay-ted MUS-el) see **skeletal muscle**

stroke volume (SV) (strohk VOL-yoom) the amount of blood that is ejected from the ventricles of the heart with each beat

structural protein (STRUK-shur-al PROH-teen) any of a category of proteins with the primary function of forming structures of the cell or tissue; contrast with **functional protein**

subcutaneous injection (sub-kyoo-TAY-nee-us in-JEK-shun) administration of substances into the subcutaneous layer beneath the skin

subcutaneous tissue (sub-kyoo-TAY-nee-us TISH-yoo) tissue below the layers of skin; made up of loose connective tissue and fat

subendocardial branch (sub-en-doh-KAR-dee-al branch) see **Purkinje fiber**

sublingual gland (sub-LING-gwal) either of a pair of salivary glands that drain saliva into the floor of the mouth

submandibular gland (sub-man-DIB-yoo-lar) either of a pair of salivary glands that drain saliva into the mouth on either side of the lingual frenulum

submucosa (sub-myoo-KOH-sah) connective tissue layer containing blood vessels and nerves in the wall of the digestive tract

sudden infant death syndrome (SIDS) (SUD-den IN-fant deth SIN-drohm) abnormal terminal condition in which an infant stops breathing

sudoriferous gland (soo-doh-RIF-er-us) sweat gland

sulcus (SUL-kus) (*pl.,* sulci) furrow or groove

superficial (soo-per-FISH-al) near the body surface

superficial fascia (soo-per-FISH-al FAH-shah) hypodermis; subcutaneous layer beneath the dermis

superior (soo-PER-ee-or) higher; opposite of inferior

superior vena cava (soo-PER-ee-or VEE-nah KAY-vah) one of two large veins returning deoxygenated blood to the right atrium

supinate (SOO-pih-nate) to turn the palm of the hand upward; opposite of pronate

supination (soo-pin-AY-shen) see **supinate**

supine (SOO-pine) used to describe the body lying in a horizontal position facing upward

supraclavicular (soo-prah-klah-VIK-yoo-lar) area above the clavicle

surfactant (sur-FAK-tant) a substance covering the surface of the respiratory membrane inside the alveolus, which reduces surface tension and prevents the alveoli from collapsing

suture (SOO-chur) immovable joint

sweat (swet) transparent, watery liquid released by glands in the skin that eliminates ammonia and uric acid and helps maintain body temperature; also known as **perspiration**

sweat gland (swet gland) exocrine gland that produces sweat

sympathetic nervous system (sim-pah-THEH-tik NER-vus SIS-tem) part of the autonomic nervous system; ganglia are connected to the thoracic and lumbar regions of the spinal cord; functions as an emergency system

sympathetic postganglionic neuron (sim-pah-THET-ik post-gang-lee-ON-ik NOO-ron) ANS neuron in which dendrites and cell body are in a sympathetic ganglion, and axon travels to a variety of visceral effectors

sympathetic preganglionic neuron (sim-pah-THET-ik pree-gang-lee-ON-ik NOO-ron) ANS neuron in which dendrites and cell body are located in the gray matter of the thoracic and lumbar segments of the spinal cord; axon leaves the cord through an anterior root of a spinal nerve and terminates in a collateral ganglion

synapse (SIN-aps) junction between adjacent neurons

synaptic cleft (sih-NAP-tik kleft) the space between a synaptic knob and the plasma membrane of a postsynaptic neuron

synaptic knob (sih-NAP-tik nob) a tiny bulge at the end of a terminal branch of a presynaptic neuron's axon that contains vesicles with neurotransmitters

synarthrosis (sin-ar-THROH-sis) a joint in which fibrous connective tissue joins bones and holds them together tightly; commonly called **suture**

synergist (SIN-er-jist) muscle that assists a prime mover

synergist muscle (SIN-er-jist MUS-el) see **synergist**

synovial fluid (sih-NOH-vee-al FLOO-id) the thick, colorless lubricating fluid secreted by the synovial membrane

synovial membrane (sih-NOH-vee-al MEM-brayn) connective tissue membrane lining the spaces between bones and joints that secretes **synovial fluid**

system (SIS-tem) group of organs arranged so that the group can perform a more complex function than any one organ can perform alone

systemic circulation (sis-TEM-ik ser-kyoo-LAY-shun) blood flow from the left ventricle to all parts of the body and back to the right atrium

systole (SIS-toh-lee) contraction of the heart muscle

systolic blood pressure (sis-TOL-ik blud PRESH-ur) force with which blood pushes against artery walls when ventricles contract

T

tachycardia (tak-ih-KAR-dee-ah) rapid heart rhythm (more than 100 beats/min)

tactile corpuscle (TAK-tyle KOR-pus-ul) large, encapsulated sensory neuron of the skin for light or discriminative touch; also known as *Meissner corpuscle*

target cell (TAR-get sel) cell acted on by a particular hormone and responding to it

tarsal (TAR-sal) relating to the ankle

tarsal bone (TAR-sal bohn) any of the seven bones of the heel and back part of the foot; the calcaneus is the largest

taste bud (tayst bud) any of the chemical receptors that generate nerve impulses, resulting in the sense of taste

T cell (tee sel) another name for **T lymphocyte**

telemetry (tel-EM-et-ree) technology by which data, such as heart activity monitored by an electrocardiograph, can be sent to a remote location through telephone wires, radio waves, or other communication pathway

telophase (TEL-oh-fayz) last stage of mitosis in which the cell divides

temporal (TEM-poh-ral) muscle that assists the masseter in closing the jaw

tendon (TEN-don) a band or cord of fibrous connective tissue that attaches a muscle to a bone or other structure

tendon sheath (TEN-don sheeth) tube-shaped structure lined with synovial membrane that encloses certain tendons

tenosynovitis (ten-oh-sin-oh-VYE-tis) inflammation of a tendon sheath

teratogen (TAYR-ah-toh-jen) any environmental factor that causes a birth defect (abnormality present at birth); common teratogens include radiation (e.g., x-rays), chemicals (e.g., drugs, cigarettes, or alcohol), and infections in the mother (e.g., herpes or rubella)

testis (TES-tis) (*pl.*, testes) pair of male gonads that produce the male sex cells or sperm

testosterone (tes-TOS-teh-rohn) male sex hormone produced by the interstitial cells in the testes; the "masculinizing hormone"

tetanic contraction (teh-TAN-ik kon-TRAK-shun) sustained contraction

tetanus (TET-ah-nus) sustained muscular contraction

thalamus (THAL-ah-muss) located just above the hypothalamus; its functions are to help produce sensations and associate sensations with emotions; plays a part in the arousal mechanism

theory (THEER-ee or THEE-uh-ree) an explanation of a scientific principle that has been tested experimentally and found to be true; compare to **hypothesis** and **law**

thermoreceptor (ther-moh-ree-SEP-tor) sensory receptor activated by heat or cold

thermoregulation (ther-moh-reg-yoo-LAY-shun) maintaining homeostasis of body temperature

third-degree burn (third deh-GREE bern) involves complete destruction of both epidermis and dermis with injury extending into subcutaneous tissue; see **full-thickness burn**

thoracic (thoh-RAS-ik) relating to the chest area of the body (upper trunk)

thoracic cavity (thoh-RAS-ik KAV-it-ee) hollow space within the larger ventral body cavity that contains the lungs (in pleural cavities) and heart (in the mediastinum)

thoracic duct (thoh-RAS-ik) largest lymphatic vessel in the body

thorax (THOR-aks) chest

threshold stimulus (THRESH-hold STIM-yoo-lus) minimal level of stimulation required to cause a muscle fiber to contract

thrombin (THROM-bin) protein important in blood clotting

thrombocyte (THROM-boh-syte) blood cell fragment that plays a central role in blood clotting; also called a *platelet*

thrombosis (throm-BOH-sis) formation of a clot in a blood vessel

thrombus (THROM-bus) (*pl.*, thrombi) stationary blood clot

thymine (THYE-meen) one of the nitrogenous bases of the nucleotides in DNA and related molecules; abbreviated *t* or *T*

thymosin (THY-moh-sin) family of hormones produced by the thymus that is vital to the development and functioning of the body's immune system, particularly the development of T lymphocytes

thymus gland (THY-muss) endocrine gland located in the mediastinum; vital part of the body's immune system; also called simply *thymus*

thyroid follicle (THY-royd FOL-lih-kul) pocket of thyroid colloid (suspended, stored form of thyroid hormone) in the thyroid gland

thyroid gland (THY-royd gland) endocrine gland located in the neck that stores its hormones until needed; thyroid hormones regulate cellular metabolism

thyroid-stimulating hormone (TSH) (THY-royd STIM-yoo-lay-ting HOHR-mohn [tee es aych]) a tropic hormone secreted by the anterior pituitary gland that stimulates the thyroid gland to increase its secretion of thyroid hormone

thyroxine (T_4) (thy-ROK-sin [tee fohr]) thyroid hormone that stimulates cellular metabolism

tibia (TIB-ee-ah) shinbone

tibialis anterior (tib-ee-AL-is an-TEER-ee-or) dorsiflexor of the foot

tidal volume (TV) (TYE-dal VOL-yoom [tee vee]) amount of air breathed in and out with each breath

tinea pedis (TIN-ee-ah PED-is) athlete's foot, a fungal infection of the skin characterized by redness and itching

tissue (TISH-yoo) group of similar cells that perform a common function

tissue fluid a dilute saltwater solution that bathes every cell in the body

tissue hormone (TISH-yoo HOHR-mohn) prostaglandins; produced in a tissue and diffuses only a short distance to act on cells within the tissue

tissue typing (TISH-yoo TYE-ping) a procedure used to identify tissue compatibility before an organ transplant

T lymphocyte (tee LIM-foh-syte) type of white blood cell that is critical to the function of the immune system, producing cell-mediated adaptive immunity

tone (tohn) see muscle tone

tonic contraction (TON-ik kon-TRAK-shen) special type of skeletal muscle contraction used to maintain posture

tonsil (TAHN-sil) mass of lymphoid tissue; protects against bacteria; three types: palatine tonsils, located on each side of the throat; pharyngeal tonsils (adenoids), near the posterior opening of the nasal cavity; and lingual tonsils, near the base of the tongue

tonsillectomy (tahn-sih-LEK-toh-mee) surgical procedure used to remove the tonsils

tonsillitis (tahn-sih-LYE-tis) an inflammation of the tonsils

total metabolic rate (TMR) (TOHT-el met-ah-BOL-ik rayt [tee em ar]) total amount of energy used by the body per day

total WBC count (TOHT-el DUB-el-yoo bee see kownt) the total number of WBCs (white blood cells) per cubic millimeter of blood

trabecula (trah-BEK-yoo-la) (*pl.*, trabeculae) tiny branchlike threads in a tissue, such as the beams of spongy (cancellous) bone, that surround a network of spaces

trachea (TRAY-kee-ah) the windpipe; the tube extending from the larynx to the bronchi

tracheostomy (tray-kee-OS-toh-mee) surgical procedure in which an opening is cut into the trachea

tract (trakt) any passageway, such as the *digestive tract, urinary tract, respiratory tract,* etc.; in nerve tissue, a single nerve pathway made up of several bundles of axons and extending through the central nervous system (compare to **nerve**)

transcellular fluid (tranz-SEL-yoo-lar FLOO-id) part of the extracellular fluid that includes cerebrospinal fluid (CSF), fluids of the eyeball, and the synovial joint fluids (but not blood plasma or interstitial fluid)

transcription (tranz-KRIP-shun) occurs when the double-stranded DNA molecules unwind and form mRNA

transfer RNA (tRNA) (TRANZ-fer ar en ay [TEE ar en ay]) RNA involved with protein synthesis; tRNA molecules carry amino acids to the ribosome for placement in the sequence prescribed by mRNA

transitional epithelium (tranz-IH-shen-al ep-ih-THEE-lee-um) type of epithelial tissue that forms membranes capable of stretching without breaking, as in the urinary bladder; cells in this type of tissue can stretch from a roughly columnar shape out to a flattened shape (squamous) and back without damage

translation (tranz-LAY-shun) the synthesis of a protein by ribosomes

transport process (TRANZ-port PROH-ses) process of carrying materials within the body, often across membranes and within fluids

transverse arch (tranz-VERS) see **metatarsal arch**

transverse canal (tranz-VERS kah-NAL) communicating canal between central (Haversian) canals that contains vessels to carry blood to the osteons; also carries nerves and lymphatic vessels; also called *Volkmann canal*

transverse colon (tranz-VERS KOH-len) division of the colon that passes horizontally across the abdomen

transverse plane (TRANZ-vers playn) horizontal plane that divides the body or any of its parts into upper and lower parts

transversus abdominis (tranz-VER-sus ab-DOM-ih-nis) the innermost layer of the anterolateral abdominal wall

trapezium (trah-PEE-zee-um) the carpal bone of the wrist that forms the saddle joint that allows the opposition of the thumb

trapezius (trah-PEE-zee-us) triangular muscle in the back that elevates the shoulder and extends the head backwards

triceps brachii (TRY-seps BRAY-kee-aye) extensor of the elbow

tricuspid (try-KUS-pid) having three points or cusps

tricuspid valve (try-KUS-ped valv) the valve located between the right atrium and ventricle

triglyceride (try-GLIS-er-yde) lipid that is synthesized from fatty acids and glycerol or from excess glucose or amino acids; stored mainly in adipose tissue cells

trigone (TRY-gon) triangular area on the wall of the urinary bladder

triiodothyronine (T_3) (try-aye-oh-doh-THY-roh-neen [tee three]) thyroid hormone that stimulates cellular metabolism

trimester (TRY-mes-ter) three-month segment of the gestation period

tropic hormone (TROH-pik HOHR-mohn) hormone that stimulates another endocrine gland to grow and secrete its hormones

true rib (troo rib) any of the first seven pairs of ribs that are attached to the sternum

tumor (TOO-mer) growth of tissues in which cell proliferation is uncontrolled and progressive

tunica adventitia (TOO-nih-kah ad-ven-TISH-ah) the outermost layer found in blood vessels

tunica albuginea (TOO-nih-kah al-byoo-JIN-ee-ah) a tough, whitish membrane that surrounds each testis and enters the gland to divide it into lobules

tunica externa (TOO-nih-kah eks-TER-nah) the outermost layer found in blood vessels; also called **tunica adventitia**

tunica intima (TOO-nih-kah IN-tih-mah) endothelium that lines the blood vessels

tunica media (TOO-nih-kah MEE-dee-ah) the muscular middle layer found in blood vessels; the tunica media of arteries is more muscular than that of veins

turbinate (TUR-bih-nayt) curving or spiral in structure; see **conchae**

T wave (tee wayv) deflection on an electrocardiogram that occurs with repolarization of the ventricles

twitch a quick, jerky response to a single stimulus

tympanic membrane (tim-PAN-ik) drumlike membrane; also called **eardrum**

type 1 diabetes mellitus (type won dye-ah-BEE-teez mell-AYE-tus) a condition resulting when the pancreatic islets secrete too little insulin, resulting in increased levels of blood glucose; formerly known as *juvenile-onset diabetes* or *insulin-dependent diabetes mellitus*

type 2 diabetes mellitus (type too dye-ah-BEE-teez mell-AYE-tus) a condition resulting when cells of the body become less sensitive to the hormone insulin and perhaps the pancreatic islets secrete too little insulin, resulting in increased levels of blood glucose; formerly known as *maturity-onset diabetes* or *insulin-independent diabetes mellitus*

U

ulcer (UL-ser) a necrotic open sore or lesion

ulna (UL-nah) one of the two forearm bones; located on the little finger side

ultrasonogram (ul-trah-SOHN-oh-gram) a technique using sound to produce images

umami (oo-MAH-mee) savory or meaty taste perceived when taste buds detect glutamate (an amino acid)

umbilical (um-BIL-ih-kul) related to the navel

umbilical artery (um-BIL-ih-kul AR-ter-ee) two small arteries that carry oxygen-poor blood from the developing fetus to the placenta

umbilical cord (um-BIL-ih-kul kord) flexible structure connecting the fetus with the placenta, which allows the umbilical arteries and vein to pass

umbilical region (um-BIL-ik-al REE-jun) center region of nine regions of the abdominopelvic cavity, as identified by a "tic-tac-toe" grid laid out over the abdominopelvic area; located beneath the umbilicus (navel)

umbilical vein (um-BIL-ih-kul vayn) a large vein carrying oxygen-rich blood from the placenta to the developing fetus

universal donor blood (yoo-neh-ver-sal DOH-nor blud) type O− blood, which can be donated to persons of any other blood type

universal recipient blood (yoo-neh-ver-sal REE-sip-ee-ahnt blud) type AB^{+} blood, which can tolerate a donation of any other blood type

upper esophageal sphincter (UES) (UP-er eh-SOF-ah-JEE-ul SFINGK-ter [yoo ee es]) ring of muscular tissue at proximal end of esophagus; helps prevent air from entering the esophagus during respiration

upper respiratory tract (UP-er res-PYE-rah-tor-ee trakt) division of respiratory tract outside the thorax that is composed of the nose, pharynx, and larynx

uracil (YOOR-ah-sil) one of the nitrogenous bases of the nucleotides in RNA and related molecules; abbreviated *u* or *U*

urea (yoo-REE-ah) nitrogen-containing waste product

uremia (yoo-REE-mee-ah) high levels of nitrogen-containing waste products in the blood; also referred to as **uremic poisoning**

uremic poisoning (yoo-REE-mik POY-zon-ing) see **uremia**

ureter (YOOR-eh-ter) long tube that carries urine from kidney to bladder

urethra (yoo-REE-thrah) passageway for elimination of urine; in males, also acts as a genital duct that carries sperm to the exterior

urinalysis (yoor-in-AL-is-is) clinical laboratory testing of urine samples

urinary bladder (YOOR-ih-nayr-ee BLAD-er) collapsible saclike organ that collects urine from the kidneys and stores it before elimination

urinary incontinence (YOOR-ih-nayr-ee in-KON-tih-nens) involuntary voiding of urine; also called *enuresis*

urinary meatus (YOOR-ih-nayr-ee mee-AY-tus) external opening of the urethra

urinary retention (YOOR-ih-nayr-ee ree-TEN-shun) condition in which no urine is voided

urinary suppression (YOOR-ih-nayr-ee supp-PRESH-un) condition in which kidneys do not produce urine

urinary system (YOOR-ih-nayr-ee) system responsible for excreting liquid waste from the body

urination (yoor-ih-NAY-shun) passage of urine from the body; emptying of the bladder

urine (YOOR-in) fluid waste excreted by the kidneys

urologist (you-ROL-uh-jist) physician specializing in treatment of the urogenital (urinary and reproductive) tract

uterine tube (YOO-ter-in toob) either of the pair of tubes that conduct the ovum from the ovary to the uterus; also called **fallopian tube**

uterus (YOO-ter-us) hollow, muscular organ where a fertilized egg implants and grows

uvula (YOO-vyoo-lah) cone-shaped process hanging down from the soft palate that helps prevent food and liquid from entering the nasal cavities

V

vagina (vah-JYE-nah) internal tube from the uterus to the vulva

vas deferens (vas DEF-er-enz) see **ductus deferens**

vasoconstriction (vay-soh-kon-STRIK-shun) reduction in vessel diameter caused by increased contraction of the muscular coat

vasomotor mechanism (vay-soh-MOH-tor MEK-ah-niz-em) factors that control changes in the diameter of arterioles by changing the tension of smooth muscles in the vessel walls
vastus (VAS-tus) wide; of great size
vein (vayn) vessel carrying blood toward the heart
ventral (VEN-tral) of or near the belly; in humans, front or anterior; opposite of dorsal or posterior
ventral body cavity (VEN-trul BOD-ee KAV-it-ee) organ-containing space in the anterior trunk of the body that includes the thoracic and abdominopelvic cavities; compare with **dorsal body cavity**
ventricle (VEN-trih-kul) small cavity, such as the pumping chambers of the heart
venule (VEN-yool) any of the small blood vessels that collect blood from the capillaries and join to form veins
vermiform appendix (VERM-ih-form ah-PEN-diks) a tubular structure attached to the cecum; composed of lymphoid tissue
vertebra (VER-teh-brah) (*pl.*, vertebrae) bone that makes up the spinal column
vertebral column (ver-TEE-bral) the spinal column, made up of a series of separate vertebrae that form a flexible, curved rod
vesicle (VES-ih-kul) any tiny membranous bubble within a cell
vestibular nerve (ves-TIB-yoo-lar) a division of the vestibulocochlear nerve (the eighth cranial nerve)
vestibule (VES-tih-byool) cavity that forms an entryway to another cavity; the *vestibule of the inner ear* is the space adjacent to the oval window between the semicircular canals and the cochlea; the *vestibule of the vulva,* between the labia, forms an entryway to the vagina
villus (VIL-us) (*pl.*, villi) fingerlike fold covering the plicae of the small intestines
visceral (VIS-er-al) relating to internal organs (viscera)
visceral effector (VIS-er-al ee-FEK-ter) see **autonomic effector**
visceral pericardium (VIS-er-al payr-ih-KAR-dee-um) the portion of serous pericardium that adheres to and covers the outside of the heart; also called **epicardium**
visceral peritoneum (VIS-er-al payr-ih-TOHN-ee-um) portion of the peritoneum that adheres to and covers organs such as the stomach and intestines
visceral pleura (VIS-er-al PLOO-rah) (*pl.*, plurae) the serous membrane that adheres to and covers the lung
vital capacity (VC) (VYE-tal kah-PAS-ih-tee [vee see]) largest amount of air that can be moved in and out of the lungs in one inspiration and expiration
vitamin (VYE-tah-min) a type of organic molecule needed in small quantities to help enzymes operate effectively
vitreous humor (VIT-ree-us HYOO-mor) the jellylike fluid found in the eye, posterior to the lens
vocal cord (VOH-kul kord) one of the bands of tissue in larynx responsible for production of sound (speech)
voiding (VOYD-ing) emptying of the bladder; also called **micturition** and **urination**
volar (VOH-lar) palm or sole
voluntary muscle (VOL-un-tayr-ee) see **skeletal muscle**
vulva (VUL-vah) external genitals of the female

W

wart raised bump that is a benign neoplasm (tumor) of the skin; caused by viruses
water (WAH-ter) compound with molecules made up of two hydrogen atoms and two oxygen atoms (H_2O); important solvent in the body
water intoxication (WAH-ter in-TOK-sih-kay-shen) potentially fatal condition of excessive water in the body
white blood cell (WBC) (wyte blud sel [DUB-el-yoo bee see]) any of several types of unpigmented blood cells that function in immunity; also called *leukocyte*
white matter nerves covered with white myelin
withdrawal reflex a reflex that moves a body part away from an irritating stimulus

Y

yellow bone marrow (YEL-oh bohn MAYR-oh) fatty tissue found inside the medullary cavity of a long bone
yolk sac (yohk sak) in humans, involved with the production of blood cells in the developing embryo

Z

zona fasciculata (ZOH-nah fas-sik-yoo-LAY-tah) middle zone of the adrenal cortex; secretes glucocorticoids
zona glomerulosa (ZOH-nah gloh-mayr-yoo-LOH-sah) outer zone of the adrenal cortex; secretes mineralocorticoids
zona reticularis (ZOH-nah reh-tik-yoo-LAYR-is) inner zone of the adrenal cortex; secretes small amounts of sex hormones
zygomatic bone (zye-goh-MAT-ik bohn) cheek bone; also called *malar bone*
zygomaticus (zye-goh-MAT-ih-kus) muscle that elevates the corners of the mouth and lips; also known as the *smiling muscle*
zygote (ZYE-goht) a fertilized ovum

Illustration/Photo Credits

Chapter 1

Opener Image, Copyright Shutterstock; 1-2, 1-6, 1-7, Courtesy Barbara Cousins; 1-4, Redrawn from Muscolino JE: *Know the body: muscle, bone, and palpation essentials,* St Louis, 2012, Mosby; Science Applications Box (Modern Anatomy)–art, Joe Kulka; Science Applications Box (Modern Anatomy)–photo, from the National Library of Medicine's Visible Human Project.

Chapter 2

2-1, From Sugimoto Y et al: Chemical identification of individual surface atoms by atomic force microscopy, *Nature* 466:64-67, 2007; Science Applications Box (Biochemistry), Joe Kulka.

Chapter 3

Opener Image, Copyright Shutterstock; 3-4A, Courtesy Charles Flickinger, University of Virginia; 3-4B, Lennart Nilsson, Albert Bonniers Forlag AB, Stockholm, Sweden; Tables 3-2, 3-3, Network Graphics; Science Applications Box (Genetics and Genomics), Joe Kulka.

Chapter 4

4-1, Adapted from Fawcett DW: *Bloom and Fawcett's a textbook of histology,* ed 11, Philadelphia, 1986, Saunders. In Garner LP, Hiatt JL: *Concise histology,* Philadelphia, 2011, Saunders; 4-2, 4-3B, 4-4B, 4-6B, 4-8B, Barbara Cousins; 4-3A, 4-4A, 4-6A, 4-8A, 4-15, Courtesy Gartner LP, Hiatt JL: *Color textbook of histology,* ed 3, Philadelphia, 2007, Saunders; 4-5, Courtesy Stanley Erlandsen, from Gartner LP, Hiatt JL: *Color textbook of histology,* ed 3, Philadelphia, 2007, Saunders; 4-7A, 4-10, 4-11, 4-12, 4-13, 4-14, 4-18, 4-19, Dennis Strete; 4-17, Edward Reschke; Science Application Box (Microscopy), Joe Kulka.

Chapter 5

5-2, 5-6, Barbara Cousins; Science Application Box (Radiography), Joe Kulka.

Chapter 6

Opener Image, Copyright Shutterstock; 6-4, Edward Reschke; 6-8A, From Rakel R: *Textbook of family medicine,* ed 7, Philadelphia, 2007, Saunders; 6-8B, From Goldman L, Ausiello D: *Cecil textbook of medicine,* ed 23, Philadelphia, 2008, Saunders; 6-8C, From Noble J: *Textbook of primary care medicine,* ed 3, Philadelphia, 2001, Mosby; 6-8D, From Townsend C, Beauchamp RD, Evers BM, Mattox K: *Sabiston textbook of surgery,* ed 18, Philadelphia, 2008, Saunders; 6-9, Barbara Cousins; 6-10A, From Kliegman RM: *Nelson textbook of pediatrics,* ed 20, Philadelphia, 2016, Elsevier; 6-10B-C, Courtesy Dr. Richard L Judd, Dwight D Ponsell, from *Mosby's first responder,* ed 2, St Louis, 1988, Mosby; Science Applications Box (Secrets of the Skin), Joe Kulka.

Chapter 7

Opener Image, Copyright Shutterstock; 7-4, 7-5, Dennis Strete; 7-6, Adapted from McCance K, Huether S: *Pathophysiology,* ed 7, St Louis, 2014, Mosby; 7-8, Network Graphics; 7-10B, 7-14, 7-25, Barbara Cousins; 7-15C, Adapted from Drake R, Vogl W, Mitchell AWM: *Gray's anatomy for students,* ed 3, Philadelphia, 2015, Churchill Livingstone; 7-16, From Hockenberry MJ, Wilson D: *Wong's essentials of pediatric nursing,* ed 9, St Louis, 2013, Mosby; 7-18C&F, 7-19, 7-20B&D, From Vidic B, Suarez FR: *Photographic atlas of the human body,* St Louis, 1984, Mosby; 7-22, Yvonne Wylie Walston; Health and Well-Being Box (The Knee Joint), Rolin Graphics; Clinical Application Box (Total Hip Replacement), From Canale ST: *Campbell's operative orthopaedics,* ed 9, St Louis, 1998, Mosby; Science Applications Box (Bone and Joints), Joe Kulka.

Chapter 8

Opener Image, Copyright Shutterstock; 8-3B, Courtesy Dr. HE Huxley; 8-5B, Courtesy Dr. Paul C. Letourneau, Department of Anatomy, Medical School, University of Minnesota, MN; 8-7A,C, 8-8A,C, Rolin Graphics; 8-10, 8-11, 8-12, John V. Hagen; Science Application Box (Muscle Function), Joe Kulka; Clinical Application Box (Muscle Injury)–photo, Courtesy Kellie White.

Chapter 9

9-2B, Dennis Strete; 9-4, Courtesy Dr. Richard Kessel, Professor of Biological Sciences, University of Iowa, Iowa City; 9-10B, 9-11, 9-12, From Vidic B, Suarez FR: *Photographic atlas of the human body,* St Louis, 1984, Mosby; Clinical Application Box (Lumbar Puncture), From Forbes CD, Jackson WD: *Color atlas and text of clinical medicine,* ed 3, London, 2003, Mosby; Clinical Application Box (Herpes Zoster, or Shingles), Courtesy TP Habif: *Clinical dermatology,* ed 5, St Louis, 2010, Mosby; Science Application Box (Neuroscience), Joe Kulka.

Chapter 10

Opener Image, Copyright Shutterstock; 10-5C, From Swartz MH: *Textbook of physical diagnosis,* ed 7, Philadelphia, 2014, Saunders; 10-7C-D, From Bingham BJG, Hawke M, Kwok P: *Atlas of clinical otolaryngology,* St Louis, 1992, Mosby-Year Book; Clinical Application Box (Color Blindness), From *Ishihara's tests for colour deficiency,* Tokyo, Japan, 1973, Kanehara Trading Co, Copyright Isshinkai Foundation; Health and Well-Being (Swimmer's Ear), From Zitelli BJ, Davis HW: *Atlas of pediatric physical diagnosis,* ed 5, Philadelphia, 2007, Elsevier. Courtesy Michael Hawke, MD; Science Applications Box (Senses), Joe Kulka.

Chapter 11

Opener Image, Copyright Shutterstock; Clinical Application Box (Growth Hormone Abnormalities)–photo A, From Gagel RF and McCutcheon IE: Pituitary gigantis, *N Engl J Med* 340:524, 1999; Clinical Application Box (Growth Hormone Abnormalities)–photo B, From Forbes CD, Jackson WF: *Color atlas and text of clinical medicine,* ed 3, Edinburgh, 2003, Mosby; Clinical Application Box (Thyroid Hormone Abnormalities)–photo A, Seidel HM, Ball JW, Dains JE, Benedict GW: *Mosby's guide to physical examination,* ed 4, St Louis, 1999, Mosby; Clinical Application Box (Thyroid Hormone Abnormalities)–photo B, Swartz MH: *Textbook of physical diagnosis,* ed 7, Philadelphia, 2014, Saunders; Clinical Application Box (Adrenal

Hormone Abnormalities), Courtesy Gower Medical Publishers; Science Applications Box (Endocrinology), Joe Kulka.

Chapter 12

Opener Image, Copyright Shutterstock; 12-1, 12-6, 12-9, Barbara Cousins; 12-2, 12-5, Courtesy Bevelander G, Ramalay JA: *Essentials of histology,* ed 8, St Louis, 1979, Mosby; 12-8, Dennis Strete; 12-10B, Copyright Dennis Kunkel Microscopy, Inc.; Science Applications Box (Hematology), Joe Kulka; Table 12-2, Adapted from Pagana KD, Pagana TJ: *Mosby's manual of diagnostic and laboratory tests,* ed 5, St Louis, 2014, Mosby.

Chapter 13

Opener Image, Copyright Shutterstock; 13-10, Barbara Cousins; Science Applications Box (Cardiology), Joe Kulka.

Chapter 14

14-1 top inset, Drake RL et al: *Grays anatomy for students,* ed 3, Philadelphia, 2015, Churchill-Livingstone; 14-4, From Ball JW, Dains JE, Flynn JA, et al: *Seidel's guide to physical examination,* ed 8, St Louis, 2015, Mosby; 14-10, From Abbas A, Lichtman A: *Cellular and molecular immunology,* ed 8, Philadelphia, 2015, Saunders; 14-11, Copyright Dennis Kunkel Microscopy Inc.; Science Applications Box (Vaccines), Joe Kulka.

Chapter 15

Opener Image, Copyright Shutterstock; 15-1, Barbara Cousins; 15-5C, From Cox JD: *Radiation oncology,* ed 9, Philadelphia, 2010, Mosby; 15-7, Network Graphics; 15-14, Clinical Application (Keeping the Trachea Open), Research, Issues, and Trends Box (Lung Volume Reduction Surgery), Courtesy Andrew P Evan, University of Indiana; Science Applications Box (Respiratory Medicine), Joe Kulka.

Chapter 16

Opener Image, Copyright Shutterstock; 16-5C, From Zitelli BJ, Davis HW: *Atlas of pediatric physical diagnosis,* ed 5, Philadelphia, 2007, Mosby; 16-12, From Vidic B, Suarez RF: *Photographic atlas of the human body,* St Louis, 1984, Mosby; 16-15, Barbara Cousins; Clinical Application Box (Gallstones), Courtesy Thompson JM, Wilson SF: *Health assessment for nursing practice,* St Louis, 1996, Mosby; Science Application Box (Gastroenterology), Joe Kulka.

Chapter 17

Opener Image, Copyright Shutterstock; 17-1, www.ChooseMyPlate.gov is hosted by the United States Department of Agriculture (USDA); Science Application Box (Food Science), Joe Kulka.

Chapter 18

Opener Image, Copyright Shutterstock; 18-1B, From Abrahams P, Marks SC, Hutchings RT: *McMinn's color atlas of human anatomy,* ed 5, Edinburgh, 2003, Mosby; 18-2B, From Abrahams PH, Spratt JD, Loukas M, van Schoor AN: *McMinn & Abrahams' clinical atlas of human anatomy,* ed 7, Edinburgh, 2013, Elsevier Ltd.; 18-4, Courtesy Andrew P Evan, University of Indiana; 18-10, From Telser A, Young J, Baldwin K: *Elsevier's integrated histology,* Philadelphia, 2008, Mosby; Clinical Application Box (Artificial Kidney), From Bonewit-West K: *Clinical procedures for medical assistants,* ed 9, St Louis, 2015, Saunders; Science Application Box (Fighting Infection), Joe Kulka.

Chapter 19

Opener Image, Copyright Shutterstock; 19-6 (photo), Copyright Kevin Patton, Lion Den, Inc., Weldon Spring, MO; 19-8, From Fritz S: *Mosby's fundamentals of therapeutic massage,* ed 5, St Louis, 2013, Mosby; 19-11, Modified from Goldman L, Schafer AI: *Goldman's Cecil medicine,* ed 24, Philadelphia, 2012, Saunders; Science Application Box (The Constancy of the Body), Joe Kulka.

Chapter 20

Science Application Box (The Body in Balance), Joe Kulka.

Chapter 21

Opener Image, Copyright Shutterstock; 21-2A, Lennart Nilsson, Albert Bonnier Forlag A, Stockholm, Sweden; 21-5A, Carolyn Coulam and John A. McIntyre; 21-6, From Abrahams PH, Spratt JD, Loukas M, van Schoor AN: *McMinn & Abrahams' clinical atlas of human anatomy,* ed 7, Edinburgh, 2013, Elsevier Ltd.; 21-7B, From Vidic B, Suarez FR: *Photographic atlas of the human body,* St Louis, 1984, Mosby; Science Application Box (Reproductive Sciences), Joe Kulka.

Chapter 22

Opener Image, Copyright Shutterstock; 22-1 (Micrograph), Lennart Nilsson, Albert Bonnier Forlag A, Stockholm, Sweden; 22-3, Courtesy Lucinda L Veeck, Jones Institute for Reproductive Medicine, Norfolk, VA; 22-5B, From Cotran R, Kumar V, Collins T: *Robbins pathologic basis of disease,* ed 6, Philadelphia, 1999, Saunders; 22-9, Barbara Cousins; 22-10, Courtesy Marjorie M Pyle for Lifecircle, Costa Mesa, CA; 22-11A, From Hockenberry MJ, Wilson D: *Wong's essentials of pediatric nursing,* ed 8, St Louis, 2009, Mosby; 22-11B, Copyright Kevin Patton, Lion Den, Inc., Weldon Spring, MO; 22-12, From Mahan LK, Escott-Stump S: *Krause's food, nutrition, and diet therapy,* ed 11, St Louis, 2004, Elsevier; Science Application Box (Embryology), Joe Kulka; Research, Issues, and Trends (Freezing Umbilical Cord Blood), Courtesy Craig Borck, St Paul Pioneer Press; Research, Issues, and Trends (Antenatal Diagnosis and Treatment), Copyright Kevin Patton, Lion Den, Inc., Weldon Spring, MO.

Appendix A

Body Mass Index Chart, Adapted from the Report of the Dietary Guidelines Advisory Committee on the Dietary Guidelines for Americans, 2000.

Index

Page numbers followed by *b*, *t*, and *f* indicate boxes, tables, and figures, respectively.

C

D

N

Q

R